Chronic Obstructive Pulmonary Disease

Neil S. Cherniack, M.D.

Professor of Medicine and
Professor of Physiology and Biophysics;
Dean, School of Medicine;
Vice President for Medical Affairs

Case Western Reserve University
Cleveland, Ohio

1991
W.B. SAUNDERS COMPANY
Harcourt Brace Jovanovich, Inc.
Philadelphia London Toronto Montreal Sydney Tokyo

W. B. SAUNDERS COMPANY
Harcourt Brace Jovanovich, Inc.

The Curtis Center
Independence Square West
Philadelphia, PA 19106

Library of Congress Cataloging-in-Publication Data

Cherniack, Neil S.

Chronic obstructive pulmonary disease/Neil S. Cherniack.—1st ed.
p. cm.

ISBN 0–7216–2300–X

1. Lungs—Diseases, Obstructive. I. Title.

RC776.03C45 1991

616.2′4—dc20 90-8693

Editor: W. B. Saunders Staff
Designer: Paul Fry
Production Manager: Ken Neimeister
Manuscript Editor: Karen Neff
Illustration Coordinator: Cecelia Kunkle
Indexer: Angela Holt
Cover Designer: Bill Donnelly

Chronic Obstructive Pulmonary Disease ISBN 0–7216–2300–X
First edition

Printed in the United States of America

Last digit is the print number: 9 8 7 6 5 4 3 2 1

CONTRIBUTORS

MURRAY D. ALTOSE, M.D.
Professor of Medicine and Associate Dean for Veterans Affairs, Case Western Reserve University School of Medicine, Cleveland, Ohio. Chief of Staff, Cleveland Veterans Administration Medical Center, Cleveland.
EFFECTS OF COPD ON BEHAVIORAL CONTROL OF BREATHING

NICHOLAS R. ANTHONISEN, M.D.
Professor of Medicine, University of Manitoba Faculty of Medicine, Health Sciences Centre, Winnipeg, Manitoba, Canada.
SYMPTOMS AND SIGNS OF COPD

MICHAEL A. BAUER, M.D.
Assistant Clinical Professor of Medicine, Columbia University, College of Physicians and Surgeons, New York, New York. Attending Physician, The Mary Imogene Bassett Hospital, Cooperstown, New York.
EFFECTS OF AIR POLLUTION ON COPD

LINDA BOGAR
Research Specialist, University of Illinois, Chicago, Illinois.
THE EFFECTS OF COPD ON AIRWAY SECRETIONS AND LUNG CLEARANCE

A. BRANCATISANO, Ph.D.
Research Fellow, Thoracic Medicine Unit, Department of Medicine, Westmead Hospital, Westmead, New South Wales, Australia.
UPPER AIRWAY FUNCTION IN COPD

MARGARET C. BRUCE, Sc.D.
Assistant Professor, Department of Pediatrics, Case Western Reserve University School of Medicine, Cleveland, Ohio.
THE EXTRACELLULAR MATRIX OF THE LUNG: IMPLICATIONS IN COPD

CLEMENT CAHAN, M.D.
Pulmonary and Critical Care Fellow, University Hospitals of Cleveland, Cleveland, Ohio.
HEMATOLOGIC MANIFESTATIONS OF COPD

JEROME O. CANTOR, M.D.
Assistant Professor of Pathology, Columbia University College of Physicians and Surgeons. Attending Pathologist and Research Associate, St. Luke's–Roosevelt Hospital Center, New York.
ANIMAL MODELS OF EMPHYSEMA

NEIL S. CHERNIACK, M.D.
Professor of Medicine and Professor of Physiology and Biophysics; Vice President for Medical Affairs and Dean, School of Medicine; Case Western Reserve University, Cleveland, Ohio.
CONTROL OF BREATHING IN COPD; EFFECTS OF COPD ON BEHAVIORAL CONTROL OF BREATHING

TATSUYA CHONAN, M.D.
Assistant, First Department of Internal Medicine, Tohoku University School of Medicine, Sendai, Japan.
EFFECTS OF COPD ON BEHAVIORAL CONTROL OF BREATHING

ALAN M. COHEN, M.D.
Associate Professor of Radiology, Case Western Reserve University School of Medicine, Cleveland, Ohio. Chief of Diagnostic Radiology, MetroHealth Medical Center, Cleveland.
IMAGING IN COPD

ALLEN B. COHEN, M.D., Ph.D.
Professor of Medicine and Biochemistry, Executive Associate Director, The University of Texas Health Center at Tyler, Texas.
TREATMENT OF ALPHA$_1$-ANTITRYPSIN DEFICIENCY AND OTHER FORMS OF EMPHYSEMA

JOEL D. COOPER, M.D.
Professor of Surgery, Head, Section of Thoracic Surgery, Division of Cardiothoracic Surgery, Washington University School of Medicine, St. Louis, Missouri. Barnes Hospital, St. Louis.
LUNG TRANSPLANTATION

GERARD J. CRINER, M.D.
Assistant Professor of Medicine, Pulmonary Division, Temple University School of Medicine, Philadelphia, Pennsylvania. Director, Medical Intensive Care Unit; Director, Chronic Ventilator Care Unit, Temple University Hospital, Philadelphia.
REHABILITATION OF PATIENTS WITH COPD

ANNE LOGAN DAVIS, M.D.
Associate Professor of Clinical Medicine, Division of Pulmonary and Critical Care Medicine, New York University School of Medicine, New York, New York. Attending Physician; Assistant Director, Chest Service; Director, Chest Clinic; Bellevue Hospital, New York.
BRONCHIECTASIS

PAMELA B. DAVIS, M.D., Ph.D.
Professor of Pediatrics, Case Western Reserve University School of Medicine, Cleveland, Ohio. Chief, Pediatric Pulmonary Division, Rainbow Babies and Children's Hospital, Cleveland.
RELATIONSHIP OF NEONATAL AND CHILDHOOD LUNG DISEASE TO ADULT COPD; CYSTIC FIBROSIS: A MAJOR CAUSE OF OBSTRUCTIVE AIRWAYS DISEASE IN THE YOUNG

THOMAS E. DICK, Ph.D.
Assistant Professor of Medicine, Physiology and Biophysics, and of Neurosciences, Case Western Reserve University School of Medicine, Cleveland, Ohio.
NEUROMUSCULAR PHYSIOLOGY OF COUGH AND OTHER RESPIRATORY TRACT REFLEXES

MICHAEL DONAHOE, M.D.
Assistant Professor of Medicine, and Director, Medical Intensive Care Unit, Presbyterian-University Hospital, Pittsburgh, Pennsylvania.
LABORATORY EVALUATION OF THE PATIENT WITH COPD

PAUL M. DORINSKY, M.D.
Associate Professor of Medicine, Ohio State University College of Medicine, Columbus, Ohio. Associate Professor, Division of Pulmonary and Critical Care Medicine, Ohio State University Hospitals, Columbus.
BRONCHIOLITIS OBLITERANS

JEFFREY M. DRAZEN, M.D.
Professor of Medicine, Harvard Medical School, Boston, Massachusetts. Associate Physician, Brigham and Women's Hospital, Boston. Physician, Beth Israel Hospital, Boston. Chief, Pulmonary Division, Beth Israel/Brigham and Women's Hospital, Boston.
NEUROPEPTIDES, PLATELET-ACTIVATING FACTOR, AND EICOSANOID ACTIONS IN COPD

NORMAN H. EDELMAN, M.D.
Professor of Medicine and Dean, University of Medicine and Dentistry of New Jersey, Robert Wood Johnson Medical School, Piscataway, New Jersey.
BRAIN BLOOD FLOW

ELLEN H. ELPERN, R.N., M.S.N.
Assistant Professor, Rush University, College of Nursing, Chicago, Illinois. Respiratory Clinical Specialist, Rush-Presbyterian/St. Luke's Medical Center, Chicago.
BEHAVIOR MODIFICATION IN COPD

LUDWIG A. ENGEL, M.B., B.S., Ph.D.
Senior Staff Specialist, Head of Thoracic Medicine, Westmead Hospital, Westmead, New South Wales, Australia.
UPPER AIRWAY FUNCTION IN COPD

GARY R. EPLER, M.D.
INVASIVE DIAGNOSTIC PROCEDURES IN COPD

MARK O. FARBER, M.D.
Professor of Medicine, Indiana University, Indianapolis, Indiana. Veterans Administration Medical Center, Indianapolis.
SODIUM AND WATER METABOLISM IN COPD

VLADIMIR FENCL, M.D.
Associate Professor of Medicine, Harvard Medical School, Boston, Massachusetts. Physician, Brigham and Women's Hospital, Boston.
DIURETICS IN THE TREATMENT OF COPD

STANLEY B. FIEL, M.D.
Professor of Medicine; Deputy Chief, Pulmonary Disease and Critical Care Section of Temple University School of Medicine; Director, Lung Transplantation Service, Cystic Fibrosis Program, Temple University Hospital, Philadelphia, Pennsylvania.
LUNG TRANSPLANTATION

DAVID C. FLENLEY, Ph.D., F.R.C.P.
Professor of Respiratory Medicine, University of Edinburgh, Edinburgh, Scotland, United Kingdom. Honorary Consultant Physician, City Hospital, Edinburgh.
THE DIAGNOSIS OF EMPHYSEMA; OXYGEN THERAPY IN THE TREATMENT OF COPD

JAMES E. GADEK, M.D.
Professor of Medicine, Ohio State University College of Medicine, Columbus, Ohio. Professor of Medicine, Director, Division of Pulmonary and Critical Care Medicine, Ohio State University Hospitals, Columbus.
BRONCHIOLITIS OBLITERANS

BARBARA M. GALKO, M.D.
Staff Physician, Doctors Hospital, Toronto, Ontario, Canada.
BRONCHODILATORS IN THE TREATMENT OF BRONCHITIS AND EMPHYSEMA; RESPIRATORY STIMULANTS IN THE TREATMENT OF COPD

CHRISTOPHER S. GARRARD, M.A., D.Phil., M.B., B.S., M.R.C.P.
Clinical Lecturer in Intensive Care, Oxford University, Oxford, England, United Kingdom. Consultant Physician, Intensive Therapy Unit, John Radcliffe Hospital, Oxford.
MUCOLYTICS AND EXPECTORANTS IN THE TREATMENT OF COPD

D. GEORGOPOULOS, M.D.
University of Thessaloniki; General Hospital G. Papanicolaou, Pulmonary Clinic, Thessaloniki, Greece.
SYMPTOMS AND SIGNS OF COPD

NORMA P. GERARD, Ph.D.
Associate Professor, Harvard Medical School, Boston, Massachusetts. Department of Medicine, Beth Israel Hospital, Boston.
NEUROPEPTIDES, PLATELET-ACTIVATING FACTOR, AND EICOSANOID ACTIONS IN COPD

DANIEL M. GOODENBERGER, M.D.
Assistant Professor of Medicine; Program Director, Pulmonary Disease; Associate Program Director, Internal Medicine, Washington University School of Medicine, St. Louis, Missouri. Assistant Physician and Director, Pulmonary Consultation Service, Barnes Hospital, St. Louis.
INVASIVE DIAGNOSTIC PROCEDURES IN COPD

DAVID E. GRIFFITH, M.D.
Assistant Professor of Medicine, The University of Texas Health Center at Tyler, Tyler, Texas.
PSYCHOLOGIC, NEUROPSYCHOLOGIC, AND SOCIAL ASPECTS OF COPD

NICHOLAS J. GROSS, M.D., Ph.D.
Professor, Departments of Medicine and Biochemistry, Stritch School of Medicine, Loyola University, Chicago, Illinois. Acting Chief of Pulmonary Diseases, Hines Veterans Administration Hospital, Hines, Illinois.
ANTICHOLINERGIC AGENTS IN THE TREATMENT OF COPD

JOHN R. HOIDAL, M.D.
Professor of Medicine, Chief, Division of Respiratory, Critical Care and Occupational Medicine, University of Utah Health Sciences Center, Salt Lake City, Utah.
OXIDATIVE DAMAGE AND COPD

FREDERIC G. HOPPIN, Jr., M.D.
Professor of Medicine and Physiology, Brown University, Providence, Rhode Island. Memorial Hospital of Rhode Island, Pawtucket.
PULMONARY FUNCTION TESTS FOR DIAGNOSIS AND EVALUATION OF COPD

ROLF D. HUBMAYR, M.D.
Associate Professor of Medicine, Mayo Medical School, Rochester, Minnesota. Consultant, Mayo Associated Hospitals, Rochester.
CELLULAR EFFECTS AND PHYSIOLOGIC RESPONSES: LUNG MECHANICS

LEONARD D. HUDSON, M.D.
Professor of Medicine, University of Washington School of Medicine, Seattle, Washington. Head, Division of Respiratory Diseases and Critical Care Medicine, Harborview Medical Center, University Hospital, Seattle.
ACUTE EXACERBATIONS IN COPD PATIENTS

RICHARD W. HYDE, M.D.
Professor of Medicine and Toxicology, University of Rochester School of Medicine and Dentistry, Rochester, New York. Attending Physician, Strong Memorial Hospital, Rochester.
EFFECTS OF AIR POLLUTION ON COPD

STEVEN IDELL, M.D., Ph.D.
Associate Professor of Medicine and Chief, Pulmonary Division, The University of Texas Health Center at Tyler, Texas.
TREATMENT OF ALPHA$_1$-ANTITRYPSIN DEFICIENCY AND OTHER FORMS OF EMPHYSEMA

NORMAN L. JONES, M.D., F.R.C.P., F.R.C.P.(C)
Professor of Medicine, McMaster University, Hamilton, Ontario, Canada; Director, Ambrose Cardiorespiratory Unit, Chedoke-McMaster Hospitals, Hamilton.
LIMITATION OF EXERCISE IN CHRONIC AIRWAY OBSTRUCTION

RICHARD E. KANNER, M.D.
Associate Professor of Medicine, University of Utah School of Medicine, Salt Lake City, Utah. Attending Physician, University of Utah Hospital, Salt Lake City.
PRECLINICAL COPD: DESCRIPTION, RECOGNITION, AND THERAPY

STEVEN G. KELSEN, M.D.
Professor of Medicine and Physiology; Director, Division of Pulmonary Disease and Critical Care Medicine, Temple University School

of Medicine, Philadelphia, Pennsylvania. Medical Director, Pulmonary Function Laboratory, Temple University Hospital, Philadelphia.

REHABILITATION OF PATIENTS WITH COPD

KAYE H. KILBURN, M.D.

Ralph Edgington Professor of Internal Medicine, University of Southern California School of Medicine, Los Angeles, California; Attending Staff, Los Angeles County–University of Southern California Medical Center, Los Angeles. President, Workers Disease Detection Services, Inc., San Dimas, California.

FLUID RETENTION ASSOCIATED WITH PULMONARY INSUFFICIENCY AND RESPIRATORY FAILURE; EVALUATION OF IMPAIRMENT AND DISABILITY IN PATIENTS WITH BRONCHITIS AND EMPHYSEMA

KIERAN J. KILLIAN, M.B., CH.B., F.R.C.P.(C), F.R.C.P.(I)

Associate Professor of Medicine, McMaster University, Hamilton, Ontario, Canada. Staff Respirologist, Chedoke-McMaster Hospitals, Hamilton.

LIMITATION OF EXERCISE IN CHRONIC AIRWAY OBSTRUCTION

RICHARD S. KRONENBERG, M.D.

Professor of Medicine; Chairman, Department of Medicine, The University of Texas Health Center at Tyler, Texas.

PSYCHOLOGIC, NEUROPSYCHOLOGIC, AND SOCIAL ASPECTS OF COPD

CHARLES KUHN III, M.D.

Professor of Pathology, Brown University, Program in Medicine, Providence, Rhode Island. Pathologist-in-Chief, Memorial Hospital of Rhode Island, Pawtucket.

LUNG REPAIR IN COPD

ALAN R. LEFF, M.D.

Professor and Head, Section of Pulmonary and Critical Care Medicine; Professor of Medicine, Anesthesia, and Clinical Pharmacology, Department of Medicine, The University of Chicago, Chicago, Illinois.

THE RELATIONSHIP OF COPD TO ASTHMA

RICHARD W. LIGHT, M.D.

Professor of Medicine, University of California at Irvine, Irvine, California. Associate Chief of Staff for Research, Veterans Administration Medical Center, Long Beach, California.

TREATMENT OF DYSPNEA WITH TRANQUILIZERS

MELVIN LOPATA, M.D.

Professor of Medicine and Acting Chairman, Department of Medicine, University of Illinois College of Medicine at Chicago, Chicago, Illinois.

EFFECTS OF COPD ON SLEEP

RUY V. LOURENCO, M.D.

Professor of Medicine and Physiology and Dean, University of Medicine and Dentistry of New Jersey, New Jersey Medical School, Newark, New Jersey.

THE EFFECTS OF COPD ON AIRWAY SECRETIONS AND LUNG CLEARANCE

FELICE MANFREDI, M.D.

Professor of Medicine, Indiana University School of Medicine, Indianapolis, Indiana. Veterans Administration Medical Center, Indianapolis.

SODIUM AND WATER METABOLISM IN COPD

JOHN J. MARINI, M.D.

Professor of Medicine and Director of Critical Care for the Department of Medicine, University of Minnesota, Minneapolis/St. Paul, Minnesota. Chief of Pulmonary/Critical Care, St. Paul-Ramsey Medical Center, St. Paul.

VENTILATORY MANAGEMENT OF COPD

BRUCE C. MARSHALL, M.D.

Assistant Professor of Medicine; Director, Adult Cystic Fibrosis Program, University of Utah Health Sciences Center, Salt Lake City, Utah.

OXIDATIVE DAMAGE AND COPD

RICHARD J. MARTIN, M.D.

Professor of Pediatrics, Case Western Reserve University School of Medicine, Cleveland, Ohio. Co-Director of Neonatology, Rainbow Babies and Children's Hospital, Cleveland.

RELATIONSHIP OF NEONATAL AND CHILDHOOD LUNG DISEASE TO ADULT COPD

RICHARD A. MATTHAY, M.D.

Professor of Medicine, Pulmonary Section, Yale University School of Medicine, New Haven, Connecticut. Yale-New Haven Hospital, New Haven.

TREATMENT OVERVIEW: CHRONIC HYPERCAPNIA AND COR PULMONALE

KEVIN T. MCCUSKER, M.D.

Assistant Professor of Medicine, University of Utah Health Sciences Center, Salt Lake City, Utah.

OXIDATIVE DAMAGE AND COPD

E. R. MCFADDEN, JR.

Argyl J. Beams Professor of Medicine, Case Western Reserve University School of Medicine, Cleveland, Ohio. Director, Airway Disease Center; Vice Chairman, Department of Medicine, University Hospitals, Cleveland.

AIRWAY RESPONSIVITY AND CHRONIC OBSTRUCTIVE LUNG DISEASE

WYLIE L. MCNABB, ED.D.

Assistant Professor of Medicine, University of Chicago, Chicago, Illinois. Director, Center for Research in Medical Education and Health Care, University of Chicago, Chicago.

BEHAVIOR MODIFICATION IN COPD

JOHN R. MICHAEL, M.D.

Associate Professor of Medicine, University of Utah Health Sciences Center, Salt Lake City, Utah. University of Utah Hospital, Salt Lake City.

PULMONARY VASODILATORS IN THE TREATMENT OF BRONCHITIS AND EMPHYSEMA

FLORO MIRALDI, M.D., SC.D.

Professor of Biomedical Engineering; Associate Professor of Radiology, Case Western Reserve University School of Medicine, Cleveland, Ohio. Director, Division of Nuclear Radiology, University Hospitals of Cleveland, Cleveland.

IMAGING IN COPD

CHARLES MITTMAN, M.D.

Adjunct Professor of Medicine, University of California, San Francisco, California; Department of Medicine, Valley Medical Center of Fresno, Fresno, California.

PREOPERATIVE EVALUATION AND PERIOPERATIVE CARE

W. K. C. MORGAN, M.D.

Professor of Medicine, University of Western Ontario, London, Ontario, Canada. Director, Chest Diseases Unit, University Hospital, London, Ontario.

CHRONIC AIRFLOW LIMITATION AND OCCUPATION

MICHAEL L. NOCHOMOVITZ, M.D.

Assistant Professor, Case Western Reserve University School of Medicine, Cleveland, Ohio. Medical Director, Pulmonary Treatment Center; Medical Director, Integrated Health Systems, University Hospitals of Cleveland, Cleveland.

RESPIRATORY CARE IN THE HOME

JAMES OSMANSKI, D.O.
Senior Resident in Internal Medicine, The Miriam Hospital, Providence, Rhode Island.
ACUTE EXACERBATIONS IN COPD PATIENTS

RICHARD L. PARDY, M.B., F.R.C.P.(C), F.R.A.C.P., F.C.C.P.
Associate Professor, Respiratory Division, Department of Medicine, University of British Columbia, Vancouver, British Columbia, Canada. Respiratory Division, Department of Medicine, St. Paul's Hospital, Vancouver.
LONG-TERM CARE OF PATIENTS WITH CHRONIC BRONCHITIS AND EMPHYSEMA

JOHN A. PIERCE, M.D.
Selma and Herman Seldin Professor of Pulmonary Medicine, Washington University School of Medicine, St. Louis, Missouri. Attending Physician, Barnes Hospital, St. Louis. Staff Physician, John Cochrane Veterans Administration Medical Center, St. Louis.
LUNG REPAIR IN COPD

GIUSEPPE G. PIETRA, M.D.
Professor of Pathology, University of Pennsylvania School of Medicine, Philadelphia, Pennsylvania. Director of Anatomic Pathology, Hospital of the University of Pennsylvania, Philadelphia.
PATHOLOGY OF THE PULMONARY VASCULATURE AND HEART

N. V. RAO, M.Sc., Ph.D.
Research Assistant and Professor, University of Utah Health Sciences Center, Salt Lake City, Utah.
OXIDATIVE DAMAGE AND COPD

ANTHONY S. REBUCK, M.D.
Professor of Medicine; Director, Asthma Center of The Toronto Hospital, Toronto, Ontario, Canada.
RESPIRATORY STIMULANTS IN THE TREATMENT OF COPD

SUSAN REDLINE, M.D., M.P.H.
Assistant Professor of Medicine, Brown Medical School, Providence, Rhode Island. Roger Williams General Hospital, Providence.
THE EPIDEMIOLOGY OF COPD

R. B. REGER, Ph.D.
Associate Professor of Occupational Medicine, West Virginia University School of Medicine, Morgantown, West Virginia.
CHRONIC AIRFLOW LIMITATION AND OCCUPATION

W. DARLENE REID, B.M.R.(P.T.), Ph.D.
Assistant Professor, School of Rehabilitation Medicine, University of British Columbia, Vancouver, British Columbia, Canada.
LONG-TERM CARE OF PATIENTS WITH CHRONIC BRONCHITIS AND EMPHYSEMA

HERBERT Y. REYNOLDS, M.D.
Professor of Medicine; Chairman, Department of Medicine. Attending Physician; The Pennsylvania State University Hospital, The Milton S. Hershey Medical Center, Hershey, Pennsylvania.
ANTIBIOTIC TREATMENT OF BRONCHITIS AND CHRONIC LUNG DISEASE

ELIZABETH A. RICH, M.D.
Assistant Professor of Medicine, Case Western Reserve University School of Medicine, Cleveland, Ohio. Department of Medicine, Pulmonary/Critical Care Division, University Hospitals of Cleveland, Cleveland.
THE ROLE OF IMMUNE ABNORMALITIES AND INFLAMMATION IN CAUSING AND PERPETUATING COPD

DUDLEY F. ROCHESTER, M.D.
E. Cato Drash Professor of Medicine, University of Virginia School of Medicine, Charlottesville, Virginia. Head, Division of Pulmonary and Critical Care Medicine; Department of Internal Medicine, University of Virginia Health Sciences Center, Charlottesville.
EFFECTS OF COPD ON THE RESPIRATORY MUSCLES

JOSEPH R. RODARTE, M.D.
Professor of Medicine and Physiology, Baylor College of Medicine, Houston, Texas. Adjunct Professor of Mechanical Engineering and Materials Science, Rice University, Houston. Chief of the Pulmonary Service, Methodist Hospital, Houston.
CELLULAR EFFECTS AND PHYSIOLOGIC RESPONSES: LUNG MECHANICS

ROBERT M. ROGERS, M.D.
Professor of Medicine, University of Pittsburgh School of Medicine; Chairman, Division of Pulmonary/Critical Care Medicine, Department of Medicine, Pittsburgh, Pennsylvania.
LABORATORY EVALUATION OF THE PATIENT WITH COPD

STEVE H. SALZMAN, M.D.
Director, Pulmonary Function Laboratory, Beth Israel Medical Center, New York, New York. Assistant Professor of Medicine, Mt. Sinai School of Medicine, New York.
BRONCHIECTASIS; THE RELATIONSHIP OF COPD TO BRONCHIECTASIS

JONATHAN M. SAMET, M.D.
Professor of Medicine; Chief, Pulmonary Division, Department of Medicine, University of New Mexico School of Medicine, Albuquerque, New Mexico.
THE RELATIONSHIP OF SMOKING TO COPD

PHILIP L. SCHIFFMAN, M.D.
Associate Professor of Medicine, University of Medicine and Dentistry of New Jersey, Robert Wood Johnson Medical School, New Brunswick, New Jersey. Medical Director, Medical Intensive Care Unit; Medical Director, Respiratory Services, Robert Wood Johnson University Hospital, New Brunswick.
ACID-BASE DISORDERS IN COPD

CHARLES B. SHERMAN, M.D.
Assistant Professor of Medicine, Brown University, Program in Medicine, Providence, Rhode Island. Director, Pulmonary Division, The Miriam Hospital, Providence.
ACUTE EXACERBATIONS IN COPD PATIENTS

STEPHANIE A. SHORE, Ph.D.
Assistant Professor, Department of Environmental Science and Physiology, Harvard School of Public Health, Boston, Massachusetts.
NEUROPEPTIDES, PLATELET-ACTIVATING FACTOR, AND EICOSANOID ACTIONS IN COPD

KINGMAN P. STROHL, M.D.
Professor of Medicine, Case Western Reserve University School of Medicine, Cleveland, Ohio. Chief, Pulmonary and Critical Care Medicine, University Hospitals of Cleveland, Cleveland.
HEMATOLOGIC MANIFESTATIONS OF COPD

J. PETER SZIDON, M.D.
Professor of Medicine, Rush Medical College, Chicago, Illinois. Rush-Presbyterian–St. Luke's Medical Center, Chicago.
THE EFFECT OF COPD ON PULMONARY CIRCULATION

WILLIAM M. THURLBECK, M.D., F.R.C.P.(C)
Professor of Pathology, University of British Columbia, Vancouver, British Columbia, Canada. Pathologist, Children's Hospital, Vancouver. Consultant Pathologist, University Hospital, Vancouver.
PATHOLOGY OF CHRONIC AIRFLOW OBSTRUCTION

GERARD M. TURINO, M.D.

Professor of Medicine, College of Physicians and Surgeons, Columbia University, New York, New York. Director of Medicine, St. Luke's—Roosevelt Hospital, New York.

ANIMAL MODELS OF EMPHYSEMA

MARK J. UTELL, M.D.

Professor of Medicine and Toxicology, University of Rochester School of Medicine and Toxicology, University of Rochester School of Medicine and Dentistry, Rochester, New York. Attending Physician, Strong Memorial Hospital, Rochester.

EFFECTS OF AIR POLLUTION ON COPD

ERIK VAN LUNTEREN, M.D.

Assistant Professor of Medicine and of Neurosciences, Case Western Reserve University School of Medicine, Cleveland, Ohio. Medical Director of Pulmonary Function Laboratory, University Hospital of Cleveland, Cleveland.

NEUROMUSCULAR PHYSIOLOGY OF COUGH AND OTHER RESPIRATORY TRACT REFLEXES

PETER D. WAGNER, M.D.

Professor of Medicine, University of California, School of Medicine San Diego, California.

EFFECTS OF COPD ON GAS EXCHANGE

WILLIAM WEISS, M.D.

Emeritus Professor of Medicine, Hahnemann University, Philadelphia, Pennsylvania.

COPD AND LUNG CANCER

STEVEN R. WHITE, M.D.

Assistant Professor of Medicine, Section of Pulmonary and Critical Care Medicine, Department of Medicine, The University of Chicago, Chicago, Illinois.

THE RELATIONSHIP OF COPD TO ASTHMA

HERBERT P. WIEDEMANN, M.D.

Head, Section of Medical Intensive Care, Department of Pulmonary Disease, Cleveland Clinic Foundation, Cleveland, Ohio.

TREATMENT OVERVIEW: CHRONIC HYPERCAPNIA AND COR PULMONALE

ROBERT A. WISE, M.D.

Associate Professor of Medicine, Division of Pulmonary and Critical Care Medicine, Johns Hopkins University School of Medicine, Baltimore, Maryland. Associate Director, Division of Pulmonary and Critical Care Medicine; Director, Pulmonary Function Laboratories, Johns Hopkins Hospital, Francis Scott Key Medical Center, Baltimore.

COPD AND THE PERIPHERAL CIRCULATION

INTRODUCTION

Chronic obstructive pulmonary disease (COPD) is a disease that affects the respiratory tract, produces persistent airflow limitation, and may eventually cause breathlessness and inadequate oxygenation. It is one of the most common conditions seen by physicians, occurring throughout the world. It is a major cause of death and disability in adults. Smoking causes most cases of COPD, but other factors, such as air pollution, occupational exposure to injurious material, and infections contribute to the occurrence and progression of the disease. Abstinence from smoking will stop COPD, but will not reverse the condition. However, new ways of treating COPD patients who have the disease at varying levels of severity are continually being reported.

These new therapies include agents with improved efficacy and fewer side effects; new methods of drug administration; and more novel methods of drug administration developed from recent studies of the cellular and subcellular mechanisms underlying COPD, and from investigations of the respiratory muscles and neurons.

The main function of the respiratory system is the transfer of O_2 and CO_2 from the body to the atmosphere. This process is vulnerable to injury at many points. Gas exchange takes place in alveoli, which are encased in muscular bellows driven by neurons in the medulla. The supply of air to the alveoli depends on the motion of these bellows. Air and blood are conveyed to the alveoli by a branching system of delicate and rather compliant tubes that enlarge and shrink with the movement of the bellows. Because the bellows themselves are mounted on the extremities, gas exchange must continue as the extremities move and must remain compatible with the changing metabolic demands created by contraction of the muscles that power the extremities. Breathlessness occurs when the metabolic demands of these muscles are not satisfied. The air brought into the lungs is contaminated with chemicals and microbes that can injure them, but elaborate defenses are in place in the respiratory tract to filter and remove these dangerous elements. In addition, white blood cells in the blood (e.g., polymorphonucleocytes, macrophages, and lymphocytes), which secrete antibodies and enzymes, can be mobilized in times of need to defend the respiratory tract. However, the defensive reactions themselves, unless controlled, can lead to lung injury.

COPD is the disease that most frequently produces long-term derangements in gas transfer. Although emphysema and bronchitis are the commonest forms of COPD, a number of other diseases, such as asthma, bronchiectasis, and cystic fibrosis, can also affect airway caliber and produce airflow limitation. Because these diseases differ considerably in their treatment and prognosis from emphysema and bronchitis, it is important to accurately diagnose them and distinguish them from COPD. This may be difficult at times, because the effects of neither emphysema nor bronchitis are anatomically uniform, and thus each can cause the patient to present with a wide range of symptoms and functional abnormalities.

Humans differ in their susceptibility to respiratory injury. For example, only about 15 per cent of smokers develop significant airflow limitation. This range in vulnerability can be partially attributed to a genetic basis. Molecular techniques promise to provide accurate methods for detecting individuals who are particularly likely to develop respiratory injury, and they offer hope for the development of techniques that can compensate for genetically based increased susceptibility.

Because levels of CO_2 and O_2 are important to the operation of all organs and not just to the lungs, severe COPD can have serious systemic effects, affecting the heart, kidneys, and brain, and ultimately most organs of the body. Conversely, diseases of the heart, kidney, and brain can exacerbate the effects of COPD on the respiratory system and further worsen gas exchange.

COPD is a treatable illness. There are many possible interventions that can help to prevent progression of the disease and relieve the adverse consequences of COPD. These include regimens that promote health, such as improved nutrition, physical training, and methods to relieve psychological stress. But there are also specific measures to widen airways, accelerate ciliary action, relieve the effects of inadequate oxygenation on the heart and pulmonary vasculature, and correct acid-base balance. Although it may not be possible to completely restore the airways and the alveoli to their normal state, carefully planned treatment will benefit most patients with COPD.

This volume brings together contributions from experts in different disciplines and is intended to present a comprehensive view of COPD, its causes, prevention, effects on the body, and current therapy. Each chapter presents a different facet of the disease and its relation to other diseases.

In addition to thanking the contributors, we would particularly like to acknowledge here the unflagging assistance of Ms. Anne W. Miller in all aspects of compiling and editing the contributions to this volume, and without whose help this book would never have reached completion.

CONTENTS

Section I

PATHOLOGY OF CHRONIC OBSTRUCTIVE PULMONARY DISEASE

Chapter 1

PATHOLOGY OF CHRONIC AIRFLOW OBSTRUCTION

William M. Thurlbeck

Airflow may be obstructed in the lung at several different sites, and at each site various lesions may be present. In any one patient there may be a combination in site, type, and severity of lesion.[108] It is thus a serious error to think that patients with chronic airflow obstruction can be neatly classified as having "chronic bronchitis," "small airways disease," or "emphysema." In many patients, perhaps the majority, the obstruction may be dominantly at one site; in a minority it may be limited to one site. In general, a wide spectrum of airway and parenchymal lesions is present in patients with symptomatic chronic airflow obstruction. For example, chronic productive cough (chronic bronchitis) increases in frequency as emphysema gets more severe; some 90% of patients with severe emphysema have chronic productive cough.[151]

RELEVANT NORMAL AIRWAY ANATOMY

For convenience of classification, it is appropriate to consider three major sites of chronic airflow obstruction: the large airways or bronchi, the small airways or bronchioles, and the gas-exchanging part of the lung, which is known as the acinus. Bronchi, by definition, are those airways that have cartilage in their walls, and they usually also have mucus-secreting glands deep into the surface epithelium. The important quantitative aspects of bronchi include that they have a modest number of generations (about four to ten, with a mean of seven), their length averages about 10 cm, and their total cross-sectional area increases from 2 cm^2 at the tracheal carina to 10 cm^2 where they terminate.[161] Another feature is that bronchi contain much smooth muscle, although proportionately this is less than in the succeeding airways. These are the membranous bronchioles that do not have cartilage in their walls, nor do they exchange gas since they have no alveoli in their walls. The number of divisions of airways in different bronchiolar pathways varies greatly.

In airways that traverse a long distance from the main bronchus to the periphery—axial pathways—there may be up to 25 bronchial and bronchiolar generations. An example of such a pathway would be to the parenchyma of the posterior basal segment. Other pathways have only a short distance to traverse, such as to the parenchyma of the medial aspect of the lung and these have as few as 10. These are known as spiral pathways.

The average summed length of bronchioles is approximately 1.8 cm and the total cross-sectional area increases from about 13.9 cm^2 to 281 cm^2.[161] The increase in total cross-sectional area of bronchioles has the important consequence that normally bronchioles contribute relatively little resistance to flow in the lungs. At one time it was thought that bronchioles contributed only 10% to 20% of total airflow resistance.[57] This had the important corollary that severe disease could be present in the bronchioles without making a serious impact on total flow resistance. The often-quoted example is that if half of the peripheral airways were obliterated, their resistance would double, but this would increase total airway resistance by only about 20%. Later data have suggested that resistance in the small airways probably contributes about 40% of total resistance[61, 68, 163]; this is in keeping with the model of asymmetric dichotomy of airways used for the quantitative data quoted here.[62] Weibel's model of symmetric dichotomy[164] produces data more consistent with the very low level of peripheral airway resistance first mentioned. This difference of opinion is of more than theoretic interest. The very low level of airflow resistance first quoted led to the notion that standard tests of pulmonary function, such as the forced expiratory volume in one second (FEV_1), might be normal in the presence of extensive peripheral airways disease. This possibility led to the proliferation of "tests of small airway function." The higher estimate of normal peripheral airway resistance suggested that these tests are of little relevance and that the FEV_1 adequately reflects abnormalities in peripheral airways.

CHRONIC AIRFLOW OBSTRUCTION AND MORPHOLOGIC CORRELATES

The term chronic airflow obstruction (CAO) is not intended to replace the term chronic obstructive pulmonary disease and has a different meaning. Chronic airflow obstruction is a simple physiologic abnormality, chronic diminished loss of expiratory flow defined in a particular way. Chronic obstructive pulmonary disease replaced the older term "chronic nonspecific lung disease," which comprised those conditions that are often, but not always, associated with CAO.[25] These conditions include chronic bronchitis, emphysema, bronchiolitis, bronchiectasis, asthma, and now rare but specific entities, such as rheumatoid bronchiolitis.

This chapter attempts to correlate various morphologic abnormalities in bronchi, bronchioles, and the acinus with chronic airflow obstruction (Table 1–1). Difficulty with interpretation of data should be recognized. Structural-functional correlations have been done mostly in three types of studies: (1) cases of patients with documented severe CAO, (2) lungs obtained at surgery for lung cancer, and (3) lungs subjected to post-mortem functional tests. Patients with lungs from the second group often have no CAO and seldom have more than

TABLE 1–1. Lesions Associated with CAO in COPD

SITE	LESION
Central Airways (Bronchi)	Mucous gland enlargement Smooth muscle hyperplasia Cartilage atrophy Inflammation Bronchial wall thickening and encroachment on lumen
Peripheral (small) Airways (Bronchioles)	Bronchiolar obliteration Bronchiolar narrowing Bronchiolar tortuosity and diminished alveolar attachments Goblet-cell metaplasia Inflammation Fibrosis Increase in smooth muscle Mucus plugging Pigmentation
Parenchymal (acinar) Airways	Respiratory bronchiolitis Emphysema

mild CAO because surgery would not be undertaken if this were not so.

Structural-Functional Correlates

These may be very different in the two groups. Figure 1–1 shows the frequency distribution of the FEV_1 of autopy findings in the National Institutes of Health (NIH) Intermittent Positive-Pressure Breathing (IPPB) clinical trial[108] and in a large series of patients whose lobes or lungs were resected for lung cancer at St. Paul's Hospital, Vancouver. Patients in the Vancouver series were reviewed in numerous structure-function correlation studies.[167–175] Very little overlap occurs between the two. Study of severe CAO using autopsy tissue has the disadvantage that long periods of time may elapse between functional investigations and study of tissue. The data may be retrospective. This was not the case in the NIH IPPB trial.

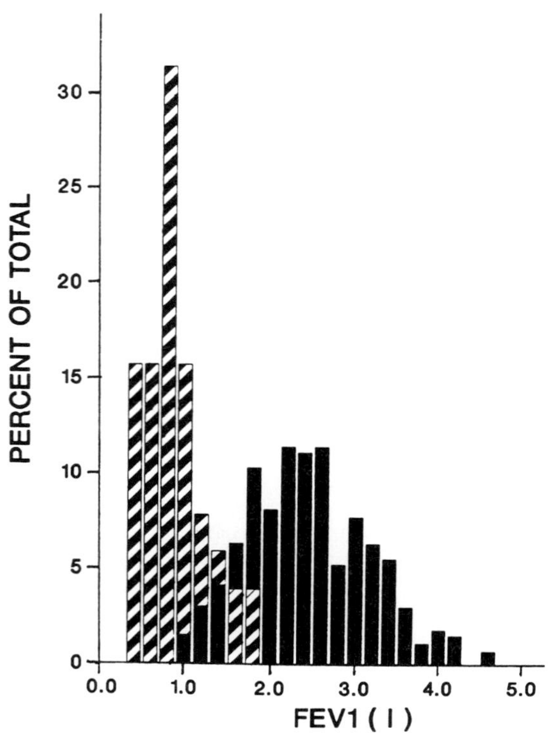

Figure 1–1. The distribution of the forced expiratory volume in one second (FEV_1) in cases studied at autopsy in the National Institutes of Health (NIH) intermittent positive-pressure breathing (IPPB) trial (hatched columns) is contrasted to that found in patients whose lungs were studied following lung surgery, mostly for lung cancer (solid columns).

The delay and retrospective nature of data are greatly obviated in surgical material, but this material has three disadvantages: a highly selected group is studied, lung cancer may affect the functional studies, and often only lobes and, occasionally, even segments are used. Given the varied topography of emphysema, assessment of lobes is theoretically fraught with error in the assessment of emphysema in the entire lung, but this may not be a major source of error in practice.[173]

Lobar differences in severity of bronchiolitis is a controversial matter, with some observers finding that the lesions were worse in the upper lobes,[29] others that they were worse in the lower lobes,[15] and yet others that there were no interlobar differences.[172] Lungs subjected to post-mortem function studies have a short interval between functional and structural analyses. They also do not have the handicap of great biases to normality or abnormality of airflow. However, the clinical data are retrospective and an artificial functional system is used.

CENTRAL AIRWAY LESIONS

Chronic bronchitis is the paradigm of lesions of the central airways. However, it should be recognized immediately that chronic bronchitis is defined as a functional abnormality and many, including myself, believe that this term's usefulness has now come to an end. It became apparent to perceptive observers in the 1950s that the term chronic bronchitis was used by British physicians to describe the same condition in patients that was described by United States physicians as emphysema. The term chronic obstructive pulmonary disease (COPD) has generally superseded these usages. Because of the confusion between the terms "chronic bronchitis" and "emphysema," a landmark symposium was held at which a number of definitions were proposed.[25] Chronic bronchitis was defined as chronic or recurrent excess secretion of mucus. Because no way existed, or exists, of accurately measuring mucus secretion, a simple, empiric clinical definition was adopted. Chronic bronchitis was defined as chronic production of sputum. Chronic was defined as occurring on most days for 3 or more months in the year, for 2 or more successive years. Further, the excess sputum production should not be due to specific diseases, such as tuberculosis or bronchiectasis. This definition led to much clarification of thought and to a proper understanding of the epidemiology of chronic bronchitis, so defined. However, there are three important reasons why the term "chronic bronchitis" could be dropped profitably. First, chronic bronchitis and "COPD" are still used interchangeably in Britain. Second, a whole spectrum of functional abnormalities may be found in patients with chronic bronchitis—from no airflow obstruction to fatal chronic airflow obstruction. In the latter, it is tempting to use the term chronic obstructive bronchitis,[97] perhaps implying that the airflow obstruction is due to hypersecretion of mucus. Third, and perhaps most importantly, a symptom, chronic sputum production, is viewed as a disease. It would clarify thinking if the term chronic sputum production replaced chronic bronchitis, and when associated with chronic cough, as is usually the case, the term chronic productive cough was used.

Asthma is another important disease of the large airways,

although a high proportion of patients with asthma also have obstruction of peripheral airways.[35] It usually has been regarded as separate from COPD, but many now believe that it is impossible to discuss the two conditions separately.[20] It has become apparent in the last decade that a significant proportion of patients with otherwise typical COPD may have wheezing or a diagnosis of asthmatic bronchitis or asthma. Airflow obstruction in these patients may be partially reversible with bronchodilators, and a proportion of these patients also exhibit methacholine sensitivity. The problem is that the criteria for the diagnosis of asthma or reversible airflow obstruction have never been defined or agreed on. The difficulty of the diagnosis of asthma in epidemiologic surveys was stressed in 1987 by Enarson and colleagues,[40] who found that the incidence of clinical asthma varied from 2.7% to 13.4% in a group of 1392 workers in various industries, depending on the criteria used. In the same group, methacholine sensitivity of less than 8 mg/ml was present in 16.5%, less than 2 mg/ml in 4.7%, and less than 0.5 mg/ml in 0.6%. In a very well-defined epidemiologic study of patients with CAO (average age 63 years, average FEV_1 48.2% predicted, and criterion for entry FEV_1 less than 60% predicted), Burrows and co-workers (1987)[20] found that 44.4% had a clinical diagnosis of asthma, 65.8% had "attacks of shortness of breath and wheeze," and 76.9% "wheezing or whistling in the chest." They were able to define a group of patients who had "asthmatic bronchitis" (23.1% of the group) and patients who were nonatopic smokers without a history of asthma ("emphysema" 38.5%), and a mixed group (38.5%). The major goals of this study were to underline the significance of "asthma" in a group of patients with CAO and point out that this group had a much better 10-year survival (85% predicted from age and FEV_1) compared with nonatopic smokers.[41] The mean decline in FEV_1 was 5 ml per year in the group of asthmatic bronchitic patients but 70 ml per year in the "emphysema" patients.

The reason for introducing the relationship of COPD and asthma is related to the significance of increased muscle in the central airways.

Mucous Gland Enlargement

The morphologic counterpart of chronic sputum production is enlargement of the compound tracheobronchial mucous glands. These lie in the submucosa and are connected to the surface by a duct through which the secretions reach the lumen of the airways. The glands consist of branching tubules that on histologic sections resemble glands and are therefore often referred to as "acini." The tubules are lined by two types of cells—paler cells, called mucous cells, and darker, granular cells, called "serous cells," which are found at the end of the tubules. Both types of cells secrete mucosubstances. The enlargement of mucous glands associated with chronic sputum production has been well studied, and several measurements have been devised to determine the enlargement. The first described method, and the easiest one to perform, is the Reid index, or gland-to-wall ratio.[126] In this technique, the thickness of the mucous glands is compared with the thickness of the bronchial wall defined as the distance from the epithelial basal lamina to the inner perichondrium. As the glands enlarge, their thickness increases and thus the Reid index increases because gland thickness is the numerator of the equation.

Other measurements, such as the area or volume proportion of glands and size of tubules, have also been used. These measurements have consistently shown an increase in patients with chronic sputum production, with occasional exceptions.[105] Mullen and co-workers measured mucous gland size on "intrapulmonary airways"; other studies have been on main or lobar bronchi. In general, the increase in size of mucous glands has been found to be modest.

More importantly, a considerable overlap in size occurs between those with chronic sputum production and those without. Indeed, the distribution curve of the Reid index and other measurements of gland size is unimodal.[6, 50, 95, 132, 136, 156] There are two consequences of this. First, the Reid index is a poor predictor of the presence of chronic sputum production except at high and low levels of the index. Second, and more importantly, a gradual transition from normal to abnormal occurs. This is in direct contrast to the epidemiologic definition of chronic bronchitis, which divides the population sharply into two groups—those with disease and those without. This is an empiric definition and the true concept is that chronic bronchitis is hypersecretion of mucus. Inability to measure secretion of mucus leads to the clinical definition. It seems likely that if mucus secretion could be measured it would also show a unimodal distribution. The clearest analogy is to blood pressure in which there is clearly "a transition between health and disease."[87]

If blood pressure could not be recorded, hypertension might be clinically defined as stroke. Surprisingly little research has been done concerning the fundamental nature of mucous gland enlargement. It is primarily due to hyperplasia of mucous gland cells,[36] but some hypertrophy, as evidenced by enlargement of tubules, also occurs.[126] A higher ratio of mucous to serous cells exists,[126] but this could not be confirmed by us,[144, 145] and there is a shift to secretion of acid glycoproteins.[33] The nature and course of these cellular changes have never been studied, nor has there been a fundamental study of the rate and control of cellular multiplication of the glands.

Numerous studies have been made of the relationship between mucous gland enlargement and expiratory flow rates. A majority of studies has shown a relationship between diminished expiratory flow rates and mucous gland enlargement, but the correlations have been weak, and a substantial number of studies have not shown a relationship (for review, see Thurlbeck 1985[153]). This is not surprising, because most studies have been on patients with severe chronic airflow limitation. As will be shown, emphysema becomes important in such patients and this may complicate or obscure the relationship between mucous gland enlargement and reduced expiratory flow. However, a study has shown no relationship, even in patients who had mild CAO and who had undergone carefully done prospective tests of expiratory flow and quantitation of morphologic changes.[104, 105] In a group of coal miners with a wide range of severity of CAO, Ruckley and colleagues[130] found that an increased Reid index was associated with a diminished FEV_1. The mechanism of flow limitation in mucous gland enlargement may be due to narrowing of the lumen because of increased mucosal thickness or to intralumenal mucus.

Muscle Hyperplasia

The exact status of increase in airway muscle is controversial. Some observers have claimed that increased amounts of muscle are invariably present in patients with chronic sputum production[63]; others claim that it does not occur.[37] Our own experience was that increased muscle occurred in occasional patients with chronic sputum production and that such patients had clinically evident episodes of wheezing.[145] We have shown that patients with moderate or severe CAO have, on the average, increased muscle, but a substantial number of patients fall within the normal range.[108] Similarly, an increase in mean amount of muscle has been described in patients with chronic productive cough and mild CAO.[105] It has also been suggested that the increase in muscle is not generalized but occurs most obviously in the left lower lobe bronchus.[22] As in the case of mucous gland enlargement, the growth in muscle mass in both chronic bronchitis and asthma is due to hyperplasia of muscle cells rather than hypertrophy.[63, 53]

The natural hypothesis is that enlarged muscle is a reflection of airflow reversibility because increased bronchial muscle is a consistent finding in patients with severe or fatal asthma.[64, 37, 145] However, no relationship has been shown between fluctuations in flow rates or reversibility with bronchodilator in one study[109] and methacholine sensitivity in another.[105] However, in the first study, patient selection excluded patients with a diagnosis of asthma. In the other (those undergoing resection for lung cancer) patients with marked airway reversibility were not likely to have been included.

One study has shown a deleterious effect on the FEV_1 and residual volume of increased muscle in patients with moderate CAO.[111] This study referred to prebronchodilator values. Airway reactivity was not studied.

Cartilage Atrophy

Atrophy of bronchial cartilage has been shown to occur in emphysematous lungs, even in mild emphysema, if special techniques are used to assess the amount of cartilage.[158] A strong association between mucous gland enlargement and cartilage atrophy was described.[146] Conversely, an increased amount of cartilage has been found in patients with chronic productive cough and mild CAO.[105] A descriptive study has claimed atrophy of all components of the bronchial wall in patients with severe emphysema.[175] Studies of random sections of bronchi have not found cartilage deficiency in either chronic sputum production or emphysema.[150]

Cartilage atrophy has been described as most prominent in the subsegmental bronchi and beyond.[158] These findings suggest that flow limitation may occur in chronic mucus hypersecretion or emphysema, or both, owing to cartilage atrophy in the same way that flow limitation has been ascribed to absence of cartilage in the syndrome of congenital lobar overinflation.[143] However, physiologic and radiologic evidence suggests that flow limitation does not occur at the subsegmental level,[85, 86] and that these airways actually dilate rather than collapse during expiration. Indeed, I was able to study one of these cases. Flow limitation and collapse occurred in the bronchus to the basal segments of the lower lobe but no cartilage atrophy was present there. However, Maisel and colleagues (1968, 1972),[89, 90] using post-mortem bronchography, suggested that bronchial atrophy, exact nature not specified, led to expiratory bronchial collapse. Whether this was flow limiting or not is unclear. Thus, the role of cartilage atrophy appears enigmatic and insufficiently studied.

Inflammation

Evidence of inflammation in bronchi has not been found consistently in older studies of patients with chronic sputum production or mucous gland enlargement.[150] Both inflammatory cells and eosinophils have been described as appearing in chronic bronchitis. The basis of the diagnosis was not described, but the importance of this observation was that the difference between chronic bronchitis and asthma is a quantitative rather than a qualitative one.

A later, useful study[105] is available that specifically addresses the question of inflammation in major airways in patients with chronic productive cough who underwent upper lobar or lung resection for carcinoma. This study showed an increase in inflammation of the mucosa, presumably the epithelium, in chronic bronchitis in cartilaginous airways 2 mm or more in greater diameter. Mucous gland enlargement, assessed by either the Reid index or the volume proportion of mucous glands, was not significantly related to inflammation.

We could not show a relationship among bronchial inflammation, eosinophilia, and fluctuations of expiratory flow rate in response to bronchodilation.[109] Another study in resected specimens could show no difference between methacholine sensitivity and bronchial inflammation.[105]

Bronchial Wall Thickening and Encroachment on the Bronchial Lumen

Surprisingly, very few studies have been made concerning thickening of the bronchial wall and narrowing of the lumen in patients with chronic sputum production. A theoretic analysis by Moreno and associates[102] suggests that thickening of bronchial walls would lead to a large increase in airway resistance. Calculations from most series suggest that the increase in bronchial wall thickness and encroachment upon the lumen due to mucous gland enlargement are modest,[156] although some studies have shown quite considerable absolute increase in gland size.[126] McKenzie and colleagues[95] showed that there was thickening of bronchial walls and loss of radius of the lumen in patients with chronic bronchitis and severe airflow obstruction. They found that the ratio of bronchial width internal to the cartilage/lumen radius approximately doubled in patients with severe obstruction, compared with patients without obstruction. This ratio showed a significant correlation ($r = 0.75$) with loss of FEV_1.

BRONCHIOLITIS: "SMALL AIRWAY" OR PERIPHERAL AIRWAY LESIONS

Bronchiolitis in Patients with COPD

That peripheral airway lesions exist in patients with COPD has been recognized for more than 30 years.[96, 124, 142] The original emphasis on these lesions was more on the pathogenesis of emphysema than as a cause of CAO. Hogg and coworkers[57] showed by direct experimentation that the major site of airflow obstruction was in the peripheral airways, as Dayman had surmised in 1951.[32] Many different types of lesions may be observed in bronchioles in patients with CAO and these are discussed subsequently in further detail. Many of the lesions may be regarded as inflammatory in origin. Since the inflammatory process is a continuous one, it may be that the lesions causing CAO may differ depending on the stage of inflammation. For example, early on there may be only inflammation as evidenced by increased numbers of inflammatory cells. At a later stage, there may be fibrosis and perhaps consequent narrowing. An important concept should be introduced at this point: the clear difference between *mild* and *early* disease. Early implies a temporal relationship; most young patients may have early disease, but most older patients may have late disease. Mild implies a quantitative, not a temporal, phenomenon and mild disease may or may not be early. The best example is the study of CAO in patients who have had lung resection. In general these patients have mild disease; otherwise they would not be suitable for resection. However, their disease is not early. Typically, their average age is 63 years, 90% are smokers or ex-smokers, and the smokers have a 36 pack–year history.[171] Thus, the process should be considered late, as in patients of the same age and with a similar history with severe CAO.

Another variable to consider, although perhaps obvious, is cause and effect. Emphasis has been placed on alveolar attachments to bronchiolar walls,[3] and there is evidence that loss of these attachments may be associated with mild CAO[133] and loss of elastic recoil.[115] However, loss of attachments really is a manifestation of emphysema. The observed CAO may thus be due to emphysema, or narrowing of bronchioles associated with loss of attachments.[133, 115]

A number of rare causes of bronchiolar obstruction are known, and the best known are a consequence of viral infection or chemical inhalation. Other causes include rheumatoid arthritis,[44, 45] graft-versus-host reaction following bone marrow transplantation,[129, 154] and heart-lung transplantation.[176] In other instances, bronchiolitis may be cryptogenic and not associated with any known cause.[162] These conditions are dealt with only briefly, as they are not part of the main thrust of this chapter. Thus, the lesions found in patients with typical CAO are dealt with first.

Bronchiolar Obliteration

Bronchiolar and peripheral bronchial obliteration have been best documented in bronchiectasis[123] and are mainly responsible for the CAO that patients with bronchiectasis sometimes exhibit. Bronchiectasis was a significant factor in older series of patients with CAO. For example, in the classic study by Burrows and colleagues (1966),[21] six of the 30 patients had extensive bronchiectasis and it was a significant associated feature in patients with type B ("blue bloater") CAO. In our own series,[157] three of 48 patients had extensive bronchiectasis. With the advent of measles and pertussis vaccines and antibiotic therapy, bronchiectasis has become an uncommon cause of CAO.

Bronchiolar obliteration has been described in patients with usual COPD and severe CAO.[92, 96, 124] However, in our hands, the extent of obliteration was slight and inconsistent in patients with severe emphysema.[92] In patients with severe CAO, airway casts have shown absence of filling of small bronchi,[34] as have post-mortem bronchograms.[138] In the last study, lack of filling was associated with right ventricular hypertrophy.[137, 138] Both casts and bronchograms have the obvious disadvantage that lack of filling may represent either an artifact or occlusion by mucous plugs. Using bronchography, Reid (1955)[125] showed that when lack of airway filling was preceded by tapered, narrowed airways, these were obliterated. When bronchial filling stopped suddenly with square ends, secretion within the airways was the cause. Examination of the bronchograms and the airway casts referred to suggests that secretions were the major cause of lack of filling. Bronchograms in surgically derived lungs from patients with mild CAO showed little or no evidence of bronchiolar obliteration.[125]

Bronchiolar obliteration is not as likely to be a cause of CAO as is bronchiolar narrowing. On the one hand, obliteration of half the airways will only double airflow resistance. Narrowing to half, on the other hand, will increase resistance to the fourth power (2^4 or 16 times). We were unable to show a relationship between loss of expiratory flow and bronchiolar obliteration in patients in the NIH IPPB clinical trial.[109]

Bronchiolar Narrowing

Bronchiolar narrowing has been observed in patients with known or surmised mild[14, 93, 114] and severe CAO.[92, 137] For the reason mentioned, narrowing is likely to be a potent cause of CAO. Mean bronchiolar diameter may not have the most significant relationship with CAO. Several studies[18, 49, 109] have indicated that a better relationship to CAO is with the proportion of very narrowed airways (less than 0.35 mm or 0.4 mm in diameter). Of special interest, this marked narrowing may be particularly associated with hypoxemia and right ventricular hypertrophy.[17, 18, 66, 109]

Loss of Alveolar Attachments and Bronchiolar Deformity

Pratt and colleagues[120, 121] and Anderson and Foraker[3] originally pointed out that emphysema was accompanied by loss of radial, alveolar attachments to bronchioles and suggested the hypothesis that bronchioles would collapse more readily on expiration. Anderson and Foraker[3] observed that bronchiolar narrowing, as measured in fully distended lungs, accompanied loss of alveolar attachments. Detailed studies by Linhartova and her colleagues[78–81] showed that loss of alveolar attachments was accompanied by distortion and tortuosity of bronchioles. Nagai and coworkers[108] also showed a relationship between bronchiolar deformity and emphysema and a significant correlation between expiratory airflow obstruction and bronchiolar deformity in patients with moderate and severe CAO.[109] As indicated previously, Saetta and colleagues[134] found that diminished alveolar attachments were associated with mild CAO, and Petty and colleagues[115] found an association between airflow obstruction and loss of attachments. Both studies found a relationship between airway narrowing and loss of attachments.

The mechanism of airflow obstruction is less certain; it may be due to associated narrowing. Airway dimensions have been measured on fully inflated lungs. As indicated, the older view was that expiratory airway collapse ensued. However, the notion of expiratory collapse as a cause of diminished expiratory flow is challenged by the old observation of Hogg and associates[57] that resistance to flow in the peripheral airways was the same on inspiration as on expiration. However, these studies were not limited to patients with severe emphysema; in many, emphysema was relatively slight and fixed airway lesions, including mucus plugging, were significant findings. In comparison, Wilson and coworkers[166] noted that focal areas of narrowing, such as might occur in loss of alveolar attachments, narrowed more on expiration than did other airways. In addition, Berend and coworkers,[14] studying pressure-flow curves, found that emphysematous lungs showed diminished flow, compared with non-emphysematous lungs having the same airway diameter. Berend and Thurlbeck[12] measured maximum flow at a transpulmonary pressure of 5 cm H_2O and found that flow was diminished in emphysematous lungs, compared with nonemphysematous lungs that had the same airway dimensions at full inflation. These observations suggest that perhaps airways in emphysematous lungs narrow unduly on expiration, which may reflect diminished alveolar attachments. Thus, there is good evidence that alveolar support is abnormal in emphysema, and that this is associated with bronchiolar deformity and with flow obstruction; but the mechanism remains controversial.

Goblet-Cell Metaplasia

First described by Karpick and colleagues[69] in patients in an intensive care unit, most of whom later died of respiratory failure, goblet-cell metaplasia is now recognized as a cause of CAO. Normally, less than 1% of the cells lining bronchioles are goblet cells; the surface cells are nearly all ciliated cells, in which cilia beat in the mucociliary blanket, which in turn is covered by a visible[46] and functional[88] surfactant layer. When goblet-cell metaplasia occurs, airflow obstruction may result because of one, or both, of two reasons. One reason is that excess mucus is secreted and this may form obstructing plugs. The hypothesis that goblet-cell metaplasia may result in displacement of the surfactant layer by mucus is more interesting. This causes instability of the airways, which now close more easily and open with more difficulty. A variant of this hypothesis was made by Ebert and Terracio,[37] who studied bronchioles in smokers and found a loss of Clara cells. These are thought by some to secrete surfactant for the airways.[43, 139] Thus, this loss would lead to bronchiolar instability. Studies have shown goblet-cell metaplasia to be a cause of a mild reduction in flow rates, including the patients in the NIH IPPB clinical trials.[94, 109, 170, 171] In this last group of patients, goblet-cell metaplasia was an important cause of obstruction of expiratory flow in those with the least emphysema. One post-mortem functional study did not show a relationship between goblet-cell metaplasia and airflow obstruction.[117] Goblet-cell metaplasia should be regarded as a manifestation of inflammation—the response of mucous membranes to irritation is increased mucus secretion—and is significantly related to cigarette smoking.[171]

Inflammation

One of the most interesting observations is that inflammation of the bronchioles per se may be responsible for mild airflow obstruction. Cosio and his colleagues[28] compared a variety of tests of expiratory flow with bronchiolar lesions in patients whose lungs were resected for cancer. The investigators found that inflammation was the most important cause contributing to the composite score of eight lesions in airways that was related to mild CAO. They suggested that the volume at isoflow—the volume at which expiratory flow is the same breathing helium-oxygen as air—and closing capacity were the tests best related to bronchiolar lesions. The FEV_1 to forced vital capacity (FVC) ratio was for practical purposes related to abnormalities of peripheral airways. This observation, in retrospect, casts serious doubt on the idea that peripheral airways normally contribute a minimal resistance to flow. The importance of inflammation has been confirmed by others.[7, 117, 170] These functional abnormalities confirm the supposition made by Niewoehner and colleagues[110] that bronchiolitis would be an important cause of mild CAO. They studied smokers under the age of 40—exactly those subjects who classically show mild CAO—dying suddenly of violence and found that bronchiolitis was a common lesion in them. All but the observations of Berend and colleagues[14] carry with them the defect that no measurements were made of airway diameter. Cosio and associates[29] noted that young smokers at autopsy had an increased proportion of airways less than 0.4 mm in diameter. Thus, inflammation may still be an epiphenomenon as a cause of airflow obstruction and the lesion really responsible is consequent airway narrowing.

Two mechanisms have been suggested for the effect of bronchiolitis per se on expiratory flow. Petty and colleagues[117] and Baile and coworkers[5] have proposed the hypothesis that the inflammatory exudate in the bronchioles displaces the surfactant layer, rendering them unstable, as in the case of goblet-cell metaplasia discussed previously. Berend and colleagues[7] suggested that bronchiolitis may lead to functional bronchiolar constriction by release of mediators of inflammation that may act on bronchiolar smooth muscle directly or reflexly via the vagus. The evidence they presented included the observation that bronchiolar diameters were smaller in surgically derived lungs as opposed to autopsy lungs, suggesting that muscle tone had been lost in the last group. In surgically derived lungs, progressive narrowing of airways with increasing inflammation was noted, but this was not the case in autopsy lungs (Table 1–2). Increased airway reactivity has been found in association with bronchiolitis.[104]

When the bronchioles of patients in the NIH IPPB clinical trial with moderate and severe CAO were examined, no relationship between bronchiolitis and abnormalities of expiratory flow was observed.[109] This observation suggests that other mechanisms of flow obstruction override inflammation per se and that in these patients inflammation had progressed to produce other lesions in the airways.

Fibrosis

Cosio and coworkers (1978)[28] found that fibrosis was an important contributor to the composite score associated with mild airflow obstruction. This has since been confirmed by others using surgically derived lungs[170, 172] but not by those using autopsy lungs.[114, 117] Thickening of the walls of bronchioles less than 0.4 mm in diameter and of respiratory bronchioles has also been shown to be associated with mild CAO[168]; this is presumably due to fibrosis. Fibrosis, however, was not associated with flow obstruction in the NIH IPPB clinical trial; rather, it was associated with beneficial effects on expiratory flow and clinical features, including blood gases.[109] These investigators speculated that fibrosis ameliorated bronchiolar deformity, which they regarded as the most important bronchiolar lesion associated with CAO.

Increased Muscle

Increased muscle was an important contributor to the total pathologic score and mild CAO in the study by Cosio and coworkers (1978)[28]; this was confirmed by others[117] and was associated with mild CAO. However, other studies have not found an association between increased muscle and mild CAO.[94, 114, 170] In the NIH IPPB trial, increased muscle appeared not to be associated with airflow obstruction but rather was beneficial.[109] In that study, decreased bronchiolar muscle appeared to be a concomitant of normal aging, and patients in the trial had, on the average, increased muscle. A substantial number of patients fell within the normal range. The meaning of the increased muscle is difficult to understand; unlike fibrosis, it is not an obvious sequela to inflammation. Increased airway muscle has been described in emphysema and asthma and has been attributed to flow obstruction.[64, 77] Perhaps it is more related to increased work associated with airway hyperreactivity.

Mucus Plugging

Bronchographic abnormalities suggestive of mucus plugging have been described in patients with mild[125] and severe[138] CAO. Using simple subjective observation, mucus plugging was considered an important cause of airflow obstruction in patients dying of CAO.[57] Quantitative studies in autopsy lungs showed increased intrabronchiolar mucus in cases with chronic bronchitis but no emphysema[93] and even more mucus in patients with chronic bronchitis and emphysema, most of whom had severe CAO.[92] However, occlusion by mucus plugs did not contribute to mild airflow obstruction in surgically derived lungs[28] and has been ignored or not found in subsequent studies in such lungs. One study in post-mortem lungs in patients with mild CAO found that intralumenal mucus was related to the slope of phase III.[117] Aikawa and colleagues (1989)[1] measured mucus at autopsy and found increased amounts in patients with severe CAO in which 50 to 100 ml of mucus was produced daily. No increase was found in cases with a similar degree of airflow obstruction who were thought to have emphysema and produced 5 to 10 ml of sputum per day. Thus, it seems possible that increased intralumenal mucus is mainly a terminal event and that patients submitted to surgery who have preoperative parasympathetic blockers and

TABLE 1–2. Comparison of Bronchiolar Diameters

	GROUP I	GROUP II	GROUP III	GROUP IV
IB (autopsy lungs) (mm)	0.79 ± 0.03	0.82 ± 0.03	0.87 ± 0.06	0.72
IB (resected lobes) (mm)	0.61 ± 0.09	0.59 ± 0.03	0.42 ± 0.04	0.40 ± 0.06

IB = Internal bronchiolar diameter. Groups I–IV are ranked by severity of inflammation.[7] Mean ± 1 standard error of the mean.

perhaps also respiratory therapy have no increased intra-airway mucus. It thus seems probable that intralumenal mucus is not an important cause of flow obstruction, although it seems unlikely to be a benefit.

Pigmentation

A significant negative correlation was found in the NIH IPPB trial between bronchiolar pigmentation and expiratory flow rates.[109] An obvious cause and effect relationship is not apparent and it is easiest to ignore this association. A positive correlation between pigmentation and emphysema has been noted,[108] and it was postulated that this association was responsible for loss of flow rates with excess pigmentation. Pigmentation may also be a marker of heavy smoking.

Special Forms of Bronchiolitis

We have dealt with lesions in the bronchioles that are commonly encountered in patients with typical COPD. However, bronchiolitis may occur in specific situations and the clinical features of patients under these circumstances may be different and distinctive (Table 1–3). These features will be dealt with only briefly since they are not directly relevant to the main thrust of this chapter. They have been reviewed in detail elsewhere.[99, 154]

Viral Infections

Bronchiolitis is a common feature of viral infections of the lung. Occasionally, the inflammation may be severe and may lead to permanent bronchiolar narrowing and obliteration. The viruses that are particularly involved include paramyxovirus, causing measles, and adenovirus. Bronchiolar obliteration may lead to bronchiectasis, the Swyer-James syndrome (see subsequent discussion), and to chronic airflow obstruction with overinflation. When the patient presents at an early age, the diagnosis may be obvious, but at a later age it is likely to be difficult.

Irritants and Chemicals

Notable examples are oxides of nitrogen, ammonia, and smoke, but high concentrations of substances such as sulfur dioxide have also been implicated. In general terms, very high doses result in pulmonary edema and very low doses result in minor functional abnormalities. Significant bronchiolar obliteration usually follows an acute, significant exposure and symptoms date from that time. Thus, diagnosis is not often a problem.

TABLE 1–3. Special Forms of Bronchiolitis

1. Viral infections
2. Toxic chemicals and gases
3. Rheumatoid arthritis
4. Diffuse panbronchiolitis
5. Graft-versus-host disease
6. Heart/lung transplantation
7. Follicular bronchitis/bronchiolitis
8. Mineral dust airways disease
9. Cryptogenic bronchiolitis
10. Bronchiolitis obliterans and organizing pneumonia

Rheumatoid Bronchiolitis

First recognized by Geddes and coworkers in 1977,[44] rheumatoid bronchiolitis is now a well-documented condition. The initial cases were described in middle-aged nonsmoking women, five of whom had classic rheumatoid arthritis and the sixth positive antinuclear factor. Clinically, the patients were characterized by rapidly developing expiratory airflow obstruction and a course which lasted 5 to 18 months. Chest radiographs showed greatly overinflated lungs without arterial deficiency, and the diffusing capacities were normal as were volume-pressure curves. The lesions consisted of occlusion of small bronchi and bronchioles by loose, fibrous tissue and were irregularly distributed through the lungs. It has since become apparent that airflow obstruction, presumably due to similar lesions, is quite common in rheumatoid arthritis, and the degree of obstruction is more often relatively mild and the course more benign than the original case.[45]

Diffuse Panbronchiolitis

This condition appears to be limited to Japan and is relatively common, with more than 1000 cases collected in a three-year period.[60] Males are more commonly affected than females, and the usual age at presentation is in the sixth decade, with a range of 20 to 60 years. No predisposing causes were apparent. Chronic cough and expectoration were usual and two of three had sinusitis. Radiologically diffuse panbronchiolitis was characterized by overinflated lungs with diffuse fine nodularity, which was most prominent in the lower zones. Functionally, the patients had progressive airflow obstruction terminating in respiratory failure. The airway lesions are diagnostic morphologically. There is chronic inflammation of proximal respiratory bronchioles and distal bronchioles. The inflammatory cells are usually mononuclear, and clear, presumably lipid-filled macrophages are prominent. There is fibrosis of the bronchiolar walls. The more proximal bronchioles dilate and become tortuous. With progression, the inflammation extends more proximally. Japanese physicians are perplexed by the apparent lack of the disease in other countries and have speculated that cases may be regarded in other countries as "chronic obstructive disease of small airways" or bronchiectasis.[60]

Graft-versus-Host Bronchiolitis

Since first described by Roca and colleagues in 1982,[129] bronchiolitis has become a well-recognized complication of graft-versus-host reaction.[99] Florid chronic airflow obstruction is relatively infrequent, but the majority of patients with graft-versus-host reaction following bone marrow transplantation have lymphocytic bronchitis and bronchiolitis. Patients have evidence of graft-versus-host reaction elsewhere and develop progressive airflow obstruction. They generally respond to treatment for graft-versus-host disease.

Heart-Lung Transplantation

Chronic inflammation, ulceration, and bronchiolar obliteration have been described in five of 16 heart-lung transplant patients who survived the immediate postoperative period.[176] Extensive bronchiectasis also has been described in some of the patients, together with pleural and interstitial fibrosis. Clinically, the patients had repeated bronchopulmonary infections and developed CAO. The etiology is unknown but it has been speculated that repeated bronchopulmonary infections, denervation, drug treatment, interruption of the bronchial blood supply, and ciliary dyskinesia all may play a part. Rejection may not be important, since similar lesions are not seen in lung transplant patients.

Follicular Bronchitis/Bronchiolitis

This condition was first recognized in a review of surgical biopsy consultations.[177] It consists of a heavy lymphocytic infiltrate with follicle formation in bronchi and bronchioles. It occurs in a wide age range, from infancy to middle age, and females are more commonly affected than males. The investigations placed their patients in three categories: collagen-vascular disease, mainly rheumatoid arthritis, involving slightly less than half the cases; immunodeficiency syndromes, both congenital and acquired, accounting for about a third; and the remainder, allergic. In the third group, blood eosinophilia was found in nearly all the patients in whom these data were available.

Mineral Dust Airways Disease

A distinctive lesion has been observed in the airways of workers exposed to mineral dust, referred to as mineral dust airways disease.[23, 24] A similar appearance has been noted in asbestos workers.[167] The lesion consists of dense fibrosis and heavy pigmentation of respiratory bronchioles. The more proximal bronchioles also had extensive fibrosis. The lesions were widespread in the airways.[24, 167] They were found in about a fourth of workers exposed to dust and in less than 1% of those not exposed. The patients with mineral dust airways disease showed expiratory flow obstruction, generally mild, and abnormalities of the single-breath nitrogen test. Although the data are to some extent controversial, there is evidence that airflow obstruction does occur in mineral dust–exposed workers (for review, see Churg and associates, 1985[24]). Churg and colleagues[24] pointed out that since only a minority of workers developed mineral dust airways disease, a survey of workers as a whole might not detect many cases of airflow obstruction.

Cryptogenic Bronchiolitis

Turton and coworkers[162] reviewed all patients with CAO, defined as having an FEV_1 of less than 60% predicted, seen in the pulmonary function laboratory at the Brompton Hospital, London, England. They excluded all known causes of CAO, such as emphysema, chronic bronchitis, asthma, smoking, and specific lung diseases, e.g., lung cancer. Of the more than 2000 patients reviewed, only ten remained, five of whom had rheumatoid arthritis and five who had no known cause. Presumably, in the latter, bronchiolitis was due to unrecognized viral infections or environmental agents.

Bronchiolitis Obliterans and Organizing Pneumonia

This interesting condition, delineated by Epler and colleagues[41] and Katzenstein and colleagues,[70] is mentioned only to be dismissed. Its major feature is morphologic intra-alveolar exudate (the British term is "cryptogenic organizing pneumonia").[31] Clinically, it is generally an example of infiltrative lung disease and restrictive lung disease,[48, 70, 106] and belongs in the differential diagnosis of these conditions.

LESIONS WITHIN THE ACINUS

The most important condition in the acinus is emphysema, which is characterized by destruction and enlargement of the acinus. The acinus is the unit of the lung in which gas exchange takes place. It is thus the structure beyond the terminal bronchiole (Fig. 1–2), the last purely conducting airway. Alveoli become evident in the subsequent airways that contain both alveoli and nonalveolated epithelium, which is mainly ciliated in humans. These are respiratory bronchioles, the transitional zone, and they contain more alveoli in succeeding generations. In the classic model of the acinus there are three orders of respiratory bronchioles. Alveolar ducts follow respiratory bronchioles; their walls are entirely alveolated. They in turn lead into the terminal structures of the acinus, alveolar sacs, likewise entirely lined by alveoli. The average distance between the terminal bronchiole and the end of the alveolar sac is small, 6.2 mm, and there is a rapid increase in surface area so that the gas-exchanging surface area is 50 to 100 m^2.[161] The transitional zone is at the respiratory bronchiolar level, where tidal volume meets resident gas and where gas transfer takes place by diffusion rather than flow.

Emphysema is classified in terms of how the acinus is enlarged and destroyed. At this time, a number of concepts and observations should be introduced. Emphysema is the most important cause of clinically assessed CAO and the most important cause of physiologically documented severe CAO.[101, 109, 165] Its significance in mild CAO still has to be explored thoroughly; conflicting data[168, 169, 174] on surgically derived lungs are available. In coal miners with a wide range of CAO, a correlation between emphysema and loss of FEV_1 was noted in an autopsy study.[130]

What has become apparent is that severity of emphysema is

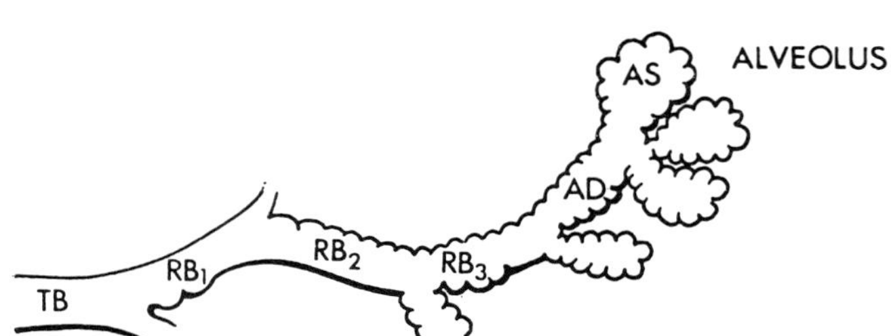

Figure 1–2. The acinus is the gas-exchanging unit of the lung and is subtended by the terminal bronchiole (TB). The acinus consists of, in sequence, respiratory bronchioles (RB) with increasing numbers of alveoli in their walls, alveolar ducts (AD), and alveolar sacs (AS). (Modified from Thurlbeck WM, Chronic Airflow Obstruction in Lung Disease. Philadelphia: W.B. Saunders Company, 1976.)

more important than type, and it is severity that determines flow reduction in CAO. An important relationship is the one between loss of elastic recoil and reduction in flow. In the simplest of terms, flow can be reduced only if airways are obstructed (narrowed), or if the driving force to expiratory flow is reduced.[84] The force that drives flow is elastic recoil, and thus flow may theoretically be limited, as opposed to obstructed, because of loss of recoil. Therefore, Macklem and Permutt (1979)[87] suggested that the term "chronic airflow limitation" be used rather than CAO.

An inherent assumption is that emphysema is the cause of loss of elastic recoil and that these two are closely related. It follows from this concept that airflow may be chronically limited by only two conditions: airway lesions and emphysema. This turns out to be an unduly simple concept that is dealt with more fully later. It has also become apparent that inflammation of respiratory bronchioles may be associated with abnormalities of expiratory flow; this will be described subsequently.

Respiratory Bronchiolitis

Wright and her colleagues[170] have shown that inflammation of respiratory bronchioles is related to a diminished FEV_1; they also found that increased muscle was positively related to the FEV_1. When the FEV_1 was normal, respiratory bronchiolitis and fibrosis were more important than membranous bronchiolar inflammation. This finding is surprising, because the total cross-sectional area at the respiratory bronchiolar level is extremely large, and, thus far, narrowing has not been described as a feature of respiratory bronchiolitis.

As has been mentioned, at this level gas exchange is more dependent on diffusion than flow. It may be that bronchiolar inflammation greatly alters the volume-pressure characteristics of these structures so that they narrow markedly on expiration. Whatever the explanation, this is an intriguing finding and suggests that respiratory bronchiolitis is more than just a predecessor to centrilobular emphysema. This lesion was first described in those patients likely to have mild CAO.[110] Some patients with respiratory bronchiolitis present with a clinical picture that resembles infiltrative lung disease.[107] These patients may be extreme examples of the cases reported by Guerry-Force and colleagues[48] concerning older smokers whose lungs were resected for lung cancer. Those reported by Myers and coworkers[107] concerned young patients, all under 40 years of age, who were very heavy smokers. Clinically, they were considered examples of patients with infiltrative lung disease with radiologic features that were consistent with this diagnosis, and, functionally, a restrictive as well as an obstructive lung pattern was seen in some cases.

Emphysema

Definition

Emphysema is defined as a permanent, abnormal enlargement of any part of the gas-exchanging structures of the lung, i.e., the acinus, accompanied by destruction of respiratory tissue, i.e., alveoli.[25, 2] This definition, long used, begs the meaning of destruction, and it was only in 1985 that this problem has been examined in detail. An NIH workshop committee[140] defined the destruction in emphysema as "nonuniformity in the pattern of respiratory airspace enlargement so that the orderly appearance of the acinus and its components is disturbed and may be lost."

In addition, it was believed that airspace enlargement accompanied by fibrosis, such as in fibrosing alveolitis (usually interstitial pneumonia), might qualify for the definition of emphysema unless fibrosis was excluded. Further, conditions associated with widespread granulomas of the lung, for example, eosinophilic granuloma, sarcoid, tuberculosis, and silicosis, might be associated with airspace enlargement (see subsequent discussions of irregular emphysema and paracicatricial emphysema).

However, the clinical, radiologic, and functional features of such patients are very different from those of the usual patients with emphysema. Since it was believed that fibrosis was not usually an evident part of emphysema, the committee concluded that airspace enlargement associated with, and probably due to, fibrosis should be excluded. Thus, the final definition becomes the following: "Emphysema is a condition of the lung characterized by permanent, abnormal enlargement of airspaces, such that the orderly appearance of the acinus is altered and may be lost and is not accompanied by obvious fibrosis."

The consequences of changing this definition are not great. The recognition of emphysema still remains a subjective one, and usually can be recognized by the naked eye. Irregular or paracicatricial emphysema disappears as an example of emphysema and becomes an example of airspace enlargement with fibrosis. Emphysema has become a subset of respiratory airspace enlargement, defined as "an increase in airspace size as compared with the airspaces of normal lungs. The term applies to all varieties of airspace enlargement distal to the terminal bronchioles, whether occurring with or without fibrosis or destruction."[140] Classification of respiratory airspace enlargement is shown in Table 1–4. The more important forms of airspace enlargement that are not emphysema are discussed in further detail later, but the implications and significance of the classification are discussed briefly.

The status of age changes in the lung becomes uncertain. An increase in airspace size occurs with increasing age in nonemphysematous lungs. However, this increase, compared with the values in young subjects, affects most, if not all, lungs.[149] Thus, the enlargement may not be abnormal. Both Down's syndrome[26] and congenital lobar overinflation have been included as examples of congenital simple airspace enlargement. It can be argued whether this is correct or not. The airspace enlargement of Down's syndrome is a postnatal event and probably represents defective alveolar multiplication in this period.[27] Although not present at birth, the defect is genetic in origin. Congenital lobar overinflation is not genetically determined but occurs most commonly in the immediate postnatal period and is discussed further later. Airspace enlargement, most commonly associated with fibrosis, is irregularly distributed within the acinus as a direct consequence of

TABLE 1–4. Respiratory Airspace Enlargement

SIMPLE AIRSPACE ENLARGEMENT
Congenital
Congenital lobar overinflation
Down's syndrome
Acquired
Secondary to loss of lung volume
Associated with aging
EMPHYSEMA
Proximal acinar (centriacinar) emphysema
Panacinar emphysema
Distal acinar emphysema
Bullae
AIRSPACE ENLARGEMENT WITH FIBROSIS
Irregular airspace enlargement
Other
Honeycomb lung

scarring. In general, this enlargement differs from that seen in "honeycomb" (end-stage) lung. In the end-stage lung, the airspaces are often lined by bronchiolar epithelium and the abnormality is best referred to as "bronchiolectasis." At other times, panacinar emphysema may result from scarring, although the emphysema itself is not accompanied by fibrosis.

Since the NIH workshop was published, workers at the Meakins-Christie laboratory in Montreal have described the "destructive index" (DI), using histologic slides of the lung[134]; they raised the question whether a redefinition of emphysema should be considered. The DI has three components: "obvious emphysema," abnormal breaks in alveolar walls, and fibrosis. Although not explicitly stated, the implications are that the DI might be the best way of recognizing emphysema, that it might be an appropriate definition of emphysema, and that the recognition of abnormal breaks in the alveolar wall might be a more sensitive and objective assessment of the disease. These investigators also showed that the DI was related to smoking and loss of pulmonary function. Another interesting observation was that the destructive index could be abnormal in smokers even when airspace size was within what they considered normal limits. Thus, the criterion of airspace enlargement might become unnecessary in the definition of emphysema, and destruction of airspace wall the only criterion. In our hands,[91, 135] obvious emphysema was by far the largest component of the DI, and the DI was not better related to pulmonary function abnormalities than the naked-eye assessment of emphysema.

Emphysema and Loss of Elastic Recoil

Another implication of the DI is that it might relate much better to loss of recoil than do the conventional assessments of emphysema, i.e., by gross or dissecting microscopic examination of inflated slices of lung or paper-mounted whole-lung sections. Although it is true that recoil is lost even in lungs with mild or trivial emphysema, compared with subjects without emphysema,[113, 116] when emphysema and volume-pressure curves have been compared, close correlations have not been found, no matter how the volume-pressure curves have been expressed.[153, 165]

As indicated, an often-made assumption is that emphysema and loss of elastic recoil are directly and closely related. It is quite clear that such is not the case. Hogg and colleagues[58] measured the compliance of centrilobular emphysematous spaces and found that, in the range equivalent to residual volume and total lung capacity, the compliance was actually decreased, but the compliance in the surrounding lung was increased. Indirect evidence from morphometry suggested increased total lung capacity in very mildly emphysematous lungs.[148] Emphysema in these lungs was so slight that average airspace size should not have been abnormal. Instead, average size was increased, suggesting overinflation of the whole lung. Direct measurements of post-mortem lung volumes, both formalin-fixed and air-filled, showed an increase in equivocal or mild emphysema,[11, 113, 152] and loss of recoil has also been observed in such lungs.[8, 13]

Perhaps the most convincing studies were those of the volume-pressure characteristics of excised human lungs.[9, 10] These studies showed that lower lobes were less compliant than upper lobes in nonemphysematous lungs. However, when lobes were compared in which emphysema was worse in the upper lobes, which is usually the case, the lower lobes lost more recoil and became more compliant than the upper lobes. All these observations have led to what has been referred to colloquially as the "doughnut hypothesis," i.e., loss of recoil in emphysematous lungs occurs in the apparently normal lung ("in the doughnut and not the hole"). Three explanations exist. First, the surrounding lung may be emphysematous, using conventional criteria, but is not recognized as such. The observer's attention is distracted by the obvious lesions, and the remaining lung is not examined adequately. In this regard, it is worth observing that in their original, classic study of centrilobular emphysema, Leopold and Gough,[75] pointed out that diffuse emphysema, i.e., panacinar emphysema or widespread airspace enlargement of the acinus, occurred in lungs with centrilobular emphysema. Second, obvious conventional emphysema might be absent but the DI, now affected only by alveolar wall breaks, might be present. These breaks reflect alterations in lung structure and are accompanied by loss of recoil. Third, the change in the lung parenchyma may be very subtle and changes in the collagen-elastin network, together with proteoglycans, may occur.

These alternatives can all be examined. Good evidence exists that there is morphologic alteration in the surrounding lung parenchyma, including the observations of Leopold and Gough[75] and the increased airspace in size in mildly emphysematous lungs. The second is easily examined by measuring breaks in the lung parenchyma; these might also be visualized using scanning electron microscopy. Observations using scanning electromicroscopy[30] have suggested that abnormal holes may be seen in the "near part," i.e., the alveoli in and adjacent to respiratory bronchioles. Those that are adjacent are distal and are "far" in the acinus. These holes correlate with loss of flow and loss of recoil. It is not clear whether these abnormal holes correspond to conventional emphysema. A detailed quantitative and qualitative study of the transmission microscopic appearance of the lung parenchyma may disclose very subtle structural abnormalities, and quantitative and qualitative biochemical measurements of the lung parenchyma may also disclose abnormalities. At this time, it is not clear which, if any, of these alternatives is the correct one.

Epidemiology of Emphysema

Numerous surveys of the frequency of emphysema have been done, and these have been reviewed elsewhere.[141, 150] Considerable discrepancies have been recorded, probably representing both interobserver variation and true differences. However, there is a general consensus from investigators whose studies are centered on populations of industrial cities about the following: in the usual population, based on studies at autopsy, average age about 60 years with predominance of males, obvious emphysema is seen in about 50% of the cases, but, on very careful examination, when airspace enlargement associated with fibrosis is included, the incidence rises to almost 100%.

About two thirds of males have emphysema and about one fourth of females. Emphysema is quite uncommon in people under the age of 40, rising in frequency till the seventh decade, and then declining. Smoking is accompanied by a dramatic increase in the frequency of emphysema. Another approach has been to examine the average severity of emphysema, because this has greater interobserver reproducibility.[155] The results were similar—average severity is greater in males than females, there is a rapid increase in average severity from the fifth to the seventh decade and then a decline. Smokers have a higher average severity, but emphysema is found in nonsmokers, particularly in the eighth and ninth decades.[159] The study also showed a greater average severity in Cardiff, Wales, compared with that in Malmö, Sweden; this was true of both men and women, smokers and nonsmokers.

Etiology and Pathogenesis of Emphysema

It has become conventional wisdom to invoke the "protease-antiprotease" hypothesis of emphysema.[67] In its simplest form, the hypothesis indicates that the structural proteins of the lung, notably collagen and elastin, are continually being synthesized and broken down, and that there are mechanisms that prevent excess breakdown. This hypothesis has its origin in two almost simultaneous, but equally serendipitous, observations. Gross and colleagues[47] were testing the hypothesis that the proteolytic enzyme papain would ameliorate the fibrosis of experimental silicosis. Instead, they made the astute observation that emphysema resulted instead.

A separate line of investigation[42, 73] noted that patients with reduced alpha$_1$-globulin levels on serum electrophoresis had an increased frequency of emphysema; this was familial. Subsequent investigations[67] showed that elastase was a potent cause of experimental emphysema, but that collagenase was not. The alpha$_1$-globulin defect was related to alpha$_1$-trypsin deficiency, and alpha$_1$-globulin had a significant antielastase activity. Smokers were found to have increased numbers of macrophages and polymorphonuclear leukocytes (PMNs) in bronchoalveolar lavage fluid. The macrophages were metabolically highly active and contained elastase and other proteolytic enzymes. Smokers were also shown to have diminished antiprotease activity, although this remains controversial. Support for this theory has also been found from a study on human lungs.

Saetta and coworkers (1985)[133] found an association between loss of alveolar attachments to airways and inflammation of the airways. In its now expanded form, the protease-antiprotease hypothesis states that the normal balance between proteolysis and antiproteolysis may be disturbed, and when proteolysis dominates, emphysema ensues. This usually occurs in tobacco smoking owing to increased inflammation, with release of proteolytic enzymes from inflammatory cells. In turn, the antiproteolytic mechanisms are defective in smokers. When antiproteolytic mechanisms are depressed, such as in congenital antiprotease deficiency, emphysema may occur spontaneously and is then much aggravated by tobacco smoking.

The hypothesis is not without defects, however. Macrophages are the dominant cell in both bronchoalveolar lavage fluid and respiratory bronchiolitis, but the elastase they contain is relatively ineffective. Serine elastase in PMNs is much more potent, and PMNs form only a small proportion of the inflammatory cells and occur in a higher proportion in airway lumina than in lung parenchyma.[174] Although increased numbers of PMNs are found in the blood and alveolar walls of smokers, there is no increase in the walls of the patients with emphysema.[83] Although airway inflammation was greater in smokers and ex-smokers than in nonsmokers, no difference in airway inflammation was present in emphysematous lungs compared with nonemphysematous lungs.[174] If PMNs are ablated experimentally, cadmium chloride plus beta-aminopropionitrile is still equally effective in producing emphysema.[59] It is also true that experimental emphysema is hard to produce by tobacco, and such models are not convincing replicas of human emphysema. Further, it is also not clear why tobacco smoking produces centrilobular emphysema in some parts of the lung and panacinar in others. Thus, although the protease-antiproteinase hypothesis is a convincing one, it contains specific defects.

Classification of Emphysema

Emphysema severity is more important than emphysema type, and it is clear that many aspects of emphysema can be discussed without resorting to classification (as mentioned earlier). However, no discussion of emphysema is complete without a consideration of classification. Many forms of emphysema exist, and broad generalizations will contain simplifications, errors, and defects. Classification leads to a closer examination of the etiology and pathogenesis of emphysema as well as clinicopathologic correlations. However, considerable interobserver variations occur in the classification of emphysema. This is particularly apparent when emphysema is severe.[155, 100] The morphology and clinical associations of emphysema have been reviewed in detail elsewhere.[150, 153, 154]

CENTRIACINAR (PROXIMAL ACINAR) EMPHYSEMA

In proximal acinar emphysema, the proximal part of the acinus—the respiratory bronchioles—is dominantly or selectively involved. Two forms are recognized.

Proximal Acinar Emphysema Due to Dust (Simple Coal Pneumoconiosis, Simple Pneumoconiosis, Focal Emphysema)

First and best described in coal miners,[54] proximal acinar emphysema may also occur with other nonfibrogenic dusts, and perhaps also in urban dwellers owing to soot.[51, 52] It is characterized by much pigment, and generally there is only a slight increase in the size of respiratory bronchioles. When cut transversely, the dilated spaces with adjacent pigment have been described as "spidery macules." The lesion is thought to be due to weakening of respiratory bronchiolar muscle, and dilatation dominates over destruction. Considerable controversy exists as to its functional significance, but contemporary evidence suggests that, whereas functional abnormalities can be identified, these are generally mild.[103]

Proximal Acinar, Nonindustrial Emphysema (Centrilobular Emphysema, CLE)

This is the commonest form of emphysema, and the common form of emphysema associated with the clinical syndrome of emphysema. It is virtually found only in smokers. As in dust-related emphysema, the lesions involve respiratory bronchioles, but these are primarily destructive. Pigmentation is usually only modest and may be absent. Centrilobular emphysema occurs most commonly and gets worse in the upper lobe and superior segment of the lower lobe. There is usually evidence of inflammation of the supplying bronchiole, which is narrowed in some 60% of instances. Characteristically, it is very irregular in severity, with considerable variation from lobule to lobule and even within lobules. Usually, the acinus peripheral to the spaces at the alveolar ducts and sacs, is normal. As has been pointed out, subtle airspace enlargement may often be present, and in many instances there may be encroachment on the peripheral part of the acinus. It is this feature that has led to controversy. As CLE gets worse, encroachment on the remaining acinus becomes more apparent. Some workers believe that this sort of encroachment obviates the diagnosis of CLE and that the diagnosis panacinar emphysema should be used.[127] Most observers believe that nonindustrial emphysema, which dominantly, but not solely, involves the proximal acinus, should be referred to as CLE.

PANACINAR (PANLOBULAR) EMPHYSEMA (PLE)

The term panacinar emphysema is applied when the acinus is more or less uniformly enlarged and destroyed. Panacinar emphysema has been reported in a variety of different situations; as in the case of proximal acinar emphysema, it should not be regarded as a single entity. All of the associations of PLE are to some extent controversial.

ALPHA$_1$-ANTITRYPSIN (PROTEINASE INHIBITOR) DEFICIENCY AND FAMILIAL EMPHYSEMA

Alpha$_1$-antitrypsin deficiency is discussed in detail elsewhere in this book (see Chapter 54). The amount and type of alpha$_1$-

antitrypsin, more properly called proteinase inhibitor (Pi), is determined by a pair of codominant alleles indicated by capital letters. PiM is the normal phenotype. PiZ is associated with an increased prevalence of emphysema, much more so in smokers. Symptomatic emphysema occurs in relatively young patients. The diagnosis should always be strongly suspected in patients with clinical emphysema who are younger than 40 years of age, and even in those who are in their forties. Chronic sputum production is less frequent than in the usual patient with severe emphysema. Clinically, the patient more frequently has "type A" COPD. Radiologically, the patient has greatly enlarged lung volume and pulmonary arterial deficiency, which is most marked in the lower zones of the lung. With one dissenting vote,[122] the emphysema has been regarded as panacinar in type. Severe pure panacinar emphysema is a relatively uncommon finding at autopsy, and this finding should suggest Pi deficiency.

PANACINAR EMPHYSEMA IN THE LOWER ZONES OF THE LUNG, WITH UPPER ZONAL CLE

This appearance is not infrequently seen in patients with significant CAO and at least moderate emphysema. These patients have similar clinical characteristics to those of CLE, namely male predominance, with a history of smoking and chronic sputum production. The argument exists whether this form of panacinar emphysema is in reality CLE that has progressed to PLE. This argument cannot be proved or disproved; it is much more logical to note this association of panacinar emphysema and regard it as a particular entity. Considerable interobserver variation occurs concerning the type of emphysema when emphysema is severe. The controversy usually occurs between panacinar emphysema and CLE in such cases.

PANACINAR EMPHYSEMA ASSOCIATED WITH BRONCHIAL AND BRONCHIOLAR ATRESIA

Swyer-James or Macleod Syndrome. This condition is most properly described as unilateral pulmonary transradiancy and is also sometimes referred to as unilateral pulmonary emphysema. The patients often give a history of severe bronchopulmonary infection in childhood, and the condition is usually recognized from a routine chest radiograph made in young adult life. Most or all of one lung appears transradiant. On expiration, the affected lung traps air and is then much larger than the contralateral lung. There is also increased blood flow through the contralateral lung and at times it may be regarded as abnormal because of the apparently increased markings. The air trapping is due to extensive bronchial and bronchiolar obliteration resulting from early childhood infection. The nature of the bronchiolar obliteration is such that the lung remains expanded owing to collateral ventilation. More usually, collapse of lung parenchyma ensues, following bronchial and bronchiolar obliteration. Patients then have typical bronchiectasis. Unilateral pulmonary transradiancy has been referred to as "bronchiectasis without atelectasis."

Few specimens have been studied,[128] but in them limited panacinar emphysema has been observed. Airflow obstruction is due to bronchiolar obliteration, not emphysema. It should be observed that the condition may not be strictly bilateral and that the lung is often not uniformly involved on one side.

Occasionally, localized bronchiolar obliteration with associated panacinar emphysema may be recognized as an incidental finding at autopsy.[150]

Another condition that may contribute to the understanding of one of the pathogeneses of panacinar emphysema is *congenital bronchial atresia.* Most commonly seen in the apicoposterior segment of the left upper lobe, the affected lung is overinflated, traps air, and shows panacinar emphysema. A distinctive radiologic feature is accumulation of mucus immediately distal to the atretic bronchus; this may present radiologically as a mass. No convincing explanation has been given for the occurrence of panacinar emphysema distal to obstructed airways. The most usual one is that intra-alveolar pressure exceeds pulmonary capillary pressure, especially on expiration, and ischemic atrophy of alveolar walls results.

PANACINAR EMPHYSEMA ASSOCIATED WITH OLD AGE. As subsequently described, a predictable set of morphologic changes affects all, or nearly all, human lungs. In addition, however, a small proportion of older, nonsmoking patients develop emphysema. This is mild and panacinar in type and is usually found along the margins of the lower lobes. It is asymptomatic.

DISTAL ACINAR (PARASEPTAL) EMPHYSEMA. Emphysema occasionally may involve, selectively, the distal part of the acinus, which includes the alveolar ducts and sacs and as such may involve the periphery of the lobule and abut on pleura, lobular septa, and bronchovascular bundles. It is usually limited in extent and is an isolated finding but may occur in conjunction with centrilobular emphysema.[52, 150, 151] It has been suggested that it is the type of emphysema that is associated with spontaneous pneumothorax in young adults.[39] This seems a logical feature of distal acinar emphysema because of its subpleural location and because it tends to involve the superior part of the lung. It is thus exposed to maximum stress due to high negative intrapleural pressures, and rupture may occur easily. Most parenchymal lesions in spontaneous pneumothorax are nonspecific, however, and associated with obvious fibrosis and inflammation.[76, 112] In addition to the association with spontaneous pneumothorax, Edge and colleagues[39] described a patient with widespread distal acinar emphysema with clinical features similar to those described by Laurenzi and coworkers[74] in patients with "bullous disease of the lung." These patients were relatively young and showed numerous radiologic bullae. Airflow obstruction was slight unless they developed significant bronchial infection.

Emphysema-Like Conditions

AIRSPACE ENLARGEMENT WITH FIBROSIS. As indicated, obvious fibrosis excludes the diagnosis of emphysema. In usual interstitial pneumonia, or fibrosing alveolitis, there is enlargement of airspaces. These enlarged airspaces mainly represent bronchiolectasis,[118] but other enlarged spaces in usual interstitial pneumonia may be lined by alveolar epithelium and thus may resemble emphysematous spaces. Isolated scars of the lung are extremely common, and adjacent airspaces are usually enlarged and destroyed. Airspace enlargement usually involves the acinus irregularly, hence the older terms "irregular emphysema" and "paracicatricial emphysema." These lesions are asymptomatic. Occasionally there may be widespread scarring in the lung accompanied by quite extensive airspace enlargement. This may be seen in some cases of sarcoidosis, eosinophilic granuloma, silicosis, and chronic infections such as tuberculosis and histoplasmosis. These patients differ from the usual patients with CAO in that whether they smoke is irrelevant, the underlying disease is usually evident, radiologically they have increased linear or nodular markings, or both, and a restrictive pattern of pulmonary function may dominate over an obstructive one.

THE AGING LUNG. With age, a predictable set of changes occur in the lung. Grossly, the anteroposterior diameter increases more than cephalocaudal dimension, and the lung thus "rounds out."[4] The airspaces become larger; in particular, alveolar ducts increase in diameter and alveoli flatten. This change has been referred to as ductectasia.[131] Morphometrically, the average interalveolar wall distance, or mean linear intercept, increases, and the gas-exchanging surface area decreases. The proportion that alveolar walls form of the total lung decreases from about 11% to 7%; this may be due to actual loss of alveoli.[19] These changes affect most, if not all, aged lungs, and thus are "normal." They therefore currently do not qualify as falling into the category of airspace enlargement. Because the orderly appearance of the acinus is not altered, the term emphysema cannot be applied. These structural changes are accompanied by minimal functional alterations, particularly when careful prospective studies are made in nonsmokers. The functional changes include a small decrement in FEV_1 and vital capacity and a slight increase in functional residual capacity and residual volume. Diffusing capacity decreases. The changes in elastic properties are small and include loss of elastic recoil.

OVERINFLATION. If the lung is acutely overinflated, such as in asthma or acute atelectasis, or chronically, such as following pneumonectomy, the remaining lung overinflates to fill much of the available space. Airspaces are enlarged but only slightly. Linear changes vary with the cube root of changes in volume. Thus, doubling lung volume increases linear dimensions by 26%, and this change may not be recognized because of the wide normal variation. No destruction occurs; thus, the alteration is not emphysema.

One special category of overinflation that requires brief mention is *infantile lobar overinflation.* In this condition, a lobe or part of the lobe rapidly overinflates, usually in early infancy. It most commonly involves the left upper lobe and is frequently associated with congenital cardiac anomalies. It may be life-threatening because of compression of the remaining lung, and therapeutic intervention may be necessary. About one half of cases are thought to be due to deficiency of airway cartilage leading to progressive overinflation.[143] Once again, there is no destruction of airspace walls, so the condition is not emphysema. Some patients with this condition do not have enlarged alveoli but rather have an increased number of small alveoli, called "polyalveolar lobe."[55] However, the normative data used in the reported study were small and poorly defined. It is now recognized that many more alveoli are present at birth[56, 72] than previously thought and that there is a very wide range. It may be that polyalveolar lobe represents a variant of the normal lobe. In any event, it is clinically indistinguishable from nonpolyalveolar congenital lobar emphysema.[147]

BLEBS. Blebs are collections of air within the pleura, do not involve the acinus, and are therefore not a form of emphysema. Interstitial emphysema is a collection of air within the interstitium of the lung. It may involve the lobular septa, bronchovascular bundles, and pleura. If the definition of blebs were broadened to include collections of air in the interstitium as well as the pleura, interstitial emphysema could be referred to more properly as multiple blebs. It is of historical interest that Laennec separated "emphysema proper," what we understand as emphysema today, from other collections of air in the lung. Emphysema until that time was thought of as being analogous to subcutaneous emphysema, corresponding to interstitial emphysema. Pulmonary interstitial emphysema is seen in adults as an occasional complication of assisted ventilation or when tissue emphysema from other sites dissects backward into the lung. Pulmonary interstitial emphysema (PIE) is a common and important complication of assisted ventilation in the neonatal period in premature infants.

Special Forms of Emphysema

Bullae are a form of emphysema and have been defined as airspaces within the lung parenchyma that are more than 1 cm in diameter in the distended state.[25] Such spaces are not uncommonly seen radiologically but pathologically are much less common. Most airspaces that are radiologically visible contain lung parenchyma pathologically and are not true cystic spaces. Some radiologically visible upper zonal bullae are large CLE spaces.[160] In the lower lobe, bullae usually represent greatly attenuated lung parenchyma, bordered by lobular septa, which form the margins as seen radiologically.

Bullae are classified into three types.[127] Type I bullae occur subpleurally in the lung and occur in the absence of widespread emphysema. They have a narrow base and in excised lungs protrude in a mushroom-like fashion from the exterior of the lung. In life, these bullae are limited by the chest wall and are thus depressed within the substance of the lung. Type II bullae have a broad base, are subpleural in position, and are usually associated with emphysema within the rest of the lung. Type III bullae are the same as type II bullae, but occur in the substance of the lung. They are quite frequently diagnosed on chest radiographs thought to show emphysema.

An occasional, but important, clinical problem is the distinction between type I bullae and types II and III. Type I bullae may compromise lung function because of their compressive effect on normal lung tissue, and surgical excision may cure this. Types II and III bullae are complications of widespread emphysema, and while they may compromise lung function per se, the remaining lung makes a variable contribution to pulmonary dysfunction. The clinical distinction between solitary bullae and bullae associated with emphysema is usually not difficult. In the former, the patient may not have the usual clinical background of COPD, and the pulmonary defect may be restrictive, with minimal evidence of airflow obstruction. In the classic examples of the latter, bullae are an incidental finding on a chest radiograph of a patient with emphysema and classic COPD. However, a group of patients remain in which the diagnosis is difficult, in that they have bullae, CAO, and evidence of at least mild emphysema. A clinical judgement has to be made, and it involves a balance between the estimate of the improvement of function likely to follow bullectomy and recognition of the severity of underlying disease, which is not likely to improve. Computed tomography may have a role to play in such decisions; this is discussed subsequently.

Recognition of the Severity of Emphysema

Considerable effort was made to correlate the severity of emphysema and pulmonary function test results in the 1960s and, to a lesser extent, subsequently. Earlier literature[150] and subsequent information[153] have been reviewed in detail. There is general agreement that emphysema is the most important association of clinically apparent severe CAO[101, 150] and that increasing severity of emphysema is associated with increasing frequency of clinically diagnosed severe CAO.[151] It should be noted, however, that up to one third of cases with severe emphysema at autopsy may not have had obvious evidence of clinical CAO.[151] As emphysema gets worse, so do pulmonary function test results. These include diminution of FEV_1, forced expiratory flow between 25% and 75% of vital capacity (FEF_{25-75}), increased residual volume, functional residual capacity, and total lung capacity (TLC), decreased diffusing capacity, and loss of elastic recoil. Most functional abnormalities, however, are poorly related to the severity of emphysema, although significantly related statistically. Correlation coefficients of 0.4 to 0.5 are usual. The best single correlate of emphysema has generally been found to be the diffusing capacity for carbon monoxide, either single-breath or steady-state. Total lung capacity was poorly or not at all correlated with emphysema in the older studies, but since then a much better correlation has been observed.[165] This improvement has been attributed to the plethysmographic measurement of TLC in the last study, as opposed to the use of helium dilution in the earlier ones. Helium dilution underestimates TLC in patients with severe emphysema.

Numerous correlations have been reported between the severity of emphysema noted at autopsy and the radiologic diagnosis of emphysema; these have been controversial.[150, 160] Part of the controversy has stemmed from the different criteria used for the radiologic diagnosis of emphysema[119] and part from lack of clarity of what is meant by the radiologic diagnosis of emphysema. The radiologic diagnosis in most studies was "all or none," and this was applied to cases with varying degrees of emphysema at autopsy. The idea of assessing the severity of emphysema was first used with conventional radiography,[82] and this showed an approximately 75% sensitivity, specificity, and accuracy when moderately severe radiologic emphysema was compared with a similar degree of emphysema in lung specimens. Pratt[119] has provided a comprehensive review of the efficacy of the radiologic diagnosis of emphysema.

Computed tomography (CT) has necessitated a quantitative approach on radiographs and shown very good correlations between CT-estimated severity and pathologic severity of the emphysema.[16] Emphysema can also be localized more precisely with CT scanning and may be important in patients with radiographically apparent bullae that require an assessment of the degree of parenchymal change in the rest of the lung. The most recent study[98] has confirmed the good correlation between morphologic emphysema and CT scans and has the advantage that the specimens were cut in the same plane as were the CT scans. Thus, direct comparisons could be made. The CT diagnosis is highly specific, but a significant number of cases were found in which there was obvious mild morphologic emphysema, which could not be recognized on the scan. In general, CT assessments of extent and severity were less than in the corresponding pathology slices. This study reviews previous CT-pathology correlative studies.

We have repeatedly emphasized the need for an integrated clinical approach in prediction of the amount of emphysema.[150, 153, 157] At the simple clinical level, history is important. A suitable age, a history of chronic productive cough, and cigarette smoking are important positive features. The more abnormal the pulmonary function data, the more likely is emphysema to be present and severe. The greater importance of TLC in predicting emphysema suggests a more significant role for radiology, since an increased TLC is reflected by radiologic "overinflation." Furthermore, TLC can be estimated accurately from chest radiographs[152]; computer-assisted digitizers make this measurement simple, very quick, and clearly cheaper than plethysmographically determined TLC. All patients with CAO undergo chest radiographs; it now becomes important that these should be taken at full inspiration. As indicated, the diffusing capacity for carbon monoxide (D_{CO}) has been widely recognized as a good predictor of emphysema. The single-breath method is simple, cheap, and quick. Thus, the algorithm consists of clinical circumstances, a chest radiograph, and measurement of diffusing capacity. The more the patient fits, in a quantitative sense, the more likely is he or she to have significant emphysema; the reverse is true as the patient fits less well.

TABLE 1–5. Functional Correlates of Lesions

LESIONS	CORRELATES
Bronchi	
Mucous gland enlargement	Sputum production, diminished flow rates
Smooth muscle hyperplasia	?Airway hyperreactivity, diminished flow rates
Cartilage atrophy	?Nil, ?expiratory collapse
Inflammation	Nil
Airway thickening and luminal encroachment	?Probable flow reduction
Bronchioles	
Bronchiolar obliteration	Peripheral flow obstruction, e.g., bronchiectasis, and special forms of bronchiolitis
Bronchiolar narrowing	Flow obstruction in mild and severe CAO
Bronchiolar tortuosity and loss of alveolar attachments	Flow obstruction in mild and severe CAO
Goblet-cell metaplasia	Flow obstruction in mild and severe CAO
Inflammation	Flow obstruction in mild CAO
Fibrosis	Flow obstruction in mild CAO; beneficial in severe CAO
Muscle increase	?Flow obstruction in mild CAO; beneficial in severe CAO
Mucus plugging	?Terminal event; insignificant in mild CAO
Pigmentation	Coincidental association with CAO
Acinus	
Respiratory bronchiolitis	Mild CAO
	Occasional cause of clinical interstitial lung disease
Emphysema	Clinical CAO, reduction in flow rates, altered lung volumes, diminished D_{CO}, abnormal chest radiograph

SUMMARY

This chapter has reviewed lesions in the airways and gas-exhanging tissue of the lung that may be associated with CAO. In each instance, the reported functional correlates have been reviewed, and these are summarized in Table 1–5. For convenience, airways were divided into bronchi and bronchioles. The major lesions that have been described in the former are mucous gland enlargement, muscle hyperplasia, and cartilage atrophy. The first corresponds approximately to chronic sputum production and is probably associated with airflow obstruction. The second is the major correlate of obstruction in patients with asthma. In patients with mild CAO, inflammation of the bronchioles is a significant lesion, as are fibrosis and goblet-cell metaplasia. Narrowing of airways has not been extensively studied in such patients. In severe CAO, other than for goblet-cell metaplasia, these lesions become less important, and fibrosis and increased muscle appear beneficial. Distortion of the shape of airways and increase in proportion of very narrowed airways become more significant. In patients with severe CAO, emphysema assumes a dominant role. It is not closely associated with loss of elastic recoil, and it may have a direct effect on airway deformity and diameter. The precise diagnosis of the lesions responsible for the obstruction in patients with CAO is often difficult. In the average patient various lesions of differing severity are present in all parts of the airways and lung parenchyma. A single lesion is not usually the sole cause. Severity of emphysema can often be assessed in living subjects with CAO with reasonable accuracy.

One topic has not been addressed: the diagnosis of mild emphysema. This is now of more than theoretic interest. The elastase model of emphysema is shown to be progressive after one intratracheal injection.[71] In the human, emphysema may also be progressive and almost certainly so in continuing smokers. Therapeutic intervention may be a possibility; alpha$_1$-antitrypsin is now available through genetic engineering and could conceivably play a role in treatment of nonfamilial emphysema. In any event, the history of medicine indicates that therapeutic agents appear often quite unexpectedly. Thus, the diagnosis of mild emphysema is an important challenge.

Although definitive information is not available it can be speculated that mild emphysema can be recognized using clinical, functional, and radiologic criteria (see "Recognition of Severity of Emphysema," earlier). Definitive data should become available from study of surgically derived lungs.

A cautionary note should be restated. A large number of correlative studies have been made to predict pathology from function. These studies are mostly derived from one of two sources: autopsy lungs from cases of known severe CAO or patients whose lungs have been surgically resected for cancer. In the former group, observed lesions are likely to be associated with pulmonary dysfunction. Lesions that are not associated with severe pulmonary dysfunction may be more interesting in this group.

Patients whose lungs are studied at surgery are from a restricted group; they nearly all have lung cancer and seldom have significant pulmonary dysfunction since they would otherwise not be operated on. In this group, lesions associated with more severe grades of CAO become of particular interest. It is not appropriate to project data derived from either source to the population at large. Although an anatomic, clinical, and functional study on such a population would be extremely interesting, it is not feasible at the present time and may never be.

REFERENCES

1. Aikawa T, Shimura S, Sasaki H, et al. Morphometric analysis of intraluminal mucus in airways in chronic obstructive pulmonary disease. Am Rev Respir Dis 1989; 140:477–482.
2. American Thoracic Society. Chronic bronchitis, asthma and pulmonary emphysema. A statement by the committee on diagnostic standards for nontuberculous respiratory diseases. Am Rev Respir Dis 1962; 85:762–768.
3. Anderson AE, Foraker AG. Relative dimensions of bronchioles and parenchymal spaces in lungs from normal subjects and emphysematous patients. Am J Med 1962; 32:218–226.
4. Anderson WF, Anderson AE Jr, Hernandez JA, Foraker AG. Topograph of aging and emphysematous lungs. Am Rev Respir Dis 1964; 90:411–423.
5. Baile EM, Wright JL, Pare PD, Hogg JC. The effect of acute small airway inflammation on pulmonary function in dog. Am Rev Respir Dis 1982; 126:298–301.
6. Bath JC, Yates PA. Clinical and pathologic correlations in chronic airways obstruction—observation on patients with pulmonary resection. In: Current Research in Chronic Airways Obstruction. Ninth Aspen Emphysema Conference, 293–308. Public Health Service Publication 1717, 1968.
7. Berend N. Lobar distribution of bronchiolar inflammation in emphysema. Am Rev Respir Dis 1981; 124:218–220.
8. Berend N, Skoog C, Thurlbeck WM. Pressure-volume characteristics of excised human lungs: effects of sex, age and emphysema. J Appl Physiol 1980; 49:558–565.
9. Berend N, Skoog C, Thurlbeck WM. Lobar pressure-volume characteristics of excised human lungs. Thorax 1981; 36:290–295.
10. Berend N, Skoog C, Thurlbeck WM. Exponential analysis of lobar pressure-volume characteristics. Thorax 1981; 36:452–455.
11. Berend N, Skoog C, Waskiewicz L, Thurlbeck WM. Maximum volumes in excised human lungs: effects of age, emphysema and formalin inflation. Thorax 1980; 35:859–864.
12. Berend N, Thurlbeck WM. Correlation of maximum expiratory flow with small airway dimensions and pathology. J Appl Physiol 1982; 52:346–351.
13. Berend N, Thurlbeck WM. Exponential analysis of pressure-volume relationship in excised human lungs. J Appl Physiol 1982; 52:838–844.
14. Berend N, Woolcock AJ, Marlin GE. Correlation between the function and structure of the lung in smokers. Am Rev Respir Dis 1979; 119:695–705.
15. Berend N, Wright JL, Thurlbeck WM, et al. Small airways disease: Reproducibility of measurement and correlation with lung function. Chest 1981; 79:263–268.
16. Bergin C, Müller N, Nichols DM, et al. The diagnosis of emphysema. A computed tomographic pathologic correlation. Am Rev Respir Dis 1986; 133:541–546.
17. Bignon J, Andre-Bougeran J, Brouet G. Parenchymal, bronchiolar and bronchial measurements in centrilobular emphysema. Relation to weight of right ventricle. Thorax 1970; 25:556–567.
18. Bignon J, Khoury F, Even P, et al. Morphometric study in chronic obstructive bronchopulmonary disease. Am Rev Respir Dis 1969; 99:669–695.
19. Brody JS, Thurlbeck WM. Development, growth, and aging of the lung. In: Macklem PT, Mead J, eds. Handbook of Physiology. Section 3. The Respiratory System. Volume III. Mechanics of Breathing, part I. Bethesda, MD: American Physiological Society, 1986, 335–386.
20. Burrows B, Bloom JW, Traver GA, Cline MG. The course and prognosis of different forms of chronic airways obstruction in a sample from the general population. N Engl J Med 1987; 317: 1309–1314.
21. Burrows B, Fletcher CM, Heard BE, et al. The emphysematous and bronchial types of chronic airways obstruction: a clinicopathological study of patients in London and Chicago. Lancet 1966; i:830–835.
22. Carlile A, Edwards C. Structural variations in the named bronchi of the left lung. A morphometric study. Br J Dis Chest 1983; 77:344–348.
23. Churg A, Wright JL. Small-airway lesions in patients exposed to nonasbestos mineral dusts. Hum Pathol 1983; 14:688–693.
24. Churg A, Wright JL, Wiggs B, et al. Small airways disease and mineral dust exposure. Am Rev Respir Dis 1985; 131:139–143.
25. Ciba Guest Symposium Report: Terminology, definitions and classification of chronic pulmonary emphysema and related conditions. Thorax 1959; 14:286–299.
26. Cooney TP, Thurlbeck WM. Pulmonary hypoplasia in Down's syndrome. N Engl J Med 1982; 307:1170–1173.
27. Cooney TP, Wentworth P, Thurlbeck WM. Diminished radial count is found only postnatally in Down's syndrome. Pediatr Pulmonol 1988; 5:204–209.
28. Cosio MG, Ghezzo H, Hogg JC, et al. The relations between structural changes in small airways and pulmonary-function tests. N Engl J Med 1978; 298:1277–1281.
29. Cosio MG, Hale KA, Niewoehner DE. Morphologic and morphometric effects of prolonged cigarette smoking on the small airways. Am Rev Respir Dis 1980; 122:265–271.
30. Cosio MG, Shiner RJ, Saetta M, et al. Alveolar fenestrae in smokers. Relationship with light microscopic and functional abnormalities. Am Rev Respir Dis 1986; 133:126–131.
31. Davison AG, Heard BE, McAlistair WAC, Turner-Warwick MEH. Cryptogenic organizing pneumonia. Q J Med 1983; 52:382–394.
32. Dayman H. Mechanics of airflow in health and disease. J Clin Invest 1951; 30:1175–1190.
33. De Haller R, Reid L. Adult chronic bronchitis. Morphology, histochemistry, and vascularisation of the bronchial mucous glands. Med Thorac 1965; 22:549–567.
34. Depierre A, Bignon J, Lebeau A, Brouet G. Quantitative study of parenchyma and small conductive airways in chronic nonspecific lung disease. Use of histologic stereology and bronchial casts. Chest 1972; 62:699–708.
35. Despas PJ, Leroux M, Macklem PT. Site of airways obstruction in asthma as determined by respiratory maximal expiratory flow breathing air and a helium-oxygen mixture. J Clin Invest 1972; 51:3235–3243.
36. Douglas AN. Quantitative study of bronchial mucus gland enlargement. Thorax 1980; 35:198–201.
37. Dunnill MS, Massarella GR, Anderson JA. A comparison of the quantitative anatomy of the bronchi in normal subject, in *status asthmaticus* in chronic bronchitis and in emphysema. Thorax 1969; 24:176–179.
38. Ebert RV, Terracio MJ. The bronchiolar epithelium in cigarette smokers. Am Rev Respir Dis 1975; 111:4–11.
39. Edge J, Simon G, Reid L. Peri-acinar (paraseptal) emphysema: its clinical, radiological and physiologic features. Br J Dis Chest 1966; 60:10–18.
40. Enarson DA, Vedal S, Schulzer M, et al. Asthma, asthmalike symptoms, chronic bronchitis, and the degree of bronchial hy-

perresponsiveness in epidemiologic surveys. Am Rev Respir Dis 1987; 136:613–617.
41. Epler GR, Colby TV, McLoud TC, et al. Idiopathic bronchiolitis obliterans with organising pneumonia. N Engl J Med 1985; 312:152–159.
42. Eriksson S. Studies in alpha$_1$-antitrypsin deficiency. Acta Med Scand 1965; 177(Suppl 432):1–85.
43. Etherton JE, Conning DM, Corrin B. Autoradiographical and morphological evidence for apocrine secretion of dipalmitoyl lecithin in the terminal bronchiole of the mouse lung. Am J Anat 1973; 138:11–19.
44. Geddes DM, Corrin B, Brewerton DA, et al. Progressive airway obliteration in adults and its association with rheumatoid disease. Q J Med 1977; 46:427–444.
45. Geddes DM, Webley M, Emerson PA. Airways obstruction in rheumatoid arthritis. Ann Rheum Dis 1979; 38:222–225.
46. Gil J, Weibel ER. Extracellular lining of bronchioles after perfusion fixation of rat lungs for electron microscopy. Anat Rec 1971; 169:185–199.
47. Gross P, Pfitzer EA, Toker E, et al. Experimental emphysema: its production with papain in normal and silicotic rats. Arch Environ Health 1965; 11:50–58.
48. Guerry-Force ML, Müller NL, Wright JL, et al. A comparison of bronchiolitis obliterans with organizing pneumonia, usual interstitial pneumonia and small airways disease. Am Rev Respir Dis 1987; 135:705–712.
49. Hale DA, Niewoehner DE, Cosio MG. Morphologic changes in the muscular pulmonary arteries: Relationship to cigarette smoking, airways disease and emphysema. Am Rev Respir Dis 1980; 122:273–278.
50. Hayes JA. Distribution of bronchial gland measurements in a Jamaican population. Thorax 1969; 24:619–622.
51. Heard BE. A pathological study of emphysema of the lungs with chronic bronchitis. Thorax 1958; 13:136–149.
52. Heard BE. Further observations on the pathology of pulmonary emphysema in chronic bronchitis. Thorax 1959; 14:58–70.
53. Heard BE, Hossain S. Hyperplasia of bronchial muscle in asthma. J Pathol 1973; 110:319–331.
54. Heppleston AG. The pathological anatomy of simple pneumokoniosis in coal workers. J Pathol Bacteriol 1953; 66:235–246.
55. Hislop A, Reid L. New pathological findings in emphysema of childhood: 1. Polyalveolar lobe with emphysema. Thorax 1970; 25:682–690.
56. Hislop A, Wigglesworth JS, Desai R. Alveolar development in the human fetus and infant. Early Hum Dev 1986; 13:1–11.
57. Hogg JC, Macklem PT, Thurlbeck WM. Site and nature of airway obstruction in chronic obstructive lung disease. N Engl J Med 1968; 278:1355–1360.
58. Hogg JC, Nepszy SJ, Macklem PT, Thurlbeck WM. Elastic properties of the centrilobular emphysematous space. J Clin Invest 1969; 48:1306–1312.
59. Hoidal JR, Niewoehner DE, Rao NV, Hibbs MS. The role of neutrophils in the development of cadmium chloride–induced emphysema in lathyrogen-fed hamsters. Am J Pathol 1985; 120:22–29.
60. Homma H, Yamanaka A, Tanimota S, et al. Diffuse panbronchitis. A disease of the transitional zone of the lung. Chest 1983; 83:63–69.
61. Hoppin FG, Green M, Morgan MS. The relationship of central and peripheral airway resistance to lung volume in dogs. J Appl Physiol 1978; 44:728–737.
62. Horsfield K, Cumming G. Morphology of the bronchial tree in man. J Appl Physiol 1968; 24:373–383.
63. Hossain S, Heard BE. Hyperplasia of bronchial muscle in chronic bronchitis. J Pathol 1970; 101:171–184.
64. Huber HL, Koessler K. The pathology of bronchial asthma. Arch Intern Med 1922; 30:689–760.
65. Jamal K, Cooney TP, Fleetham JA, Thurlbeck WM. Chronic bronchitis: correlation of morphological findings in sputum production and flow rates. Am Rev Respir Dis 1984; 129:719–722.
66. Jamal K, Fleetham JA, Thurlbeck WM. Cor pulmonale: correlations with central airway lesions, peripheral airway lesions, emphysema and control of breathing. Am Rev Respir Dis, In press, 1990.
67. Janoff A. State of the art. Elastases and emphysema. Current assessment of the protease-antiprotease hypothesis. Am Rev Respir Dis 1985; 132:417–433.
68. Kappos AD, Rodarte JR, Lai-Fook SJ. Frequency dependence and partitioning of respiratory impedance in dogs. J Appl Physiol 1981; 51:621–629.
69. Karpick RJ, Pratt PC, Asmundsson T, Kilburn KH. Pathological findings in respiratory failure. Ann Intern Med 1970; 72:189–197.
70. Katzenstein A-LA, Myers JL, Prophet WD, et al. Bronchiolitis obliterans and usual interstitial pneumonia. A comparative clinicopathologic study. Am J Surg Pathol 1986; 10:373–381.
71. Kuhn C III, Tavassoli F. The scanning electron microscopy of elastase-induced emphysema. Lab Invest 1976; 34:2–9.
72. Langston C, Kida K, Reed M, Thurlbeck WM. Human lung growth in late gestation and in the neonate. Am Rev Respir Dis 1984; 129:607–613.
73. Laurell CB, Eriksson S. The electrophoretic alpha–1-globulin pattern in alpha–1-antitrypsin deficiency. Scand J Clin Invest 1963; 15:132–140.
74. Laurenzi GA, Turino GM, Fishman AP. Bullous disease of the lung. Am J Med 1962; 32:361–378.
75. Leopold JG, Gough J. The centrilobular form of hypertrophic emphysema and its relation to chronic bronchitis. Thorax 1957; 12:219–235.
76. Lichter I, Gwynne JF. Spontaneous pneumothorax in young subjects. Thorax 1971; 26:409.
77. Liebow AA, Loring WE, Felton WL II. The musculature of the lungs in chronic pulmonary disease. Am J Pathol 1953; 29:885–912.
78. Linhartova A, Anderson AE Jr, Foraker AG. Radial traction and bronchiolar obstruction in pulmonary emphysema. Arch Pathol 1971; 92:384–391.
79. Linhartova A, Anderson AE, Foraker AG. Non-respiratory bronchiolar deformities. Graphic assessment in normal and emphysematous lungs. Arch Pathol Lab Med 1973; 95:45–47.
80. Linhartova A, Anderson AE, Foraker AG. Topology of non-respiratory bronchioles of normal and emphysematous lungs. Hum Pathol 1974; 5:729–735.
81. Linhartova A, Anderson AE, Foraker AG. Further observations on luminal deformity and stenosis of non-respiratory bronchioles in pulmonary emphysema. Thorax 1977; 32:53–59.
82. Lohela P, Sutinen S, Pääkkä P, et al. Diagnosis of emphysema on chest radiographs. ROFO 1984; 141:395–402.
83. Ludwig PW, Schwartz BA, Hoidal JR, Niewoehner DE. Cigarette smoking causes accumulation of polymorphonuclear leukocytes in alveolar septum. Am Rev Respir Dis 1985; 131:828–830.
84. Macklem PT. Airway obstruction and collateral ventilation. Physiol Rev 1971; 51:368–436.
85. Macklem PT, Fraser RG, Bates DV. Bronchial pressures and dimensions in health and obstructive airway disease. J Appl Physiol 1963; 18:669–706.
86. Macklem PT, Fraser RG, Brown WG. Bronchial pressure measurements in emphysema and bronchitis. J Clin Invest 1965; 44:897–905.
87. Macklem PT, Permutt S. The Lung in Transition Between Health and Disease. New York: Marcel Dekker Inc., 1979.
88. Macklem PT, Proctor DF, Hogg JC. The stability of peripheral airways. Respir Physiol 1970; 8:191–203.
89. Maisel JC, Silvers GW, George MS, et al. The significance of bronchial atrophy. Am J Pathol 1972; 67:371–386.
90. Maisel JC, Silvers GW, Mitchell RS, Petty TL. Bronchial atrophy and dynamic expiratory collapse. Am Rev Respir Dis 1968; 98:988–997.
91. Matsuba K, Ikeda T, Nagai A, Thurlbeck WM. The National Institutes of Health Intermittent Positive-Pressure Breathing trial. Pathology studies. Am Rev Respir Dis 1989; B9:1439–1445.
92. Matsuba K, Thurlbeck WM. The number and dimensions of small airways in emphysematous lungs. Am J Pathol 1972; 67:265–275.
93. Matsuba K, Thurlbeck WM. Disease of the small airways in chronic bronchitis. Am Rev Respir Dis 1973; 107:552–558.
94. Matsuba K, Shirakusa T, Kuwano K, et al. Small airways disease in patients without chronic airflow limitation. Am Rev Respir Dis 1987; 136:1106–1111.
95. McKenzie HI, Glick M, Outhred KG. Chronic bronchitis in coal miners: ante-mortem/post-mortem comparisons. Thorax 1969; 24:527–535.

96. McLean KH. The pathogenesis of pulmonary emphysema. Am J Med 1958; 25:62–74.
97. Medical Research Council. Definition and classification of chronic bronchitis for clinical and epidemiological purposes. A report to the Medical Research Council by their committee on the aetiology of chronic bronchitis. Lancet 1965; i:775–779.
98. Miller RR, Müller NL, Vedal S, et al. Limitations of computed tomography in the assessment of emphysema. Am Rev Respir Dis 1989; 139:980–983.
99. Miller RR, Thurlbeck WM. Diffuse diseases of the lungs. In: Silverberg S, ed. Principles and Practice of Surgical Pathology, 2nd ed. New York: Wiley and Sons, 1989,
100. Mitchell RS, Silvers GW, Goodman N, et al. Are centrilobular emphysema and panlobular emphysema two different diseases? Hum Pathol 1970; 1:433–441.
101. Mitchell RS, Stanford RE, Johnson JM, et al. The morphologic features of the bronchi, bronchioles and alveoli in chronic airway obstruction. Am Rev Respir Dis 1976; 114:137–145.
102. Moreno RM, Hogg JC, Pare PD. Mechanisms of airway narrowing. Am Rev Respir Dis 1986; 133:1171–1180.
103. Morgan WKC, Seaton A. Occupational Lung Diseases, 2nd ed. Philadelphia: WB Saunders Company, 1984.
104. Mullen JBM, Wiggs BR, Wright JL, et al. Non-specific airway reactivity in smokers. Relationship to airway pathology and baseline lung function. Am Rev Respir Dis 1986; 133:120–125.
105. Mullen JBM, Wright JL, Wiggs BR, et al. Reassessment of inflammation of airways in chronic bronchitis. Br Med J 1985; 291:1235–1239.
106. Müller NL, Guerry-Force ML, Staples CA, et al. Differential diagnosis of bronchiolitis obliterans with organizing pneumonia and usual interstitial pneumonia: clinical, functional, and radiologic findings. Radiology 1987; 162:151–156.
107. Myers JL, Veal CF, Shin MS, Katzenstein A-LA. Respiratory bronchiolitis causing interstitial lung disease. Am Rev Respir Dis 1987; 135:880–884.
108. Nagai A, West WW, Paul JL, Thurlbeck WM. The National Institutes of Health Intermittent Positive-Pressure Breathing trial: pathology studies. I. Inter-relationship between morphologic lesions. Am Rev Respir Dis 1985; 132:937–945.
109. Nagai A, West WW, Thurlbeck WM. The National Institutes of Health Intermittent Positive-Pressure Breathing trial: pathology studies. II. Correlation between morphologic findings, clinical findings, and evidence of expiratory air-flow obstruction. Am Rev Respir Dis 1985; 132:946–953.
110. Niewoehner DE, Kleinerman J, Rick DP. Pathologic changes in the peripheral airways of young cigarette smokers. N Engl J Med 1974; 291:755–758.
111. Oberholzer M, Dalquen P, Rohr HP. Morphologic findings in central bronchi correlated to lung function data in obstructive airways disease. Pathol Res Pract 1979; 164:58–67.
112. Ohata M, Suzuki H. Pathogenesis of spontaneous pneumothorax with special reference to the ultrastructure of emphysematous bullae. Chest 1980; 77:771–776.
113. Petty TL, Silvers GW, Stanford RE. Functional correlations with mild and moderate emphysema in excised human lungs. Am Rev Respir Dis 1981; 124:700–704.
114. Petty TL, Silvers GW, Stanford RE. Small airway dimension and size distribution in human lungs with an increased closing capacity. Am Rev Respir Dis 1982; 125:535–539.
115. Petty TL, Silvers GW, Stanford RE. Radial traction and small airways disease in excised human lungs. Am Rev Respir Dis 1986; 133:132–135.
116. Petty TL, Silvers GW, Stanford RE. Mild emphysema is associated with reduced elastic recoil and increased lung size but not with airflow limitation. Am Rev Respir Dis 1987; 136:867–871.
117. Petty TL, Silvers GW, Stanford RE, et al. Small airway pathology is related to increased closing capacity and abnormal slope of phase III in excised human lungs. Am Rev Respir Dis 1980; 121:449–456.
118. Pimental JG. Tridimensional photographic reconstruction in a study of the pathogenesis of honeycomb lung. Thorax 1967; 22:444–452.
119. Pratt PC. Role of conventional chest radiography in diagnosis and exclusion of emphysema. Am J Med 1987; 82:998–1006.
120. Pratt PC, Haque A, Klugh GA. Correlation of postmortem function and structure in normal and emphysematous lungs. Am Rev Respir Dis 1961; 83:856–865.
121. Pratt PC, Jutabha O, Klugh GA. Quantitative relationship between structural extent of centrilobular emphysema and postmortem volume and flow characteristics of lungs. Med Thorac 1965; 22:197–209.
122. Pratt PC, Kilburn KH. A modern concept of the emphysemas based on correlations of structure and function. Hum Pathol 1970; 1:443–453.
123. Reid LMcA. Reduction in bronchial subdivision in bronchiectasis. Thorax 1950; 5:233–247.
124. Reid LMcA. Pathology of chronic bronchitis. Lancet 1954; i:275–278.
125. Reid LM. Correlation of certain bronchographic abnormalities seen in chronic bronchitis with the pathological changes. Thorax 1955; 10:199–204.
126. Reid L. Measurement of the bronchial mucous gland layer: a diagnostic yardstick in chronic bronchitis. Thorax 1960; 15:132–141.
127. Reid L. The Pathology of Emphysema. London: Lloyd-Luke, 1967, 22–28.
128. Reid L, Simon G. Unilateral lung transradiancy. Thorax 1962; 17:230–239.
129. Roca J, Granena A, Rodrigues-Roison R, et al. Fatal airway disease in an adult with graft-versus-host disease. Thorax 1982; 57:77–78.
130. Ruckley VA, Fernie JM, Campbell SJ, Cowie HA. Causes of disability in coal miners: a clinico-pathological study of emphysema, airways obstruction and massive fibrosis. Report No TM/89/05. CEC Contract 7248/81/030. Edinburgh: Institute of Occupational Medicine, 1989, 150.
131. Ryan SF, Vincent TN, Mitchell RS, et al. Ductectasia: an asymptomatic pulmonary change related to age. Med Thorac 1965; 22:181–187.
132. Ryder RC, Lyons JP, Campbell H, Gough J. Bronchial mucous gland status in coal workers' pneumoconiosis. Ann NY Acad Sci 1972; 200:370–380.
133. Saetta M, Ghezzo H, Kim WD, et al. Loss of alveolar attachments in smokers. A morphologic correlate of lung function impairment. Am Rev Respir Dis 1985; 132:894–900.
134. Saetta M, Shiner RG, Angus GE, et al. Destructive index: a measurement of lung parenchymal destruction in smokers. Am Rev Respir Dis 1985; 131:764–769.
135. Saito K, Cagle P, Berend N, Thurlbeck WM. The "destructive index" in nonemphysematous and emphysematous lungs. Am Rev Respir Dis 1989; 139:308–312.
136. Scott KWM. An autopsy study of bronchial mucous gland hypertrophy in Glasgow. Am Rev Respir Dis 1973; 107:239–245.
137. Scott KWM. A pathological study of the lungs and heart in fatal and non-fatal chronic airway obstruction. Thorax 1976; 31:70–79.
138. Scott KWM, Steiner GM. Post mortem assessment of chronic airways obstruction by tantalum bronchography. Thorax 1975; 30:405–414.
139. Smith P, Heath D, Moosavi H. The Clara cell. Thorax 1974; 29:147–163.
140. Snider GL, Kleinerman J, Thurlbeck WM, Bengali ZK. The definition of emphysema. Report of a National Heart, Lung and Blood Institute, Division of Lung Disease Workshop. Am Rev Respir Dis 1985; 132:182–185.
141. Sobonya RE, Burrows B. The epidemiology of emphysema. Clin Chest Med 1983; 4:351–358.
142. Spain DM, Kaufman G. The basic lesion in chronic pulmonary emphysema. Am Rev Tubercul 1953; 68:24–30.
143. Stovin PG. Congenital lobar emphysema. Thorax 1959; 14:254–262.
144. Takizawa T, Thurlbeck WM. A comparative study of four methods of assessing the morphologic changes in chronic bronchitis. Am Rev Respir Dis 1971; 103:774–783.
145. Takizawa T, Thurlbeck WM. Muscle and mucous gland size in the major bronchi of patients with chronic bronchitis, asthma and asthmatic bronchitis. Am Rev Respir Dis 1971; 104:331–336.
146. Tandon MK, Campbell AH. Bronchial cartilage in chronic bronchitis. Thorax 1969; 24:607–612.
147. Tapper T, Schuster S, McBride J, et al. Polyalveolar lobe: anatomic and physiologic parameters and their relationship to congenital lobal emphysema. J Pediatr Surg 1980; 15:931–936.
148. Thurlbeck WM. Internal surface area and other measurements in emphysema. Thorax 1967; 22:483–496.

149. Thurlbeck WM. The internal surface area of non-emphysematous lungs. Am Rev Respir Dis 1967; 95:765–773.
150. Thurlbeck WM. Chronic Airflow Obstruction in Lung Disease. Philadelphia: W.B. Saunders Company, 1976.
151. Thurlbeck WM. Aspects of chronic airflow obstruction. Chest 1977; 72:341–349.
152. Thurlbeck WM. Postmortem lung volumes. Thorax 1979; 34:735–739.
153. Thurlbeck WM. Chronic airflow obstruction: correlation of structure and function. In: Petty TL, ed. Chronic Obstructive Lung Disease. 2nd ed. New York: Marcel Dekker Inc, 1985, 129–204.
154. Thurlbeck WM. Chronic airflow obstruction. In: Thurlbeck WM, ed. Pathology of the Lung. Stuttgart: Thieme Medical Publishers Inc, 1988, chapter 21.
155. Thurlbeck WM, Anderson AA, Janis M, et al. A co-operative study of certain measurements of emphysema. Am Rev Respir Dis 1968; 98:217–228.
156. Thurlbeck WM, Angus GE. A distribution curve for chronic bronchitis. Thorax 1964; 19:436–442.
157. Thurlbeck WM, Henderson JA, Fraser RG, Bates DV. Chronic obstructive lung disease. A comparison between clinical, roentgenologic, functional and morphologic criteria in chronic bronchitis, emphysema, asthma and bronchiectasis. Medicine 1970; 49:81–145.
158. Thurlbeck WM, Pun R, Toth J, Fraser RG. Bronchial cartilage in chronic obstructive lung disease. Am Rev Respir Dis 1974; 109:73–80.
159. Thurlbeck WM, Ryder RC, Sternby N. A comparative study of the severity of emphysema in necropsy populations in three different countries. Am Rev Respir Dis 1974; 109:239–248.
160. Thurlbeck WM, Simon G. Radiographic appearance of the chest in emphysema. Am J Roentgenol 1978; 130:429–440.
161. Thurlbeck WM, Wang NS. The structure of the lungs. In: Widdicombe JG, ed. MTP International Review of Science. Physiology Series I, Vol. 2, Respiratory Physiology. Baltimore: University Park Press, 1974.
162. Turton CW, Williams G, Green M. Cryptogenic obliterative bronchiolitis in adults. Thorax 1981; 36:805–810.
163. Van Brabandt H, Cauberghs M, Verbeken E, et al. Partitioning of pulmonary impedance in excised human and canine lungs. Functional-structural relationship. J Appl Physiol 1983; 55:1733–1742.
164. Weibel ER. Morphometry of the Human Lung. New York: Academic Press Inc, 1963.
165. West WW, Nagai A, Hodgkin JE, Thurlbeck WM. The National Institute of Health Intermittent Positive-Pressure Breathing trial—pathology studies. III. The diagnosis of emphysema. Am Rev Respir Dis 1987; 135:123–129.
166. Wilson AG, Massarella GR, Pride NB. Elastic properties of airways in human lungs post-mortem. Am Rev Respir Dis 1974; 110:716–729.
167. Wright JL, Churg A. Morphology of small-airway lesions in patients with asbestos exposure. Hum Pathol 1984; 15:68–74.
168. Wright JL, Hobson J, Wiggs BR, et al. Effect of cigarette smoking on structure of the small airways. Lung 1987; 165:91–100.
169. Wright JL, Hobson J, Wiggs BR, Hogg JC. Comparison of inflammatory cells in bronchoalveolar fluid to those in the lumen and tissue of the peripheral airways and alveolar airspace. Lung 1988; 166:75–83.
170. Wright JL, Lawson L, Pare PD, et al. The detection of small airways disease. Am Rev Respir Dis 1984; 129:989–994.
171. Wright JL, Lawson LM, Pare PD, et al. Morphology of peripheral airways in current smokers and ex-smokers. Am Rev Respir Dis 1983; 127:474–477.
172. Wright JL, Wiggs BJ, Hogg JC. Airway disease in upper and lower lobes in lungs of patients with and without emphysema. Thorax 1984; 39:282–285.
173. Wright JL, Wiggs BJ, Pare PD, Hogg JC. Ranking the severity of emphysema on whole lung slices. Concordance of upper lobe, lower lobe, and entire lung ranks. Am Rev Respir Dis 1986; 133:930–931.
174. Wright JL, Hobson JE, Wiggs B, et al. Airway inflammation and peribronchial attachments in the lungs of nonsmokers, current and ex-smokers. Lung 1988; 166:277–286.
175. Wright RR. Bronchial atrophy and collapse in chronic obstructive pulmonary emphysema. Am J Pathol 1960; 37:63–77.
176. Yousem SA, Burke CM, Billingham ME. Pathologic pulmonary alterations in long term human heart-lung transplantation. Hum Pathol 1985; 16:911–923.
177. Yousem SA, Colby TV, Carrington CB. Follicular bronchitis/bronchiolitis. Human Pathol 1985, 16:700–706.

Chapter 2

PATHOLOGY OF THE PULMONARY VASCULATURE AND HEART

Giuseppe G. Pietra

This chapter reviews the cardiac and pulmonary vascular pathology in patients with chronic obstructive pulmonary disease (COPD) due to emphysema, chronic bronchitis, and chronic bronchiolitis. Obstruction to airflow due to other diseases, e.g., asthma, bronchiectasis, and cystic fibrosis, is not considered.

Essential and preliminary to an understanding of the pathology of the pulmonary vasculature is a knowledge of the normal microanatomy of the pulmonary and bronchial circulations.

THE NORMAL PULMONARY VASCULAR SYSTEM

The Pulmonary Circulation

In postnatal life, the structure of the pulmonary vascular bed reflects the hemodynamic conditions of a low-pressure and low-resistance system capable of accommodating large increases in blood flow with little increase in pressure. Although no sudden change occurs from one segment to another, the pulmonary arterial bed can be subdivided, morphologically and functionally, into three components: elastic arteries, muscular arteries, and arterioles.

The pulmonary elastic arteries include the main pulmonary trunk, the right and left pulmonary arteries, and their intrapulmonary branches down to vessels 1 mm in diameter. Although the pulmonary arteries divide in company with the airways, they also give off supernumerary branches at right angles to supply adjacent lung tissue. The pulmonary elastic arteries are compliant conduits for blood flow, characterized by several layers of perforated elastic membranes in the media. In contrast to elastic systemic arteries, the elastic membranes in pulmonary vessels are less regularly arranged, fewer in number, and separated by abundant collagenous matrix. As these vessels extend into lung periphery, the elastic membranes are gradually replaced by circular or nearly circular layers of smooth muscle. Eventually, a point is reached where vessels approximately 1 mm in diameter have a completely muscular medial coat.

Muscular pulmonary arteries are mainly intralobular vessels with a diameter slightly smaller than that of the adjacent airways. These are the vessels that modulate pulmonary vascular resistance by active contraction and relaxation of the medial coat.[2, 6] They range in size from about 0.1 to 1 mm and are characterized by a media composed of circular or nearly circular layers of smooth muscle bound by internal and external elastic laminae. In comparison to systemic arteries of the same caliber, the media is relatively thin, occupying less than 10 percent of the cross-sectional area (Fig. 2–1*A*). In the smaller arteries the muscle fibers, instead of being arranged in circular rings, are spirally wound and gradually taper off. Thus, in cross section, these vessels will appear partially muscularized, with muscle fibers present in only one segment of their circumference, or entirely nonmuscular (Fig. 2–1*B*). Nonmuscular precapillary vessels, 70 μm in diameter or less, are endothelial tubes with an outer coat of pericytes and connective tissue and a single spirally wound elastic lamina. They cannot be distinguished from veins of the same caliber unless their origin from a parent vessel can be traced.

Although arterial vessels less than 100 μm in diameter have been designated as arterioles, the transition from one vessel type to another does not correlate well with external diameter. Hence, Reid[27] has recommended classifying small pulmonary arteries as muscular, partially muscular, and nonmuscular on the basis of the presence or absence of medial muscle rather than on the basis of external diameter.

The pulmonary capillaries are involved in gas and liquid exchange. They are endothelium-lined tubes supported by a continuous basal lamina, surrounded by a wide-meshed network of pericytes. They course eccentrically within the alveolar walls, subdividing the alveolar interstitial space into thin and thick regions, with the nuclear regions of the endothelium and the pericytes located in the thick regions. Normally, most capillaries in the lung are closed, but they can easily open to accommodate an increased blood flow without appreciable increase in pulmonary vascular resistance.

The postcapillary veins are lined by endothelium closely applied to a single elastic lamina. As mentioned previously, they are indistinguishable from precapillary arterioles unless their origin from a parent vessel can be traced. Larger veins can be readily identified because of their location within the interlobular septa at the periphery of the lobules and the presence of a prominent collagenous media and elastic fibers. The media may also contain smooth muscle fibers.

The Bronchial Circulation

The human bronchial arteries usually originate from the aorta at the level of the carina. They follow the bronchi down to the level of the respiratory bronchioli and supply arterial blood to the bronchi and the vasa vasorum of the large

Acknowledgments. The skillful help of Ruth Krakower is gratefully appreciated. Grant support in parts: Grants HL-32482/03 and HR-14000.

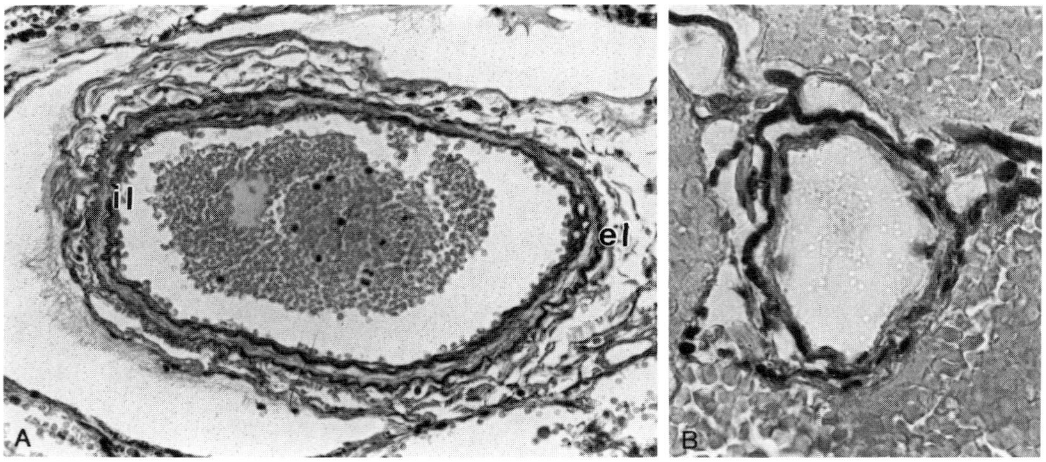

Figure 2–1. Light micrographs of muscular (*A*) and nonmuscular (*B*) pulmonary arteries from a 21-year-old healthy male. Note the relatively thin muscular medial coat bound by internal (il) and external (el) elastic laminae. In *B*, note the lack of medial coat between the intima and the single elastic lamina (Verhoeff–van Gieson; *A* ×320; *B* ×500).

pulmonary vessels.[19] The lobar bronchi are accompanied by two bronchial arteries. The segmental and subsegmental bronchi have two to four bronchial arteries. These vessels are located in the peribronchial connective tissue, in proximity to nerves and bronchial glands, and send perforating branches to the bronchial submucosa.[19] The bronchial arteries have rather small lumens and thick, muscular media with a well-developed internal elastica and absent or poorly developed external elastica. Frequently, thick bundles of longitudinal smooth muscle are contained in the intima (Fig. 2–2).

The bronchial capillaries are lined by continuous endothelium and basal lamina, except in proximity to the bronchial glands, where the endothelium is fenestrated.[25] The capillaries merge with a network of anastomosing small venules located in the bronchial submucosa and in the peribronchial connective tissue.[19, 25] This capillary-venular system plays an important role in heat and fluid exchange in the bronchi.[25]

In the lung periphery, the bronchial veins drain into the pulmonary veins, whereas in the proximal bronchi blood is drained by bronchial veins, which are part of the azygos system. The two segments of the bronchial venous circulation are extensively anastomosed,[23] resulting in a source of venous admixture to oxygenated blood in the normal lung.

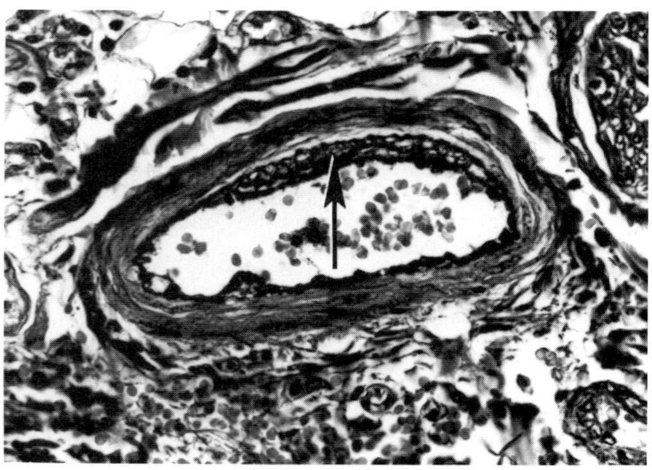

Figure 2–2. Light micrograph of a bronchial artery showing bundles of intimal longitudinal muscle (arrow) and the single elastic lamina (Verhoeff–van Gieson; ×320).

Bronchopulmonary Vascular Anastomoses

The existence in normal adult lungs of anastomoses between the pulmonary and bronchial arteries or the bronchial arteries and pulmonary veins is still controversial. The preponderance of evidence indicates that bronchopulmonary vascular anastomoses are present in fetal life but disappear during childhood; they are readily re-established in regions of the lung where the pulmonary flow is diminished.[16]

Age Changes in the Pulmonary Vessels

With increasing age, changes occur in the intima, media, and adventitia of pulmonary vessels, which at times may be difficult to distinguish from pathologic processes complicating COPD. The large pulmonary arteries, with age, show an increasing fibrous thickening of the intima and fragmentation of elastic fibers in the media. In older individuals, atheromatous intimal plaques are common, without apparent relationship to the presence of cardiac or pulmonary diseases. In muscular pulmonary arteries, intimal fibrosis is common in the elderly and is particularly striking in arteries of the upper lobes. Patchy or circumferential intimal hyalinization of veins is a universal finding in old individuals. Although small veins may become distinctly narrowed by this process, the change is not associated with detectable impairment of venous flow.

GENERAL FEATURES OF HYPERTENSIVE ARTERIOPATHY IN COPD

Pulmonary artery hypertension in COPD is characterized by lesions of the intima and media of muscular arteries and arterioles. The various lesions are considered individually in the following sections, notwithstanding that several or all may coexist in the same vessel.

Lesions of the Intima

Proliferation and fibrosis are the commonly observed intimal lesions in pulmonary muscular arteries and in arterioles. Three

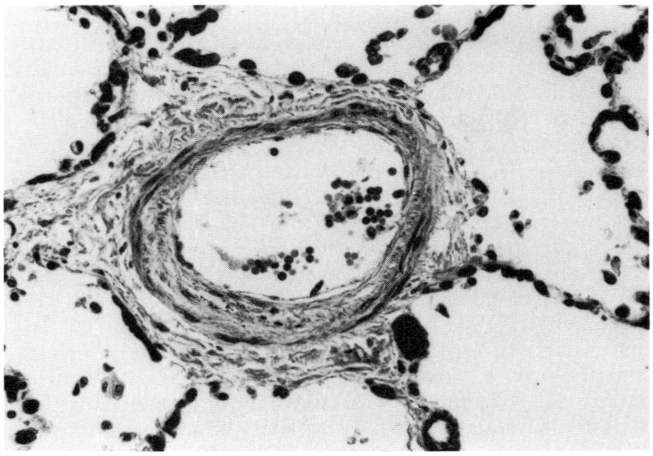

Figure 2–3. Eccentric intimal fibrosis in a muscular pulmonary artery (trichrome, ×100).

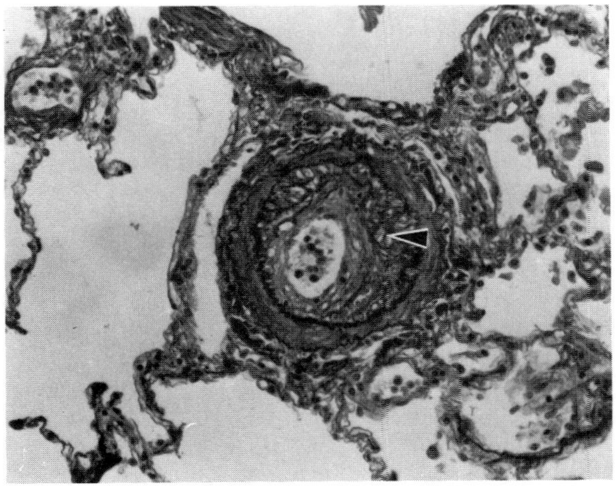

Figure 2–5. Medial hypertrophy, longitudinal intimal muscle (arrowhead), and concentric nonlaminar fibrosis in a small pulmonary artery (Verhoeff–van Gieson; ×200).

types of intimal lesions are recognized: eccentric fibrosis, concentric nonlaminar fibrosis, and longitudinal muscle formation.[10, 11, 15, 29, 31, 36, 38]

Eccentric intimal fibrosis is characterized by intimal cushions that are composed of myofibroblasts, connective tissue fibers, and proteoglycans (Fig. 2–3). Irregular elastic fibers may appear within the thickened intima (fibroelastosis). Below the acellular fibrous thickening of the intima reduplication of the internal elastic lamina may occur. Concentric nonlaminar intimal fibrosis is observed only in small muscular pulmonary arteries and it may be so extensive as to obliterate the arterial lumen completely (Fig. 2–4). Both eccentric and concentric nonlaminar fibrosis are considered potentially reversible processes, resulting in proliferation of intimal myofibroblasts, triggered either by microthromboembolism or by a variety of insults to the intima. Intimal fibrosis of small pulmonary arteries is present in the lungs of smokers who have no significant obstruction to airflow, hypoxemia, or pulmonary artery hypertension,[10, 38] suggesting that it is a primary vascular lesion rather than a change secondary to elevated arterial pressure or hypoxic vasoconstriction.

Longitudinal muscle bundles are present in fetal life and disappear in postnatal life to reappear within the thickened intima in hypoxic pulmonary hypertension. The muscle bundles may be localized to one segment of the intima or involve its entire circumference and are separated by anastomosing bands of elastic fibers (Fig. 2–5). Muscle bundles occur characteristically in small, muscularized, intra-acinar arteries in hypoxic pulmonary hypertension, regardless of its etiology.[11]

Lesions of the Media

Hypertrophy and hyperplasia of the medial muscle in pulmonary arteries and muscularization of arterioles (Figs. 2–5, 2–6) are among the most constant anatomic changes in pulmonary artery hypertension.[11, 15, 31, 38] Thickening of the medial coat of muscular arteries and muscularization of nonmuscular arterioles are probably the anatomic expression of persistent vasoconstriction. In patients with COPD the severity of medial hypertrophy is usually slight.[11] In these patients its extent and severity are best assessed by quantitative or semiquantitative analysis of histologic slides stained for visualization of elastic and smooth muscle tissues, rather than by cursory scanning of slides stained with hematoxylin eosin.

Regardless of its severity, medial hypertrophy and hyperplasia are considered potentially reversible lesions if the cause of pulmonary hypertension is removed. However, persistent elevation of pulmonary artery pressure may lead to degeneration of smooth muscle fibers and partial or total replacement of the media by connective tissue. Because this process is a gradual one, muscle hypertrophy and fibrosis may coexist in the same vessel. Eventually, atrophy of the medial muscle and fibrosis may lead to arterial dilatation and thinning of the media (dilatation lesions).

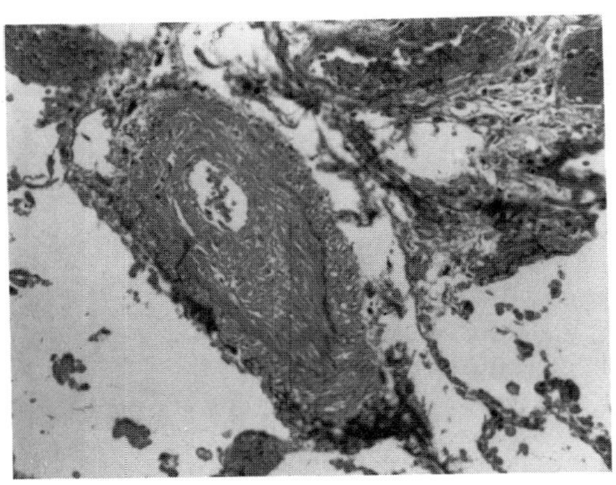

Figure 2–4. Concentric nonlaminar intimal fibrosis in a small pulmonary artery (Verhoeff–van Gieson; ×150).

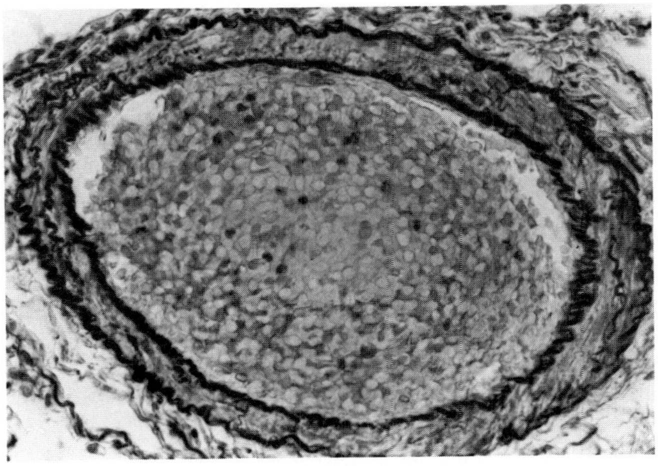

Figure 2–6. Muscular pulmonary artery with medial hypertrophy and early duplication of elastic laminae (Verhoeff–van Gieson; ×100).

Lesions of the Adventitia

In most cases of pulmonary hypertension, the adventitia remains uninvolved. Occasionally, longitudinal bundles of smooth muscle cells may develop in the adventitia of pulmonary muscular arteries in conditions characterized by chronic venous hypertension.

Lumenal Lesions

Relevant to the present discussion are recanalized thrombi or emboli, which may form cushion-like thickening of the intima or occlude the vascular lumen with endothelium-lined anastomosing channels (so-called colander lesions).

Obliteration of pre- and intra-acinar arteries and capillaries may be considerable in pulmonary fibrosis and in severe emphysema.[15] Unfortunately, the quantitative assessment of these changes is difficult and their functional implications remain not well understood.

THE BRONCHIAL CIRCULATION IN COPD

The changes in the bronchial circulation in patients with COPD are not well defined. Cudkowicz and Armstrong[5] examined the bronchial arteries in 18 patients with either panacinar or centrilobular emphysema, using angiography and histology. In 14 cases there was considerable narrowing of the bronchial arteries as they penetrated into the lung. The narrowing was caused by marked medial hypertrophy and intimal proliferation. In all cases the bronchial artery branches to the visceral pleura were obliterated. Bronchopulmonary anastomoses were present in four cases in areas of the lung where the pulmonary blood supply had been interrupted by emboli. Liebow and colleagues[16] found instead that the bronchial arteries were enlarged in patients with COPD. The dilatation did not seem to correlate with the presence of chronic bronchitis. Because very little is known about the normal physiology of the bronchial circulation,[25] the functional significance of the vascular lesions in the bronchial circulation in COPD is difficult to assess.

PATHOGENETIC MECHANISMS

About 50% of patients over age 50 with severe COPD develop pulmonary hypertension, elevated pulmonary vascular resistance, right ventricular enlargement, and failure.[12–14, 17] The development of right heart dysfunction, or cor pulmonale, in the setting of chronic obstruction to airflow contributes significantly to mortality in these patients. Thus, the 50% cumulative survival of patients with cor pulmonale and COPD is only 2.2 years, as compared with more than 5 years for patients with a similar degree of respiratory impairment but without cor pulmonale.[13, 14, 17]

Although pulmonary artery hypertension has long been recognized as the principal cause of right ventricular dysfunction in COPD, its pathogenesis is still incompletely defined. Many patients with mild COPD and no hypoxemia have an increase in pulmonary vascular resistance that is rarely demonstrable at rest but may become noticeable during exercise.[13, 38] Several factors may be responsible for the altered hemodynamics: loss of pulmonary microvascular bed, hypoxic vasoconstriction, blood volume expansion, increased transthoracic pressures, and left heart failure.[15, 17, 38]

Reduction of the pulmonary microvascular bed due to parenchymal destruction because of emphysema has been considered an important factor in reducing the cross-sectional area of the pulmonary vascular bed and increasing pulmonary vascular resistance.[15] However, the severity of emphysema correlates poorly with the weight of the right ventricle at autopsy,[3, 12, 31] and right ventricular hypertrophy may be present in individuals with mild emphysema and absent in individuals with severe emphysema.[17, 29]

Chronic hypoxia and hypoxic pulmonary vasoconstriction are generally recognized as the most important factors leading to the development of pulmonary hypertension in COPD. Although it is well established that acute hypoxia causes constriction of muscular arteries in the terminal respiratory units both by a direct effect on smooth muscle and through release of mediators,[2, 6, 22] the contribution of vasoconstriction to the anatomic pulmonary vascular changes observed in COPD remains to be elucidated. Studies in autopsy and surgical specimens from smokers with and without COPD have provided an improved understanding of the early vascular lesions in patients with COPD. Application of quantitative analysis for studying vascular lesions has shown that both the media and the intima of small pulmonary arteries and arterioles are abnormal in individuals with mild small airways disease and emphysema.[10, 38] The severity of the intimal lesions was found to increase with the severity of the emphysema.[38]

Experimental data in rats have shown that, within a few days of hypoxia, smooth muscle hypertrophy and hyperplasia in the small pulmonary arteries occurs resulting from proliferation and differentiation of precursor cells into smooth muscle cells.[27] Dogs with papain-induced emphysema develop medial hypertrophy and muscularization of arterioles but not intimal fibrosis.[28] Since intimal fibrosis is not present in pulmonary vessels of hypoxic animals but is present in smokers without hypoxemia and only mild emphysema,[10] it is likely that this vascular lesion may result from endothelial injury due to tobacco smoke rather than hypoxia. Cigarette smoke condensate has been shown to contain substances that can activate the intrinsic pathway of coagulation *in vivo*, stimulate expression of intercellular adhesion molecules on the surface of the endothelium, and activate the alternative pathway of complement.[1]

In early autopsy studies of COPD cases, right ventricular hypertrophy, medial hypertrophy, and muscularization of pulmonary arteries were found to correlate with chronic bronchitis and mucous gland enlargement rather than with severity of emphysema.[18] These anatomic findings were thought to provide the morphologic basis for the clinical observation of cor pulmonale in the "bronchitic" (blue bloater) rather than the "emphysemic" (pink puffer) type of COPD.[4]

Later observations have modified these traditional concepts and have shown little correlation between disease of the large airways and clinical indices of airflow obstruction.[9, 32, 34] Evidence is mounting that respiratory bronchiolitis is an important intermediate step in the pathogenesis of emphysema, and that emphysema is the most important factor responsible for chronic airflow obstruction.[32, 34] The severity of medial hypertrophy and intimal fibrosis of peripheral pulmonary arteries in COPD correlated best with the severity of emphysema and pulmonary artery hypertension.[38]

Although right ventricular hypertrophy at autopsy is more common in cases of severe emphysema,[3, 20, 29, 30] many individuals with right ventricular hypertrophy have only mild or moderate emphysema.[4, 17, 21, 29, 33] Thus, the link between pulmonary hypertension and emphysema appears to be an indirect one and to involve the interplay of several functional and anatomic changes. In addition to fixed vascular lesions, a disproportionate rise in alveolar pressure can increase pulmonary vascular resistance and cause pulmonary hypertension in patients with COPD.[13, 17, 38]

Patients with COPD and chronic right heart dysfunction do not always show hemodynamic improvement with supplemental oxygen therapy.[35] Hence, other factors may play a role in the persistence of pulmonary artery hypertension in these patients. Increased blood volume and polycythemia with increased blood viscosity, which develops in some patients with severe COPD, may contribute to the development of pulmonary artery hypertension and to thromboembolism. Thromboemboli are commonly found in COPD at autopsy, particularly in those who die of cardiac failure. An incidence as high as 62% has been reported in autopsy series,[17, 33] but it should be noted that the incidence of pulmonary thromboemboli noted at autopsy varies considerably, depending on the population and the expertise or interest of the prosectors. Left ventricular dysfunction and associated increase in left artrial pressure may also contribute to the development of pulmonary hypertension in some patients with COPD.[17, 26]

COR PULMONALE

As stated, pulmonary artery hypertension and increased pulmonary vascular resistance in chronic obstruction to airflow place a major burden upon the right ventricle of the heart. The term cor pulmonale was proposed to distinguish right ventricular dysfunction from lung disease. Because the term has meant different things to different workers, the World Health Organization[37] has defined cor pulmonale in terms of anatomy as "right ventricular hypertrophy resulting from disorders that affect either the function and/or the structure of the lung." In spite of this definition, many clinicians still equate cor pulmonale with overt right ventricular failure.

Estimates on the prevalence of right ventricular hypertrophy in COPD range from 10% to 40% of individuals affected.[17, 33] These wide ranges stem, in part, from the lack of a standard approach to the assessment of right ventricular hypertrophy at autopsy. Most pathologists rely on measurements of right ventricular wall thickness, a very imprecise method which is influenced by several factors, such as the degree of dilatation of the heart, the plane of sectioning, and the site of wall thickness measurements.[33] A simple and accurate method to assess right ventricular hypertrophy is to calculate the ratio of the weight of the left ventricle and septum to the weight of the right ventricle, as proposed by Fulton.[8] In right ventricular hypertrophy, the ratio is less than 2.0.[8] Others consider right ventricular hypertrophy to be present when the weight of the right ventricle is greater than 60 g.[33]

Grossly, hypertrophy of the right ventricle is characterized by increased firmness of the myocardium and increased thickness of its wall, most prominent in the pulmonary outflow tract (Fig. 2–7). The papillary muscles and the trabeculae carneae may be twice as thick as normal. The mural endocardium in the pulmonary outflow tract and the cusps of the pulmonary artery may be thickened. Straightening of the ventricular septum in severe cases of right ventricular hypertrophy may alter the shape and function of both cardiac chambers.

Microscopically, the diameter of the individual muscle fibers is thicker than normal and may approximate that of the left ventricular myofibers. The nuclei are large and distorted. In some cases there is an increase in interstitial connective tissue and loss of myofibers.

LEFT VENTRICULAR HYPERTROPHY

Autopsy studies have shown that left ventricular hypertrophy occurs in 10% to 90% of cases with COPD.[17, 24] While it is clear that left ventricular hypertrophy and dysfunction occur in COPD, controversy exists concerning pathogenesis. Several potential mechanisms for left ventricular failure in COPD have been proposed, although conclusive evidence for any of these hypotheses is lacking. Among the several factors the following have been implicated:[17, 26] systemic hypoxemia, acidosis, coronary artery or valvular heart disease, systemic hypertension, bulging of the interventricular septum into the ventricular cavity, alterations in intrathoracic pressures, and increased shunt volume by bronchopulmonary anastomoses. Regardless of the etiology, when left ventricular dysfunction occurs, it may severely aggravate the right heart dysfunction by increasing pulmonary blood volume and edema formation.

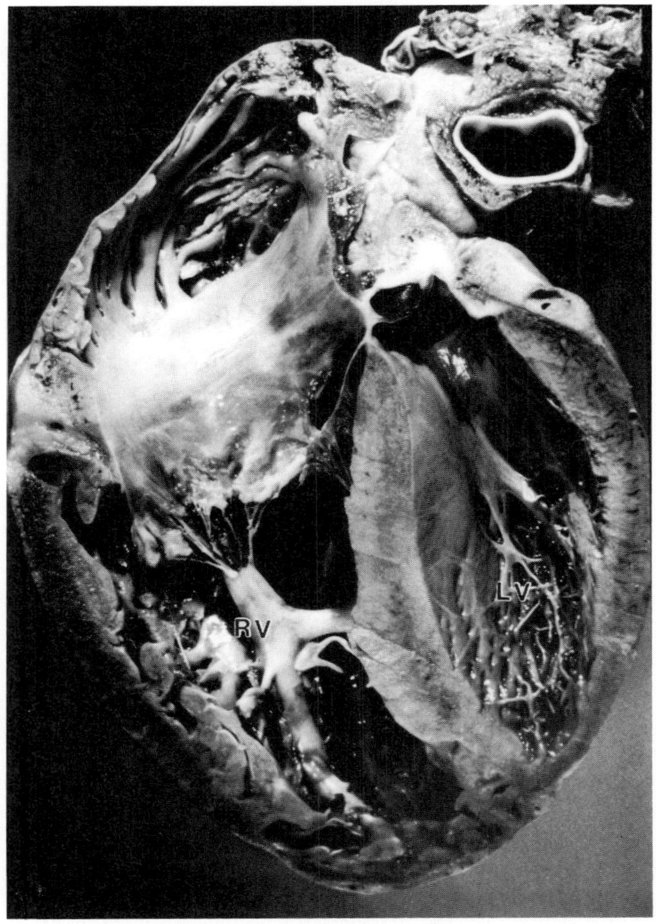

Figure 2–7. Cor pulmonale. This coronal section reveals the marked dilatation of the right ventricle (RV) and the hypertrophy of its wall. Note the relative small size of the left ventricle (LV).

Left ventricular atrophy has been demonstrated at autopsy in some cases of severe emphysema.[7] This observation is likely to reflect the fact that patients with severe emphysema are frequently emaciated and have low cardiac output.

SUMMARY

Despite advances in the understanding of the pathogenesis of COPD, pulmonary hypertension and cor pulmonale remain frequent and important contributing factors in the morbidity and mortality associated with this disease. Detection of early structural changes and their correlation with functional derangements may be helpful in filling some of the gaps in our understanding of pathogenetic mechanisms and may provide new directions for treatment.

REFERENCES

1. Becker CG. Immunologic aspects of vessel injury and thrombosis. Adv Exp Med Biol 1987; 214:131–143.
2. Bergofsky EH. Mechanisms underlying vasomotor regulation of regional pulmonary blood flow in normal and disease states. Am J Med 1974; 57:378–394.
3. Bignon J, Andre-Bougaran J, Brouet G. Parenchymal, bronchiolar, and bronchial measurements in centrilobular emphysema. Relation to weight of right ventricle. Thorax 1970; 25:556–567.
4. Burrows B, Fletcher CM, Heard BE, et al. The emphysematous and bronchial types of chronic airways obstruction: A clinicopathological study of patients in London and Chicago. Lancet 1966; i:830–835.
5. Cudkowicz L, Armstrong JB. The bronchial arteries in pulmonary emphysema. Thorax 1953; 8:46–58.
6. Fishman AP. Hypoxia on the pulmonary circulation. How and where it acts. Circ Res 1976; 38:220–231.
7. Foraker AG, Bedrossian CWM, Anderson AE Jr. Myocardial dimensions and proportions in pulmonary emphysema. Arch Pathol 1970; 90:344–347.
8. Fulton RM, Hutchinson EC, Jones, AM. Ventricular weight in cardiac hypertrophy. Br Heart J 1952; 14:413–420.
9. Greaves IA, Colebatch JJH. Observations on the pathogenesis of chronic airflow obstruction in smokers: implications for the detection of "early" lung disease. Thorax 1986; 41:81–87.
10. Hale KA, Ewing SL, Gosnell BA, Niewoehner DE. Lung disease in long-term cigarette smokers with and without chronic air-flow obstruction. Am Rev Respir Dis 1984; 130:716–721.
11. Hasleton PS, Heath D, Brewer DB. Hypertensive pulmonary vascular disease in states of chronic hypoxia. J Pathol Bacteriol 1968; 95:431–440.
12. Hicken P, Heath D, Brewer D. The relation between the weight of the right ventricle and the percentage of abnormal air space in the lung in emphysema. J Pathol Bacteriol 1966; 92:519–527.
13. Keller CA, Shepard JW Jr, Chun DS, et al. Pulmonary hypertension in chronic obstructive pulmonary disease. Multivariate analysis. Chest 1986; 90:185–192.
14. Langloh P, Brandli O, Schnieper R. Uberlebenswahrscheinlichkeit und prognostische Faktoren der chronischen obstruktiven Lungenkrankheit. Schweiz Med Wochenschr 1982; 112:1841–1846.
15. Liebow AA. Pulmonary emphysema with special reference to vascular changes. Am Rev Respir Dis 1959; 80:67–91.
16. Liebow AA. Broncho-pulmonary venous collateral circulation with special reference to emphysema. Am J Pathol 1953; 29:251–289.
17. Matthay RA, Berger HJ. Cardiovascular function in cor pulmonale. Clin Chest Med 1983; 4:269–295.
18. Millard J, Reid L. Right ventricular hypertrophy and its relationship to chronic bronchitis and emphysema. Br J Dis Chest 1974; 68:103–110.
19. Miller WS. The vascular supply of the bronchial tree. Am Rev Tuberc 1925; 12:87–93.
20. Mitchell RS, Stanford RE, Johnson JM, et al. The morphologic features of the bronchi, bronchioles, and alveoli in chronic airway obstruction: a clinicopathologic study. Am Rev Respir Dis 1976; 114:137–145.
21. Mitchell RS, Stanford RE, Silvers GW, Dart G. The right ventricle in chronic airway obstruction: A clinicopathologic study. Am Rev Respir Dis 1976; 114:147–154.
22. Moncada S, Vane JR. Arachidonic acid metabolites and the interactions between platelets and blood vessel walls. N Engl J Med 1979; 300:1142–1147.
23. Murata K, Itoh H, Todo G, et al. Bronchial venous plexus and its communication with pulmonary circulation. Invest Radiol 1986; 21:24–30.
24. Murphy ML, Adamson J, Hutcheson F. Left ventricular hypertrophy in patients with chronic bronchitis and emphysema. Ann Intern Med 1974; 81:307–313.
25. Pietra GG, Magno M. Pharmacological factors influencing permeability of the bronchial microcirculation. Fed Proc 1978; 37:2466–2470.
26. Rahlf G, Komori R. Der linke Ventrikel bei chronischem Cor pulmonale. Virchows Arch Pathol Anat 1975; 366:237–247.
27. Reid LM. The pulmonary circulation: remodeling in growth and disease. The 1978 J. Burns Amberson lecture. Am Rev Respir Dis 1979; 119:531–546.
28. Rubin LJ, Windberg P, Taylor W, Heatfield B. Pulmonary vascular structural and functional changes in papain-induced emphysema in dogs. Am Rev Respir Dis 1987; 136:704–709.
29. Scott KW. A clinicopathological study of fatal chronic airways obstruction. Thorax 1976; 31:693–701.
30. Scott KWM. A pathological study of the lungs and heart in fatal and non-fatal chronic airway obstruction. Thorax 1976; 31:70–79.
31. Semmens M, Reid L. Pulmonary arterial muscularity and right ventricular hypertrophy in chronic bronchitis and emphysema. Br J Dis Chest 1974; 68:253–263.
32. Thurlbeck WM. Small airways disease. Hum Pathol 1973; 4:150–152.
33. Thurlbeck WM. Chronic airflow obstruction in lung disease. In: Bennington JL, ed. Major Problems in Pathology, Vol V. Philadelphia: WB Saunders, 1976, 1–203.
34. Thurlbeck WM. The pathology of small airways in chronic airflow limitation. Eur J Respir Dis 1982; 121:9–18.
35. Timms RM, Khaja FU, Williams GW. Hemodynamic response to oxygen therapy in hypoxemic chronic obstructive lung disease. Ann Intern Med 1985;102:29–36.
36. Warnock ML, Kunzmann A. Muscular pulmonary arteries in chronic obstructive lung disease. Arch Pathol 1977; 101:180–186.
37. World Health Organization. Chronic cor pulmonale. Report of an expert committee. Circulation 1963; 27:594.
38. Wright JL, Lawson L, Pare PD, et al. The structure and function of the pulmonary vasculature in mild chronic obstructive pulmonary disease. The effect of oxygen and exercise. Am Rev Respir Dis 1983; 128:702–707.

Section II

CELLULAR AND BIOCHEMICAL BASIS OF CHRONIC OBSTRUCTIVE PULMONARY DISEASE

Chapter 3

THE EXTRACELLULAR MATRIX OF THE LUNG: IMPLICATIONS IN COPD

Margaret C. Bruce

Significant advances have recently been made toward increasing our understanding of the pivotal role played by the components of the extracellular matrix (ECM) in normal lung function as well as during lung development and maturation, injury, and repair. In addition to providing the structural support for an organ such as the lung, in which expansion and subsequent recoil are an integral part of normal function, ECM molecules also regulate the distribution of water, nutrients, and cytokines within lung parenchyma. The ECM components also respond to injurious substances entering the lung and play a critical role in directing lung repair after acute and chronic injury. Changes in the ECM associated with aging also contribute to changes in pulmonary function.

The ECM found in the extracellular space of most tissues is located beneath a layer of endothelial or epithelial cells and includes the basal lamina secreted by these cells. The ECM contains proteins and polysaccharides secreted by, and to some extent organized by, the cells contained within this matrix. Although usually assembled into a flexible meshwork, the ECM can also be highly organized, as in cartilage and tendons. The term "connective tissue" refers to both the ECM and the cells located within it, usually fibroblasts, macrophages, and mast cells. Between the connective tissue layer and the epithelial or endothelial cell layer are the basal lamina and the reticular lamina (Fig. 3–1).

The macromolecules found in greatest abundance in most extracellular matrices are the collagens and the glycosaminoglycans and proteoglycans. In the lung parenchyma, however, the relative proportions differ in that collagen constitutes 60% to 70%,[63] elastin 25% to 30%,[27] glycosaminoglycans and proteoglycans less than 1%,[135] and fibronectin approximately 0.5%.[18]

The ECM proteins acting in concert to maintain the functional and structural integrity of the lung include collagen, elastin, laminin, and fibronectin. Laminin is found in the basement membranes of the alveoli, vessels, and smooth muscle. Fibronectin is located in the interstitium and on the surface of collagen fibers but is generally absent from the basement membranes of the lung with the exception of low concentrations observed at sites of fusion of the endothelial and alveolar basement membranes.[59] Collagen types I, II, and III are present in the interstitium of the lung, whereas collagen type IV is located in basement membranes.

These structural fibers are embedded in a hydrated polysaccharide gel, often referred to as the ground substance, which is composed of glycosaminoglycans and proteoglycans. The aqueous phase of this gel allows for the diffusion of nutrients, metabolites, and hormones between blood and tissue and contributes to the ECM a degree of resistance against compressive forces encountered during breathing. Glycosaminoglycans and proteoglycans also influence cell movement and differentiation. Hyaluronic acid, because of its hydrophilic nature, provides a loose matrix in which cells can readily migrate and through which nutrients and mediators can diffuse to reach the cells of the developing lung. The concentration of hyaluronic acid in lung parenchyma is highest during lung development and during the initial phase of lung repair following injury.[50, 69] Cell differentiation and proliferation are associated with a decrease in the concentration of hyaluronic acid and an increase in the concentration of chondroitin sulfate and other sulfated glycosaminoglycans.[150]

In addition to providing a hydrated matrix, glycosaminoglycans and proteoglycans also contribute to lung structure. Hyaline cartilaginous rings surround the trachea and larger bronchi, becoming smaller and less regular with increasing distance from the hilum. Elastic and collagen fibers are also important structural components of the airways. These fibers are found in close association throughout the lung. Collagen fibers add strength and organization to the ECM whereas elastic fibers confer resilience. Type I collagen fibers are arranged in both small and large bundles in concentric rings around the major airways. Most of the elastic fiber bundles are longitudinal in orientation in the larger bronchi and are occasionally interlaced with thin elastic fibers arranged circumferentially. As airway size decreases, the density of elastic fibers around the circumference of the airway increases. Distal to the respiratory bronchioles, the elastic fiber bundles are replaced by circular and helical arrangements at the mouths of the alveolar ducts and in the alveoli. In the pulmonary vessels, elastic fibers are prominent in the media and present to a lesser extent in the intima and adventitia. Elastic fibers form a continuum that connects alveoli, bronchi, interlobular septa, and pleura with pulmonary arteries. The net effect of this continuum is to distribute any force applied to the parenchyma throughout the lung.[171]

The structural and functional integrity of the lung is dependent on the presence of intact ECM molecules. The structure of the collagen and elastic fibers, the absolute concentrations of the ECM components, and the ratios of one ECM component to another all appear to be important in maintaining normal lung function. Each of these proteins is vulnerable to proteolytic degradation associated with lung injury and inflammation. The extent to which damage to any one of these molecules impacts on the function of other ECM molecules and of the lung continues to be a topic of considerable interest.

This work was supported in part by NIH Grant HL-31172 from the Public Health Service.

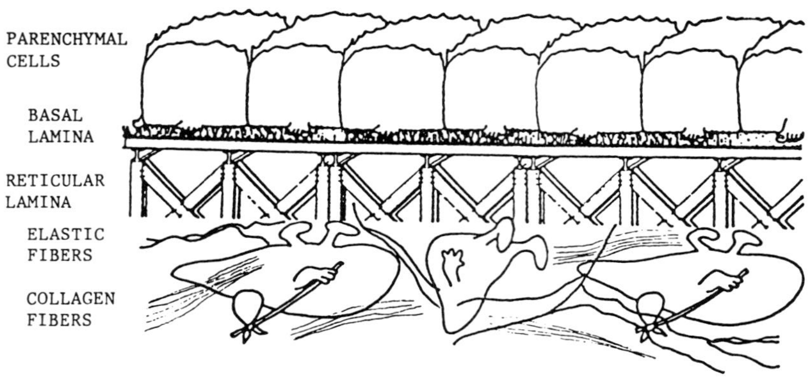

Figure 3–1. In this cartoon, the parenchymal cells are shown to adhere closely to the basal lamina, which is derived from these cells. The cellular components of the extracellular matrix, such as fibroblasts, macrophages, and mast cells, associate with but are not anchored to the reticular lamina. The reticular lamina is a scaffolding of dense connective tissue produced by the cells in the extracellular matrix. The reticular lamina is absent in the alveolar capillary basement membrane of the lung. The basement membrane is composed of both the basal and reticular lamina, which are closely linked. The basement membrane provides a boundary between the parenchymal and extracellular matrix cell populations and a substratum to which the cells may be anchored or on which they can move. (Modified from Bernfield, M: Introduction. In: Porter R, Whelan J, eds. Basement Membranes and Cell Movement, Ciba Foundation Symposium 108. London: Pitman Publishing Ltd, 1984.)

MAJOR CLASSES OF MACROMOLECULES PRESENT IN THE EXTRACELLULAR MATRIX OF THE LUNG

Glycosaminoglycans and Proteoglycans

MOLECULAR STRUCTURE AND PHYSICAL PROPERTIES OF GLYCOSAMINOGLYCANS AND PROTEOGLYCANS

Glycosaminoglycans (GAGs) are long, unbranched polysaccharide chains consisting of repeated disaccharide units in which one of the sugar residues is an amino sugar (*N*-acetylglucosamine or *N*-acetylgalactosamine). Glycosaminoglycan molecules are highly charged owing to the presence of carboxyl or sulfate groups, or both. There are four major categories of GAGs: (1) hyaluronic acid, (2) chondroitin sulfate/dermatan sulfate, (3) heparin/heparan sulfate, and (4) keratan sulfate. Each GAG chain is a polymer of a specific disaccharide unit. In heparin, heparan sulfate and hyaluronic acids GAGs, the disaccharide unit consists of *N*-acetylglucosamine and uronic acid. In chondroitin sulfate and dermatan sulfate the disaccharide unit consists of *N*-acetylgalactosamine and uronic acid. Keratan sulfate contains *N*-acetylglucosamine and galactose. Glycosaminoglycans also differ with respect to the number and position of sulfate groups. Hyaluronic acid, also referred to as hyaluronan, is made up of repeating disaccharide units that do not contain sulfates.

Proteoglycans (PGs) are large molecules consisting of a protein backbone, also referred to as a core protein, to which N- or O-linked oligosaccharides, or both, and GAG chains are covalently attached. The GAG chains are covalently bound to a link trisaccharide, which is bound to serine or threonine on the core protein. A proteoglycan molecule is similar in appearance to a long-bristled brush where the GAGs (bristles) are attached to the protein core (brush handle). Proteoglycans are grouped together on the basis of their GAG content rather than on the basis of size, molecular weight, or core protein. The GAG components of proteoglycans determine to a significant extent the behavior of the PG molecule. The sizes of core proteins characterized thus far range from 11,000 to 220,000 daltons, and the number of GAG chains attached to a core protein varies from 1 to 100.[17, 41] Hyaluronic acid differs from the other GAGs in that it is not linked to a core protein molecule. In addition, the hyaluronic GAG chain is generally much longer than GAG chains in proteoglycan molecules.

The physical properties of GAGs are such that the molecules lack the flexibility to form compact, globular molecules; instead, they adopt a highly extended random coil configuration, which occupies a much larger volume per unit mass than would a globular molecule with a similar molecular weight. Because of their hydrophilic nature, GAGs attract sufficient water molecules to form a hydrated gel, even at low concentrations. Because GAGs bind a large volume of water, they can occupy much more space with respect to their molecular weight than other molecules. The resulting osmotic pressure enables the ECM to resist compressive forces. In addition, water-soluble molecules diffuse readily through the hydrated gel, allowing for rapid transit of nutrients, cytokines, and metabolites.

Because of their uronic acid and sulfate content, GAG molecules contain a high density of negative charges. This charge density appears to be a major factor in determining the extent to which GAG molecules will interact with other ECM molecules.[130] Heparin, the most highly sulfated of the GAGs, binds more avidly to other ECM molecules than do other GAGs.[126] Heparan sulfate and dermatan sulfate contain fewer sulfate groups and have a somewhat lower binding affinity. Chondroitin sulfate has the fewest sulfate groups and the lowest binding affinity for heparin-binding ligands.[87] In addition to charge density, size is also an important factor. Large GAG chains tend to interact to a greater extent than small ones.[85]

DISTRIBUTION OF GLYCOSAMINOGLYCANS AND PROTEOGLYCANS WITHIN THE LUNG

Proteoglycans (PGs) have been localized within the mouse lung by electron microscopic analysis of tissue in which the GAGs were preserved by staining with cuprolinic blue.[157] Cuprolinic blue–positive filaments, thought to represent individual PG monomers, were observed in the alveolar basement membranes of types I and II epithelial cells, in the basement membrane of capillary endothelial cells, and in close contact with collagen fibrils. The results of enzyme and nitrous acid treatments used to selectively digest or destroy individual GAGs suggest that the filaments present in the basement membranes of types I and II alveolar epithelial cells contain heparin or heparan sulfate, or both. These filaments were found to occur in single plane, forming a nearly continuous sheet. The filaments observed in the basement membrane of the capillary endothelial cells were also thought to contain heparin or heparan sulfate, or both, based on the results of enzyme digest studies.[157] If this is indeed the case, a layer of anionic PG molecules could contribute to the regulation of transport of molecules from blood to epithelium and vice versa. A similar role has been identified for heparan sulfate–containing PGs in the glomerular basement membrane of the kidney.[78]

The filaments associated with collagen fibrils in the mouse lung appeared to contain dermatan sulfate.[157] *In vitro* studies suggest that the fibroblast may be a major source of dermatan sulfate in the lung.[25, 161] Increasing the ionic strength prior to fixation of the tissue has been reported to significantly decrease the association between collagen and dermatan sulfate, suggesting that the interaction between these two components is ionic in nature.[61] Dermatan sulfate is thought to play a role in the development of collagen fibers in the lung[102, 103] and to influence the tensile strength of the collagen fibers once they are formed.[36]

SYNTHESIS AND TURNOVER OF GLYCOSAMINOGLYCANS AND PROTEOGLYCANS

In vitro studies suggest that in the lung GAGs are synthesized by fibroblasts, epithelial cells, endothelial cells, and mast cells (heparin).[69] Proteoglycan biosynthesis is initiated with the translation and N-glycosylation of the core protein in the rough endoplasmic reticulum. The core protein is then transported to the Golgi apparatus where post-translational modifications occur.[82, 92] Synthesis of the O-linked GAGs, e.g., chondroitin sulfates, dermatan sulfates, heparan sulfates, and heparin, is initiated by the addition of xylose to a serine residue in the core protein. The signal for the attachment of the GAG chain to the core protein appears to lie within a consensus sequence in the core protein.[16, 130, 132] The consensus sequence for the attachment of chondroitin sulfate/dermatan sulfate to certain core protein molecules has been shown to consist of ser-gly-x-gly preceded by several acidic amino acids. Not surprisingly, these peptide sequences are excellent receptors for xylosyltransferase that attaches the first sugar residue of the GAG chain to the core protein.[16] It is not yet known what triggers the initiation of heparin/heparan sulfate chains as they, like dermatan sulfate/chondroitin sulfate, are initiated by the same sugar residue, xylose, and only one xylosyltransferase has been identified.[123] In the Golgi apparatus, specific glycosyltransferases act in sequence to assemble glycosaminoglycans and oligosaccharides.[81, 91] Sulfotransferases add sulfate groups to the GAG chains on proteoglycan molecules, which are then packaged into secretory granules and released from the cell.[159, 176]

Synthesis of hyaluronic acid (HA) differs in several respects from synthesis of other GAGs.[140] In contrast to proteoglycan synthesis, the synthesis of hyaluronic acid does not appear to be linked to the synthesis of a core protein. Treatment with cycloheximide, a potent inhibitor of protein synthesis, does not inhibit hyaluronic acid synthesis, which suggests that a protein does not serve as a primer. In addition, hyaluronic acid synthesis differs from synthesis of other GAGs in that hyaluronic acid synthesis is not inhibited by treatment with monensin, which inhibits normal function of the Golgi apparatus and the secretory pathways.[97, 174]

CATABOLISM. The core protein of the PG molecule is susceptible to degradation by proteolytic enzymes synthesized by fibroblasts, macrophages, and neutrophils (Table 3–1). After the initial degradation of the core protein has taken place, smaller PG fragments are phagocytized and further degraded within the cell by lysosomal enzymes. Endoglycosidases then depolymerize the GAG chain. Beginning at the nonreducing terminal, specific sulfatases remove sulfate groups. Monosaccharides are removed by iduronidases, glucuronidases, *N*-acetylglucosaminidases, and *N*-acetylgalactosaminidases, reducing the GAGs to their component monosaccharide residues and free sulfates.[65]

Degradation of hyaluronic acid proceeds by a different mechanism. It is generally accepted that hyaluronidase is required for metabolic degradation and that the distribution of this enzyme within a given tissue is indicative of the sites at which degradation will occur. During the course of lung development or wound healing, tissues contain high concentrations of hyaluronic acid. After the migration and cell proliferation phases are completed, cell differentiation occurs. It is at this point that hyaluronidase appears and the amount of HA decreases, particularly in lung parenchyma. The relative amounts of enzyme and substrate vary from one tissue to another. The lung and kidney contain moderate amounts of both, the liver contains high concentrations of enzyme and relatively little HA, whereas the skin contains high concentrations of HA and relatively little hyaluronidase. In addition to on-site degradation of HA in the lung, HA also travels via lymphatics where significant degradation occurs. The remaining HA travels via the blood to the liver, where it is degraded in the sinusoidal epithelial cells.[50]

Collagen

STRUCTURE. Collagen is the structural protein present in the highest concentration in the ECM, accounting for 20% of the dry lung weight.[28] The collagen molecule consists of three polypeptide or alpha chains wound around each other into a triple helical conformation to form a stiff fibrous protein molecule that, together with other collagen molecules, plays an important role in maintaining the structural integrity of the lung. A total of 13 genetically distinct collagen alpha chains have been identified, the products of at least 23 genes.[2] Although there are numerous differences among the collagen molecules associated with different cells and tissues, all collagen molecules have in common regions of repeating amino acid sequences. Every third amino acid in these repeated sequences is a glycine, the only amino acid small enough to fit inside the small dimensions of the triple helix. The other two amino acids in the repeating triplet are variable, but usually are proline, hydroxyproline, lysine, or hydroxylysine.

Collagens can be grouped according to structural similarities. The first group consists of collagens found in most connective

TABLE 3–1. Enzymes Capable of Degrading Lung Extracellular Matrix

ENZYME	LUNG SOURCE	SUBSTRATE	INHIBITORS
Elastase	PMN	tropoelastin, fibronectin, collagen types I, III (nonhelical region), and IV, PG core protein	$alpha_1$-PI, $alpha_2$-M, BMPI
	macrophage	elastin	$alpha_2$-M (inactivates $alpha_1$-PI)
Cathepsin B	PMN	elastin	
Cathepsin L	PMN	elastin	
Cathepsin G	PMN	tropoelastin, elastin, PG core protein	$alpha_1$-PI, $alpha_2$-M, BMPI, $alpha_1$-antichymotrypsin
Collagenase	PMN, fibroblast, macrophage	collagen types I, II, and III	$alpha_2$-M, human leukocyte collagenase inhibitor, B_1-anticollagenase
Metalloendoproteinase	fibroblast	collagen type IV	TIMP

PMN = polymorphonuclear leukocytes, $alpha_1$-PI = alpha-1-proteinase inhibitor, $alpha_2$-M = alpha-2-macroglobulin, BMPI = bronchial mucous proteinase inhibitor, TIMP = tissue inhibitor of metalloendoproteinase.

tissues, with the exception of hyaline cartilage, and includes types I, III, V, and VI.[2] As is the case elsewhere in the body, type I collagen is the predominant form found in the lung, accounting for 3% of total protein synthesis in the lung[149] and roughly 65% of total lung collagen.[137] Results of *in vitro* studies suggest that the fibroblast is the major source of type I collagen in the lung; however, endothelial cells, smooth muscle cells, and alveolar type II cells may also synthesize collagen. Type III collagen, which accounts for approximately 30% of lung collagen,[137] is also synthesized by lung fibroblasts and endothelial and smooth muscle cells. The concentration of type III collagen is increased in developing lung[10] as well as in healing wounds, suggesting a unique role for this collagen.

The second group consists of collagens found primarily in cartilages and includes types II, IX, X, and XI.[2] These collagens have smaller triple helical domains than the collagens in group I. In the lung, type II collagen is present in tracheal and bronchial cartilage but is not present in the smaller bronchi and bronchioles, which lack cartilage. The collagens in the third group are nonfibrillar and, in contrast to the other two types, have helical domains that are interrupted. The collagens in this group tend to be unique to a particular cell or tissue, such as type IV collagen, which in the lung is found primarily in the basement membrane of alveoli and capillaries. Instead of forming fibrils, type IV collagen forms a meshwork.

SYNTHESIS. Collagen polypeptide chains, referred to as pro-alpha chains, are synthesized on membrane-bound ribosomes (Fig. 3–2). These large precursors are then injected into the lumen of the endoplasmic reticulum. Pro-alpha chains contain extension peptides at both the amino- and carboxyl-terminal ends and a signal peptide. The signal peptide plays a role in guiding the secreted protein through the endoplasmic reticulum.

Post-translational modification of the pro-alpha collagen chains occurs first in the endoplasmic reticulum and later in the Golgi apparatus. Some proline and lysine residues undergo hydroxylation in the endoplasmic reticulum. Hydroxylation of proline appears to be a requirement for triple helix formation, perhaps by stabilizing this conformation. Inhibition of proline hydroxylation associated with a deficiency of oxygen, iron, or ascorbic acid impairs the formation of triple helical molecules. Sites at which lysine is hydroxylated serve as subsequent sites for the glycosylation that occurs prior to secretion of the pro-alpha chains into the extracellular space. Depending on the type of collagen molecule, variable numbers of two oligosaccharide side chains are covalently linked to the hydroxyl groups of the lysine residues in the Golgi apparatus (Fig. 3–2).

After hydroxylation and glycosylation, three pro-alpha chains combine to form a hydrogen-bonded triple helical procollagen molecule, which is secreted from the cell. During exocytosis, the extension peptides of types I, II, and III pro-alpha collagen are cleaved by procollagen peptidases, converting the triple helix to a collagen molecule. The enzymes responsible for the cleavage of the extension peptides (propeptides) are specific both for the amino and the carboxyl ends of the collagen molecule as well as for the type of procollagen molecule. In the process of converting type I procollagen to collagen, the *N*-propeptide is cleaved by a procollagen *N*-proteinase and the C-propeptide is cleaved by a C-proteinase. The *N*-proteinase removes *N*-propeptides from type II as well as type I procollagen, but will not cleave *N*-propeptides from type III procollagen, in spite of the structural similarities among the three molecules. In addition, the *N*-proteinases for types I, II, and III collagen require a procollagen substrate with a native conformation (Fig. 3–2).

After cleavage of the peptides, the newly formed collagen molecule assembles with other collagen molecules in the extracellular space to form a larger collagen microfibril close to the cell surface. The presence of the extension peptides on the procollagen molecule prior to secretion prevents collagen fibril formation within the cell. These extension peptides do not appear to be removed from types IV and V collagen, which may explain why these collagen types do not assemble into fibrils but form a kind of mesh instead.

Collagen molecules are assembled into microfibrils, groups of which are organized to form a collagen fibril, which has a diameter of approximately 50 nm and can be observed at the electron microscopic level. Collagen fibers consist of a number of densely packed collagen fibrils. The periodicity of the banding pattern seen at the electron microscopic level is due to the staggered arrangement of the collagen molecules. When viewed in a horizontal plane, there is a 35 nm gap between each of the collagen molecules in a horizontal row. The collagen fibril consists of many such rows of collagen molecules. In each successive row, the end of the first collagen molecule is 67 nm from the end of the collagen molecule in the preceding row. After five such parallel rows, the gap between molecules in the sixth row lines up with the gap in the first row. The banding pattern observed at the electron microscopic level results from the intense staining of these gaps compared with the lighter staining of the rest of the molecule.

COLLAGEN GENE EXPRESSION. Type I collagen is the most abundant collagen in mammalian tissues. Tissue concentrations vary, however. Embryonic bones and tendons have high concentrations, whereas the lung, skin, and muscle have somewhat lower concentrations. In the lung, type I collagen synthesis accounts for 3% of the total protein synthesis.[149] Collagen synthesis is regulated at many levels. The amount of collagen produced is a function of (1) rate of transcription, (2) mRNA stability, (3) level of translation of cytoplasmic mRNA, and (4) post-translational modification.[2]

Type I collagen consists of two alpha$_1$(I) subunits and one alpha$_2$(I) subunit. The gene coding for the alpha$_1$(I) subunit contains approximately 18k base pairs compared with 38k base pairs in the gene coding for the alpha$_2$(I) subunit. In cultured human skin fibroblasts the alpha$_1$(I) collagen gene is transcribed twice as fast as the alpha$_2$(I) collagen gene, but the mechanism for coordinating the synthesis of these two mRNAs is unknown.[62] Post-transcriptional processing is rapid but complex, owing to the relatively large size of the gene and the number of introns to be excised. Although type I collagen is absent in hyaline cartilage, transcription of the alpha$_1$(I) and alpha$_2$(I) genes does occur. The absence of alpha$_1$(I) appears to be due to the fact that the primary transcript is not processed completely,[3] nor is it secreted into the cytoplasm.[134] The mRNA alpha$_2$(I) has a short half-life and its translation is inefficient.

There is an increase in the amount of type I collagen in fibrotic tissues. This increase in accumulated collagen is the result of both proliferation of fibroblasts and an increase in the amount of collagen synthesis per cell. Depending on cell type, increased collagen synthesis can be due to either an increased rate of transcription or an increased association of type I collagen mRNAs with ribosomes.[143]

Ascorbate, a cofactor for prolyl- and lysyl-hydroxylase, is necessary for post-translational modification of most types of collagen. In addition, *in vitro* studies conducted in a variety of fibroblast types have shown that ascorbate causes an increase in the steady-state levels of type I collagen mRNA by increasing both the rate of transcription and the stability of type I collagen mRNA.[94] Levels of type I collagen mRNA are also augmented by estradiol,[44] insulin,[32] interleukin-1,[77] and transforming growth factor B.[110, 120, 158]

Dexamethasone and cortisol have been shown to decrease synthesis of type I collagen in both *in vitro* and *in vivo* systems. The mechanisms responsible for this decrease appear to vary with cell type, however. In rat hepatocytes[164] and in chick skin

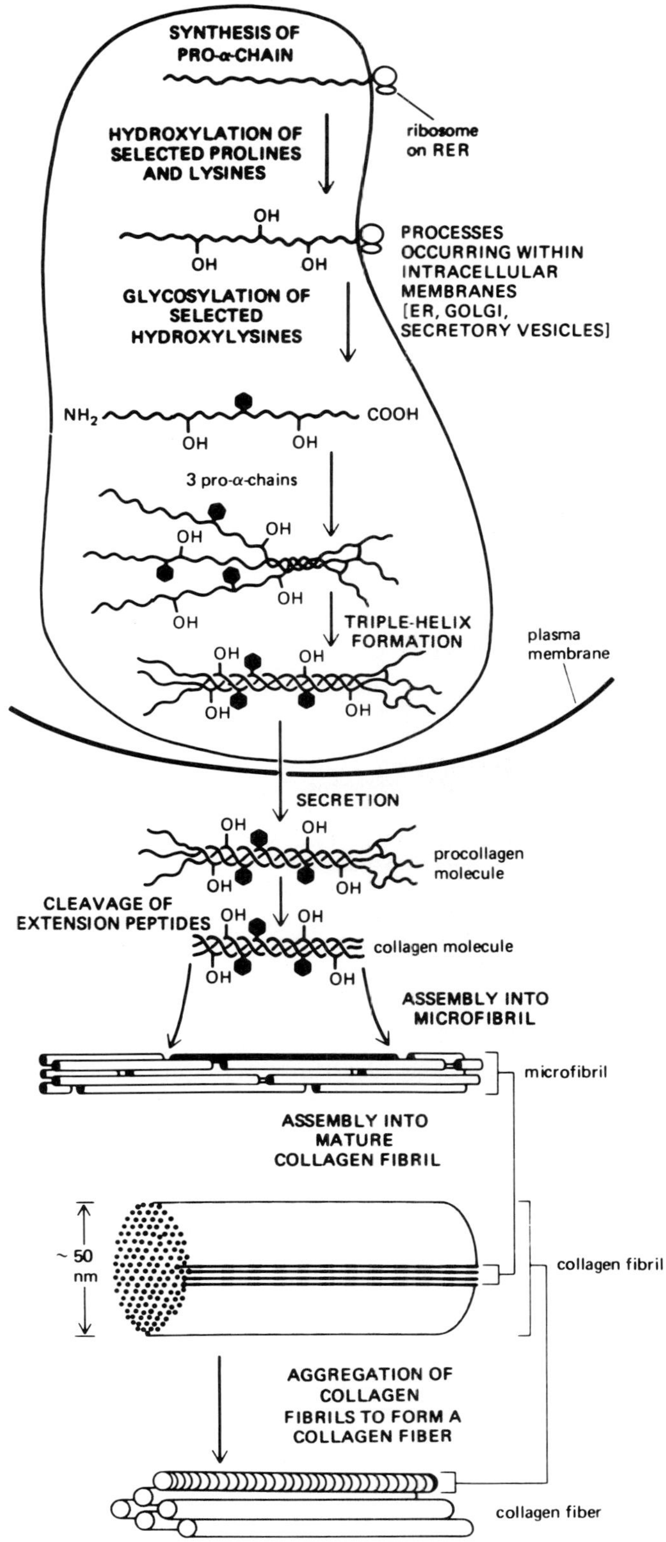

Figure 3–2. Collagen polypeptide chains (pro-alpha chains) are synthesized on ribosomes in the endoplasmic reticulum. Post-translational modifications include hydroxylation of some prolines and lysines and glycosylation of some hydroxylysines. Next, three pro-alpha chains combine, forming a triple helical procollagen molecule, which is then secreted from the cell. Procollagen peptidases cleave the extension peptides of types I, II, and III pro-alpha collagen, converting the triple helix into a collagen molecule, which then assembles with other collagen molecules to form a microfibril. Bundles of microfibrils form collagen fibrils. Collagen fibers contain many collagen fibrils. (From cell-cell adhesion and the extracellular matrix, p 700, In: Alberts B, Bray D, Lewis J, et al., eds. Molecular Biology of the Cell. New York: Garland Publishing Inc., 1983.)

fibroblasts,[30] transcription rate is decreased but stability of mRNA is unaffected. In rat[119] and human[62] skin fibroblasts, decreased collagen synthesis is the result of reduction in mRNA stability. The rate of type I collagen transcription is unaffected by glucocorticoids. It is currently thought that the therapeutic efficacy of steroids in some disease states characterized by excessive collagen production is due at least in part to a reduction in the steady state levels of type I collagen mRNA.[2] Dexamethasone has been reported to modulate increased type I collagen gene expression in hepatic fibrosis associated with murine schistosomiasis.[163] However, keloid fibroblasts and rheumatoid synovial cells are refractory to down regulation by hydrocortisone, suggesting that abnormal glucocorticoid regulation may be a feature of some fibrotic disease.[131]

Elastin

The elastic properties of the pulmonary parenchyma and vasculature are largely attributable to the presence of elastic fibers in the extracellular matrix. Elastic fibers can be stretched to 140% of their resting length in contrast to collagen fibers, which can be stretched only 2%.[141] The protein elastin is the primary constituent of elastic fibers. When reviewed at the electron microscopic level, the elastic fiber is seen to consist of two components: an amorphous inner core and a peripheral microfibrillar component.[45, 60, 80] The amorphous component comprises 90% or more of the fiber and is responsible for the elastic properties. The microfibrillar portion of the fiber contains small fibrils approximately 10 to 12 nm in diameter. Neither the composition nor the function of these microfibrils has been established. The chemical composition of elastin is similar to that of collagen. However, in contrast to collagen, elastin contains little hydroxyproline and no hydroxylysine. The majority of the amino acids are nonpolar, e.g., glycine (33%), proline (10% to 13%), alanine (24%), valine, phenylalanine, isoleucine, and leucine.[108]

STRUCTURE OF THE ELASTIN GENE. The entire human elastin gene, including the 5′ flanking sequences, has been cloned.[9] All available evidence indicates that, in spite of the reported sequence variability, only one elastin gene exists per genome. A single locus has been identified on the long arm of chromosome 2.[42] The gene contains approximately 45 kb and has an intron to exon ratio of 15 to 1, indicating that it is one of the most dispersed genes reported thus far. Collagen alpha$_2$(I), also a highly dispersed gene, has an intron to exon ratio of 8 to 1.[15, 124]

There are 34 exons in the human elastin gene. These exons have been shown to be segregated into functionally distinct domains, the hydrophobic domains and the potential cross-linking domains. The variability observed in the sequence of the translated portion of tropoelastin mRNA results from alternative splicing of the primary transcript. Exons 22, 23, 24, 26, 32, and 33 have been shown to undergo alternative splicing.[46, 47, 74] Although there is some evidence that splicing varies with age,[175] it is not known whether tissue or disease state has any influence on patterns of splicing. Transcription can be initiated at three major and four minor sites but there is no evidence of an association between site of transcript initiation and the pattern of alternative splicing.[9] Regulation of elastin gene expression varies with both age and type of tissue. Although expression of the gene appears to be controlled by the steady state level of elastin mRNA, the rate of transcription of the gene might not be the sole determinant of the steady state level of mRNA. In addition, the significance of multiple initiation sites with respect to rate of gene transcription has yet to be determined.[10]

SYNTHESIS OF TROPOELASTIN. Tropoelastin, the soluble precursor of elastin, has a molecular size of approximately 70 kD and contains approximately 750 amino acids. The hydrophobic domains of the tropoelastin molecule, which are rich in proline, glycine, and valine, alternate with the putative crosslink regions containing alanine and lysine. The primary sequence of human tropoelastin is encoded by a 3.5 kb mRNA. Tropoelastin is synthesized on ribosomes of the rough endoplasmic reticulum and secreted into the cisternae of the endoplasmic reticulum where the signal peptide is cleaved and proline residues are hydroxylated. Tropoelastin is then transported to the Golgi apparatus where it is packaged into vesicles, which later fuse with the cell membrane. Synthesis and secretion of a tropoelastin molecule requires approximately 20 minutes.[124] In contrast to collagen synthesis, tropoelastin synthesis is not decreased by either inhibition of peptidyl proline hydroxylation or substitution of hydroxyproline for proline. However, compounds that depolymerize microtubules, such as colchicine, significantly impair the secretion of tropoelastin (Fig. 3–3).[124]

Electron microscopic studies have suggested that elastic fibers are assembled along folds or indentations on the surface of the cell. The microfibrillar component appears first outside the cell and the tropoelastin appears later on the surface of the developing fiber. Thus, the initial location of the microfibrillar component has the potential for playing a role in determining the final orientation of the elastic fiber.[45, 80, 124]

Once secreted from the cell, the copper-dependent enzyme lysyl oxidase reacts with the epsilon amino groups on most of the 37 lysine residues in the tropoelastin molecule, forming highly reactive alpha-aminoadipic semialdehydes, allysines, which condense, forming Schiff bases and aldol condensation crosslinks between adjacent tropoelastin molecules. These crosslinks isomerize over a period of several days to form the stable quaternary pyridinium ring structures, desmosine, and isodesmosine.[141] The formation of the crosslinking amino acids, desmosine and isodesmosine, confers on the insoluble elastin molecule the ability to perform as a true elastomer. In many tissues, including that in the lung, elastic fibers are oriented in such a way that they take advantage of the ability of the meshwork of fibers to undergo considerable extension and still recoil such that the fibers return to their original dimensions and configuration (see Fig. 3–3).

TURNOVER OF ELASTIN. In the developing lung, the rate of tropoelastin synthesis is greatest during the period of alveolar septal formation, days 4 through 13 in the rat.[125] Once formed, however, elastin does not undergo extensive remodeling in the absence of inflammatory processes. In contrast, synthesis of lung collagen continues into adulthood. In the absence of disease processes, lung collagen content does not increase after the period of lung development, indicating that the rate of degradation of lung collagen must approximate the rate of synthesis.[28, 63] Studies involving quantitation of elastin peptides in blood and desmosines excreted in the urine have indicated that less than 1% of the total elastin in the body is turned over in the course of a year.[37] Degradation of elastin is greatly accelerated in many disease states, however. In cystic fibrosis patients, urinary excretion of desmosines has been shown to be correlated with the severity of lung disease.[22] Elastic fibers observed at autopsy in the chronically infected lungs of these individuals were thick, tortuous, and often fragmented, reminiscent of the elastic fibers observed in the lungs of animals who received intratracheal instillations of elastase.[22, 89]

Fibronectin

The fibronectins are a group of high molecular weight glycoproteins that exist in a soluble form in high concentrations

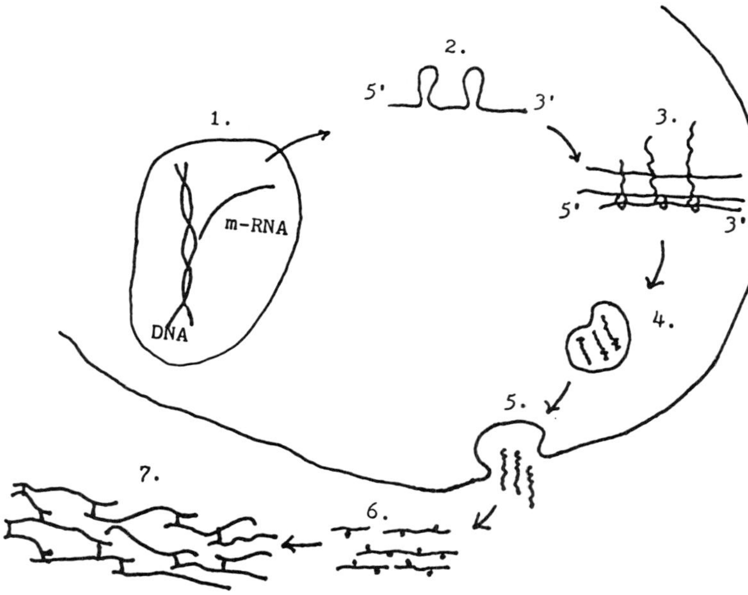

Figure 3–3. BIOSYNTHESIS OF ELASTIN
1. **Transcription of mRNA for soluble elastin.**
2. **Alternative splicing of mRNA.**
3. **Translation of mRNA and modifications including the removal of the signal peptide and proline hydroxylation.**
4. **Packaging of the soluble tropoelastin into vesicles.**
5. **Secretion of tropoelastin.**
6. **Assembly of the tropoelastin molecules on the microfibrillar component.**
7. **Lysyl oxidase catalyzes the crosslinking of tropoelastin to form insoluble elastin.**

in the plasma (300 μg/ml) and in an insoluble form in the extracellular matrix. In the lung, fibronectin is present in both the extracellular matrix and the basal lamina of the capillaries and the alveolar epithelial cells. Fibronectin has been observed surrounding smooth muscle cells and in alveolar septa, bronchioles, and blood vessels.[28] Plasma fibronectin is synthesized by hepatocytes in the liver, whereas cellular fibronectin is synthesized by fibroblasts, endothelial cells, and alveolar macrophages.[129] In addition to the cellular fibronectin synthesized by cells in the lung, it is possible that plasma fibronectin also contributes to the total lung fibronectin content because plasma fibronectin has been shown to be incorporated into basement membranes.[104]

Fibronectin promotes cell attachment by serving as a ligand between cells and extracellular matrix proteins.[84] Fibronectin has also been implicated in the regulation of cell polarity, migration, and differentiation, as well as cytoskeletal organization, neoplastic transformation, and wound healing.[72] In addition to its ability to bind to cells, fibronectin also has the capacity to bind to other proteins, including collagen, glycosaminoglycans, and proteoglycans.[43, 53, 111, 142] Fibronectin is also an important opsonin, enhancing both the adherence and ingestion of microorganisms.[138]

STRUCTURE AND SYNTHESIS. The fibronectin molecule consists of two subunits, approximately 230 kD and 250 kD, which are joined near their carboxy-termini by a pair of disulfide bonds. The fibronectin dimer is formed inside the cell. Once it is secreted, fibronectin binds to the cell surface.[127] Evidence suggests that the fibronectin molecule, although flexible, is folded such that the length to width ratio is 1 to 1.6.[122]

Fibronectin has three internal repeats, types I, II and III, each of which is the product of a different exon. There are 12 type I repeats, each 45 to 50 amino acids long, which are found at the amino- and carboxy-terminal ends of the polypeptide. The two type II repeats, each 60 amino acids long, are located within a row of nine type I repeats at the NH_2-terminal. Type III segments, of which there are 15 to 17, approximately 90 amino acids long, are found in the middle of the polypeptide. Domains homologous to types I and II repeats have been identified in other proteins, suggesting that the fibronectin gene might have evolved from exon shuffling of domains from other genes, some of which have similar functional properties.[109] Homologies to the type III segment have not yet been found in other proteins.

The two subunits of the dimeric fibronectin molecule contain a series of globular domains, each of which binds to specific extracellular matrix proteins or cells. The NH_2-terminal domain contains one binding site each for fibrin, heparin, and staphylococci, and one site for transglutaminase-catalyzed crosslinking to other proteins.[126, 136, 173] The binding of fibronectin to fibrin could be important in wound healing in that this molecular interaction could direct fibronectin into the blood clot where fibronectin could facilitate adhesion and migration of cells into the wound area.[129] Additional binding sites, each in separate domains, also exist for gelatin (denatured type I collagen), cells, heparin, fibrin, DNA, and another site for transglutaminase-catalyzed crosslinking to other proteins.

FIBRONECTIN GENE EXPRESSION. Many growth factors and hormones increase the expression of the fibronectin gene either by increasing transcription or by influencing post-transcriptional events. Transcription is stimulated by cAMP, epidermal growth factor (EGF), gamma-interferon, platelet-derived growth factor (PDGF), and transforming growth factor B.[14, 38] Glucocorticoids appear to act by increasing the stability of fibronectin mRNA.[39]

At least 20 variants of the fibronectin molecule are generated by differences in mRNA splicing. Plasma and cellular fibronectin differ in that, as a result of alternative splicing of the fibronectin transcript, the plasma fibronectin lacks one type III repeat. The differences in structure between plasma and cellular fibronectin do not, however, appear to explain the difference between the two types of fibronectin.[129] Alternative splicing might alter the functional properties of other variants of the fibronectin molecule, however. It has been suggested that the fibronectin splicing pattern may be determined by the splicing pattern required for another protein more critical for a particular cell.[129]

FIBRONECTIN RECEPTOR. Fibronectin receptors, members of a large family of related matrix receptors, have been identified on the surface of a variety of cell types, including fibroblasts, platelets, and mononuclear phagocytes.[23, 57, 66, 71] These receptors recognize the cell attachment site on the fibronectin molecule that contains the sequence arginine-glycine-asparagine-serine (RGDS). A cell containing a fibronectin receptor on its surface can attach to another surface to which fibronectin is bound as a result of the interaction between the fibronectin receptor on the cell surface and the RGDS sequence in the fibronectin molecule.[114, 128] The fibronectin receptor found on mammalian cells consists of two glycoprotein subunits of approximately 120 and 160 kD. It is currently thought that both of these subunits are involved in the binding of the RGDS attachment site.[129] The interaction between the cell surface receptor and the cell adhesion site on fibronectin occurs more readily in solid phases such as extracellular matrix, blood clots, and opsonized particles than in solutions, such as blood, where fibronectin is present in high concentrations. These receptors also possess a transmembrane domain and a cytoplasmic domain. The latter allows for the interaction with components of the cytoskeleton.[4, 5, 48, 68, 83, 95, 98, 116–118, 144, 145]

Basement Membrane

The basement membrane is a thin sheet of structured extracellular matrix located between parenchymal cells and the connective tissue layer. The basement membrane has two important functions. First, it defines the boundaries of the connective tissue. Second, it provides a substrate to which the parenchymal cells can attach by hemidesmosomes or anchoring filaments or by receptor-ligand interactions between the basal lamina and plasma membrane molecules. It acts as a barrier between connective tissue cells and parenchymal cells while allowing passage of granulocytes, lymphocytes, and monocytes.[12] Viewed at the electron microscopic level, this sheet appears to consist of three layers. The first, the lamina lucida or lamina rara lies adjacent to the plasma membranes of the parenchymal cell layer. The next layer, in close contact with the first, is the lamina densa, also referred to as the basal lamina or the basement membrane. The third layer, the reticular lamina, lies beneath the lamina densa. The first two layers are derived from the parenchymal cells, whereas the reticular lamina is derived from the connective tissue layer. The reticular lamina is absent in the alveolar capillary basement membrane and in other regions such as the glomerulus, where the transit of molecules is closely regulated (see Fig. 3–1).[12]

The lung parenchyma is somewhat unique in that the basement membranes for both the respiratory epithelium and the capillary endothelium are in close proximity. The epithelial basement membrane is homogeneous and compact and has a layer of heparan sulfate proteoglycans facing the epithelial cells. The endothelial basement membrane is fibrillar in appearance, with proteoglycans scattered throughout.[154, 155]

The basement membrane contains high concentrations of laminin and type IV collagen, proteins not found in significant concentrations elsewhere in the body. In addition, heparan sulfate proteoglycans and entactin/nidogen are present but, in contrast to other biologic membranes, the basement membrane contains little, if any, lipid.

LAMININ. Laminin is the most abundant glycoprotein in the basement membrane. The primary effect of this molecule is on cells of epithelial origin. Like fibronectin, laminin plays a role in the assembly of the extracellular matrix and can also influence cell adhesion, chemotaxis, migration, and differentiation.[86] Laminin binds to other extracellular matrix proteins, including type IV collagen, heparan sulfate proteoglycan, entactin, nidogen, and heparin.[147, 148, 168] The laminin molecule (Mr = 850,000) is a cross-shaped structure consisting of one long and three short arms. Each of the short arms contains two globular and two rodlike structures. Current evidence suggests that the three short arms (chains A, B1, and B2) intersect at the center of the cross where they are linked by disulfide bonds. The three extensions of the "short" arms are thought to run in parallel, sometimes coiling, to form the rigid, rod-like segment of the long arm.

Laminin is synthesized by many cell types. It appears that the B1 and B2 chains form a disulfide dimer.[31, 99, 112] The subsequent addition of the A chain to the dimer, prior to secretion, appears to be the rate-limiting step. Variable degrees of glycosylation of the B chains occur, but glycosylation does not appear to be a requirement for either assembly or secretion of the laminin molecule.[70]

TYPE IV COLLAGEN. Type IV collagen is the most abundant collagenous constituent of the basement membrane. The primary function of this protein is to provide mechanical stability to the basement membrane. The molecule is a trimer consisting of two $alpha_1$(IV) chains and one $alpha_2$(IV) chain, which contain 1669 and 1712 amino acids, respectively. Four structural and functional domains have been identified for the type IV collagen monomer: (1) a long triple helix located in the center of the molecule; (2) a shorter triple helical rod located at the N-terminal end of the molecule referred to as the 7S region; (3) a very short nonhelical region connecting the two helical regions, thought to act as a flexible hinge; and (4) a globular, noncollagenous domain at the C-terminal end of the molecule. In contrast to types I, II, and III collagen, which exist in a continuous triple helix, the triple helical region of type IV collagen contains frequent interruptions by noncollagenous sequences that lack the Gly-X-Y sequences required for triple helix formation.[151] These interruptions are thought to contribute to the flexibility of type IV collagen.[81]

Type IV collagen also differs from the interstitial collagens in that post-translational modification is more extensive, extracellular processing is less, and type IV collagen is more susceptible to proteolytic degradation.[115] In addition, instead of forming the cross-striated fibrils characteristic of the interstitial collagens, type IV collagen molecules self-assemble to form an irregular polygonal meshwork.[177] The results of *in vitro* experiments have shown that type IV collagen is secreted into the medium primarily in monomer form. The subsequent formation of tetramers is concentration dependent.[6] These tetramers are stabilized by the formation of disulfide bridges within the 7S domains and nonreducible crosslinks. Dimers are also formed by interactions of the globular noncollagenous region (NC1 domain).

PROTEOLYTIC ENZYMES THAT DEGRADE STRUCTURAL PROTEINS OF THE LUNG

Elastases (Neutrophil, Macrophage, Bacterial)

The soluble tropoelastin molecule is susceptible to proteolytic degradation by trypsin, chymotrypsin, cathepsin G, thermolysin, thrombin, kallikrein, and pronase in addition to elastase. In contrast, the mature crosslinked elastin fiber is degraded only by elastases. Elastases can also degrade proteins other than elastin, e.g., fibronectin, proteoglycan core proteins, and types III and IV collagen. The neutrophil is a major source of elastase, containing up to 3 $\mu g/10^6$ cells. Neutrophil elastase, a serine protease that readily degrades elastin, is inhibited by both $alpha_1$-proteinase inhibitor ($alpha_1$-PI) and $alpha_2$-macroglobulin (see Table 3–1). Macrophages also contain an elastase. This enzyme is a metalloproteinase that is inhibited by $alpha_2$-macroglobulin but not by $alpha_1$-proteinase inhibitor.[7]

Other sources of elastase include the fibroblast, platelet, smooth muscle cell, and pancreas.[141] In addition, bacteria also produce elastases. One of those most relevant to human lung disease is the elastase produced by *Pseudomonas aeruginosa.* This enzyme, also a metalloproteinase, is inhibited by $alpha_2$-macroglobulin and actually inactivates $alpha_1$-proteinase inhibitor. *P. aeruginosa* elastase is inhibited to a limited extent by the bronchial mucous protease inhibitor. However, this inhibitor is found predominantly in the upper respiratory tract.[166, 167] Therefore patients who are susceptible to *P. aeruginosa* infection, e.g., those who have cystic fibrosis and are immunocompromised, are at risk for proteolytic destruction of tissue in the lower respiratory tract. Although neutrophil elastase has been found in most studies to be the predominant enzyme in the lung secretions of cystic fibrosis patients, the presence of even low concentrations of *P. aeruginosa* elastase could well exacerbate the situation by inactivating alpha$_1$-PI.

Connective Tissue Metalloproteinases

Connective tissue metalloproteinases are zinc-containing enzymes, active at a neutral pH, that are capable of degrading proteins in the extracellular matrix (see Table 3–1).[100, 121, 170] These metalloproteinases are members of a multigene family that share a number of structural similarities. One of these enzymes, collagenase, is unique in that it is the only enzyme that can initiate degradation of native interstitial collagens (types I, II, and III) at a neutral pH.[100] Collagenase produced by synovial fibroblasts that line joints is thought to be responsible for the significant joint destruction in rheumatoid arthritis. Another of these metalloproteinases, stromelysin, degrades proteoglycans, laminin, and fibronectin.

Collagenase has been difficult to localize in specific cell types because of its lability. The enzyme appears to be localized in the perinuclear region of the cell.[169] With the exception of the collagenase produced by polymorphonuclear leukocytes (PMNs), collagenase has not been observed to exist in storage pools or granules within cells, suggesting that this enzyme is synthesized and released only when needed. Fibroblasts, macrophages, and PMNs are likely sources of collagenase within the lung.

Tissue collagenase is synthesized in a latent form, procollagenase. The mechanisms by which procollagenase is activated *in vivo* are not yet well understood, although numerous *in vitro* studies have provided some information. Studies suggest that plasmin first removes 81 residues from the amino-terminal portion of the collagenase molecule, resulting in the formation of a 42 kD fragment, which is then subject to further degradation at the carboxyl-terminal end of the molecule by stromelysin, after which the collagenase molecule is fully activated.[64]

Upon activation, collagenase is capable of cleaving the native triple helical region of collagen to form an N-terminal three-quarter fragment and a C-terminal one-quarter fragment. Cleavage can occur only at one collagenase-specific region consisting of the sequence Gly-Ile-Ala or Gly-Leu-Ala. Cleavage occurs at the Gly-Ile or Gly-Leu bonds and although these bonds occur elsewhere in the molecule, helix stability is lowest in the region of the collagen molecule where cleavage actually occurs.[67]

The synthesis of collagenase is stimulated by a number of cytokines, including interleukin-1, tumor necrosis factor, substance P, epidermal growth factor, and platelet-derived growth factor. Transforming growth factor B has been shown to decrease collagenase activity both by decreasing the synthesis of procollagenase and by increasing the synthesis of two collagenase inhibitors, tissue inhibitor of metalloproteinases (TIMP) and endothelial-type plasminogen activator inhibitor (PAI-1).[107] Type IV collagen is degraded by a protease found in tumor cells[148] that does not degrade the interstitial collagens. Type IV collagen is also degraded by PMN elastase.[153]

ENDOGENOUS INHIBITORS OF PROTEOLYTIC ENZYMES: FACTORS INFLUENCING CONCENTRATION AND FUNCTION

The proteinase inhibitors present in the lung are, in general, capable of inactivating proteolytic enzymes released as a result of phagocytosis or cell death and preventing significant proteolytic destruction of lung tissue. This does not, however, preclude the possibility that within the normal lung, foci may exist where there is a proteinase/antiproteinase imbalance.

The inhibitor that plays the major role in protecting the lower respiratory tract is alpha$_1$-PI. A relatively low molecular weight protein (52 kD), alpha$_1$-PI, enters the lung primarily by transudation from the serum, but it is also synthesized in the lung by mononuclear cells.[75, 156] Although alpha$_1$-PI inhibits a broad spectrum of enzymes, including trypsin, chymotrypsin, cathepsin G, plasmin, thrombin, tissue kallikrein, factor Xa, and plasminogen, human neutrophil elastase (HNE) is the only significant substrate for this inhibitor *in vivo*.[152] The association rate constant for alpha$_1$-PI and HNE is 25 times greater than that for other proteases. In addition, once formed, the alpha$_1$-PI:HNE complex is essentially irreversible.[13, 152]

A second plasma proteinase inhibitor, alpha$_2$-macroglobulin, forms a tight 2:1 complex with neutrophil elastase.[40, 105] Unfortunately, the large size of alpha$_2$-macroglobulin (725 kD) precludes serum transudation of this inhibitor. In the intact mature lung, less than 0.5% of the molar content of elastase inhibitory activity in the lower respiratory tract is attributable to alpha$_2$-macroglobulin.[55] Alpha$_2$-macroglobulin is present in the secretions of the injured adult lung, however,[56] and has also been detected in the lung secretions of ventilated premature infants.[20] A third inhibitor, the bronchial mucous protease inhibitor, is concentrated primarily in the upper airways, both in the nonciliated bronchial epithelial cells and in the serous cells of the central airways.[49, 162, 166] This inhibitor is also found to a lesser extent in the peripheral lung in the Clara and goblet cells of the bronchioles[162] and in airway walls and alveolar septa in association with elastin fibers.[167, 170]

Collagenase is inhibited by both the leukocyte collagenase inhibitor and by B-1-anticollagenase. The latter is present in human blood[169, 170] and the low molecular weight of this inhibitor (33 kD) suggests that it may be present in lung secretions as well.

Although alpha$_1$-PI is normally present in sufficient quantities to protect the lung against proteolytic insult, there are two notable exceptions, hereditary alpha$_1$-PI deficiency and oxidative inactivation of alpha$_1$-PI.

Alpha$_1$-Proteinase Inhibitor Deficiency

The importance of alpha$_1$-PI for the protection of the lung against proteolytic destruction was first recognized by Laurell and Eriksson,[90] who observed that emphysema in young adults was associated with an inherited deficiency of alpha$_1$-PI. The recent cloning of the alpha$_1$-PI gene has enhanced significantly our understanding of the molecular basis for the major alpha$_1$-PI deficiency states.[33] The alpha$_1$-PI gene consists of 12.2 kb, contains 7 exons and 6 introns, and has been localized to chromosome 14. The protein coding region starts on exon II and ends on exon V.[93] The carbohydrate attachment sites are encoded by exons II and III and the active site is encoded by exon V.

Alpha$_1$-proteinase inhibitor is highly polymorphic. The variants, 75 of which have been identified thus far, can be separated into four major categories based on the serum concentration of alpha$_1$-PI and the functional activity of the inhibitor: normal, deficient, dysfunctional, and Null. Classification of the alpha$_1$-PI phenotype is based on the migration of the inhibitor on isoelectric focusing of plasma between pH 4.2 and 4.9. The most common form, M, is so designated because of its migration to the middle of the gel. Although there are approximately 47 different M alleles, there is no evidence to date that any of these are abnormal.[33] In normal individuals the serum concentration of alpha$_1$-PI ranges from 20 to 48 μM.[165]

The mutant forms most commonly associated with the deficiency state are Z and S. The S variant is the more common of the two.[54] Individuals with these deficiency states are not at risk for either emphysema or liver disease.[33] The genetic defect is attributable to a difference of one base resulting in an amino acid substitution. Although transcription proceeds at a normal rate, the newly synthesized alpha$_1$-PI is unstable and 60% is destroyed within the cell.[34] The Z variant is also caused by a difference of one base and an amino acid substitution. Although these Z-variant molecules appear to be processed normally until glycosylation, there is significant aggregation after glycosylation and only a fraction of the alpha$_1$-PI molecules are translocated to the Golgi apparatus and secreted.[160] The alpha$_1$-PI that is secreted has a lower than normal association rate constant with neutrophil elastase.[33] The only dysfunctional variant described thus far, alpha$_1$-$AT_{pittsburgh}$, has an active site that is similar to that of antithrombin III. This variant is a good inhibitor of thrombin but a poor inhibitor of HNE.[33]

In the fourth category, the Null state, the serum is completely devoid of alpha$_1$-AT. Individuals in this category are at high risk for developing pulmonary emphysema between 30 and 40 years of age.[34, 51, 58, 101, 133, 146] There are six known Null mutations attributable to the deletion, insertion or substitution of one or more nucleotides. The $Null_{bellingham}$ mutation is due to the substitution of a base in a coding exon, which results in a premature stop codon.[58, 133] $Null_{granite\ falls}$,[101] $Null_{bolton}$,[51] and $Null_{hong\ kong}$ mutations are due to deletions of one or two bases resulting in premature stop codons. $Null_{procida}$ results from the deletion of all four coding exons, and $Null_{mattawa}$[34] is caused by an insertion mutation resulting in a premature stop codon. The risk for developing pulmonary emphysema is associated primarily with the inheritance of two Null alleles, certain combinations of deficiency alleles, or a Null allele plus specific deficiency alleles.[33]

Functional proteinase inhibitor deficiency can also result from the oxidative inactivation of the methionine residue in the active site of alpha$_1$-PI. After oxidation, alpha$_1$-PI can no longer inhibit porcine pancreatic elastase, human plasmin, or thrombin, and the rate association constant for HNE is decreased by a factor of 2000.[13] Methionine sulfoxide peptide reductase, an enzyme present in PMNs,[24] has been reported to be able to reduce oxidized alpha$_1$-PI.[1]

Results of *in vitro* studies have demonstrated that reactive species such as H_2O_2 and O_2 released by activated phagocytic cells can inactivate alpha$_1$-PI. These cells also produce myeloperoxidase, which, in the presence of H_2O_2 and Cl^-, can oxidize alpha$_1$-PI.[76, 96] There is little doubt that smoking increases the risk of proteinase/antiproteinase imbalance in the lung; however, considerable controversy has surrounded the question of whether or not cigarette smoke per se inactivates alpha$_1$-PI. Although *in vivo* exposure to cigarette smoke does not appear to be particularly efficient in oxidizing alpha$_1$-PI,[172] components of cigarette smoke decrease the rate association constant for alpha$_1$-PI and HNE.[91] In addition, smokers tend to have higher concentrations of activated macrophages in their lung secretions, and it is likely that oxidants from these phagocytic cells inactivate alpha$_1$-PI in smokers, contributing further to the overall risk for lung injury associated with cigarette smoking.[13]

Evidence also exists that alpha$_1$-PI is inactivated in inflammatory sites, such as synovial fluids from joints of arthritic patients and lung secretions of adult respiratory distress syndrome (ARDS) patients.[29] In addition, inactivated alpha$_1$-PI has been detected in the lung secretions of premature infants ventilated with concentrations of inspired oxygen $> 60\%$ for 6 or more days.[19] The diminished functional activity of alpha$_1$-PI present in the lungs of both the ventilated infants and the ARDS patients is likely to be due to the combined effects of hyperoxic exposure, phagocytic cell oxidants, and complex formation with HNE.

FACTORS INFLUENCING THE CONCENTRATION, FUNCTION, AND STRUCTURE OF LUNG EXTRACELLULAR MATRIX

Effects of Aging

With increasing age, total lung collagen content decreases, whereas lung elastin content tends to increase. Pierce and Ebert[113] conducted a biochemical quantitation of lung collagen and elastin in lung tissue obtained from 18 individuals without any evidence of acute or chronic lung disease who ranged in age from 9 to 76 years. Collagen concentrations in parenchymal, pleural, vascular, and bronchial compartments of the 70- to 76-year-olds were 84%, 85%, 59%, and 49%, respectively, of values obtained from the lungs of 9- to 18-year olds. In the same age groups, elastin content increased 141% in the parenchyma, 223% in the pleura, 137% in the vessels, and 103% in the bronchi in the 70- to 76-year-old group versus the 9- to 18-year-old group.

Scanning and transmission electron microscopic evaluation of changes in skin elastin and collagen fibers have demonstrated changes in both the arrangement and structure of these connective tissue fibers associated with aging.[73] Elastin fibers in the superficial fascia of the 2-week-old rat were observed to be thin and straight. Fibers were arranged in layers with the orientation varying somewhat in succeeding layers, giving the appearance of parallelograms. As the animals got older, the parallelograms formed by the elastin fibers were observed to increase in size until, by 2 years of age, there was no longer an apparent pattern to the meshwork of elastin fibers. Individual fibers, originally thin and straight, became increasingly distorted and tortuous. Collagen fibers became straighter and thicker as the animals got older. The observed changes in tortuosity of the elastic fibers suggest that these fibers may have lost some of their original elasticity. If similar changes occur in the lung with increasing age, the compliance of the lung could be decreased as a result.

The total glycosaminoglycan/proteoglycan content of the lung (expressed as mg/gm dry defatted tissue) was found by Schmid and coworkers[135] to change from 5.6 in fetal lung (26 to 32 weeks gestational age) to 3.15 at 8 years, 3.98 at 22 years, 4.59 at 39 years, and 4.85 at 70 years. The concentration of glycosaminoglycans/proteoglycans increased with age in the alveoli, veins, and arteries, remained relatively unchanged in the pleura and peripheral bronchi, and decreased dramatically from 5.4 in 8-year-olds to 2.4 in 22-year-olds in the central bronchi. In the mature lung, dermatan sulfate was found in greatest abundance in the pleura, the alveoli contained more heparan sulfate and dermatan sulfate, and the central bronchi contained primarily chondroitin-6-sulfate. In the peripheral bronchi, veins, and arteries, dermatan sulfate predominated in the 8- and 22-year-olds. Chondroitin-6-sulfate was present in the highest concentrations in these tissue compartments in the lungs of the 39- and 70-year-olds. Hyaluronic acid, known to be present in high concentrations in the ECM of organs in which cell migration or proliferation, or both, occur, accounted for 48% of the total in fetal lungs, followed by chondroitin-6-sulfate (38%), dermatan sulfate (9%), and heparan sulfate (5%).[135]

Effects of Inflammation on Connective Tissue Proteins

Proteolytic degradation of the proteins and polysaccharides, which constitute the extracellular matrix and basal laminae, can have profound physiologic and pathologic effects on the lung. The severity of the injury is largely a function of the intensity and duration of the proteolytic insult and the ability of the host antiproteinase defense system to inactivate these enzymes. Polymorphonuclear leukocytes and alveolar macrophages, the primary sources of these degradative enzymes in the lung, enter the lung in increased numbers as a result of infection or exposure to irritants, such as cigarette smoke and high concentrations of oxygen, nitrogen dioxide, or sulfur dioxide. An imbalance between PMN elastase and elastase inhibitors within the lung is now accepted as a major factor in the etiology of pulmonary emphysema.

ACUTE INFLAMMATORY RESPONSE. Connective tissue changes in response to acute lung inflammation have been evaluated extensively in studies in which a bolus of porcine pancreatic elastase or human neutrophil elastase is instilled into the trachea of an experimental animal. Although elastin is the primary substrate for elastase, other ECM proteins are also subject to degradation.[79] Intratracheal administration of porcine pancreatic elastase to the hamster has been shown to cause an acute response characterized by hemorrhage, which is followed by an inflammatory response. By 21 days, the structural and physiologic changes in the hamster lung were equivalent to those observed in patients with panlobular emphysema. Abnormal restructuring of the lung, including airspace enlargement and distortion, progressed beyond day 21 in spite of the fact that uninhibited elastase was no longer detectable.

After elastase instillation, a dramatic change was observed in the lung elastin content, which decreased to 50% of control level within 1 day.[79] After this initial decrease, lung elastin gradually increased until control levels were reached within 3 weeks. Lung elastin content continued to increase and remained significantly greater than that in the control animals until day 360. The rate of collagen synthesis was also increased when compared with the control animals, but the total amount of lung collagen was not greater than that in the controls, suggesting that degradation was also elevated in the elastase-treated hamsters. *In vitro* studies of lung explants from these animals indicated that during the inflammatory phase there was an increase in both glucosamine incorporation into GAGs and total GAG content, largely attributable to an increase in chondroitin-6-sulfate, during the inflammatory phase. By day 21, both the rates of GAG synthesis and the total amounts of GAG subtypes had returned to normal.

Undoubtedly, many differences exist between the effects of an acute inflammatory response following the intratracheal instillation of a bolus of elastase to an experimental animal and the lung inflammation associated with chronic disease in humans. In animal models of acute lung injury, for example, repair processes are not hampered by continual elastolytic insult as is frequently the case in human lung disease. In spite of the differences, there are likely to be some similarities with respect to the initial phases of both the acute and the chronic processes that will enhance the understanding of some of the factors involved in the etiology of chronic lung disease.

ROLE OF CONNECTIVE TISSUE DESTRUCTION IN THE ETIOLOGY OF CHRONIC OBSTRUCTIVE PULMONARY DISEASE

Pathologic Evidence of Elastic and Collagen Fiber Destruction in Pulmonary Emphysema

Substantial evidence exists that elastic fibers have undergone proteolytic destruction in the lungs of pulmonary emphysema patients.[171] The effects of inflammation and subsequent proteolysis on lung elastin content and elastic fiber structure have been evaluated far more extensively than have inflammatory changes in any other connective tissue protein. Structural alterations in elastic fibers from emphysematous lungs were observed by Orsós in 1907.[106] Subsequent studies have confirmed and extended these observations in the lungs of patients with emphysema as well as in other acute and chronic inflammatory conditions. Wright[171] compared the three-dimensional architecture of 200- to 300-μm thick sections of normal and emphysematous lungs and observed that elastic fibers were attenuated, separated from each other, and retracted at the unattached ends. Damaged elastic fibers were generally associated with alveolar wall fenestrae, loss of capillaries, and presence of a slight increase in fibrous tissue. Dense aggregations of frayed, attenuated fibers were often observed in the thickened, fibrous walls of bullae.

Fukuda and coworkers,[52] using an antibody to elastin that penetrated only the periphery of the amorphous component, described four distinct types of abnormal elastic fibers in emphysematous lungs. In the lungs from a patient with panacinar emphysema resulting from alpha$_1$-proteinase inhibitor deficiency, fragmented fibers were observed frequently in alveolar walls and occasionally in bronchioles. At the electron microscopic level, the amorphous component of the elastic fiber appeared disrupted, with a fine granularity and a diminished electron density after tannic acid staining when compared with normal elastic fibers. Elastic fibers observed in the lungs from three patients with severe anthracosis and centriacinar emphysema were found to contain vacuolar changes along with deposits of an electron-dense granular material and small, round deposits of the amorphous component adjacent to microfibril bundles. The lungs of the patients with centriacinar emphysema contained few of the disrupted elastic fibers observed frequently in the patient with panacinar emphysema. In addition, lungs from the centriacinar emphysema patients also contained dense, irregular masses of amorphous component.

In further support of the protease-antiprotease hypothesis for the etiology of emphysema, Damiano and coworkers[35] used ultrastructural immunohistochemical techniques to localize elastase in lung tissue obtained from eight patients undergoing lobectomy. Seven of the eight patients were smokers and all eight had lung cancer. The investigators reported a correlation between the presence of elastase observed in contact with interstitial elastic fibers and the severity of emphysematous changes in the same regions as evidenced by an increased mean alveolar size. Lesions were more severe and elastase concentrations tended to be higher in the upper lobes than those in the lower lobes. Although the immunoreactivity of elastase cannot be equated with enzymatic activity, elastase complexed to alpha$_1$-proteinase inhibitor does not selectively bind to elastin,[139] suggesting that the elastase observed to be bound to parenchymal elastin was active at the time that binding occurred.

Additional evidence for the destruction of lung elastin in acute and chronic pulmonary inflammation has been provided by the quantitation of urinary excretion of the crosslinking amino acids unique to elastin, desmosine, and isodesmosine. Urinary desmosine excretion is not affected by dietary intake of elastin, all of which is excreted in the feces. Desmosines excreted in the urine reflect degradation of endogenous elastin. Urinary excretion of desmosines has been found to be significantly correlated with the severity of lung disease in cystic fibrosis patients.[22] In addition, premature infants ventilated with high concentrations of oxygen who ultimately developed the chronic lung disease bronchopulmonary dysplasia excreted significantly more desmosine in the urine at the end of the first week of life than did infants ventilated with lower concentrations of oxygen who did not develop chronic lung disease.[21] Although urinary desmosine excretion is not specific for lung injury, the low basal levels of elastin turnover in the body as a whole allow dramatic increases in sites such as the lung to be detected.

Considerably less attention has been devoted to the description of alterations in collagen fibers in emphysematous lungs. Some of this apparent lack of interest in the role of collagen fiber injury in the etiology of pulmonary emphysema undoubtedly stems from experimental observations that animal models of emphysema could be produced only by the intratracheal instillation of elastolytic enzymes. Ultrastructural changes in collagen fibers have, however, been documented in the lungs of patients with both mild and severe emphysema. Belton and coworkers[11] reported that collagen fibers observed in areas with minimal emphysematous changes were no longer arranged in parallel and that collagen fibers seen in areas of severe emphysema were enlarged and swollen.

SEQUELAE OF PROTEOLYTIC DESTRUCTION OF LUNG EXTRACELLULAR MATRIX PROTEIN

Although lung content of extracellular matrix (ECM) proteins is essentially normal after repair, the structure of some of these proteins may be altered to such an extent that their function is severely impaired. After elastolytic insult, collagen fibers are coarser and their orientation is deranged. Significant changes are also seen in elastic fibers in spite of the fact that the amino acid content of the new fibers is normal.[89] Thin, wavy elastic fibers are replaced by thick, tortuous fibers that are tangled and disorganized. Perhaps most relevant to normal lung function is that the newly formed elastic fibers are not attached to what was once a continuum of elastic fibers connecting alveolar septa, airways, pleura, and vessels.[88]

Although the extent of the interdependence of the ECM proteins has yet to be determined, it is becoming increasingly apparent that alterations in the structure or concentration of any one ECM protein are likely to have an impact on other components of the ECM. Results of developmental studies have emphasized the role of specific GAGs in regulating cell migration, proliferation, and differentiation. Similarities between the response of the ECM to development and repair suggest that the relative concentrations of ECM proteins may well be critical for lung repair as well. Karlinski and coworkers[79] have shown that the ratios of GAGs, collagen, and elastin are altered after elastolytic injury to the hamster lung and suggest that the observed abnormal restructuring of the lung parenchyma might have been influenced by altered ratios of ECM proteins. These studies and others involving animal models have made significant contributions to the understanding of the response of ECM molecules to acute lung inflammation. At the other end of the spectrum, the pathologic changes that occur in the fibrous ECM proteins, collagen and elastin, have been well described in the lungs of older patients with emphysema. A large gap, however, remains in the knowledge of the sequence of events occurring at the molecular level in the chronically inflamed lung.

REFERENCES

1. Abrams WR, Weinbaum C, Weissbach L, et al. Enzymatic reduction of oxidized alpha$_1$-proteinase inhibitor restores biological activity. Proc Natl Acad Sci USA 1981; 78:7483–7486.
2. Adams SL. Collagen gene expression. Am J Respir Cell Mol Biol 1989; 1:161–168.
3. Allebach ES, Boettiger D, Pacifici M, Adams S. Control of types I and II collagen and fibronectin gene expression in chondrocytes delineated by viral transformation. Mol Cell Biol 1985; 5:1002–1008.
4. Argraves WS, Pytela R, Suzuki S, et al. cDNA sequences from the alpha subunit of the fibronectin receptor predict a transmembrane domain and a short cytoplasmic peptide. J Biol Chem 1986; 261:12922–12924.
5. Argraves WS, Suzuki S, Arai H, et al. Amino acid sequence of the human fibronectin receptor. J Cell Biol 1987; 105:1183–1190.
6. Bächinger HP, Fessler LI, Fessler JH. Mouse procollagen IV. Characterization and supramolecular association. J Biol Chem 1982; 257:9796–9803.
7. Banda MJ, Werb Z. Mouse macrophage elastase. Biochem J 1981; 193:589–605.
8. Bartholomew JS, Lowther DA, Handley CJ. Changes in proteoglycan biosynthesis following leukocyte elastase treatment of bovine articular cartilage in culture. Arth Rheum 1984; 27:905–912.
9. Bashir MM, Indik Z, Yeh H, et al. Characterization of the complete human elastin gene. Delineation of unusual features in the 5′-flanking region. J Biol Chem 1989; 264:8887–8891.
10. Bateman E, Turner-Warwick M, Adelmann-Grill BC. Immunohistochemical study of collagen in human foetal lung and fibrotic lung disease. Thorax 1981; 36:645–653.
11. Belton JC, Crise N, McLaughlin RF, Tueller ET. Ultrastructural alterations in collagen associated with microscopic foci of human emphysema. Hum Pathol 1977; 8:669–677.
12. Bernfield M. In: Porter R, Whelan J, eds. Basement Membranes and Cell Movement. Ciba Foundation Symposium 108, London: Pitman Publishing Ltd., 1984, 1–5.
13. Bieth JG. Elastases: Catalytic and biological properties. In: Mecham R, ed. Biology of the Extracellular Matrix: Regulation of Matrix Accumulation. Orlando: Academic Press, Inc, 1986, 217–320.
14. Blatti SP, Foster DN, Ranganathan G, et al. Induction of fibronectin gene transcription and mRNA is a primary response to growth factor stimulation of AKR-2B cells. Proc Natl Acad Sci USA 1988; 85:1119–1123.
15. Boedtker H, Fuller F, Tate V. The structure of collagen genes. Int Rev Connect Res 1983; 10:1–63.
16. Bourdon MA, Krusius T, Campbell S, et al. Identification and synthesis of a recognition signal for the attachment of glycosaminoglycans to proteins. Proc Natl Acad Sci USA 1987; 84:3194–3198.
17. Bourdon MA, Oldberg A, Pierschbacher M, Ruoslahti E. Molecular cloning and sequence analysis of a chondroitin sulfate proteoglycan cDNA. Proc Natl Acad Sci USA 1985; 82:1321–1325.
18. Bray BA. Cold-isoluble globulin (fibronectin) in connective tissues of adult human lung and in trophoblast basement membrane. J Clin Invest 1978; 62:745–752.
19. Bruce M, Boat T, Martin R, et al. Protease inhibitors and inhibitor inactivation in neonatal airways secretions. Chest 1982; 81(Suppl):44S–45S.
20. Bruce MC, Martin RJ, Boat TF. Concentrations of alpha$_1$-proteinase inhibitor in serum and lung secretions of intubated infants. Pediatr Res 1984; 18:35–40.
21. Bruce MC, Poncz L, Klinger JD, et al. Biochemical and pathologic evidence for proteolytic destruction of lung connective tissue in cystic fibrosis. Am Rev Respir Dis 1985; 132:529–535.
22. Bruce MC, Wedig K, Jentoft N, et al. Altered urinary excretion of elastin crosslinks in premature infants who developed bronchopulmonary dysplasia. Am Rev Respir Dis 1985; 131:568–572.

23. Buck CA, Horwitz AF. Cell surface receptors for extracellular matrix molecules. Ann Rev Cell Biol 1987; 3:179–205.
24. Carp H, Janoff A, Abrams W, et al. Human methionine sulfoxide-peptide reductase, an enzyme capable of reactivating oxidized $alpha_1$-proteinase inhibitor *in vitro*. Am Rev Respir Dis 1983; 127:301–305.
25. Castor CW, Heiss PR, Gray RM, Seidman JC. Connective tissue formation by lung fibroblasts *in vitro*. Am Rev Respir Dis 1979; 120:107–119.
26. Choi MG, Hynes RO. Biosynthesis and processing of fibronectin in NIL.8 hamster cells. J Biol Chem 1979; 254:12050–12055.
27. Chrzanowski P, Keller S, Cerreta JM, et al. Elastin content of normal and emphysematous lung parenchyma. Am J Med 1980; 69:351–359.
28. Clark JG, Kuhn C, McDonald JA, Mecham RP. Lung connective tissue. Int Rev Connect Tissue Res 1983; 10:249–318.
29. Cochrane CG, Spragg R, Revak SD. Pathogenesis of adult respiratory distress syndrome: Evidence of oxidant activity in bronchoalveolar lavage fluid. J Clin Invest 1983; 71:754–761.
30. Cockayne D, Sterling KM, Shull S, et al. Glucocorticoids decrease the synthesis of type I procollagen mRNAs. Biochemistry 1986; 25:3202–3209.
31. Cooper AR, Kurkinen M, Taylor A, Hogan BLM. Studies on the biosynthesis of laminin by murine parietal endoderm cells. Eur J Biochem 1981; 119:189–197.
32. Craig RG, Rowe DW, Petersen DN, Kream BE. Insulin increases steady-state levels of procollagen mRNA in the osteoblast-rich segment of fetal rat calvaria. Endocrinology 1989; 125:1430–1437.
33. Crystal RG, Brantly ML, Hubbard RC, et al. The $alpha_1$-antitrypsin gene and its mutations: clinical consequences and strategies for therapy. Chest 1989; 95:196–208.
34. Curiel D, Brantly ML, Curiel E, et al. $Alpha_1$-antitrypsin deficiency caused by the $alpha_1$-antitrypsin Null mattawa-subscript gene: an insertion mutation rendering the $alpha_1$-antitrypsin gene incapable of producing $alpha_1$-antitrypsin. J Clin Invest 1989; 83:1144–1152.
35. Damiano VV, Tsang A, Kucich U, et al. Immunolocalization of elastase in human emphysematous lungs. J Clin Invest 1986; 78:482–493.
36. Danielsen CC. Mechanical properties of reconstituted collagen fibrils. Influence of a glycosaminoglycan: dermatan sulfate. Connect Tissue Res 1982; 9:219–225.
37. Davidson JM, Giro MG. Control of elastin synthesis: Molecular and cellular aspects. In: Mecham RP, ed. Biology of the Extracellular Matrix: Regulation of Matrix Accumulation. New York: Academic Press, 1986.
38. Dean DC, Newby RF, Bourgeois S. Regulation of fibronectin biosynthesis by dexamethasone, transforming growth factor-B, and cAMP in human cell lines. J Cell Biol 1988; 106:2159–2170.
39. Dean DC. Expression of the fibronectin gene. Am J Respir Cell Mol Biol 1989; 1:5–10.
40. Delshammar M, Ohlsson K. Isolation and partial characterization of elastase from dog granulocytes. Eur J Biochem 1976; 69:125–131.
41. Doege K, Sasaki M, Horigan E, et al. Complete primary structure of the rat cartilage proteoglycan core protein deduced from cDNA clones. J Biol Chem 1987; 262:17757–17767.
42. Emanuel BS, Cannizzaro L, Ornstein-Goldstein N, et al. Chromosome localization of the human elastin gene. Am J Hum Genet 1985; 37:873–882.
43. Engvall E, Ruoslahti E. Binding of soluble form of fibroblast surface protein, fibronectin, to collagen. Int J Cancer 1977; 20:1–5.
44. Ernst M, Schmid C, Froesch ER. Enhanced osteoblast proliferation and collagen gene expression by estradiol. Proc Natl Acad Sci USA 1988; 85:2307–2310.
45. Fahrenbach WH, Sandberg LB, Cleary EG. Ultrastructural studies on early elastogenesis. Anat Rec 1966; 155:563–576.
46. Fazio MJ, Olsen DR, Kauh EA, et al. Cloning of full-length elastin cDNAs from a human skin fibroblast recombinant cDNA library: Further elucidation of alternative splicing utilizing exon-specific oligonucleotides. J Invest Dermatol 1988; 91:458–464.
47. Fazio MJ, Olsen DR, Kuivaniemi H, et al. Isolation and characterization of human elastin cDNAs and age-associated variation in elastin gene expression in cultured skin fibroblasts. Lab Invest 1988; 58:270–277.
48. Fitzgerald LA, Steiner B, Rall SC Jr, et al. Protein sequence of endothelial glycoprotein IIIa derived from a cDNA clone. Identity with platelet glycoprotein IIIa and similarity to "integrin." J Biol Chem 1987; 262:3936–3939.
49. Franken C, Kramps JA, Meijer C, Dijkman JH, et al. Localization of a low molecular weight protease inhibitor in the respiratory tract. Bull Eur Physiopathol Respir 1980; 16(Suppl):231–236.
50. Fraser JRE, Laurent TC. Turnover and metabolism of hyaluronan. In: Evered D, Whelan J, eds. The Biology of Hyaluronan: Ciba Foundation Symposium. Chichester, UK: John Wiley and Sons, 1989.
51. Frazier G, Harrold TR, Siewertsen M, Cox DW. Deletion/frameshift mutation in the $alpha_1$-antitrypsin null allele, PI*QO bolton. Am J Hum Genet 1988; 43(Suppl):A183.
52. Fukuda Y, Masuda Y, Ishizaki M, et al. Morphogenesis of abnormal elastic fibers in lungs of patients with panacinar and centriacinar emphysema. Hum Pathol 1989; 20:652–659.
53. Furcht LT. Structure and function of the adhesive glycoprotein fibronectin. Mod Cell Biol 1983; 1:53–117.
54. Gadek JE, Crystal RG. $Alpha_1$-antitrypsin deficiency. In: Stanbury JB, Wyngaarden JB, Frederickson DS, et al., eds. Metabolic Basis of Inherited Disease. New York: McGraw-Hill, 1982, 1450–1467.
55. Gadek JE, Fells GA, Zimmerman RL, Rennard SI. Antielastases of the human alveolar structures: Implications for the protease-antiprotease theory of emphysema. J Clin Invest 1981; 68:889–898.
56. Gadek JE, Klein HG, Holland PV, Crystal RG. Replacement therapy of $alpha_1$-antitrypsin deficiency. Reversal of protease-antiprotease imbalance within the alveolar structures of PiZ subjects. J Clin Invest 1981; 68:1158–1165.
57. Gardner JM, Hynes RO. Interaction of fibronectin with its receptor on platelets. Cell 1985; 42:439–448.
58. Garver RI Jr, Mornex J-F, Nukiwa T, et al. $Alpha_1$-antitrypsin deficiency and emphysema caused by homozygous inheritance of non-expressing $alpha_1$-antitrypsin genes. N Engl J Med 1986; 314:762–766.
59. Gil J, Martinez-Hernandez A. The connective tissue of the rat lung: Electron immunohistochemical studies. J Histochem Cytochem 1984; 32:230–238.
60. Greenlee TK, Ross R, Hartman JL. The fine structure of elastic fibers. J Cell Biol 1966; 30:59–71.
61. Greenwald RA, Schwartz CE, Cantor JO. Interaction of cartilage proteoglycans with collagen-substituted agarose gels. Biochem J 1975; 145:601–605.
62. Hamalainen L, Oikarinen J, Kivirikko KI. Synthesis and degradation of type I procollagen mRNAs in cultured human skin fibroblasts and the effect of cortisol. J Biol Chem 1985; 260:720–725.
63. Hance AJ, Crystal RG. Collagen. In: Crystal RG, ed. The Biochemical Basis of Pulmonary Function. vol II: Lenfant C, ed. Lung Biology in Health and Disease. New York: Marcel Dekker, 1976, 213–257.
64. He C, Wilhelm SM, Pentland AP, et al. Tissue cooperation in a proteolytic cascade activating human interstitial collagenase. Proc Natl Acad Sci USA 1989; 86:2632–2636.
65. Heinegård D, Paulsson M. Structure and metabolism of proteoglycans. In: Piez KA and Reddi AH, eds. Extracellular Matrix Biochemistry. New York: Elsevier, 1984.
66. Hemler ME, Huang C, Schwarz L. The VLA protein family. Characterization of five distinct cell surface heterodimers each with a common 130,000 molecular weight beta subunit. J Biol Chem 1987; 262:3300–3309.
67. Highberger JH, Corbett C, Gross J. Isolation and characterization of a peptide containing the site of cleavage of the chick skin collagen $alpha_1$ (I) chain by animal collagenases. Biochem Biophys Res Commun 1979; 89:202–208.
68. Horwitz A, Duggan K, Greggs R, et al. The cell substrate attachment (CSAT) antigen has properties of a receptor for laminin and fibronectin. J Cell Biol 1985; 101:2134–2144.
69. Horwitz AL, Crystal RG. Content and synthesis of glycosaminoglycans in the developing lung. J Clin Invest 1975; 56:1312–1318.
70. Howe CC, Dietzschold B. Structural analysis of three subunits of laminin from teratocarcinoma-derived parietal endoderm cells. Dev Biol 1983; 98:385–391.

71. Hynes R. Integrins: A family of cell surface receptors. Cell 1987; 48:549–454.
72. Hynes RO. Fibronectin and its relation to cellular structures and behavior. In: Hay ED, ed. Cell Biology of Extracellular Matrix. New York: Plenum Press, 1983, 295–334.
73. Imayama S, Braverman IM. A hypothetical explanation for the aging of skin. Chronologic alteration of the three-dimensional arrangement of collagen and elastic fibers in connective tissue. Am J Pathol 1989; 134:1019–1025.
74. Indik Z, Yeh H, Ornstein-Goldstein N, et al. Alternative splicing of human elastin mRNA indicated by sequence analysis of cloned genomic and complementary DNA. Proc Natl Acad Sci USA 1987; 84:5680–5684.
75. Isaacson P, Jones DB, Millward-Sadler GH, et al. Alpha$_1$-antitrypsin in human macrophages. J Clin Pathol 1981; 34:982–990.
76. Janoff A. Biochemical links between cigarette smoking and pulmonary emphysema. J Appl Physiol 1983; 55:285–293.
77. Kahari V-M, Heino J, Vuorio E. Interleukin 1 increases collagen production and mRNA levels in cultured skin fibroblasts. Biochim Biophys Acta 1987; 929:142–147.
78. Kanwar YS, Hascall VC, Farquhar MG. Partial characterization of newly synthesized proteoglycans isolated from the glomerular basement membrane. J Cell Biol 1981; 90:527–532.
79. Karlinski J, Fredette J, Davidovits G, et al. The balance of lung connective tissue elements in elastase-induced emphysema. J Lab Clin Med 1983; 102:151–162.
80. Karrer HE, Cox J. Electron microscopic study of developing chick embryo aorta. J Ultrastruct Res 1960; 4:420–454.
81. Kilcherr E, Hoffman H, Steigemann W, Engel J. Structural model of the collagen-like region of C1q comprising the kink region and the fibre-like packing of the six triple helices. J Mol Biol 1985; 186:403–415.
82. Kimura JH, Lohamnder LS, Hascall VC. Studies on the biosynthesis of cartilage proteoglycan in a model system of cultured chondrocytes from the swarm rat chondrosarcoma. J Cell Biochem 1984; 26:261–278.
83. Kishimoto TK, O'Connor K, Lee A, et al. Cloning of the beta subunit of the leukocyte adhesion proteins: Homology to an extracellular matrix receptor defines a novel supergene family. Cell 1987; 48:681–690.
84. Klebe RJ, Mock PJ. Effect of glycosaminoglycans on fibronectin-mediated cell attachment. J Cell Physiol 1982; 112:5–9.
85. Klebe RJ. Isolation of a collagen-dependent cell attachment factor. Nature 1974; 250:248–251.
86. Kleinman HK, Cannon FB, Laurie GW, et al. Biological activities of laminin. J Cellular Biochem 1985; 27:317–325.
87. Koda JE, Bernfeld M. Heparan sulfate proteoglycans from mouse mammary epithelial cells. J Biol Chem 1984; 259:11763–11770.
88. Kuhn C, Slodkowska J, Smith T, Starcher B. The tissue response to exogenous elastase. Bull Eur Physiopath Respir 1980; 16(suppl):127–137.
89. Kuhn C, Yu SY, Chraplyvy M, et al. The induction of emphysema with elastase. II. Changes in connective tissue. Lab Invest 1976; 34:372–380.
90. Laurell C-B, Eriksson S. The electrophoretic alpha$_1$-globulin pattern of serum in alpha$_1$-antitrypsin deficiency. Scand J Clin Lab Invest 1963; 15:132–140.
91. Laurent P, Bieth JG. There is no solid evidence that oxidative inactivation of alpha$_1$-proteinase inhibitor is important in smokers' emphysema. Biochem Biophys Res Commun 1985; 126:275–281.
92. Lohmander LS, Hascall VC, Yanagashita M, et al. Posttranslational events in proteoglycan synthesis: Kinetics of synthesis of chondroitin sulfate and oligosaccharides on the core protein. Arch Biochem Biophys 1986; 250:211–227.
93. Long GL, Chandra T, Woo SLC, et al. Complete sequence of the cDNA for human alpha$_1$-antitrypsin and the gene for the S variant. Biochemistry 1984; 23:4828–4837.
94. Lyons BL, Schwarz RI. Ascorbate stimulation of PAT cells causes an increase in transcription rates and a decrease in degradation rates of procollagen mRNA. Nucleic Acids Res 1984; 12:2569–2579.
95. Malinoff HL, Wicha MS. Isolation of a cell surface receptor protein for laminin from murine fibrosarcoma cells. J Cell Biol 1983; 96:1475–1479.
96. Matheson NR, Janoff A, Travis J. Enzymatic oxidation of alpha$_1$-proteinase inhibitor in abnormal tissue turnover. Mol Cell Biochem 1982; 45:65–71.
97. Mitchell D, Hardingham T. Monensin inhibits synthesis of proteoglycan, but not hyaluronate, in chondrocytes. Biochem J 1982; 202:249–254.
98. Mollenhauer J, von der Mark K. Isolation and characterization of a collagen-binding glycoprotein from chondrocyte membranes. EMBO J 1983; 2:45–50.
99. Morita A, Sugimoto E, Kitigawa Y. Post-translational assembly and glycosylation of laminin subunits in parietal endoderm-like F-9 cells. Biochem J 1985; 229:259–264.
100. Murphy G, Nagase H, Brinckerhoff CE. Relationship of procollagenase activator, stromelysin and matrix metalloproteinase 3. Coll Relat Res 1988; 8:389–391.
101. Nukiwa T, Takahashi H, Brantly M, et al. Alpha$_1$-antitrypsin Null granite falls, a nonexpressing alpha$_1$ antitrypsin gene associated with a frameshift to stop mutation in a coding exon. J Biol Chem 1987; 262:1199–2004.
102. Obrink B. A study of the interactions between monomeric tropocollagen and glycosaminoglycans. Eur J Biochem 1973; 33:387–400.
103. Obrink B. The influence of glycosaminoglycans on the formation of fibres from monomeric tropocollagen *in vitro*. Eur J Biochem 1973; 34:129–137.
104. Oh E, Pierschbacher M, Ruoslahti E. Deposition of plasma fibronectin in tissues. Proc Natl Acad Sci USA 1981; 78:3218–3221.
105. Ohlsson K, Olsson I. The neutral proteases of human granulocytes: Isolation and partial characterization of granulocyte elastases. Eur J Biochem 1974; 42:519–527.
106. Orsós F. Über das elastische Gerüst der normalen und der emphysematosen Lunge. Beitr Pathol Anat 1907; 41:95–121.
107. Overall CM, Wrana JL, Sodek J. Independent regulation of collagenase, 72-kDa progelatinase, and metalloendoproteinase inhibitor expression in human fibroblasts by TGF-B. J Biol Chem 1989; 264:1860–1869.
108. Partridge SM. Elastin. In: Anfinsen CB Jr, Anson ML, Bailey KJ, Edsall JT, eds. Advances in Protein Chemistry. New York: Academic Press, 1962.
109. Patel RS, Odermatt E, Schwarzbauer JE, Hynes RO. Organization of the fibronectin gene provides evidence for exon shuffling during evolution. EMBO J 1987; 6:256–572.
110. Penttinen R, Kobayashi S, Bornstein P. Transforming growth factor B increases mRNA for matrix proteins both in the presence and in the absence of changes in mRNA stability. Proc Natl Acad Sci USA 1988; 85:1105–1108.
111. Perkins ME, Ji TH, Hynes RO. Cross-linking of fibronectin to sulfated proteoglycans at the cell surface. Cell 1979; 16:941–952.
112. Peters BP, Hartle RJ, Krzesicki RF, et al. The biosynthesis, processing, and secretion of laminin by human choriocarcinoma cells. J Biol Chem 1985; 260:14732–14742.
113. Pierce JA, Ebert RV. Fibrous network of the lung and its change with age. Thorax 1965; 20:469–476.
114. Pierschbacher MD, Ruoslahti E. Cell attachment activity of fibronectin can be duplicated by small synthetic fragments of the molecule. Nature 1984; 309:30–33.
115. Pihlajaniemi T, Tryggvason K, Myers JC, et al. cDNA clones coding for the pro-11(IV) chain of human type IV procollagen reveal an unusual homology of amino acid sequences in two halves of the carboxy-terminal domain. J Biol Chem 1985; 260:7681–7687.
116. Pytela R, Pierschbacher MD, Ginzberg MH, Plow E. Platelet membrane glycoprotein IIb/IIIa: Member of a family of Arg-Gly-Asp-specific adhesion receptors. Science 1986; 231:1559–1562.
117. Pytela R, Pierschbacher MD, Ruoslahti E. A 125/115-kDa cell surface receptor specific for vitronectin interacts with the arginine-glycine aspartic acid adhesion sequence derived from fibronectin. Proc Natl Acad Sci USA 1985; 82:5766–5770.
118. Pytela R, Pierschbacher MD, Ruoslahti E. Identification and isolation of a 140 kd cell surface glycoprotein with properties expected of a fibronectin receptor. Cell 1985; 40:191–198.
119. Raghow R, Gossage D, Kang AH. Pretranslational regulation of type I collagen, fibronectin and a 50 kilodalton noncollagenous extracellular protein by dexamethasone in rat fibroblasts. J Biol Chem 1986; 261:4677–4684.

120. Raghow R, Postlewaite AE, Keski-Oja J, et al. Transforming growth factor B increases steady state levels of type I procollagen and fibronectin messenger RNAs posttranscriptionally in cultured human dermal fibroblasts. J Clin Invest 1987; 79:1285–1288.
121. Reddi AH. Extracellular Matrix: Structure and Function. New York: Alan R. Liss, Inc., 1985.
122. Rocco M, Infusini E, Daga MG, et al. Models of fibronectin. EMBO J 1987; 6:2343–2349.
123. Roden L, Koerner T, Olson C, Schwartz NB. Mechanisms of chain in the biosynthesis of connective tissue polysaccharides. Fed Proc 1985; 44:373–380.
124. Rosenbloom J. Elastin: An overview. In: Cunningham LW, ed. Biochemistry of the Major Components of the Extracellular Matrix, Methods in Enzymology. Orlando: Academic Press, Inc., 1987, 172–304.
125. Rucker RB, Dubick MA. Elastin metabolism and chemistry: potential roles in lung development and structure. Environ Health Perspect 1984; 55:179–191.
126. Ruoslahti E, Engvall E, Hayman E. Fibronectin: Current concepts of its structure and functions. Coll Relat Res 1981; 1:95–128.
127. Ruoslahti E, Engvall E. Complexing of fibronectin, glycosaminoglycans and collagen. Biochim Biophys Acta 1980; 361:350–358.
128. Ruoslahti E, Pierschbacher MD. Arg-Gly-Asp: A versatile cell recognition site. Cell 1986; 44:517–518.
129. Ruoslahti E. Fibronectin and its receptors. Ann Rev Biochem 1988; 57:375–413.
130. Ruoslahti E. Structure and biology of proteoglycans. Ann Rev Cell Biol 1988; 4:229–255.
131. Russell SB, Trupin JS, Myers JC, et al. Differential glucocorticoid regulation of collagen mRNAs in human dermal fibroblasts: Keloid-derived and fetal fibroblasts are refractory to down regulation. J Biol Chem 1989; 264:13730–13735.
132. Sant AJ, Cullen SE, Giacoletto KS, Schwartz BD. Invariant chain is the core protein of the Ia-associated chondroitin sulfate proteoglycan. J Exp Med 1985; 162:1916–1934.
133. Satoh K, Nukiwa T, Brantly M, et al. Emphysema associated with complete absence of alpha$_1$-antitrypsin in serum and the homozygous inheritance of stop codon in an alpha$_1$-antitrypsin coding exon. Am J Hum Genet 1988; 42:77–83.
134. Saxe SA, Lukens LN, Pawlowski PJ. Changes in the nuclear and cytoplasmic levels of type I and type II collagen RNAs during growth of chondrocytes in 5-bromo-2′-deoxyuridine. J Biol Chem 1985; 260:3812–3819.
135. Schmid K, Grundboeck-Jusco G, Kimura A, et al. The distribution of the glycosaminoglycans in the anatomic components of the lung and the changes in concentration of these macromolecules during development and aging. Biochim Biophys Acta 1982; 716:178–187.
136. Sekiguchi K, Fukuda M, Hakomori S-I. Domain structure of hamster plasma fibronectin. J Biol Chem 1981; 256:6452–6462.
137. Seyer JM, Hutcheson ET, Kang AH. Collagen polymorphism in idiopathic chronic pulmonary fibrosis. J Clin Invest 1976; 57:1498–1507.
138. Simpson AW, Boughton BJ. Fibronectin as an opsonic regulator of monocyte phagocytosis. J Clin Pathol 1984; 37:787–789.
139. Sloan B, Abrams WR, Meranze DR, et al. Emphysema induced *in vitro* and *in vivo* in dogs by a purified elastase from homologous leukocytes. Am Rev Respir Dis 1981; 123:295–301.
140. Spooner BS, Thompson-Pletscher HA. Matrix accumulation and the development of form. In: Mecham RP ed. Biology of Extracellular Matrix: Regulation of Matrix Accumulation. Orlando: Academic Press, 1986.
141. Starcher B. Elastin and the lung. Thorax 1986; 41:577–585.
142. Stathakis NE, Mosesson MW. Interactions among heparin, cold-insoluble globulin and fibronectin in the formation of the heparin-precipitable fraction of plasma. J Clin Invest 1977; 60:855–865.
143. Sterling KM Jr., Harris MJ, Mitchell JJ, Cutroneo KR. Bleomycin treatment of chick fibroblasts causes an increase of polysomal type I procollagen mRNAs. J Biol Chem 1983; 258:14438–14444.
144. Suzuki S, Argraves WS, Arai H, et al. Amino acid sequence of the vitronectin receptor alpha subunit and comparative expression of adhesion receptor mRNAs. J Biol Chem 1987; 262:14080–14085.
145. Suzuki S, Argraves WS, Pytela R, et al. cDNA and amino acid sequences of the cell adhesion protein receptor recognizing vitronectin reveal a transmembrane domain and homologies with other adhesion protein receptors. Proc Natl Acad Sci USA 1986; 83:8614–8618.
146. Talamo RC, Langley CE, Reed CE, Makino S. Alpha$_1$-antitrypsin deficiency: A variant with no detectable alpha$_1$-antitrypin. Science 1973; 181:70–71.
147. Timpl R, Dziadek M, Fujware S, et al. Nidogen: A new self-aggregating basement membrane protein. Eur J Biochem 1983; 137:455–465.
148. Timpl R, Dziadek M. Structure, development and molecular pathology of basement membranes. Int Rev Exp Pathol 1986; 29:1–112.
149. Tolstoshev P, Haber R, Trapnell BC, Crystal RG. Procollagen messenger RNA levels and activity and collagen synthesis during the fetal development of sheep lung, tendon and skin. J Biol Chem 1981; 256:9672–9679.
150. Toole BP, Gross J. The extracellular matrix of the regenerating newt limb: synthesis and removal of hyaluronate prior to differentiation. Dev Biol 1971; 25:57–77.
151. Traub W, Piez KA. The chemistry and structure of collagen. Adv Protein Chem 1971; 25:243–252.
152. Travis J, Salvesen GS. Human plasma protease inhibitors. Annu Rev Biochem 1983; 52:655–709.
153. Uitto VJ, Schwartz D, Veis A. Degradation of basement membrane collagen by neutral proteases from human leukocytes. Eur J Biochem 1980; 105:409–417.
154. Vaccaro C, Brody JS. Structural features of the alveolar wall basement membrane in the adult rat lung. J Cell Biol 1981; 91:427–437.
155. Vaccaro C, Brody JS. Ultrastructural localization and characterization of proteoglycans in the pulmonary alveolus. Am Rev Respir Dis 1979; 120:901–910.
156. Van Furth R, Kramps JA, Diesselhof-Den Dulk MMC. Synthesis of alpha$_1$-antitrypsin by human monocytes. Clin Exp Immunol 1983; 51:551–557.
157. Van Kuppevelt THMSM, Domen JGW, Cremers FPM, Kuyper CMA. Staining of proteoglycans in mouse lung alveoli. I. Ultrastructural localization of anionic sites. Histochem J 1984; 16:657–669.
158. Varga J, Rosenbloom J, Jimenez SA. Transforming growth factor B causes a persistent increase in steady-state amounts of type I and type III collagen and fibronectin mRNAs in normal human dermal fibroblasts. Biochem J 1987; 247:597–604.
159. Velasco A, Hidalgo J, Perez-Vilar J, et al. Detection of glycosaminoglycans in the Golgi complex of chondrocytes. Eur J Cell Biol 1988; 47:241–250.
160. Verbanac KM, Heath EC. Synthesis and processing of M and Z variant alpha$_1$-antitrypsin. Biol Chem 1986; 261:9979–9989.
161. Vogel KG, Peterson DW. Extracellular, surface, and intracellular proteoglycans produced by human embryo lung fibroblast in culture. (IMR-90) J Biol Chem 1981; 256:13235–13242.
162. DeWater R, Willems LN, VanMuijen GN, et al. Ultrastructural localization of bronchial antileukoprotease in central and peripheral human airways by a gold-labeling technique using monoclonal antibodies. Am Rev Respir Dis 1986; 133:882–890.
163. Weiner FR, Czaja MJ, Giambrone M-A, et al. Transcriptional and post-transcriptional effects of dexamethasone on albumin and procollagen messenger RNAs in murine schistosomiasis. Biochemistry 1987; 26:1557–1562.
164. Weiner FR, Czaja MJ, Jefferson DM, et al. The effects of dexamethasone on *in vitro* collagen gene expression. J Biol Chem 1987; 262:6955–6958.
165. Wewers MD, Casolaro MA, Sellers SE, et al. Replacement therapy for alpha$_1$-antitrypsin deficiency associated with emphysema. N Engl J Med 1987; 316:1055–1062.
166. Willems LNA, Kramps JA, DeWater R, et al. Evaluation of antileukoprotease in surgical lung specimens. Eur J Respir Dis 1986; 69:242–247.
167. Willems LNA, Otto-Verberne CJM, Kramps JA, et al. Detection of antileukoprotease in connective tissue of the lung. Histochemistry 1986; 86:165–168.
168. Woodley DT, Rao CN, Hassell JR, et al. Interactions of basement membrane components. Biochim Biophys Acta 1983; 761:278–283.
169. Woolley DE, Brinckerhoff CE, Mainardi CL, et al. Collagenase production by rheumatoid synovial cells: Morphological and

immunohistochemical studies of the dendritic cell. Ann Rheum Dis 1979; 38:262–270.
170. Woolley DE, Evanson JM. Present status and future prospects in collagenase research. In: Woolley DE, Evanson JM, eds. Collagenase in Normal and Pathological Connective Tissues. Chichester, UK: John Wiley and Sons, 1980.
171. Wright RR. Elastic tissue of normal and emphysematous lungs. A tridimensional histologic study. Am J Pahthol 1961; 39:355–363.
172. Wyss A, Virca GD, Schnebli HP. Cigarette smoke components are not very effective in directly inactivating alpha$_1$-proteinase inhibitor. Hoppe-Seyler's Z Physiol Chem 1984; 365:511–516.
173. Yamada KM. Cell surface interactions with extracellular materials. Ann Rev Biochem 1983; 52:761–799.
174. Yanagishita M, Hascall VC. Metabolism of proteoglycans in rat ovarian granulosa cell culture. Multiple intracellular degradative pathways and the effect of chloroquine. J Biol Chem 1984; 259:10270–10283.
175. Yeh H, Anderson N, Ornstein-Goldstein N, et al. Structure of the bovine elastin gene and S1 nuclease analysis of alternative splicing of elastin mRNA in the bovine nuchal ligament. Biochemistry 1989; 28:2365–2370.
176. Young RW. The role of the Golgi complex in sulfate metabolism. J Cell Biol 1973; 57:175–189.
177. Yurchenco PD, Ruben GC. Basement membrane structure *in situ:* Evidence for lateral associations in the type IV collagen network. J Cell Biol 1987; 105:2559–2568.

Chapter 4

OXIDATIVE DAMAGE AND COPD

John R. Hoidal Kevin T. McCusker
Bruce C. Marshall N. V. Rao

The theme of this chapter is oxidative damage and chronic obstructive pulmonary disease (COPD). The review focuses primarily on the potential role of oxidizing radicals or oxidized halogens as a mechanism of emphysema. The possible role of these agents in the development of chronic bronchitis is examined briefly.

Cigarette smoking is firmly established as the primary environmental risk factor associated with emphysema. The mechanism by which smoking causes emphysema is not known. Contemporary thinking has championed the protease pathogenesis hypothesis, which holds that emphysema is caused by damage to elastic fibers due to an imbalance between elastase and antielastases in the lung. Elastase causes emphysema experimentally, and its relative excess is the likely basis for disease in individuals with alpha$_1$ protease inhibitor (alpha$_1$-PI) deficiency. However, uncertainty exists about the role of elastase in cigarette smokers without alpha$_1$-PI deficiency. Studies suggest that the increased risk of emphysema associated with cigarette smoking may be partially due to the effect of oxidants on the lung. This chapter reviews highlights of the experimental evidence supporting a role for oxidants. The four general areas reviewed include (1) the physicochemical properties of oxyradicals and related species; (2) the source and characterization of oxidant burden in the lungs of cigarette smokers; (3) the probable mechanisms of oxidant-mediated lung injury; and (4) the antioxidant protective mechanisms in the lung.

PHYSICOCHEMICAL PROPERTIES OF OXIDANTS

Oxidants are highly reactive electron acceptors capable of removing electrons from a variety of molecules. The process of oxidation may reversibly or irreversibly damage compounds of all chemical classes, including nucleic acids, proteins and free amino acids, lipids and lipoproteins, and carbohydrates. In this regard, oxidants can damage cells and extracellular matrix components critical for normal lung function.

The oxidant species of primary interest in the pathogenesis of COPD are listed in Table 4–1. Relevant molecules include free radicals, which are any species with one or more unpaired electrons, including oxygen itself, and molecules that contain only paired electrons and therefore are not free radicals, which include oxidized halogens, i.e., hypochlorous acid (HOCl). Appreciable variation occurs in the reactivities and lifetime of these molecules. Some of them, e.g., the peroxyl radical and hydrogen peroxide (H_2O_2), are sufficiently stable so that they can probably diffuse considerable distance from their origin. Thus, damage by these agents may be remote from the site of generation. Others, such as the hydroxyl radical (•OH), react with extremely high rate constants with almost every type of molecule. Hence, these agents likely react within 1 to 5 molecular diameters of their origin,[1] and thus the damage produced by them will be "site specific" to the locus of their generation.[2] As pointed out by Halliwell and Gutteridge,[2] this

TABLE 4–1. Oxidants and Related Species Implicated in the Pathogenesis of Emphysema

SPECIES	SYMBOL	PROBABLE SOURCE
Superoxide anion	O_2^-	a, c
Hydrogen peroxide	H_2O_2	a, c
Hydroxyl radical	·OH	a, b, and c
Hypochlorous acid	HOCl	a
Monochloramine	NH_2Cl	a
Taurine monochloramine	TauNCl	a
Nitrogen dioxide	NO_2	b
Semiquinone radical	HQ·	c
Peroxyl radical	ROO·	b

a = Phagocyte respiratory burst.
b = Gas phase of cigarette smoke.
c = Tars of cigarette smoke.

concept has important implications in biologic systems. First, it means that the actual chemical reactions taking place *in vivo*, particularly of the highly reactive site-specific oxidants, are not necessarily predictable from the chemistry of these species in free solution, but are highly dependent on the chemical milieu of their origin. Second, the effect of scavengers on the site-specific oxidants will not necessarily be what is expected from chemically determined rate constants, because site-specific reactions may occur at locations relatively inaccessible to the antioxidant scavenger, an important consideration in designing therapeutic strategies.

Oxidants are ubiquitous in living organisms. Reactive oxygen species, such as superoxide anion (O_2^-), H_2O_2, and •OH are intermediates in a number of physiologic reactions and are generated *in vivo* during normal metabolism. Even though an elaborate cellular and extracellular antioxidant system has evolved to keep this ongoing oxidant burden in check, this defense system is not complete. Random cell changes resulting from oxidant attack are produced continuously throughout living systems. For example, the number of oxidative hits on DNA has been estimated to be greater than 10^3 per day for each of the body's 6×10^{13} cells.[3] These hits may cause cumulative oxidative alterations of long-lived molecules, such as elastin, and thus may be responsible for the age-related decline in pulmonary function and other alterations associated with normal aging.

SOURCE AND CHARACTERIZATION OF THE OXIDANT BURDEN IN CIGARETTE SMOKERS

The lungs of cigarette smokers are subject to an enhanced oxidant burden. The primary sources of this burden are cigarette smoke itself and activated lung phagocytes. By convention, two phases of cigarette smoke are defined, a gas phase and a tar phase. Fresh, undiluted gas phase cigarette smoke is remarkable in containing more than 10^{17} reactive oxyradicals per puff.[4] Undiluted cigarette smoke also contains several hundred ppm of oxides of nitrogen[5]; in contrast, polluted air generally contains less than 1 ppm. While mostly in the form of nitric oxide (NO), appreciable amounts of the more potent oxidant, nitrogen dioxide (NO_2), have been demonstrated.[6] Ongoing generation of NO_2 is possible because NO can be slowly oxidized to NO_2.[4] Nitrogen dioxide can interact with H_2O_2 to generate O_2^- and •OH.[7] Thus, these free radicals may be continuously formed and destroyed as a result of these gas-phase reactions.

Cigarette tar contains several exceptionally stable radical species. The predominant radical species in tar is semiquinone held in a polymeric tarry matrix rich in hydroquinones and quinones.[8] This tar radical can reduce molecular O_2 to O_2^- and H_2O_2.[9] Transition metals, particularly iron, catalyze the production of •OH from H_2O_2. Cigarette tar contains large amounts of iron, which is likely intimately involved in the cigarette tar production of •OH.[10]

Phagocytes, the other important source of oxidants, accumulate in the lungs of cigarette smokers precisely at the sites of the airflow obstruction. Clusters of pigmented alveolar macrophages (AMs) lodge in the respiratory bronchioles of smokers prior to the development of COPD[11] and persist as tissue destruction and airflow obstruction progress.[12] The alveolar septa of cigarette smokers also contain increased numbers of polymorphonuclear leukocytes (PMNs) compared with those of nonsmokers.[13] In contrast to the peripheral airways and gas exchange units, no persistent increase in the number of inflammatory cells in the large airways of cigarette smokers is evident.[14] However, during acute exacerbations in patients with chronic bronchitis, these large airways become loaded with PMNs.[15]

Phagocytes from smokers generate more oxidants than do phagocytes from nonsmokers. The oxidants fall into two classes. Oxidizing radicals are formed from sequential transfer of single electrons to oxygen and include O_2^- and •OH. H_2O_2, although not a radical, is a central species in this monovalent reduction pathway. Oxidized halogens, the second class of phagocyte-derived oxidants, result from modification of H_2O_2 by peroxidases, primarily myeloperoxidase, and include HOCl and its major metabolites, monochloramine (NH_2Cl) and taurine monochloramine. Alveolar macrophages and PMNs from cigarette smokers release more O_2^- and H_2O_2 *in vitro* than do cells from nonsmokers.[16, 17] These differences may be amplified *in vivo* where repetitive stimulation by inhaled particulates likely provides almost constant stimulation of the AM respiratory burst.[18] Moreover, the lung parenchyma of cigarette smokers contains more iron,[19] which may potentiate the generation of •OH. Polymorphonuclear leukocytes from some smokers also generate more oxidants than are generated by nonsmokers. Luminol-enhanced luminescence, which presumably reflects generation of oxidized halogens by PMNs,[20] is increased in smokers with persistent elevations of peripheral blood leukocyte counts,[17] the group most susceptible to COPD.[21]

Although it is currently not possible to determine the exact concentrations of reactive oxygen species in the lungs of human smokers, available evidence suggests that it is substantial. Chance and colleagues, using luminescence techniques, have demonstrated 3×10^{-8}M H_2O_2 in the exhaled breath from nonsmokers and a 3-to-4-fold increase in smokers.[22, 23] Hydrogen peroxide is readily diffusible, and these concentrations represent "leakage" into breath. Concentrations at sites of synthesis may be much greater. Thus, substantial H_2O_2 is present in lungs of smokers for generation of •OH or HOCl. Prerequisite iron and myeloperoxidase (MPO) are also available, particularly during periods of superimposed acute inflammation. Micromolar quantities of iron bound to low molecular weight chelating agents have been detected in human extracellular fluids and inflammatory exudates.[24] Up to 45 u/ml active MPO accumulates extracellularly in experimental models of inflammation.[25] In contrast to the intracellular environment, the extracellular milieu is relatively deficient in antioxidant enzymes required to limit the accumulation of reactive oxygen species, *vide infra*. It seems entirely plausible that sufficient amounts of •OH or HOCl may be present extracellularly to participate in destruction of lung matrix components.

PROBABLE MECHANISMS OF OXIDANT-MEDIATED LUNG INJURY

Although direct evidence linking an enhanced oxidant burden to the pathogenesis of COPD is lacking, circumstantial evidence supporting this notion is mounting. Most studies to date have focused on the role of oxidants in the development of emphysema. Two mechanisms are proposed by which oxidants could cause matrix destruction and resultant emphysema: First, they might facilitate destruction of lung matrix proteins by proteases. Second, oxidants could directly degrade lung matrix constituents.

The notion that oxidants promote protease-mediated destruction of lung matrix molecules has received considerable attention. One suggested mode is by stimulating recruitment of phagocytes to the lung and thus increasing the protease burden. Multiple potential chemotactic factors have been identified in the lungs of oxidant-exposed animals. During hyperoxic exposure, PMN chemotactic factors appear in the alveolar lavage fluids of rats or rabbits.[26, 27] The AM has been proposed as the source of the chemotactic activity.[27] In addition, cigarette smoke inhalation is capable of activating the alternate complement pathway within the airways.[28, 29] Whether this effect is directly due to the oxidants in cigarette smoke is not known. Finally, degraded lung connective tissue fragments, including collagen and elastin peptides, are potent chemotaxins.[30, 31]

A second mechanism by which oxidants may facilitate protease-mediated matrix destruction is oxidative inactivation of alpha$_1$-PI. The major inhibitor of serine proteases in the lower respiratory tract[32] acts as a pseudosubstrate for serine proteases by combining at its reactive methionine^{358}-serine^{359} site with the target protease.[33] The methionine residue at the active site can be oxidized readily by triggered phagocytes and possibly by cigarette smoke.[34] As a result, the association rate constant for PMN elastase diminishes by more than three orders of magnitude.[35] The potential pathophysiologic significance of this finding was demonstrated by experiments in which dogs were treated with chloramine-T, which reduced the elastase inhibitory capacity of alpha$_1$-PI to essentially zero; emphysema developed.[36]

The critical issue of the functional status of alpha$_1$-PI within the alveolar space and interstitium of cigarette smokers remains unresolved. Initial studies that demonstrated oxidative inactivation and methionine oxidation of alpha$_1$-PI recovered by bronchoalveolar lavage from smokers[37, 38] have not been confirmed by other investigators.[39, 40] Additional rigorously designed studies assessing the functional status of alpha$_1$-PI at sites within the gas exchange units will be necessary to resolve this issue.

Oxidative inactivation of antiproteases may also play a role in the pathogenesis of chronic bronchitis. Intratracheal instillation of leukocyte proteases into the hamster causes chronic bronchial injury, including secretory cell metaplasia.[41] This finding suggests that the protease-antiprotease balance may be important in maintaining the integrity of the bronchial epithelium. The major antiprotease protecting the mucus-lined airways against the destructive effects of leukocyte proteases is bronchial mucous protease inhibitor (BMPi). Bronchial mucous protease inhibitor can be inactivated by oxidants contained in cigarette smoke or released by PMNs.[42] Antioxidants prevent this effect. The functional activity of BMPi is significantly reduced in aspirates of human smokers compared with that of nonsmokers.[42]

Increasing alveolar epithelial permeability is another mechanism by which oxidants may enhance protease-mediated degradation of lung matrix, by facilitating fluxes of proteases, or, agents that amplify protease activity, into the interstitium. To cause emphysema, instilled proteases residing within the airspaces must travel across the alveolar epithelium and into the interstitium. The tight junctions between adjacent cells form nearly impermeable seals. Both cigarette smoke and NO_2 enhance alveolar epithelial permeability[43–45] and augment porcine pancreatic elastase-induced emphysema.[46] The relevance of these observations to the pathogenesis of human COPD is not certain because it remains to be determined whether the alveolar space is an important source of proteases for the interstitium.

A further mechanism by which oxidants may enhance protease-mediated degradation of lung matrix is by modifying the matrix molecules, making them more susceptible to protease attack. A well-established precedent exists in degradation of intracellular proteins. Numerous examples of oxidatively modified proteins being rapidly and selectively degraded by proteolytic systems are reviewed.[47] The question of whether oxidants alter long-lived extracellular matrix molecules, making them susceptible to proteolytic degradation, has received little attention. Weiss and Regiani demonstrated that oxidants and proteases released by stimulated PMNs cooperate by degrading subendothelial matrices.[48] However, the facilitating role of oxidants appeared to be inactivation of alpha$_1$-PI rather than alteration of the matrix molecules. Campbell and coworkers found no cooperation by PMN-derived oxidants and proteases in hydrolysis of fibronectin.[49] In contrast, Curran and coworkers demonstrated that brief exposure to ozone modifies the type I collagen molecule, making it more susceptible to protease attack.[50] Fligiel and colleagues observed that pretreatment by H_2O_2 facilitated subsequent protease-mediated degradation of basement membrane.[51] In our laboratory, we have found that pretreatment of elastin with lipophilic chloramines enhances the subsequent degradation by human leukocyte elastase. Thus, a complex interplay of PMN oxidants and proteinases may take place, the net effect of which is likely an important determinant of the pattern and extent of connective tissue injury.

The concept that oxidants directly degrade matrix molecules is germane because, as mentioned, these agents are likely generated in large quantities in proximity to the structural proteins and basement membranes in the lungs of smokers. The oxidants of primary interest are oxidizing free radicals, e.g., O_2^- and •OH, and oxidized halogens. The chemistry of oxidizing free radicals supports their ability to react with lung matrix molecules. Compelling evidence has been obtained that •OH can initiate depolymerization of polysaccharides. Initial studies used pulse radiolysis or electrolysis cells, and depolymerization was demonstrated by altered functional properties.[52, 53] Subsequent studies confirmed this finding and showed that reactive oxygen species could mediate degradation of tissue glycosaminoglycans, including hyaluronate.[54] Balazs and colleagues, using electron paramagnetic resonance, suggested that •OH attacked hyaluronate at the glycosidic bond and at the C_5 hydrogen of the pyranose ring.[55] Greenwald and Moy provided direct evidence of •OH-mediated degradation of hyaluronate by demonstrating shift in chromatographic profiles to lower molecular weights.[56]

The •OH may also modify protein constituents, including peptide bonds, free amino and sulfhydryl groups, and aromatic residues.[57, 58] Studies also have demonstrated that •OH or related oxidants can initiate nonenzymatic degradation of type I collagen. Initially, Greenwald and Moy observed that •OH inhibited collagen gelation.[59] Subsequently, Curran and colleagues provided direct chromatographic evidence of ozone-mediated degradation of soluble collagen.[50] Monboisse and coworkers demonstrated degradation of microfibrillar collagen by O_2^-.[60] In addition, desmosine and isodesmosine, the cross-linking amino acids responsible for the insolubility of elastin, are degraded by photooxidation,[61] a probable •OH-mediated process.

The chemistry of oxidized halogens also supports their ability to degrade lung matrix components. The classic study by Baker demonstrated that one peptide link of native egg albumin was broken for every 2.9 molecules of OCl^- reduced.[62] HOCl also reacts rapidly with sulfhydryls, thioethers, and a wide variety of nitrogen-containing compounds.[63] Degradative oxidation of proteins may result. Tyrosine, an aromatic amino acid which is vulnerable to oxidation by HOCl, is immediately adjacent to desmosine residues in elastin.[64] Thus, the stability of this important crosslinkage may be jeopardized by HOCl attack. Chloramines formed by interaction of HOCl with amines are more restricted in reactivity than HOCl but are longer lasting.[65] Of note is that proteins with no methionine, such as elastin, are particularly prone to incorporate chloramines.[66] Studies have also demonstrated oxidation of lysine side chains of elastin by oxidized halogens.[67] These data provide a biochemical basis for oxidative changes in lung matrix proteins, which may bear directly on the pathogenesis of emphysema.

ANTIOXIDANT PROTECTIVE MECHANISMS IN THE LUNG

The importance of oxidants in the pathogenesis of COPD is dependent on the status of the antioxidant defense. Aerobic organisms have evolved an elaborate system of antioxidant defense that is sufficient to keep a reasonable check on the normal oxidant burden. Within cells, antioxidant enzymatic and nonenzymatic defenses prevent the accumulation of oxy-radicals and peroxides. Intracellular O_2^- concentrations are kept at 10^{-11}M or less by superoxide dismutases, which include a 33,000 dalton, copper- and zinc-dependent form present in the cytoplasm and a 85,000 dalton, manganese-dependent form in mitochondria.[68, 69] Hydrogen peroxide is eliminated by the hemoprotein catalase and glutathione peroxidase. Catalase is most effective against high concentrations of H_2O_2.[70] Glutathione peroxidase is more effective against low concentrations of H_2O_2 and in contrast to catalase requires the presence of a reductant, glutathione (GSH).[71] Nonenzymatic antioxidants associated with cells include alpha-tocopherol, which is the major lipid-soluble chain-breaking antioxidant, ascorbate, and GSH.[72]

In extracellular fluids, superoxide dismutase activity and catalase activity are low and GSH peroxidase is essentially absent. A major extracellular antioxidant defense is to keep iron from participating in radical forming reactions.[73] Agents that inhibit radical reactions by sequestering metals include transferrin, uric acid, and haptoglobin.[73] Ceruloplasmin is an important serum antioxidant primarily due to its ability to keep iron in the Fe^{+++} state.[74] Albumin provides the primary protective effect in serum from myeloperoxidase-catalyzed oxidative inactivation of alpha$_1$-PI.[75] It is viewed as a "sacrificial antioxidant" because it is irreversibly modified during the reaction.[73]

The epithelial surface of the respiratory tract is particularly well equipped to protect itself against oxidants. By direct measurement, Snyder and colleagues estimated that the ascorbate concentration of alveolar lining fluid of rats was 6.3 mM, considerably higher than the 0.1 mM in normal rat serum.[76] Similarly, the GSH concentration in alveolar lining fluid in humans was 140-fold higher than that in plasma.[77] Transferrin concentration is also relatively increased in alveolar lavage fluid when compared with serum.[78] In addition, the surface epithelium of the respiratory tract is covered by mucus glycoproteins that react efficiently with H_2O_2 and •OH and thus should protect underlying cells and matrix from oxidative damage.[79]

Although not extensively studied to date, the antioxidant mechanisms in the lungs of cigarette smokers appear to be more activated, perhaps in response to the oxidant stress. Superoxide dismutase and catalase activities in AMs of cigarette smokers are twice those of nonsmokers.[80] Ascorbate and alpha-tocopherol levels are also substantially elevated in AM from cigarette smokers compared with nonsmokers.[81] Moreover, cigarette smokers have 180% higher concentration of GSH in alveolar lining fluid than do nonsmokers; however, alpha-tocopherol concentrations are decreased.[77, 82] The effectiveness of the selective increases in antioxidant defenses in limiting the oxidant-mediated lung damage in cigarette smokers is not currently known.

In summary, the protease pathogenesis concept remains dominant in current understanding of the pathogenesis of COPD. However, as pointed out in this chapter, this concept may represent too narrow a focus. The role of oxidants and other potentially important factors merit consideration and further study in order to define the basis for the disorder.

REFERENCES

1. Pryor WA. Oxy-radical and related species: their formation, lifetime and reactions. Ann Rev Physiol 1986; 48:657–667.
2. Halliwell B, Gutteridge JMC. Oxygen-free radicals and iron in relation to biology and medicine: some problems and concepts. Arch Biochem Biophys 1986; 246:501–514.
3. Cross CE, Halliwell B, Borish ET, et al. Oxygen radicals and human diseases. Ann Intern Med 1987; 107:526–545.
4. Pryor WA, Prier DG, Church DF. An electron-spin resonance study of mainstream and sidestream cigarette smoke: the nature of the free radicals in gas-phase smoke and in cigarette tar. Environ Health Prospect 1983; 47:345–355.
5. Guerin MR. Chemical composition of cigarette smoke. In: Gori GB and Bock FG, eds. Banbury Report: A Safe Cigarette? Cold Springs Harbor, New York: Cold Springs Harbor Laboratory, 1980, 191–204.
6. Jenkins RA, Gill BE. Determination of oxides of nitrogen (NO_2) in cigarette smoke by chemiluminescent analysis. Anal Chem 1980; 52:925–928.
7. Dooley MM, Pryor WA. Free radical pathology: inactivation of human alpha$_1$-proteinase inhibitor by products from the reaction of nitrogen dioxide with hydrogen peroxide and the etiology of emphysema. Biochem Biophys Res Commun 1982; 106:981–987.
8. Church DF, Pryor WA. Free-radical chemistry of cigarette smoke and its toxicological implications. Environ Health Perspect 1985; 64:111–126.
9. Nakayama T, Kodama M, Nagata C. Generation of hydrogen peroxide and superoxide anion radical by cigarette smoke. Gann 1984; 75:95–98.
10. VanDunnen BL, Goldschmidt BM. Cocarcinogenic and tumor promoting agents in tobacco carcinogenesis. J Natl Cancer Inst 1976; 56:1237–1242.
11. Niewoehner DE, Kleinerman J, Rice DB. Pathologic changes in the peripheral airways of young cigarette smokers. N Engl J Med 1974; 291:755–758.
12. Cosio MG, Hale KA, Niewoehner DE. Morphologic and morphometric effects of prolonged cigarette smoking on the small airways. Am Rev Respir Dis 1980; 122:265–271.
13. Ludwig PW, Schwartz BA, Hoidal JR, Niewoehner DE. Cigarette smoking causes accumulation of polymorphonuclear leukocytes in lung parenchyma. Am Rev Respir Dis 1985; 131:828–830.
14. Sobonya RE, Kleinerman J. Morphometric study of bronchi in young smokers. Am Rev Respir Dis 1972; 105:768–775.
15. Spencer H, ed. Pathology of the Lung. Oxford: Pergamon Press, 1985, 131–166.
16. Hoidal JR, Fox RB, LeMarbe PA, et al. Altered oxidative metabolic responses *in vitro* of alveolar macrophages from young asymptomatic cigarette smokers. Am Rev Respir Dis 1981; 123:85–92.
17. Ludwig PW, Hoidal JR. Alterations in leukocyte oxidative metabolism in cigarette smokers. Am Rev Respir Dis 1982; 126:977–980.

18. Richter AM, Abboud RT, Johal SS, Ferra TA. Acute effect of smoking on superoxide production by pulmonary alveolar macrophages. Lung 1986; 164:233–242.
19. McGowan SE, Murray JJ, Parrish MG. Iron binding, internalization and fate in human alveolar macrophages. J Lab Clin Med 1983; 108:587–595.
20. Dahlgren C, Stendahl O. Role of myeloperoxidase in luminol-dependent chemiluminescence of polymorphonuclear leukocytes. Infect Immun 1983; 39:736–741.
21. Sparrow D, Glynn RJ, Cohen M, Weiss ST. The relationship of the peripheral leukocyte count and cigarette smoking to pulmonary function among adult men. Chest 1984; 86:383–386.
22. Boveris A, Cadenas A, Chance B. Ultraweak chemiluminescence: a sensitive assay for oxidative radical reactions. Fed Proc 1981; 40:195–198.
23. Williams MD, Leigh JS Jr, Chance B. Hydrogen peroxide in human breath and its probable role in spontaneous breath luminescence. Ann NY Acad Sci 1982; 386:478–483.
24. Halliwell B, Gutteridge JMC. Oxygen toxicity, oxygen radicals, transition metals and disease. Biochem J 1984; 219:1–14.
25. Bradley PB, Christensen RD, Rothstein G. Cellular and extracellular myeloperoxidase in pyogenic inflammation. Blood 1982; 60:618–622.
26. Fox RB, Hoidal JR, Brown DM, Repine JE. Pulmonary inflammation due to oxygen toxicity: involvement of chemotactic factors and polymorphonuclear leukocytes. Am Rev Respir Dis 1987; 123:521–523.
27. Harada RN, Vatter AE, Repine JE. Macrophage effector function in pulmonary oxygen toxicity: hyperoxia damages and stimulates alveolar macrophages to make and release chemotaxins for polymorphonuclear leukocytes. J Leukocyte Biol 1984; 35:373–383.
28. Kew RR, Ghebrehiwet B, Janoff A. Cigarette smoke can activate the alternative pathway of complement *in vitro* by modifying C_3. J Clin Invest 1985; 75:1000–1007.
29. Kew RR, Ghebrehiwet B, Janoff A. The role of complement in cigarette smoke–induced chemotactic activity of lung fluids. Am Rev Respir Dis 1986; 133:478–481.
30. Postlethwaite AE, Seyer JM, Kang AH. Collagen and collagen peptide–induced chemotaxis of human blood monocytes. J Exp Med 1976; 143:1299–1307.
31. Senior RM, Griffin GL, Mecham RP. Chemotactic activity of elastin-derived peptides. J Clin Invest 1980; 66:859–862.
32. Gadek JE, Fells GA, Zimmerman RL, et al. Antielastases of the human alveolar structure. Implications for the protease-antiprotease theory of emphysema. J Clin Invest 1981; 68:889–898.
33. Johnson D, Travis J. Structural evidence for methionine at the reactive site of human alpha$_1$-proteinase inhibitor. J Biol Chem 1978; 253:7142–7145.
34. Tsan M, Chen JW. Oxidation of methionine by human polymorphonuclear leukocytes. J Clin Invest 1980; 65:1041–1050.
35. Beatty K, Bieth J, Travis J. Kinetics of association of serine proteinases with native and oxidized alpha$_1$-proteinase inhibitor and alpha$_1$-antichymotrypsin. J Biol Chem 1980; 255:3931–3934.
36. Abrams WR, Cohen AB, Damiano VV, et al. A model of decreased functional alpha$_1$-proteinase inhibitor. Pulmonary pathology of dogs exposed to chloramine T. J Clin Invest 1981; 68:1132–1139.
37. Gadek JE, Fells GA, Crystal RG. Cigarette smoking induces functional antiprotease deficiency in the lower respiratory tract of humans. Science 1979; 206:1315–1316.
38. Carp H, Miller F, Hoidal JR, Janoff A. Potential mechanism of emphysema: alpha$_1$-proteinase inhibitor recovered from lungs of cigarette smokers contains oxidized methionine and has decreased elastase inhibitory capacity. Proc Natl Acad Sci USA 1982; 29:2041–2045.
39. Stone PJ, Calore JD, McGowan SE, et al. Functional alpha$_1$-proteinase inhibitor in the lower respiratory tract is not decreased. Science 1983; 221:1187–1189.
40. Boudier C, Pelletier A, Pauli G, Bieth JG. The functional acitivity of alpha$_1$-proteinase inhibitor in bronchoalveolar lavage fluids from healthy smokers and nonsmokers. Clin Chim Acta 1983; 132:309–315.
41. Snider GL, Lucey EC, Christensen TG, et al. Emphysema and bronchial secretory cell metaplasia induced in hamsters by human neutrophil products. Am Rev Respir Dis 1984; 129:155–160.
42. Carp H, Janoff A. Inactivation of bronchial mucous proteinase inhibitor by cigarette smoke and phagocyte-derived oxidants. Exp Lung Res 1980; 1:225–237.
43. Jones JG, Minty BD, Lawler P, et al. Increased alveolar epithelial permeability in cigarette smokers. Lancet 1980; i:66–68.
44. Simani AS, Inoue S, Hogg JC. Penetration of the respiratory epithelium of guinea pigs following exposure to cigarette smoke. Lab Invest 1984; 31:75–81.
45. Gordon RE, Case BW, Kleinerman J. Acute NO_2 effect on penetration and transport of horseradish peroxidase in hamster respiratory epithelium. Am Rev Respir Dis 1983; 128:528–533.
46. Hoidal JR, Niewoehner DE. Cigarette smoke inhalation potentiates elastase-induced emphysema. Am Rev Respir Dis 1983; 127:478–481.
47. Davies KJA. Protein damage and degradation by oxygen radicals: general aspects. J Biol Chem 1982; 262:9895–9901.
48. Weiss SJ, Regiani S. Neutrophils degrade subendothelial matrices in the presence of alpha$_1$-proteinase inhibitor. Cooperative use of lysosomal proteinases and oxygen metabolites. J Clin Invest 1984; 73:1297–1303.
49. Campbell EJ, Senior RM, McDonald JA, Cox DL. Proteolysis by neutrophils. Relative importance of cell-substrate contact and oxidative inactivation of proteinase inhibitors *in vitro*. J Clin Invest 1982; 70:845–852.
50. Curran SF, Amoruso MA, Goldstein BD, Berg RA. Degradation of soluble collagen by ozone or hydroxyl radicals. FEBS Lett 1984; 176:155–160.
51. Fligiel SEG, Lee EC, McCoy JP, et al. Protein degradation following treatment with hydrogen peroxide. Am J Pathol 1984; 115:418–425.
52. Richards T, Herp A, Pigman W. The kinetics of depolymerization of hyaluronic acid by L-ascorbic acid, and the inhibition of this reaction by anions of the lyotropic series. J Polym Sci 1967; Al-5:931–934.
53. Harris MJ, Herp A, Pigman W. Depolymerization of polysaccharides through the generation of free radicals at a platinum surface: a novel procedure for the controlled production of free-radical oxidation. Archiv Biochem Biophys 1971; 142:615–622.
54. Moore JS, Phillips GO, Davis JV, Dodgson KS. Reactions of connective tissue and related polyanions with hydrated electrons and hydroxyl radicals. Carbohydr Res 1970; 12:253–260.
55. Balazs EA, Davis JV, Phillips GO, Young MD. Transient intermediates in the radiolysis of hyaluronic acid. Radiation Res 1967; 31:243–255.
56. Greenwald RA, Moy WW. Inhibition of collagen gelatin by the action of superoxide radical. Arthritis Rheum 1979; 22:251–259.
57. Freeman BA, Crapo JD. Free radicals and tissue injury. Lab Invest 1982; 47:412–426.
58. Trelstad RL, Lawley KR, Holmes LB. Nonenzymatic hydroxylations of proline and lysine by reduced oxygen derivatives. Nature 1981; 289:310–312.
59. Greenwald RA, Moy WW. Effect of oxygen derived free radicals on hyaluronic acid. Arthritis Rheum 1980; 23:455–463.
60. Monboisse JC, Braquet P, Randoux A, Borel JP. Non-enzymatic degradation of acid-soluble calf skin collagen by superoxide: protective effects of flavinoids. Biochem Pharmacol 1983; 32:53–58.
61. Baurain R, Larochelle SF, Lamy F. Photolysis of desmosine and isodesmosine by ultraviolet light. Eur J Biochem 1976; 67:155–164.
62. Baker RWR. Studies on the reaction between sodium hypochlorite and proteins. Biochem J 1947; 41:337–342.
63. Aldrich JM, McCarthy CA, Hurst JK. Biological reactivity of hypochlorous acid: implications for microbicidal mechanisms of leukocyte myeloperoxidase. Proc Natl Acad Sci USA 1981; 78:210–214.
64. Foster JA, Rubin L, Kagan HM, et al. Isolation and characterization of cross-linked peptides from elastin. J Biol Chem 1974; 249:6191–6196.
65. Weiss SJ, Lampert MB, Test ST. Long-lived oxidants generated by human neutrophils: characterization and bioactivity. Science 1983; 222:625–628.
66. Thomas EL, Jefferson MM, Graham MB. Myeloperoxidase catalyzed incorporation of amines into proteins: role of hypochlorous acid and dichloramines. Biochemistry 1982; 21:6299–6308.
67. Clark RA, Szot S, Williams MA, Kagan HM. Oxidation of lysine side-chains of elastin by the myeloperoxidase system and by stimulated human neutrophils. Biochem Biophys Res Commun 1986; 135:451–457.
68. Tyler DD. Polarographic assay and intracellular distribution of superoxide dismutase in rat liver. Biochem J 1975; 147:493–504.

69. Fridovich I. Superoxide dismutases. Ann Rev Biochem 1975; 44:147–159.
70. Agar NS, Sadrzadeh SMH, Hallaway PE, Eaton JW. Erythrocyte catalase. A somatic oxidant defense. J Clin Invest 1986; 77:319–321.
71. Cohen G, Hochstein P. Glutathione peroxidase: the primary agent for the elimination of hydrogen peroxide in erythrocytes. Biochemistry 1963; 2:1420–1428.
72. Junod AF. Data on oxidants and antioxidants. Bull Eur J Pathophysiol Respir 1986; 22:253S–255S.
73. Halliwell B, Gutteridge JMC. Oxygen-free radicals and iron in relation to biology and medicine: some problems and concepts. Arch Biochem Biophys 1986; 246:501–514.
74. Dormandy TL. Free-radical oxidation and antioxidants. Lancet 1978; i:647–650.
75. Wasil M, Halliwell B, Hutchison DCS, Baum H. The antioxidant action of human extracellular fluids. Biochem J 1987; 243:219–223.
76. Snyder A, Skoza L, Kikkawa Y. Comparative removal of ascorbic acid and other airway substances by sequential bronchoalveolar lavage. Lung 1983; 161:111–121.
77. Cantin AM, North SL, Hubbard RC, Crystal RG. Normal alveolar epithelial lung lining fluid contains high levels of glutathione. J Appl Physiol 1987; 63:152–157.
78. Bell DY, Haseman JA, Spock A, et al. Plasma proteins of the bronchoalveolar surface of the lungs of smokers and nonsmokers. Am Rev Respir Dis 1981; 124:72–79.
79. Cross CE, Halliwell B, Allen A. Antioxidant protection: a function of tracheobronchial and gastrointestinal mucus. Lancet 1984; i:1328–1330.
80. McCusker K, Hoidal J. Selective increase of antioxidant enzyme activity in alveolar macrophages from cigarette smokers and smoke-exposed hamsters. Am Rev Respir Dis 1990; 141:678–682.
81. McGowan SE, Parenti CM, Hoidal JR, Niewoehner DE. Ascorbic acid and accumulation by alveolar macrophages from cigarette smokers and nonsmokers. J Lab Clin Med 1984; 104:127–134.
82. Pracht ER, Kaseki H, Mohammed JR, et al. Deficiency of vitamin E in the alveolar fluid of cigarette smokers: influence on alveolar macrophage cytotoxicity. J Clin Invest 1986; 77:789–796.

Chapter 5

LUNG REPAIR IN COPD

Charles Kuhn III John A. Pierce

Soon after any injury, tissues respond by inflammation and repair, processes that are distinguished from each other for didactic purposes but that commonly take place concurrently. During repair, damaged cells are replaced by others of the same class, while structural defects are filled by the deposition of connective tissue. Replacement of damaged cells may aid adaptation to the injurious agent by selecting a population more resistant to the agent or better able to cope with it, but the new cells are not always optimally differentiated to fulfill the functions of those they replace.

Patients with chronic obstructive lung disease have heterogeneous and often subtle histopathologic changes in the central airways, bronchioles, and acini.[1] These changes reflect not only different susceptibilities of these tissues to damage by particular agents and different repertoires of inflammatory cells and mediators but also their unique responses to damage. Thus, chronic airflow obstruction in cigarette smokers and others chronically exposed to respiratory irritants may result from the repair of low grade or repetitive injury at various levels of the respiratory tract.

BRONCHI

Hyperplasia of bronchial mucous glands and mucus-producing cells in the surface epithelium are classic histologic features in cigarette smokers. The severity of mucous gland hyperplasia correlates with cough and volume of sputum production but not with intensity of airflow limitation.[1] Squamous metaplasia and varying degrees of atypism of the surface epithelium are also common.[2] These metaplastic changes are studied because they may be stages in lung carcinogenesis, but they are important for COPD because they disrupt orderly mucociliary clearance and predispose the patient to bronchial infection.

Studies in animals using both thymidine incorporation and mitotic inhibitors to study replication of airway epithelium indicate that both the secretory cells and the basal cells divide but ciliated cells do not, even following injury. Instead of dividing, ciliated cells are replaced by differentiation of other epithelial cells. Although traditionally the basal cells have been regarded as stem cells for the replacement of various columnar cell types, studies over the past ten years have challenged this view, suggesting that mucous and serous secretory cells beget other types of columnar cells, but basal cells produce only basal cells.[2A] In fact, both columnar cells and cloned basal cells have the capacity to give rise to all the major cell types of the bronchial epithelium,[3] so it seems probable that the stem cell for repair depends on the severity of the injury. When the injury is mild and sufficient columnar cells persist, division of the columnar secretory cells is the predominant mode of repair.[4] With more severe injury, such as often occurs in viral infections and in asthma, wholesale sloughing of the columnar cells occurs but many basal cells persist and serve as important stem cells for repair. With such severe injury that even basal cells are lost, the airway lining is repopulated by outgrowth of epithelium from the ducts of the mucous glands.[5]

Temporary squamous metaplasia occurs early during the repair of severe injury to airway epithelium when flattened cells that have migrated onto the damaged airway surface continue to divide, leading to an epithelium two or three cells thick.[6] Chronic squamous metaplasia occurs by differentiation of mucous cells.[7,8]

The signals that trigger the proliferation of airway epithelium are largely unknown. Several soluble factors might be involved. One candidate is a 27-amino acid peptide, called gastrin-releasing peptide (GRP), produced by bronchial neuroendocrine cells. Gastrin-releasing peptide is sometimes called mammalian bombesin because of its homology to the 14-amino acid amphibian peptide, bombesin, with which it shares nine of ten carboxy-terminal amino acids. Gastrin-releasing peptide is mitogenic for airway epithelial cells in culture.[9] Cigarette smoke produces proliferation of GRP-containing endocrine cells in animals.[10] In humans, levels of a GRP-like peptide are elevated in bronchial washings from smokers.[11]

Epidermal growth factor (EGF), the classic epithelial mitogen, has been found in developing airway epithelium at sites where cell proliferation is rapid. It is most abundant in the bronchial glands, whence it could play a role in gland development or be secreted onto the airway mucosa. During the repair of damaged airways in newborns, EGF has been identified immunohistochemically in flattened epithelium migrating over the denuded airway surface, strongly suggesting that it is an important signal for epithelial repair.[5]

Fibronectin plays an important role in tissue repair. It circulates in plasma as a 440-kilodalton dimer of two almost identical subunits but occurs in tissues in slightly higher molecular weight form as a result of alternative splicing of the primary gene transcript. Each subunit contains specific sites for the binding of heparin and other proteoglycans, for collagen, for fibrinogen, and for specific cell-surface receptors called integrins. Fibronectin is present in the lung extracellular matrix and can be synthesized by different lung cells, including fibroblasts, epithelial cells, endothelial cells, and macrophages. Fibronectin's production by tracheobronchial epithelium has been demonstrated. It is chemotactic for several cell types, including airway epithelium *in vitro,* which suggests that it might be a signal for the migration of bronchial epithelium during the repair of airway injury.[12]

Many irritants stimulate a relative increase in goblet cells in experimental animals, accompanied by a shift toward a more acidic, highly sulfated mucus.[13] Among these irritants are tobacco smoke, sulfur dioxide, nitrogen dioxide, and ozone. The factors that control epithelial differentiation are complex and include sex hormones[14]; retinoids; composition of the extracellular matrix; and probably soluble mediators, including beta-adrenergic agonists.[13] Because drugs that inhibit arachidonic acid cyclo-oxygenase also prevent goblet-cell hyperplasia, it is likely that arachidonic acid products are involved in the goblet-cell response to irritants. A single exposure to proteolytic enzymes of neutrophil or other origin elicits a long-lasting increase in goblet cells, suggesting that secretion of proteases by phagocytes during airway inflammation is another mechanism to produce goblet-cell hyperplasia.[15]

PERIPHERAL AIRWAYS

The peripheral airways are major contributors to the airflow obstruction of cigarette smokers and others chronically exposed to respiratory irritants. Anatomic abnormalities of both the epithelium and bronchiolar walls are associated with small-airway dysfunction.

Normal small airways are lined by an epithelium composed of two main cell types: ciliated cells and nonciliated secretory cells, i.e., Clara cells, that synthesize surfactant proteins, protease inhibitors, and other specific proteins, but not mucus.[16,17] Physiologists believe that small airways narrow markedly and even close at the end of expiration, particularly in the dependent portions of the lung. The caliber of the airways during the ventilatory cycle depends in part on the properties of the airway lining fluid, including its surface activity.[18] The repair of epithelial injury in peripheral airways replaces some Clara cells by mucus-secreting cells. Abnormal bronchiolar secretions and even plugging of the bronchiolar lumen by mucus result.

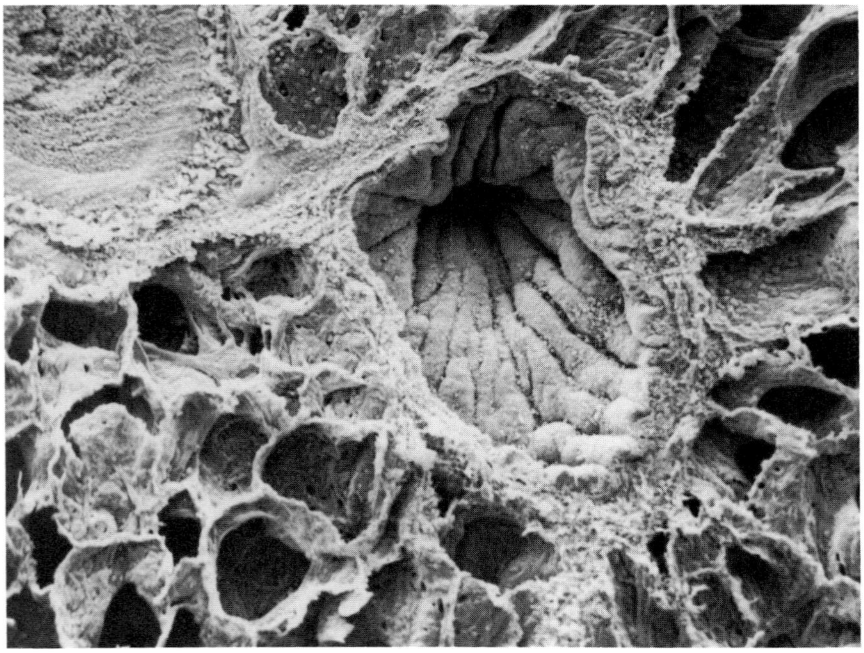

Figure 5–1. Distortion and narrowing of a small airway due to intramural fibrosis. Patient with chronic airflow obstruction and mild centriacinar emphysema. Scanning electron micrograph × 75.

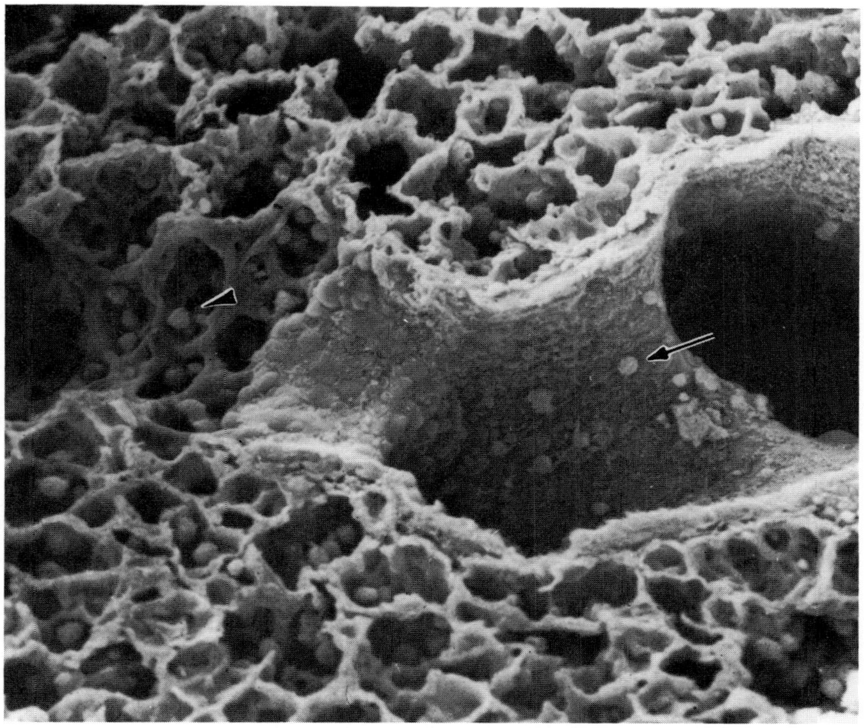

Figure 5–2. Bronchiolar-alveolar junction in the lung of a hamster exposed to a mixture of urban air pollutants, including ozone and NO_2, for two months. Note the presence of macrophages on the mucosal lining of the bronchiole (arrow) as well as nearby alveoli (arrow head). Scanning electron micrograph × 330.

Our most detailed knowledge of the repair of injury to peripheral airways comes from the study of rodent lungs, which differ in important respects from human airways. Injury by inhaled particles or by poorly soluble irritant gases such as ozone and NO_2 is concentrated near the bronchiolar-alveolar junction. Exposure of animals to near-ambient levels results in acute injury to the epithelium of the bronchioles and proximal alveolar ducts and inflammation in their walls. Ciliated cells and type I alveolar epithelial cells are particularly susceptible, and many undergo necrosis and slough. The epithelial damage is repaired by a burst of proliferation by both type II alveolar cells and Clara cells as well as by distal migration of the bronchiolar epithelium into neighboring alveoli.[19–21] Replacement of ciliated cells and type I cells occurs by differentiation of Clara cells and type II cells, respectively. The cell proliferation subsides after 3 to 4 days, even in the presence of continued exposure to the irritant.[20, 21] The resultant epithelium is much more resistant to injury, either because of replacement of susceptible cells by resistant ones or because of adaptive metabolic changes in the surviving cells. In rodents this process produces morphologically abnormal, poorly differentiated Clara cells,[22] but in humans some Clara cells must differentiate into goblet cells.

Study of the regulation of repair in small airways is in its infancy. Clara cells have been shown to have the capacity to give rise to a complete bronchiolar-type epithelium.[23] As in more central airways, EGF is present in repairing epithelial cells of injured bronchioles in newborns, suggesting that autocrine or paracrine signals are involved.[5]

Increased thickness of bronchiolar walls, tortuosity, and reduction in the lumen are well established morphologic changes that correlate with airflow obstruction (Fig. 5–1). Fibrosis in both bronchioles and adjacent centriacinar airways is found in humans with airflow obstruction and in animals exposed to irritant gases. The limited biochemical information available concerning the fibrotic response of the lung to oxidant gases suggests that the kinetics are quite different from those of epithelial repair. In contrast to the brief peak of proliferative activity in the epithelium in the first days of exposure, collagen synthesis remains continuously elevated during a prolonged exposure and indeed only slowly subsides after the cessation of exposure.[24, 25]

Macrophages have a central role in orchestrating the tissue response in wound healing. Alveolar macrophages accumulate in the respiratory bronchioles of smokers[26] and in the terminal bronchiolar-alveolar duct junction region of animals exposed to dust, tobacco smoke, or oxidant air pollutants (Fig. 5–2). Their role in the regulation of tissue repair in this region remains to be defined, but they secrete factors that could be involved in several aspects of the response to injury. Macrophages modulate fibrin deposition by their production of procoagulants and plasminogen activators.[27, 28] They synthesize fibronectin, a chemoattractant for fibroblasts.[29, 30] Macrophages secrete transforming growth factor alpha to regulate epithelial repair, as well as transforming growth factor beta, homologues of platelet-derived growth factor, fibroblast growth factor, interleukin-1, insulin-like growth factor 1, prostaglandins, and biochemically undefined suppressive factors with diverse effects on fibroblast function.[31–42] Macrophages are a source for the connective tissue–degrading proteases used in connective tissue remodeling.[43–45B]

EMPHYSEMA

Historical Background

Laennec proposed that emphysema resulted from overdistention of alveoli with septal rupture due to a one-way valve type of bronchial obstruction produced by catarrh.[45A] The explanation proved accurate for tension cysts but not for generalized emphysema. After World War II, Gough recognized that localized forms of emphysema resulted from inflammation, but there was still no sound theory about the cause of generalized emphysema.[45B] Attention had begun to focus on the connective tissue of the lung when two observations signalled the importance of proteolysis. Laurell and Eriksson discovered an inherited deficiency of alpha$_1$-antitrypsin in 1963 that was regularly associated with severe respiratory impairment due to premature pulmonary emphysema.[46, 47] Soon afterward, emphysema was produced in animals by a single intratracheal injection of the powerfully elastolytic enzyme, papain.[48]

The concept evolved that maintenance of normal lung architecture requires a balance between proteinase inhibitors in the lung and elastolytic enzymes that might be released interstitially.[49] By now, abundant evidence has suggested that degradation of connective tissue is an essential step in the development of emphysema. More specifically, it is necessary to interrupt the elastic fibers, because all animal models to date have required elastolysis, and because attempts to produce emphysema with intratracheal instillation of collagenase have not been successful.

Lung Extracellular Matrix

The lung connective tissue network is complex, containing several types of proteoglycans, five types of collagen, elastin, microfibrils, fibronectin, and several basal lamina glycoproteins. The major components of the fibrous skeleton of the lung are types I and III collagen, which convey great strength, and elastin, which permits long-range deformation. These fibrous proteins are organized in different patterns in different interstitial compartments. Alternate sheet-like layers of collagen and elastin reinforce the pleura, the interlobular, and interlobar septa. The airways, arteries, and veins contain single or multiple layers of elastin interspersed with smooth muscle, whereas collagen predominates in the adventitia. Stresses in the parenchyma are borne by a looping system of linear elastin-rich bundles of connective tissue fibers, which wind down alveolar ducts, form rings at the mouths of alveoli, and send supporting struts through bends in the primary septa of the alveolar ducts.[50] Between these bundles the alveolar interstitium consists mainly of closely woven collagen fibers, with only a few small elastic fibers. Although the inter- and intramolecular cross-linking amino acids have been characterized for both collagen and elastin, the precise location and type of physical attachments between collagen and elastin remain obscure. The parenchymal connective tissue is about two-thirds collagen and one-third elastin. As people grow older, the collagen content of the lung tends to remain constant, but the amount of elastin increases.[51, 52] The increase in elastin does not occur in the parenchyma but is localized to the sheet-like configurations found in the pleura, the vessels, and the bronchi. Under normal circumstances, the turnover of the proteins of the parenchymal collagenous and elastic fiber networks is extremely slow and can be considered negligible.[53, 54]

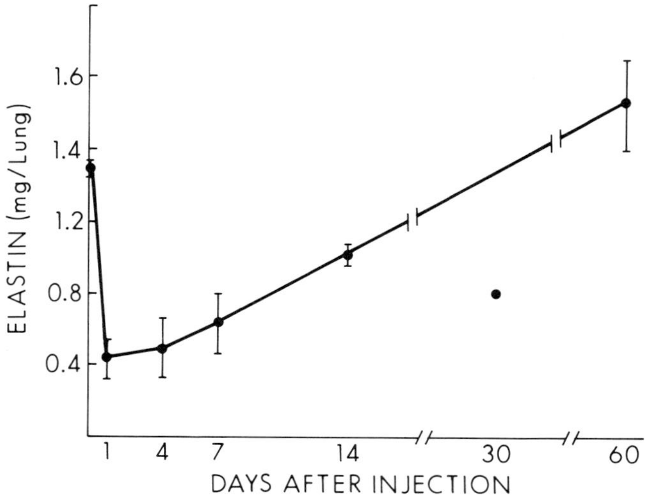

Figure 5–3. Changes in the elastin content of hamster lungs following intratracheal injection of 25 units of pancreatic elastase.[53]

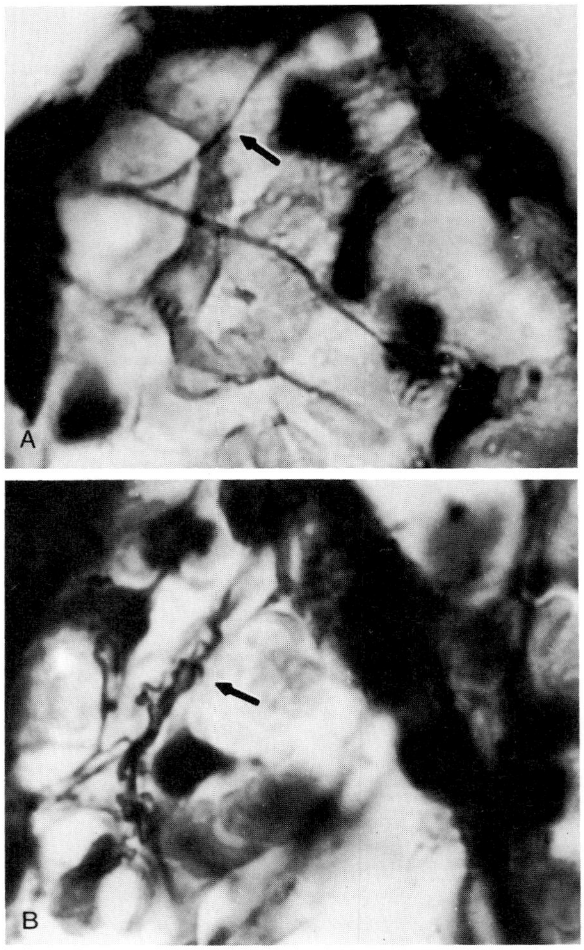

Figure 5–4. ***A,*** **Twenty-micron thick section of healthy hamster lung stained for elastin. An alveolar wall, viewed en face, is crossed by uniform smoothly curved elastic fibers (arrow).** ***B,*** **Lung of a hamster with emphysema induced by an injection of elastase 2 months earlier. Elastic fibers in the wall of an emphysematous space are tangled and irregular (acid orcein-Verhoef stain × 1200).**

Repair of Proteolytic Injury

When a large dose of an elastolytic enzyme is instilled into the lung of an animal to produce emphysema, the lung responds with a burst of connective tissue synthesis, which results in replacement of the destroyed elastin (Fig. 5–3) and small increases in the collagen and glycosaminoglycan content of the lung.[55, 56] The repaired elastin takes the form of a disorganized network of elastic fibers (Fig. 5–4), much as healing of a fracture results in disorganized bone trabeculae or the healing of a skin wound in disorderly dermal collagen. The total elastin content of emphysematous human lungs at autopsy is normal by biochemical measurements and by morphometry, but the fiber network is disorganized and the fibers are ultrastructurally abnormal.[57–60] These findings suggest that cycles of damage and repair to elastic tissue also occur in humans, spread over many years. Techniques are currently being developed to measure the turnover of human lung elastin, which will enable investigators to determine directly whether elastin degradation in humans produces disruption of the elastic fiber network or also stimulates the synthesis of elastin.[61]

Very little information is currently available about the regulation of connective tissue synthesis in response to proteolytic damage. In other types of lung injury, collagen deposition is regulated both by transcription and by post-translational events. Normally there is a measurable baseline level of procollagen synthesis in lung tissue, but it seems that much of the collagen is rapidly degraded intracellularly and never incorporated into extracellular matrix.[62–64] In response to fibrogenic damage, collagen gene transcription is accelerated[65] but, in addition, intracellular degradation decreases.[63] In the response to elastase, turnover of collagen increases,[55] although synthesis must increase to a greater degree than degradation, because the collagen content of the lung is slightly increased.

The synthesis of elastin is transcriptionally regulated during lung development and in a fibrogenic-type lung injury.[62, 63] Analysis of gene expression in experimental emphysema has not been reported. The soluble precursor of elastin, tropoelastin, is very susceptible to proteolytic degradation, but it is unlikely that intracellular degradation is important in regulation of elastin deposition.[67]

The deposition of collagen and elastin in extracellular matrix requires post-translational modifications of the initial translation products, including hydroxylation of proline and oxidation of lysine residues involved in formation of crosslinks. The enzyme activities responsible for these reactions rise during enzyme-induced emphysema.[55, 68]

Very little is known of the signals that trigger connective tissue repair during the development of emphysema. Soluble products released by proteolysis of collagen and elastin can be sensed by fibroblasts and other cells by receptor-mediated mechanisms,[68, 70] but this recognition has not been shown to alter biosynthesis. Connective tissue synthesis by smooth muscle cells and fibroblasts responds to mechanical stimuli and to a variety of soluble factors, including peptide growth factors, prostaglandins, steroid hormones, and cyclic nucleotides.[67, 71, 72]

Interventions in animals to prevent collagen and elastin synthesis suggest that connective tissue deposition mitigates the effects of elastolysis. Inhibition of the crosslinking of newly synthesized collagen and elastin exacerbates enzyme-induced emphysema, alters the response to $CdCl_2$ from fibrosis to emphysema, and interacts with NO_2 in the production of emphysema.[73, 74] Sequential administration of elastase and trypsin also impairs elastin resynthesis and results in more severe emphysema than elastase does alone.[75]

If, as these animal experiments suggest, the severity of emphysema is determined by the balance between elastin degradation and resynthesis, the resynthesis is a potential target for environmental agents. Cigarette smoke can inhibit lysyl oxidase, the enzyme that catalyzes the first step in crosslinking elastin or collagen,[68, 76] and could easily influence other steps in the process of connective tissue synthesis. Thus emphysema may be promoted by smoke-related inhibition of lung repair.

Our present understanding of the pathogenesis of emphysema is surely naive and oversimplified. Any hypothesis of the pathogenesis of emphysema must explain the epidemiologic observations. Emphysema occurs commonly in smokers but is exceedingly rare in nonsmokers. But many smokers do not develop symptoms of airflow limitation and some have no lesions of emphysema at autopsy even after a lifetime of smoking. Variation in plasma protease inhibitors, leukocyte elastase levels, and cigarette dosage explain only part of the variation in pulmonary function between subjects.[77, 78] Individual differences in the pattern and efficiency of the repair of injury could also be important. Identifying such differences is a challenge for future research.

REFERENCES

1. Thurlbeck WM. Chronic airflow obstruction. In: Thurlbeck WM, Ed. Pathology of the Lung. New York: Thieme Medical Publishers, 1988, 519–575.
2. Auerbach O, Stout AP, Hammond EC, et al. Changes in bronchial epithelium in relation to cigarette smoking and in relation to lung cancer. N Engl J Med 1961; 245:253–267.

2A. Evans MJ, Plopper CG. The role of basal cells in adhesion of columnar epithelium to airway basement membrane. Am Rev Respir Dis 1988; 138:481–483.

3. Inayama Y, Hook GE, Brody AR, et al. *In vitro* and *in vivo* growth and differentiation of clones of tracheal basal cells. Am J Pathol 1989; 134:539–550.
4. Evans MJ, Shami SG, Cabral-Anderson LG, Dekker NP. Role of nonciliated cells in renewal of the bronchial epithelium of rats exposed to NO_2. Am J Pathol 1986; 123:126–133.
5. Stahlman MT, Orth DN, Gray, ME. Immunocytochemical localization of epidermal growth factor in the developing human respiratory system and in acute and chronic lung disease in the neonate. Lab Invest 1989; 60:539–547.
6. Keenan KP, Combs JW, McDowell EM. Regeneration of hamster tracheal epithelium after mechanical injury. I. Focal lesions. Virchows Arch (Cell Pathol) 1982; 41:193–214.
7. Becci PJ, McDowell EM, Trump BF. The respiratory epithelium. IV. Histogenesis of epidermoid metaplasia and carcinoma-in-situ in the hamster. J Natl Cancer Inst 1978; 61:577–586.
8. Trump BF, McDowell EM, Glavin F, et al. The respiratory epithelium. III. Histogenesis of epidermoid metaplasia and carcinoma-*in-situ* in the human. J Natl Cancer Inst 1978; 61:563–575.
9. Willey JC, Lechner JR, Harris CC. Bombesin and the C-terminal tetradecapeptide of gastrin-releasing peptide are growth factors for normal human bronchial epithelial cells. Exp Cell Res 1984; 153:246–248.
10. Tabassian AR, Nylen ES, Linnoila RI, et al. Stimulation of hamster pulmonary neuroendocrine cells and associated peptides by repeated exposure to cigarette smoke. Am Rev Respir Dis 1989; 140:436–440.
11. Aguayo SM, Kane MA, King TE, et al. Increased levels of bombesin-like peptides in the lower respiratory tract of asymptomatic cigarette smokers. J Clin Invest 1989; 84:1105–1113.
12. Shoji S, Ertl RF, Linder J, et al. Bronchial epithelial cells produce chemotactic activity for bronchial epithelial cells: possible role for fibronectin in airway repair. Am Rev Respir Dis 1990; 141:218–225.
13. Reid L, Jones R. Bronchial mucosal cells. Fed Proc 1979; 38:191–196.
14. Hayashi M, Huber GL. Quantitative differences in goblet cells in the tracheal epithelium of male and female rats. Am Rev Respir Dis 1977; 115:595–599.
15. Snider GL, Lucey EC, Christensen TG, et al. Emphysema and bronchial secretory cell metaplasia induced in hamsters by human neutrophil products. Am Rev Respir Dis 1984; 129:155–160.
16. Walker SR, Williams MC, Benson B. Immunocytochemical localization of the major surfactant apoproteins in type II cells, Clara cells and alveolar macrophages of rat lung. J Histochem Cytochem 1986; 34:1137–1148.
17. Singh G, Katyal SL, Ward SM, et al. Secretory proteins of the lung in rodents. J Histochem Cytochem 1985; 33:564–568.
18. Macklem PT, Proctor DF, Hogg JC. The stability of peripheral airways. Respir Physiol 1970; 8:191–203.
19. Nettesheim P, Szakal AK. The morphogenesis of alveolar bronchiolization. Lab Invest 1972; 26:210–219.
20. Evans MJ, Cabral LJ, Stephens RJ, Freeman G. Renewal of

alveolar epithelium in the rat following exposure to NO_2. Am J Pathol 1973; 70:175–198.
21. Evans MJ, Johnson LV, Stephens RJ, Freeman G. Renewal of the terminal bronchiolar epithelium in the rat following exposure to NO_2 or O_3. Lab Invest 1976; 35:246–257.
22. Evans MJ, Cabral-Anderson LF, Freeman G. The role of the Clara cell in renewal of the bronchiolar epithelium. Lab Invest 1978; 38:648–653.
23. Hook GER, Brody AR, Cameron GS, et al. Repopulation of denuded tracheas by Clara cells isolated from the lungs of rabbits. Exp Lung Res 1987; 12:311–330.
24. Last JA, Greenberg DB, Castleman WL. Ozone-induced alterations in collagen metabolism of rat lungs. Toxicol Appl Pharmacol 1979; 51:247–258.
25. Last JA, Reiser KM, Tyler WS, Rucker RB. Long-term consequences of exposure to ozone. I. Lung collagen content. Toxicol Appl Pharmacol 1984; 72:111–118.
26. Niewoehner DE, Kleinerman J, Rice DB. Pathologic changes in the peripheral airways of young cigarette smokers. N Engl J Med 1974; 291:755–758.
27. Helen H. Macrophage procoagulant factors, mediators of inflammatory and neo-plastic tissue lesions. Med Biol 1986; 64:167–176.
28. Chapman HA, Bertozzi P, Reilly JJ. Role of enzymes mediating thrombosis and thrombolysis in lung disease. Chest 1988; 93:1256–1263.
29. Rennard SI, Hunninghake GW, Bitterman PB, Crystal RG. Production of fibronectin by the human alveolar macrophage: Mechanism for the recruitment of fibroblasts to sites of tissue injury in interstitial lung diseases. Proc Natl Acad Sci USA 1981; 78:7147–7151.
30. Villiger B, Kelley DG, Engleman W, et al. Human alveolar macrophage fibronectin: synthesis, secretion and ultrastructural localization during gelatin latex binding. J Cell Biol 1981; 90:711–720.
31. Madtes DK, Raines EW, Sokariassen KS, et al. Induction of transforming growth factor alpha in activated human alveolar macrophages. Cell 1988; 53:285–293.
32. Assoian RK, Fleurdelys BE, Stevenson HC, et al. Expression and secretion of type B transforming growth factor by activated human macrophages. Proc Natl Acad Sci USA 1987; 84:6020–6024.
33. Shimokado K, Raines EW, Madtes DK, et al. A significant part of macrophage-derived growth factor consists of at least two forms of PDGF. Cell 1985; 43:277–286.
34. Mornex J-F, Martinet Y, Yamauchi K, et al. Spontaneous expression of the c-sis gene and release of a platelet-derived growth factor-like molecule by human alveolar macrophages. J Clin Invest 1986; 78:61–66.
35. Baird A, Mormede P, Bohlen P. Immunoreactive fibroblast growth factor in cells of peritoneal exudate suggests its identity with macrophage-derived growth factor. Biochem Biophys Res Commun 1985; 126:358–364.
36. Schmidt JA, Oliver CN, Lepe-Zuniga JL, et al. Silica-stimulated monocytes release fibroblast proliferation factors identical to interleukin 1. J Clin Invest 1984; 73:1462–1472.
37. Postlewaite AE, Raghow R, Stricklin GP, et al. Modulation of fibroblast functions by interleukin 1: Increased steady state accumulation of type I procollagen messenger RNAs and stimulation of other functions but not chemotaxis by human recombinant interleukin$_1$-alpha and -beta. J Cell Biol 1988; 106:311–318.
38. Rom WN, Basset P, Fells GA, et al. Alveolar macrophages release an insulin like growth factor I-type molecule. J Clin Invest 1988; 82:1685–1693.
39. Jimenez SA, McArthur AW, Rosenbloom J. Inhibition of collagen synthesis by mononuclear cell supernatants. J Exp Med 1979; 150:1421–1431.
40. Korn JH, Halashka PV, LeRoy EC. Mononuclear cell modulation of connective tissue function. Suppression of fibroblast growth by stimulation of endogenous prostaglandin production. J Clin Invest 1980; 65:543–554.
41. Clark JG, Kostal KM, Marino BA. Bleomycin-induced pulmonary fibrosis in hamsters. An alveolar macrophage product increases fibroblast prostaglandin E_2 and cyclic adenosine monophosphate and suppresses fibroblast proliferation and collagen production. J Clin Invest 1983; 72:2082–2091.
42. Clark JG, Greenberg J. Modulation of the effects of alveolar macrophages on lung fibroblast collagen production rate. Am Rev Respir Dis 1987; 135:52–56.
43. Chapman HA, Stone OL. Comparison of live neutrophil and alveolar macrophage elastolytic activity *in vitro*. Relative resistance of macrophage elastolytic activity to serum and alveolar proteinase inhibitors. J Clin Invest 1984; 74:1693–1700.
44. Welgus HG, Campbell EJ, Bar-Shavit Z, et al. Human alveolar macrophages produce a fibroblast-like collagenase and collagenase inhibitor. J Clin Invest 1985; 76:219–224.
45. Senior RM, Connolly NL, Cury JD, et al. Elastin degradation by human alveolar macrophages. A prominent role of metalloproteinase activity. Am Rev Respir Dis 1989; 139:1251–1256.
45A. Laennec RTH. A Treatise on Diseases of the Chest and on Mediate Auscultation, 3rd ed., translated by Farber J. New York: S and W Wood, 1938.
45B. Leopold JG, Gough J. The centrilobular form of hypertrophic emphysema and its relation to chronic bronchitis. Thorax 1957; 12:219–235.
46. Laurell CB, Eriksson S. The electrophoretic alpha$_1$-globulin pattern of serum in alpha$_1$-antitrypsin deficiency. Scand J Clin Invest 1963; 15:132–140.
47. Eriksson S. Studies of alpha$_1$-antitrypsin deficiency. Acta Med Scand 1965; 177:(Suppl) 432:1–85.
48. Gross P, Pfitzer EA, Toker E, et al. Experimental emphysema. Its production with papain in normal and silicotic rats. Arch Environ Health 1965; 11:50–58.
49. Janoff A. Elastases and emphysema. Current assessment of the protease-anti-protease hypothesis. Am Rev Respir Dis 1985; 132:417–433.
50. Kuhn C, Oldmixon EH. The interstitium of the lung. In: Schraufnagel D, ed. The Electron Microscopy of the Lung. New York: Marcel Dekker, 1990; 177–214.
51. Pierce JA, Hocott JB. Studies on the collagen and elastin content of the human lung. J Clin Invest 1960; 39:8–14.
52. Pierce JA, Ebert RV. Fibrous network of the lung and its change with age. Thorax 1965; 20:429–476.
53. Dubick MA, Rucker RB, Cross CE, Last JA. Elastin metabolism in rodent lung. Biochem Biophys Acta 1981; 672:303–306.
54. Last JA, Reiser KM. Biosynthesis of collagen crosslinks III. *In vivo* labeling and stability of lung collagen in rats with bleomycin-induced pulmonary fibrosis. Am J Respir Cell Molec Biol 1989; 1:111–118.
55. Kuhn C, Yu S-Y, Chraplyvy M, Linder HE, Senior RM. The induction of emphysema with elastase. II. Changes in connective tissue. Lab Invest 1976; 34:372–380.
56. Karlinsky J, Fredette J, Davidovits G, et al. The balance of lung connective tissue elements in elastase-induced emphysema. J Lab Clin Med 1983; 102:151–162.
57. Pierce JA, Hocott JB, Ebert RV. The collagen and elastin content of the lung in emphysema. Ann Intern Med 1961; 55:210–221.
58. Niewoehner DE, Kleinerman J. Morphometric study of elastic fibers in normal and emphysematous human lungs. Am Rev Respir Dis 1977; 115:15–21.
59. Wright RR. Elastic tissue of normal and emphysematous lungs. A tridimensional histologic study. Am J Pathol 1961; 39:355–367.
60. Fukuda Y, Masuda Y, Ishizaki M, et al. Morphogenesis of abnormal elastic fibers in lungs of patients with panacinar and centriacinar emphysema. Human Pathol 1989; 20:652–659.
61. Shapiro SD, Pierce JA, Endicott SK, Campbell EJ. Marked longevity of human lung elastin fibers deduced from aspartic acid racemization. Am Rev Respir Dis 1989; 139:A229.
62. Bienkowski RS, Cowan MJ, McDonald JA, Crystal RG. Degradation of newly synthesized collagen. J Biol Chem 1978; 253:4356–4363.
63. Laurent GJ, McAnulty RJ. Protein metabolism during bleomycin induced pulmonary fibrosis in rabbits: *in vivo* evidence for collagen accumulation because of increased synthesis and decreased degradation of newly synthesized collagen. Am Rev Respir Dis 1983; 128:82–88.
64. Berg RA. Intracellular turnover of collagen. In: Mecham RP, ed. Regulation of Matrix Accumulation. New York: Academic Press, 1986; 29–52.
65. Raghow R, Lurie S, Seyer JM, Kang AH. Profiles of steady state levels of messenger RNAs coding for type I procollagen, elastin, and fibronectin in hamster lungs undergoing bleomycin-induced interstitial pulmonary fibrosis. J Clin Invest 1985; 76:1733–1739.
66. Davidson JM, Shibahara S, Boyd C, et al. Elastin mRNA levels during foetal development of sheep nuchal ligament and lung. Biochem J 1984; 220:653–663.

67. Prosser IW, Mecham RP. Regulation of extracellular matrix accumulation: A short review of elastin biosynthesis. In: Self-Assembling Architecture. New York: Alan R. Liss, Inc., 1988; 1–23.
68. Osman M, Cantor JO, Roffman S, et al. Cigarette smoke impairs elastin resynthesis in lungs of hamsters with elastase-induced emphysema. Am Rev Respir Dis 1985; 132:640–643.
69. Mecham RP, Hinek A, Entwistle R, et al. Elastin binds to a 67-kilodalton multifunctional peripheral membrane protein. Biochemistry 1989; 28:3716–3722.
70. Senior RM, Griffin GL, Mecham RP, et al. Val-Gly-Val-Pro-Gly, a repeating peptide in elastin is chemotactic for fibroblasts and monocytes. J Cell Biol 1984; 99:870–874.
71. Leung DYM, Glagov S, Matthews MB. A new *in vitro* system for studying cell response to mechanical stimulation. Exp Cell Res 1977; 109:285.
72. Davidson JM, Giro GM. Control of elastin synthesis: molecular and cellular aspects. In: Mecham RP, ed. Regulation of Matrix Accumulation. New York: Academic Press, 1986; 177–216.
73. Kuhn C, Starcher BC. The effect of lathyrogens on the evolution of elastase-induced emphysema. Am Rev Respir Dis 1980; 122:453–460.
74. Niewoehner DE, Hoidal JR. Lung fibrosis and emphysema: Divergent responses to a common injury. Science 1982; 217:359–360.
75. Osman M, Keller S, Hosannah Y, et al. Impairment of elastin resynthesis in the lungs of hamsters with experimental emphysema induced by sequential administration of elastase and trypsin. J Lab Clin Med 1985; 105:524–528.
76. Laurent P, Janoff A, Kagan HM. Cigarette smoke blocks cross-linking of elastin *in vitro*. Am Rev Respir Dis 1983; 127:189–192.
77. Galdston M, Melnick EL, Goldring RM, et al. Interaction of neutrophil elastase serum trypsin inhibitory activity and smoking history as risk factors for chronic obstructive pulmonary disease in patients with MM MZ and ZZ phenotypes for alpha$_1$-antitrypsin. Am Rev Respir Dis 1977; 116:837.
78. Silverman EK, Pierce JA, Province MA, et al. Variability of pulmonary function in alpha$_1$-antitrypsin deficiency: clinical correlates. Ann Intern Med 1989; 111:982–991.

Chapter 6

NEUROPEPTIDES, PLATELET-ACTIVATING FACTOR, AND EICOSANOID ACTIONS IN COPD

Norma P. Gerard Stephanie A. Shore Jeffrey M. Drazen

One of the clinical problems in patients with chronic obstructive pulmonary disease (COPD), regardless of whether it is of the emphysematous or bronchitic variety, is intermittent episodes of acute reversible airway obstruction, which are engrafted on fixed components of airway narrowing. The pathobiology of these episodes is unknown, but the airway inflammation, which is a hallmark of at least the bronchitic form of COPD, represents a possible mechanism that could lead to airway obstruction through either the formation of bronchoactive mediators or alterations in the metabolism of bronchoactive peptides. In this chapter, we broadly review how three distinct, but interrelated, effector systems have the capacity to alter the luminal area available for airflow in inflammatory conditions. These effector systems are the neuropeptides, including substance P and neurokinin A, platelet-activating factor (PAF), and the sulfidopeptide leukotrienes. Because of the paucity of data available from human subjects, we include in our review appropriate data from lower animals as well as data from studies conducted in human subjects.

Supported in part by NIH Grants HL 36162, HL 39827, and HL 41587. Dr. N.P. Gerard is the recipient of NIH Research Career Development Award, HL 01777.

A NEUROGENIC MECHANISM FOR COPD

Intensive research over the past several years has identified a new mechanism, based on established mediators and cell types, that is hypothesized to play a role in the general category of inflammatory pulmonary diseases, including those that may lead to COPD. Central to this hypothesis is the release from sensory nerve endings in the lungs and airways of a group of neuropeptides, their actions in concert with eicosanoids and PAF. The possible mechanisms by which these peptides may contribute to tissue destruction, bronchoconstriction, hypertrophy, and increased mucus secretion all may be of importance in the pathobiology of COPD. A hypothetic scenario is depicted schematically in Figure 6–1.

Irritant stimulation, resulting from either an exogenous or an endogenous source, stimulates bronchopulmonary sensory C fibers to release neuropeptides. These neuropeptides exert a broad spectrum of biologic activities, which can result in airway narrowing, edema formation, increased mucus production, and stimulation of inflammatory and immune cells. These actions, in turn, result in release of secondary mediators, including PAF and eicosanoids, and a variety of other nonlipid substances. These secondary mediators amplify the lung injury

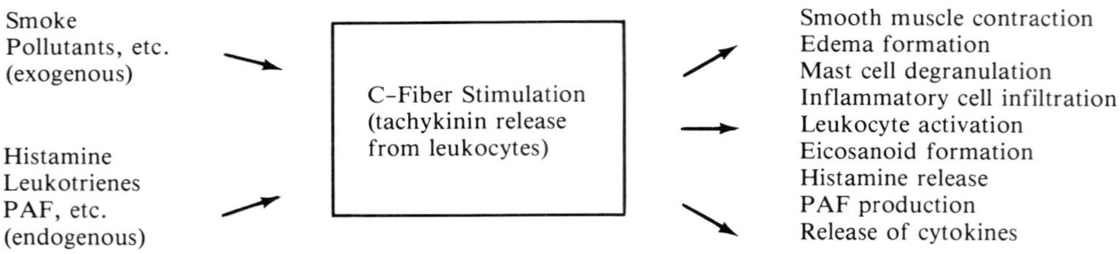

Figure 6–1. Schematic representation of a possible mechanism for tackykinin-mediated lung injury.

produced by stimulating additional mediator release and by triggering other neuropeptide-containing C fibers in the vicinity of the inflammatory process, creating a progressively spreading injury. Under normal conditions, in the absence of lung disease, this sequence of events is held in check by inactivation of neuropeptides by epithelial and endothelial enzymes, as detailed later. However, in the face of ongoing disease, such as viral infection[1] or environmental injury,[2] neuropeptide control may be severely diminished. This scenario may progress relatively unchecked, resulting in much more extensive injury.

The Neuropeptides of C Fibers

The neuropeptide contents of C fibers include the tachykinins, peptides with the common carboxy-terminal amino acid sequence -Phe-X-Gly-Leu-Met-NH_2,[3, 4] such as substance P,[5] neurokinin A (substance K),[6, 7] neurokinin B,[8, 9] and neuropeptide K.[10] Immunohistochemical studies indicate that another, structurally unrelated peptide, calcitonin gene–related peptide (CGRP),[11] is also present in the same C fibers.[12–15] Substance P also has been localized in murine eosinophils from granulomas caused by *Schistosoma mansoni*,[16] and CGRP is found in neuroendocrine cells in the lung.[17] The amino acid sequences of each of these peptides are shown in Figure 6–2.

The sensory neurons that contain these peptides have been identified, mostly by using immunohistochemical techniques, staining for substance P or CGRP. They are found in the lung within and just beneath the airway epithelium, around blood vessels and ganglia, and surrounding smooth muscle bundles within airways.[18–20] They extend far out into the peripheral regions of the lung in humans and in many animal species studied.[20] These neurons are sensitive to capsaicin,[21] the pungent ingredient of hot peppers, and release their peptide contents in a calcium-dependent manner following exposure to this agent.[22] They also respond to cigarette smoke[23, 24] and other environmental pollutants[25] in addition to endogenous mediators, such as PAF,[26] sulfidopeptide leukotrienes,[27] bradykinin, and histamine.[28]

Actions of the Neuropeptides in Experimental Animals and Humans

In experimental animals, substance P and related tachykinins have been shown to induce both the cough[29] and mucus hypersecretion[30–33] that are hallmarks of COPD. These peptides also cause airway smooth muscle constriction and acute bronchoconstriction following intravenous or aerosol administration.[34–37] Administration of tachykinins results in increased bronchopulmonary vascular permeability,[38–41] which may lead to airway edema. The tachykinins also have been shown to alter the secretion of ions across the airway epithelium[42, 43] and to alter the integrity of the epithelial barrier.[44] All of these actions constitute mechanisms whereby airway narrowing can occur. In humans, inhalation of capsaicin causes cough and a dose-dependent decrease in specific airway conductance,[45] but neither inhaled nor intravenous substance P has any profound effect on airway narrowing,[46] perhaps as a result of degradation of peptide before it can act on airway smooth muscle (see subsequent discussion).

Calcitonin gene–related peptide released coincidentally with the tachykinin contents of C fibers is also a vasodilator, both in the lung and in the skin,[40, 47] and several reports indicate potentially important interactions between these peptides. Calcitonin gene–related peptide potentiates the increases in vascular permeability induced by substance P,[48, 49] suggesting a possible synergy between these neuropeptides. In contrast, the bronchoconstriction induced by continuous vascular infusion of substance P is reduced if CGRP is coinfused with this peptide.[50]

Substance P: Arg-Pro-Lys-Pro-Gln-Gln-Phe-Phe-Gly-Leu-Met-NH_2

Neurokinin A: His-Lys-Thr-Asp-Ser-Phe-Val-Gly-Leu-Met-NH_2

Neurokinin B: Asp-Met-His-Asp-Phe-Phe-Val-Gly-Leu-Met-NH_2

Neuropeptide K (porcine):

Asp-Ala-Asp-Ser-Ser-Ile-Glu-Lys-Gln-Val-Ala-Leu-Leu-Lys-Ala-Leu-Tyr-Gly-His-

Gly-Gln-Ile-Ser-His-Lys-Arg-His-Lys-Thr-Asp-Ser-Phe-Val-Gly-Leu-Met-NH_2

CGRP (human):

Ala-Cys-Asp-Thr-Ala-Thr-Cys-Val-Thr-His-Arg-Leu-Ala-Gly-Leu-Ser-Arg-Ser-Gly-

Gly-Val-Val-Lys-Asn-Asn-Phe-Val-Pro-Thr-Asn-Val-Gly-Ser-Lys-Ala-Phe-NH_2

Figure 6–2. Amino acid sequences for the tachykinins, substance P, and neurokinins A and B, neuropeptide K, and calcitonin gene–related peptide (CGRP).

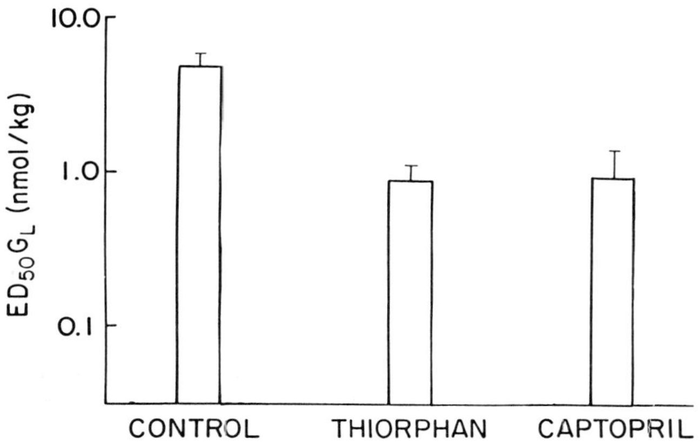

Figure 6–3. Airway responses to rapid intravenous infusions of substance P in anesthetized, mechanically ventilated guinea pigs treated with saline dimethylsulfoxide (control, n = 22), thiorphan (0.5 mg/animal, n = 13), or captopril (1.7 mg/animal, n = 5). Median effective dose ($ED_{50}G_L$) is the dose of substance P required to decrease pulmonary conductance to 50% of baseline. Bars indicate mean ± SE. Both thiorphan and captopril caused a significant decrease in $ED_{50}G_L$ ($P<0.001$).

The bronchoconstrictor action of intravenously administered substance P is markedly potentiated by inhibitors of neutral endopeptidase (phosphoramidon or thiorphan) and angiotensin-converting enzyme (captopril) (Fig. 6–3).[51] Neurokinin A, or substance K, is approximately ten times more potent than substance P, with or without neutral endopeptidase inhibitors, but bronchoconstrictor responses to this tachykinin are not altered by captopril.[52] The potency of substance P following aerosol administration is much more pronounced in the presence of thiorphan than in the presence of captopril in the guinea pig, suggesting a more important role for neutral endopeptidase than angiotensin-converting enzyme in the bronchoconstrictor response to this peptide when release occurs on the airway side of the lungs.[53] Mucus production induced by substance P in the ferret is also potentiated by inhibitors of neutral endopeptidase but not by angiotensin-converting enzyme inhibitors.[32]

The proposed mechanisms of these neuropeptide actions in the lung are somewhat varied and appear to depend on the animal species studied as well as the route of administration. In the rabbit, cat, and ferret, substance P appears to act at least in part by a presynaptic mechanism to promote local release of acetylcholine.[36, 54–56] The guinea pig and human do not appear to share this mechanism;[57–60] this likely reflects differences in the neuroanatomy of the lungs between these species or in the distribution of neurokinin receptors. In lung tissues isolated from the guinea pig, contractile responses induced by substance P and neurokinin A are mediated, at least in part, by prostaglandin production,[61] although a similar role of arachidonic acid metabolites is not observed in the intact animal.[59] Carstairs and Barnes[62] have provided evidence for direct action of substance P on smooth muscle in guinea pig lung, and it is possible that action on this cell type predominates in humans as well in the bronchoconstriction caused by this peptide.

The bronchoconstrictor activity of substance P in the guinea pig appears to require an intact carboxy-terminal sequence, because studies using truncated molecules show substance P 1-9 to be totally devoid of this action.[63] In contrast, substance P 5-11 is actually more potent than the intact peptide.[63] It has been suggested that CGRP coreleased with substance P may potentiate the action of the tachykinin,[48, 64] either by blocking degradation of the intact peptide or by preserving one or more of the more active amino terminally degraded fragments.

Neuropeptide Activities on Isolated Cells

As indicated previously, the evidence for action of neuropeptides with smooth muscle cells in the lung is very strong.[62] This cell type may be responsible for neurokinin-induced prostaglandin production, which mediates contractile responses of some tissues.[61] In addition, a receptor protein for neurokinin A was cloned from a bovine stomach,[65] confirming its expression on smooth muscle. Unfortunately, the expression of neurokinin receptors is rapidly lost when airway smooth muscle cells are placed in culture (NP Gerard, unpublished data), likely due to de-differentiation of this cell type.

A variety of other cell types present in the lung have been reported to respond to substance P, including mast cells,[66, 67] monocytes,[68, 69] macrophages,[70] and lymphocytes.[71] Although evidence for their role in producing bronchoconstriction is not overwhelming, the actions of neurokinins on these cell types may contribute to airway narrowing and other symptoms of COPD by release of PAF, eicosanoids, cytokines, and other secondary mediators. Interestingly, the influx of neutrophils into the airways associated with COPD may also play an important role in modulating responses to tachykinins or tachykinin-induced mediator release, as these cells express a membrane-bound, neutral endopeptidase.[72]

PLATELET-ACTIVATING FACTOR: A POTENTIAL ROLE IN COPD

Platelet-activating factor was originally identified as a unique, ether-linked phospholipid, 1-O-hexadecyl- (or octadecyl-) 2-acetyl-sn-glyceryl-3-phosphorylcholine (Fig. 6–4)[73, 74] that is released following IgE-dependent activation of basophils.[75] Platelet-activating factor is now known to consist of a number of related molecular species[76, 77] and is produced by and released from a wide variety of cell types.[75, 78–84] In addition to its actions on platelets, PAF has effects on many other cell types present in the lung, and the potential for involvement of this mediator in illnesses such as COPD and asthma is quite high[85–87].

Actions of Platelet-Activating Factor on Isolated Lung Tissues and Cells

Platelet-activating factor contracts isolated parenchymal tissues from guinea pig, rat, rabbit, and human lung in a highly specific and concentration-dependent manner.[88–91] Isolated tracheal tissues do not respond similarly, and this result, coupled with the extreme sensitivity of most species' platelets to the phospholipid, led investigators to believe that PAF-induced bronchoconstriction was an indirect result of action on platelets

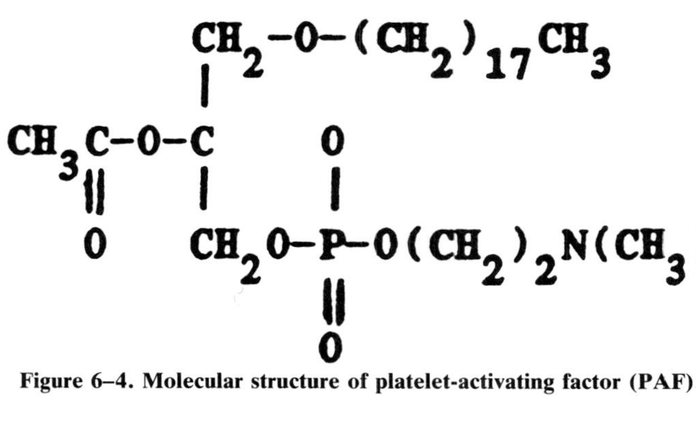

Figure 6–4. Molecular structure of platelet-activating factor (PAF).

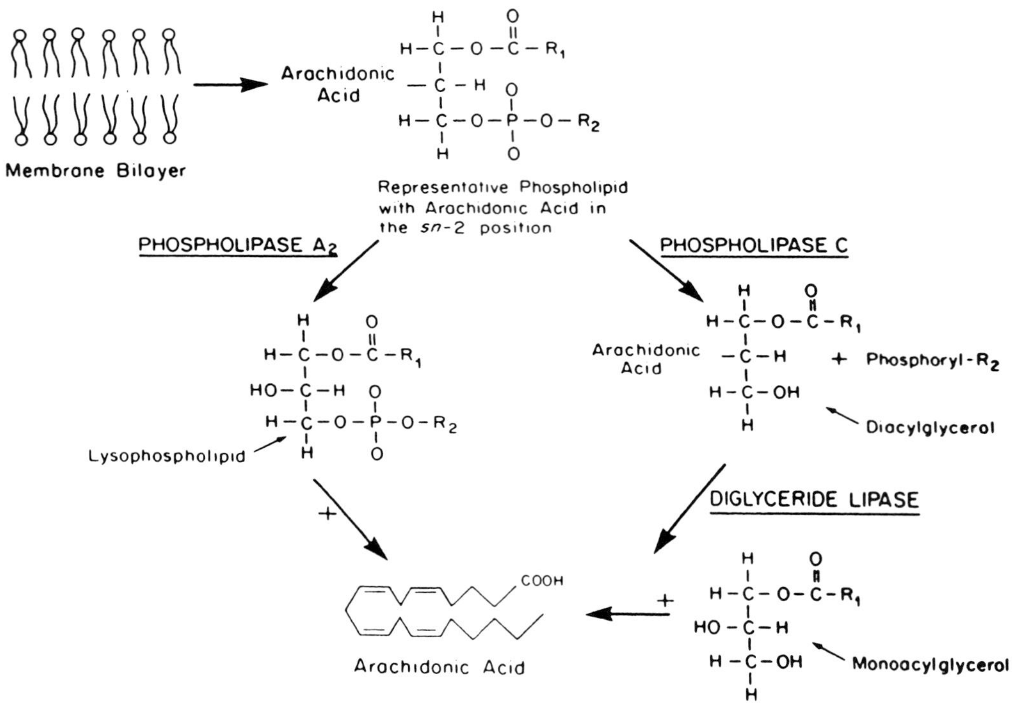

Figure 6–5. Biochemical pathways leading to the release of arachidonic acid from membrane phospholipids. Details of the pathway are discussed in the text.

remaining in the tissue.[92] Subsequent studies demonstrated that, although the actions of PAF on platelets can elicit contractions of airway smooth muscle,[93, 94] a platelet-independent mechanism is evident as well.[89, 95]

It is not certain which or how many cell types in the lung are targets for PAF. The phospholipid is extremely potent for stimulating release of eicosanoids from lung tissue, including thromboxane A_2 (TxA_2), prostaglandins, and variable amounts of the peptidoleukotrienes, LTC_4 and LTD_4.[61, 89, 96–98] Responses of macrophages and endothelial cells are potentially responsible for this release. In addition, the phospholipid acts on parasympathetic neurons in the lung in a local reflex mechanism to stimulate release of acetylcholine[96, 99, 100] and on irritant C fibers to release substance P and most likely other neuropeptides.[26]

Effects of Platelet-Activating Factor *in Vivo*

In vivo, the effects of PAF generated in or administered to the intravascular space are dominated by the results of activation of platelets and neutrophils,[101] and include bronchospasm, hypotension, thrombocytopenia, and neutropenia.[101–103] However, when PAF is not generated in the blood, the physiologic changes observed are reflected by the responses of the cell types affected.[102] Administration by aerosol to dogs, guinea pigs, and humans results in acute bronchospasm, which appears to be mediated by actions on other cell types.

In the dog, *in vivo* injection into the tracheal artery after platelets were maximally removed revealed acetylcholine-mediated contraction of the trachealis muscle.[100] The response was blocked by atropine but not hexamethonium, indicating parasympathetic stimulation via a local reflex. This response was also blocked by an H-1 antihistamine or by methysergide, an antagonist of serotonin. Thus, it is not clear whether the antihistamine and methysergide-blocked reflexive release of acetylcholine was because of weak anesthetic effects, or whether release of histamine or serotonin, or both, caused subsequent parasympathetic responses. Because no precedent exists for the last mentioned responses, we interpreted the finding as indicating that PAF stimulates parasympathetic neurons in the dog as well as in the guinea pig, and we hypothesize that it may do so in humans as well.

In addition to causing acute bronchospasm *in vivo,* PAF also causes nonspecific airway hyper-responsiveness, which can last several days.[104] Indeed, it is this action of the phospholipid that leads many investigators to propose a major role for PAF in asthma.[17, 104, 105]

THE PEPTIDOLEUKOTRIENES: A ROLE IN COPD

The leukotrienes are derived from eicosatetraenoic acid, or arachidonic acid, a 20-carbon polyunsaturated fatty acid that is a common constituent of the phospholipids composing mammalian cell membranes. Under resting conditions, most of the arachidonic acid is found esterified at the sn-2 position of these phospholipids[106] (Fig. 6–5) and can be released by the action of phospholipase A_2[107] or phospholipase C and diglyceride lipase.[108] Phospholipase A_2 is activated by a variety of stimuli, which also result in cellular activation.[107] This enzyme is a component of neutrophils and other inflammatory cells. Phospholipase C is a relatively ubiquitous enzyme and activates in the process of activation of membrane receptors.[108] This enzyme removes the polar head group of phospholipids to form diacylglycerols, and the subsequent action of diglyceride lipase results in the formation of a monoacylglycerol and free arachidonic acid.

The arachidonic acid released by these processes can then enter a number of metabolic pathways. The action of cyclo-oxygenase and subsequent cyclo-oxygenase pathway enzymes first results in the formation of the unstable metabolites, prostaglandins (PG) G_2 and H_2. These compounds are then converted to TxA_2 or more stable prostaglandins, PGD_2, PGE_2, $PGF_{2\alpha}$, or PGI_2.[109] Alternatively, metabolism by 5-lipoxygenase results initially in the formation of 5-hydroperoxyeicosatetraenoic acid (5-HPETE), which is relatively unstable in aqueous solutions. This substance is converted either to 5-hydroxyeicosatetraenoic acid (5-HETE), or to leukotriene A_4 (LTA_4). Leukotriene A_4 can then serve as a substrate for LTA_4 epoxide hydrolase and results in the formation of LTB_4. Alternatively, LTA_4 can undergo nonenzymatic degradation to 5,12-diHETEs or it can be metabolized by LTC_4 synthase and result in formation of leukotriene C_4 by the addition of glutathione at the C-6 position. Leukotriene D_4 and LTE_4 are subsequently formed by sequential removal of glutamic acid and glycine from the glutathione side chain.[110]

In order to produce LTC_4, a cell not only needs a source of free arachidonic acid but must also express the enzymes 5-lipoxygenase and LTC_4 synthase. 5-Lipoxygenase is widely distributed in tissues;[111] however, LTC_4 synthase is found in relatively few tissues and cell types. Mast cells,[112] alveolar macrophages,[113] and eosinophils[114, 115] are among the cell types that contain both enzymes and can produce LTC_4 when appropriately activated. Polymorphonuclear leukocytes (PMNs) contain 5-lipoxygenase but lack LTC_4 synthase. Thus, they can synthesize LTB_4 but not the peptidoleukotrienes. They are, however, capable of providing LTA_4 for other cells, such as vascular endothelial cells, which do contain LTC_4 synthase and can form LTC_4 from substrate donated by PMNs.[116] Other examples of cell-to-cell interactions of this type may exist as well. Airway epithelial cells also produce LTC_4 and may be an important focus of inflammatory reactions in COPD.[117]

Clearly, many of the cell types that are known to infiltrate the lung in chronic bronchitis possess the capability, either alone or in concert with other cell types, to produce bronchoactive leukotrienes. Furthermore, this disease process may alter the metabolism of arachidonic acid by inflammatory cells through both the lipoxygenase and the cyclo-oxygenase pathway; reports indicate important differences in the production of LTB_4,[118] 5-HETE,[118] and prostaglandins[119] in alveolar macrophages from smokers and nonsmokers. Finally, leukotrienes have been detected in the sputum of patients with COPD.[120]

In Vitro Studies With Isolated Pulmonary Tissues

The contractile responses of normal human lung tissues, obtained from resection for bronchial carcinoma, to leukotrienes have been studied by a number of investigative teams. The ED_{50} for LTC_4-mediated contractions of 2- to 4-mm airways occurs at tissue bath concentrations on the order of 10 nM, approximately 3000 times less than the concentration required for a similar response to histamine in this tissue. Similar responses are observed for LTD_4 and LTE_4.[121–123] Leukotriene D_4 can also contract isolated human lung parenchymal strips at similar concentrations.[124]

The leukotrienes appear to exert their effects through specific receptor molecules; however, the number and type of these molecules remain controversial. Data obtained using the leukotriene receptor antagonist FPL55712 to block contractile responses of isolated guinea pig lung tissues stimulated by LTC_4 or LTD_4 suggest that leukotrienes have distinct receptors in this tissue.[125, 126] The metabolic relationship of these molecules makes an analysis of receptor types complex. However, when appropriate precautions are taken to prevent conversion of LTC_4 to LTD_4, the distinction between contractile responses caused by the two leukotrienes is more clearly evident. In the presence of serine borate, an inhibitor of LTC_4 degradation, contractions induced by this leukotriene are not effectively blocked by beta-adrenergic agonists, whereas contractions of similar magnitude induced by LTD_4 are inhibited.[127, 128] These data suggest the possible existence of distinct leukotriene receptor types in guinea pig lungs.

Systematic studies of the responses of human airway tissues to the leukotrienes have yielded somewhat different results.[129, 130] In these tissues, the responses elicited by LTC_4 and LTD_4 were both inhibited to a similar degree by FPL55712, and the analogous substances LY171883[131] and SKF104353,[130] under conditions in which metabolic conversion of LTC_4 to LTD_4 was blocked by serine borate. These findings suggest that normal human airways contain only a single leukotriene receptor type that can be activated by both LTC_4 and LTD_4, which is similar to the guinea pig LTD_4 receptor in its antagonism by LTD_4 receptor antagonists. Although these experiments were performed using relatively normal lung tissues, the extent of possible alterations due to the presence of tumor and the surgical procedure cannot be evaluated. Further, it is not known whether tissues isolated from individuals with chronic bronchitis, asthma, or emphysema would behave similarly.

In addition to their effects on airway contraction, leukotrienes have been shown to cause increases in the secretion of both macromolecules and ions from isolated airways. Explants of human airways incubated with ^{3}H-glucosamine release high molecular weight ^{3}H-labeled glycoproteins into the culture fluid following stimulation with LTC_4 or LTD_4.[132, 133] Repeated exposure results in a decrement in the amount of radiolabeled product released, suggesting that the leukotrienes stimulate secretion of mucous glycoprotein rather than an increase in synthesis. The peptidoleukotrienes also induce an increase in the short-circuit current and chloride flux and enhance the fluid formation in the isolated canine tracheal epithelium.[134, 135] The combined effect of these responses *in vivo* could be manifested as a thickening of the mucus gel layer and a decrease in tracheal mucus velocity due to physical inability of the epithelial cilia to penetrate the thickened liquid layer. If these changes occurred as a result of leukotriene production, it would likely result in a decrease in the clearance.

In Vivo Studies in Experimental Animals and Humans

It is well established that the peptidoleukotrienes are potent bronchoconstrictor agonists in a number of species *in vivo*.[111] The guinea pig is one of the most sensitive and frequently used for these studies. In this species, inhalation of aerosolized LTC_4 or LTD_4 in concentrations of 1 to 10 μg/ml results in substantial bronchospasm. These substances also cause increases in pulmonary arterial pressure in sheep, rabbits, and guinea pigs.[111] These findings are likely because of constriction of postcapillary venules. The pressure increase is associated with a transient increase in lung weight in isolated perfused lungs, without an increase in filtration fraction.

When aerosols of leukotrienes are inhaled by normal humans, airway obstruction is evident as a decrease in flow rates during a forced exhalation.[136–146] Both LTC_4 and LTD_4 are potent bronchoconstrictor agonists, each being approximately 3000-fold more potent than histamine. The mechanism of their response appears to reflect a predominant action directly on airway muscle as opposed to an indirect effect resulting from generation of prostaglandins.[136, 147] The time course of the response in normal subjects to inhaled LTC_4 is relatively slow compared with that for LTD_4.[140] This finding is consistent with a requirement for conversion of LTC_4 to LTD_4 prior to induction of bronchospasm in normal subjects.

Asthmatics require lower concentrations of LTD_4 than do healthy individuals to achieve an equivalent degree of bronchoconstriction consistent with the nonspecific airway hyperresponsiveness associated with this disease.[141, 142, 144–146] However, the degree of hyperresponsiveness to LTD_4 is less than that found for histamine or methacholine. It has been proposed that this finding is due to selective tachyphylaxis to the leukotrienes in asthmatics, an alteration in the receptor distribution, or a minimal induction of hyperresponsiveness to leukotrienes relative to other agonists in this disease. Most of these studies in asthmatics have been conducted using LTD_4 and, although comparisons are of interest, there is relatively little information on the effects of inhaled LTC_4 in these subjects.[144, 148]

In addition to the differences in responsiveness of asthmatics and healthy individuals to the peptidoleukotrienes, there also may be a difference in the mechanisms of action of these substances in these groups. Adelroth and colleagues[144] and Roberts and coworkers[148] have shown a differential effect of the calcium channel blocker verapamil on the responses to LTD_4 in normal, compared with asthmatic, subjects. These investigators suggested that the mechanism coupling leukotriene-mediated receptor stimulation to airway narrowing is abnormal in asthmatics. At this time, there are no data on the effects and potency of inhaled leukotrienes on airway function in patients with COPD. However, because there appear to be distinctions between normal and asthmatic subjects, it seems reasonable that there may also be distinctions in COPD.

SUMMARY

Each of the classes of mediators considered has the capacity to induce airway obstruction through a number of mechanisms. These include muscular constriction, secretion of mucous glycoproteins, and alteration in the integrity of the vascular endothelial barrier. The former two mechanisms will result in direct obstruction of the lumen, while the latter can result in thickening of the airway and peribronchiolar space, which will result in indirect obstruction of the lumen. Importantly, the availability of each of the classes of mediators reviewed can be influenced by the cell populations known to infiltrate the airway in chronic bronchitis. Even though the exact pathophysiologic role for each of these closely related systems has yet to be established, the data available to date certainly indicate a pivotal role for these substances in the airway obstruction of COPD.

REFERENCES

1. Jacoby DB, Tamaoki J, Borson DB, Nadel JA. Influenza infection causes airway hyperresponsiveness by decreasing enkephalinase. J Appl Physiol 1988; 64:2653–2658.
2. Sheppard D, Scypinski L. A tachykinin receptor antagonist inhibits and an inhibitor of tachykinin metabolism potentiates toluene diisocyanate-induced airway hyperresponsiveness in guinea pigs. Am Rev Respir Dis 1988; 138:547–551.
3. Erspamer V. The tachykinin peptide family. Trends Neurosci 1981; 4:267–269.
4. Pernow B. Substance P. Pharmacol Rev 1983; 35:85–141.
5. Chang MM, Leeman SE, Niall HD. Amino acid sequence of substance P. Nature New Biol 1971; 432:86.
6. Nawa H, Hirose T, Takashima H, et al. Nucleotide sequences of cloned cDNAs for two types of bovine brain substance P precursor. Nature 1983; 306:32–36.
7. Kimura S, Goto K, Ogawa T, et al. Pharmacological characterization of novel mammalian tachykinins, neurokinin alpha and neurokinin beta. Neurosci Res 1983; 2:97–104.
8. Kangawa K, Minamino N, Fukuda A, Matsuo H. Neuromedin K: a novel mammalian tachykinin identified in porcine spinal cord. Biochem Biophys Res Commun 1983; 114:533–559.
9. Theodorsson-Norheim E, Norheim I, Oberg K, et al. Neuropeptide K: a major tachykinin in plasma and tumor tissues from carcinoid patients. Biochem Biophys Res Commun 1985; 131:77–83.
10. Tatemoto K, Lundberg JM, Jornvall H, Mutt V. Neuropeptide K: isolation, structure and biological activities of a novel brain tachykinin. Biochem Biophys Res Commun 1985; 128:947–953.
11. Rosenfeld MG, Mermod J-J, Amara SG, et al. Production of a novel neuropeptide encoded by the calcitonin gene via tissue-specific RNA processing. Nature 1983; 304:129–135.
12. Cadieux A, Springall DR, Mulderry PK, et al. Occurrence, distribution and ontogeny of CGRP-immunoreactivity in the rat lower respiratory tract: effect of capsaicin treatment and surgical denervations. Neuroscience 1986; 19:605–627.
13. Lundberg JM, Franco-Cereceda A, Hua X-Y, et al. Co-existence of substance P and calcitonin gene-related peptide immunoreactivities in sensory nerves in relation to cardiovascular and bronchoconstrictor effects of capsaicin. Eur J Pharmacol 1985; 108:315–319.
14. Martling C-R, Saria A, Fischer J, et al. Calcitonin gene-related peptide and the lung: co-existence with substance P, release by capsaicin and vasodilatory effects. Regul Pept 1988; 20:125–139.
15. Palmer JBD, Cuss FMC, Mulderry PK, et al. Calcitonin gene-related peptide is localised to human airway nerves and potentially constricts airway smooth muscle. Br J Pharmacol 1987; 91:95–101.
16. Weinstock JV, Blum A, Walder J, Walder R. Eosinophils from granulomas in murine schistosomiasis mansoni produce substance P. J Immunol 1988; 141:961–966.
17. Barnes PJ, Chung KF, Page CP. Inflammatory mediators and asthma. Pharmacol Rev 1988; 40:49–84.
18. Lundberg JM, Hokfelt T, Martling C-R, et al. Sensory substance P-immunoreactive nerves in the lower respiratory tract of various mammals including man. Cell Tissue Res 1984; 235:251–261.
19. Lundblad L, Lundberg JM, Brodin E, Anggard A. Origin and distribution of sensory substance P nerves in the nasal mucosa. Acta Otolaryngol 1983; 96:485–493.
20. Polak JM, Bloom SR. Peripheral localization of regulatory peptides as a clue to their function. J Histochem Cytochem 1980; 28:918–924.
21. Lundberg JM, Brodin E, Saria A. Effects and distribution of vagal capsaicin-sensitive substance P neurons with special reference to the trachea and lungs. Acta Physiol Scand 1983; 119:243–252.
22. Saria A, Theodorsson-Norheim E, Gamse R, Lundberg JM. Release of substance P and substance K-like immunoreactivities from the isolated perfused guinea pig lung. Eur J Pharmacol 1985; 106:207–208.
23. Lundberg JM, Saria A. Capsaicin-induced desensitization of airway mucosa to cigarette smoke, mechanical and chemical irritants. Nature 1983; 302:251–253.
24. Lundberg JM, Martling C-R, Saria A, et al. Neuroscience 1983; 10:1361–1368.
25. Thompson JE, Scypinski LA, Gordon T, Sheppard D. Tachykinins mediate the acute increase in airway responsiveness caused by toluene diisocyanate in guinea pigs. Am Rev Respir Dis 1987; 136:43–49.
26. Braquet P, Rola-Pleszczynski M. Platelet-activating factor and cellular immune responses. Immunol Today 1987; 8:345–352.
27. Stewart AG, Thompson DC, Fennessy MR. Involvement of capsaicin-sensitive afferent neurones in a vagal-dependent interaction between leukotriene D_4 and histamine on bronchomotor tone. Agents Actions 1984; 15:500–508.
28. Saria A, Martling C-R, Yan Z, et al. Release of multiple tachykinins from capsaicin-sensitive sensory nerves in the lung by bradykinin, histamine, dimethylphenyl piperazinium, and vagal nerve stimulation. Am Rev Respir Dis 1988; 137:1330–1335.
29. Khrogi H, Graf PD, Sekizawa K, et al. Neutral endopeptidase (enkephalinase, E.C. 3.4.24.11) inhibitor potentiates substance P– and capsaicin-induced cough in awake guinea pigs. FASEB J 1988; 2:A1383.
30. Baker AP, Hillegass LM, Holden DA, Smith WJ. Effect of kallidin, substance P and other basic polypeptides on the production of respiratory macromolecules. Am Rev Respir Dis 1977; 115:811–817.
31. Gashi AA, Borson DB, Finkbeiner WE, et al. Neuropeptides degranulate serous cells of ferret tracheal glands. Am J Physiol 1986; 251:C223–C229.

32. Borson DB, Corrales R, Varsano S, et al. Enkephalinase inhibitors potentiate substance P–induced secretion of $^{35}SO_4$-macromolecules from ferret trachea. Exp Lung Res 1987; 12:21–36.
33. Coles SJ, Neill KH, Reid LM. Potent stimulation of glycoprotein secretion in canine trachea by substance P. J Appl Physiol 1988; 251:C223–C229.
34. Andersson P, Persson H. Effect of substance P on pulmonary resistance and dynamic pulmonary compliance in the anesthetized cat and guinea pig. Acta Pharmacol Toxicol 1977; 41:444–448.
35. Joos G, Kips J, Pauwels R, van der Straeten M. The effect of tachykinins on the conducting airways of the rat. Arch Int Pharmacodyn Ther 1986; 280:176–190.
36. Grunstein MM, Tanaka DT, Grunstein JS. Mechanism of substance P–induced bronchoconstriction in maturing rabbit. J Appl Physiol 1984; 57:1238–1246.
37. Hua X, Lundberg JM, Theodorsson-Norheim E, Brodin E. Comparison of cardiovascular and bronchoconstrictor effects of substance P, substance K and other tachykinins. Naunyn-Schmiedeberg's Arch Pharmacol 1984; 328:196–201.
38. Laitinen LA, Laitinen A, Widdicombe JG. Effects of inflammatory and other mediators on airway vascular beds. Am Rev Respir Dis 1987; 135:S67–S70.
39. Saria A, Lundberg JM, Skofitsch G, Lembeck F. Vascular protein leakage in various tissues induced by substance P, capsaicin, bradykinin, serotonin, histamine and by antigen challenge. Naunyn-Schmiedeberg's Arch Pharmacol 1983; 324:212–218.
40. Aursudkij B, Barnes PJ, Belvisi MG, et al. Effect of substance P, neurokinins and calcitonin gene-related peptide on microvascular permeability in guinea pig airways. J Physiol 1988; 398:51P.
41. Lundberg JM, Saria A, Brodin E, et al. A substance P antagonist inhibits vagally induced increases in vascular permeability and bronchial smooth muscle contraction in the guinea pig. Proc Natl Acad Sci 1983; 80:1120–1124.
42. Tamaoki J, Ueki IF, Widdicombe JH, Nadel JA. Stimulation of Cl secretion by neurokinin A and neurokinin B in canine tracheal epithelium. Am Rev Respir Dis 1988; 137:899–902.
43. Al-Bazzaz FJ, Kelsey JG, Kaage WD. Substance P stimulation of chloride secretion by canine tracheal mucosa. Am Rev Respir Dis 1985; 131:86–89.
44. Persson CGA, Erjefalt I, Andersson P. Leakage of macromolecules from guinea pig tracheobronchial microcirculation. Effects of allergen, leukotrienes, tachykinins and anti-asthma drugs. Acta Physiol Scand 1986; 127:95–105.
45. Fuller RW, Dixon CMS, Barnes PJ. Bronchoconstrictor response to inhaled capsaicin in humans. J Appl Physiol 1985; 58:1080–1084.
46. Fuller RW, Maxwell DL, Dixon CMS, et al. Effect of substance P on cardiovascular and respiratory function in subjects. J Appl Physiol 1987; 62:1473–1479.
47. Brain SD, Williams TJ, Tippins JR, et al. Calcitonin gene-related peptide is a potent vasodilator. Nature 1985; 313:54–56.
48. Brain SD, Williams TJ. Inflammatory oedema induced by synergism between CGRP and mediators of increased vascular permeability. Br J Pharmacol 1985; 86:855–860.
49. Gamse R, Saria A. Potentiation of tachykinin-induced plasma proteinextravasation by calcitonin gene-related peptide. Eur J Pharmacol 1985; 114:61–66.
50. Gatto C, Lussky RC, Erickson LW, et al. Calcitonin and CGRP block bombesin- and substance P-induced increases in airway tone. J Appl Physiol 1989; 66:573–577.
51. Shore SA, Stimler-Gerard NP, Coats SR, Drazen JM. Substance P–induced bronchoconstriction in guinea pig. Enhancement by inhibitors of neutral metalloendopeptidase and angiotensin converting enzyme. Am Rev Respir Dis 1988; 137:331–336.
52. Shore SA, Drazen JM. Enzymatic degradation of neurokinin A modulates its bronchoactive properties: comparison with other neuropeptides. Am Rev Respir Dis 1988; 137(Suppl):200.
53. Dusser DJ, Umeno E, Graf PD, et al. Airway neutral endopeptidase-like enzyme modulates tachykinin-induced bronchoconstriction *in vivo*. J Appl Physiol 1988; 65:2585–2591.
54. Joos GF, Pauwels RA, van der Straeten M. The mechanism of tachykinin induced bronchoconstriction in the rat. Am Rev Respir Dis 1988; 137:1038–1044.
55. Sekizawa K, Tamaoki J, Graf PD, et al. Enkephalinase inhibitor potentiates mammalian tachykinin-induced contraction in ferret trachea. J Pharm Exp Ther 1987; 243:1211–1217.
56. Sekizawa K, Tamaoki J, Nadel JA, Borson DB. Enkephalinase inhibitor potentiates substance P and electrically induced contraction in ferret trachea. J Appl Physiol 1987; 63:1401–1405.
57. Lundberg JM, Saria A. Bronchial smooth muscle contraction induced by stimulation of capsaicin-sensitive sensory neurons. Acta Physiol Scand 1982; 116:473–476.
58. Goel V, Biggs DF. Comparison of the bronchoconstrictor and cardiovascular effects of some tachykinins in guinea pigs. Life Sci 1987; 40:1007–1015.
59. Shore SA, Drazen JM. Enhanced airway responses to substance P after repeated challenge in the guinea pig. J Appl Physiol 1989; 66:955–961.
60. Martling CR, Theordosson-Norheim E, Lundberg JM. Occurrence and effects of multiple tachykinins: substance P, neurokinin A and neuropeptide K in human lower airways. Life Sci 1987; 40:1633–1643.
61. Gerard NP. Characterization of substance P contractile activity on isolated guinea pig lung tissues. J Pharm Exp Ther 1987; 243:901–906.
62. Carstairs JR, Barnes PJ. Autoradiographic mapping of substance P receptors in lung. Eur J Pharmacol 1986; 127:295–296.
63. Shore SA, Drazen JM. Airway responses to substance P and substance P fragments in the guinea pig. Pulmonary Pharmacol 1988; 1:113–118.
64. LeGreves P, Nyberg F, Terenius L, Hokfelt T. Calcitonin gene-related peptide is a potent inhibitor of substance P degradation. Eur J Pharmacol 1985; 115:309–311.
65. Masu Y, Nakayama K, Tamaki H, et al. cDNA cloning of bovine substance K receptor through oocyte expression system. Nature 1987; 329:836–838.
66. Foreman JC, Jordan CC, Oehme P, Renner H. Structure-activity relationships for some substance P-related peptides that cause wheal and flare reactions in human skin. J Physiol 1983; 335:449–465.
67. Barnes PJ, Brown MJ, Dollery CT, et al. Histamine is released from skin by substance P but does not act as the final vasodilator in the axon reflex. Br J Pharmacol 1986; 88:741–745.
68. Payan DG, McGillis JP, Goetzl EJ. Neuroimmunology. In: Dixon FJ, Austen KF, Hood L, Uhr JW, eds. Advances in Immunology. New York: Academic Press, 1986; 299–323.
69. Lotz M, Vaughan JH, Carson DA. Effect of neuropeptides on production of inflammatory cytokines by human monocytes. Science 1988; 241:1218–1221.
70. Hartung H-P, Wolters K, Toyka KV. Substance P: Binding properties and studies on cellular responses in guinea pig macrophages. J Immunol 1986; 136:3856–3863.
71. Payan DG, Brewster DR, Missirian-Bastien A, Goetzl EJ. Substance P recognition by a subset of human T lymphocytes. J Clin Invest 1984; 74:1532–1539.
72. Connelly JC, Skidgel RA, Schulz WW, et al. Neutral endopeptidase 24.11 in human neutrophils: cleavage of chemotactic peptide. Proc Natl Acad Sci USA 1985; 82:8737–8741.
73. Benveniste J, Tence M, Varenne P, et al. Semi-synthese et structure proposee du facteur activant les plaquettes (PAF): PAF-acether, un alkyl ether analogue de la lysophosphotidylcholine. CR Acad Sci 1979; 289:1037–1040.
74. Demopoulos CA, Pinckard RN, Hanahan DJ. Platelet-activating factor: evidence for 1-O-alkyl-2-O-acetyl-sn-glyceryl-3-phosphorylcholine as the active component (a new class of lipid mediators). J Biol Chem 1979; 254:9355–9358.
75. Benveniste J, Henson PM, Cochrane CG. Leukocyte dependent histamine release from rabbit platelets: the role of IgE, basophils, and a platelet activating factor. J Exp Med 1972; 136:1356–1377.
76. Satouchi J, Pinckard RN, McManus LM, Hanahan DJ. Modification of the polar head group of acetyl glyceryl ether phosphorylcholine and subsequent effects upon platelet activation. J Biol Chem 1981; 256:4425–4432.
77. Ludwig JC, Pinckard RN. Diversity in the chemical structures of neutrophil-derived platelet activating factors. In: Winslow CM, Lee ML, eds. New Horizons in Platelet Activating Factor Research. New York, John Wiley & Sons Inc., 1987, 59–65.
78. Chap H, Mauco G, Simon MF, et al. Biosynthetic labelling of platelet activating factor from radioactive acetate by stimulated platelets. Nature 1981; 289:312–314.
79. Camussi G, Aglietta M, Malavasi, F., et al. The release of platelet activating factor from human endothelial cells in culture. J Immunol 1983; 131:2397–2403.

80. Betz SJ, Henson PM. Production and release of platelet activating factor (PAF): Dissociation from degranulation and superoxide production in the human neutrophil. J Immunol 1980; 125:2756–2763.
81. Muller HW, O'Flaherty JT, Wykle RL. Biosynthesis of platelet activating factor in rabbit polymorphonuclear neutrophils. J Biol Chem 1983; 258:6213–6218.
82. Lee T-C, Lenihan DJ, Malone BT, et al. Increased biosynthesis of platelet activating factor in activated human eosinophils. J Biol Chem 1984; 259:5526–5530.
83. Mencia-Huerta JM, Roubin R, Morgat L-L, Benveniste J. Biosynthesis of platelet activating factor (PAF-acether). III. Formation of PAF-acether from synthetic substrates by stimulated murine macrophages. J Immunol 1982; 129:804–808.
84. Prescott SM, Zimmerman GA, McIntyre TM. Human endothelial cells in culture produce platelet activating factor (1-alkyl-2-acetyl-sn-glycero-3-phosphocholine) when stimulated with thrombin. Proc Natl Acad Sci USA 1984; 81:3534–3538.
85. Morley J, Page CP, Sanjar S. Pulmonary responses to platelet-activating factor. Prog Resp Res 1985; 19:117–123.
86. Braquet P, Rola-Pleszczynski M. Platelet-activating factor and cellular immune responses. Immunol Today 1987; 8:345–352.
87. Barnes PJ, Chung KF, Page CP. Inflammatory mediators in asthma. Pharmacol Rev 1988; 40:49–84.
88. Stimler NP, Bloor CM, Hugli TE, et al. Anaphylactic actions of platelet-activating factor. Am J Pathol 1981; 105:64–69.
89. Stimler NP, O'Flaherty JT. Spasmogenic properties of platelet-activating factor: evidence for a direct mechanism in the contractile response of pulmonary tissues. Am J Pathol 1983; 113:75–84.
90. Camussi G, Montruccio G, Antro C, et al. Platelet-activating factor-mediated contraction of rabbit lung strips: pharmacologic modulation. Immunopharmacology 1983; 6:87–96.
91. Stimler NP, Gerard C, O'Flaherty JT. Contraction of human lung tissues by platelet-activating factor (AAGPC). In: Benveniste J, Arnoux B, eds. Platelet-Activating Factor, INSERM Symp. No. 23. New York: Elsevier Science Publishing Co. Inc. B.V., 1983, 195–204.
92. Vargaftig BB, Lefort J, Chignard M, Benveniste J. Platelet-activating factor induces a platelet-dependent bronchoconstriction unrelated to the formation of prostaglandin derivatives. Eur J Pharmacol 1980; 65:185–192.
93. Cerrina J, Raffestin B, Labat C, et al. Effects of PAF-acether on isolated muscle preparations from the rat, guinea pig and human lung. In: Benveniste J, Arnoux B eds. Platelet-Activating Factor, INSERM Symp. No. 23. New York: Elsevier Science Publishing Co. Inc. B.V., 1983, 205–212.
94. Schellenberg RR. Airway responses to platelet-activating factor. Am Rev Respir Dis 1987; 136:S28–S31.
95. Lefort J, Rotilio D, Vargaftig BB. The platelet-independent release of thromboxane A_2 by PAF-acether for guinea pig lungs involves mechanisms distinct from those for leukotriene C_4 and bradykinin. Br J Pharmacol 1984; 82:525–531.
96. Stimler-Gerard NP. Parasympathetic stimulation as a mechanism for PAF-induced contractile responses in the lung. J Pharmacol Exp Ther 1986; 237:209–213.
97. Voelkel NF, Worthen S, Reeves, JT, et al. Nonimmunological production of leukotrienes induced by platelet-activating factor. Science 1982; 218:286–288.
98. Bonnet J, Thibaudeau D, Bessin P. Dependancy of PAF-acether induced bronchospasm on the lipoxygenase pathway in the guinea pig. Prostaglandins 1983; 26:457–466.
99. Stimler-Gerard NP. Parasympathetic action of platelet activating factor in lung. In: Winslow CM, Lee ML, eds. New Horizons in Platelet Activating Factor Research. New York: John Wiley and Sons Inc., 1987; 269–275.
100. Leff AR, White SR, Munoz NM, et al. Parasympathetic mediation of PAF–induced contraction in canine trachealis *in vivo*. J Appl Physiol 1987; 62:599–605.
101. Vargaftig BB, Lefort J, Chignard M, Benveniste J. Platelet-activating factor induces a platelet-dependent bronchoconstriction unrelated to the formulation of prostanoid derivatives. Eur J Pharmacol 1980; 65:185–192.
102. Handley DA, Van Valen RG, Melden MK, Saunders RN. Evaluation of dose and route effects of platelet activating factor–induced extravasation in the guinea pig. Thromb Haemost 1984; 52:34–36.
103. Vargaftig BB, Lefort J, Wal F, et al. Non-steroidal anti-inflammatory drugs if combined with anti-histamine and anti-serotonin agents interfere with the bronchial and platelet effects of 'platelet-activating factor' (PAF-acether). Eur J Pharmacol 1982; 82:121–130.
104. Barnes PJ, Chung KF. PAF closely mimics pathology of asthma. Trends Pharmacol Sci 1987; 8:285–287.
105. Barnes PJ, Chung KF, Page CP. Inflammatory mediators and asthma. Pharmacol Rev 1988; 40:49–84.
106. Lewis RA, Austen KF. The biologically active leukotrienes. Biosynthesis, metabolism, receptors, functions, and pharmacology. J Clin Invest 1984; 73:889–897.
107. Blackwell GJ, Flower RJ. Inhibition of phospholipase. Br Med Bull 1983; 39:260–264.
108. Abdel-Latif AA. Calcium-mobilizing receptors, polyphosphoinositides, and the generation of second messengers. Pharmacol Rev 1986; 38:227–272.
109. Robinson C, Hardy CC, Holgate ST. Pulmonary synthesis, release and metabolism of prostaglandins. J Allergy Clin Immunol 1985; 76:265–271.
110. Aharony D, Dobson PT, Krell RD. *In vitro* metabolism of (3H)-peptide leukotrienes in human and ferret lung: a comparison with the guinea pig. Biochem Biophys Res Commun 1985; 131:892–889.
111. Shore S, Austen KF, Drazen JM. Eicosanoids and the lung. In: L'Enfant C, Massaro D, eds. Lung Biology in Health and Disease: Lung Cell Biology. New York: Marcel Dekker Inc., in press.
112. MacGlashan DW, Schleimer RP, Peters SP, et al. Generation of leukotrienes by purified human lung mast cells. J Clin Invest 1982; 70:747–751.
113. Rankin JA, Hitchock M, Merrill WW, et al. IgE immune complexes induce immediate and prolonged release of leukotriene C_4 (LTC_4) from rat alveolar macrophages. J Immunol 1984; 132:1993–1999.
114. Weller PF, Lee CW, Foster DW, et al. Generation and metabolism of 5-lipoxygenase pathway leukotrienes by human eosinophils: predominant production of leukotriene C_4. Proc Natl Acad Sci USA 1983; 80:7626–7630.
115. Hodges MK, Weller PF, Gerard NP, et al. Variability of leukotriene C_4 production by eosinophils from asthmatic and normal subjects. Am Rev Respir Dis 1988; 138:799–804.
116. Feinmark SJ, Cannon PJ. Endothelial cell leukotriene C_4 synthesis results from intercellular transfer of leukotriene A_4 synthesized by polymorphonuclear leukocytes. J Biol Chem 1986; 261:16466–16472.
117. Eling TE, Danilowicz RM, Henke DC, et al. Arachidonic acid metabolism by canine tracheal epithelial cells. Product formation and relationship to chloride secretion. J Biol Chem 1986; 261:12841–12849.
118. Laviolette M, Coulombe S, Holzgrefe H, Fitzpatrick F. Decreased leukotriene B_4 synthesis in smokers' alveolar macrophages *in vitro*. J Clin Invest 1986; 77:54–60.
119. Laviolette M, Chang J, Newcombe DS. Human alveolar macrophages: a lesion in arachidonic acid metabolism in cigarette smokers. Am Rev Respir Dis 1981; 124:397–401.
120. O'Driscoll BR, Cromwell O, Kay AB. Sputum leukotrienes in obstructive airways diseases. Clin Exp Immunol 1984; 55:397–404.
121. Dahlen SE, Hedqvist P, Hammarstrom S, Samuelsson B. Leukotrienes are potent constrictors of human bronchi. Nature 1980; 288:484–486.
122. Hanna CJ, Bach MK, Pare PD, Schellenberg RR. Slow reacting substances (leukotrienes) contract human airway and pulmonary vascular smooth muscle *in vitro*. Nature 1981; 290:343–344.
123. Jones TR, Davis C, Daniel EE. Pharmacological study of the contractile activity of leukotriene C_4 and D_4 on isolated human airway smooth muscle. Can J Physiol Pharmacol 1982; 60:638–643.
124. Chagon M, Gentile J, Gladu M, Sirois P. The mechanism of action of leukotrienes A_4, C_4 and D_4 on human lung parenchyma *in vitro*. Lung 1985; 163:55–62.
125. Drazen JM, Austen KF, Lewis RA, et al. Comparative airway and vascular activities of leukotrienes C_1 and D *in vivo* and *in vitro*. Proc Natl Acad Sci USA 1980; 77:4354–4358.
126. Krell RD, Osborn R, Vickery L, et al. Contraction of isolated airway smooth muscle by synthetic leukotrienes C_4 and D_4. Prostaglandins 1981; 22:387–409.

127. Charette L, Jones TR. Effects of L-serine borate on antagonism of leukotriene C_4-induced contractions of guinea-pig trachea. Br J Pharmacol 1987; 91:179–188.
128. Hay DW, Muccitelli RM, Wilson KA, et al. Functional antagonism by salbutamol suggests differences in the relative efficacies and dissociation constants of the peptidoleukotrienes in guinea pig trachea. J Pharmacol Exp Ther 1988; 244:71–78.
129. Buckner CK, Krell RD, Laravuso RB, et al. Pharmacological evidence that human intralobar airways do not contain different receptors that mediate contractions to leukotriene C_4 and leukotriene D_4. J Pharmacol Exp Ther 1986; 237:558–562.
130. Hay DW, Muccitelli RM, Tucker SS, et al. Pharmacologic profile of SK&F 104353: a novel, potent, and selective peptidoleukotriene receptor antagonist in guinea pig and human airways. J Pharmacol Exp Ther 1987; 243:474–481.
131. Fleisch JH, Rinkema LE, Haisch KD, et al. LY171883, 1-less than 2-hydroxy-3-propyl-4-less than 4-(1H-tetrazol-5-yl) butoxy greater than phenyl greater than ethanone, an orally active leukotriene D_4 antagonist. J Pharmacol Exp Ther 1985; 233:148–157.
132. Coles SJ, Neill KH, Reid LM, et al. Effects of leukotrienes C_4 and D_4 on glycoprotein and lysozyme secretion by human bronchial mucosa. Prostaglandins 1983; 25:155–170.
133. Marom Z, Shelhamer JH, Sun F, Kaliner M. Human airway monohydroxyeicosatetraenoic acid generation and mucus release. J Clin Invest 1983; 72:122–127.
134. Leikauf GD, Ueki IF, Widdicombe JH, Nadel JA. Alteration of chloride secretion across canine tracheal epithelium by lipoxygenase products of arachidonic acid. Am J Physiol 1986; 250:F47–F53.
135. Johnson HG, McNee ML, Johnson MA, Miller MD. Leukotriene C_4 and dimethylphenylpiperazinium-induced responses in canine airway tracheal muscle, contraction and fluid secretion. Int Arch Allergy Appl Immunol 1983; 71:214–218.
136. Weiss JW, Drazen JM, McFadden ER Jr, et al. Airway constriction in normal humans produced by inhalation of leukotriene D: potency, time course, and effect of acetylsalicylic acid. JAMA 1983; 249:2814–2817.
137. Davidson AB, Lee TH, Scanlon PD, et al. Bronchoconstrictor effects of leukotriene E_4 in normal and asthmatic individuals. Am Rev Respir Dis 1987; 135:333–337.
138. Holroyde MC, Altounyan REC, Cole M, et al. Bronchoconstriction produced in man by leukotrienes C and D. Lancet 1981; ii:17–18.
139. Weiss JW, Drazen JM, Coles N, et al. Bronchoconstrictor effects of leukotriene C in humans. Science 1982; 216:196–198.
140. Barnes NC, Piper PJ, Costello JF. Comparative effects of inhaled leukotriene C_4, leukotriene D_4 and histamine in normal human subjects. Thorax 1984; 39:500–504.
141. Smith LJ, Greenberger PA, Patterson R, et al. The effect of inhaled leukotriene D_4 in humans. Am Rev Respir Dis 1985; 131:368–372.
142. Bisgaard H, Groth S, Masden F. Bronchial hyperreactivity to leukotriene D_4 in exogenous asthma. Br Med J 1985; 290:1468–1471.
143. Roberts SA, Giembycz MA, Raeburn D, et al. *In vitro* and *in vivo* effect of verapamil on human airway responsiveness to leukotriene D_4. Thorax 1986; 41:12–16.
144. Adelroth E, Morris MM, Hargreave FE, O'Byrne PM. Airway responsiveness to leukotrienes C_4 and D_4 and to methacholine in patients with asthma and normal controls. N Engl J Med 1986; 315:480–484.
145. Bisgaard H, Groth S, Dirksen H. Leukotriene D_4 induces bronchoconstriction in man. Allergy 1983; 38:441–443.
146. Bisgaard H, Poulsen L, Sondergaard I. Nebulization and selective deposition of LTD_4 in human lungs. Allergy 1987; 42:336–342.
147. Smith LJ, Kern R, Patterson R, et al. Mechanism of leukotriene D_4-induced bronchoconstriction in normal subjects. J Allergy Clin Immunol 1987; 80:340–347.
148. Roberts JA, Rodger IW, Thomson NC. Effect of verapamil and sodium cromoglycate on leukotriene D_4 induced bronchoconstriction in patients with asthma. Thorax 1986; 41:753–758.

Chapter 7

ANIMAL MODELS OF EMPHYSEMA

Jerome O. Cantor Gerard M. Turino

Although animal models of emphysema have achieved success as a research tool only within the last two decades, they are not a new phenomenon. Efforts to construct an experimental form of the disease date back more than a century. The crudeness of the early models reflected the very limited understanding of emphysema that then existed. Mechanical obstruction of airways was tried, for example, in the belief that the disease was primarily due to a blockage of airflow. This approach achieved localized distention of air spaces but did not satisfactorily reproduce the physiologic characteristics of emphysema. Development of more representative models of the disease awaited the recognition that enzyme-induced damage to pulmonary connective tissue components, particularly elastic fibers, was of critical importance in the destruction of alveolar walls (Fig. 7–1). Papain and, later, elastase were used to produce lesions that more closely approximated the morphologic and physiologic features of emphysema. A number of other methods were subsequently devised to induce similar lung changes. Despite these advances, however, models of emphysema still bear little resemblance to the actual disease in terms of pathogenesis and must be viewed as analogues rather than equivalents of the human entity.

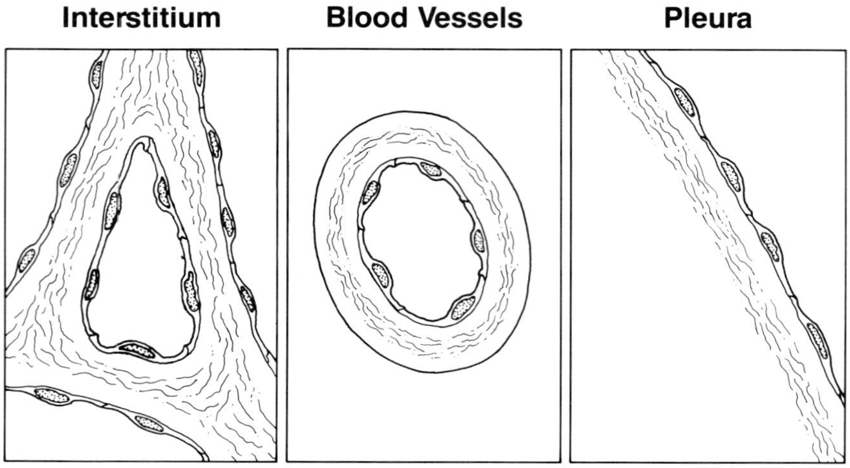

Figure 7–1. Elastic fibers, which account for approximately 25% of the connective tissue mass of the lung, are an important component of alveolar walls, blood vessels, and pleura. The fibers have the ability to undergo a several-fold linear expansion and return to their original configuration. Consequently, they influence the efficiency of air movement through the lung. Loss of elastic fibers causes distention and rupture of alveoli and may lead to severe respiratory dysfunction. (Reproduced with permission from Cantor JO, Turino GM. Elastin and elastases in lung disease. In: Robert L, Hornbeck W, eds. Elastin and Elastases. Boca Raton: CRC Press, 1989, 159.)

EMPHYSEMA PRODUCED BY EXOGENOUS PROTEASES

Papain-Induced Emphysema

The use of papain to induce emphysema was a breakthrough in the development of animal models of the disease. Originally intended as a possible treatment for pulmonary fibrosis, intratracheal instillation of the enzyme was instead found to produce prominent air space enlargement.[1] Introduction of the papain model had added significance because it came at a time when the role of alpha$_1$-antiprotease was just being understood. These two findings firmly established the importance of proteolysis in the pathogenesis of emphysema.

Morphologically, papain-induced lung lesions resemble human panacinar emphysema. Air space enlargement is accompanied by increases in total lung capacity, functional residual capacity, and compliance.[2, 3] This injury is additionally associated with damage to lung elastic fibers, which remain disrupted despite undergoing resynthesis.[4, 5] Consequently, there is no restoration of lung recoil.

By providing insight into the relationship between elastic fibers and alveolar wall destruction, papain-induced emphysema paved the way for development of models that utilized either pancreatic or leukocyte elastase to induce air space enlargement. Such was the advantage of using mammalian elastases rather than the plant-derived papain that the new models soon eclipsed their predecessor. The pancreatic elastase model has gained a particularly strong foothold in emphysema research due to its efficacy and cost-effectiveness.

Elastase-Induced Emphysema

Introduction of either pancreatic or leukocyte elastase into the lung causes rapid destruction of elastic fibers, resulting in diffuse air space enlargement (Fig. 7–2).[6–8] Although lesions resulting from neutrophil elastase tend to be less severe, the enzyme may initially cause greater hemorrhage and cell damage than its pancreatic counterpart.[7]

Biochemically, degradation of lung elastic fibers is reflected by a large increase in urinary desmosine crosslinks during the first 24 hours following instillation of pancreatic elastase.[9] Marked resynthesis of the fibers occurs almost immediately[10] and, by 3 weeks, their content in the lung has returned to normal.[11] Tissue damage is irreversible, however, and may progress for months, despite the fact that nearly all of the instilled elastase is quickly cleared from the extracellular compartment.[12, 13] With regard to physiologic alterations, increases in total lung capacity, functional residual capacity, and compliance are observed, along with a reduction in arterial oxygen tension.[12, 14]

Comparing this model with the actual disease, differences clearly exist with regard to the nature of the injury and its rate of development. Nevertheless, the simplicity of the model and its morphologic and physiologic resemblance to human panacinar emphysema have resulted in its widespread use in the study of this disorder.

EMPHYSEMA PRODUCED BY ENDOGENOUS PROTEASES

Cadmium Chloride/Beta-Aminopropionitrile-Induced Emphysema

While intratracheal instillation of cadmium chloride induces lung disease that is morphologically similar to interstitial pulmonary fibrosis, concomitant administration of the crosslink inhibitor, beta-aminopropionitrile (BAPN), results in injury that more nearly resembles emphysema.[15] This complex response is produced by at least two separate actions on the pulmonary extracellular matrix. Initially, cadmium chloride–induced inflammation causes the release of enzymes that degrade the matrix. Then, BAPN impairs proper assembling of newly synthesized collagen and elastin, causing eventual rupture of alveolar walls.

Breakdown of pulmonary elastin and collagen begins shortly after instillation of cadmium chloride. Within 24 hours, the amount of desmosine and hydroxyproline in the parenchyma is substantially decreased.[16] The damage coincides with migration of large numbers of neutrophils to the lung. After the first week, this reaction subsides and is replaced by a sustained influx of mononuclear cells.

The inflammation is accompanied by diffuse enlargement of air spaces and formation of thin-walled, subpleural bullae, which are prone to rupture. A substantial number of animals indeed die from pneumothorax during the first month. Those that survive show significant increases in lung volume and compliance.[16]

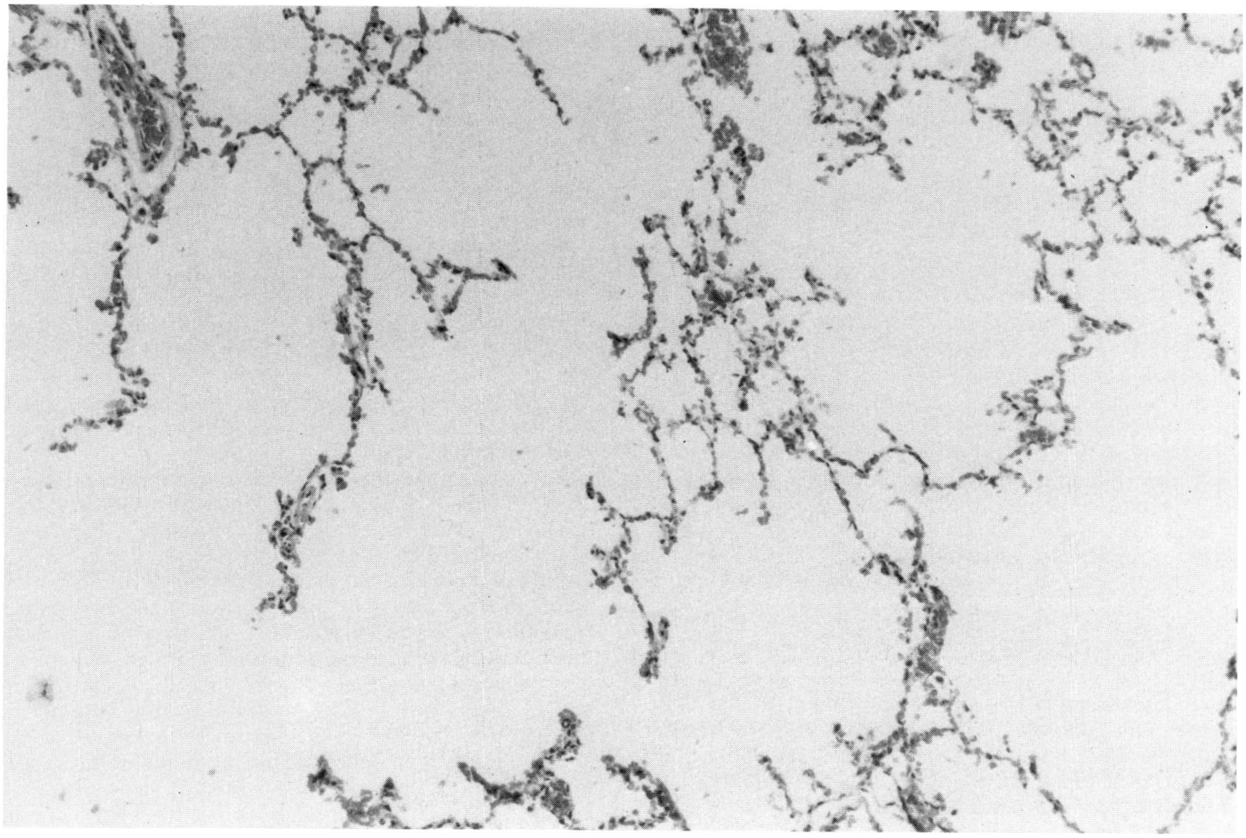

Figure 7–2. Photomicrograph of a hamster lung 5 weeks after intratracheal instillation of porcine pancreatic elastase. Marked enlargement of air spaces results from rupture of alveolar septa.

By virtue of its reliance on endogenous proteases to effect lung damage, cadmium chloride/BAPN-induced emphysema may be more representative of the actual disease process than the previously discussed intratracheal elastase model. It is particularly suited to evaluating the role of inflammatory cells in degrading elastin and other matrix constituents.

Nitrogen Dioxide-Induced Emphysema

Prolonged inhalation of as little as 30 ppm of nitrogen dioxide causes focal air space enlargement.[17] Injury is largely confined to the terminal bronchioles and alveolar ducts, producing lesions that most closely resemble centriacinar emphysema. The disease is believed to result mainly from the release of elastase by neutrophils migrating into the lung. Studies suggest, however, that nitrogen dioxide may also interfere with elastic fiber repair.[18]

Endotoxin-Induced Emphysema

Administration of endotoxin initiates an acute inflammatory reaction that degrades the pulmonary extracellular matrix.[19] The resultant increase in air space size is relatively small, however, and occurs only after repeated infusion of the material.[20] Despite these limitations, the model has been used to demonstrate the importance of alpha$_1$-antiprotease in preventing lung injury. By injecting galactosamine to disrupt synthesis of this inhibitor in the liver, the severity of endotoxin-induced emphysema is increased.[21] The finding also suggests that elastase is at least partly responsible for the changes that occur in the lung.

EMPHYSEMA PRODUCED BY IMPAIRED ELASTOGENESIS

Copper Deficiency-Induced Emphysema

Emphysema may also be induced by restricting the intake of copper during lung development.[22] The underlying mechanism of injury is believed to be inhibition of lysyl oxidase, the enzyme responsible for elastin and collagen crosslinking. Although the disease may be produced postnatally, a more severe form results when the deficiency occurs *in utero*.

As a result of a low-copper diet, generalized air space enlargement develops along with subpleural and intraparenchymal bullae. Increases in both lung volume and compliance are also observed. Surprisingly, there is no significant alteration in lung elastic fiber content.[23] This finding suggests that the underlying mechanism of injury in the copper deficiency model may be more complex than previously thought.

Emphysema in the Blotchy Mouse

Diffuse air space enlargement occurs spontaneously in the blotchy mouse as a result of a genetically induced loss of lysyl oxidase activity, though a secondary abnormality in macrophage function may contribute to the injury.[24, 25] Alveolar distention is seen very shortly after birth and becomes progressively worse as the animal matures. Both lung volume and compliance are increased. Although the changes in lung mechanics suggest that damage to elastic fibers has occurred, this needs to be confirmed biochemically.[24]

MODELS OF UNCERTAIN PATHOGENESIS

Starvation-Induced Emphysema

Starvation of newborn animals causes generalized impairment of organ growth, including a marked reduction in lung volume and weight.[26, 27] Maturing animals, in contrast, develop less severe lung disease characterized by an increase in alveolar size.[28] Although the cause of the air space enlargement has not been determined, it may conceivably result from an insufficient repair response to normal degradative processes. Similar lung changes may be induced by restricting the intake of specific nutrients, such as lysine.[29]

Emphysema in the Tight-Skin Mouse

Another genetic model of emphysema involves the tight-skin mouse. Alveolar dilatation develops 6 to 8 weeks after birth and is associated with increases in both lung volume and compliance.[30, 31] The underlying biochemical abnormality in these animals remains unclear, however.

THE IMPORTANCE OF ANIMAL MODELS IN EMPHYSEMA RESEARCH

Determining Mechanisms of Injury

OVERVIEW. Although research on emphysema has primarily focused on the role of elastolytic enzymes, the use of animal models has permitted identification of additional mechanisms that may be involved in the disease process. Several studies have shown, for example, that the amount of damage caused by elastase is influenced by the rate of elastic fiber resynthesis. Other investigations suggest that the extent of injury may also be related to the activity of free radicals. As a clearer picture of the causes of emphysema emerges, the likelihood of developing more effective forms of therapy greatly increases.

THE ROLE OF ELASTASES. The ability of exogenously administered elastase to induce emphysema provided strong support for its role in the pathogenesis of the disease. The importance of elastase was further confirmed by the inability of collagenase and other proteolytic enzymes to cause similar injury.[32, 33] The source of the elastase responsible for human emphysema nevertheless remains uncertain.

Neutrophil elastase is currently considered to be the most important contributor to matrix injury in human emphysema. When instilled into the lung, it produces the same types of changes as pancreatic elastase, albeit to a lesser degree. Certain animal investigations, however, point to only a limited role for neutrophil elastase in the development of emphysema. In endotoxin injury, migration of large numbers of neutrophils into the lung does not readily induce air space enlargement.[20] Furthermore, inhibition of neutrophil influx does not alter the severity of cadmium chloride/BAPN-induced emphysema.[34]

Alternatively, elastic fiber damage may be caused by the macrophage. Unlike neutrophils, these cells remain abundant in the lung in the absence of disease. Studies show that it is possible to induce a mild form of emphysema by intratracheal instillation of macrophage homogenates.[35] An important question to be answered, however, is which of the several macrophage enzymes with elastolytic activity contribute to lung injury.

THE ROLE OF ELASTIC FIBER RESYNTHESIS. Following degradation of elastic fibers, there is a rapid upsurge in their synthesis.[10] The importance of this response is clearly demonstrated in the cadmium chloride/BAPN model, where inhibition of crosslinking is directly responsible for the development of emphysema.[15] In lung injury produced by intratracheal instillation of elastase, the role of elastic fiber resynthesis is less evident because of the overwhelming damage caused by the large excess of enzyme. It is nevertheless possible to enhance the severity of emphysema in this model by interfering with repair. Administration of BAPN to elastase-treated animals results in a significant increase in air space size.[11] Likewise, enzymatic disruption of the microfibrillar component of elastic fibers, which may facilitate crosslinking, causes a marked decrease in new desmosine formation and a worsening of the disease (Fig. 7–3).[33]

THE ROLE OF FREE RADICALS. Despite a number of experiments that indicate that free radicals are capable of degrading components of the extracellular matrix, the importance of these molecules in the pathogenesis of emphysema is unclear. Certain studies point to a rather limited role of free radicals in the disease process. Exposure of the lung to radicals generated by high levels of oxygen, for example, causes only a mild degree of air space enlargement and no decrease in the total amount of desmosine cross-links.[36]

Nevertheless, evidence suggests that free radicals, especially those present in cigarette smoke, contribute to the development of emphysema. Tobacco smoke both increases the dam-

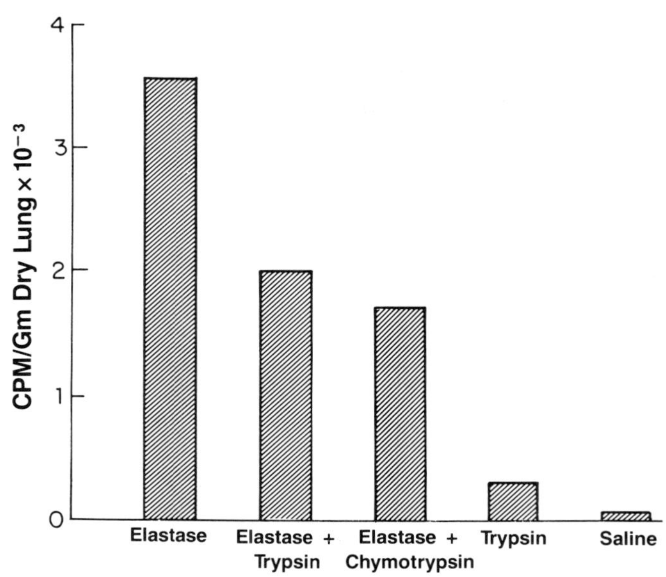

Figure 7–3. The graph depicts incorporation of ^{14}C-lysine into the desmosine crosslinks of hamster lung elastic fibers 1 week following intratracheal instillation of various enzymes. When compared with animals receiving elastase alone, those given either trypsin or chymotrypsin, 24 hours postelastase, showed diminished uptake of the radioactive label. (Animals instilled only with trypsin or saline served as negative controls.) The results suggest that secondary injury to extracellular matrix components other than elastin, such as neighboring microfibrils, adversely affects the crosslinking process. (Reproduced with permission from Cantor JO, Turino GM. Elastin and elastases in lung disease. In: Robert L, Hornbeck W, eds. Elastin and Elastases. Boca Raton: CRC Press, 1989, 159.)

age caused by intratracheal instillation[37] of elastase and inhibits elastic fiber cross-linking (Fig. 7–4).[38, 39] Radicals formed within the smoke are believed to interfere with the activity of alpha$_1$-antiprotease,[40] and might similarly affect lysyl oxidase or other components involved in maintaining the integrity of elastic fibers.

OTHER MECHANISMS. Mechanical processes may also play a role in the development of emphysema, particularly the centriacinar form. Evidence in favor of this concept is seen in studies of cadmium chloride–induced lung injury (without BAPN).[41] Interstitial scarring and atelectasis following administration of the agent induce a pattern of residual air space enlargement. Although the lesions are much less pronounced than those observed with concomitant BAPN administration, they nevertheless serve as an example of air space enlargement caused primarily by stresses in the lung parenchyma.

Therapeutic Intervention

Animal models are ideally suited to evaluating the effects of various agents on the progression of emphysema (Fig. 7–5). Although the results of such studies may not be directly applicable to the clinical setting, they nevertheless suggest possible approaches to designing better forms of treatment for patients with the disease.

Attempts to reduce the severity of emphysema have mostly involved the administration of elastase inhibitors. Alpha$_1$-antiprotease and lower molecular weight compounds have been used to mitigate the damage caused by intratracheal instillation of elastase.[42, 43] Most of these agents are effective

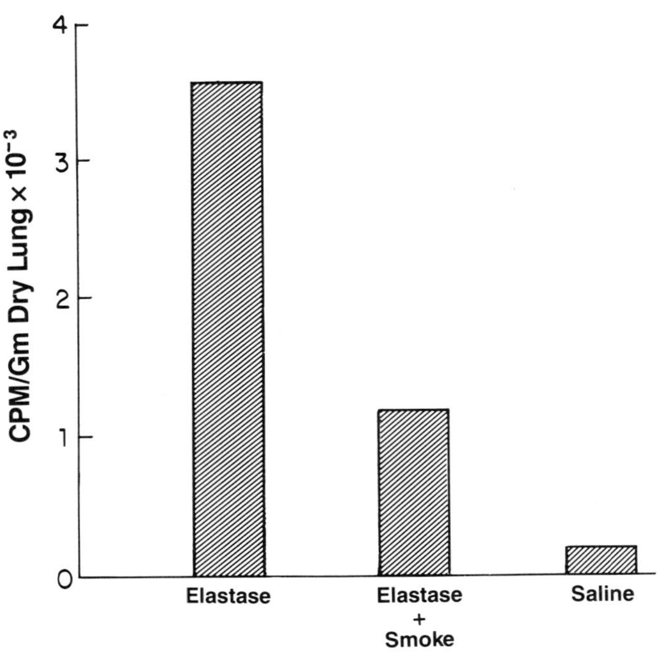

Figure 7–4. The graph depicts incorporation of ^{14}C-lysine into the desmosine crosslinks of hamster lung elastic fibers 1 week following intratracheal instillation of elastase. Animals treated with elastase and continuously exposed to cigarette smoke showed decreased uptake of the radioactive label compared with those given the enzyme and allowed to breathe room air. (Saline-instilled animals served as negative controls.) A reduction in lysyl oxidase activity was also observed,[38] suggesting that elements in the tobacco smoke, possibly free radicals, are directed against this enzyme. (Reproduced with permission from Cantor JO, Turino GM. Elastin and elastases in lung disease. In: Robert L, Hornbeck W, eds. Elastin and Elastases. Boca Raton: CRC Press, 1989, 159.)

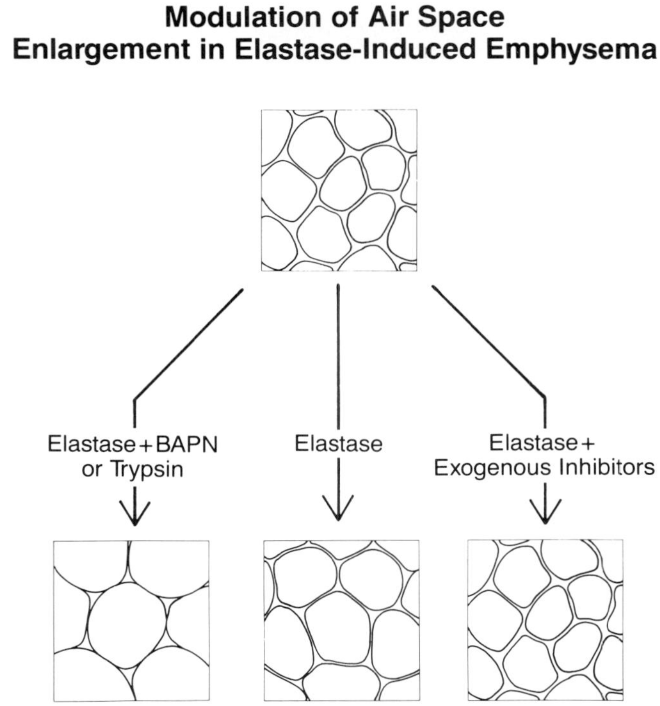

Figure 7–5. Animal models of emphysema may be used to evaluate the effects of different agents on the disease process. In the intratracheal elastase model, air space size may be increased or diminished, depending on the type of substance administered. Compounds that bind to elastase prevent damage to alveolar walls, whereas those that impair elastic fiber neosynthesis enhance injury.

only when given immediately before or after exposure to the enzyme. This finding is probably due to their rapid clearance from the body. Attaching these compounds to larger molecular weight carriers might prolong their usefulness. Furthermore, such inhibitors may have greater efficacy in models of emphysema that do not involve an extreme excess of elastase.

Although control of elastolysis is an important therapeutic goal, it is of limited value in an advanced case of emphysema, where much of the lung is already destroyed. Greater benefit might be derived from development of a means to resynthesize functional elastic fibers, thus increasing air movement through the lung and preventing further distention and rupture of alveolar septa. The ability to devise this type of treatment, however, will require much greater insight into the factors that regulate the assembly of elastic fibers.

CONCLUSIONS

Our understanding of pulmonary emphysema is becoming increasingly tied to animal models. Many of the newer ideas about the causes and potential treatment of the disease have evolved from studies that have utilized the models described in this chapter (Fig. 7–6). Whereas it was once possible to think of emphysema mainly in terms of the balance between neutrophil elastase and alpha$_1$-antiprotease, it is now necessary to consider the roles of lysyl oxidase, free radicals, and other elastolytic enzymes.

In assessing the relative contributions of these various mechanisms of lung injury, it will be necessary to develop animal models of emphysema that more faithfully represent the human disease. These models would also permit more meaningful testing of therapeutic agents. Perhaps enough is now known about elastic fiber damage and repair to begin designing new

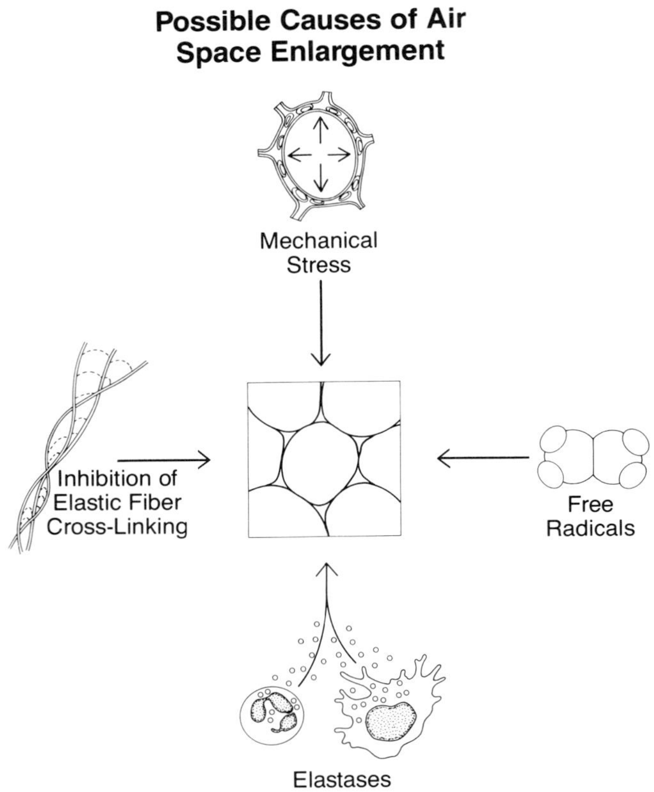

Figure 7–6. Animal models provide an important tool for investigating the various mechanisms of injury depicted. The intratracheal elastase model has been especially useful for studying the factors that influence elastic fiber repair. Cadmium chloride/beta–aminopropionitrile (BAPN)–induced emphysema is well suited for determining the cellular sources of elastase-mediated lung damage. Although these models do not accurately represent the human disease process, they nevertheless provide a means of studying analogous morphologic, physiologic, and biochemical changes under controlled, reproducible conditions.

models that combine the best features of those that already exist. The attempt to produce a more complex and subtle form of experimental injury may, itself, teach us a great deal about the intricacies of pulmonary emphysema.

REFERENCES

1. Gross P, Babyak MA, Tolker E, Kaschak M. Enzymatically produced pulmonary emphysema: a preliminary report. J Occup Med 1964; 6:481.
2. Giles RE, Finkel MP, Leeds R. The production of an emphysema-like condition in rats by the administration of papain aerosol. Proc Soc Exp Biol Med 1970; 134:157.
3. Pushpakom R, Hogg JC, Woolcock AJ, et al. Experimental papain-induced emphysema in dogs. Am Rev Respir Dis 1970; 102:778.
4. Goldring IP, Greenburg L, Ratner IM. On the production of emphysema in Syrian hamsters by aerosol inhalation of papain. Arch Environ Health 1968; 16:59.
5. Osman M, Keller S, Cerreta JM, et al. Effect of papain-induced emphysema on canine pulmonary elastin. Proc Soc Exp Biol Med 1980; 164:471.
6. Janoff A, Sloan B, Weinbaum G, et al. Experimental emphysema induced with purified human neutrophil elastase: tissue localization of the instilled protease. Am Rev Respir Dis 1977; 115:461.
7. Senior RM, Tegner H, Kuhn C, et al. The induction of pulmonary emphysema with human leukocyte elastase. Am Rev Respir Dis 1977; 116:469.
8. Kaplan PD, Kuhn C, Pierce JA. The induction of emphysema with elastase: the evolution of the lesion and the influence of serum. J Lab Clin Med 1973; 82:349.
9. Kuhn C III, Engleman W, Chraplyvy M, Starcher BC. Degradation of elastin in experimental elastase-induced emphysema measured by a radioimmunoassay for desmosine. Exp Lung Res 1983; 5:115.
10. Osman M, Kaldany RRJ, Cantor JO, et al. Stimulation of lung lysyl oxidase activity in hamsters with elastase-induced emphysema. Am Rev Respir Dis 1985; 131:169.
11. Kuhn C III, Starcher BC. The effect of lathyrogens on the evolution of elastase-induced emphysema. Am Rev Respir Dis 1980; 122:453.
12. Snider GL, Sherter CB. A one-year study of the evolution of elastase-induced emphysema in hamsters. J Appl Physiol 1977; 43:721.
13. Morris SM, Stone PJ, Snider GL, et al. Autoradiographic study of ^{3}H-methylated elastase in hamster lungs. Anat Rec 1983; 206:31.
14. Pereira W Jr, O'Brien J, Snider GL. Arterial blood gases in awake normal and emphysematous hamsters [abstract]. Clin Res 1977; 25:421A.
15. Niewoehner DE, Hoidal JR. Lung fibrosis and emphysema: divergent responses to a common injury? Science 1982; 217:359.
16. Hoidal JR, Niewoehner DE, Rao NV, Marshall BC. Cadmium chloride-induced emphysema in lathyrogenic hamsters. In: Cantor JO, ed. Handbook of Animal Models of Pulmonary Disease. Boca Raton: CRC Press, 1989, 159.
17. Kleinerman J, Ip MPC. Effects of nitrogen dioxide on elastin and collagen contents of lung. Arch Environ Health 1979; 34:228.
18. Blank J, Glasgow JE, Pietra GG, et al. Nitrogen-dioxide-induced emphysema in rats: lack of worsening by beta-aminopropionitrile treatment. Am Rev Respir Dis 1988; 137:376.
19. Blackwood RA, Cantor JO, Moret J, et al. Glycosaminoglycan synthesis in endotoxin-induced lung injury. Proc Soc Exp Biol Med 1983; 174:343.
20. Guenter CA, Coalson JJ, Jacques J. Emphysema associated with intravascular leukocyte sequestration: comparison with papain-induced emphysema. Am Rev Respir Dis 1981; 123:79.
21. Blackwood RA, Moret J, Mandl I, Turino GM. Emphysema induced by intravenously administered endotoxin in an alpha$_1$-antitrypsin-deficient rat model. Am Rev Respir Dis 1984; 130:231.
22. O'Dell BL, Kilburn KH, McKenzie WN, Thurston RJ. The lung of the copper-deficient rat: a model for developmental pulmonary emphysema. Am J Pathol 1978; 91:413.
23. Soskel NT, Watanabe S, Hammond E, et al. A copper-deficient, zinc-supplemented diet produces emphysema in pigs. Am Rev Respir Dis 1982; 126:316.
24. Fisk DE, Kuhn C. Emphysema-like changes in the lungs of the blotchy mouse. Am Rev Respir Dis 1976; 113:787.
25. Ranga V, Kleinerman J. Lung injury and repair in the blotchy mouse: effects of nitrogen dioxide inhalation. Am Rev Respir Dis 1981; 123:90.
26. Lechner AJ. Growth retardation and mortality in guinea pigs following perinatal starvation. Nutr Rep Int 1984; 30:1435.
27. Lechner AJ. Perinatal age determines the severity of retarded lung development induced by starvation. Am Rev Respir Dis 1985; 131:638.
28. Sahebjami H, Wirman JA. Emphysema-like changes in the lungs of starved rats. Am Rev Respir Dis 1981; 124:619.
29. Kerr JS. Lung injury induced by nutritional restriction. In: Cantor JO, ed. Handbook of Animal Models of Pulmonary Disease. Boca Raton: CRC Press, 1989, 159.
30. Szapiel SV, Fulmer JD, Hunninghake GW, et al. Hereditary emphysema in the tight-skin (Tsk/+) mouse. Am Rev Respir Dis 1981; 123:680.
31. Kueppers F. Animal models of emphysema. In: Taylor JC, Mittman C, eds. Pulmonary Emphysema and Proteolysis: 1986. Orlando: Academic Press, 1987, 485.
32. Johanson WG Jr, Pierce AK. Effects of elastase, collagenase, and papain on structure and function of rat lungs *in vitro*. J Clin Invest 1972; 51:288.
33. Osman M, Keller S, Hosannah Y, et al. Impairment of elastin resynthesis in the lungs of hamsters with experimental emphysema induced by sequential administration of elastase and trypsin. J Lab Clin Med 1985; 104:254.
34. Hoidal JR, Niewoehner DE, Rao NV, Hibbs MS. The role of

neutrophils in the development of cadmium-chloride-induced emphysema in lathyrogen-fed hamsters. Am J Pathol 1985; 120:22.
35. Mass B, Ikeda T, Meranze DR, et al. Induction of experimental emphysema: cellular and species specificity. Am Rev Respir Dis 1972; 106:384.
36. Riley DJ, Kramer MJ, Kerr JS, et al. Damage and repair of lung connective tissue in rats exposed to toxic levels of oxygen. Am Rev Respir Dis 1987; 135:441.
37. Hoidal JR, Niewoehner DE. Cigarette smoke inhalation potentiates elastase-induced emphysema in hamsters. Am Rev Respir Dis 1983; 127:478.
38. Osman M, Cantor JO, Roffman S, et al. Cigarette smoke impairs elastin resynthesis in lungs of hamsters with elastase-induced emphysema. Am Rev Respir Dis 1985; 132:640.
39. Laurent P, Janoff A, Kagan HM. Cigarette smoke blocks cross-linking of elastin in-vitro. Am Rev Respir Dis 1983; 127:189.
40. Pryor WA. The free radical chemistry of cigarette smoke and the inactivation of alpha$_1$-proteinase inhibitor. In: Taylor JC, Mittman C, eds. Pulmonary Emphysema and Proteolysis: 1986. Orlando: Academic Press, 1987, 369.
41. Snider GL, Lucey EC, Faris B, et al. Cadmium-chloride-induced air-space enlargement with interstitial pulmonary fibrosis is not associated with destruction of lung elastin. Am Rev Respir Dis 1988; 137:918.
42. Martorana PA, Share NN. Effect of human alpha$_1$-antitrypsin on papain-induced emphysema in the hamster. Am Rev Respir Dis 1976; 113:607.
43. Snider GL, Lucey EC, Stone PJ. Animal models of emphysema. Am Rev Respir Dis 1986; 133:149.
44. Cantor JO, Turino GM. Elastin and elastases in lung disease. In: Robert L, Hornebeck W, eds. Elastin and Elastases. Boca Raton: CRC Press, 1989, 159.

Section III

PHYSIOLOGIC RESPONSES TO CHRONIC OBSTRUCTIVE PULMONARY DISEASE

Chapter 8

EFFECTS OF COPD ON GAS EXCHANGE

Peter D. Wagner

This chapter primarily addresses the ways in which chronic obstructive pulmonary disease (COPD) leads to disturbances of gas exchange, arterial partial pressure of oxygen (Po_2) and partial pressure of carbon dioxide (Pco_2) in particular. Abnormalities in arterial blood gases are common to a host of pulmonary diseases, however, so an attempt has been made to delve deeper into the relationships between structure and function in an effort to provide an understanding of how the pathophysiologic changes of COPD lead to disturbances of gas exchange. This is closely related to the question of what gas exchange measurements can tell us about the functional significance of pathophysiologic abnormalities in COPD, which is also discussed.

The relationships among pathologic change, functional deterioration, and clinical status are still somewhat unclear. We all have come to recognize the "pink puffer" and "blue bloater" of Burrows and colleagues,[3] and one's first instinct is to associate the former with emphysema and the latter with chronic bronchitis, both of which are in themselves reasonably well understood in pathologic terms. However, Flenley and colleagues[6] suggest a different possible basis for these two clinical types, namely, an inherent difference in ventilatory response to chemical and other stimuli: the blue bloaters fail to respond normally to chemical or other stimuli for respiration. A major objective of this chapter is to relate the gas exchange picture to clinical type and, by hypothesis, to the underlying pathology.

Another issue addressed is the importance of each of the classic causes of hypoxemia in COPD, both at rest and during exercise.

The majority of this chapter focuses on patients with advanced disease not only because the structure-function relationships become more apparent as disease progresses, but also because most data so far accumulated pertain to advanced disease. Finally, because arterial Po_2 and Pco_2 are determined by both intrapulmonary and extrapulmonary factors, much of the most insightful data obtained to date are based on direct measurements of ventilation-perfusion ($\dot{V}_A/\dot{Q}$) inequality made with the multiple inert elimination technique[5, 19] together with simultaneous measurements of overall variables such as ventilation, blood flow, flow of oxygen ($\dot{V}o_2$), and carbon dioxide output ($\dot{V}co_2$) and arterial blood gases.

ARTERIAL BLOOD GAS PATTERNS IN COPD

Every medical student is taught that COPD produces arterial hypoxemia and may also lead to hypercapnia. The range of values encompassed is very broad and relates poorly to the degree of airflow obstruction as measured by conventional approaches, such as forced spirometry. Figure 8–1, from a study of 23 patients with advanced COPD, shows this dissociation well.[18] Clearly, patients with advanced disease can have well-preserved arterial blood gas values, whereas those with more abnormal arterial Po_2 and Pco_2 are not necessarily those with the most severe disease by spirometric criteria.

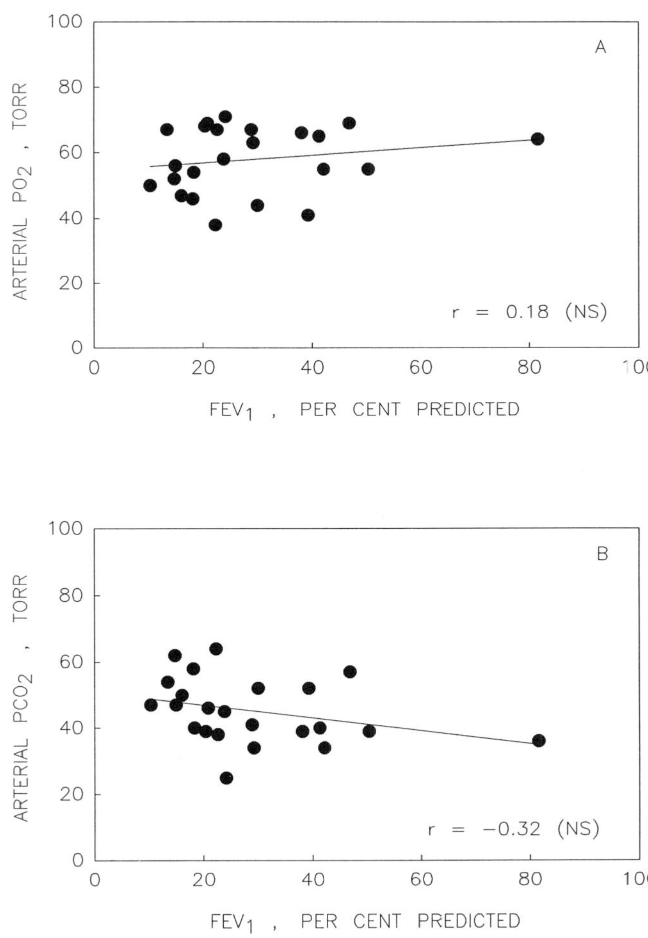

Figure 8–1. Relationship between *(A)* arterial partial pressure of oxygen (Po_2) and forced expired volume in 1 second (FEV_1) (percent predicted) and *(B)* arterial partial pressure of carbon dioxide (Pco_2) and FEV_1 (percent predicted). No significant relationships are apparent, indicating that it is not possible to predict the degree of hypoxemia or hypercapnia from such spirometric indices. (From Wagner PD, et al. Am Rev Respir Dis 1978; 118:511–524.)

This work was supported by NIH grant HL 17731. I also wish to thank Tania Davisson for her assistance in its preparation.

As discussed subsequently, the explanation for this at first puzzling lack of good correlation is probably not obscure. Firstly, the degree of severity and the pattern of the $\dot{V}_A/\dot{Q}$ distribution are not closely related to forced expiratory volume in 1 second (FEV_1), yet $\dot{V}_A/\dot{Q}$ relationships play a large role in determining arterial Po_2, as known for many years.[21, 23] Secondly, the total alveolar ventilation varies greatly among patients; this has considerable additional effect on arterial blood gases, Pco_2 in particular. Those patients with greater ventilation have less hypoxemia and less, or no, hypercapnia, all other factors aside. Thirdly, when subnormal, the cardiac output has yet another independent influence on arterial Po_2 because a reduction in cardiac output leads to a lower mixed venous Po_2, which may depress arterial Po_2.

Taken together, these three factors can explain an individual's arterial blood gas findings. In other words, for a given (1) pattern and degree of severity of $\dot{V}_A/\dot{Q}$ relationships, (2) total alveolar ventilation, and (3) cardiac output, the arterial Po_2 and Pco_2 of an individual patient are not difficult to understand. The obvious questions in the present context are, therefore, (1) how does lung pathologic change alter $\dot{V}_A/\dot{Q}$ distribution; (2) what sets total (alveolar) ventilation in any one patient; and (3) what determines cardiac output in each patient?

THE VENTILATION-PERFUSION RATIO DISTRIBUTION IN COPD

That $\dot{V}_A/\dot{Q}$ inequality is of great significance in COPD is beyond dispute; this has been recognized for many years. Briscoe and colleagues[2] put much effort into analyzing the N_2 washout patterns and the response of arterial Po_2 to elevated fractional inspired oxygen (FIO_2) in patients with COPD and clearly showed the presence of $\dot{V}_A/\dot{Q}$ inequality. The N_2 washout technique also showed gross inequality of specific ventilation, i.e., the distribution of ventilation per unit lung volume, such that it was very clear that some lung units had a very low ratio of alveolar ventilation to lung volume. The Briscoe approach cannot rigorously associate blood flow with such poorly ventilated units, so their $\dot{V}_A/\dot{Q}$ ratio is not known. Typical analyses according to the Briscoe scheme, involving assumptions about the matching of compartmental blood flow to ventilation, are shown in Figure 8–2, taken from King and Briscoe.[10] Their technique also does not permit rigorous identification of $\dot{V}_A/\dot{Q}$, as opposed to diffusion-perfusion abnormalities, as responsible for the hypoxemia. Various combinations of both forms of gas exchange interference can be found to fit the measured data.

The multiple inert gas elimination technique,[5, 19] in contrast, cannot shed light on gas volume distribution but does relate ventilation to blood flow and permit distinction of $\dot{V}_A/\dot{Q}$ inequality and reduced rates of diffusion equilibration as determinants of hypoxemia.[15, 22]

Figure 8–3 shows the three typical patterns of $\dot{V}_A/\dot{Q}$ mismatch observed in patients with advanced COPD (FEV_1 <30% of predicted).[16] For reference purposes, the typical pattern observed in young (20- to 40-year old), healthy subjects at rest would appear like the $\dot{V}_A/\dot{Q}$ mode centered on a $\dot{V}_A/\dot{Q}$ ratio of about 1 in panels A and B, i.e., without the additional modes of high or low $\dot{V}_A/\dot{Q}$ regions. All three panels present "frequency function"–type information, showing the relative amount of ventilation and blood flow associated with the various regions of the $\dot{V}_A\dot{Q}$ spectrum from zero (unventilated lung or shunt) through normal $\dot{V}_A/\dot{Q}$ ratios (roughly 0.2 to 5.0) to infinite (unperfused lung or dead space).[19] The data are obtained by computer-assisted analysis of the pattern of elimination of a set of six inert gases of differing blood

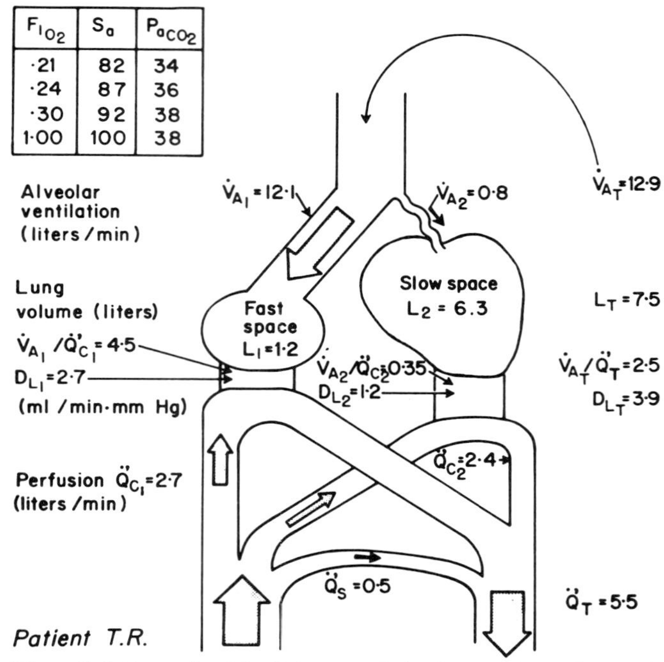

Figure 8–2. Example of the Briscoe analysis of gas exchange in chronic obstructive lung disease. Based on the response of arterial partial pressure of oxygen (Po_2) to increasing concentrations of inspired oxygen, and also on the results of a multibreath nitrogen washout, the lung is divided into two compartments: a well-ventilated fast space and poorly ventilated slow space. See text for further discussion. (From King TKC, et al. J Appl Physiol 1967; 23:672–682.)

solubilities, which are administered dissolved in 5% dextrose by constant intravenous infusion.[5, 16, 20] These patterns are shown in the left-hand panels as retention (R) and excretion (E) plots.

The distribution seen in healthy subjects is narrow (log SD, the 2nd moment of the distribution about its mean on a log $\dot{V}_A/\dot{Q}$ scale is usually about 0.3) and is centered on a mean $\dot{V}_A/\dot{Q}$ of about 1.

By comparison, panels A, B, and C show marked abnormalities in the pattern and extent of $\dot{V}_A/\dot{Q}$ mismatch. Panel A shows a separate population of high $\dot{V}_A/\dot{Q}$ areas in the $\dot{V}_A/\dot{Q}$ range 10 to 100, but *no* clear group of low $\dot{V}_A/\dot{Q}$ areas. Note that because virtually all of the cardiac output but only about half of the ventilation perfuses the left-hand population of units, its mean $\dot{V}_A/\dot{Q}$ ratio is less than the normal value of about 1, at about 0.6. Structurally, panel A is most likely to reflect two major populations of lung units: (1) those whose perfusion has been greatly reduced in the presence of continued ventilation, thus producing the high $\dot{V}_A/\dot{Q}$ mode, and (2) the rest of the lung with somewhat subnormal $\dot{V}_A/\dot{Q}$ ratios secondary to the redistribution of blood flow away from the first group of units. The possible pathologic basis for this pattern is discussed later in this chapter.

Panel B shows the second common pattern of $\dot{V}_A/\dot{Q}$ distribution in COPD, a mirror image of that in panel A. Two populations of units are noted, but now one has $\dot{V}_A/\dot{Q}$ ratios in the normal range and the other is a mode of very low $\dot{V}_A/\dot{Q}$ units. These $\dot{V}_A/\dot{Q}$ values lie in the range of 0.01 to 0.1 or thereabouts. We would interpret the genesis of this pattern as a situation in which considerable airway obstruction has attenuated local alveolar ventilation while perfusion has been maintained, at least in part, thus giving rise to portions of the lung with a very low $\dot{V}_A/\dot{Q}$ ratio. Again, the mode of normal $\dot{V}_A/\dot{Q}$ units presumably reflects those areas not subject to dramatic airway obstruction.

In both panels A and B it is necessary to involve the concept of nonuniform pathologic changes in the COPD-affected lung

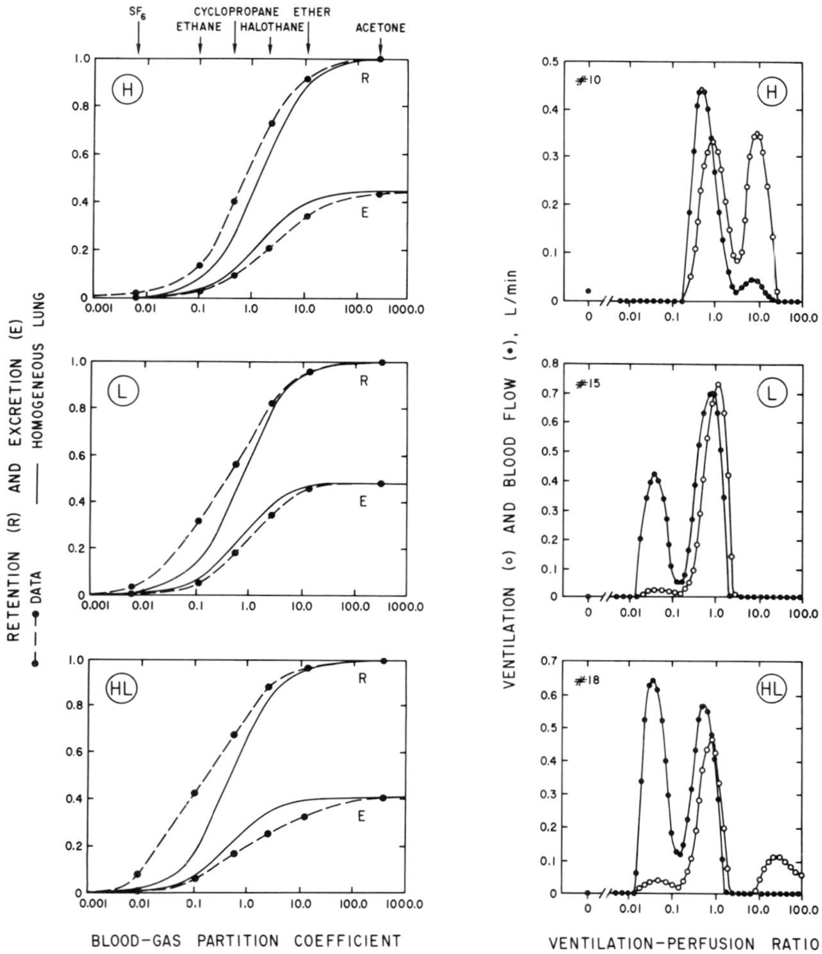

Figure 8–3. Patterns of ventilation-perfusion ratio distribution in chronic obstructive lung disease. These were obtained with the multiple inert gas elimination technique based on the steady state retention (R) and excretion (E) of 6 different inert gases infused intravenously under steady state conditions (left panels). The right panels show the corresponding ventilation-perfusion ($\dot{V}_A/\dot{Q}$) distributions and indicate the three stereotyped patterns (labeled H, L, and HL) generally observed in advanced COPD. The interpretation and presumed pathophysiologic basis of these distributions are discussed in the text. (From Wagner PD, et al. J Clin Invest 1977; 59:203–216.)

whereby some areas are relatively unaffected in terms of gas exchange and others are considerably abnormal. The presumed pathologic basis of the changes in panel B is discussed later in this chapter.

Panel C shows the third pattern seen in advanced COPD; it is the simultaneous presence of the two patterns in panels A and B and thus presumes the same pathologic bases as discussed previously in each case.

That such clear-cut patterns of $\dot{V}_A/\dot{Q}$ distribution have been observed in COPD has been confirmed by several investigators using the multiple inert gas elimination technique in patients with similarly advanced disease.[4, 11, 13] Of special note is the virtual absence of significant amounts of true shunt in patients with stable COPD. For example, only two of 23 patients in our original study had more than 4% right-to-left shunt, and in the remaining 21, shunt averaged only 0.7% of the cardiac output.[16]

This observation at first sight would seem to conflict with the traditional finding that arterial P_{O_2} on 100% O_2 in such patients often fails to reach values of more than 400 torr, suggesting that a sizable shunt is present. The explanation for the apparent discrepancy lies in the observations of Briscoe and colleagues[2] of the presence of lung units in which N_2 turnover is very slow. Thus, 30 minutes of O_2 breathing does not fully eliminate alveolar N_2, keeping alveolar and hence arterial P_{O_2} from rising rapidly. In other words, a 30-minute N_2 washout is insufficient for the purposes of shunt measurement in patients with advanced COPD.

Patterns of $\dot{V}_A/\dot{Q}$ shown in panels A and B do not merely reflect different levels of total ventilation. If alveolar ventilation in panel A were reduced in every $\dot{V}_A/\dot{Q}$ unit, the whole distribution would be displaced leftward as each unit $\dot{V}_A/\dot{Q}$ were reduced and eventually would look very much like the example in panel B. Because of the log $\dot{V}_A/\dot{Q}$ scale in Figure 8–3, completely unphysiologic reductions in ventilation of two orders of magnitude would be required for this to happen, but this cannot be. Consequently, panels A and B may reflect fundamentally different pathophysiologic processes and not simply modulation by extrapulmonary variables.

Figure 8–4 demonstrates that the pattern of $\dot{V}_A/\dot{Q}$ mismatch per se as shown in Figure 8–3 is poorly related to arterial blood gas values, although trends are apparent in our particular group of subjects. It is not only pattern, but severity combined with extrapulmonary factors, e.g., total ventilation and blood flow, that together explain arterial P_{O_2} in each patient.

Figure 8–5 shows that FEV_1 is also poorly related to the $\dot{V}_A/\dot{Q}$ pattern per se. Although the format of Figure 8–5 does not incorporate severity of $\dot{V}_A/\dot{Q}$ inequality, the figure does emphasize that degree of airflow obstruction does not permit prediction of the $\dot{V}_A/\dot{Q}$ pattern. The best explanation for the lack of this relationship would seem to be that reductions in FEV_1 in COPD are produced by various mechanisms that may vary among patients. As covered previously in more detail, obstruction due to loss of elastic recoil and thus to lack of support of peripheral airways may not give rise to low $\dot{V}_A/\dot{Q}$ areas. Conversely, obstruction due to airway distortion, luminal secretions, or wall thickening is presumed more likely to give rise to low $\dot{V}_A/\dot{Q}$ regions, just as in asthma.[17]

Figure 8–6 shows the relationship between clinical type A or B according to the Burrows and Fletcher[3] scheme and the

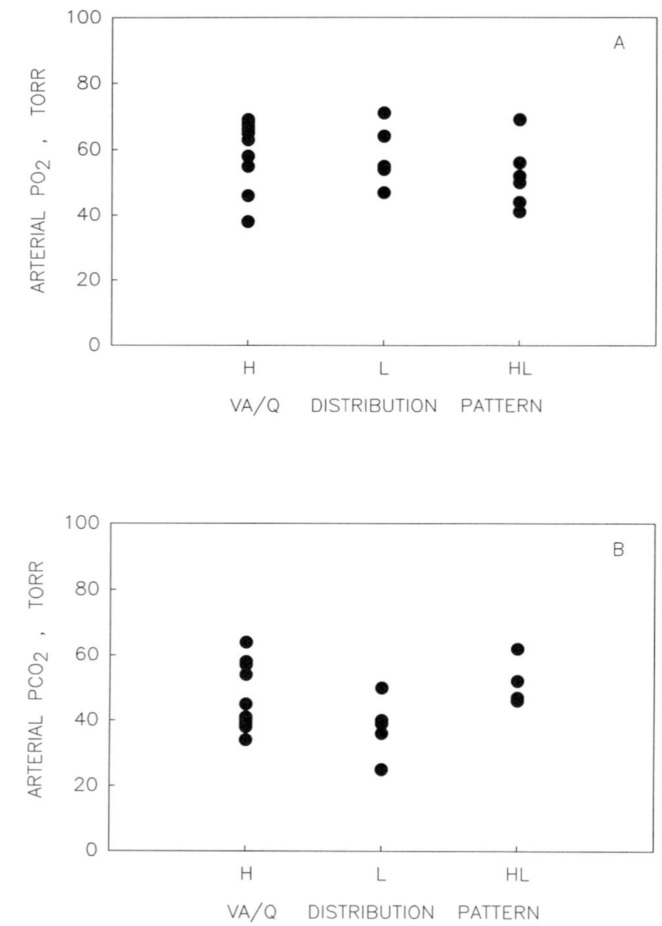

Figure 8–4. Relationship between arterial P_{O_2} and the pattern of ventilation-perfusion ratio ($\dot{V}_A/\dot{Q}$) distribution as defined in Figure 8–3. There is no clear-cut relationship between the degree of hypoxemia and the pattern of distribution, indicating that additional factors must be in part responsible for arterial partial pressure of oxygen (P_{O_2}). Similar interpretation applies to the determinants of arterial partial pressure of carbon dioxide (P_{CO_2}) as shown in the lower panel.

$\dot{V}_A/\dot{Q}$ pattern. The two panels in Figure 8–6 reflect the same data plotted two different ways. A clear-cut relationship between type A and the high $\dot{V}_A/\dot{Q}$ pattern is seen. Thus, ten of 11 patients of type A or mixed type had high $\dot{V}_A/\dot{Q}$ regions. Presumably there is a rational basis for the association between high $\dot{V}_A/\dot{Q}$ areas and emphysema, i.e., emphysema expected to be present on the basis of increased compliance, hyperinflation, and increased alveolar ventilation. The work of Barberá and associates[1] supports this notion. Barberá and associates used the multiple inert gas elimination technique in patients prior to lobectomy for solitary lesions and subsequently determined the degree of pathologic emphysema in the excised lobe. They found a significant relationship between the prevalence of high $\dot{V}_A/\dot{Q}$ regions and the severity of emphysema.

The relationships among $\dot{V}_A/\dot{Q}$ patterns and clinical type are not so clear-cut in type B patients. However, Figure 8–6 does show that most type B or mixed-category patients have low $\dot{V}_A/\dot{Q}$ areas (ten of 15). Thus, simultaneous presence of high $\dot{V}_A/\dot{Q}$ and low $\dot{V}_A/\dot{Q}$ areas in some type B patients may reflect the presence of emphysema and chronic bronchitis, the former being notably difficult to document in life, especially if chronic bronchitis is present.

Figures 8–4, 8–5, and 8–6 are summarized in the subsequent list. Relationships among gas exchange, spirometry, clinical presentation, and pattern of $\dot{V}_A/\dot{Q}$ distribution are certainly complex, but logical threads in these relationships suggest some order in what is apparent chaos. These conclusions are, however, tentative.

1. Areas of high $\dot{V}_A/\dot{Q}$ ratio probably reflect destroyed alveoli, and hence alveolar capillaries, in which air spaces remain ventilated, i.e., emphysema.
2. Areas of low $\dot{V}_A/\dot{Q}$ ratio probably reflect airways obstruction on the basis of distortion, wall thickening and luminal secretions, i.e., chronic bronchitis, and not dynamic compression.
3. The degree of arterial hypoxemia is not difficult to understand even while there is little apparent relationship to other manifestations and abnormalities of COPD; it is the integrated result of the severity and pattern of $\dot{V}_A/\dot{Q}$ mismatch, total alveolar ventilation, and cardiac output. Much the same applies to hypercapnia.
4. Clinical type (A or B) probably reflects both the relative importance of emphysema versus bronchitis and the overall level of alveolar ventilation. Thus, patients with more emphysema and less bronchitis who maintain alveolar ventilation become type A. Patients with more bronchitis who fail to maintain ventilation become type B.
5. The lack of relationship between FEV_1 and arterial blood gases or $\dot{V}_A/\dot{Q}$ pattern may reflect the relative importance of dynamic compression versus the other mechanisms of obstruction such that emphysema, causing dynamic compression, does not produce low $\dot{V}_A/\dot{Q}$ areas. Chronic bronchitis, having different mechanisms of obstruction, does often lead to low $\dot{V}_A/\dot{Q}$ regions.
6. Type B patients with high $\dot{V}_A/\dot{Q}$ areas presumably have emphysema as well as chronic bronchitis. Type A patients with low $\dot{V}_A/\dot{Q}$ areas are rarely encountered (1 of 11 patients only).

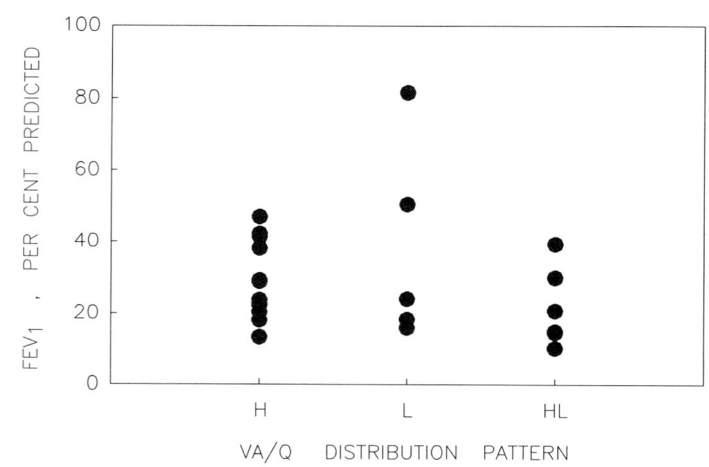

Figure 8–5. Relationship between percent predicted FEV_1 and the pattern of the ventilation-perfusion ratio ($\dot{V}_A/\dot{Q}$) distribution. As with gas exchange variables, there is no clear relationship between the degree of airway obstruction and the pattern of $\dot{V}_A/\dot{Q}$ distribution as discussed in the text.

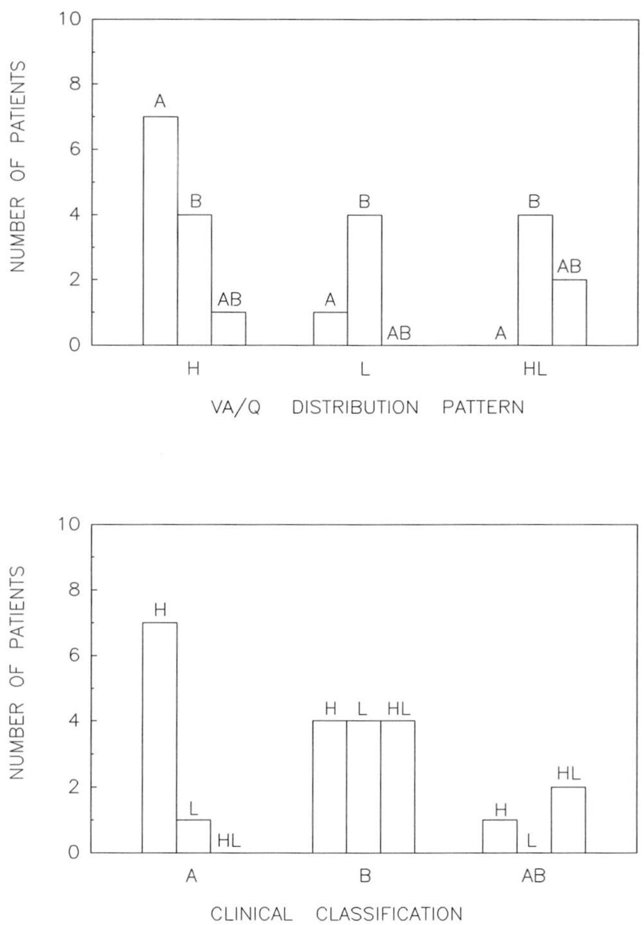

Figure 8–6. Relationship between the ventilation-perfusion ratio ($\dot{V}_A/\dot{Q}$) distribution pattern (H, L, or HL, as in Figure 8–3) and the clinical classification of the patients according to the Burrows and Fletcher criteria (A, B, or mixed [AB]). Note that 10 of 11 patients with type A characteristics possessed areas of high ventilation-perfusion ratio, and only one type A patient did not show such areas. Ten of 15 patients with type B characteristics had areas of low $\dot{V}_A/\dot{Q}$ ratio and only five did not. See text for more complete discussion of these associations.

PHYSIOLOGIC BASIS OF HYPOXEMIA IN COPD

As discussed previously, despite the apparently poor relationships among spirometric changes, $\dot{V}_A/\dot{Q}$ patterns, and hypoxemia in COPD, some order is apparent. With direct estimates of the $\dot{V}_A/\dot{Q}$ distribution made by the multiple inert gas elimination technique and simultaneous measurement of total ventilation and blood flow, it is a relatively straightforward matter to compute the arterial P_{O_2} expected to result from the interaction of all these variables. This is done by computer-assisted analyses,[23, 25] employing numeric algorithms describing the O_2 and CO_2 dissociation curves such as those of Kelman.[8, 9] Figure 8–7 shows that for the group of 23 patients in our study,[16] such predicted values of arterial P_{O_2} match those obtained by conventional arterial sampling and measurement by blood gas electrodes. This agreement (the regression line is not different from the identity line) demonstrates that under the operating values for total ventilation and blood flow, the degree of $\dot{V}_A/\dot{Q}$ inequality completely accounts for observed hypoxemia over a wide range, a finding that has been confirmed by others.[4, 11] In turn, these data exclude other potential causes of hypoxemia, notably shunting in almost all outpatients studied to date, and diffusion limitation of pulmonary O_2 transfer. Shunting is excluded simply by its absence according to the multiple inert gas elimination technique; diffusion limitation is excluded because of the agreement between measured and predicted arterial oxygen pressure (Pa_{O_2}).[22] Thus, if diffusion limitation had been a significant factor, it would have been manifested by measured arterial P_{O_2} values that were systematically lower than those predicted by the inert gas technique. This is because inert gases are essentially invulnerable to diffusion limitation in the lungs,[7, 16] in contrast to O_2, which can be diffusion-limited under certain conditions.[14, 18, 21]

Although not evident from Figure 8–7, another factor is of relevance in determining arterial P_{O_2}, i.e., the mixed venous P_{O_2}, where in the context of shunts the effect has been clearly pointed out.[12] Thus, for a given degree of $\dot{V}_A/\dot{Q}$ mismatch, a reduction in mixed venous P_{O_2} decreases the arterial P_{O_2}. This is taken into account in the predictions of Figure 8–7, but a quantitative analysis of the importance of this effect has not been included herein.

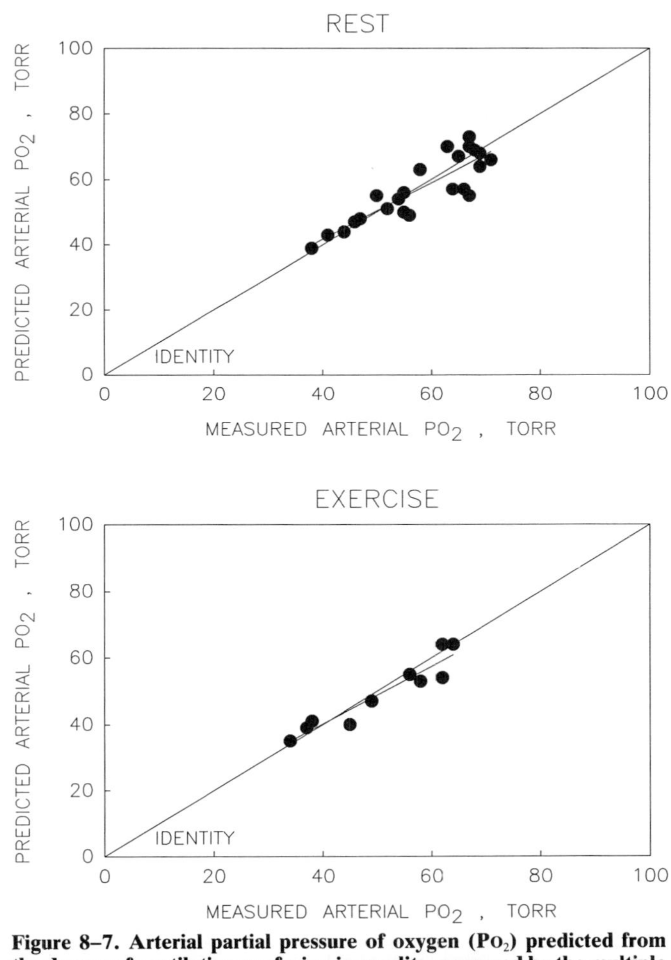

Figure 8–7. Arterial partial pressure of oxygen (P_{O_2}) predicted from the degree of ventilation-perfusion inequality measured by the multiple inert gas elimination technique compared with measured arterial P_{O_2}. The relationships for both rest and exercise are shown and are not different from the identity line. This indicates that hypoxemia both at rest and at exercise is fully explained by the measured amounts of ventilation blood flow mismatch. In particular, alveolar-capillary diffusion equilibration is complete, and therefore diffusion limitation is not a factor in the hypoxemia of these patients. (From Wagner PD, et al. J Clin Invest 1977; 59:203–216.)

GAS EXCHANGE DURING EXERCISE IN COPD

The final topic addressed in this chapter is the changes in gas exchange in COPD observed during exercise. The data discussed pertain to advanced disease in the main, and in patients so affected, the achievable increase in oxygen uptake ($\dot{V}O_2$) above resting levels is not great—from 280 to 620 ml/min in our patients.[16] Thus, to exercise in a relatively steady state for some 5 to 8 minutes, $\dot{V}O_2$ levels are generally less than 1 L/min, with total ventilation increasing from 11 L/min at rest to 21 L/min in our group. At the same time, cardiac output increased from 5.6 L/min to only 8.7 L/min. These small changes should be contrasted with those of normal subjects who can mount a $\dot{V}O_2$ in excess of 3 L/min at levels of ventilation well over 100 L/min and of cardiac output of 25 L/min or so. It should not be surprising that the effects of these low exercise levels in patients with COPD are modest.

In terms of arterial blood gas levels, PO_2 may fall, remain unchanged, or even rise. We noted a mean fall of 7 torr from 58 to 51 torr. Likewise, arterial carbon dioxide pressure ($PaCO_2$) may fall, remain the same, or rise; we found a 5 torr rise. Direct measurements of the degree of $\dot{V}_A/\dot{Q}$ mismatch show no significant changes,[4, 16] and, as at rest, shunts are of negligible proportions. Again, as at rest, no evidence of alveolar-capillary O_2 diffusion limitation is found during exercise.[4, 16] This finding is demonstrated in the lower panel of Figure 8–7. However, in all patients, just as in normal subjects, mixed venous PO_2 falls because the relative increase in $\dot{V}O_2$ from rest exceeds the relative increase in cardiac output. In those subjects for whom all of the aforementioned general findings are true, explanation of blood gas changes during exercise is generally simple. Thus, changes in arterial PCO_2 reflect the change in the ratio of alveolar ventilation to $\dot{V}CO_2$, comparing rest with exercise. If exercise produces a lesser relative increase in alveolar ventilation than in $\dot{V}CO_2$, arterial PCO_2 will rise. If alveolar ventilation were to rise relatively more than $\dot{V}CO_2$, arterial PCO_2 would fall, other factors unchanged. Similarly, arterial PO_2 will be affected by the relative changes in alveolar ventilation and $\dot{V}O_2$. However, through the effect of cardiac output on mixed venous PO_2, arterial PO_2 may also be affected by changes in the ratio of cardiac output to $\dot{V}O_2$ from rest to exercise. Thus, if $\dot{V}O_2$ rises relatively more than blood flow, as normally happens, mixed venous PO_2 must fall; all other factors unchanged, this fall in mixed venous PO_2 will cause a fall in arterial PO_2.

Thus, given the very limited exercise of which COPD patients are capable, arterial blood gas alterations on exercise are determined mostly by extrapulmonary factors: $\dot{V}O_2$, $\dot{V}CO_2$, alveolar ventilation, and cardiac output, and in particular by the ratios of $\dot{V}O_2$ and $\dot{V}CO_2$ to ventilation and $\dot{V}O_2$ to blood flow. Individual patients may not fit this simple paradigm in that changes in $\dot{V}_A/\dot{Q}$ relationships, either improvement or deterioration, may also occur.

SUMMARY

Although it is known that COPD can produce hypoxemia and sometimes hypercapnia, the relationships among blood gas values, $\dot{V}_A/\dot{Q}$ distribution, spirometric indices of airways obstruction, and clinical profile at first sight appear poor. Considerable sense can be made out of apparent chaos by recognizing that: (1) the $\dot{V}_A/\dot{Q}$ pattern probably depends on dominant pathologic changes, i.e., emphysema produces high $\dot{V}_A/\dot{Q}$ areas and chronic bronchitis low $\dot{V}_A/\dot{Q}$ areas; (2) the overall level of ventilation independently modulates arterial PO_2 and PCO_2, and it may have as much to do with clinical profile as do the pathologic changes per se, and as much to do with abnormal blood gases as does the $\dot{V}_A/\dot{Q}$ pattern per se; (3) there are several mechanisms of airway obstruction, in particular, dynamic compression in emphysema and airway distortion or luminal encroachment in chronic bronchitis, and it appears that dynamic compression does not cause a reduction in $\dot{V}_A/\dot{Q}$ ratio in the corresponding segment of lung. Thus, despite similar degrees of reduction in FEV_1, different obstructive mechanisms may produce different $\dot{V}_A/\dot{Q}$ abnormalities. Although some of these statements are supported by data as shown herein, some remain speculative. There is much room for further clarification of the physiologic basis of these relationships, and ultimately we will need to directly relate structure to function in these most unfortunate patients to achieve such an understanding.

REFERENCES

1. Barberá JA, Ramirez J, Roca J, et al. Lung structure and gas exchange in mild chronic obstructive pulmonary disease. Am Rev Respir Dis (in press, 1990).
2. Briscoe WA, Cree EM, Filler S, et al. Lung volume, alveolar ventilation and perfusion interrelationships in chronic pulmonary emphysema. J Appl Physiol 1960; 15:785–795.
3. Burrows B, Fletcher CM, Heard BE, et al. The emphysematous and bronchial types of chronic airways obstruction. A clinicopathological study of patients in London and Chicago. Lancet 1966; i:830–835.
4. Dantzker DR, D'Alonzo GE: The effect of exercise on pulmonary gas exchange in patients with severe chronic obstructive pulmonary disease. Am Rev Respir Dis 1986; 134:1135–1139.
5. Evans JW, Wagner PD: Limits on $\dot{V}_A/\dot{Q}$ distributions from analysis of experimental inert gas elimination. J Appl Physiol 1977; 42:889–898.
6. Flenley DC, Franklin DH, Millar JS: The hypoxic drive to breathing in chronic bronchitis and emphysema. Clin Sci 1970; 38:503–518.
7. Forster RE: Exchange of gases between alveolar air and pulmonary capillary blood: pulmonary diffusing capacity. Physiol Rev 1957; 37:391–452.
8. Kelman GR: Digital computer subroutine for the conversion of oxygen tension into saturation. J Appl Physiol 1965; 21:1375–1376.
9. Kelman GR: Computer programs for the production of O_2-CO_2 diagrams. Respir Physiol 1968; 4:260–269.
10. King TKC, Briscoe WA: Blood gas exchange in emphysema: an example illustrating method of calculation. J Appl Physiol 1967; 23:672–682.
11. Marthan R, Castaing I, Manier G, Guenard H: Gas exchange alterations in patients with chronic obstructive lung disease. Chest 1985; 87:470–475.
12. Pontopiddan H, Geffin B, Lowenstein E: Acute Respiratory Failure in the Adult. Boston: Little, Brown and Co., Inc., 1973.
13. Roca J, Montserrat JM, Rodriguez-Roisin R, et al. Gas exchange response to naxolone in chronic obstructive pulmonary disease with hypercapnic respiratory failure. Bull Eur Physiopathol Respir 1987; 23:249–254.
14. Torre-Bueno J, Wagner PD, Saltzman HA, et al. Diffusion limitation in normal humans during exercise at sea level and simulated altitude. J Appl Physiol 1985; 58:989–995.
15. Wagner PD: Diffusion and chemical reaction in pulmonary gas exchange. Physiol Rev 1977; 57:257–312.
16. Wagner PD, Dantzker DR, Dueck R, et al. Ventilation-perfusion inequality in chronic obstructive pulmonary disease. J Clin Invest 1977; 59:203–216.
17. Wagner PD, Dantzker DR, Iacovoni VE, et al. Ventilation-perfusion inequality in asymptomatic asthma. Am Rev Respir Dis 1978; 118:511–524.
18. Wagner PD, Gale GE, Moon RE, et al. Pulmonary gas exchange in humans exercising at sea level and simulated altitude. J Appl Physiol 1986; 60:260–270.

19. Wagner PD, Laravuso RB, Uhl RR, West JB. Continuous distributions of ventilation-perfusion ratios in normal subjects breathing air and 100% O_2. J Clin Invest 1974; 54:54–68.
20. Wagner PD, Naumann PF, Laravuso RB. Simultaneous measurement of eight foreign gases in blood by gas chromatography. J Appl Physiol 1974; 36:600–605.
21. Wagner PD, Sutton JR, Reeves JT, et al. Operation Everest. II: pulmonary gas exchange during a simulated ascent of Mt. Everest. J Appl Physiol 1988; 63:2348–2359.
22. Wagner PD, West JB: Ventilation-perfusion relationships. In: West JB, ed. Pulmonary Gas Exchange. Vol. I. New York: Academic Press, 1980, 219–262.
23. West JB: Ventilation-perfusion inequality and overall gas exchange in computer models of the lung. Respir Physiol 1969; 7:88–110.
24. West JB. Ventilation/Bloodflow and Gas Exchange, 4th edition. Philadelphia: J.B. Lippincott Co., 1985.
25. West JB, Wagner PD. Pulmonary gas exchange. In: West JB, ed. Bioengineering Aspects of the Lung. New York: Marcel Dekker, 1980, 361–457.

Chapter 9

CELLULAR EFFECTS AND PHYSIOLOGIC RESPONSES: LUNG MECHANICS

Rolf D. Hubmayr Joseph R. Rodarte

The physiologic hallmark of chronic obstructive pulmonary disease (COPD) is a reduction of maximal expiratory flow. For the purpose of this chapter we define COPD as a group of related pathologic conditions of the lung parenchyma, intrathoracic airways, or both, that cause a chronic reduction of maximal expiratory flow. Several distinct pathologic entities described in detail elsewhere in this volume reduce maximal flow and thus produce overlapping clinical syndromes. Most patients have more than one pathologic lesion. It is not possible in an individual to determine precisely how much each lesion contributes to the observed functional impairment.

PATHOLOGY

The conditions considered in this chapter affect either the lung parenchyma, e.g., emphysema, or the airways, e.g., chronic bronchitis. Other diseases of the lung parenchyma associated with airway lesions that also reduce maximal flow, e.g., sarcoidosis or lymphangiomyomatosis, are not discussed. Asthma, which produces acute and completely reversible airways obstruction, also is not considered separately from generalized chronic airway disease. Whether or not asthma is a risk factor for the development of chronic irreversible disease is controversial. Most patients with COPD have an increased sensitivity to bronchoconstrictor agents by criteria developed for normal subjects.[17] Many COPD patients have frequent acute exacerbation of airway obstruction as a prominent manifestation of the disease. Clinicians refer to this condition as asthmatic bronchitis but have not agreed on objective clinical or pathologic criteria for this syndrome.

Lungs

AIRWAYS. Chronic bronchitis is a clinical diagnosis. Standards adopted by the American Thoracic Society require that the patient have a daily cough productive of sputum for at least 3 months of the year for 2 consecutive years in the absence of other diseases that produce this symptom.[1] Most long-term cigarette smokers have a "smoker's cough" and meet these criteria. In North America and Europe, most individuals with chronic bronchitis are cigarette smokers. Chronic bronchitis is associated with well-defined pathologic lesions of the airways.

Many individuals with chronic bronchitis do not have COPD when it is defined as a decrease in maximal expiratory flow below the 95% confidence limits derived from populations of asymptomatic nonsmokers.[5] Similarly, many patients with chronic bronchitis do not have a rate of decline of lung function that exceeds the range established for healthy subjects. In spite of these observations from epidemiologic studies, it is extremely difficult to find anyone who has smoked more than 40 pack-years who has normal lung function.

It is not clear whether the pathology of chronic bronchitis, when associated with airways obstruction, differs qualitatively or only quantitatively from chronic bronchitis with normal lung function. In chronic bronchitis associated with COPD, there are marked mucosal thickening, which reduces the airway lumen; tenacious mucus, which obstructs the already reduced lumen; and destruction of the cartilage plates of the conducting airways, which produces increased airway compliance. Airway compliance is an important determinant of maximal flow (see Fig. 9–5).

A generally accepted concept supported by only modest evidence is that the most significant lesions in the initial pathogenesis of COPD from chronic bronchitis are confined to the small (<2 mm in diameter) conducting airways.[23, 35]

Smokers have a high incidence of bronchiolitis with mucus plugging, fibrosis, and remodeling of the peripheral airways. In lung tissue specimens removed at operation for other diseases, the severity of these lesions is correlated with abnormalities of lung function.[7, 58] Unfortunately, central airways were not always sampled in these studies. The correlation between severity of pathology and results of lung function tests thought to be specific for lesions of the peripheral airways has been distressingly poor, perhaps because of the important influence of uncontrolled variables, such as central airway function. In only one study was the degree of central airway inflammation compared with the degree of airways obstruction, but no correlation could be established.[40]

PARENCHYMA. In the context of this chapter, emphysema is defined as destruction of the gas-exchanging parenchyma distal to the terminal bronchioles, resulting in enlarged airspaces. Other conditions associated with enlarged airspaces, such as those occurring in the remaining lung after pulmonary resection or with aging, are not considered.

A number of different pathologic types of emphysema are described. The different types and distributions of the lesions in various forms of emphysema may be associated with distinct physiologic abnormalities, but no data are available on this subject. Centrilobular emphysema is most common, but because of its association with cigarette smoking it rarely occurs in the absence of chronic bronchitis. Because lesions are not uniformly distributed in the lung, the severity of centrilobular emphysema would be difficult to assess from biopsy specimens obtained in clinical studies of patients with small airway disease.

Alpha$_1$-antitrypsin deficiency produces panlobular emphysema.[16] Most of our understanding of the physiologic sequelae of emphysema is derived from nonsmokers with alpha$_1$-antitrypsin deficiency who have no symptoms of airway disease[8] and from animal models of elastase-induced emphysema.[56] As discussed subsequently, these patients and animal models clearly demonstrate how airway obstruction can occur in anatomically normal airways.

VASCULATURE. The capillary bed of the pulmonary circulation is in the alveolar wall. The destruction of alveolar walls in emphysema reduces the capillary bed and, thus, decreases the pulmonary gas-exchange surface. The capillaries contribute a relatively small portion of the pulmonary vascular resistance. Enough reserve is present that can be recruited so that pulmonary hypertension at rest occurs only late in the natural history of emphysema.[22]

When hypoxia and hypoxic vasoconstriction, along with reduction in the cross-sectional area of the capillary bed, become severe enough, pulmonary hypertension develops. Pulmonary hypertension is associated with muscular hypertrophy and intimal changes of the pulmonary arteries and causes secondary changes in the right side of the heart.[21]

For reasons not completely understood, when equal reductions in maximal expiratory airflow are present, obstructive bronchitis is associated with worse hypoxemia than is emphysema.[15] Chronic hypoxemia ultimately results in fixed pulmonary hypertension and cor pulmonale. The pulmonary vasculature is not believed to be directly involved in the pathogenesis of obstructive bronchitis. The bronchial vessels that supply the airways are hypertrophied in chronic bronchitis and in chronic asthma, which may contribute to the pathophysiology of these conditions.

Chest Wall

Patients with COPD breathe at higher lung volumes than do healthy subjects. It is suspected that this causes structural changes in the thorax. In hamsters, chronic hyperinflation causes a reduction in the number and length of sarcomeres of the diaphragm, which adapts to a shorter operating length.[18, 26] Presumably this effect also occurs in patients with COPD.

Theoretically, the increased work of breathing with COPD should cause hypertrophy of the respiratory muscles; however, this effect has been difficult to demonstrate. The maximal inspiratory pressure that can be produced at residual volume (RV) is not increased in patients with COPD.[10] In part, this finding may be because of the increased RV, since maximal inspiratory pressure decreases with increasing lung volume. It is unclear whether the geometry of the diaphragm and of the respiratory system has a volume-independent effect on the maximal inspiratory pressure in these patients. In some postmortem studies of individuals who had severe COPD, hypertrophy of the diaphragm has not been demonstrated. In fact, these patients suffered from terminal inanition and generalized muscle atrophy that does not seem to spare the diaphragm.[4]

The abdominal muscles are the major expiratory muscles. Although patients with severe COPD frequently recruit abdominal muscles during expiration, the mechanical demands on these muscles during breathing are small compared with those that occur during a change in posture or during a cough.[44] Chronic obstructive pulmonary disease patients with severe cough may produce sustained increases in pleural pressure (Ppl) sufficient to impede cerebral perfusion and to produce syncope.[33] We are unaware of any study in which expiratory muscle strength of COPD patients has been compared with that of subjects belonging to a control group matched for other activities that would increase the use of the abdominal muscles.

FUNCTION

Mechanical Derangement in COPD

STATICS. The rib cage and abdomen/diaphragm, which form the chest wall, and the lungs can be considered elastic bodies with mechanical properties defined by their pressure-volume (PV) curves (Fig. 9–1, upper panel). The static PV curve of the lung is approximately a monoexponential function between functional residual capacity (FRC) and total lung capacity (TLC). The compliance at FRC is proportional to body size and in a 70-kg adult male it averages about 0.25 L/cm H_2O. The chest wall PV curve is more linear than that of the lung and does not approach a plateau near TLC. The chest wall PV curve of healthy individuals has not been defined above normal TLC because it is not considered safe to passively inflate the lungs above TLC.

The intersection of the lung and chest wall PV curves represents the relaxation point of the respiratory system. At rest, healthy, seated subjects usually have no respiratory muscle activity at end expiration, and they breathe at a frequency that provides sufficient time to exhale to this relaxation point. Therefore, end expiratory lung volume is statically determined. Many physiologists use the term "functional residual capacity" for both end expiratory lung volume and relaxation volume, with the implied assumption that they are equal. Functional residual capacity is little affected by standing but is influenced by the position of the shoulders and spine, i.e., slouched versus standing at attention. In the supine position FRC is reduced because the gravity has less inspiratory effect on the abdominal contents. These effects are caused almost entirely by changes in the chest wall PV curve, although evidence suggests that lung elastic recoil is significantly changed by posture as well.[2]

Emphysema causes a marked reduction in the lung elastic

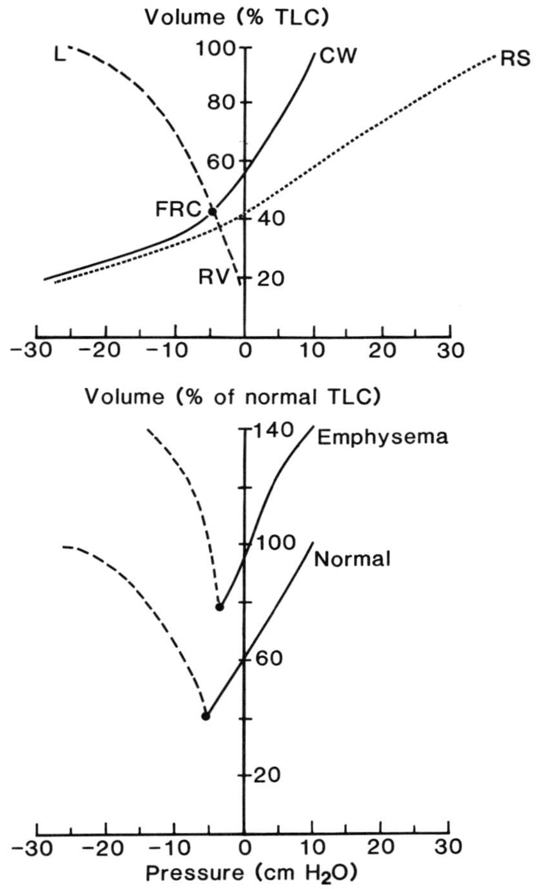

Figure 9–1. ***Upper panel.*** **Pressure-volume curves of the lung (L, dashed line), chest wall (CW, solid line), and respiratory system (RS, dotted line) in the healthy individual. Volume is expressed as percent of total lung capacity (TLC). The relevant recoil pressures for the respiratory system and the chest wall represent airway and intrathoracic (esophageal) pressures, respectively, when measured during relaxation against a closed mouth shutter. The transpulmonary, or lung recoil, pressure is derived by subtraction of the contribution of the chest wall from the respiratory system curve. Functional residual capacity (FRC) is determined statically at a volume at which the recoil pressures of the lung and chest wall are equal. RV refers to residual volume.** ***Lower panel.*** **Pressure-volume curves in healthy individuals compared with those in patients with emphysema. Volume is expressed as percent predicted normal TLC. Note the increased lung compliance (greater slope) and the reduction in pulmonary recoil pressure at TLC in emphysema. Although in emphysema the compliance of the chest wall remains normal, the chest wall curve is shifted to the left, which results in a marked increase in FRC to volumes near normal TLC. (Adapted with permission from Sharp JT, et al. Am J Med 1968; 44:39–46.)**

recoil and a change in the shape of the lung PV curve. This change produces an increase in FRC (Fig. 9–1, lower panel). At least in anesthetized paralyzed patients with COPD, the compliance of the thorax remains normal even at lung volumes above normal TLC.[55] Compared with that in normal subjects, the chest wall curve is shifted to the left to higher lung volumes, suggesting that the thorax adapts to chronic hyperinflation. If the inspiratory muscles were able to produce a normal maximal inspiratory pressure, the reduced elastic recoil of the emphysematous lung and the loss in chest wall recoil would allow a considerable increase in maximal lung volume. Although TLC is invariably increased in severe emphysema, the pressure-generating capacity of inspiratory muscles is sufficiently reduced to prevent lung inflation to normal recoil pressures. As a case in point, the PV curve in Figure 9–1, lower panel, for emphysema was constructed during mechanical inflation of the respiratory system, whereas the TLC, which patients were able to achieve during a maximal inspiration, was invariably lower, for instance, near 120% of normal TLC.[55]

The horizontal separation between the lung and chest wall PV curves represents the elastic energy stored in the respiratory system (see Fig. 9–1). At volumes above FRC, this elastic recoil produces expiratory flow unless retarded by persistent inspiratory muscle activity, glottic narrowing, or both. In emphysema, this elastic recoil is reduced because of the steepness of the lung PV curve.

A patient with a clinical diagnosis of chronic bronchitis also has an increased TLC. The lung retractive force at observed (elevated) TLC is normal.[20] This finding means that the lung retractive force at predicted (normal) TLC is reduced, suggesting that, in fact, there is some loss of lung elastic recoil. It is difficult to demonstrate the presence of mild emphysema *in vivo*. In addition, longitudinal studies of lung volumes and respiratory system mechanics in patients with "pure chronic bronchitis" (absence of emphysema) have not been carried out. Therefore, whether chronic bronchitis by itself can cause a loss of lung elastic recoil without emphysema will likely remain an enigma for some time.

Asthmatic patients reputedly have large increases in TLC during severe attacks.[9] Because plethysmographically determined TLC can be artifactually high during severe airways obstruction, this finding must be re-evaluated.[57] It is exceedingly difficult to determine valid PV curves during severe respiratory distress, so it is not known whether the increased TLC during asthma, if it occurs, is associated with decreased lung recoil.

Thus far we have considered the chest wall as a single homogeneous structure. It is more appropriately viewed as a two-compartment system, consisting of the rib cage and abdomen, which can operate with two degrees of freedom.[30] That is, lung volume can be changed by displacement of the rib cage or of the diaphragm, which, because the abdominal contents are incompressible, displaces the anterior abdominal wall. The volume displacements of the two compartments are conventionally assessed with magnetometers, which measure changes of linear dimensions, or inductance coils, which measure changes of cross-sectional area. The displacement of the free wall of the abdomen underestimates the volume swept by the diaphragm because the upper part of the abdominal contents lies beneath the lower ribs and expands with the rib cage.[37] For example, if a subject inspires by elevating the rib cage and keeps the free wall of the abdomen fixed, the part of the abdomen beneath the rib cage expands and the diaphragm must shorten and descend to prevent the abdominal free wall from displacing inward.

With this caveat, the contributions of the rib cage and abdomen to the passive chest wall PV curve can be estimated from measurements of displacements of the body surface (Fig. 9–2). Healthy individuals who are breathing quietly in a sitting position displace their chest wall very near their passive rib cage/abdomen relationship. It is now recognized that the coordinated contraction of many muscles of inspiration is required to drive the respiratory system along its relaxation configuration.[14] When the diaphragm is the only active muscle, as in quadriplegic patients, the upper rib cage moves paradoxically inward during inspiration.[42]

At high lung volumes (see Fig. 9–2) the ratio of rib cage-to-abdominal volume displacement increases. Presumably this is because of a greater abdominal impedance at high lung volumes. During breathing at high volumes, the force-generating capacity of the shortened diaphragm is reduced. In addition, the mechanical advantage of the flattened diaphragm is decreased. The latter is probably of great significance in COPD. In dogs in which the lungs have been passively inflated

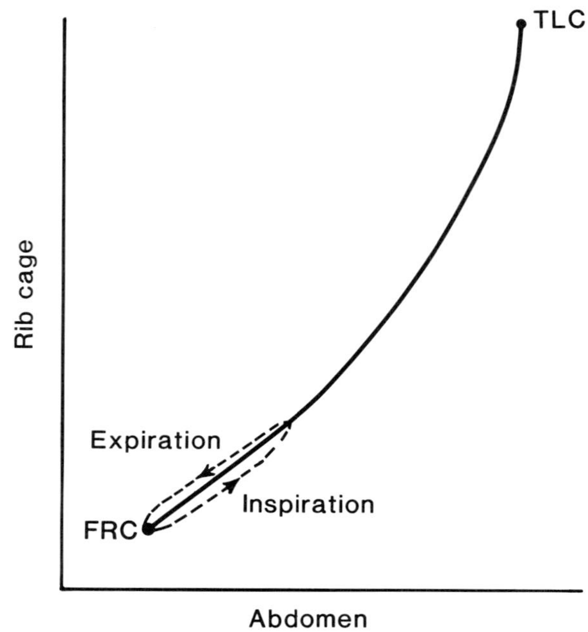

Figure 9–2. Relative dimensions of rib cage and abdomen during relaxation between functional residual capacity (FRC) and total lung capacity (TLC) (solid line). During quiet breathing (dashed line), seated healthy subjects displace their chest walls in a pattern similar to that seen during relaxation.

to near TLC, phrenic stimulation produces an increase rather than a decrease in Ppl, indicating that the flattened diaphragm has an expiratory rather than an inspiratory action on the lungs.[39]

Chronic obstructive pulmonary disease patients with marked hyperinflation breathe with a much greater ratio of rib cage-to-abdominal displacement than normal subjects and may even have a paradoxic inward displacement of the abdomen during inspiration.[54] This finding is consistent with the hypothesis that the flattened diaphragm is virtually ineffectual at displacing volume. The classic clinical sign corresponding to these observations is Hoover's sign, a paradoxic inward displacement of the lower rib cage along the insertion of the diaphragm in a patient with severe COPD and hyperinflation.[24]

DYNAMICS

Airway Resistance. If, in patients with emphysema, the loss of lung elastic recoil had no effect on the dynamic properties of the respiratory system, the effort required to breathe would be reduced. However, COPD is characterized by an increased work of breathing because of the direct and indirect effects of increased airway resistance. The fluid mechanics of flow in the airways are complex. Traditionally, physiologists think of flow as laminar or turbulent, depending on whether the pressure drop is proportional to gas viscosity and flow or to gas density and flow squared.[53] Almost certainly, neither flow type exists in a pure form in any region of the tracheobronchial tree. In general, the pressure-flow curve in the lung periphery is linear, and the slope is determined predominantly by gas viscosity, i.e., laminar flow. In the central airways, the pressure-flow relationship is nonlinear and the local slope is determined predominantly by gas density, especially at high flow, i.e., turbulent flow. In addition to these frictional pressure losses, there is a pressure drop due to convective acceleration. A marked decrease occurs in total airway cross-sectional area between the most peripheral and the most central airways. For a given expiratory flow, the mean velocity must increase in proportion to the reduction in cross-sectional area. The pressure required to accelerate the gas as it moves into smaller areas is given by the Bernoulli equation:

Equation 1: $$P = \frac{1}{2} \rho \dot{V}^2/A^2$$

where ρ = gas density, $\dot{V}$ is volume flow, and A is local airway cross-sectional area.

With respect to airway resistance, it is important to recognize that the pressure drop related to frictional resistance and convective acceleration is inversely proportional to the luminal radius to the fourth power. A 10% reduction in luminal radius can cause a 52% increase in resistance.

In normal subjects, inspiratory resistive work is only a small fraction of the elastic work of breathing. In contrast, in patients with chronic bronchitis, resistive work frequently exceeds elastic work of breathing.[11]

The airways are elastic tubes, the diameter of which is determined by transmural pressure. During embryologic development, the airways bud off the foregut and invade the primordial lung parenchyma. They can be thought of as invaginating the pleura as they invade the lung to form the bronchovascular sheath that surrounds the airways and pulmonary arteries. During inspiration, this sheath expands proportional to the lung, as the hole in an inner tube would expand as the tube is inflated. The airways are coupled to the lung parenchyma by a pressure close to Ppl. Airway diameter can be determined by the difference between intraluminal pressure and Ppl.

If the airways had the same mechanical properties as the lung, their radii would vary with lung volume to the one-third power ($V^{1/3}$). Because the airways extend from the hilum to all areas in the lung, airway length must also vary with $V^{1/3}$. Therefore, conductance, G, the reciprocal of resistance, should be a linear function of lung volume.

Equation 2: $$G \cong r^4/1 \sim V^{4/3}/V^{1/3} \sim V$$

This is an approximate but not completely accurate prediction. The airways do not remain patent at low lung volumes. However, above RV, conductance is a monotonic function of lung volume and transpulmonary pressure.

The increased resistance seen in patients with emphysema without airway pathology is explained by the dependence of bronchial diameter on transpulmonary pressure. Even though FRC is increased in emphysema, lung elastic recoil is reduced and G is appropriate for that lung recoil. The hyperinflated emphysema patient breathes with a mean lung recoil and airway resistance similar to that of a healthy subject near RV. Only near TLC can he or she develop the lung recoil and conductance of a healthy subject at FRC (Fig. 9–3).

Maximal Expiratory Flow. A characteristic of the lungs of all terrestrial mammals that have been studied is expiratory flow limitation; once a threshold in expiratory effort is exceeded, expiratory flow remains constant.[19] Understanding the mechanics of normal flow limitation is helpful in appreciating the pathophysiology of COPD.

The classic observations of Fry and Hyatt[19] are illustrated in Figure 9–4. A healthy subject performs a series of inspiratory and expiratory vital capacity (VC) maneuvers with increasing effort. Increasing effort is reflected by progressive deviation of the Ppl from the static lung PV curve (stippled line) (Fig. 9–4, left panel). Greater inspiratory effort results in monotonic increases of inspiratory flow (Fig. 9–4, center panel). In contrast, once a modest threshold of expiratory effort has been exceeded, there is no further increase in expiratory flow. That is, at a given lung volume, once a critical pressure (P*) is reached, further increases in pressure merely cause an increase in resistance with no increase in flow (Fig. 9–4, right panel).

This process of expiratory flow limitation has been likened by earlier investigators to a waterfall,[49] and this analogy is

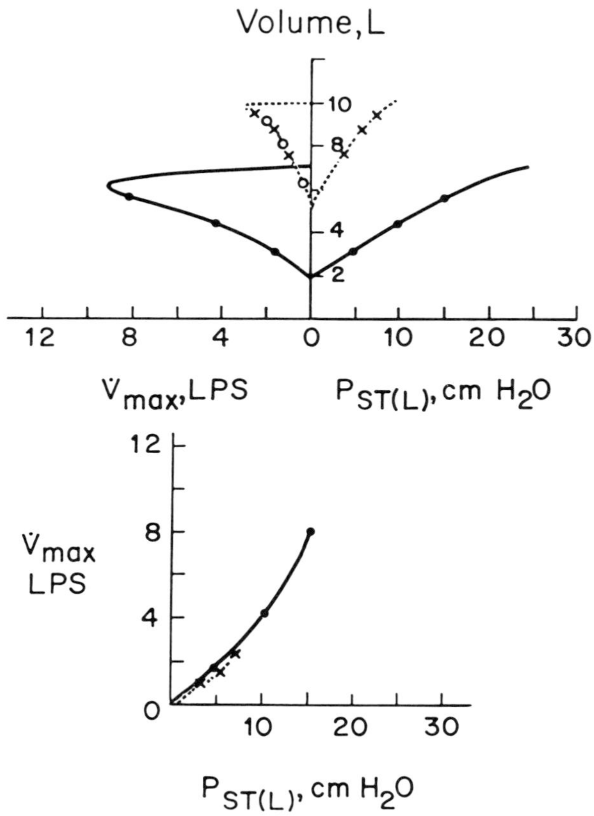

Figure 9–3. Derivation of maximal flow static recoil (MFSR) curves (lower panel) from pressure-volume (PV) and flow-volume (FV) curves (upper panel). The solid lines represent data from a normal subject; the broken lines, a patient with emphysema. Note that in emphysema maximal respiratory flow ($\dot{V}_{max}$) is severely reduced at all volumes, but that it is normal with respect to lung recoil ($P_{ST(L)}$). (Reproduced with permission from Black et al. Am Rev Respir Dis 1972; 105:891–899.)

more apt than they may have appreciated. The flow of water over a waterfall is influenced by conditions in the riverbed above the waterfall, but it is not influenced by conditions below it. In other words, damming the river downstream and reducing the height of the waterfall have no effect on the flow of water. In the airways, once the effort necessary to achieve maximal flow is exerted, a "waterfall," now commonly referred to as a choke point, is established, and lowering the pressure downstream collapses the downstream airways but cannot increase flow through the choke. Expiratory effort increases pleural and alveolar pressures equally. Because the airways are exposed to Ppl on their outer surface, increasing expiratory effort is equivalent to reducing pressure at the airway opening.

At any lung volume, the transmural pressure of the intrathoracic airways is approximately determined by the difference between alveolar and pleural pressures, i.e., static lung recoil, minus the pressure losses produced by the flow of gas. It was originally thought that once transmural pressure at some point in the airway became negative because the pressure loss in the airways exceeded the static lung recoil ($P_{ST(L)}$), the airways downstream of that point collapsed.[19] Once this occurred, further increases in effort could not affect flow. Under conditions of maximal expiratory flow, the airway could be divided into two regions, one above and one below the point where intraluminal pressure had decreased to equal Ppl, or, equal pressure point, and transmural pressure was zero. The equal pressure point defined the demarcation of an upstream segment with a resistance of $P_{ST(L)}/\dot{V}_{max}$, in which the pressure losses were independent of effort and the airway transmural pressures were positive, and of a downstream segment, in which airway transmural pressures were negative and pressure losses increased to dissipate greater expiratory effort. The equal pressure point formulation does not explain the mechanism of flow limitation; it has been helpful in defining the concepts of airway segments upstream and downstream of the flow-limiting point and in defining the importance of lung recoil and resistance of the upstream segment in determining expiratory flow.

Current understanding of the mechanisms of flow limitation is shown schematically in Figure 9–5. For simplicity, assume that the airway upstream of the segment shown has no frictional resistance and that pressure losses are all produced by convective acceleration (see Equation 1). The solid isopleths are plots of Equation 1 for increasing flows; they represent the pressure loss associated with accelerating gas at various flows from the lung periphery with its large cross-sectional area to the areas shown on the abscissa. Intraluminal pressure must also satisfy the pressure-diameter behavior of the airway, shown in Figure 9–5 as the broken line. The simultaneous solutions for these equations are the intersections of the airway and fluid mechanics curves. For example, at a flow of 2 liters per second (L/s), the equations are satisfied at pressure of −1 cm H_2O. A flow of 6 L/s does not intersect the airway curve; therefore, it could not occur. A flow of 5 L/s is just tangent at a pressure of −10 cm H_2O and is the highest flow, i.e., maximal flow, that can be achieved in that airway.

The conditions of tangency mean that the area (A) in the Bernoulli equation at the critical pressure equals that of the airway and that the slopes are identical. That is, the compliance of the airway dA/dP must equal the derivative of the Bernoulli equation.

$$dP/dA = \rho\dot{V}^2/A^3$$

Solving for flow gives the equation for $\dot{V}_{max}$.

Equation 3: $$\dot{V}_{max} = (A^3/\rho^* \, dA/dP)^{1/2}$$

This concept was understood for many years by physiologists and engineers, but it was not clear why, when transmural pressure was decreased further, e.g., to −17 cm H_2O, flow did not decrease to 4 L/s as predicted by the graphic solution in Figure 9–5. This is what usually happens when gas is sucked through soft rubber tubes.

Dawson and Elliott[13] were the first to recognize that Equation 3 is also the formula for wavespeed in an elastic tube. The speed of propagation of a disturbance of fluid in a tube with a compliance greater than the compressibility of the fluid is determined by the compliance of the tube, its cross-sectional area, and the density of fluid. When a disturbance, such as a pressure change, occurs in a fluid-filled tube, it is propagated at a rate determined by the wave speed. If there is flow in the tube, the rate of propagation upstream is the difference between wave speed and the fluid velocity. Because the fluid velocity at maximal flow defined by Equation 3 is the wave speed, the upstream propagation is zero, and a decreased pressure downstream cannot traverse the choke point and influence flow in the upstream segment. Therefore, the condition of a pressure of −17 cm H_2O in Figure 9–5 cannot occur.

The model in Figure 9–5 assumes that there is no frictional pressure loss between alveolus and choke point. This is a reasonable assumption when flow limitation occurs in peripheral airways where the total cross-sectional area for flow is large. The presence of frictional pressure loss causes a leftward shift of the flow isopleths, causing a further reduction in $\dot{V}_{max}$.

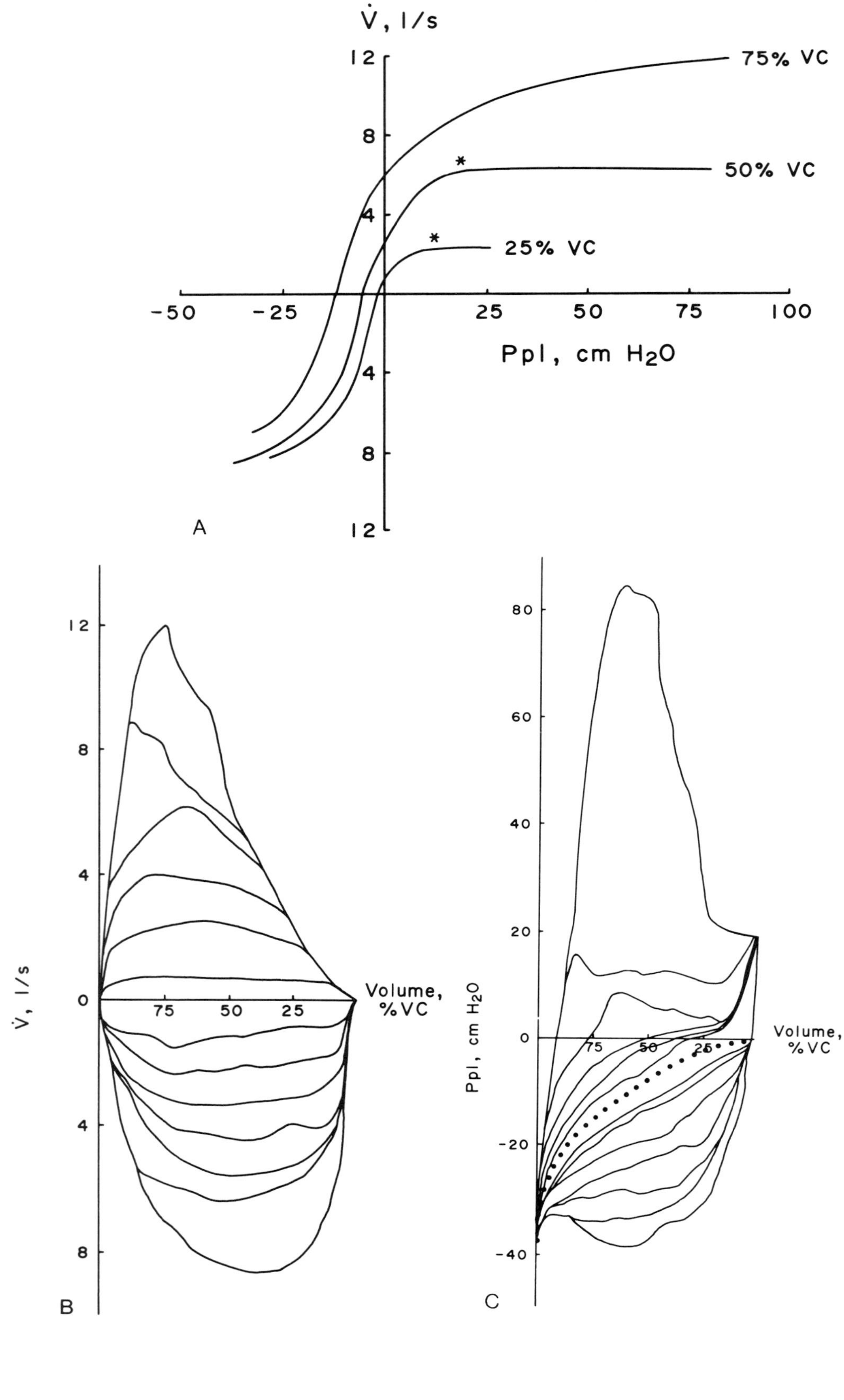

Figure 9–4. *A*, Relationships between pleural pressure (Ppl) and expiratory flow (V̇) at three lung volumes (expressed as percent vital capacity, VC). The asterisk * indicates the threshold in effort (critical Ppl) above which V̇ remains constant. *B*, Flow-volume relationships during graded inspiratory efforts (below abscissa) and expiratory efforts (above abscissa). *C*, Relationships between pleural pressure and lung volume derived from the values shown in the left and center panels. The dotted line indicates the static pressure-volume curve of the lung. For further explanation, see text. (Reproduced with permission from Rodarte JR, Rehder K. Dynamics of respiration. In: Geiger S, ed. Handbook of Physiology, Vol III, section 3 [part 1], The Respiratory System. Bethesda: American Physiological Society, 1986, 131–144.)

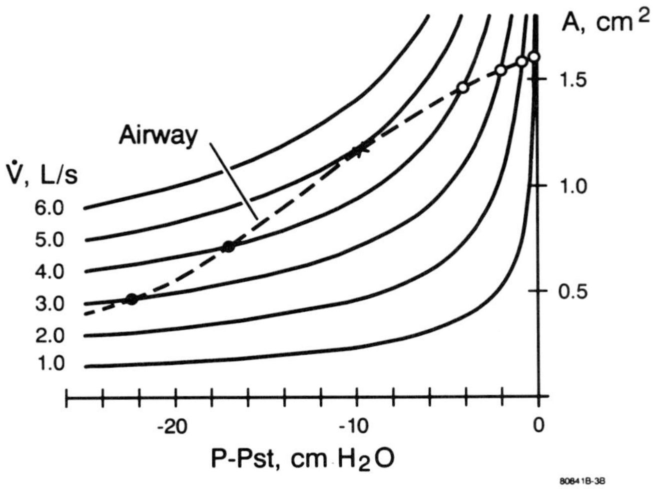

Figure 9–5. Graphic solution of maximal flows. The solid lines show the pressure/area relationship computed from the Bernoulli equation (Eq. 1) at flows between 1 and 6 L/s. The broken line indicates the static transmural pressure/cross-sectional area relationship for an nth-generation bronchus. As is explained in the text, maximal flow has been reached when conditions of tangency (cross) between the fluid dynamics and airway curve are satisfied.

The analysis in Figure 9–5 also illustrates that the determinant of maximal flow is lung elastic recoil, not lung volume per se. Patients with pure emphysema have low conductance and flows for their lung volume, but the values are normal when related to the lung elastic recoil.[8] In principle, it is possible to distinguish airway obstruction due to emphysema from that due to airway disease by determining if the patient's low maximal flows and conductances at a given lung volume are normal for the elastic recoil (see Fig. 9–3). Patients with isolated bullae or a pneumothorax, whose lungs are small for a given intrathoracic gas volume and thus have a low elastic recoil, are indistinguishable by conventional physiologic tests from patients with diffuse emphysema.

The wave speed equation indicates that $\dot{V}_{max}$ at the choke point is inversely proportional to the square root of gas density. However, if frictional losses upstream to the choke point are large and independent of density, the increase in flow achieved by breathing a gas of reduced density may be negligible.

Equation 3 also indicates that $\dot{V}_{max}$ is inversely proportional to the square root of airway compliance. Thus, the increased airway compliance occurring with the chondromalacia of chronic bronchitis may be of major significance in reducing maximal flow.

A computer model has been established that uses estimates of airway geometry and compliance, determines the pressure losses in each generation, solves coupled equations for frictional and convective losses, adjusts airway areas for each incremental pressure loss, and determines the site in the airway and the flow at which wavespeed first occurs.[32] Model predictions agree well with observations in excised human lungs. At high lung volumes the choke point occurs in central airways and $\dot{V}_{max}$ increases when helium is substituted for air. At low volumes the choke point is in more peripheral generations of the bronchial tree. Frictional upstream losses are dominant, and $\dot{V}_{max}$ does not increase when the respired gas is helium.

Regional Nonuniformities. In diseased lungs, areas with differing degrees of abnormality will empty nonuniformly. In patients with COPD the inhomogeneous ventilation can be demonstrated by inert gas washout or equilibration, as well as by various indices of the dispersion of regional ventilation-to-perfusion ratios.[59] Regional nonuniformity also affects overall mechanical behavior. As regions with lower airway resistance empty faster, their elastic recoil pressure also decreases more rapidly than that of more diseased regions. This causes differences in emptying rates to diminish with time. When a forced expiratory maneuver is begun from TLC, more normal areas empty preferentially and are at lower relative volumes by 50% VC than more diseased areas and, thus, have low maximal flows. This is one reason why the flow-volume (FV) curve of COPD patients is more convex to the volume axis than in healthy subjects. Flow interdependence acts in addition to lung parenchymal interdependence to diminish discrepancies in regional parenchymal expansion.[60]

The terminal portion of the flow-volume curve is believed to reflect emptying of the most diseased regions. If a forced exhalation is begun at 50% VC, normal lung regions contain a larger volume of gas than they would have at 50% VC during a forced expiratory maneuver from TLC. Therefore, maximal expiratory flows are higher in the first instance. This effect may be so pronounced that in patients with severe COPD, the FV loop during quiet breathing may be above the FV curve for a maximal effort (Fig. 9–6). This phenomenon is observed in FV curves obtained in a body plethysmograph and is accentuated by the gas-compression artifact discussed subsequently.

Pulmonary Function Tests

In this section we discuss how the mechanical derangements in COPD alter parameters that are commonly measured in a pulmonary function laboratory. The conduct and interpretation of pulmonary function tests are covered in Chapter 39.

LUNG VOLUMES. The most commonly performed test of pulmonary function is the VC. There is not a unique set of determinants for the VC; it should be thought of as the

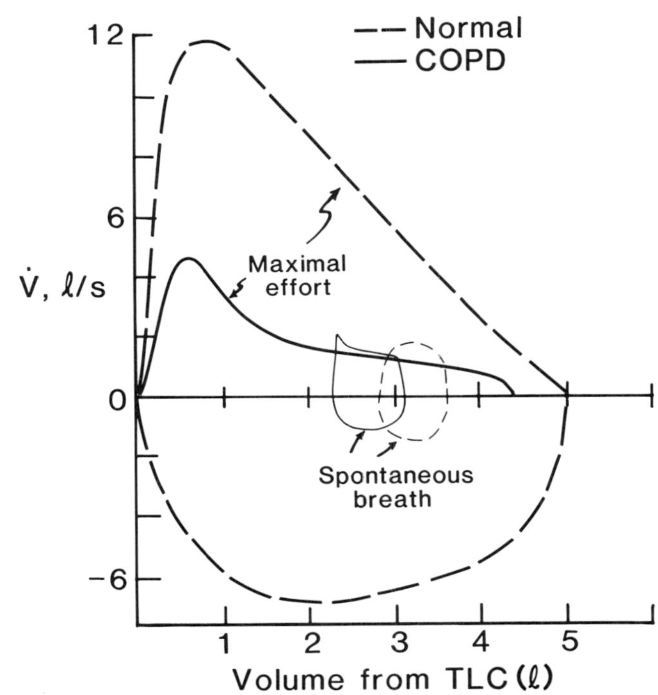

Figure 9–6. Flow-volume loops from a patient with chronic obstructive pulmonary disease (COPD) (solid line) during forced expiration from total lung capacity (TLC) and during spontaneous breathing. Loops from a healthy subject are shown as a reference (dashed line). Inspiratory flow has been assigned a negative value. Note the substantial reserve for expiratory flow in healthy individuals compared with those who have COPD.

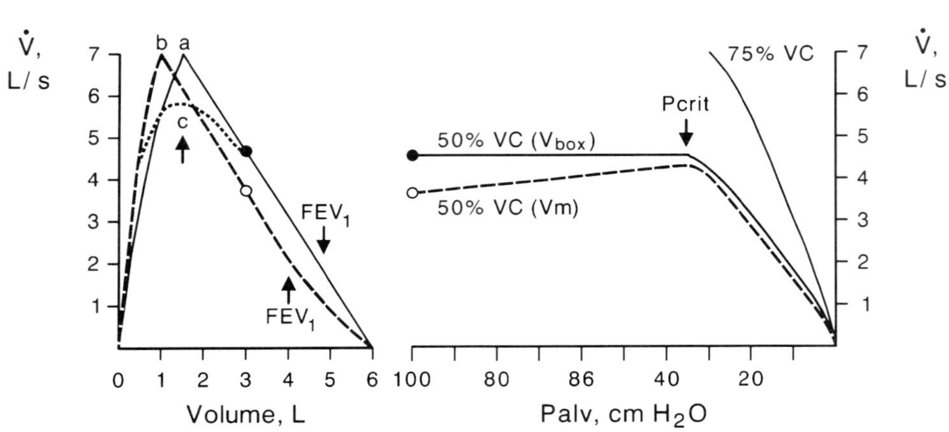

Figure 9–7. Illustration of the "gas compression artifact" on maximal expiratory flow at 50% of vital capacity (VC). The solid lines show the flow($\dot{V}$)-volume (V) (*a*) and alveolar pressure (P_{alv})-flow relationship when thoracic gas volumes are measured in a body plethysmograph; that is, the volume of compressed gas is accounted for. The line of long dashes (*b*) shows the same relationships when thoracic gas volumes are calculated from TLC minus expired volume; that is, intrathoracic gas compression is assumed to be negligible. The finely stippled line (*c*) on the flow-volume loop represents a submaximal expiratory effort with minimal gas compression. (Reproduced with permission from Krowka MJ, et al. Am Rev Respir Dis 1987; 136:829–833.)

difference between TLC and RV. A disproportionate change in either of these results in a change of the VC. Total lung capacity is determined by the balance between the inspiratory pressure generated by the respiratory muscles and the inward elastic recoil of the lung and chest wall. The decreased lung elastic recoil in emphysema produces an increase in TLC, as discussed previously.

In individuals less than 25 years old, RV is determined by the ability of the expiratory muscles to compress the chest wall.[34] The lung volumes at which lung recoil decreases to near zero and airways collapse, precluding further emptying, increase monotonically with age. By the age of 25, this volume exceeds the minimum volume to which the chest wall can be compressed, and RV is now determined by lung mechanics. In healthy individuals, maximal flow decreases linearly with expired volume so that a few seconds' expiration is sufficient to reach the volume at which no more air can be expressed from the lungs.

With the development of COPD, there are poorly ventilated regions that continue to empty at a low, but essentially constant, rate for long periods of time. This has two effects. First, the lung volume at which flow decreases to low levels (< 0.1 L/s) occurs at a much higher volume than the normal RV and patients can continue to exhale at this rate for long periods (20 to 30 seconds). In such patients RV is determined by their breath-holding ability, which is reduced in the presence of pre-existing hypoxemia, and by their motivation to continue this uncomfortable activity.

In many patients with airway disease, expiring to low lung volumes provokes coughing that cannot be voluntarily suppressed, thus limiting the patient's ability to maintain a continuous expiratory effort for long periods. Rarely will a patient with well-established COPD be able to exhale sufficiently to achieve a normal RV. This "effort dependence" of RV produces an effort dependence of VC that contributes significantly to the variability of instantaneous flows measured at certain fractions of the VC, such as the maximal expiratory flow at 50% VC or the maximal mid-expiratory flow. It also contributes to the variability of normalized timed expired volumes, such as the traditional forced expiratory volume in one second-to-forced vital capacity (FEV_1/FVC) ratio. Therapeutic response to a bronchodilator may produce a modest increase in maximal flow that is minimally dependent on lung volume. Therefore, over most of the VC, there is a small increase in flow. At low lung volumes this small absolute increase in flow represents a relatively large fractional change from baseline and, when integrated over time, produces a substantial increase in FVC. This explains why, in spite of minor improvements in isovolume flow with a bronchodilator, the flow between 25% and 75% VC may appear to have paradoxically decreased.

Another problem with measurements of maximal expiratory flow is the gas-compression artifact.[31] Figure 9–7 shows an isovolume pressure-flow curve for a constant absolute lung volume as determined in a volume-displacement body plethysmograph. The change in volume during measurement of a FVC has two components: the first is produced by the volume of gas expired and the second is related to the compression of intrathoracic gas. Virtually all clinical pulmonary function testing is done using measurement of expired volume; that is, gas compression is neglected. When a subject exerts the minimal effort required to achieve maximal flow, there is little gas compression, and expired volume accurately reflects absolute volume relative to TLC. However, with maximal expiratory effort at the same expired volume, absolute lung volume and, thus, maximal flow are significantly reduced. The decrease in absolute flow at a constant expired volume can be computed from Equation 4, in which P_B is barometric pressure, P_{alv} is alveolar pressure, and the subscript m identifies exhaled volume and flows.

Equation 4: $$d\dot{V}_m = (P_{alv}/P_B)\,(TLC - V_m)\,(d\dot{V}_{max}/dV)$$

This difference in flow can be substantial even in patients with moderate COPD and forceful expiratory efforts.[12] These patients are usually men and therefore have reasonably strong expiratory muscles. Because of the force-velocity relationships of skeletal muscles, their reduced maximal expiratory flows allow them to produce higher alveolar pressures than normal. This means that the fractional decrease in absolute lung volume may be substantial (for example, $P_{alv}/P_B = 0.15$).

Because of hyperinflation, the volume change produced by gas compression is larger. If the FV curve is convex to the volume axis, its slope at 50% VC may not be significantly reduced (for example, $d\dot{V}_m/dV = 2\ s^{-1}$). The values in this example would produce a difference in flow of 1.8 L/s at 50% VC between a maximal effort FVC with volume measured at the mouth and measured with the body plethysmograph. A difference of similar magnitude would occur between maximal flow at 50% VC measured at the mouth during maximal expiratory effort compared with one in which the effort was a minimum required to achieve maximal expiratory flow. When these flow differences are integrated over time, the absence of gas compression more than makes up for the diminished peak flows seen in Figure 9–7. Because of gas compression, the FEV_1 produced by submaximal effort can exceed that produced by a maximal effort. This difference is accentuated by the use of back extrapolation for the measurement of FEV_1, as is currently recommended by the American Thoracic Society.[3] With severe chronic obstructive lung disease, this artifact becomes less significant because even though volume change due to gas compression is greater, maximal expiratory flow is virtually independent of lung volume; therefore, it is little affected by alveolar gas compression.

At high lung volumes in healthy individuals, the choke point resides in the central airways and much of the pressure loss upstream is due to convective acceleration. A modest increase in frictional resistance in the smaller airways should have minimal effect on maximal expiratory flow. In contrast, at low lung volume where maximal expiratory flows are lower and viscosity-dependent resistance in the small airways makes up a greater portion of the upstream pressure losses, maximal flow should be more sensitive to increased resistance in the small airways. Consistent with this reasoning, computer models predict that flows at low lung volumes should be more sensitive to small airway disease than flows at high lung volumes.[32] This reasonable hypothesis is not supported by definitive clinical investigation, perhaps because the range of normal values for flow at low lung volumes is quite large. Furthermore, in most studies flow has been measured at volumes expressed as a certain percentage of VC rather than TLC, so that the diminution in flows at absolute volume may be obscured by the increase in RV.

Similarly, there is discouraging evidence about the specificity of measurements of maximal expiratory flow while breathing helium.[38] In fact, patients with tracheal chondromalacia due to polychondritis, e.g., variable intrathoracic major airway obstruction, can have spirometric abnormalities not different from those observed in patients with diffuse COPD.[41]

The measurement of lung static elastic recoil pressure-volume curves is an exacting research tool for which there is probably no role in clinical pulmonary function testing. In the presence of anatomic emphysema, a correlation exists between severity of emphysema and loss of elastic recoil.[43] Although the diffusing capacity for carbon monoxide is frequently thought of as a test of parenchymal thickening in interstitial lung disease, in reality, it is a test of the diffusivity of the surface area product of the alveolar capillary membrane and, thus, is also decreased by the parenchymal destruction that occurs in emphysema.[58] In patients with alpha$_1$-antitrypsin deficiency a good correlation exists between loss of elastic recoil at high lung volume and reduced diffusing capacity for carbon monoxide.[8] Although the diffusing capacity for carbon monoxide is undoubtedly influenced by maldistribution of ventilation with regard to perfusion, it is less so than the arterial oxygen tension and, therefore, is a more specific test for lung parenchymal integrity.

FUNCTIONAL CONSEQUENCES OF ALTERED LUNG MECHANICS IN COPD

Like many body systems, the respiratory system of healthy individuals has tremendous reserve, and its function can be substantially impaired by disease before the condition becomes life-threatening. In even the most highly trained athletes, it appears that the cardiovascular rather than the respiratory component of the oxygen delivery system limits maximal work capacity. The pathologic processes underlying COPD and the consequent mechanical derangements of the respiratory system increasingly limit aerobic work capacity until, in the terminal stages of disease, the maximum oxygen delivery capacity equals basal metabolic requirements. In the following scenario, there are only quantitative rather than qualitative differences between the pathophysiologic abnormalities that can be demonstrated by stress testing in the early stages of the disease and those limitations that ultimately become life-threatening.

Effect of Altered Gas Exchange on Ventilatory Requirements

The focal nature of the pathologic features of chronic obstructive lung disease produces an increased nonuniformity of ventilation distribution. Regional hypoxic vasoconstriction is inadequate to restore a normal ventilation-to-perfusion ratio. The increased dispersion of ventilation-to-perfusion ratios produces inefficient gas exchange and mandates an increase in total ventilation in order to achieve a normal oxygen uptake and carbon dioxide elimination. Frequently, an adequate oxygen uptake and carbon dioxide production are achieved only at the cost of hypoxia and sometimes hypocapnia. Later, when the work of breathing becomes excessive, many patients accommodate by employing alveolar hypoventilation. Nevertheless, total ventilation required for any level of metabolic demand is abnormally high.

Similarly, for any level of ventilation, the work of breathing is increased because of the high airway resistance and the greater elastic work mandated by dynamic hyperinflation.[28] Elastic work performed on the respiratory system during inspiration is available to drive expiration. In healthy individuals, continued inspiratory muscle activity during expiration occurs in order to prevent expiring to FRC before it is time to take the next breath.[50] With increasing airway resistance and decreased elastic recoil, the expiratory flow rate produced by a passive expiration progressively decreases, and the need for inspiratory muscle breaking during expiration progressively decreases. When passive expiratory flow is insufficient to reach FRC, mean inspiratory flow rate is increased to allow more time for expiration at the same respiratory rate. This is why spirometric tracings during quiet breathing of patients with COPD are different from the near-sinusoidal tracings seen in healthy individuals. The reduction of metabolic demand on the inspiratory muscles from the absence of expiratory breaking is far less than the increased inspiratory work produced by the increased resistance and the increased mean inspiratory flow rate.

When passive expiratory flow is inadequate to reach FRC during the allotted expiratory time, the subject may recruit expiratory muscles, but in the presence of COPD the ability to increase expiratory flow is sharply diminished. In severe disease, maximal and passive expiratory flows may be equal.[25] The physiologic consequences of reduced maximal expiratory flow are at least as important as the increased work of inspiration.

The maximal inspiratory and expiratory FV loop may be thought of as a maximal performance envelope within which a subject must operate. Figure 9–6 illustrates the tremendous flow reserve of normal individuals, which increases ventilation to meet rising metabolic demands, e.g., during exercise. In contrast, patients with COPD rapidly impinge on the maximal expiratory FV curve. Once this event occurs and FRC is maintained, the time required to expire a given tidal volume (V_T) is fixed. A larger V_T requires more expiratory time; therefore, the only way to increase ventilation at constant end expiratory lung volume is by disproportionate increases in maximal inspiratory flow. This is illustrated by Equation 5:

Equation 5: $$\dot{V}_i = V_T/T_{tot} - T_e$$

where $\dot{V}_i$ is equal to mean inspiratory flow rate, V_T is tidal volume, T_i is inspiratory time, T_e is expiratory time, and T_{tot} is the total duration of the breath. If an individual who is breathing on his or her maximal expiratory envelope attempts to increase respiratory frequency without changing V_T, T_{tot} approaches T_e, and mean inspiratory flow rate must approach infinity. Because of the shape of the FV curve, an increase in

V_T causes a less than proportionate increase in T_e. If a subject achieves maximal expiratory flow and keeps end expiratory lung volume constant, an increase in ventilation must be achieved by disproportionate increases in inspiratory flow. However, patients with COPD do not maintain normal end expiratory lung volumes, as is discussed subsequently.

Healthy subjects at the limit of their exercise capacity maintain an end expiratory lung volume below their normal FRC and an end inspiratory volume near TLC.[62] That is, their V_T may approach 50% TLC or 60% VC and expiratory flows are near maximal throughout expiration. However, healthy subjects do not generate expiratory pressures in excess of those required to achieve maximal expiratory flow. End expiratory lung volume remains between FRC and RV.

In contrast, patients with COPD have a disproportionate reduction in expiratory flow compared with inspiratory flow. Faced with the necessity of increasing ventilation, they can raise mean expiratory flow rates substantially only by increasing end expiratory lung volume. How frequently they generate expiratory pressures in excess of those required to achieve maximal flow and, thus, "waste the effort" by producing dynamic compression of the airways is not clear.[48] Because of the reduced expiratory flows, expiratory time is inadequate to return to a normal FRC. Muscular effort must be expended to stop expiratory flow, to overcome the expiratory elastic recoil of the respiratory system, and to initiate inspiration. Even though the elastic recoil of the respiratory system in COPD patients may be reduced compared with healthy individuals, the elastic inspiratory work of breathing is increased when ventilatory demand, and with it high respiratory rates, mandate dynamic hyperinflation to volumes near TLC. The high respiratory frequency and the greater inspiratory resistance require an increase in the resistive work of breathing. Intrinsic positive end expiratory pressure (PEEP), i.e., the elastic recoil pressure at end expiration, and dynamic hyperinflation have been of considerable interest in patients requiring mechanical ventilation in respiratory intensive care units.[46] This same pathophysiology occurs in patients with less severe COPD during the metabolic demands produced by exercise.

With more severe COPD, the metabolic demands of a sedentary existence may tax the ventilatory capacity to the utmost. A subject who has a maximal expiratory flow of 0.2 L/s over most of the VC would require 50 seconds to exhale 10 L. In order to achieve a minute ventilation of 10 L, such a patient must produce a mean inspiratory flow rate of 1 L/s. In order to raise ventilation to 11 L/min, he or she must achieve a mean inspiratory flow of 2.2 L/s. A ventilation of 12 L/min cannot be achieved with that expiratory flow rate.

When patients with moderate-to-severe COPD attempt to exercise and produce expiratory pressures in excess of those required to achieve maximal flow, the increased Ppl during a prolonged expiration impedes the venous return and impairs cardiac output.[47] Similarly, the negative Ppl required to produce rapid inspirations at high lung volumes, although enhancing venous return, produces a significant afterload on the left ventricle. The large amplitude oscillations in Ppl occurring even at rest in patients with COPD and the associated cardiovascular reflexes are responsible for pulsus paradoxus. The effect on cardiovascular performance of the increased frequency and amplitude oscillations occurring during exercise is not known.

Inspiratory Muscle Function

Virtually all pathophysiologic factors considered so far have an adverse impact on the inspiratory muscles. Inefficient gas exchange increases the ventilation required to meet metabolic oxygen requirements. Expiratory flow limitation increases the mean inspiratory flow rate required to achieve a given level of ventilation. The greater airway resistance and increased lung volume at which breathing occurs increase the resistive and elastic work of breathing. Higher lung volume has two additional adverse effects on inspiratory muscle function. Inspiratory muscle length decreases with increased lung volume.[51] This limits the force-generating capacity unless there is substantial remodeling and adjustment of the optimal lengths. Furthermore, the inspiratory muscles have a mechanical disadvantage at high lung volumes.[36] The Laplace relationship for a curved membrane states that the transmembrane pressure is directly proportional to the tension in the membrane and is inversely proportional to the radius of the curvature. Thus, as the diaphragm descends and flattens at high lung volumes the tension that is generated is less effective in producing a transdiaphragmatic pressure. Also, the orientation of the muscle fibers with respect to the chest wall becomes more horizontal and less vertical. Therefore, in extremely hyperinflated patients, contraction of the diaphragm may produce little lowering of the intrathoracic pressure. Because the diaphragm may become totally ineffectual as an inspiratory muscle at high lung volumes, patients with severe COPD must depend on other muscles to act directly on the rib cage.

RESPIRATORY FAILURE

Many patients with severe COPD ultimately succumb to hypercapnic respiratory failure. This is frequently defined as an arterial carbon dioxide partial pressure (P_{CO_2}) of greater than 50 mm Hg. Many patients live outside the hospital for considerable periods of time with this degree of hypoventilation. Exacerbations of the disease leading to decompensation are usually attributed to events that worsen the severity of the airways obstruction. Yet, in contrast to patients with acute lung injury, it is nearly always possible to achieve adequate levels of ventilation with a mechanical ventilator. This suggests that, although the underlying cause of the ventilatory failure is lung disease, the immediate cause is respiratory pump failure. Such a hypothesis has led to the suggestion that respiratory muscle fatigue may play a major role in the genesis of ventilator-dependent respiratory failure and in the failure to wean from mechanical ventilation.[52]

This hypothesis has provoked interest in muscle physiology among investigators interested in chronic obstructive lung disease. The hypothesis raises questions about the role of respiratory muscle training in the treatment of ambulatory patients with COPD and in the design of treatment regimens for ventilator-dependent COPD patients that provide rest to fatigued muscles while avoiding disuse atrophy. The role of the respiratory muscles in COPD is the topic of another chapter.

DYSPNEA

One might question whether a discussion of dyspnea should be in the purview of a chapter on the effects of COPD on lung mechanics. Yet, it is difficult to consider the effects of altered lung mechanics on patients without discussing this cardinal symptom of their disease. All pulmonary clinicians are struck with the poor correlation between single objective measures of functional impairment and symptoms. This discordance persists even after making allowance for the patient's personality, mood, and other psychosocial factors that obviously bear on the severity of symptomatology in any chronic disease. It is difficult to study the genesis of dyspnea for a number of reasons. This symptom is a subjective sensation that is difficult to quantify objectively even though there are quite reproducible psychologic scaling techniques. However, some investigators in this field quantify the perception of increased respiratory effort, whereas others differentiate this perception from a sensation of unpleasantness. Also, it is almost certainly naive to think that a single physiologic abnormality causes this symptom. There may be many factors that sum to reach a threshold of conscious awareness. For example, altered mechanics that may not be associated with a sensation of dyspnea during normoxia may well be during hypoxia.

In spite of these caveats, there are several intriguing observations in patients with COPD regarding the genesis of dyspnea. The first involves the expiratory phenomena. One hypothesis suggests that, when patients exert expiratory pressures in excess of those required to achieve maximal expiratory flow and produce dynamic compression of the airways, this is somehow perceived as and associated with a sensation of dyspnea.[45, 61] Another observation focuses on inspiratory events. When the Ppl generated by patients during inspiration reaches about two thirds of the maximum that they are able to generate over that lung volume and at that flow rate, many patients complain of dyspnea.[27] Repetitive efforts at about two thirds maximal are usually above the threshold that causes respiratory muscle fatigue.[6]

These two observations may not be at all incompatible. Both of these situations associated with dyspnea occur when ventilatory demands are high relative to capacity. In the absence of experimental variables, such as inspiratory resistive loading, if a spontaneously breathing subject were inspiring with a muscular effort that was two-thirds maximal, he or she would probably also be achieving maximal expiratory flow because this requires minimal expiratory effort. Therefore, it is not unlikely that the acutely dyspneic COPD patient may be making expiratory efforts that produce dynamic airway compression and inspiratory efforts that produce inspiratory muscle fatigue simultaneously. The cause-and-effect relationship of these associated phenomena is not yet clear.

REFERENCES

1. A Statement by the Committee on Diagnostic Standards for Nontuberculous Respiratory Diseases. American Thoracic Society. Chronic bronchitis, asthma, and pulmonary emphysema. Am Rev Respir Dis 1962; 85:762–769.
2. Abel MD, Grinton SF, Rehder K, Hyatt RE. Effect of postural reduction in lung volume on maximum flow-static recoil relationship. FASEB J 1985; A175.
3. American Thoracic Society. Snowbird workshop on standardization of spirometry. Am Rev Respir Dis 1979; 119:831–838.
4. Arora NS, Rochester DF. COPD and human diaphragm muscle dimensions. Chest 1987; 91:719–724.
5. Bates DV. The fate of the chronic bronchitic: a report of the ten-year follow-up in the Canadian Department of Veteran's Affairs Coordinated Study of Chronic Bronchitis. Am Rev Respir Dis 1973; 108:1043–1065.
6. Bellemare F, Grassino A. Force reserve of the diaphragm in patients with chronic obstructive pulmonary disease. J Appl Physiol 1983; 55:8–15.
7. Berend N, Woolcock AJ, Marlin GE. Correlation between the function and structure of the lung in smokers. Am Rev Respir Dis 1979; 119:695–705.
8. Black LF, Hyatt RE, Stubbs SE. Mechanism of expiratory airflow limitation in chronic obstructive pulmonary disease associated with α_1-antitrypsin deficiency. Am Rev Respir Dis 1972; 105:891–899.
9. Brown R, Ingram RH Jr, McFadden ER Jr. Problems in the plethysmographic assessment of changes in total lung capacity in asthma. Am Rev Respir Dis 1978; 118:685–692.
10. Byrd RB, Hyatt RE. Maximal respiratory pressures in chronic obstructive lung disease. Am Rev Respir Dis 1968; 98:848–856.
11. Campbell EJM. The Respiratory Muscles and the Mechanics of Breathing. Chicago: Year Book Medical Publishers, 1958.
12. Charan NB, Hildebrandt J, Butler J. Alveolar gas compression in smokers and asthmatics. Am Rev Respir Dis 1980; 121:291–295.
13. Dawson SV, Elliott EA. Wave-speed limitation on expiratory flow—a unifying concept. J Appl Physiol 1977; 43:498–515.
14. De Troyer A, Estenne M. Functional anatomy of the respiratory muscles. Clin Chest Med 1988; 9:175–193.
15. Dornhorst AC. Respiratory insufficiency. Lancet 1955; i:1185–1187.
16. Eriksson S. Studies in alpha$_1$-antitrypsin deficiency. Acta Med Scand 1965; 177(Suppl):1–85.
17. Fanta CH, Ingram RH Jr. Airway responsiveness and chronic airway obstruction. Med Clin North Am 1981; 65:473–487.
18. Farkas GA, Roussos C. Adaptability of the hamster diaphragm to exercise and/or emphysema. J Appl Physiol 1982; 53:1263–1272.
19. Fry DL, Hyatt RE. Pulmonary mechanics: A unified analysis of the relationship between pressure, volume and gas flow in the lungs of normal and diseased human subjects. Am J Med 1960; 29:672–689.
20. Gibson GJ, Pride NB. Lung distensibility. The static pressure-volume curve of the lungs and its use in clinical assessment. Br J Dis Chest 1976; 70:143–184.
21. Hasleton PS, Heath D, Brewer DB. Hypertensive pulmonary vascular disease in states of chronic hypoxia. J Pathol Bacteriol 1968; 95:431–440.
22. Hicken P, Brewer D, Heath D. The relation between the weight of the right ventricle of the heart and the internal surface area and number of alveoli in the human lung in emphysema. J Pathol Bacteriol 1966; 92:529–546.
23. Hogg JC, Macklem PT, Thurlbeck WM. Site and nature of airway obstruction in chronic obstructive lung disease. N Engl J Med 1968; 278:1355–1360.
24. Hoover CF. The diagnostic significance of inspiratory movements of the costal margins. Am J Med Sci 1920; 159:633–646.
25. Hyatt RE. The interrelationships of pressure, flow, and volume during various respiratory maneuvers in normal and emphysematous subjects. Am Rev Respir Dis 1961; 83:676–683.
26. Kelsen SG, Wolanski T, Supinski GS, Roessmann U. The effect of elastase induced emphysema on diaphragmatic muscle structure in hamsters. Am Rev Respir Dis 1983; 127:330–334.
27. Killian KJ, Campbell MEJ. Dyspnea. In: Roussos C, Macklem PT, eds. The Thorax, Part B. New York: Marcel Dekker, 1985, 787–828.
28. Kimball WR, Leith DE, Robins AG. Dynamic hyperinflation and ventilator dependence in chronic obstructive pulmonary disease. Am Rev Respir Dis 1982; 126:991–995.
29. Knudson RJ, Lebowitz MD. Maximal mid-expiratory flow ($FEF_{25-75\%}$): Normal limits and assessment of sensitivity [letter]. Am Rev Respir Dis 1978; 117:609–610.
30. Konno K, Mead J. Measurement of the separate volume changes of rib cage and abdomen during breathing. J Appl Physiol 1967; 22:407–422.
31. Krowka MJ, Enright PL, Rodarte JR, Hyatt RE. Effect of effort on measurement of forced expiratory volume in one second. Am Rev Respir Dis 1987; 136:829–833.
32. Lambert RK. Sensitivity and specificity of the computational model for maximal expiratory flow. J Appl Physiol 1984; 57:958–970.
33. Leith DE. Cough. In: Brain JD, Proctor DF, Reid LM, eds. Respiratory Defense Mechanisms, Vol 5, Part II. New York: Marcel Dekker, 1977, 545–592.
34. Leith DE, Mead J. Mechanisms determining residual volume of the lungs in normal subjects. J Appl Physiol 1967; 23:221–227.
35. Macklem PT, Mead J. Resistance of central and peripheral airways measured by a retrograde catheter. J Appl Physiol 1967; 22:395–401.
36. Marshall R. Relationships between stimulus and work of breathing at different lung volumes. J Appl Physiol 1962; 17:917–921.
37. Mead J. Functional significance of the area of apposition of diaphragm to rib cage [Proceedings]. Am Rev Respir Dis 1979; 119:31–32.
38. Meadows JA III, Rodarte JR, Hyatt RE. Density dependence of maximal expiratory flow in chronic obstructive pulmonary disease. Am Rev Respir Dis 1980; 121:47–53.
39. Minh V-D, Dolan GF, Konopka RF, Moser KM. Effect of hyperinflation on inspiratory function of the diaphragm. J Appl Physiol 1976; 40:67–73.
40. Mitchell RS, Stanford RE, Johnson JM, et al. The morphologic

features of the bronchi, bronchioles, and alveoli in chronic airway obstruction: a clinicopathologic study. Am Rev Respir Dis 1976; 114:137–145.
41. Mohsenifar Z, Tashkin DP, Carson SA, Bellamy PE. Pulmonary function in patients with relapsing polychondritis. Chest 1982; 81:711–717.
42. Mortola JP, Sant'Ambrogio G. Motion of the rib cage and the abdomen in tetraplegic patients. Clin Sci 1978; 54:25–32.
43. Niewoehner DE, Kleinerman J, Liotta L. Elastic behavior of postmortem human lungs: effects of aging and mild emphysema. J Appl Physiol 1975; 39:943–949.
44. Ninane V, Gilmartin JJ, De Troyer A. Changes in abdominal muscle length during breathing in supine dogs. Respir Physiol 1988; 73:31–42.
45. O'Donnell DE, Sanii R, Anthonisen NR, Younes M. Effect of dynamic airway compression of breathing pattern and respiratory sensation in severe chronic obstructive pulmonary disease. Am Rev Respir Dis 1987; 135:912–918.
46. Pepe PE, Marini JJ. Occult positive end-expiratory pressure in mechanically ventilated patients with airflow obstruction: the auto-PEEP effect. Am Rev Respir Dis 1982; 126:166–170.
47. Permutt S, Wise RA, Sylvester JT. Interaction between the circulatory and ventilatory pumps. In: Roussos C, Macklem PT, eds. The Thorax, Part B. New York: Marcel Dekker, 1985, 701–735.
48. Potter WA, Olafsson S, Hyatt RE. Ventilatory mechanics and expiratory flow limitation during exercise in patients with obstructive lung disease. J Clin Invest 1971; 50:910–919.
49. Pride NB, Permutt S, Riley RL, Bromberger-Barnea B. Determinants of maximal expiratory flow from the lungs. J Appl Physiol 1967; 23:646–662.
50. Richter DW, Ballantyne D. A three phase theory about the basic respiratory pattern generator. In: Schläfke ME, Koepchen HP, eds. Central Neurone Environment and the Control Systems of Breathing and Circulation. Berlin: Springer-Verlag, 1983, 164–174.
51. Road J, Newman S, Derenne JP, Grassino A. *In vivo* length-force relationship of canine diaphragm. J Appl Physiol 1986; 60:63–70.
52. Rochester DF, Arora NS. Respiratory muscle failure. Med Clin North Am 1983; 67:573–597.
53. Rodarte JR, Rehder K. Dynamics of respiration. In: Geiger SR, ed. Handbook of Physiology, Vol III, section 3 (part 1), The Respiratory System. Bethesda: American Physiological Society, 1986, 131–144.
54. Sharp JT, Goldberg NB, Druz WS, et al. Thoracoabdominal motion in chronic obstructive pulmonary disease. Am Rev Respir Dis 1977; 115:47–56.
55. Sharp JT, Van Lith P, Nuchprayoon CV, et al. The thorax in chronic obstructive lung disease. Am J Med 1968; 44:39–46.
56. Snider GL, Lucey EC, Stone PJ. Animal models of emphysema. Am Rev Respir Dis 1986; 133:149–169.
57. Stanescu DC, Rodenstein D, Cauberghs M, Van de Woestijne KP. Failure of body plethysmography in bronchial asthma. J Appl Physiol 1982; 52:939–948.
58. Thurlbeck WM, Henderson JA, Fraser RG, Bates DV. Chronic obstructive lung disease: A comparison between clinical, roentgenologic, functional and morphologic criteria in chronic bronchitis, emphysema, asthma and bronchiectasis. Medicine (Baltimore) 1970; 49:81–145.
59. Wagner PD, Dantzker DR, Dueck R, et al. Ventilation-perfusion inequality in chronic obstructive pulmonary disease. J Clin Invest 1977; 59:203–216.
60. Wilson TA, Fredberg JJ, Rodarte JR, Hyatt RE. Interdependence of regional expiratory flow. J Appl Physiol 1985; 59:1924–1928.
61. Wood LDH, Bryan AC. Exercise ventilatory mechanics at increased ambient pressure. J Appl Physiol 1978; 44:231–237.
62. Younes M, Kivinen G. Respiratory mechanics and breathing pattern during and following maximal exercise. J Appl Physiol 1984; 57:1773–1782.

Chapter 10

AIRWAY RESPONSIVITY AND CHRONIC OBSTRUCTIVE LUNG DISEASE

E. R. Mc Fadden, Jr.

This chapter deals with the airway physiology and airway responsivity of patients with chronic obstructive lung disease. The human tracheobronchial tree is not a series of rigid tubes. Rather, it is a dynamic structure that is capable of changing its size and activity in response to a variety of internal and external stimuli. For example, in circumstances of increased oxygen demands, such as in exercise, the airways dilate to facilitate greater airflow. In contrast, in a hostile environment, such as a smoke-filled room, bronchoconstriction, cough, and mucus production can all occur in an effort to limit exposure of and damage to the lungs. This ability of the airways to respond to stimuli is referred to as "airway reactivity" and is a normal aspect of pulmonary physiology. In some of the chronic obstructive syndromes, airway reactivity rises to pathologic levels and the tracheobronchial tree becomes hyperactive to minor stimuli such that symptomatic episodes of cough, dyspnea, and wheezing are induced. The purpose of this chapter is to explore the mechanisms for heightened airway

Supported in part by SCOR Grant HL-37117, Program Project Grant HL-25830, and General Clinical Research Center Grant MO1RR-00080-25 from the National Institutes of Health.

responsiveness and to examine the relationship between this factor and disease activity.

DEFINITIONS

The chronic obstructive pulmonary syndromes that occur in adult patients are chronic bronchitis, emphysema, and bronchial asthma. Chronic bronchitis is a condition associated with excessive sputum production sufficient to cause cough with expectoration for at least 3 months of the year for 2 consecutive years.[1] This illness is associated with hyperplasia and hypertrophy of the mucus-producing glands in the submucosa of the large cartilaginous airways. In the periphery of the lung, goblet-cell hyperplasia, mucosal, and submucosal inflammation and edema, peribronchial fibrosis, and increased smooth muscle are characteristically found.[1]

Emphysema is a pathologic diagnosis and is defined as distention of the air spaces distal to the terminal bronchi, with destruction of the alveolar septa.[1] Two types of emphysema are commonly described: centriacinar and panacinar. In the former, the destructive process involves the respiratory ducts and respiratory bronchioles in the center of the acinus. In the latter, both the central and peripheral portions of the acinus are involved. Thus, the entire acinus is destroyed.

Bronchial asthma is a disease of the airways that is characterized by increased responsiveness of the tracheobronchial tree to a multiplicity of stimuli.[1] Asthma is manifested physiologically by widespread narrowing of the air passages, which may be relieved spontaneously or as a result of therapy. From a clinical standpoint, asthma is manifested by paroxysms of cough, dyspnea, and wheezing, interspersed with symptom-free periods. Asthma is associated with hypertrophy of the bronchial smooth muscle, mucosal edema, denudation of the surface epithelium, pronounced thickening of the basement membrane, and eosinophilic infiltration of the bronchial wall.[2] In patients dying from this disease, widespread mucus plugging is characteristic.

PREVALENCE AND SOCIOECONOMIC IMPACT

It has been estimated that approximately 20% of adult males have chronic bronchitis; however, only a minority are clinically disabled. Males are affected more often than females. Cigarette smoking is the single most important etiologic factor in producing the illness, but exposure to environmental and occupational pollutants may also contribute.

The precise prevalence of emphysema in life is unknown. However, in post-mortem studies it is rare to find adult lungs that are completely free of this disease. Approximately two thirds of males and one fourth of females will have well-defined changes characteristic of emphysema. Usually the changes are limited in scope and are found in individuals who were either free of symptoms or only mildly symptomatic during life.

Prevalence figures for bronchial asthma on a worldwide basis are difficult to assess because of the lack of reliable population-based data that have been determined through uniform diagnostic criteria. However, it is generally believed that 3% to 4% of the population of the United States suffers from this illness. Similar figures have been reported from other countries, particularly Western Europe.

As indicated by the aforementioned information, the chronic obstructive pulmonary syndromes are extremely common conditions. According to Public Health Service data,[3,4] these disorders afflict a total of 15 to 20 million Americans and account for approximately 60,000 deaths annually. As a group, they are the fourth most common cause of morbidity and the fifth most common cause of mortality in the United States. In addition, the social and economic impacts of the illnesses are enormous. Patients with advanced degrees of obstructive lung disease are unable to work and frequently cannot even participate in the daily activities of life. Even in milder cases, activities often are restricted, considerable time is lost from school and job, and work is limited to those activities that are not physically demanding or that reduce exposure of the individual to stimuli that would exacerbate his or her illness.

From an economic standpoint, the total cost of all obstructive lung diseases runs into billions of dollars each year. It is estimated that asthma and other forms of airway obstruction result in over 6 million lost work days annually and that asthma alone accounts for 90.5 million days of restricted activity per year. Moreover, the Federal Government pays over $400 million yearly to patients with acute and chronic airway disorders. Families with affected members may spend as much as 18% of their total income on treatment.

PATHOPHYSIOLOGY

Although all of the chronic obstructive syndromes produce airflow limitation, each does so through different mechanisms. With chronic bronchitis the obstruction is believed to result from acute and chronic inflammatory changes that slowly develop within the bronchioles. Because of the extremely large cross-sectional area of the small peripheral airways, their contribution to overall pulmonary resistance in the normal lung is quite small, and considerable obstruction has to be present in them before it can be detected.[5,6] Direct and reflex constriction of the smooth muscle can be present throughout the tracheobronchial tree. In some patients with combined chronic bronchitis and emphysema a loss of elasticity can also contribute to the airway narrowing (see subsequent discussion).

In emphysema, the major cause of increased airflow resistance is a loss of radial support produced by a decrease in elastic recoil.[6] The intrapulmonic airways are tethered to the lung parenchyma. Any process associated with a destruction of alveolar septa reduces the lateral pull on the bronchi and bronchioles, causing them to narrow. As the airways move toward their resting diameter, resistance rises. The reduction in resting airway size that occurs with emphysema need not be associated with symptoms. Intrinsic airway disease may be required to make this patient symptomatic. A good example of this phenomenon is provided by individuals with homozygous alpha$_1$-antitrypsin deficiency. Affected patients have severe emphysema but may not develop symptoms of cough or dyspnea unless they smoke or have some other form of airway pathology.

The causes of obstruction in asthma are multiple. Smooth muscle constriction, direct and reflex, mucosal and submucosal edema, and failure of mucociliary transport mechanisms with retention of secretions all contribute.[7] In some instances, a transient loss of elastic recoil can occur as well.[8] In asthma the obstruction tends to be more dynamic than in other conditions, and at any given time a patient can be normal from both functional and clinical standpoints, asymptomatic with abnormal mechanics, or symptomatic with varying degrees of obstruction.[7]

FUNCTIONAL DEFECTS

Both chronic bronchitis and emphysema result in airway narrowing. Thus, the test results of pulmonary mechanics are usually abnormal. In the early stages of chronic bronchitis, in which the changes are confined to the periphery of the lung, standard test results may not be affected, and techniques such as closing volumes, flows in the mid-vital capacity, and testing of frequency dependency of compliance and resistance may be required for detection.[9] As the disease advances, alterations in the pressure-flow and pressure-volume relationships of the lungs become more marked, and airway resistance and lung volumes rise while specific conductance and forced expiratory volumes and flow rates fall.[10, 11] As a direct consequence of these changes, the work of breathing is increased, particularly at high levels of ventilation.

In addition to changes in mechanics, there are major abnormalities in gas exchange.[10–13] In those individuals in whom alveolar septa have been destroyed, the diffusing capacity is low; otherwise it tends to be normal. However, maldistribution of inspired air with mismatched ventilation-perfusion relationships is an invariable finding. Although arterial hypoxemia is a universal finding, not all patients develop hypercapnia. The degree of arterial desaturation and the presence of carbon dioxide retention depend on the patient's ability to compensate for mechanical aberrations by changing the responsivity of his or her ventilatory drive. Those patients who maintain reasonable values for arterial oxygen and who have low or normal carbon dioxide tensions appear to have an increased ventilatory responsivity and therefore hyperventilate. Alternatively, in those with severe hypoxemia and hypercarbia, the ventilatory drive is sometimes diminished. As gas exchange deteriorates, pulmonary arterial pressures rise in response to the severe hypoxemia, and in untreated cases, cor pulmonale can eventually develop.[10, 13]

As indicated previously, the functional abnormalities in asthma are evanescent, and patients whose disease is quiescent may have perfectly normal lung function when tested. When their illness is active, however, the changes that occur in pulmonary mechanics are similar to those that occur in chronic bronchitis. The pressure, flow, and volume relationships of the lungs are all disturbed, resulting in hyperinflation, increased resistance to airflow, decreased forced expiratory flow rates, elevated work of breathing, and mismatched ventilation-perfusion relationships.[7] Unlike the situation in the other chronic obstructive syndromes, however, the functional abnormalities are reversible.

In asthma, severe hypoxemia and hypercapnia are relatively rare occurrences.[14–16] During acute exacerbations (e.g., breathing air at sea level), arterial oxygen tensions are usually greater than 50 torr and the vast majority of patients have hypocarbia. In contrast, in patients with chronic bronchitis, emphysema, or both, who are admitted to the hospital in acute distress, the oxygen tension is typically less than 30 torr, whereas the carbon dioxide tension is 60 torr or greater.[17, 18] As the obstruction becomes more severe in asthma, the carbon dioxide normalizes; thus, the finding of a normal value for this variable in a symptomatic asthmatic patient indicates impending suffocation and should be treated as such. Hypercapnia is seen in less than 10% of cases and is invariably associated with extremely severe obstruction or with the use of sedative or tranquilizing drugs.

AIRWAY REACTIVITY

Two of the major advances in the understanding of the chronic obstructive syndromes that have occurred in the last 25 years have been the recognition that the bronchial tree has the capability of hyperreacting to a variety of stimuli and that this phenomenon can contribute significantly to the morbidity and mortality of airway disease. The human tracheobronchial tree can respond to noxious stimuli in a variety of fashions. Ciliary activity can increase or decrease, the volume and character of the secretions can change, cough can develop, or the airways can decrease in size. This ability of the airways to reversibly alter their diameters in response to stimuli has been given the notation airway reactivity. This term tends to be used synonymously with smooth muscle contraction; however, one must keep in mind that more than one pathologic process can result in airway narrowing. Mucosal edema with or without inflammatory cellular infiltrate, increased secretion with or without changes in clearance, alterations in parenchymal elasticity, loss of stability of distal bronchioles, and changes in airway vasculature can all contribute or interact to cause a reduction in the size of the airway lumen. The dominant response depends on such variables as the nature of the offending agent, its distribution within the tracheobronchial tree, the duration and intensity of the exposure, and the responsivity of the host.

Changes in airway caliber can result from exposure to a variety of heterogenous stimuli, e.g.:

1. pharmacologic and immunologic aerosols (e.g., methacholine, histamine, propranolol, prostaglandin F_2, leukotrienes, and antigens);
2. physical-chemical agents (e.g., ozone, sulfur dioxide, nitrogen dioxide, distilled water, and hypertonic solutions);
3. thermal factors (e.g., exercise, hyperventilation, and cold air);
4. infections (e.g., common cold, influenza, and other viruses); and
5. emotions.

In addition, many of these stimuli can interact and so amplify the airway response. As a group, asthmatic patients tend to be hyperresponsive to these stimuli,[19, 20] and this increased reactivity usually correlates with many clinical features of the illness. Hence, the phenomenon of heightened airway reactivity in asthmatics can be used in clinical practice not only to diagnose the presence of the disease but also to help assess its severity and expected treatment requirements.

Heightened airway reactivity is a cardinal feature of asthma.[1] It is also found in asymptomatic first-degree relatives of asthmatic patients who are free of the disease[21] and in some individuals with chronic bronchitis, rhinitis, and cystic fibrosis.[22–27] It has not been reported as a feature of emphysema. When airway reactivity is high, symptoms are more severe and persistent, the acute response to bronchodilators is larger, and the amount of therapy required to control the patient's symptoms increases.[20]

AIRWAY REACTIVITY AND CHRONIC BRONCHITIS

Most of the work on airway reactivity has been performed on asthmatic patients, and it is clear that a relationship exists between this facet of the illness and the patient's symptoms. In the other types of chronic obstructive lung disease this relationship has been harder to prove, particularly in established disease. However, in the early stages of chronic bronchitis, heightened airway responses may play an important role in the initiation and progression of the illness. Although conflicting data exist, evidence is mounting that chronic cigarette smoking, a major cause of chronic bronchitis, may induce airway hyperreactivity and an accelerated loss of lung function.[28–39] In one study, cigarette smokers were found to be four times as likely to develop bronchoconstriction in response to hyperventilation of cold air as were nonsmokers.[39] In addition, this study showed that among current and ex-smokers, those individuals with increased airway responsiveness had a 15%

to 45% greater frequency of respiratory symptoms than did those with normal airway reactivity. Barter and Campbell[32] reported that the progression of functional abnormalities in smokers is closely related to their degree of bronchial responsiveness to methacholine or isoproterenol. In this study, even minimal tobacco consumption led to serious ventilatory deterioration over time in people whose airway reactivity was high, whereas heavy smoking produced little decrease in mechanics in those whose airway reactivity was slight. Furthermore, other data indicate that adults with heightened airway reactivity or pre-existing airway disease, or both, may also be more susceptible to the adverse effects of even passive exposure to sidestream smoke.[40]

In the main, the airway responsivity of bronchitic patients is not as high as that seen in asthmatic patients; however, most studies indicate that it is greater than that found in normal individuals and that it probably contributes to the patient's complaints.[24, 26, 27] For example, the clinical course of chronic bronchitis is frequently punctuated by acute transient attacks of cough, dyspnea, and wheezing, and it has been suggested that these symptoms are the result of increased periods of responsivity leading to episodic bouts of bronchoconstriction.[24, 25] Moreover, data indicate that airway reactivity to nonspecific stimuli in patients with chronic bronchitis can be reduced by treatment.[41] It remains to be determined if such maneuvers will influence the course of the disease.

AIRWAY REACTIVITY AND ASTHMA

In both normal and asthmatic subjects, airway reactivity is known to rise during viral respiratory tract infections and following exposure to air pollutants, such as ozone and nitrogen dioxide.[42–44] Sulfur dioxide does not appear to possess this ability.[45] In asthmatic patients, the inhalation of specific antigen not only increases responsivity within minutes, but, depending on dose, can also initiate a situation in which acute episodes of obstruction may occur daily for a prolonged period.[20] Other stimuli, such as exercise, do not produce this effect.[46] Part of the mechanism for the increase in reactivity with antigen may be related to the activity of platelet-activating factor generated from arachidonic acid. Inhalation of this compound by normal subjects results in a heightened airway responsivity that can last for several weeks (see subsequent discussion).[47]

When airway reactivity rises in asthmatic patients, lung function becomes more unstable, presumably because the airways are now reacting to stimuli that previously had no effect on them. One of the most subtle, yet clinically most important, manifestations of this phenomenon is an increase in circadian variation in airway function.

In the human tracheobronchial tree, airway caliber decreases at night and increases during the day.[48–50] In healthy individuals the day-to-night changes are quite small and typically account for only 5% to 10% difference in flow rates. In asthmatic patients, however, an overnight fall in peak flows of 50% or more can occur, and the timing of the decrease tends to correlate with episodes of nocturnal dyspnea. The magnitude of the change in bronchial diameter is related to the state of reactivity of the patient's airways, which in itself varies rhythmically.[51–53] The more active the underlying illness, the greater the airway lability and the larger the diurnal fluctuations of lung function become. The less active the asthma, the smaller the nocturnal changes. In addition to reductions in airway caliber, asthmatic patients also have nocturnal increases in the susceptibility of their airways to provocational stimuli.[52, 53] During sleep, less of a given stimulus is required to evoke airway narrowing, and so airway lability rises. The net result of all of these changes is the production of nocturnal bronchoconstriction.

In the usual course of events, airway function tends to improve during the day following nocturnal problems. Hence, a patient who suffered a moderately severe episode of asthma in the middle of the night may come to the physician's office or pulmonary laboratory the following day and have normal findings on physical examination, with pulmonary mechanics well within the predicted normal range. If the circadian nature of airway obstruction is not considered, the significance and seriousness of the patient's complaints may go unrecognized.

For many years it was believed that the increased bronchial responsiveness of asthmatic patients was a permanent feature of the illness. This belief, in turn, led to the concept that the airways of patients with this disease would always remain more sensitive to nonspecific stimuli than would those of healthy individuals. Obviously, if such a phenomenon were true, it would not make sense to treat this aspect of the illness. Thus, asthmatic patients were believed to represent a unique population in whom little was to be gained by attempting to control their response to inhaled irritants or allergens, and so forth. Therapy was limited to treating acute episodes as they arose, and the only effective form of prophylaxis was thought to be the complete avoidance of known, or suspected, precipitants.

As simple and reliable means of assessing and quantitating airway responsivity began to be applied to large groups of patients under different clinical circumstances, these beliefs began to be modified. Epidemiologic studies demonstrated that the range of airway responsiveness in humans has a normal distribution, with asthmatic patients representing the most sensitive.[54] Hence, asthmatic patients are not a separate population but rather part of a continuum. Further, instead of being a static marker denoting only the presence of respiratory illness, airway reactivity was found to be a dynamic phenomenon capable of great change, the expression of which could profoundly influence clinical manifestations.[20, 51] Consequently, the reduction of airway responsiveness has become an important therapeutic goal.

MECHANISMS FOR AIRWAY HYPERREACTIVITY

A number of causes for increased airway reactivity have been postulated. The basic mechanism remains unknown, however. Abnormalities in airway smooth muscle, airway inflammation, axon reflexes, and vascular pathology have all been implicated, and it is likely that more than one process may be involved.

Abnormalities in Airway Smooth Muscle

One postulate that has been studied for a number of years suggests that acquired or congenital increases in the intrinsic contractile apparatus of the airway smooth muscle play a prominent role in this phenomenon.[19] Although there are data in animal models to support this possibility, *in vitro* physiologic examination of the smooth muscle of asthmatic airways does not uniformly confirm this finding. Whereas some investigators have found an increase in responsivity,[55] others have found asthmatic bronchial smooth muscle to be no more reactive to constrictor stimuli than is muscle taken from normal individuals.[56] Still others have observed hyperresponsivity to some stimuli but not all.[57] Hence, this issue remains unsettled.

Airway Inflammation

One of the most popular hypotheses is that the changes in reactivity in asthmatic airways derive from a chronic inflammatory process.[58, 59] Accumulating data suggest that, on exposure to initiating stimuli, mast cells, basophils, and perhaps macrophages may be activated to release mediators that directly, and acutely, evoke bronchoconstriction, increase capillary permeability, produce edema, increase mucus production, and decrease mucociliary transport. In addition, the elaboration of mediators with chemotactic and chemokinetic effects calls forth a secondary reaction, characterized by a cellular infiltrate composed of eosinophils, neutrophils, and lymphocytes. Each of these cell types contains the necessary enzymatic machinery to produce significant damage to the airway surface epithelium. This damage, in turn, causes the release of more mediators, which may enhance the immediate effect. The damaged epithelium is shed into the airway lumen and adds to the already overburdened mucociliary escalator, thereby worsening the lumenal narrowing.

A series of interactions between a multitude of chemical mediators may be required to produce the aforementioned reaction sequence. The metabolites of arachidonic acid appear to be particularly important in this regard.[60, 61] The approximately 40 cell types that are resident in normal lungs, as well as the inflammatory leukocytes that can infiltrate the airways and parenchyma in airway disease, all contain phospholipids as a major component of their plasma membranes. When stimulated appropriately by either immunologic or nonimmunologic events, each cell type can release arachidonic acid, which can undergo oxidative metabolism to form prostaglandins, thromboxanes, hydroxyeicosatetraenoic acids (HETEs), platelet-activating factor, and leukotrienes.

Some leukotrienes are powerful chemotactic agents, whereas others are potent spasmogens. These agents also increase vascular permeability and mucus formation in human airways and interact synergistically with other mediators. Some of the prostaglandins are also potent bronchoconstrictor agents with chemokinetic effects. In addition, they cause increased secretions from submucosal glands and are potent vasodilators. Hence, the metabolic products of arachidonic acid have the capability of producing the majority of the physiologic effects seen in acute and chronic asthma.

It has been argued that the secondary or "late reaction" was necessary to produce an increase in airway reactivity following antigen exposure.[62] This view no longer appears tenable. Airway reactivity is known to rise long before the late reaction begins.[63] Further, administration of cromolyn after the immediate response to antigen blocks the increase in reactivity but has no effect on the late reaction.[64] Hence, the data in these two studies dissociate the late reaction from the production of secondary effects in reactivity.

Axon Reflex

One of the pathologic features that is characteristic of bronchial asthma is damage and denudation of the surface epithelium of the airways.[2, 65] This phenomenon can elevate airway responsivity in several ways. For example, the epithelium, in many species, is known to contain a "relaxing factor" that protects against bronchoconstriction from many contractile agents.[66] The loss of this agent may permit exaggerated responses. Perhaps more importantly, denudation may expose sensory nerve endings. In the skin, evidence is mounting that the wheal and flare reaction seen with antigen injection is an axon reflex in which antidromic conduction down sensory pathways results in retrograde release of various neuropeptides, such as substance P, calcitonin gene-related peptide, and neurokinin A. If a similar situation developed in the airways, many of the features of asthma could be duplicated, as these neuropeptides are potential spasmogens that also increase vascular permeability and mucus production.[67]

Bronchial Microvasculature

In the past, major research on the pathogenesis and pathophysiology of asthma has focused on the bronchial smooth muscle. However, some of the most striking pathologic features are edema of the mucosa and submucosa and increased capillary density. Because of these observations, a number of investigators have begun to explore whether the bronchial microvasculature may make a contribution to the airway responses in this disease.

In theory, the bronchial circulation may play a significant role in the pathophysiology of airway obstruction from multiple vantage points.[68, 69] This vascular bed is critically situated anatomically to exert a modulating influence on airway geometry. Vascular engorgement or thickening of the mucosa from edema might readily produce obstruction in and of itself or might amplify the effects of airway smooth muscle constrictive stimuli. This circulation might also hypertrophy in response to multiple stimuli, such as a reduction in pulmonary blood flow, chronic inflammation, and obstructive airway disease. Under these circumstances, further acute increases in vascular size or changes in permeability might have dramatic effects on airway caliber.

In humans, the pulmonary venous hypertension that occurs in left-sided cardiac dysfunction is associated with engorgement of bronchial circulation. This, in turn, may produce wheezing and airflow obstruction.[70] These conditions can develop and evolve quickly and are presumed to be secondary to engorgement of the blood vessels within the confines of the bronchovascular sheath and thickening of the airway mucosa and submucosa from edema. For example, during experimentally induced myocardial ischemia, airway conductance rapidly falls and rises in concert with changes in left ventricular end diastolic pressures.[71] In addition, within the first several days following myocardial infarction, closing volumes rise and forced expiratory volumes and flow rates fall in association with elevations of pulmonary wedge pressure.[71–73] These mechanical decrements in lung function are not reversible by beta-agonist inhalation but do improve with the administration of diuretics, suggesting that vascular engorgement rather than smooth muscle contraction is the etiologic factor.

Bronchovascular engorgement and airway wall edema may also be important in the production of bronchial hyperresponsivity to nonspecific stimuli. Researchers[74] have found that patients with chronic impairment of left ventricular function and congestion of the bronchial vessels have airway responses to methacholine in the same range as patients with asthma. In these circumstances, beta-adrenergic agonists are only partially effective in reversing the obstruction. However, the vasoconstriction produced by an agonist prevents obstruction from developing. Similarly, rapid intravenous infusion of saline in normal subjects not only produces significant decrements in lung function but also reduces the provocative dose of methacholine required to cause a 35% fall in specific conductance.[75, 76]

Evidence for the role of bronchial circulation in the production of airway obstruction in certain aspects of asthma is growing. Data suggest that the airway obstruction in exercise-induced asthma derives from a vascular hyperemia with edema of the airway wall.[77–79] It is now recognized that the critical determinant for the development of airway narrowing with thermal stimuli, such as exercise or hyperventilation, is the magnitude of the temperature gradient that exists within the airways at the end of the challenge and immediate recovery period. The larger the gradient, the more rapid the rewarming and the more severe the obstruction.[77] Asthmatic patients have a larger bronchial vascular bed than healthy individuals and are known to rewarm the airways two to three times more quickly for any given gradient.[78] As this hyperemia develops, airway narrowing follows. If rewarming is blocked or reduced the obstruction follows suit.

REFERENCES

1. American Thoracic Society. Definitions and classifications of chronic bronchitis, asthma and pulmonary emphysema. Am Rev Respir Dis 1962; 85:762.
2. Dunill MS. The pathology of asthma with special reference to changes in the bronchial mucosa. J Clin Pathol 1960; 13:27–33.
3. NIAID Task Force on Asthma and Allergic Diseases. NIH Publications 79–387.
4. Respiratory Disease: Task Force Report on Prevention Control and Education, NHLBI, DHEW Publication 77–1248.
5. Hogg JC, Macklem PT, Thurlbeck WM. Site and nature of airway obstruction in chronic obstructive lung disease. N Engl J Med 1968; 278:1355–1360.
6. Thurlbeck WM. A pathologist's approach to clinical bronchitis and emphysema. In: Update: Fishman AP, Ed. Pulmonary Diseases and Disorders. New York: McGraw Hill, 1982, 137–148.
7. McFadden ER Jr. Asthma: airway dynamics, cardiac function and clinical correlates. In: Middleton E Jr, Reed CE, Ellis EF, et al., eds. Allergy: Principles and Practice. St. Louis: C.V. Mosby Company, 1988, 1018–1036.
8. Gold WM, Kaufman HS, Nadel JA. Elastic recoil of the lungs in chronic asthmatic patients before and after therapy. J Appl Physiol 1967; 23:483.
9. McFadden ER Jr, Ingram RH. Peripheral airway obstruction. JAMA 1976; 235:259–260.
10. Ingram RH, McFadden ER Jr. Pulmonary performance in chronic bronchitis and emphysema. In: Fishman AP, ed. Pulmonary Diseases and Disorders, New York: McGraw Hill, 1983, 542–548.
11. Thurlbeck WM, Henderson JA, Fraser RG, Bates DV. Chronic obstructive lung disease. A comparison between clinical, roentgenologic, functional and morphologic criteria in chronic bronchitis, emphysema, asthma and bronchiectasis. Medicine 1970; 49:81–145.
12. Levine G, Housley F, MacLeod P, Macklem PT. Gas exchange abnormalities in mild bronchitis and asymptomatic asthma. N Engl J Med 1970; 282:1277–1282.
13. McFadden ER Jr, Braunwald E. Cor pulmonale. In: Braunwald E, ed. Heart Disease. Philadelphia: W.B. Saunders Company, 1988, 1597–1616.
14. McFadden ER Jr, Lyons HA. Arterial blood gas tensions in asthma. N Engl J Med 1968; 278:1027.
15. Tri E, Reed J. Blood gas tensions in bronchial asthma. Lancet 1967; i:644.
16. Wong TR, Langer HM, Featherby EA, Levinson H. Arterial blood gas tensions and acid-base balance in symptomatic and asymptomatic asthma in childhood. Am Rev Respir Dis 1970; 101:274.
17. Kung TK, Briscoe WA. Abnormalities of blood gas exchange in COPD. Postgrad Med 1973; 54:101–108.
18. McNicol MW, Campbell EJ. Severity of respiratory failure. Arterial blood gases in untreated patients. Lancet 1965; i:336–338.
19. Boushey HA, Holtzman MJ, Sheller JR, Nadel JA. Bronchial hyperreactivity. Am Rev Respir Dis 1980; 121:389–413.
20. Hargreave FE, Ryan G, Thomson NC, et al. Bronchial responsiveness to histamine or methacholine in asthma: measurement and clinical significance. J Allergy Clin Immunol 1981; 68:347–355.
21. Konig P, Godfrey S. Prevalence of exercise-induced bronchial lability in families of children with asthma. Arch Dis Child 1973; 48:513–518.
22. Deal EC Jr, McFadden ER Jr, Ingram RH Jr, et al. Airway responsiveness to cold air and hyperpnea in normal subjects and in those with hay fever and asthma. Am Rev Respir Dis 1980; 121:621–628.
23. Silverman M, Hobbs FDR, Gordeon IRS, Carswell F. Cystic fibrosis, atopy and airway lability. Arch Dis Child 1978; 53:873–877.
24. Ramsdell JW, Nachtwey FS, Moser KM. Bronchial hyperreactivity in chronic obstructive bronchitis. Am Rev Respir Dis 1982; 126:829–832.
25. Astin TW. Reversibility of airways obstruction in chronic bronchitis. Clin Sci 1972; 42:725–733.
26. Simonsson BG, Jacobs FM, Nadel JA. Role of autonomic nervous system and the cough reflex in the increased responsiveness of airways in patients with obstructive airway disease. J Clin Invest 1967; 46:1812–1818.
27. DeVries K, Boois-Nsord H, Goei JT, et al. Hyperreactivity of the bronchial tree to drugs, chemical and physical agents. In: Orie NGM, Sluiter HJ, eds. Bronchitis II. An International Symposium. The Netherlands: Royal van Goreum, 1964, 167–180.
28. Payne CE, Chester EH, Hsi BP. Airway responsiveness in chronic obstructive pulmonary disease. Am J Med 1967; 42:554–566.
29. Light RW, Summe WR, Luchsinger PC. Response of patients with chronic obstructive lung disease to the regular administration of nebulized isoproterenol: a double-blind crossover study. Chest 1975; 67:634–639.
30. Ramsdell JW, Nachtwey FJ, Moser KM. Bronchial hyperreactivity in chronic obstructive bronchitis. Am Rev Respir Dis 1982; 126:829–832.
31. Gerrard JW, Cockcroft DW, Mink JT, et al. Increased nonspecific bronchial reactivity in cigarette smokers with normal lung function. Am Rev Respir Dis 1980; 122:577–581.
32. Barter CE, Campbell AH. Relationship of constitutional factors and cigarette smoking to decrease in 1-second forced expiratory volume. Am Rev Respir Dis 1976; 113:305–314.
33. Kabiraj MV, Simonsson BG, Groth S, et al. Bronchial reactivity, smoking, and alpha$_1$-antitrypsin: a population-based study of middle-aged men. Am Rev Respir Dis 1982; 126:864–869.
34. Buczko GB, Day A, Vanderdoelen JL, et al. Effects of cigarette smoking and short-term smoking cessation on airway responsiveness to inhaled methacholine. Am Rev Respir Dis 1984; 129:12–14.
35. Malo JL, Filiatrault S, Martin RR. Bronchial responsiveness to inhaled methacholine in young asymptomatic smokers. J Appl Physiol 1982; 52:1464–1470.
36. Brown NE, McFadden ER, Ingram RH. Airway response to inhaled histamine in asymptomatic smokers and non-smokers. J Appl Physiol 1977; 42:508–513.
37. Cockcroft DW, Berscheid BA, Murdock KY. Bronchial response to inhaled histamine in asymptomatic young smokers. Eur J Respir Dis 1983; 64:207–211.
38. McIntyre EL, Ruffin RE, Alpers JH. Lack of short-term effects of cigarette smoking on bronchial sensitivity to histamine and methacholine. Eur J Respir Dis 1982; 63:535–542.
39. Welty C, Weiss JF, Tager IB, et al. The relationship of airways responsiveness to cold air, cigarette smoking, and atopy to respiratory symptoms and pulmonary function in adults. Am Rev Respir Dis 1984; 130:198–203.
40. Dahms TE, Bolin JF, Slavin RG. Passive smoking: effects on bronchial asthma. Chest 1981; 80:530–534.
41. Numeroso R, Della Torre F, Radaelli C, et al. Effect of long-term treatment with sodium cromoglycate in non-specific bronchial hyperreactivity in non-atopic patients with chronic bronchitis. Respiration 1983; 44:109–117.
42. Empey DW, Laitinen LA, Jacobs L, et al. Mechanisms of bronchial hyperreactivity in normal subjects after upper respiratory tract infection. Am Rev Respir Dis 1976; 113:131–139.
43. Holtzman MI, Cunningham JH, Sheller JR, et al. Effect of ozone on bronchial reactivity in atopic and non-atopic subjects. Am Rev Respir Dis 1979; 120:1059–1067.
44. Orehek J, Massari JP, Gayrard P, et al. Effect of short-term, low-level nitrogen dioxide exposure on bronchial sensitivity of asthmatic patients. J Clin Invest 1976; 57:301–307.
45. Sheppard D, Epstein J, Bethel RA, et al. Tolerance to sulfur dioxide–induced bronchoconstriction in subjects with asthma. Environ Res 1983; 30:412–419.
46. Zawadski DK, Lenner KA, McFadden ER Jr. Effects of exercise on non-specific airway reactivity in asthmatics. J Appl Physiol 1988; 64:812–816.
47. Cuss FM, Dixon CMS, Barnes PJ. Effects of inhaled platelet activating factor on pulmonary function and bronchial responsiveness in man. Lancet 1986; ii:189–192.
48. Smolensky MH, Barnes PJ, Reinberg A, McGovern JP. Chronobiology and asthma. I. Day-night differences in bronchial patency and dyspnea and circadian rhythm dependencies. J Asthma 1986; 23:321–343.
49. Turner-Warwick M. On observing patterns of airflow obstruction in chronic asthma. Br J Dis Chest 1977; 71:73–86.

50. Hetzel MR, Clark TJH. Comparison of normal and asthmatic circadian rhythms in peak expiratory flow rate. Thorax 1980; 35:732–738.
51. Boulet LP, Cartier A, Thomson NC, et al. Asthma and increases in nonallergic bronchial responsiveness from seasonal pollen exposure. J Allergy Clin Immunol 1983; 71:399–406.
52. De Vries K, Goei JT, Booy-Noord H, Orie NGM. Changes during 24 hours in the lung function and histamine hyperreactivity of the bronchial tree in asthmatic and bronchitic patients. Int Arch Allergy Appl Immunol 1962; 20:93–101.
53. Gervais P, Reinberg A, Gervais C, et al. Twenty-four hour rhythm in the bronchial hyperreactivity to house dust in asthmatics. J Allergy Clin Immunol 1977; 59:207–213.
54. Weiss ST, Tager IB, Weiss JW, et al. The distribution of airways responsiveness in a population sample of adults and children. Am Rev Respir Dis 1981; 123:130 (abstract).
55. DeJongste JC, Mons H, Bonta IL, Kerrebijn KF. *In vitro* responses of airways from an asthmatic patient. Eur J Respir Dis 1987; 71:23–29.
56. Goldie RG, Spina D, Henry PJ, et al. *In vitro* responsiveness of human asthmatic bronchus to carbachol, histamine, beta-adrenergic agonists and theophylline. Br J Clin Pharmacol 1986; 22:669–676.
57. Schellenberg RR, Foster A. *In vitro* responses of human asthmatic airway and pulmonary vascular smooth muscle. Int Arch Allergy Appl Immunol 1984; 75:237–241.
58. Chung KF. Role of inflammation in the hyperreactivity of the airways in asthma. Thorax 1986; 41:657–662.
59. Nadel JA. Inflammation and asthma. J Allergy Clin Immunol 1984; 73:651–653.
60. Henderson WR Jr. Lipid-derived and other chemical mediators of inflammation in the lung. J Allergy Clin Immunol 1987; 79:543–553.
61. Drazen JM, Austen KF. Leukotrienes and airway responses. Am Rev Respir Dis 1987; 136:985–998.
62. Cartier A, Thompson NC, Frith PA, et al. Allergen-induced increases in bronchial responsiveness to histamine: Relationship to the late asthmatic response and change in airway caliber. J Allergy Clin Immunol 1982; 70:170–177.
63. Thorpe JE, Steinberg D, Bernstein IL, Murlas CG. Bronchial reactivity increases soon after the immediate response in dual-responding asthmatic subjects. Chest 1987; 91:21–25.
64. Mattoli S, Foresi A, Corbo GM, et al. Effects of two doses of cromolyn on allergen-induced late asthmatic response and increased responsiveness. J Allergy Clin Immunol 1987; 79:747–754.
65. Laitinen LA, Heino M, Laitinen A, et al. Damage of the airway epithelium and bronchial reactivity in patients with asthma. Am Rev Respir Dis 1985; 131:599–606.
66. Flanahan NA, Aarhus LL, Rimele TJ, Vanhoutte PM. Respiratory epithelium inhibits bronchial smooth muscle tone. J Appl Physiol 1985; 58:834–838.
67. Barnes PJ. Asthma as an axon reflex. Lancet 1986; i:242–245.
68. Baier H, Long WM, Wanner A. Bronchial circulation in asthma. Respiration 1985; 48:199–205.
69. Laitinen LA, Laitinen A, Widdicombe J. Effects of inflammatory and other mediators on airway vascular beds. Am Rev Respir Dis 1987; 135:S67–S70.
70. McFadden ER Jr, Ingram RH Jr. Relationship between diseases of the heart and lungs. In: Braunwald E, ed. Heart Disease. Philadelphia: WB Saunders Company, 1988, 1870–1882.
71. Pepine CJ, Wiener L. Relationship of an anginal symptom to lung mechanics during myocardial ischemia. Circulation 1972; 46:863–869.
72. Light RW, George RB. Serial pulmonary function in patients with acute heart failure. Arch Intern Med 1983; 143:429–433.
73. Hales CA, Kazemi H. Small airways dysfunction in myocardial infarction. N Engl J Med 1974; 290:761–763.
74. Gabanes LR, Weber SN, Matran R, et al. Bronchial hyperresponsiveness to methacholine in patients with impaired left ventricular function. N Engl J Med 1989; 320:1317–1322.
75. Rolla G, Bucca C, Polizzi S, et al. Site of airway obstruction after rapid saline infusion in healthy subjects. Respiration 1983; 44:90–96.
76. Rolla G, Scappaticci E, Baldi S, Bucca C. Methacholine inhalation challenge after rapid saline infusion in healthy subjects. Respiration 1986; 50:18–22.
77. McFadden ER Jr, Lenner KA, Strohl KP. Post-exertional airway rewarming and thermally induced asthma. J Clin Invest 1986; 78:18–25.
78. Gilbert IA, Fouke JM, McFadden ER Jr. Heat and water flux in the intrathoracic airways and exercise induced asthma. J Appl Physiol 1987; 63:1681–1691.
79. Gilbert IA, Fouke JM, McFadden ER Jr. Intra-airway thermodynamics during exercise and hyperventilation in asthmatics. J Appl Physiol 1988; 64:2167–2174.

Chapter 11

UPPER AIRWAY FUNCTION IN COPD

A. Brancatisano Ludwig A. Engel

Interest in the upper airway as a respiratory organ active in ventilatory control naturally has raised the question as to its function in respiratory disease states. In neonates, the upper airway plays a prominent role in the control of expiratory flow and lung volume. In healthy adults its contribution is probably minor. However, clinical observations in patients with airflow obstructions have for a long time suggested that the upper airway is in some way involved in the behavioral or physiologic adjustments, or both, that these individuals make to their ventilatory impairment.

In this chapter we attempt to identify and discuss the anatomic and functional aspects of the upper airway that are important in patients with airflow obstruction.

SIZE AND DIMENSIONS

Among the earliest measurements of upper airway resistance in patients with chronic airflow limitation were those of Campbell and colleagues,[8] who studied individuals with noticeably noisy respiration and harsh breath sounds on auscultation over the larynx. These investigators noted that during quiet tidal breathing, upper airway resistance was significantly greater in these patients compared with healthy subjects. The main difference was due to a greater than two-fold increase in expiratory resistance that the authors attributed to enhanced glottic narrowing.

Subsequently, Higenbottam and Payne[22] measured the width of the vocal cords from photographs taken through a fiberoptic bronchoscope in a larger group of patients with chronic obstructive pulmonary disease (COPD). The patients were grouped on the basis of severity of disease, as indicated by the forced expiratory volume in 1 second (FEV_1), and demonstrated a relationship between glottic width and FEV_1 during quiet tidal breathing (Fig. 11–1). After correction for age and weight, the greater the reduction in FEV_1 the smaller were the glottic dimensions. Although the largest changes were at the onset of expiration, inspiratory glottic size also appeared to correlate with FEV_1.

Computed tomography (CT) of the upper airways in a group of 32 patients with severe COPD (FEV_1 < 1.5 L) indicated that in those with hypercapnia the cross-sectional area of the upper airways was approximately half of that measured in the age-matched eucapnic patients.[10] No significant difference was observed in age, FEV_1, degree of hyperinflation, or gas exchange capacity (DL_{CO}) between the two groups. However, the hypercapnic patients had significantly greater cigarette and alcohol consumption. In another group of patients with severe COPD and obstructive sleep apnea (OSA), the upper airway cross-sectional area (measured by CT scanning) was found to be substantially smaller in the hypercapnic patients relative to the eucapnic patients.[11] The patients with hypercapnia and small upper airway dimensions had a greater alcohol consumption. No significant difference in FEV_1 or the apnea index occurred between the two groups.

DYNAMIC RESPONSES

In healthy subjects voluntary panting results in a wider glottic aperture, with minimal variability between two phases of panting.[7] Relative to quiet breathing, the changes are exclusively due to the abolition of the glottic narrowing during expiration. In contrast, in patients with COPD the response of the glottis depends on the severity of the airflow limitation.[22] In those with FEV_1 above 80% predicted, the glottis responds normally. However, in patients with FEV_1 less than 60% predicted, expiratory glottic narrowing persists during panting. Indeed, relative to the dimensions during quiet breathing a narrowing of the glottis occurs during both phases of respiration.

During a forced expiration the glottis widens maximally in healthy subjects.[5, 12] In contrast, in patients with chronic airflow obstruction the glottis remains narrowed,[22] without any changes as a function of lung volume.

In healthy subjects, as well as in anesthetized and unanesthetized animals, the expiratory glottic narrowing and laryngeal resistance are diminished during hyperventilation induced by hypercapnia.[18, 20, 33, 34] However, in patients with severe chronic airflow obstruction this does not appear to be the case. Kelly and colleagues[28] measured glottic and supraglottic dimensions from a fluoroscopic image in a group of patients with an FEV_1 36% predicted. During hyperoxic hypercapnia, although ventilation increased from 12 to 21 L/min (corresponding to 73% of maximum), the expiratory narrowing of the glottis was not reduced (Table 11–1). No change in supraglottic dimensions was observed. Similarly, 10 cm H_2O continuous positive airway pressure (CPAP) at the mouth also failed to reduce the marked expiratory glottic narrowing.[28] This finding contrasted with the results in asthmatic patients with induced bronchoconstriction, in whom the expiratory glottic and supraglottic narrowing during expiration was reversed by CPAP.[14, 15]

FUNCTIONAL IMPLICATIONS

Airflow Regulation in Normal Subjects

It has been suggested that the expiratory glottic narrowing during tidal breathing in healthy subjects constitutes a mechanism for braking expiratory flow and thereby controlling the

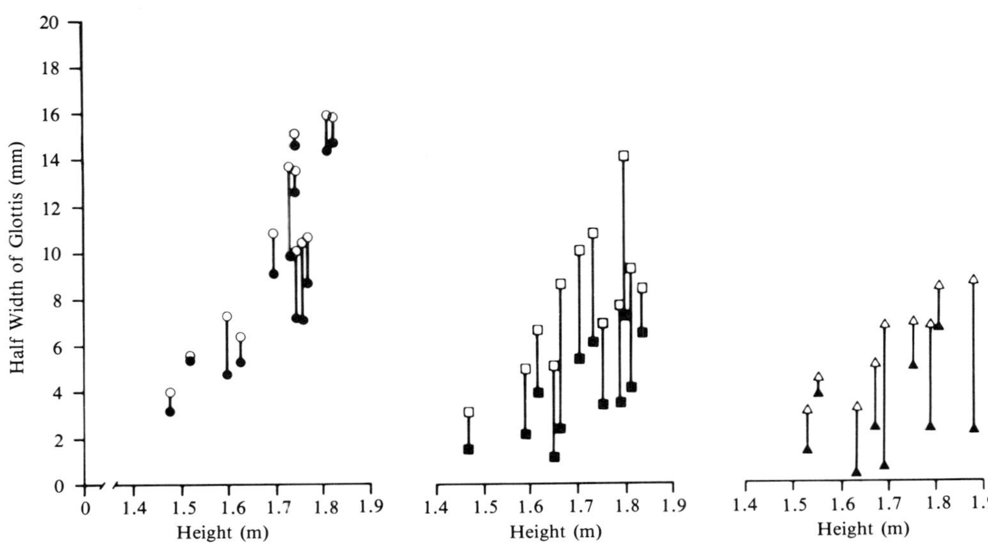

Figure 11–1. Mean values for half-width of the glottis plotted against height in patients with chronic airflow limitation. Circles: FEV_1 > 80% predicted. Squares: FEV_1 60% to 80% predicted. Triangles: FEV_1 < 60% predicted. Open symbols: mean values on inspiration. Closed symbols: values during expiration. Note that the greater the degree of airflow obstruction the narrower the glottis. (Reproduced with permission from Higenbottam TW, Payne J. Am Rev Respir Dis 1982; 125:746.)

TABLE 11–1. Upper Airway Dimensions and Ventilatory Parameters in Patients with COPD*

	$\dot{V}_E$ (L/min)	$FeCO_2$ (%)	Dgi (mm)	Dge (mm)	Dsgi (mm)	Dsge (mm)
QB n=13	2.3 (1.3)	4.8 (0.3)	7.7 (0.4)	4.2† (0.5)	12.2 (1.0)	8.5† (1.0)
CPAP n=8	15.4 (1.5)	4.8 (0.3)	8.7 (0.5)	5.6† (0.6)	14.6 (1.3)	11.2† (1.2)
RB n=8	20.7 (1.5)	7.8 (0.1)	8.5 (0.9)	3.0† (0.5)	12.7‡ (1.0)	8.6 (1.1)

*Glottic and supraglottic lateral diameters (Dg and Dsg) at mid-tidal inspiration (i) and expiration (e), at the stated ventilation ($\dot{V}_E$), and expired CO_2 concentration ($FeCO_2$) during quiet breathing (QB), continuous positive airway pressure (CPAP), and hyperoxic hypercapnia (n = no. of patients; mean ± SE).

†$p<0.02$ (relative to Di).

‡$p<0.02$ (relative to QB).

(Adapted from Kelly W, Tully A, Brancatisano A, Engel LA. Thorax 1987; 40:727.)

time course of lung emptying.[2, 6, 20] This narrowing is reduced during hyperpnea induced by hypoxia, hypercapnia, or exercise[4, 18] as well as during voluntary panting and forced expiratory maneuvers. These dimensional changes are reflected in corresponding decreases in upper airway resistance at the higher flow rates.[1, 2, 29, 34]

Implicit in the regulatory role attributed to the upper airway is the compensatory change in dimensions expected when pulmonary resistance increases. In this context, the enhanced expiratory glottic narrowing in patients with COPD is paradoxical, as it does not compensate for the increase in resistance. A similar paradox applies to induced bronchoconstriction, both in patients with bronchial asthma and healthy subjects.[14, 19, 23] Brancatisano and Engel[6] suggested that the expiratory upper airway narrowing may be recruited as a mechanism for maintaining lung volume and hyperinflation in patients with airflow obstruction. This is similar to the role of the glottis in young infants in whom endotracheal intubation, bypassing this mechanism, results in a decreased lung volume and impaired gas exchange.[21] Supportive evidence for this concept in adults has been obtained by Collett and colleagues[14] who studied the glottic and supraglottic expiratory narrowing in asthmatic patients with induced bronchoconstriction. When CPAP was applied at the mouth, the expiratory narrowing was reversed. This is what would have been expected if the upper airway served to decrease expiratory flow, maintain hyperinflation, or both. Presumably, the CPAP took the place of the upper airway mechanism. However, extension of this mechanism to patients with COPD is complicated by the fact that application of CPAP to such patients does not reduce the expiratory glottic and upper airway narrowing.[28] Whether the failure to abolish the expiratory upper airway narrowing by CPAP reflects an adaptation to chronic hyperinflation or whether the changes in the upper airway reflect some other physiologic mechanism is not certain.

Relationship to Pursed-Lip Breathing

Many patients with chronic airflow limitations breathe with their lips pursed during expiration, during and immediately after exertion, or even at rest. We have studied the upper airways in several such patients by visualization through bronchoscopy and by fluoroscopy. In each case it was our impression that the pursing of the lips and the upper airway narrowing were synchronous and part of a single functional process.

Thomson and coworkers[35] measured the effects of pursed-lip breathing at rest in patients with airflow limitation and found that it slowed expiratory flow and breathing frequency and increased tidal volume. Other investigators have reported similar findings and showed that gas exchange was improved.[31, 36] However, the beneficial effect on gas exchange could be reproduced by modifying the temporal pattern of breathing without pursing the lips.[30] Therefore, it is not the pursed-lip breathing per se that improves gas exchange.

In contrast, Ingram and Schilder[24] proposed that pursed-lip breathing minimizes the collapse of intrapulmonary airways during expiration. Because airway collapse or deformation may stimulate airway afferents, thereby creating unpleasant respiratory sensations, a mechanism for slowing expiratory flow, thus avoiding such stimuli, seems plausible. A reduction in intrathoracic airway pressure, achieved by upper airway narrowing, may diminish airway collapse downstream of the flow-limiting segment without a reduction in expiratory flow. A reduction in peak expiratory flow by upper airway narrowing will also diminish airway collapse and should be energetically advantageous over alternative mechanisms, such as the post-inspiratory activity of the inspiratory muscles. Thus, it is possible, though speculative, that pursed-lip breathing constitutes an outward manifestation of an integrated upper airway process aimed at minimizing airway collapse and maintaining hyperinflation by an endogenous positive end-expiratory pressure.

Implications of Inspiratory Upper Airway Narrowing

In contrast to the potentially beneficial effects of expiratory upper airway narrowing on regulating flow and maintaining lung volume, it is difficult to conceive of a mechanism by which an increase in inspiratory upper airway resistance could be of benefit. In patients with airflow limitation, the smaller laryngeal dimensions during inspiration constitute an additional resistance in series to that of the lung,[22] to be overcome by the inspiratory muscles. Similarly, during sleep, partial upper airway obstruction, associated with snoring, constitutes an added load. Even in the absence of obstructive sleep apnea this load may result in hypoventilation that in healthy individuals may be associated with minor changes in arterial hemoglobin desaturation. However, in patients with chronic airflow limitation and some degree of hypoxemia in the awake state, the added inspiratory obstruction may result in periods of substantial hypoxemia.

It is not known how sleep influences the expiratory upper airway narrowing and the consequent modulation of lung volume. It is possible that impaired regulation of lung volume and hypoventilation due to increased inspiratory resistance combine to disadvantage the patient with chronic airflow limitation during sleep. The role of excessive alcohol consumption, addressed by Chan and colleagues,[10] may result in a vicious cycle of increased snoring causing soft tissue edema with further inspiratory obstruction and hypoventilation. As suggested by these investigators, this mechanism may be important in the development of chronic hypercapnic respiratory failure in such patients.

Implications for Measurement of Intrapulmonary Airway Function

Measurement of intrapulmonary airway function either by indices derived from a forced expiration or by airway/pulmonary resistance carries the implicit assumption that the resistance in the upper airway is a small component of the total.

Indeed, in healthy individuals the glottic dilatation during forced expiration, panting, or hyperpnea insures that this is the case. However, in a patient with airflow obstruction, in whom the glottis fails to dilate during such maneuvers or even narrows further, the intrapulmonary airflow obstruction may be overestimated. Additional studies are needed to determine to what degree and under what circumstances this overestimate is important.

CLINICAL VARIANTS

A number of clinical conditions exist in which fixed or variable narrowing of the upper airways gives rise to symptoms of dyspnea and exercise limitation. Although laryngotracheal obstruction can be suspected from a careful history and physical examination, it often mimics diffuse airway obstruction. Furthermore, routine pulmonary function tests may fail to identify the true site of the obstructive process.

Chronic upper airway obstruction can be caused by a wide variety of conditions and the following list is by no means complete: vocal cord paralysis, carcinoma of the pharynx and larynx, subglottic stenosis, goiter, extrinsic compression of the trachea, and tracheomalacia. However, certain physiologic features are common in these conditions and form the bases for detecting and differentiating upper airway obstruction from more peripheral intrapulmonary obstruction using the flow-volume loop.[27]

DETECTION OF UPPER AIRWAY OBSTRUCTION

Because intraluminal pressures are positive during a forced expiration, the extrathoracic portion of the airway is exposed to expanding transmural forces. In contrast, during a rapid inspiration, the pressure drop between the mouth (or nose) and alveoli results in negative transmural pressures along the extrathoracic airway. Consequently, a variable extrathoracic obstruction (e.g., due to bilateral vocal cord paralysis or carcinoma of the larynx) will be marked by a relatively greater reduction of maximum inspiratory flow, with a relatively flat inspiratory limb of the maximum flow-volume loop. Depending on the severity of the obstruction, the expiratory flow may also be decreased. However, differentiation from intrapulmonary airflow obstruction is often possible, as in the latter case flow reduction is greatest at the low lung volumes, whereas in upper airway obstruction flow at high lung volumes is most affected. Nevertheless, in patients with severe COPD marked expiratory flow limitation during a forced expiration can mask even moderately severe upper airway obstruction.

During a forced expiration the intrathoracic portion of the trachea narrows. This effect reflects the relatively more positive pleural pressure due to the pressure drop within the airway between the alveoli and the trachea. Consequently an intrathoracic lesion of the trachea or major bronchus (e.g., endobronchial tumor) results in a relatively greater reduction of flow on the expiratory limb of the flow-volume loop, especially at the higher lung volumes. However, coexistence of the more peripheral airway narrowing of COPD with such a lesion may mask the central airway obstruction. The clinical symptoms may be wrongly attributed to irreversible COPD.

Expiratory Tracheobronchial Collapse

Whereas normal tracheal dynamics include a small caliber change with respiration and a one-half or less diameter collapse with coughing in the anteroposterior plane,[25] in some individuals marked expiratory narrowing of the trachea and mainstem bronchi may give rise to a special type of intrathoracic large airway obstruction. The condition is well described but poorly defined and its etiology not understood. In contrast to localized tracheal collapse secondary to surgical intervention (e.g., tracheostomy) or localized pathology extrinsic to the trachea, the etiology of most cases of expiratory tracheal collapse is not known. Even the semantics of the term "tracheomalacia," frequently applied to this condition, are misleading. Indeed, Baxter and Dunbar[3] attributed the abnormality to weakness of the tracheal wall from softening of the supporting cartilage as well as hypotonia of the myoelastic elements. However, most endoscopic observations indicate that the pars membranacea is widened and flattened, resulting in the invagination of the posterior wall into the lumen with relatively slight increases of intrathoracic pressure. In one patient in whom histologic examination of the trachea was performed, the number of longitudinal elastic fibers in the pars membranacea was clearly reduced throughout the whole trachea, but no differences were found in the amount of collagen, mucopolysaccharides, and elastin in the cartilages of the trachea and bronchi relative to healthy control subjects.[26]

Although the condition is diagnosed endoscopically or fluoroscopically, the symptomatology attributable to the expiratory tracheal collapse is not clear. In most studies an association with COPD was inferred and the same etiologic factors were implicated.[9, 26]

Most investigators associated expiratory tracheal collapse with a cough that was frequently paroxysmal and persistent, and in some cases had a barking or honking quality. Exertional dyspnea was present in many cases but differentiation from the associated COPD was difficult. In at least one study in which tracheal closure on coughing was demonstrated by fluoroscopy in a group of otherwise fit relatively young patients, no other respiratory illness appeared to be present.[16] Interestingly, a repeat study in two patients in whom symptoms resolved showed persistence of the abnormality.

Management of the condition is complicated by its poorly understood nature. In patients with persistent cough, symptomatic therapy may be helpful. In cases of marked expiratory flow limitation, relaxed exhalation or breathing with lips pursed reduces the peak expiratory flows and the degree of tracheal collapse. In very severe cases, surgical stabilization of the posterior, membranous wall of the trachea has been performed with claims of substantial improvement. The condition in adults differs from congenital tracheomalacia in infants, which appears to be self-limiting and resolves after the age of 2 years.

Laryngeal Wheeze

In some individuals, marked expiratory glottic narrowing may appear as a primary abnormality. These patients present with wheeze and dyspnea and are usually diagnosed as suffering from bronchial asthma. However, the wheezing is loudest over the larynx and pulmonary function test results, including those of flow-volume loops, are generally normal. Rodenstein and colleagues[32] studied such a patient in detail and observed that during the wheezing attack end-expiratory lung volume was displaced toward residual volume, with forced expiration at low lung volumes. Inhalation challenge test findings with histamine and methylcholine were all negative. In another study, when patients with laryngeal wheezing were asked to pant or were mildly sedated, the wheezing ceased.[17] However, at least in one well-documented case, the expiratory glottic narrowing continued during general anesthesia,[13] so that the term "emotional laryngeal wheezing" applied to this condition by Rodenstein and colleagues may not be entirely appropriate.[32]

CONCLUSIONS

The realization that the upper airway is not merely a passive conduit to the lung but constitutes an active mechanism relevant to ventilatory control has altered the way we view this part of the respiratory system both in health and disease. Observations in patients with chronic airflow obstruction suggest that significant changes in function related to respiration take place in these conditions. Some of these changes appear well defined (e.g., expiratory glottic narrowing and pursed-lip breathing), although the exact functional benefit is not yet clear. Other changes appear to contribute to the load borne by the respiratory system and do not appear to serve any useful function. Snoring, although not limited to patients with airflow obstruction, falls into this category and may have more adverse effects than in the healthy population. Clearly, further work is required to understand the mechanism and the consequences of inspiratory upper airway obstruction in patients, particularly during sleep.

REFERENCES

1. Bartlett D Jr. Effects of hypercapnia and hypoxia on laryngeal resistance to airflow. Respir Physiol 1979; 37:293.
2. Bartlett D Jr, Remmers JE, Gautier H. Laryngeal regulation of respiratory airflow. Respir Physiol 1973; 18:194.
3. Baxter JD, Dunbar JS. Tracheomalacia. Ann Otol 1963; 72:1012.
4. Brancatisano A, Dodd DS, Engel LA. Responses of the posterior cricoarytenoid and alae nasi muscles to increased chemical drive in man. Respir Physiol 1986; 64:177.
5. Brancatisano A, Collett PW, Engel LA. Respiratory movements of the vocal cords. J Appl Physiol 1983; 54:1269.
6. Brancatisano A, Engel LA. Role of the upper airway in the control of respiratory flow and lung volume in humans. In: Mathew O, Sant'Ambrogio G, eds. Respiratory Function of the Upper Airway. New York: Marcel Dekker, 1988, 477.
7. Brancatisano A, Dodd DS, Engel LA. Respiratory activity of posterior cricoarytenoid muscle and vocal cords in humans. J Appl Physiol 1984; 57:1143.
8. Campbell AH, Imberger H, Jones B McC. Increased upper airway resistance in patients with airway narrowing. Br J Dis Chest 1976; 70:58.
9. Campbell AH, Young IF. Tracheobronchial collapse, a variant of obstructive respiratory disease. Br J Dis Chest 1963; 57:174.
10. Chan CS, Bye PTP, Woolcock AT. Hypercapnic COPD: The role of the upper airway. Aust NZ J Med 1988; 18:529.
11. Chan CS, Sullivan CE. Obstructive sleep apnea with severe COPD: Hypercapnic versus eucapnic. Aust NZ J Med 1988; 18:528.
12. Clement J, Stanescu DG, Van De Woestijne KP. Glottis opening and effort-dependent part of the isovolume pressure-flow curves. J Appl Physiol 1973; 34:18.
13. Cohen JI, ed. Upper airway obstruction in asthma. Johns Hopkins Med J 1980; 147:233.
14. Collett PW, Brancatisano A, Engel LA. Changes in the glottic aperture during bronchial asthma. Am Rev Respir Dis 1983; 128:719.
15. Collett PW, Brancatisano A, Engel LA. Upper airway dimensions and movements in bronchial asthma. Am Rev Respir Dis 1986; 133:1143.
16. Delohery JF, Allen DH, Vandenberg RA. Tracheomalacia and its association with persistent barking cough in fit young patients. Aust NZ J Med 1983; 13:549.
17. Downing ET, Braman SS, Fox MJ, Carrao WM. Factitious asthma: Physiological approach to diagnosis. JAMA 1982; 248:2878.
18. England SJ, Bartlett D Jr, Knuth SL. Comparison of human vocal cord movements during isocapnic hypoxia and hypercapnia. J Appl Physiol 1982; 53:81.
19. England SJ, Ho V, Zamel N. Laryngeal constriction in normal humans during experimentally induced bronchoconstriction. J Appl Physiol 1985; 58:352.
20. Gautier H, Remmers JE, Bartlett D Jr. Control of the duration of expiration. Respir Physiol 1973; 18:205.
21. Harrison VC, Heese H de V, Klein M. The significance of grunting in hyaline membrane disease. Pediatrics 1968; 41:549.
22. Higenbottam TW, Payne J. Glottis narrowing in lung disease. Am Rev Respir Dis 1982; 125:746.
23. Higenbottam TW. Narrowing of glottis opening in humans associated with experimentally induced bronchoconstriction. J Appl Physiol 1980; 49:403.
24. Ingram RH, Schilder DP. Effect of pursed-lips expiration on the pulmonary pressure-flow relationship in obstructive lung disease. Am Rev Respir Dis 1967; 96:381.
25. Johnson TH, Mikita JHJ, Wilton RJ, Feist JH. Acquired tracheomalacia. Radiology 1973; 109:577.
26. Jokinen K, Palva T, Sutinen S, Nuutinen J. Acquired tracheomalacia. Ann Clin Res 1977; 9:52.
27. Jordanoglou J, Price NB. A comparison of maximum inspiratory and expiratory flow in health and in lung disease. Thorax 1968; 23:38.
28. Kelly W, Tully A, Brancatisano A, Engel LA. Respiratory changes in laryngeal dimensions in patients with chronic airflow limitation (CAL). Thorax 1987; 42:727.
29. McCaffrey TV, Kern EB. Laryngeal regulation of airway resistance, I: Chemoreceptor reflexes. Ann Otol Rhinol Laryngol 1980; 89:209.
30. Motley HL. The effects of slow deep breathing on the blood gas exchange in emphysema. Am Rev Respir Dis 1963; 88:485.
31. Mueller RE, Petty TL, Filley GF. Ventilation and arterial blood gas changes induced by pursed-lips breathing. J Appl Physiol 1970; 28:784.
32. Rodenstein DO, Francis D, Stanescu DC. Emotional laryngeal wheezing: A new syndrome. Am Rev Respir Dis 1983; 127:354.
33. Sekizawa K, Yanai M, Sasaki H, Takishima T. Control of larynx during loaded breathing in normal subjects. J Appl Physiol 1986; 60:1887.
34. Spann RW, Hyatt RE. Factors affecting upper airway resistance in conscious man. J Appl Physiol 1971; 31:708.
35. Thomson RL, Stocker CL, Ross JC. The efficacy of pursed lips breathing in patients with chronic obstructive pulmonary disease. Am Rev Respir Dis 1966; 93:100.
36. Tiep BL, Burns M, Kao D, et al. Pursed-lips breathing training using ear oximetry. Chest 1986; 90:218.

Chapter 12

THE EFFECT OF COPD ON PULMONARY CIRCULATION

J. Peter Szidon

PULMONARY VASCULAR RESISTANCE

The pulmonary circulation is a low-resistance circuit that can accommodate ten-fold increases in cardiac output while requiring a driving pressure of almost an order of magnitude less than the systemic circulation. The large aggregate cross-sectional area of the pulmonary circulation is the primary reason for this low resistance. Among its anatomic counterparts are the relative sparsity of smooth muscle in the walls of pulmonary resistance vessels and the large capacity and recruitment potential of the capillary bed.

The concept of resistance to flow through the pulmonary circulation has been applied to investigate potential mechanisms of pulmonary hypertension and to assess changes in the properties of blood vessels in the lungs of patients with COPD and in animal models of emphysema. Some of the properties that are believed to be contributory have included the anatomic decrease in cross-sectional area of the circulation, presumably caused by either destruction of the vascular bed due to emphysema or the decrease in lumen area of arteries secondary to proliferation of components of the vessel wall; the effects of increase in viscosity of blood; the quantitation of vasomotor activity secondary to changes in alveolar gas composition or to the administration of vasoactive agents; and the effects of lung inflation and increased alveolar pressures.

The relationship among pulmonary vascular resistance (R), pulmonary blood flow (cardiac output, $\dot{Q}$), and the pressure drop across the pulmonary circulation (ΔP) is given by the expression

$$R = \frac{\Delta P}{\dot{Q}}$$

which is the linear hydraulic equivalent of Ohm's law. If the vascular resistance is elevated, the favorite interpretation given is that vessels are vasoconstricted. However, if a change in resistance is to be equated with a change in vascular caliber, the rigorous application of Ohm's law would require that flow be laminar, viscosity unchanging, and vessels be otherwise rigid, i.e., that little or no vascular geometric change be associated with alterations in lung volume or in left atrial pressure. If one wished to take into consideration the presence of pulsatile blood flow and pressure in the pulmonary circulation, a series of additional complexities for interpretation would have to be added.[46] Methods to measure pulsations and to describe the propagation of oscillatory pressures and flows across the pulmonary circulation are available.[66] The theoretic bases for the interpretation of measurements of vascular impedance[50] or for describing how the oscillatory hydraulic energy imparted by the right ventricle is dissipated in its passage through the pulmonary circulation have been published.[62] However, the applicability of these methodologies to clinical situations, such as chronic obstructive pulmonary disease (COPD), remains to be tested.

The basic usefulness of the calculation of pulmonary vascular resistance is limited to its ability to provide information about the magnitude of the pressure gradient required to drive a unit of volume flow across the lung vasculature. In order to understand the interpretation of the mechanisms underlying changes in pulmonary vascular resistance, it is necessary to examine the behavior of pressure-flow curves over a full range. If pressure-flow curves were not so difficult to obtain, calculation of vascular resistance would probably be unnecessary. All pertinent information is contained in pressure-flow curves without having to deal with some of the potential pitfalls described subsequently. The choice of the type of circuit with which to model the relationship between pressure and flow determines the nature of the inferences that can be made. To exemplify this point, we consider two circuit models and examine the effects of changes in blood flow and in outflow pressure on vascular resistance calculated according to the formula shown previously. The circuit on Figure 12–1 consists of an indistensible tube. The outflow pressure is left atrial (LA) and inflow pressure pulmonary arterial (PA). The relationship between the pressure drop (PA-LA) and flow ($\dot{Q}$) is constant and can be established by measuring any single point

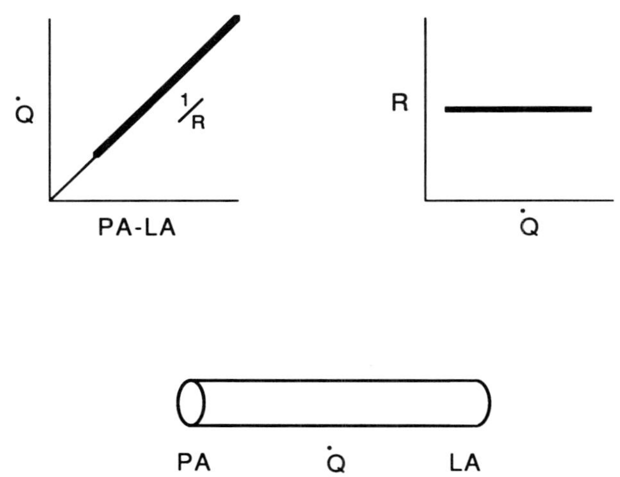

Figure 12–1. Diagrammatic representation of the relationship among pressure gradient (PA-LA), flow ($\dot{Q}$), and resistance (R) in a rigid tube model.

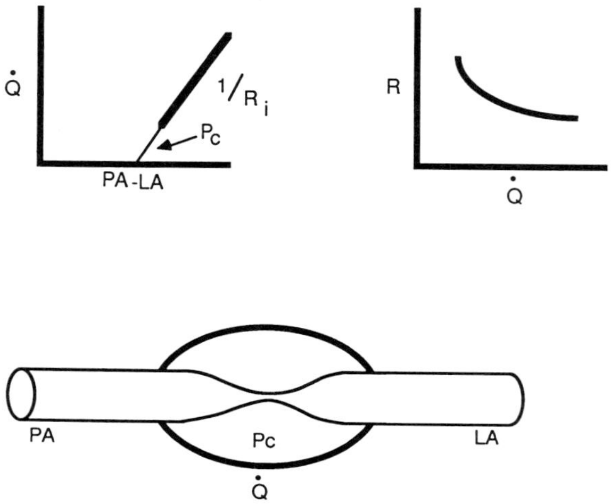

Figure 12–2. Diagrammatic representation of the relationship among pressure gradient (PA-LA), flow ($\dot{Q}$), critical closing pressure (Pc), "ohmic" resistance (R), and incremental resistance (Ri) in a Starling resistor model.

on the line. The origin of the line, by extrapolation, passes through zero. Increases in outflow pressure do not change the slope. If a similar rigid tube of smaller caliber is substituted, there will be a larger value of R and a corresponding decrease in the slope of the pressure-flow line, which will tilt toward the pressure axis, whereas the origin will still pass through zero. This is the model that accounts for the calculation of resistance according to Ohm's law.

The model depicted in Figure 12–2, the Starling resistor, contains a segment of collapsible tubing enclosed in a rigid chamber. The pressure in this chamber (Pc) is sufficient to collapse the tubing. Under these circumstances, flow will not begin until the pressure in PA is made to exceed Pc. If we assume that the outflow pressure LA is less than Pc, the line describing the relationship between PA-LA and $\dot{Q}$ will intercept the abscissa at a point equal to Pc. The inverse slope of this line (1/Ri) is different from the 1/R calculated according to the hydraulic equivalent of Ohm's law using the same set of data. In analogy to electrical circuits with nonlinear voltage/current relationships, Ri can be called an "incremental resistance" and it reflects the unit change in pressure per unit change in flow. A change in the magnitude of Pc will cause an equivalent parallel shift in the position of the pressure-flow line, but there will be no change in incremental resistance. Replacing the rigid portion of the tube upstream from Pc with another of smaller caliber will be associated with a change in slope, as in the first model, but the intercept of the pressure-flow line will continue to cross the abscissa at Pc.

Figure 12–2 also illustrates that if calculations of "ohmic" resistance are done in the Starling resistor circuit, e.g., for the hypothetic situation of constant LA, Pc larger than LA, there will be a progressive decline in R with increasing values of PA-LA and $\dot{Q}$ along their linear relationship even though neither the slope nor the position of the line has changed. This point is better illustrated numerically in the right hand columns of Figure 12–3 (A, B, and C). On the left-hand columns (B_1, B_2, and B_3) another example of progressive decline in R without change in Ri is given, this time for the case of increases in LA going from zero to just below Pc, whereas PA and $\dot{Q}$ are constant. It is clear that now a smaller pressure gradient is required to drive the unit of volume flow through the circuit, but "vasodilation" does not need to be invoked.

It should be apparent from these examples that the slope and the intercept of pressure-flow lines can provide significant information regarding the nature of changes in the vasculature. In contrast, the calculation of vascular resistance using the hydraulic equivalent of Ohm's law in a setting where a significant level of Pc is suspected or known to be present can lead to potential misinterpretation of the mechanism of change in R. The reasons for elaborating on models for the pressure-flow relationship of the pulmonary vasculature will become evident later. The pulmonary circulation in COPD seems to have a high value of Pc, which apparently increases during exercise. This effect greatly limits the use of the "ohmic" calculation of pulmonary vascular resistance as an index of cross-sectional area.

Pressure-flow curves obtained in a variety of experimental animals both in excised lungs[51] and *in vivo*[63] consistently show an intersection of the abscissa at values that exceed alveolar and outflow pressures (Fig. 12–4). This is especially evident in preparations in which zone II conditions, i.e., alveolar pressure greater than outflow pressure, are created. Even though a variety of mechanical models can be used to account for the behavior of pressure-flow curves under various experimental conditions, the concept of a vascular bed represented by an array of Starling resistors in parallel each with its own critical closing pressure Pc is particularly appealing and is both elegant and simple.[40] In addition, the application of this model seems to have provided unique insights into mechanisms underlying

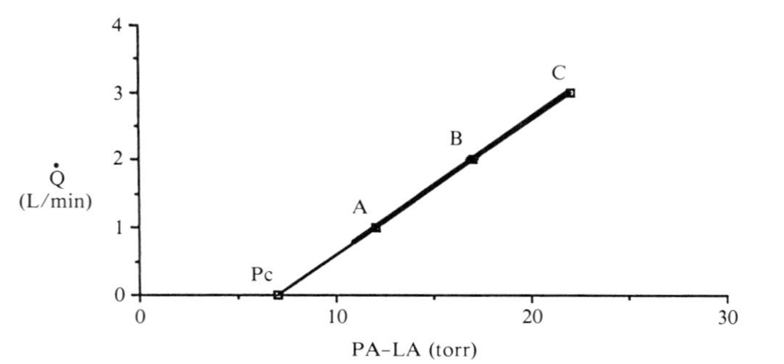

B_1	B_2	B_3	A	B	C
$\dot{Q}$ = 2.0	$\dot{Q}$ = 2.0	$\dot{Q}$ = 2.0	$\dot{Q}$ = 1.0	$\dot{Q}$ = 2.0	$\dot{Q}$ = 3.0
PA = 22	PA = 22	PA = 22	PA = 17	PA = 22	PA = 27
LA = 0	LA = 5	LA = 7	LA = 5	LA = 5	LA = 5
Ri = 5	Ri = 5	Ri = 5	Ri = 5	Ri = 5	Ri = 5
R = 11	R = 8.5	R = 7.5	R = 12	R = 8.5	R = 7.3

Figure 12–3. Numeric examples of the behavior of ohmic resistance in a Starling resistor model. In points A, B, and C, a progressive rise in pressure gradient and flow with a drop in ohmic resistance occurs while incremental resistance does not change. In points B_1, B_2, and B_3, ohmic resistance falls as LA pressure rises from zero to just below the critical closing pressure while incremental resistance does not change.

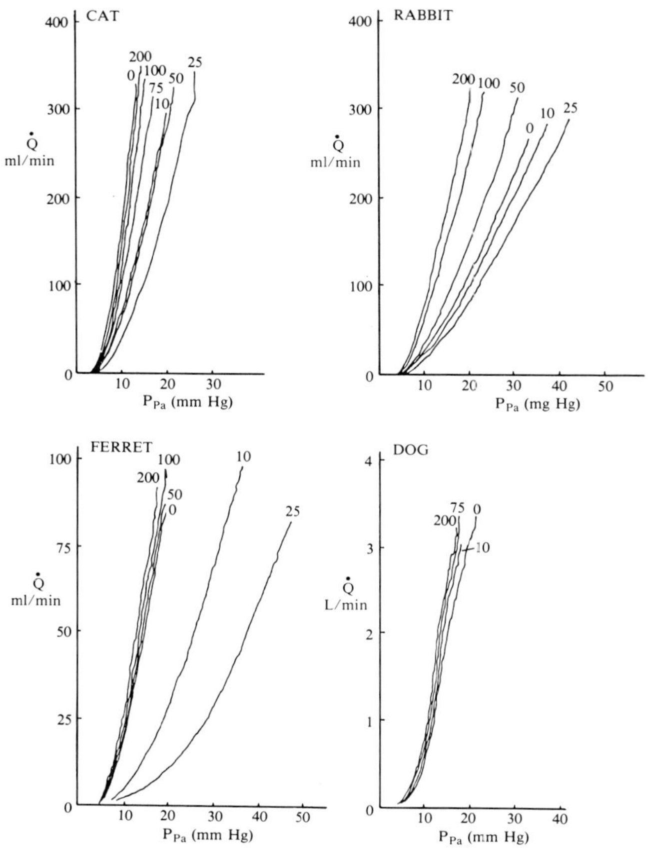

Figure 12–4. Examples of pulmonary artery pressure (Ppa) and flow (Q̇) plots in four different species. Except in the low range of flow data all plots are rectilinear. The extrapolation of the linear portion intersects the pressure axis in all cases. The numbers above each curve represent partial pressure of oxygen (Po_2). (Reproduced with permission from Peake MD, Harabin AL, Brenna NJ, Sylvester JT. J Appl Physiol 1981; 51:1214–1219.)

the effects of acute alveolar hypoxia and increased alveolar pressure,[56] both of which are thought to play a substantial role in the impact of COPD on the pulmonary circulation.

The assessment of pressure-flow relationships in the pulmonary circulation of humans is difficult and cumbersome. The only direct information in this regard comes from the type of measurement devised by Harris and associates.[27] These investigators occluded the right main branch of the pulmonary artery using a balloon-tipped catheter, thereby diverting cardiac output to the left lung. Measurements of inflow and outflow pressures and blood flow to the left lung before and after occluding the right pulmonary artery could, thus, provide two points of the pressure-flow relationship of the left lung and approximate information on the magnitude of incremental resistance and pressure intercept. Pressure and flow points during exercise, occluded and nonoccluded, were found by Harris and colleagues to lie in the approximate position or the linear extension of the pressure-flow points at rest both in healthy subjects and in patients with mitral valve disease. This finding suggested that, at least in these subjects, in whom left atrial pressures were high and in whom hyperinflation was not expected to occur in exercise, pressure and flow data obtained in succession during progressively increasing levels of exercise intensity might provide an acceptable means of describing the pressure-flow relationship of the human pulmonary circulation. This possibility still awaits direct demonstration.

The data points of Harris and colleagues formed a linear relationship that extrapolated to zero. This finding would imply that, at least in humans, ohmic pulmonary vascular resistance should be constant during exercise and that the value of Pc, if present, might be normally less than LA. An analogous observation was made by Janicki and coworkers,[33] who used multiple determinations of pressure and flow during progressively increasing treadmill exercise to exhaustion both in healthy subjects and in patients with a variety of cardiovascular diseases. The relationship between pressures and flows was linear over the entire range studied in all patients. Again, as in Harris's data, with few exceptions, in diseased patients and healthy subjects the zero flow extrapolation of the PA versus Q̇ relationship had a value smaller than the wedge pressure (Fig. 12–5). Ducas and coworkers,[14] however, warned against equating the extrapolated intercept of the PA versus Q̇ relationship to Pc in circumstances such as exercise in cardiac patients when the left atrial pressure varies with increasing cardiac output.[14] This practice would lead to an erroneous estimation of Pc. Among the data supporting the existence of significant levels of critical closing pressures in healthy humans are the observations of Emirgil and associates,[18] who used Harris's technique of balloon occlusion to investigate the effect of aging on pulmonary vascular pressure and flow relationships of healthy subjects. The extrapolated intercept of the pressure-flow line intersected the abscissa at values approximately 5 torr higher than the left atrial pressure. The data by Ekelund and Holmgren,[17] obtained during progressively increasing exercise in healthy subjects, also support this argument but may have underestimated Pc, given the caveat of Ducas.[14] Pressure and flow data on all subjects intersected the pressure axis at closing pressures in healthy subjects of approximately 3 torr higher than the wedge pressure. The example in Figure 12–6

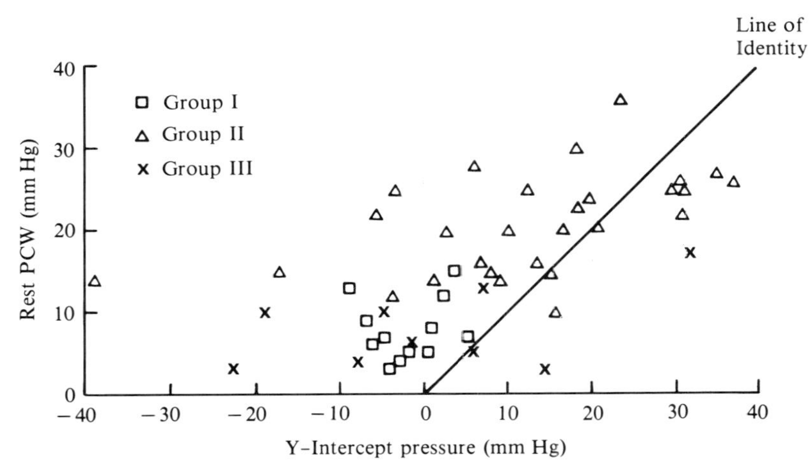

Figure 12–5. Plots of capillary wedge pressures (PCW) obtained at rest and the extrapolated intercept (Y-intercept) of the pulmonary artery pressure and cardiac output relationship during exercise. Most points fall at or below the line of identity. (Reproduced with permission from Janicki JS, Weber KT, Likoff MS, Fishman AP. Circulation 1985; 72:1270–1278.)

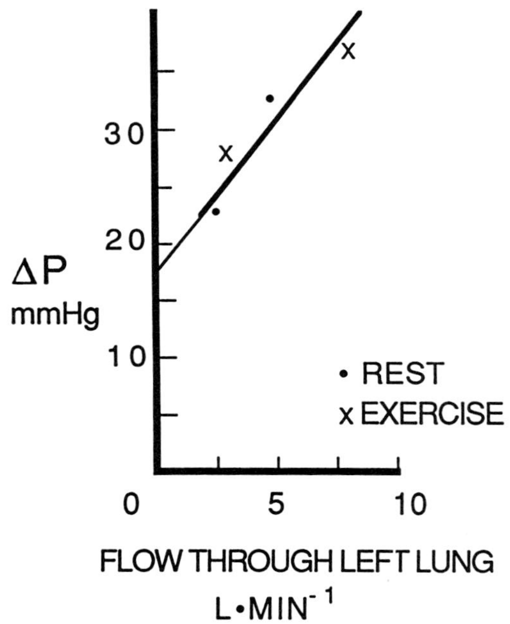

Figure 12–6. Pressure gradient (ΔP) versus flow plot in a subject with pulmonary hypertension secondary to multiple emboli to illustrate the presence of a large critical closing pressure. (Redrawn from Harris P, and Heath D. The Pulmonary Circulation. 2nd ed. London: Churchill Livingstone, 1977, 552, Figure 35–1.)

shows a substantial level of critical closing pressure observed in a patient with multiple pulmonary emboli.[29]

Given the current difficulties in routinely obtaining pressure-flow curves on the pulmonary circulation of humans, it is likely that the magnitude or even the existence of critical closing pressures in healthy individuals will remain uncertain for some time. However, it is our opinion that substantial values of critical closing pressures are likely to be present in pulmonary hypertensive states. The interpretation of changes in "ohmic" vascular resistance should take this possibility into account.

THE EFFECT OF EXERCISE AND HYPERINFLATION ON THE PULMONARY CIRCULATION IN PATIENTS WITH COPD

The response of the pulmonary circulation of patients with COPD during exercise has been investigated many times. There is general agreement that, in study protocols employing progressive increments in exercise intensity, impaired lung mechanics are the primary factors that limit the maximum exercise workload that can be achieved.[36] In this type of protocol, exercise is terminated when ventilation approaches or slightly exceeds maximal voluntary ventilation (MVV). The cardiac output in COPD patients increases in direct proportion to increments in oxygen consumption during exercise and the relationship between these two variables is the same in patients with COPD as in healthy individuals.[64] This normal cardiac output response occurs in spite of well-described abnormalities in intrathoracic pressures and in oxygenation, which could potentially affect hemodynamics.

The heart rate response to exercise in COPD patients is abnormal, at least as shown in some studies. There is an apparent excess tachycardia relative to oxygen consumption that has not yet been satisfactorily explained.[39] The heart rate discrepancy is not sufficient in magnitude to interfere with the cardiac output response or to adversely affect exercise performance.

In most patients with COPD, exercise is associated with a fall in arterial partial pressure of oxygen (Po_2), which is roughly proportional to the intensity of exercise. In an earlier study by Jones,[35] there was an attempt to make a distinction between the response of patients with predominant emphysema and that of subjects with chronic bronchitis. Patients with chronic bronchitis failed to decrease arterial Po_2 during exercise. The mechanism of worsening of hypoxemia in COPD during exercise is related to a combination of factors: (1) in severely obstructed subjects the ventilatory response is insufficient to cope with increasing carbon dioxide production levels leading to a rise in arterial partial pressure of carbon dioxide (Pco_2) and a corresponding fall in Po_2 and (2) the adverse impact on gas exchange of the normal fall in mixed venous oxygen, causing units with low ventilation-perfusion ratios to be supplied with less oxygenated blood. Evidence for a systematic worsening of ventilation-perfusion ($\dot{V}_A/\dot{Q}$) ratios or for a diffusion defect developing during exercise in COPD is lacking.

Hyperinflation is an unavoidable consequence of the ventilatory response of patients with COPD to exercise. In COPD patients with moderate or severe airways obstruction, respiratory rates around 30 breaths per minute are typically present during exercise.[36] Respiratory frequencies in this range are associated with corresponding shortening of expiratory durations, which necessitates increases in lung volume given the greater time constants of peripheral lung units. In COPD, in spite of decreased lung elastic recoil and the shift to a higher level of the volume intersect of the chest pressure-volume curve,[61] it is likely that at sufficiently high lung volumes, as the chest wall recoils inward, considerable recoil pressures of the respiratory system can be generated. Positive pleural pressures (higher than atmospheric pressure) and elevated alveolar pressures (auto-PEEP) would be expected to be present under these circumstances, in addition to increased volumes at the end of expiration.[23] Grimby and colleagues[24] described the progressive upward shift in functional residual capacity (FRC) that occurs during exercise in patients with COPD. Increases in alveolar pressures, per se, have not been documented directly during exercise in COPD, but this situation is inferred without difficulty and should be analogous to Permutt's[53] classic descriptions of the mechanical events during induced asthmatic attacks, although the primary mechanism is not airway closure.

The pulmonary artery pressure is usually abnormally elevated during exercise in patients with COPD, an observation that has been documented several times.[12, 71] The magnitude of the elevation compared with resting levels is variable, but is by and large proportional to exercise intensity and tends to be greater if pressures are elevated at rest. The observations of Burrows and colleagues[12] suggested that patients who were more hypoxic, with the bronchitic type of COPD, tended to have a greater cardiac output than their emphysematous counterparts and had more severe pulmonary hypertension during exercise. This distinction was not sought or encountered in subsequent studies.

The mechanisms of elevation of pulmonary artery pressure have been the subject of continued debate. Although it can be argued that decreased cross-sectional area of the bed secondary to vessel destruction should play some role, this is clearly not sufficient to account for all data. Most clinical observations have used atmospheric instead of pleural pressure as the level of reference for intravascular pressures. This constitutes a potentially confounding variable, because the swings of pleural pressure in COPD during exercise can be of comparable magnitude to the actual values of pulmonary artery pressure. Pleural pressure oscillations are transmitted directly to the heart chambers and large thoracic vessels and are recorded by manometers placed within them. Permutt[53] has discussed the advantages of measuring transmural pressures. However, changes in intrathoracic pressures alone do not account for the pulmonary artery pressure changes during exercise in COPD. When vascular pressures are referred to pleural pressure, the abnormal elevations in pulmonary artery pressure during exercise still persist.[42]

Perhaps the best insight into the potential mechanisms of pulmonary hypertension during exercise comes from the observations of Harris and colleagues,[27] reproduced in Figure 12–7. Using their technique of unilateral pulmonary artery balloon occlusions, pressure-flow points were obtained in five patients with COPD at rest and in four both at rest and at exercise. If the pressure-flow points in Figure 12–7 are extrapolated to the pressure axis, incremental resistance appears to be comparable with values obtained in healthy subjects. In contrast, a large critical closing pressure, some 10 to 15 torr higher than LA, can be assumed to be present. During exercise there was an apparent shift in the pressure-flow relationship to a higher intercept. The slope of the pressure-flow line became steeper during exercise in one subject and did not change in the other. In this subject (number 3) it is quite evident that the increase in pulmonary artery pressure during exercise can be fully accounted for by the increase in critical closing pressure. This behavior of the pressure-flow curve during exercise in COPD is analogous to the effects of increases in alveolar pressure or of alveolar hypoxia in isolated perfused pig lungs, which led Mitzner and Sylvester[47] to postulate that the site of pulmonary vasoconstriction during acute hypoxia involved alveolar vessels.

All subjects of Harris and colleagues had normal oxygen saturations at rest and desaturated to about 85% during exercise. Unfortunately, the experiments were not repeated while desaturation was prevented by breathing oxygen, which might have separated the relative contributors of increased alveolar pressure and hypoxia. Instead, Harris and coworkers[28] demonstrated in a different experiment that the same type of pressure-flow shift could be induced in healthy subjects during continuous positive-pressure breathing. Similarly, during voluntary hyperpnea, patients with COPD developed increases in pulmonary artery pressure of the same order of magnitude observed during exercise but without the development of hypoxemia. Hyperpnea had no effect on the pulmonary circulation of healthy subjects. Taken together, these observations indicate that increases in alveolar pressures (the auto-PEEP effect)[38] play a significant, perhaps the most important role in causing elevations in pulmonary artery pressure during exercise in patients with COPD.

The extent to which acute hypoxic vasoconstriction developing during exercise adds to the alveolar pressure–mediated shifts in the critical closing pressure or to an increase in the steepness of the pressure-flow line is difficult to determine from data in the literature. Burrows and colleagues[12] observed a greater attenuation of the pulmonary hypertensive response during exercise in COPD patients breathing 100% oxygen than the oxygen effect on pressures at rest. Wright and colleagues[71] and Selinger and colleagues[60] have confirmed this observation. However, no effort was made in these experiments to compare pulmonary hemodynamics at the same level of ventilatory response with exercise. Because it is well known that oxygen breathing blunts the ventilatory response to exercise in COPD it is conceivable that, during oxygen breathing, subject had less ventilation for a given workload, a smaller respiratory frequency, and hence less hyperinflation than during exercise breathing room air.

In our opinion, the magnitude of the contribution of acute hypoxia in mediating pulmonary vascular hypertensive response by vasoconstriction in patients with COPD during exercise still has to be established by a more carefully controlled experiment. In contrast, we believe that the role of increased alveolar pressures is better established and probably is the predominant factor.

The behavior of the pressure-flow relationship of the pulmonary circulation during exercise or hyperpnea in COPD patients as demonstrated by Harris does not preclude the use of points of a pressure and flow relationship derived from exercise stints to calculate ohmic resistance.[27, 28] However, the interpretation of such data should take into account that this vascular bed is better represented by a model consisting of an array of Starling resistors. Several studies attempting to uncover vasodilatory effects of pharmacologic agents during exercise in COPD patients have used this approach. The interpretation of the results of these experiments is tricky, however.

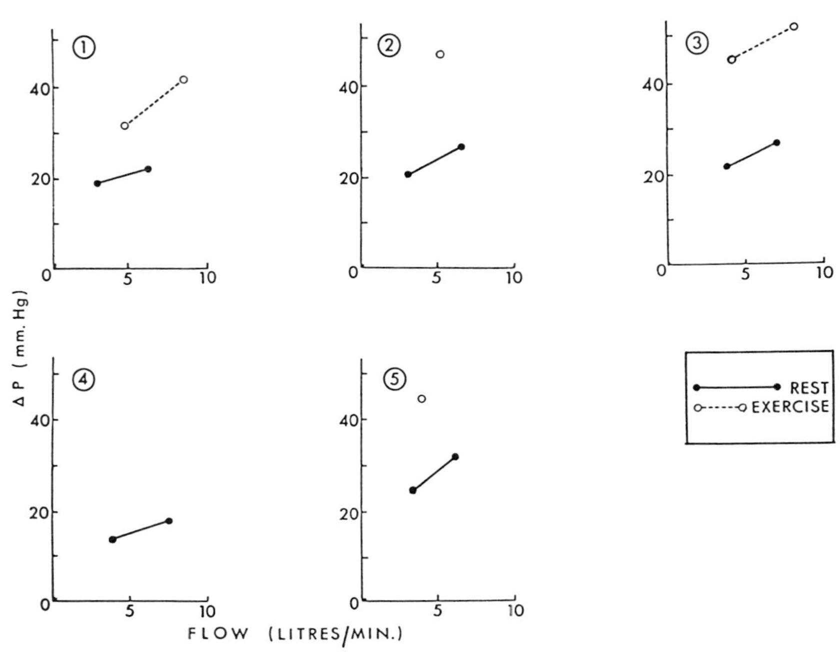

Figure 12–7. Examples of pressure-flow points from the pulmonary circulation in patients with COPD at rest and during exercise. For details see text. (Redrawn from Harris and colleagues, Cardiovasc Res 1968; 2:73–83.)

LEFT ATRIAL HYPERTENSION IN COPD

Controvery is still going on regarding the possibility that elevations in left atrial pressure secondary to left ventricular dysfunction may play a significant, if not systematic, role as contributors to the increased pulmonary artery pressures observed in COPD.

This argument gains partial support from experimental evidence, which indicates that chronic myocardial failure induced by pulmonary artery banding causes biochemical and structural changes in both ventricles.[11, 13] In addition, there are experimental settings in which the performance of the left ventricle can be shown to be affected by interventions directed primarily at modifying the performance of the right ventricle.[7, 37] The evidence in humans is less compelling. The pulmonary arterial wedge pressure of patients with COPD when recorded using atmospheric pressure as the level of reference is usually within normal range at rest. However, during exercise or during voluntary hyperpnea, it does increase abnormally in most patients, sometimes to remarkably high levels.[55] As discussed in greater detail previously, there is good reason to believe that increments in wedge pressure recorded during these maneuvers simply represent the transmission to the left atrium of elevated intrathoracic pressure and are not evidence of abnormal left ventricular function. When pleural pressure is used as the level of reference, left atrial pressures change very little with hyperpnea.[55] Furthermore, it is possible that, at least in some instances, the wedge pressure in COPD may not accurately reflect the left atrial pressure.[49]

Several clinical[6, 34] and pathologic reports[16] document the presence of left ventricular hypertrophy in post-mortem studies. There is also good evidence from cardiac catheterization studies that shows left ventricular dysfunction in some patients with COPD. The study by Jezek and Schrijen[34] is provocative in this regard because an abnormal left ventricular response to increase in afterload using angiotensin was shown to be present regularly in patients with COPD. These patients were in decompensated clinical cor pulmonale, but the response was absent in patients who had had no previous episodes of acute decompensation.

The bulk of the current evidence obtained from cardiac catheterization studies and from sophisticated noninvasive means, however, very strongly indicates the presence of little or no systematic abnormality in left ventricular function in COPD.[44] The instances in which substantial left ventricular dysfunction has been shown in these patients are best considered, as suggested by Fishman,[20] manifestations of independent disease of the left ventricle.

INCREASED BLOOD VISCOSITY

Chronic hypoxemia is a potent erythropoietic stimulus that can lead to the development of polycythemia in some patients with COPD. The polycythemic response that accompanies acclimatization of humans to altitude can be considered adaptive. Whether polycythemia is beneficial or detrimental to oxygen transport or to other physiologic mechanisms in COPD has not been determined. The subject of the relationship between hypoxia and erythropoietic stimuli in COPD is dealt with in greater detail elsewhere in this text (see chapter 24).

Because the viscosity of blood is related to the hematocrit, both *in vitro* and *in vivo,*[69] the theoretic possibility exists that increased blood viscosity might contribute to the mechanisms of pulmonary hypertension in COPD. Experiments in isolated perfused dog lungs under controlled conditions of oxygenation, perfusion pressure, and flow indicate that, in fact, changes in hematocrit value can result in changes in pulmonary vascular resistance.[48] Several clinical attempts have been made to sort out the potential effects of increased blood viscosity on pulmonary hemodynamics and oxygenation in COPD. A classic study by Segel and Bishop[59] investigated the role of reducing the hematocrit level by repeated phlebotomies in 15 stable patients with COPD. Special care was taken to replace bloodletting with saline infusions and to control associated variables. As a result, there was no change in cardiac output, wedge pressure, or arterial blood gas values. The hematocrit level was lowered from 60% to 44% and blood viscosity from 5.7 to 2.6 centipoise. A small, but significant, decline occurred in pulmonary artery pressure and pulmonary vascular resistance after venesection.

Even though, in our opinion, it is quite clear that increased viscosity can contribute to pulmonary hypertension in polycythemic patients with COPD, it does not necessarily follow that venesection should be recommended in the treatment of polycythemic patients with COPD. Other effects, immediate or long-term, may be associated with venesection, either beneficial or detrimental, which could alter the overall impact of this intervention in COPD patients. The clinical value of measures such as venesection is best established, prospectively, in controlled trials. We are not aware that such a trial has ever been performed and, currently, the magnitude of the problem is probably not sufficient to encourage this effort.

EFFECTS OF HYPOXIA ON THE PULMONARY CIRCULATION IN COPD

Acute hypoxic pulmonary vasoconstriction was first demonstrated by von Euler and Liljestrand[19] 40 years ago in the feline pulmonary circulation. Since then, it has been shown to be present in virtually all species tested, including humans, but the intensity of the response is highly variable from species to species. Evidence suggests that within the same species the propensity to respond to hypoxia with vigorous vasoconstriction can be transmitted genetically. The genetically determined propensity to exhibit intense hypoxic vasoconstriction has been used in attempting to explain why diseases causing chronic hypoxia induce more severe pulmonary hypertension in some individuals than in others.[25]

In spite of voluminous literature on the subject, the mechanism of hypoxic vasoconstriction, the relative importance of the route of hypoxia (precapillary versus alveolar), the site of its action on the vasculature of the lung, and its interaction with the hydrogen ion as a stimulus, have continued to be subjects of investigation and debate.[21, 22]

Chronic hypoxia, elicited experimentally by exposure to low oxygen atmospheres or naturally by living at high altitude or by alveolar hypoventilation, results in proliferative changes in the pulmonary vasculature. Experiments in the pulmonary circulation of rodents exposed to hypoxia for several weeks show that structural changes begin early and are completely reversible after cessation of hypoxia. This subject is reviewed in more detail elsewhere in this text (see chapter 2). The most impressive change in this remodeling process is the "de novo" muscularization of small arteries, which normally have little or no muscle in their walls.[45] The extent to which this newly formed muscle, by narrowing the lumina of vessels, can contribute to increases in vascular resistance has not yet been determined. It is also not established whether newly formed smooth muscle reacts to hypoxia in the same manner as does the pre-existing musculature. In experimental chronic hypoxia, medium-sized vessels also undergo increases in medial thickness. The anatomic counterpart in humans of these experiments is found in the morphology of the pulmonary circulation of residents of high altitudes and of subjects in chronic hypoxic states, such as severe kyphoscoliosis.[5] The pulmonary hypertension of residents of high altitude is only partially reduced by acute correction of hypoxemia, indicating that structural changes in pulmonary vessels are largely responsible for the maintenance of elevated pulmonary artery pressures. After a suitable period of residence at sea level, the pulmonary artery pressure of natives of high altitudes returns to normal sea level values.[52] The apparent complete reversibility of altitude-related pulmonary hypertension suggests that in humans, as in rodents, hypoxia-induced structural changes in pulmonary vessels are, also, completely reversible. However, this has not yet been directly verified.

In COPD, several potential mechanisms can contribute to the morphologic changes in the pulmonary vasculature, in addition to those that can be ascribed to chronic hypoxia: the effects of aging on the pulmonary circulation,[65] the inflammatory and vascular proliferative stimuli associated with cigarette smoking or chronic inflammatory changes in adjacent airways,[26] and the destruction of lung parenchyma possibly including the vessels within it.[15]

In spite of a diversity of potential mechanisms leading to reduction in cross-sectional area of the pulmonary circulation in COPD, the best correlations with pulmonary artery pressure have been those obtained with the level of arterial oxygenation, especially in the early observations of the Bellevue group.[30] These early data, showing an inverse linear relationship between pulmonary artery pressure and arterial oxygen saturation, were obviously not demonstrative of a causative role of hypoxia. They were used as the necessary basis for a well-subscribed thesis, which, in turn, provided the reasoning for therapeutic recommendations. Subsequent attempts in cross-sectional studies to demonstrate correlations with pulmonary artery pressures in COPD have found, instead, significant relationships with indices of airways obstruction.[71] However, a large multicenter European study reported by Bishop and Cross[8] involving a series of common chronic lung diseases seems to have resurrected the Bellevue group's correlation: oxygen saturation accounted for 44% of the variance in pulmonary artery pressure in a population of almost 1000 subjects.

The effect of correcting arterial hypoxemia on the pulmonary arterial pressure of patients with stable COPD is not striking.[1] There is usually a slight decrease in pulmonary artery pressure in most patients, of the order of 3 to 5 torr. In some instances, there is no change whatsoever in pressures, and in others, the fall in pulmonary artery pressure can be ascribed to a decline in cardiac output. The response to oxygen breathing is also small in patients with COPD living at high altitude in whom one might, perhaps, have expected a more pronounced reduction in pressures.[41] Although this has not been performed many times, the administration of low oxygen mixtures to patients with COPD is associated with a pulmonary hypertensive response which, in the Abraham experiment,[3] was quite brisk and not attributable to an increase in cardiac output. In contrast, the acute removal of oxygen in patients who are enrolled in continuous oxygen treatment programs is associated with a modest increase in pulmonary artery pressures.[60] Oxygen administration reduces the pulmonary hypertensive response to exercise in stable COPD patients, even in those in whom the pulmonary hypotensive effect of oxygen is small or nonexistent at rest.[12] As discussed, it is difficult to separate the relative contributions of increased alveolar pressures and of hypoxia to the pulmonary hypertensive response during exercise in COPD.

The observations described previously consistently point in the same direction: hypoxic vasoconstriction plays a minor role in the genesis of pulmonary artery pressure elevations in stable patients with chronic obstructive lung disease.

Two clinical settings occur in which the acute pulmonary hypertensive effects of hypoxia in COPD patients seem to be more consistent and less difficult to demonstrate: during the acute exacerbations of respiratory failure and the transient episodes of hypoxemia occurring in some patients during sleep. Figure 12–8, taken from Abraham and colleagues,[2] compares the pulmonary artery pressures measured daily in patients with acute respiratory failure breathing air and oxygen mixtures sequentially. In several subjects, the administration of oxygen caused consistent and substantial decreases in pulmonary artery pressures, which seemed to be superimposed on a general pattern of decline of pressures with time as they recovered. The administration of oxygen after recovery from acute respiratory failure had taken place resulted in inconsistent changes in pulmonary artery pressure, in keeping with the typical response of stable COPD patients as described previously.

Some patients with COPD can experience transient, severe episodes of nocturnal hypoxemia during sleep occurring mostly during the rapid eye movement (REM) stage. Pulmonary artery pressure elevations, sometimes of considerable magnitude, have been recorded with these episodes of hypoxemia. Pulmonary artery pressures revert to baseline levels on arousal in the morning.[10]

The long-term clinical follow-up and possibly anatomic verification of structural changes in pulmonary vessels of patients undergoing prolonged, continuous oxygen therapy have not yet been reported. The early results, after 6 months of the Nocturnal Oxygen Therapy Trials (NOTT) study,[4] indicate a slight reduction in pulmonary artery pressures of the group who used continuous oxygen compared with the group who used oxygen for 12 hours. If we speculate that hypoxia-related structural changes in pulmonary vessels have undergone involution after 6 months of oxygen use,[52] the results of the NOTT study would suggest that the vascular changes related to lung destruction and inflammation account

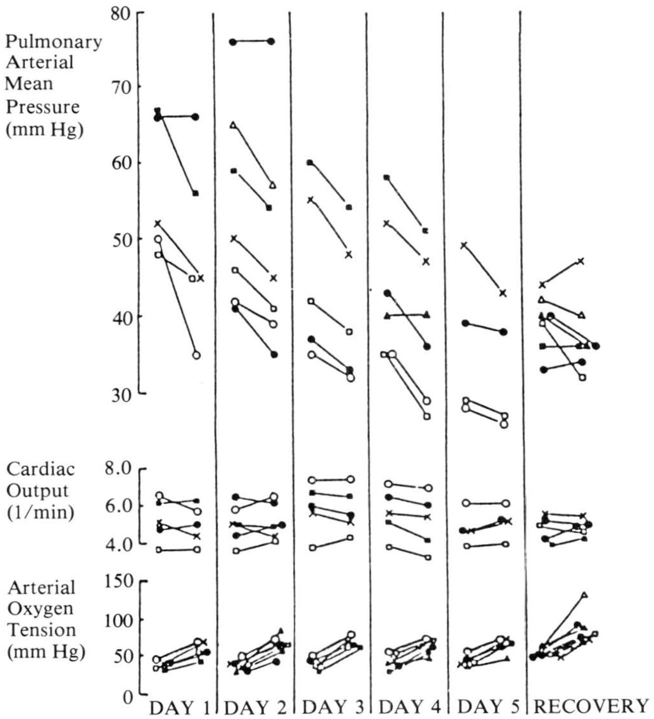

Figure 12–8. Comparison of the effect of oxygen administration on pulmonary artery pressures in subjects with acute respiratory failure during 5 consecutive days and after recovery. (Reproduced with permission from Abraham AS, Cole RB, Green ID, et al. Circ Res 1969; 23:51–60.)

for most of the pulmonary hypertension of COPD patients at rest.

EVOLUTION OF PULMONARY HYPERTENSION IN PATIENTS WITH COPD

The natural history of pulmonary artery pressure changes obtained by repeated cardiac catheterization studies in patients with COPD not receiving continuous O_2 therapy has been addressed in a rather limited number of studies. Two of these papers, by Boushy and North[9] and by Schrijen and colleagues,[58] have reported results in 136 and 35 patients, respectively, followed for 2 to 3.5 years. The characteristics, at entry, were approximately comparable; patients were mildly hypoxemic and had either normal or mildly elevated pulmonary artery pressures. The rate of progression of pulmonary artery pressures during the period of observation was minor but appeared to have clearly exceeded the expected rate of increase normally attributable to age, i.e., about 0.1 mm Hg per year.[54]

These observations, showing relative stability or chronic, gradual, mild progression, are not surprising, given the known evolutionary characteristics of the natural history of COPD. Furthermore, these kinds of studies, aiming at prolonged follow-up, would be expected to have an inherent selection feature that would preclude the enrollment of acutely ill or near-terminal patients. A different rate of progression might have been observed preterminally.

The most extensive long-term studies on pulmonary artery pressure in COPD are those of Weizenblum and associates.[67, 68] Their 1984 study reported on 93 patients who were followed for at least 5 years. The essential stability or slow progression of pulmonary artery pressures observed in the preceding studies was confirmed in this larger cohort. The rate of increase in pulmonary artery pressure, approximately 0.5 mm Hg per year, did not seem to be influenced by whether, on entry, patients had normal or elevated pulmonary artery pressures. "Hemodynamic worsening," defined as an increase in 5 mm Hg in pulmonary artery pressure during the period of observation, was seen in approximately one third of subjects (it is not clear whether this classification was part of the original study design or whether the separation was made as the result of a post hoc hypothesis). The mortality of the subset with hemodynamic worsening was significantly greater than that of the others: 70% versus 48%. The group with hemodynamic worsening became slightly but significantly more hypoxic and hypercapnic, with a P_{O_2} drop from 66 to 59 torr, whereas the other group of patients did not change oxygenation during the observation period, with P_{O_2} maintained at 65 torr. At entry, the patients who subsequently had deterioration in blood gases and increase in pulmonary artery pressures could not be distinguished from those who did not.

The data of Weizenblum and colleagues[68] could, conceivably, be used to support the speculation of a direct, causal relationship among deterioration of blood gases, development of pulmonary hypertension, and mortality. We find this simple construct highly improbable when applied to the type of patient enrolled in the studies cited. However, this reasoning continues to be used to justify exploring strategies for long-term use of pulmonary vasodilators in COPD. It is very unlikely that the increased survival associated with long-term use of oxygen is mediated directly through the reversal or prevention of the kind of long-term pulmonary hemodynamic changes described by Weizenblum and others. Anthonisen[4] reviewed the results of two controlled trials of oxygen therapy in COPD in the United States and the United Kingdom. Pulmonary hemodynamics changed very little in both trials, whereas mortality was substantially affected by the use of oxygen. In the British trial, catheterization studies were performed after 1 year of oxygen use and failed to show a significant difference in pulmonary vascular resistance between treated and untreated groups. In the North American study, the second cardiac catheterization was performed after 6 months of oxygen use. The group using oxygen for 12 hours, which served as the control group, had a significantly larger pulmonary vascular resistance, i.e., 17% higher, than the group continuously using oxygen.

During episodes of acute respiratory failure sharp increases in pulmonary artery pressure can be observed, but as a rule pulmonary artery pressures return to baseline values once the acute exacerbation of COPD subsides.[2] The same kind of reversibility has been documented with the nocturnal episodes of pulmonary hypertension that occur in some patients with COPD. On arousal in the morning, pulmonary artery pressures return to baseline levels.[10] Whether these episodes of intermittent pulmonary hypertension are associated with differences in the long-term evolution of pulmonary hypertension in COPD patients remains to be determined.

EXPERIMENTAL EMPHYSEMA IN ANIMAL MODELS AND ITS EFFECT ON THE PULMONARY CIRCULATION

From the considerations above, it should be apparent that multiple factors can contribute to the genesis of the functional changes in the pulmonary circulation of patients with COPD. It is also gradually becoming obvious that the relative contribution of given factors is probably not possible to resolve on clinical grounds alone. This awareness is now moving several investigators to evaluate the possibility of quantifying the impact of experimentally induced emphysema on physiologic and morphologic variables of the pulmonary circulation. A more detailed account of the subject of experimental emphysema in general is given elsewhere in this text (see chapter 7).

In spite of the relatively large amount of literature on this subject, few reports have focused on pulmonary vascular changes. Will and Kay[70] were the first to show that right ventricular systolic pressures were increased in rats made emphysematous by aerosols of papain. The degree of emphysema induced was slight, i.e., mean linear intercepts increased by 13%, and hypoxemia did not develop to a substantial degree. Right ventricular hypertrophy did not occur. Herget and colleagues[31] caused emphysema in rats by a combination of chronic tracheal stenosis and repeated instillations of papain intratracheally. The degree of induction of emphysema, again, was not severe. The proportion of air space to lung tissue, according to the Dunhill index, rose from 40% to 59%. Approximately half of the animals developed elevations of mean pulmonary artery pressure. However, no differences could be shown in the degree of emphysema or in the extent of increase in medial thickness between pulmonary hypertensive and normotensive rats. The investigators pointed out that a small statistical difference in arterial P_{O_2} between pulmonary hypertensive and nonhypertensive rats was present. But neither experimental groups nor control groups were hypoxemic.

Icochea and coworkers[32] induced severe emphysema in Syrian hamsters by intratracheal instillation of porcine pancreatic elastase alone or in combination with a diet containing the lathyrogen beta-aminopropionitrile. Reductions in internal surface area of lungs of the order of 40% to 50% were achieved by this procedure. The animals became severely hypoxemic (P_{O_2} 35 torr) and hypercapnic. This seems to be the only study of experimental emphysema focusing on circulatory changes in which substantial alterations in arterial blood gases were induced. Right ventricular hypertrophy did occur, and its magnitude was attenuated but not abolished when the animals were housed in a chamber ventilated with 35% O_2, even though hypoxemia was not fully corrected in all animals. Structural changes in pulmonary vessels were not studied. Hemodynamic effects were not examined. If the inference can be made that right ventricular hypertrophy developed in this experiment as a result of pulmonary hypertension, this study argues convincingly for a contribution of hypoxia in the genesis of pulmonary hypertension in COPD. Because right ventricular hypertrophy was not abolished by prevention of hypoxemia, it also suggests that substantial pulmonary hypertension, sufficient to cause right ventricular hypertrophy, can develop in experimental emphysema in the absence of hypoxia.

Experimental difficulties inherent with collecting comprehensive hemodynamic data in small animals were obviated in two studies using papain-induced emphysema in dogs. Martorana and colleagues[43] were able to achieve decreases in internal surface area of lung on the order of 18% to 25% after 6 months using two doses of aerosolized papain administered at 3-week intervals. These doses were claimed to be the maximum that could be tolerated without systematic mortality. There were neither changes in arterial blood gas levels nor development of right ventricular hypertrophy. Morphologic features in pulmonary vessels were not studied. Mean pulmonary artery pressure increased progressively with time, reaching a significantly larger level than control after 6 months. This increase could not be ascribed to changes in left ventricular end-diastolic pressure or cardiac output. A significant correlation was found between morphometric indices of emphysema and mean pulmonary artery pressure. This study showed that in experimental emphysema increases in pulmonary artery pressure can occur in the absence of hypoxia. The extent to which pulmonary hypertension could be ascribed to pulmonary vascular hypertrophy versus destruction of the vasculature was not directly addressed.

The study of Rubin and coworkers[57] was very similar in design to that of Martorana and colleagues[43] and reached basically the same conclusions, with some subtle differences. Rubin and colleagues found a significant increase in medial thickness of pulmonary arteries greater than 50 μ in dogs with emphysema, but they did not count blood vessels. The extent of emphysema was comparable in severity to that in Martorana's experiments. In spite of the apparent hypertrophy of vascular smooth muscle in medium-to-small-sized vessels, the acute hypoxic pulmonary artery pressure response was not increased in dogs with emphysema. Rubin and coworkers did not examine the effects of oxygen administration.

The evidence of pulmonary vascular structural changes and dysfunction generated by experimental models of emphysema is at an early stage. It appears that models of early, mild COPD have been successfully developed in large animals. These should be employed in attempting to correlate functional and structural evidence of airways obstruction and mechanical performance of the lung with corresponding structural and functional changes in the pulmonary vasculature. In particular, these experiments could provide comprehensive information on numbers of vessels reduced by the induction of emphysema and their caliber and the effects of such changes on hemodynamics. Questions having to do with the role of elevations in alveolar pressure during exercise or during tachypnea and the characteristics of pressure/flow curves in the pulmonary circulation seem to be particularly suitable to be addressed in these models. One special advantage of the dog model of mild emphysema is the absence of hypoxia. This model could facilitate the sorting out of the potential role of several pathophysiologic mechanisms without the confounding hemodynamic and vasomotor effects of hypoxia. However, further refinements in methodology appear to be required to develop a model of moderate to severe emphysema in a large animal in which hypoxemia and, possibly, hypercapnia are also present. It is probable that only then questions relating to the influence of hypoxic/hypercapnic vasomotor activity and vascular remodeling can be properly addressed.

REFERENCES

1. Abel GM, Harris AM, Bishop JM. The effect of acute changes in inspired oxygen concentrations on cardiac, respiratory and renal function in patients with chronic obstructive airways disease. Clin Sci 1964; 26:133–143.
2. Abraham AS, Cole RB, Green ID, et al. Factors contributing to the reversible pulmonary hypertension in patients with respiratory failure studied by serial observations during recovery. Circ Res 1969; 23:51–60.
3. Abraham AS, Hedworth-Whitty RB, Bishop JM. Effects of acute hypoxia and hypervolemia singly and together upon the pulmonary circulation in patients with chronic bronchitis. Clin Sci 1967; 33:371–380.
4. Anthonisen NR. Hypoxemia and O_2 therapy. Am Rev Respir Dis 1982; 126:729–733.
5. Arias-Stella J, Saldana M. The terminal portion of the pulmonary arterial tree in people native to high altitude. Circulation 1963; 28:915–925.
6. Baum GL, Schwartz A, Llamas R, Castillo C. Left ventricular function in chronic obstructive lung disease. N Engl J Med 1971; 285:361–364.
7. Bemis CE, Serur JR, Borkenhagen D, et al. Influence of right ventricular pressure on left ventricular pressure and dimension. Circ Res 1974; 34:498–504.
8. Bishop JM, Cross KW. Use of other physiological variables to predict pulmonary artery pressure in patients with chronic respiratory disease. Multicentre study. Eur Heart J 1981; 2:509.
9. Boushy JF, North LB. Hemodynamic changes in chronic obstructive pulmonary disease. Chest 1977; 72:565–570.
10. Boysen PG, Block AJ, Wynne JW, et al. Nocturnal pulmonary hypertension in patients with chronic obstructive pulmonary disease. Chest 1979; 76:36–42.
11. Buccino RA, Harris E, Spann JF, Sonnenblick EH. Response of myocardial connective tissues to development of experimental heart failure. Am J Physiol 1969; 216:425–428.
12. Burrows B, Kettel LJ, Niden AH, et al. Patterns of cardiovascular dysfunction in chronic obstructive lung disease. N Engl J Med 1972; 286:912–918.
13. Chidsey CA, Kaiser GA, Sonnenblick EH, et al. Cardiac norepinephrine stores in experimental heart failure in the dog. J Clin Invest 1964; 43:2386–2393.
14. Ducas J, Schick U, Girling L, Prewitt RM. Effects of altered left atrial pressure on the pulmonary vascular pressure-flow relationship. Am J Physiol (in press).
15. Dunnill MS. An assessment of the anatomical factor in cor pulmonale in emphysema. J Clin Pathol 1961; 14:246–258.
16. Edwardo CW. Left ventricular hypertrophy in emphysema. Thorax 1974; 29:75–80.
17. Ekelund LG, Holmgren A. Central hemodynamics during exercise. Circ Res 1967; 20(Suppl I):33–43.
18. Emirgil C, Sobol BJ, Campodonico S, et al. Pulmonary circulation in the aged. J Appl Physiol 1967; 23:631–640.
19. Euler US von, Liljestrand G. Observations on the pulmonary arterial blood pressure in the cat. Acta Physiol Scand 1946; 12:301–320.
20. Fishman AP. The left ventricle in chronic bronchitis and emphysema. N Engl J Med 1971; 285:402–404.
21. Fishman AP. Hypoxia and its effects on the pulmonary circulation. Circ Res 1976; 38:221–231.
22. Fishman AP. Pulmonary circulation. In: Fishman AP, Fisher AB, eds. Handbook of Physiology, section 3: The Respiratory System, vol. I. Bethesda: American Physiological Society, 1985, 93-165.
23. Fleury B, Murciano D, Talamo C, et al. Work of breathing in patients with chronic obstructive pulmonary•disease in acute respiratory failure. Am Rev Respir Dis 1985; 131:822–827.
24. Grimby G, Elgefors B, Oxhoj H. Ventilatory levels and chest

mechanics during exercise in obstructive lung disease. Scand J Respir Dis 1973; 54:45–52.
25. Grover RF, Hill DH, Reeves JT, et al. Genetic transmission of susceptibility to hypoxic pulmonary hypertension. Prog Respir Res 1975; 9:112–117.
26. Hale KA, Niewoehner D, Cosio M. Morphologic changes in muscular pulmonary arteries: relationship to cigarette smoking, airway disease and emphysema. Am Rev Respir Dis 1980; 122:273–278.
27. Harris P, Segal N, Bishop JM. The relation between pressure and flow in the pulmonary circulation in normal subjects and in patients with chronic bronchitis and mitral stenosis. Cardiovasc Res 1968; 2:73–83.
28. Harris P, Segal N, Green I, Housley E. The influence of the airways resistance and alveolar pressure on the pulmonary vascular resistance in chronic bronchitis. Cardiovasc Res 1968; 2:84–92.
29. Harris P, Heath D. The Pulmonary Circulation. 2nd ed. London: Churchill Livingstone, 1977, 552, Figure 35–1.
30. Harvey RM, Ferrer MI, Richards DW Jr, Cournand A. Influence of chronic pulmonary disease on the heart and circulation. Am J Med 1951; 10:719–738.
31. Herget J, Palacek F, Cermakova M, Vizek M. Pulmonary hypertension in rats with papain emphysema. Respiration 1979; 38:204–212.
32. Icochea A, Cooper BS, Kuhn C. The effect of oxygen on cor pulmonale in experimental emphysema induced by elastase or elastase and beta-aminopropionitrile in hamsters. Am Rev Respir Dis 1982; 126:792–796.
33. Janicki JS, Weber KT, Likoff MS, Fishman AP. The pressure-flow response of the pulmonary circulation in patients with heart failure and pulmonary vascular disease. Circulation 1985; 72:1270–1278.
34. Jezek V, Schrijen F. Left ventricular function in chronic obstructive pulmonary disease with and without cardiac failure. Clin Sci Mol Med 1973; 45:267–279.
35. Jones N. Pulmonary gas exchange during exercise in patients with chronic airway obstruction. Clin Sci 1966; 31:39–50.
36. Jones NL, Campbell EJM, Edwards RHT, Robertson DG. Clinical Exercise Testing. Philadelphia: W.B. Saunders Company, 1975.
37. Kelley DT, Spotnitz HM, Beiser GD, et al. Effects of chronic right ventricular volume and pressure loading on left ventricular performance. Circulation 1971; 44:403–412.
38. Kimball WR, Leith DE, Robins AG. Dynamic hyperinflation and ventilator dependence in chronic obstructive pulmonary disease. Am Rev Respir Dis 1982; 126:991–995.
39. Light RW, Mintz HM, Linden GS, Brown SE. Hemodynamics of patients with severe chronic obstructive pulmonary disease during progressive upright exercise. Am Rev Respir Dis 1984; 130:391–395.
40. Lopez-Muniz HM, Stephens NL, Bromberger-Barnea B, et al. Critical closure of pulmonary vessels analyzed in terms of a Starling resistor model. J Appl Physiol 1968; 24:625–635.
41. Lupi-Herrera E, Sandoval J, Seoane M, Bialostozky D. Behaviour of the pulmonary circulation in chronic obstructive pulmonary disease. Pathogenesis of pulmonary arterial hypertension at an altitude of 2,240 meters. Am Rev Respir Dis 1982; 126:509–514.
42. Mahler DA, Brent BN, Loke J, et al. Right ventricular performance and central circulatory hemodynamics during upright exercise in patients with chronic obstructive pulmonary disease. Am Rev Respir Dis 1984; 130:722–729.
43. Martorana PA, Wusten B, Van Even P, et al. A six month study of the evolution of papain-induced emphysema in the dog. A morphometric and pulmonary hemodynamic investigation. Am Rev Respir Dis 1982; 126:898–903.
44. Matthay RA, Berger HJ, Davies RA, et al. Right and left ventricular exercise performance in chronic obstructive pulmonary disease: radionuclide assessment. Ann Intern Med 1980; 93:234–239.
45. Meyrick B, Fujiwara K, Reid L. Smooth muscle myosin in precursor and mature smooth muscle cells in normal pulmonary arteries and the effect of hypoxia. Exp Lung Res 1981; 4:303–312.
46. Milnor WR. Hemodynamics. Baltimore: Williams & Wilkins, 1982.
47. Mitzner W, Sylvester JT. Hypoxic vasoconstriction and fluid filtration in pig lungs. J Appl Physiol 1981; 51:1065–1071.
48. Murray JF, Karp RB, Nadel JA. Viscosity effects on pressure-flow relations and vascular resistance in dogs' lungs. J Appl Physiol 1969; 27:336–341.
49. O'Quin R, Marini JJ. Pulmonary artery occlusion pressure: clinical physiology, measurement and interpretation. Am Rev Respir Dis 1983; 128:319–326.
50. O'Rourke MF. Vascular impedance in studies of arterial and cardiac function. Physiol Rev 1982; 62:570–623.
51. Peake MD, Harabin AL, Brenna NJ, Sylvester JT. Steady state vascular responses to graded hypoxia in isolated lungs of five species. J Appl Physiol 1981; 51:1214–1219.
52. Penaloza D, Sime I, Banchero N, et al. Pulmonary hypertension in healthy men born and living at high altitude. Am J Cardiol 1963; 11:150–157.
53. Permutt S. Some physiological aspects of asthma: Bronchomuscular contraction and airway calibre. In: Identification of Asthma. The Ciba Foundation Symposium. Edinburgh and London: Churchill & Livingstone, 1971, 63–85.
54. Perrault JL, Morinet J, Nader FA, Lockhardt A. Influence de l'age et de l'exercice physique sur les pressions dans la circulation pulmonaire de sujets normaux âgés de plus de 40 ans. Bull Eur Physiopathol Respir 1969; 5:505–522.
55. Rice DL, Awe RJ, Gaasch WH, et al. Wedge pressure measurement in chronic obstructive pulmonary disease. Chest 1974; 66:628–632.
56. Rock P, Patterson AG, Permutt S, Sylvester JT. Nature and distribution of vascular resistance in hypoxic pig lungs. J Appl Physiol 1985; 59:1891–1901.
57. Rubin LJ, Windberg P, Taylor W, Heatfield B. Pulmonary vascular structural and functional changes in papain-induced emphysema in dogs. Am Rev Respir Dis 1987; 136:704–709.
58. Schrijen F, Uffholz H, Polu JM, Poincelot F. Pulmonary and systemic hemodynamic evaluation in chronic bronchitis. Am Rev Respir Dis 1978; 117:25–31.
59. Segel N, Bishop JM. The circulation in patients with chronic bronchitis and emphysema at rest and during exercise with special reference to the influence of changes in blood viscosity and blood volume on the pulmonary circulation. J Clin Invest 1966; 45:1555–1568.
60. Selinger SR, Kennedy TP, Buescher P, et al. Effects of removing oxygen from patients with chronic obstructive pulmonary disease. Am Rev Respir Dis 1987; 136:85–91.
61. Sharp JT, Van Lith P, Nuchprayoon CV, et al. The thorax in chronic obstructive lung disease. Am J Med 1968; 44:39–46.
62. Skalak R, Wiener F, Morkin E, Fishman AP. The energy distribution in the pulmonary circulation. Phys Med Biol 1966; 11:437–449.
63. Szidon JP, Flint JF. Significance of sympathetic innervation of pulmonary vessels in response to acute hypoxia. J Appl Physiol 1977; 43:65–71.
64. Wade OL, Bishop JM. Cardiac Output and Regional Blood Flow. Philadelphia: F.A. Davis Co., 1962.
65. Warnock ML, Kunzmann A. Changes with age in muscular pulmonary arteries. Arch Pathol Lab Med 1977; 101:175–179.
66. Weiner F, Morkin E, Skalak R, Fishman AP. Wave propagation in the pulmonary circulation. Circ Res 1966; 19:834–850.
67. Weizenblum E, Loiseau A, Hirth C, et al. Course of pulmonary hemodynamics in patients with chronic obstructive pulmonary disease. Chest 1979; 75:656–662.
68. Weizenblum E, Sautegeau A, Ehrhart M, et al. Long term course of pulmonary arterial pressure in chronic obstructive pulmonary disease. Am Rev Respir Dis 1984; 130:993–998.
69. Wells RE, Merill EW. Influence of flow properties of blood upon viscosity-hematocrit relationships. J Clin Invest 1962; 41:1591–1598.
70. Will JA, Kay JM. Hypertensive pulmonary vascular disease associated with papain emphysema in rats. Respiration 1974; 31:208–220.
71. Wright JL, Lawson L, Pare PD, et al. The structure and function of the pulmonary vasculature in mild chronic obstructive pulmonary disease. Am Rev Respir Dis 1983; 128:702–707.

Chapter 13

THE EFFECTS OF COPD ON AIRWAY SECRETIONS AND LUNG CLEARANCE

Ruy V. Lourenco **Linda Bogar**

Although mucociliary clearance does not seem to be essential for the maintenance of life, it is widely considered an important defense mechanism of the lungs against inhaled particles. Several studies have attempted to define a relationship between mucociliary dysfunction and respiratory infection. Experimentally, mucociliary dysfunction impairs the clearance from the lung of aerosolized bacteria.[1, 2] For example, transient depression of mucociliary transport caused by atropine has been shown to prolong the persistence of inhaled bacteria in the trachea.[2]

In addition, mucus trapped within the airways may be a factor in carcinogenesis. In one study,[3] the depression of mucus clearance in patients with both chronic bronchitis and carcinoma of the lung was found to be significantly higher than in those with chronic bronchitis alone. It is an attractive but unproven hypothesis that decreased mucociliary clearance increases the residency time of potential carcinogens in contact with the bronchial mucosa and therefore is a factor in the development of lung cancer.

This chapter describes the mechanisms of mucociliary clearance, summarizes the most often-used methods of measurement of clearance, and examines relationships between mucociliary clearance and chronic obstructive pulmonary disease (COPD).

MECHANISMS OF MUCOCILIARY CLEARANCE

CILIA. In the larger airways, ciliated cells form a nearly continuous cover over the epithelium. In the trachea, ciliated cells outnumber goblet cells and brush cells by a ratio of 5 to 1 or more, but in the smaller airways the proportion of nonciliated to ciliated cells increases.[4] Each ciliated cell carries some 250 to 300 cilia on its luminal surface.[4, 5] The cilia are spaced along the cell surface in a hexagonal lattice interspersed with slender microvilli.[5] The length of the cilia becomes shorter with each succeeding airway generation, ranging from approximately 6 μm long in the trachea to about 3.6 μm long in the seventh airway generation.[6] Cilia range in diameter from about 0.25 μm to 0.3 μm.[5, 6] Each cilium is surrounded by an extension of the cell membrane, which constitutes the ciliary membrane. This membrane has an important role in regulating the ionic environment and the concentrations of adenosine triphosphate (ATP) essential for the production of energy necessary for the movement of the cilia. The membrane

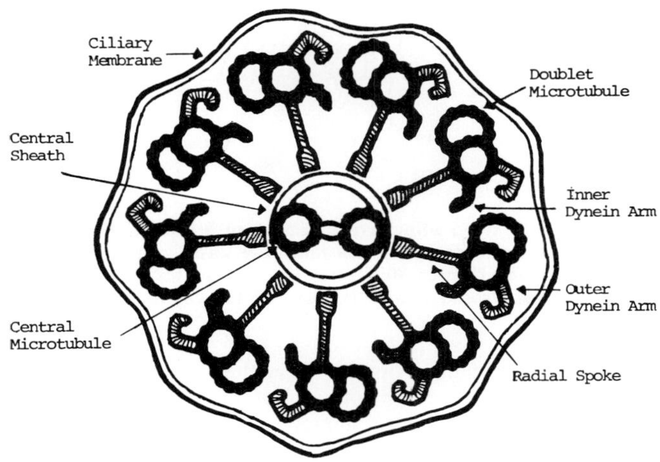

Figure 13–1. A cross-sectional view of a cilium. (Diagram by Linda Bogar.)

surrounds the axoneme, which consists of a central microtubule surrounded by nine doublet microtubules linked by dynein arms (Fig. 13–1). Both dynein arms and radial spokes play major roles in the movement of the cilia. Essentially, there is a bending movement of the axoneme as the microtubules slide against each other.[7] Dynein, an ATPase protein, uses energy from ATP to produce the sliding movements of the microtubules.[4] Radial spokes between axonemal fibrils resist the sliding movements and contribute to the formation of bends.[4] A combination of these movements accounts for the movement of the cilia. A more detailed description of the movement of cilia can be obtained from two excellent reviews (see references 4 and 5).

At the tip of the cilia there is a specialized structure called the ciliary crown, which is in direct contact with the overlying mucous blanket and probably plays an important role in the propulsion of the mucus. At the base of the cilium is the ciliary necklace, which is possibly an important attachment region for the developing cilium and may be involved in the transmission of sensory impulses during normal ciliary beating.[5] A basal foot points in the direction of the mucous flow and provides anchorage for the cilia (Fig. 13–2).[8]

Rates of ciliary beating increase from the peripheral airways toward the larynx. Thus, ciliary beat frequency in rats ranges from 360 beats per minute (b/m) in the smallest airways to 600 b/m in small bronchi and 1080 b/m in larger bronchi.[9]

LUNG SECRETIONS. Lying atop the airway epithelium are two

Supported by a grant from the National Institutes of Health (ROIHL 33461).

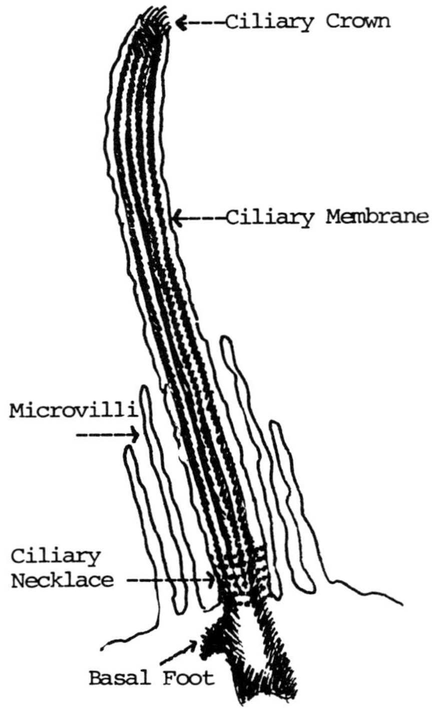

Figure 13–2. A longitudinal cross section of a cilium showing the ciliary crown, necklace, and basal foot. The basal foot points in the direction of the effective stroke (to the left in this diagram). The necklace forms strands about the base of the cilium. (Diagram by Linda Bogar.)

distinct layers of fluid. The periciliary fluid surrounds the cilia and consists of a watery solution of materials secreted by goblet cells and submucosal glands. The viscosity of this fluid is similar to that of serum. The periciliary fluid provides a base on which the mucous layer floats and allows for the efficient movement of cilia.

The mucous layer is distributed in patches over the epithelium immediately above the periciliary fluid and is propelled forward by the ciliary crowns during the effective stroke.[5] The mucous layer has been reported to vary from 2 to 5 μm thick.[76, 77] Materials may penetrate through the mucous layer into the periciliary fluid to interact with the ciliary membrane. The mucus is a viscoelastic, non-Newtonian gel that is comprised of elongated glycosylated macromolecules, a major component of which is a 500,000-dalton glycoprotein.[5] Glycoproteins appear to be the most important components conferring viscoelastic properties on the mucus. Since mucus is a non-Newtonian fluid, its viscosity decreases with applied force. Therefore, the more forcefully the cilia beat, the more easily the mucus moves.[4] Elastic properties allow mucus to return to near its original shape when stretched and released.

Elasticity seems to be more important than viscosity in relation to the efficiency of transport. Altering the mucous elasticity and viscosity independently on the frog palate demonstrated that changes in viscosity, in the presence of constant elasticity, had little effect on the rate of mucous transport.[10] Spinability is a term indicating a feature of mucus that appears to represent a combination of elasticity and cohesion and is defined as the maximum length a thread of mucus can be drawn out before breaking.[11] Measurements *in vivo* on frog palates show a direct correlation between spinability and mucous transport.[11]

INTERACTION BETWEEN CILIA AND MUCUS. Like cilia in other species, mammalian cilia beat with an effective stroke and a recovery stroke. During the effective stroke, the cilium is in its most vertical position, with the crown in contact with the mucous blanket. In this effective stroke, the cilia propels the mucus forward in the direction of the throat. In their recovery stroke, the cilia lie entirely within the periciliary fluid, which permits movement with a minimum loss of energy (Fig. 13–3).

Beating cilia influence each other through the periciliary fluid. By this mechanism, a field of cilia becomes coordinated by hydrocoupling. Each cilium is forced to beat somewhat out of phase with many of its neighbors, creating what is called a metachronal wave. The characteristics of metachronal waves are related to such factors as the length and spacing of the cilia, the pattern of the beat, and the viscosity of the mucus surrounding the cilia. Cinematographic records of cilia from the tracheal epithelium of the rabbit suggest that only a small number of cilia clustered in relatively discrete areas are beating at any given time.[12] Present evidence suggests that the quantity and composition of the mucus and periciliary fluid are more important for an efficient mucociliary clearance than is the function of the cilia. Unfortunately, there is significantly more knowledge about the cilia than about the bronchial secretions.

Although this chapter deals with mucociliary clearance, a distinction needs to be made between bronchial mucociliary clearance and alveolar clearance. Alveolar clearance is the clearance of particles that are deposited in the most peripheral areas of the lungs: the alveoli and the respiratory bronchioles. The majority of inhaled particles that are deposited within these regions cannot be removed through the process of mucociliary clearance, owing to the absence of cilia. However, while cilia may be absent in these regions, a "rope of mucus," extending from the larger airways into the alveoli, may remove some particulate matter. Particles not cleared by mucociliary clearance are primarily engulfed by macrophages or directly absorbed into the blood or lymphatic circulations. It is also possible that some particles are absorbed through the interstitium and may return back to the ciliated airways.

MEASUREMENT OF MUCOCILIARY CLEARANCE

A critical factor influencing the study of mucociliary clearance is deposition. The rate of clearance of inhaled substances from the lung is dependent on the sites of deposition of these substances. Particles deposited more centrally, in the larger

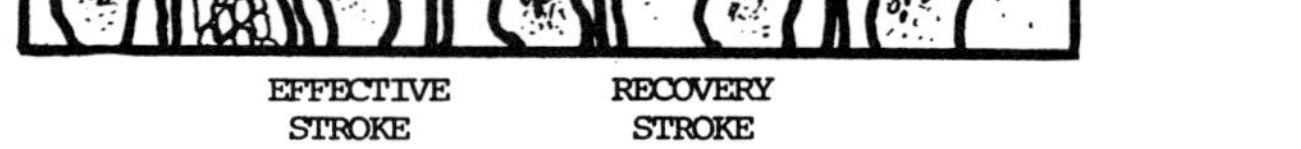

Figure 13–3. Mucus transport in the bronchial tree. Cilia transport mucus in the direction of their effective stroke (arrow). Note that the tips of the cilia come in contact with the layer of mucus while cilia are in their effective stroke to propel it forward. Cilia in their recovery stroke lie entirely within the less dense periciliary fluid, thus allowing for more energy efficient movement. In actuality, the length of the cilia may range from about 4 to 6 μm long and number approximately 250 to 300 per cell. (Diagram by Linda Bogar.)

airways of the lung, will be cleared faster than particles deposited in the peripheral airways. Any technique that attempts to quantify tracheobronchial clearance of inhaled particles in the lung must consider the deposition of the particles inhaled.[13] A number of factors influence the site of deposition: the aerodynamic diameter of the inhaled particles, derived from their diameter and density; breathing pattern during deposition; and size, shape, and degree of obstruction of the airways. Typically, a more centralized deposition of particles of the same size is found in patients with COPD than in healthy individuals if the same pattern of breathing is used.

Various techniques have been developed to study mucociliary clearance. The rate of clearance from the trachea is often measured separately from the rate of clearance from the lungs (Fig. 13–4). Since the trachea is a single tube, *tracheal mucus velocity* is considered a linear velocity measurement—expressed in millimeters per minute. The measurement of *tracheobronchial clearance* encompasses a number of clearance mechanisms for the numerous airways in the lung and is represented by a percentage of particulate matter cleared per unit of time in relation to that initially deposited.

TRACHEAL MUCUS VELOCITY. One method of measuring tracheal mucus velocity uses bronchofiberscopic techniques to observe the movement of Teflon discs deposited in the trachea.[14] Another method uses radiographic techniques to measure the movement of Teflon discs.[15] Still another technique involves the deposition of radioactive particles in the lung. The particles may be introduced into the lung through a bronchoscope or through the inhalation of an aerosol. The rate of movement of the radioactive particles is detected by a gamma camera or a specially designed multidetector probe.[16, 17] A multidetector probe compact enough to be positioned strategically in front of the trachea can be employed so that tracheobronchial clearance can be measured simultaneously.[18]

TRACHEOBRONCHIAL CLEARANCE. Techniques for the measurement of tracheobronchial clearance involve aerosolized deposition of radioactive particles. The mucociliary clearance of the deposited particles can be recorded using either a single crystal detector or a gamma camera centered over an area of interest in the chest. Generally, three major phases of clearance can be identified. The fastest phase represents tracheobronchial clearance from the heavily ciliated airways. The intermediate phase reflects mucociliary clearance in airways wherein cilia are few. The slowest phase represents alveolar clearance. Aerosol retained in the lung at 24 hours is assumed to represent aerosol initially deposited within alveoli. Although something of an oversimplification, the tracheobronchial component of the clearance curve can be obtained by subtracting the percentage of initially deposited aerosol retained at 24 hours from the whole lung clearance curve. During the clearance of radiolabeled mucus, the large bronchi of some subjects become anatomically definable through the use of a gamma camera and can be utilized to measure the velocity of the boluses within these airways.[19]

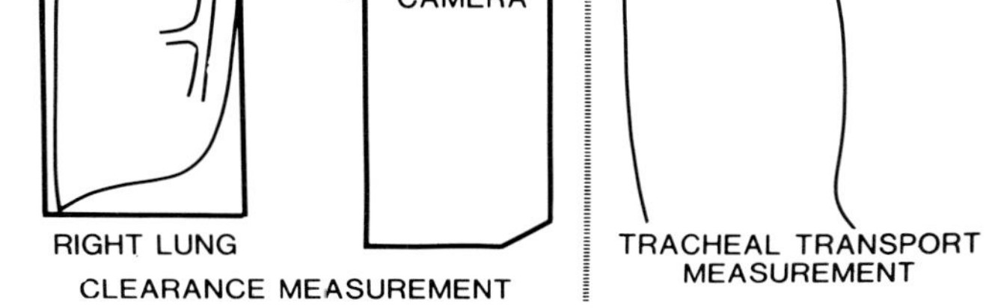

Figure 13–4. Diagrammatic representation of radioaerosol techniques for measurement of tracheobronchial clearance and tracheal mucus velocity. For both measurements a radioactive aerosol is inhaled. The clearance measurement uses a gamma camera, which quantifies the amount of radiation present in a region of interest (ROI) in the lung. The tracheal transport measurement uses a tracheal probe, which measures the velocity of boluses of radioactivity moving upwards in the trachea.

Although studies indicate that coughing does not significantly contribute to mucociliary clearance in health, it does appear that the cough mechanism can compensate for slowed mucus transport in disease states.[20] It may be that cough is not an effective aid to clearance unless there is an excess of tracheobronchial secretions.[21] In disease conditions that are characterized by excessive mucous secretions such as chronic bronchitis, cystic fibrosis, and influenza, cough moves boluses of mucus-containing radiolabeled particles from the major bronchi to the trachea.[22] Some researchers predict that cough may be effective in moving secretions down to the fourth airway generation.[23]

Various investigators have attempted to define a normal range of mucociliary clearance. Changes in the clearance rates of 19 nonsmokers under the age of 50 varying with particle penetration in the lung, inhalation flow rate, and alveolar deposition were examined.[24] The correlation between retention at 3 hours and particle penetration was statistically significant as were the correlations between retention and inhalation flow rate and retention and alveolar deposition.

We have measured deposition and clearance of inhaled particles in normal subjects.[25] Clearance began immediately after inhalation, showing faster rates for centrally deposited particles than for peripherally deposited particles. In most subjects, the fastest clearance rate occurred during the first hour (average 18.5% of initial count). Clearance slowed to rates of 7.0%, 7.1%, and 4.2% during the next 3 hours. No measurable clearance was observed in seven out of ten subjects after 5 and 6 hours.

We also measured pulmonary clearance in nine healthy males, dividing the lung into three regions varying from the most central to the most peripheral.[26] We found that bronchial and regional clearance was reproducible within subjects over the first 4.5 hours, but significant variation was observed among subjects. The coefficients of variance in mucociliary clearance, we observed, are similar to those from other reports demonstrating a variance in the 30% to 60% range.[27–30] Intersubject comparisons of mucociliary clearance indicate an uncertainty level on the order of 50%, which is comparable to that of other more commonly used measures of biologic function in humans, e.g., blood urea nitrogen (BUN) and complete blood count (CBC).

A wide range of tracheal mucus transport velocities are observed in healthy subjects. Rates have been observed ranging from less than 5 mm/min using radioaerosol bolus techniques[17] to as high as 21.5 mm/min using cinebronchoscopic techniques.[31] Data from our own laboratory based on measurements in 40 normal subjects indicate an average tracheal mucus transport velocity of 6.3 mm/min with a standard deviation of 2.4.

MUCOCILIARY CLEARANCE IN COPD

In COPD, drainage of bronchial secretions is less efficient than in normal subjects.[13] Secretions are cleared less effec-

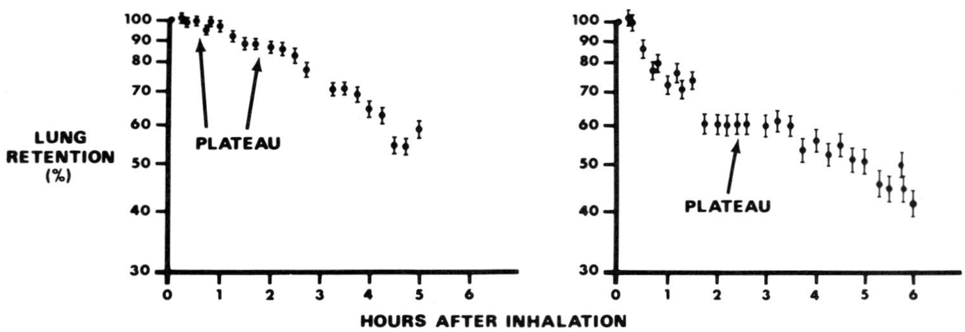

Figure 13–5. Plateaus of retention of inhaled particles in patients with chronic bronchitis. For prolonged periods of time there is no clearance from the lung of an inhaled aerosol. These findings appear only in patients with bronchial disease.

tively, owing to alterations in both the volume and rheology of the mucus.[32]

Chronic bronchitis is characterized by mucous hypersecretion resulting from hypertrophy of bronchial submucosal glands and an increase in the number of secretory cells in the surface of the epithelium.[33] Irritation from tobacco smoking is a factor in this gland hypertrophy. Cigarette smoking and environmental pollutants have been shown to be responsible for the mucous hypersecretion so characteristic of COPD. It has been demonstrated that cigarette smoke causes decreased ciliary beat, which may be a factor in slowed mucociliary clearance.[22] However, other factors, such as environmental pollutants, also contribute to hypersecretion. In fact, the areas of the bronchial tree most exposed to the environment, the segmental and subsegmental bronchi, are usually the sites of greatest hypersecretion. Although hypersecretion of mucus may cause an increase in ciliary beat, if the depth of the mucus is too great, transport is poorer and mucus may slide back down the airways.[22] In patients so affected, cough then plays an important role in augmenting the clearance mechanism.

Excess mucus trapped within the airways may be infected by bacteria or viruses, which may alter its viscoelastic properties, triggering a vicious cycle.[22] Altered viscosity and elasticity have been found in the bronchial mucus of patients with COPD[34] and are probably both a cause and a consequence of slowed mucous transport. Sputum from patients with chronic obstructive pulmonary disease usually has low elastic recoil.[35, 36] Low elasticity and, possibly, high viscosity seem to be factors contributing to the slowed mucociliary transport present in these patients.[35, 36] Purulent sputum from patients with COPD has shown lower spinability values than has nonpurulent sputum.[37]

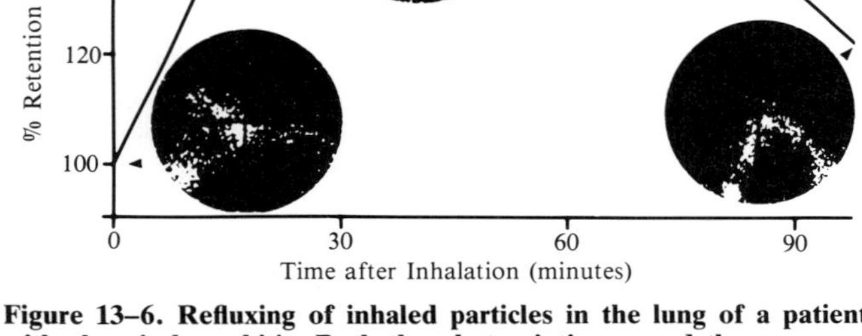

Figure 13–6. Refluxing of inhaled particles in the lung of a patient with chronic bronchitis. Both the photoscintigram and the measurement of radioactivity show an increased concentration of particles in the left lower quadrant of a region of interest (ROI) as measured between 0 and 30 minutes after inhalation of a radioactive aerosol.

Several studies demonstrate abnormalities of mucociliary clearance in patients with COPD.[13, 15, 38–40] However, rates of clearance in patients with chronic bronchitis and airway obstruction are affected by deposition patterns of the inhaled particles, which vary with the sites of airway obstruction. Obstruction in the airways may prevent the aerosol from depositing in the alveoli. In fact, a more central deposition, nearer the trachea, of aerosols may cause the rate of mucociliary transport to appear to be faster.[13]

Long periods, perhaps for as long as 4 hours, in which inhaled particles seem to be immobile, have been seen in patients with chronic bronchitis during clearance studies (Fig. 13–5). Images obtained with gamma cameras have shown reflux movement of radioactivity down larger airways, indicating a reversal of the clearance process or a retention of particles in certain areas (Fig. 13–6). In one study half of the patients exhibited either absent or side-to-side oscillatory movement of marker discs within the trachea instead of progressive movement upward.[15] Even bronchitic patients without significant airway obstruction, as demonstrated by standard pulmonary function tests, often show subnormally low mucociliary clearance.[13]

Cigarette smoking retards mucociliary clearance. Many studies have implicated chronic cigarette smoking as the most frequent exogenous factor leading to chronic bronchitis, emphysema, and bronchial carcinoma.[41–45] In fact, slowed clearance is evident in smokers with or without symptoms of airway disease and with or without abnormalities in standard pulmonary function test results.[25, 28] In subjects who smoke, the number of pack years correlates with the decreased mucociliary clearance rate.[46] In addition, mucociliary clearance is not as steady and uniform in smokers as in nonsmokers, and particle accumulations in large airways several hours after inhalation have been reported.[25] Although smokers without symptoms of chronic bronchitis have slow rates of mucociliary clearance, it is usually not as markedly abnormal as clearance in patients with COPD.[13] Mucociliary clearance may improve in those who quit smoking if symptoms of chronic bronchitis are not yet evident and cigarette consumption has not been too heavy.[46] In our laboratory we have found that ex-smokers

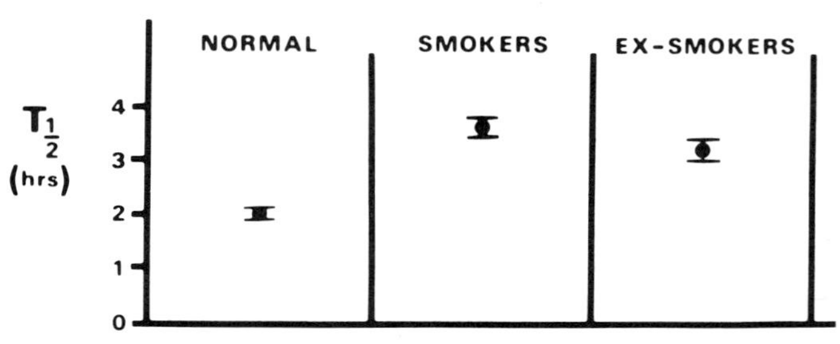

Figure 13–7. Time necessary to clear half of inhaled particles from the lung in nonsmokers, smokers for at least 10 years, and ex-smokers who have smoked for at least 10 years but have stopped smoking for at least 3 years prior to the measurement of mucociliary clearance.

improve their mucociliary clearance but usually without reaching normal values (Fig. 13–7).

Matthys and colleagues[3] assessed clearance in smokers with chronic bronchitis and smokers with bronchial carcinoma. Both groups of patients had smoked cigarettes for approximately 30 pack years. These investigators found that patients with bronchial carcinoma showed the slowest clearance, although results of pulmonary function tests did not differ significantly between the groups. Decreased clearance mechanisms of the central bronchial tree in patients with COPD may be a factor in the preferential development of bronchial cancer at these sites.[3]

In the immotile cilia syndrome, the cilia are incapable of effective transport and tracheobronchial clearance is almost completely absent.[48–50] In this syndrome, a variety of ultrastructural defects of cilia have been shown, but the most common defect is the lack of dynein arms.[47] Patients with this syndrome often have a chronic productive cough and show increased incidence of respiratory infections.[50–52] Although it is logical to suppose that abnormalities in mucociliary clearance are important in the pathogenesis of COPD,[52] many individuals with the immotile cilia syndrome fail to develop this disease.[47]

In patients with emphysema secondary to alpha$_1$-antitrypsin deficiency with no history of chronic bronchitis, tracheobronchial clearance is normal or even slightly increased.[53] Because of the frequent simultaneous incidence of chronic bronchitis with emphysema, abnormalities of clearance are frequently present in patients with both chronic bronchitis and emphysema.

In patients with bronchiectasis, if differences in deposition of aerosols are taken into consideration, mucociliary clearance is decreased.[54] This slowed mucociliary clearance quite often correlates with the severity of chronic bronchitis present and in certain patients is in large part attributed to ultrastructural defects in the cilia.[55, 56] Svartengren and colleagues[57] found that more marked, generalized airway symptoms correlated with more impaired clearances in patients with bronchiectasis. Also, patients whose symptoms began early in life exhibited slower clearances.[57] Patients with the immotile cilia syndrome frequently have bronchiectasis,[52, 58] and impaired mucociliary clearance may be of pathogenetic significance in the development of bronchiectasis. Reduced rates of mucociliary clearance have also been demonstrated in patients with cystic fibrosis.[59]

Mucociliary clearance is frequently slowed both in symptomatic[60] and asymptomatic[61] asthmatic patients despite a more centralized deposition of aerosolized particles. Patients with bronchial asthma show a decrease of mucus transport in the peripheral, bronchial, and tracheal airways, but these transport values are significantly improved by the administration of beta-adrenergic agents.[62] Decreases in tracheal transport velocity have been demonstrated in asymptomatic asthmatic patients, with a further diminution of velocity during bronchial provocation with ragweed antigen.[63]

The viscosity of mucus in asthmatic patients varies widely; mucus can be watery or increase in viscosity by as much as 80-fold.[64] But, in general, sputum from asthmatic patients tends to be more viscous than that from patients with other types of lung diseases.[34] This finding may be due to the altered water-glycoprotein structure of the mucus.[65] Additionally, it may be due to the presence of inflammatory cells in the mucus, such as eosinophils and shed epithelial cells, which may cause mucus plugging, a significant problem in patients with status asthmaticus.[66, 67] Mucus plugs are in part created by eosinophils in rows or bands that form swirls within the mucus.[68] Mucus trapped in the airways by bronchospasm and lack of clearance may slowly dehydrate, causing tenacious plugs or bronchial casts, which may be expelled by coughing[69] and may contribute to the abnormalities in distribution of ventilation present in asthmatic patients.[68]

The action of the mediators in slowing mucociliary clearance in asthma is not clear. Studies in both animals and humans, both healthy subjects and asthmatic patients, have shown that histamine stimulates mucociliary clearance.[70] Yet, various studies in animals have found that histamine does not stimulate ciliary beat frequency[71, 72] or stimulates it only slightly.[73] By contrast, leukotriene D$_4$ causes a decrease in mucociliary clearance,[74] although data *in vitro* shows that this substance increases ciliary beat frequency.[75]

REFERENCES

1. Wanner A. Is airway clearance of clinical relevance? Bull Eur Physiopathol Respir 1984; 20:477–480.
2. Whiteside ME, Lauredo I, Chapman GA, et al. Effect of atropine on tracheal bacterial counts. Bull Eur Physiopathol Respir 1984; 20:347–351.
3. Matthys H, Vastag E, Kohler D, et al. Mucociliary clearance in patients with chronic bronchitis and bronchial carcinoma. Respiration 1983; 44:329–337.
4. Sleigh MA, Blake JR, Liron N. State of Art: The propulsion of mucus by cilia. Am Rev Respir Dis 1988; 137:726–741.
5. Satir P, Dirksen ER. Function-structure correlations in cilia from mammalian respiratory tract. In: Fishman AP, Fishman AB, Geiger SR, eds. Handbook of Physiology. Bethesda, Maryland: American Physiological Society, 1985, 473–494.
6. Serafini SM, Michaelson ED. Length and distribution of cilia in human and canine airways. Bull Eur Physiopathol Respir 1977; 13:551–559.
7. Rhodin JAG. Ultrastructure and function of the human tracheal mucosa. Am Rev Respir Dis 1966; 93(Suppl):1–15.
8. Sleigh MA, Silvester NR. Anchorage functions of the basal apparatus of cilia. J Submicrosc Cytol 1983; 15:101–104.
9. Iravani J. Flimmerbewegung in den intrapulmonalen Luftwegen der Ratte. Pflugers Arch 1967; 297:221–237.
10. Gelman RA, Meyer FA. Mucociliary transference rate and mucus viscoelasticity. Dependence on dynamic storage and loss modulus. Am Rev Respir Dis 1979; 120:553–557.
11. Puchelle E, Zahm JM, Duvivier C. Spinability of bronchial mucus. Relationship with viscoelasticity and mucous transport properties. Biorheology 1983; 20:239–249.
12. Sanderson MJ, Sleigh MA. The function of respiratory tract cilia. In: Bonsignore G, Cumming G, eds. The Lung and Its Environment. New York: Plenum Publishing Corp, 1982.
13. Lourenco RV. Distribution and clearance of aerosols. Am Rev Respir Dis 1970; 101:460.
14. Sackner MA, Rosen MJ, Wanner A: Estimation of tracheal mucous velocity by bronchofiberoscopy. J Appl Physiol 1973; 34:495.
15. Goodman RM, Yergin BM, Landa JF, et al. Relationship of smoking history and pulmonary function tests to tracheal mucous velocity in nonsmokers, young smokers, ex-smokers, and patients with chronic bronchitis. Am Rev Respir Dis 1978; 117: 205.
16. Chopra SK, Taplin GV, Elam D, et al. Measurement of tracheal mucociliary transport velocity in human-smokers versus nonsmokers (preliminary findings). Am Rev Respir Dis 1979; 119:205.
17. Yeates DB, Aspin N, Levison H, et al. Mucociliary tracheal transport rates in man. J Appl Physiol 1975; 39:487–495.
18. Yeates DB, Gerrity TR, Garrard CS. Characteristics of tracheobronchial deposition and clearance in man. In: Walton WH, ed. Inhaled Particles V. New York: Pergamon Press, 1981.
19. Foster WM, Langenback EG, Bergofsky EH. Disassociation in the mucociliary function of central and peripheral airways of asymptomatic smokers. Am Rev Respir Dis 1985; 132:633–639.
20. Camner R, Mossberg B, Philipson K, Strandberg K. Elimination of test particles from the human tracheobronchial tract by voluntary coughing. Scand J Respir Dis 1979; 60:56.
21. Zahm JM, Girard F, et al. Mucociliary transport *in vivo* and *in vitro:* Relations to sputum properties in chronic bronchitis. Eur J Respir Dis 1980; 61:254.
22. Garrard CS, Lourenco RV. Mucociliary clearance. In: Montenegro HD, ed. Chronic Obstructive Pulmonary Disease. New York: Churchill Livingstone, 1984:29–48.
23. Clarke SW, Jones JG, Oliver DR. Factors affecting airflow through bronchial tubes. Bull Eur Physiopathol Respir 1972; 8:409.

24. Agnew JE, Sutton PP, Pavia D, Clarke SW. Radioaerosol assessment of mucociliary clearance: towards definition of a normal range. Br J Radiol 1986; 59:147–151.
25. Lourenco RV, Klimek MF, Borowski CJ. Deposition and clearance of 2 μm particles in the tracheobronchial tree of normal subjects—smokers and nonsmokers. J Clin Invest 1971; 50:1411–1420.
26. Wilkey D, Lee P, Hass F, et al. Mucociliary clearance of deposited particles from the human lung: intra- and inter-subject reproducibility, total and regional lung clearance, and model comparisons. Arch Environ Health 1980; 35:294–303.
27. Camner P, Philipson K. Tracheobronchial clearance in smoking-discordant twins. Arch Environ Health 1972; 25:60–63.
28. Albert RE, Lippman M, Briscoe W. The characteristics of bronchial clearance in humans and the effects of cigarette smoking. Arch Environ Health 1969; 18:738–755.
29. Thomson ML, Pavia D. Particle penetration and clearance in the human lung; results in healthy subjects and subjects with chronic bronchitis. Arch Environ Health 1974; 29:214–219.
30. Bohning DE, Albert RE, Lippmann M, Foster WM. Tracheobronchial particle deposition and clearance—a study of the effects of cigarette smoking in monozygotic twins. Arch Environ Health 1975; 30:457–462.
31. Goodman RM, Yergin BM, Landa JF, et al. Tracheal mucus velocity in nonsmokers, smokers and patients with obstructive lung disease. Fed Proc 1977; 36:607.
32. Litt M. Mucus rheology: Relevance to mucociliary clearance. Arch Intern Med 1970; 126:417–423.
33. Reid L, Bhaskar K, Coles S. Control and modulation of airway epithelial cells and their secretions. Exper Lung Res 1983; 4:157–170.
34. Charman J, Reid L. Sputum viscosity in chronic bronchitis, bronchiectasis, asthma, and cystic fibrosis. Biorheology 1972; 9:185.
35. Dulfano MJ, Adler KB. Physical properties of sputum. Am Rev Respir Dis 1975; 112:341.
36. Adler K, Dulfano MJ. The rheological factor in mucociliary clearance. J Lab Clin Med 1976; 88:22.
37. Puchelle E, Zahm JM, Petit A. Spinability and transport properties of sputum in chronic bronchitics. In: Chantler N, Elder JB, Epstein M, eds. Mucus in Health and Disease. New York: Plenum Press, 1982, 397.
38. Camner P, Mossberg B, Philipson K. Tracheobronchial clearance and chronic obstructive lung disease. Scand J Respir Dis 1973; 54:272–281.
39. Mossberg B, Strandberg K, Philipson K, Camner P. Tracheobronchial clearance and beta-adrenoreceptor stimulation in patients with chronic bronchitis. Scand J Respir Dis 1976; 57:281–289.
40. Puchelle E, Zahm JM, Girard R, et al. Mucociliary transport *in vivo* and *in vitro*. Relations to sputum properties in chronic bronchitis. Eur J Respir Dis 1980; 61:254–264.
41. Auerbach O, Hammond EC, Garfinkel L. Changes in bronchial epithelium in relation to cigarette smoking 1955–1960 vs 1970–1977. N Engl J Med 1979; 300:381.
42. Nierwoehner DE, Kleinermann J, Rice DB. Histologic changes in the peripheral airways of young cigarette smokers. N Engl J Med 1974; 291:755–758.
43. Petty TL, Ryan SF, Mitchell RS. Cigarette smoking and the lungs: relation to postmortem evidence of emphysema, chronic bronchitis and black lung pigmentation. Arch Environ Health 1967; 14:172–177.
44. Silverberg E, Holleb AJ. Cancer statistics 1974—worldwide epidemiology. Cancer 1974; 24:2–21.
45. Spain DM, Spiegel H, Bradess VA. Emphysema in apparently healthy adults: smoking age and sex. JAMA 1973; 224:322–325.
46. Vastag E, Matthys H, Kohler D, et al. Mucociliary clearance and airways obstruction in smokers, ex-smokers and normal subjects who never smoked. Eur J Respir Dis 1985; 139(Suppl 66): 93–100.
47. Mossberg B, Afzelius BA, Camner P. Mucociliary clearance in obstructive lung diseases. Correlations to the immotile cilia syndrome. Eur J Respir Dis 1986; 69(Suppl 146):295–301.
48. Mossberg B, Afzelius BA, Eliasson R, Camner P. On the pathogenesis of obstructive lung disease. A study on the immotile-cilia syndrome. Scand J Respir Dis 1978; 59:55–65.
49. Camner P, Mossberg B, Afzelius BA. Measurements of tracheobronchial clearance in patients with immotile-cilia syndrome and its value in differential diagnosis. Eur J Respir Dis 1983; 64(Suppl 127):57–63.
50. Pedersen M, Stafanger E. Bronchopulmonary symptoms in primary ciliary dyskinesia. Eur J Respir Dis 1983; 64 (Suppl 127):118–128.
51. Eliasson R, Mossberg B, Camner P, Afzelius BA. The immotile-cilia syndrome: A congenital ciliary abnormality as an etiologic factor in chronic airway infections and male sterility. N Engl J Med 1977; 297:1–6.
52. Mossberg B, Camner P, Afzelius BA. The immotile cilia syndrome compared to other obstructive lung diseases: a clue to their pathogenesis. Eur J Respir Dis 1983; 64(Suppl 127):129–136
53. Mossberg B, Philipson K, Camner P. Tracheobronchial clearance in patients with emphysema associated with alpha$_1$-antitrypsin deficiency. Scand J Respir Dis 1978; 59:1–7.
54. Lourenco RV, Loddenkemper R, Carton RW. Patterns of distribution and clearance of aerosols in patients with bronchiectasis. Am Rev Respir Dis 1972; 106:857–866.
55. Waite D, Wakefield J St J, Steele R, et al. Cilia and sperm tail abnormalities in Polynesian bronchiectatics. Lancet 1978; 2:132.
56. Pedersen H, Mygind N. Absence of axonemal arms in nasal mucosal cilia in Kartagener syndrome. Nature 1976; 262:494.
57. Svartengren M, Mossberg B, Philipson K, Camner P. Mucociliary clearance in relation to clinical features in patients with bronchiectasis. Eur J Respir Dis 1986; 69(Suppl 146):303–310.
58. Turner P, Corkey C, Lee J, et al. Clinical expressions of immotile cilia syndrome. Pediatrics 1980; 67:805.
59. Wanner A. Clinical aspects of mucociliary transport. Am Rev Respir Dis 1977; 116:73–126.
60. Foster WB, Lagenback E, Bohning D, Bergofsky EH. Quantitation of mucus clearance in peripheral lung and comparison with tracheal and bronchial mucus transport velocities in man: Adrenergics return depressed clearance and transport velocities in asthmatics to normal. Am Rev Respir Dis 1978; 117(Suppl):337.
61. Bateman JRM, Pavia D, Sheahan NF, Clarke SW. Tracheobronchial clearance in bronchial asthma: Response to beta-adrenoreceptor stimulation. Scand J Respir Dis 1976; 57:119.
62. Foster WM, Langenback EG, Bergofsky EH. Lung mucociliary function in man: interdependence of bronchial and tracheal mucus transport velocities with lung clearance in bronchial asthma and healthy subjects. Ann Occup Hyg 1982; 26:227–244.
63. Mezey RJ, Cohn MA, Fernandez RJ, et al. Mucociliary transport in allergic patients with antigen-induced bronchospasm. Am Rev Respir Dis 1978; 118:677.
64. Keal EE, Reid L. Pathologic alterations in mucus in asthma within and without the cell. In: Stein M, ed. New Directions in Asthma. Park Ridge, IL: American College of Chest Physicians, 1975, 223–239.
65. Barton AD, Powers JL, Lopata M. Biochemical characteristics affecting the consistency of bronchial secretions. Chest 1973; 63(Suppl):59.
66. Dunnill MS. The pathology of asthma, with special reference to changes in the bronchial mucosa. J Clin Pathol 1960; 13:27.
67. Sanerkin NG, Evans DMD. The sputum in bronchial asthma: pathognomonic patterns. J Pathol Bacteriol 1965; 89:535–541.
68. Jelihovsky T. The structure of bronchial plugs in mucoid impaction, bronchocentric granulomatosis and asthma. Histopathology 1983; 7:153–167.
69. Fanta C. Clinical aspects of mucus and mucous plugging in asthma. J Asthma 1985; 22(6):295–301.
70. Mussatto DJ, Garrard CS, Lourenco RV. The effect of inhaled histamine on human tracheal mucus velocity and bronchial mucociliary clearance. Am Rev Respir Dis 1988; 138:775–777.
71. Scudi JV, Kimura ET, Reinhard JF. Study of drug action on mammalian ciliated epithelium. J Pharmacol Exp Ther 1951; 102:132–137.
72. Iravani J, Melville GN. Wirkung von Pharmaka und Milieuanderungen auf die Flimmertatigkeit der Atemwege. Respiration 1975; 32:157–164.
73. Wanner A, Zarecki S, Hirsch J, Epstein S. Tracheal mucous transport in experimental canine asthma. J Appl Physiol 1975; 39:950.

74. Mussatto DJ, Lourenco RV. The effect of inhaled leukotriene-D_4 on mucociliary transport in health and asthmatic subjects. Am Rev Respir Dis 1988; 137:486 (abstract).
75. Wanner A, Sielczak M, Mella J, Abraham W. Ciliary responsiveness in allergic and nonallergic airways. J Appl Physiol 1986; 60:1967–1971.
76. Hirsch SR. The role of mucus in asthma. In: Stein M, ed. New Directions in Asthma. Park Ridge, IL: American College of Chest Physicians, 1975, 351–363.
77. Kilburn K. A hypothesis for pulmonary clearance and its implications. Am Rev Respir Dis 1968; 98, 449–463.

Chapter 14

CONTROL OF BREATHING IN COPD

Neil S. Cherniack

BACKGROUND

Impairment of the performance of the respiratory apparatus either as a pump or as a gas exchanger, such as occurs in chronic obstructive pulmonary disease (COPD), brings into play compensatory mechanisms that help preserve ventilation and arterial blood gas tensions.[12–14, 62, 64, 68]

These mechanisms include (1) the intrinsic properties of the respiratory muscles which allow them to produce greater force when their rate shortening is hindered; (2) the reflex responses arising in the lungs and airways as well as in the proprioceptors in the muscles and joints; (3) the adjustments in signals from peripheral and central chemoreceptors to the brain; and (4) the behavioral modifications that increase motor output to the respiratory muscles.[9, 12, 27]

These compensatory maneuvers in response to sudden changes in the ease with which air flows in and out of the lungs can be initiated within a breath, but as the defect in respiratory performance is maintained, change their characteristics over minutes, days, and perhaps years. These gradually occurring adaptations can cause the differences seen, for example, in the response of asthmatics versus patients with COPD to acute episodes of increased obstruction.[2, 48]

The ability of these compensations to maintain different aspects of respiration varies. Ventilation is usually very well protected, better than gas exchange. Patients with asthma as well as patients with severe chronic obstruction are able to maintain normal or even supernormal levels of minute ventilation.[68] The ability to preserve normal levels of arterial P_{CO_2} is also excellent. Usually P_{CO_2} does not increase above normal levels in COPD until the forced expiratory volume in one second (FEV_1) is reduced below 1 L.[33] In asthma, hypercapnia is even less common and usually requires reduction of the FEV_1 to less than 0.5 L.[43] In comparison, arterial P_{O_2} is poorly maintained and is decreased by even slight variations in ventilation-perfusion ratios in the lung and is not appreciably restored by increases either in minute ventilation or in depth of breathing.

Oxygen delivery to the tissues is well guarded in several ways: by the characteristics of oxyhemoglobin binding, because arterial O_2 saturation is little affected until arterial P_{O_2} falls more than 20 mm Hg from normal; by the potential of the tissues to extract more O_2 from the venous blood as arterial O_2 saturation declines; and by the ability of the heart to pump more blood and generate a higher cardiac output. It is known that the circulatory rather than the respiratory system is the primary mechanism which compensates for declines in O_2 delivery caused by reduction in arterial P_{O_2}.[10] The inability of the ventilatory control system to reverse the hypoxia caused by COPD contrasts with the ease with which increases in ventilation overcome the defective exchange of CO_2 in the lung and the rather poor capability of the circulatory system to do so.

Bronchitis and COPD are usually diseases of lifestyle initiated by the inhalation of noxious agents in the air and, most frequently, by cigarette smoking, which ultimately overwhelm the defense mechanisms of the lung. Hypersecretion, the main hallmark of bronchitis, and pulmonary tissue destruction arising from imbalance in protease-antiprotease actions in the lung, the major factor responsible for emphysema, fundamentally alter the capacity of the respiratory pump to function. The work of breathing needed to maintain a given level of ventilation is increased and a larger amount of efferent neural traffic is required if ventilation is to be preserved.[15]

Characteristic functional changes in COPD include the following:

1. Destruction of lung connective tissue reduces the tethering of the airways of the pulmonary interstitium, leads to premature collapse of the airways, and increases the unevenness of distribution of the inspired air to different regions of the lungs. All these changes hamper the transfer of CO_2 and O_2 between the blood and the alveolar air.

2. Injury and inflammation of the bronchial tubes and alveoli increase the resistance to airflow during both inspiration and expiration. More force per breath or quicker breaths are needed to maintain even normal levels of ventilation.[8, 13]

3. Increased lung compliance as a result of damage to the lung tissues and declining ability of the muscles to empty the lung completely because of airway narrowing and greater collapsibility ultimately produce hyperinflation and raise the resting end expiratory position of the lungs. Because the lung

is more expanded, the inspiratory muscles operate from a shorter initial length and like all skeletal muscles produce less force when foreshortened.[5, 56, 65]

4. Displacement and flattening of the diaphragm as a result of hyperinflation alter the vector of the forces that the muscle generates during contraction (Fig. 14–1). The more horizontally placed diaphragm is less able to lift the rib cage. Because of the adverse alignment of the diaphragm and because of the shrinkage in its initial length, the diaphragm may contract ineffectively, so that the abdomen moves inward rather than outward with each inspiration.[5, 56, 57]

5. Because of the increased demands for work output of the respiratory muscles, the energy requirement of these muscles escalates. More of the cardiac output goes to these muscles. If hypoxemia is present and there is a requirement for increased ventilation (e.g., as in exercise), the energy supply of the muscles may become inadequate, ultimately producing respiratory muscle fatigue.[5, 57, 58]

6. The expansion of the lung and thorax also misaligns the intercostal muscles and accessory respiratory muscles, such as the scalenes and the sternocleidomastoid. Special postures may be adopted by patients with COPD during breathing, such as leaning forward, to help correct this poor alignment. This is an example of a behavioral change (another is pursed-lip breathing to prevent airway collapse and retain airflow) that helps compensate for the functional effects of COPD.[5, 70]

7. Inflammation of the bronchial tubes and airways allows noxious agents in the air to reach the more deeply placed tissues in the lung and gain access to blood vessels, macrophages, mast cells, and nerves in the lung. The airways may become more irritable, producing asthmatic episodes as introduction of noxious agents causes the release of spasmogenic agents from tissue cells and nerve endings.[34]

In the remainder of the chapter we review briefly the normal operation of the respiratory control system and describe how adaptive changes which can affect the outcome of COPD occur in this system. Next we discuss the characteristics of the breathing patterns observed in patients with COPD and their possible genesis. Then we examine methods of diagnosing control system abnormalities in patients with COPD. Finally we discuss some of the therapeutic interventions that have been suggested for treating such abnormalities.

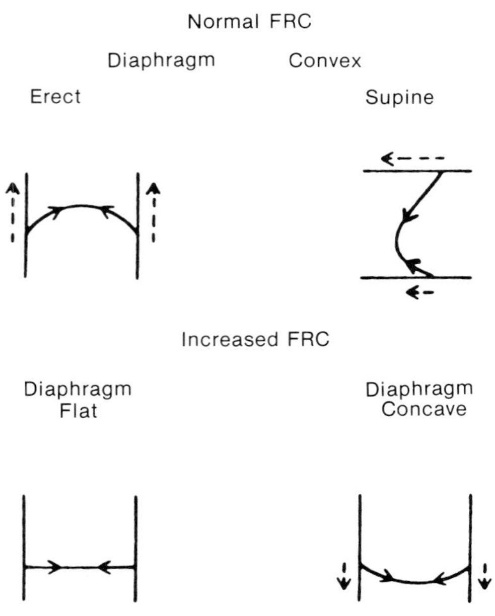

Figure 14–1. Effect of lung volume and body position on diaphragm curvature and the effect of contraction of the diaphragm on the rib cage. Broken arrows indicate direction of rib cage movement; length of arrow represents amplitude of movement (FRC = functional residual capacity). (Reproduced with permission from Cherniack NS, Altose MD. Respiratory responses to ventilatory loading. In: Hornbein TF, ed. Regulation of Breathing, vol 17, part 2. New York: Marcel Dekker, 1981, 905–964.)

CONTROL SYSTEM OPERATION

Basic Neural Organization

Respiration is a reflex act which can be modified voluntarily.[24, 25, 39, 40, 62] Breathing is controlled, and the respiratory pattern generated, formed, and shaped, by the action of a hierarchy of integrating centers located in different regions of the brain and spinal cord.[24, 39] Since the respiratory muscles also have postural, digestive, and communicative uses in addition to their function in breathing, this hierarchical control allows respiratory movements to be coordinated and integrated with complex behavioral acts. They allow us to breathe while we eat, speak, and move.[9, 12]

Despite the complexity of control, a nearly normal, albeit stereotyped, breathing pattern can be maintained in animals after separation of the lower brain stem at the level of the pons or the medulla from the rest of the brain.[39]

Three major groups of neurons in the medulla and pons are concerned with breathing:[24, 39]

1. The dorsal respiratory group (DRG) in the medulla is made up of neurons in the ventrolateral portion of the nucleus of the tractus solitarius (NTS).[24, 39] These neurons are primarily inspiratory and receive input from chemoreceptors and lung mechanoreceptors.[25, 50]

2. The ventral respiratory group (VRG) in the ventral medulla consists of neurons in the nucleus retroambiguus, parambiguus, and ambiguus, and in the nucleus retrofacialis. These neurons are both inspiratory and expiratory.[24, 39]

3. The pontine respiratory group (PRG) consists of neurons in the nucleus parabrachialis medialis and Kölliker-Fuse nucleus. These neurons are in large part phase spanning, i.e., discharge during inspiration and expiration or with a pattern that is modulated by respiration, but overlaps portions of the inspiratory and expiratory phases of breathing. This group seems primarily to be concerned with adjustments in the duration of the phases of breathing and the rate of respiration.[24, 39]

These three groups of neurons are heavily interconnected and receive multiple respiratory inputs and afferent signals from the cardiovascular, somatic, and visceral afferent systems.

The DRG and VRG contain premotor neurons that actuate phrenic and intercostal motor units in the spinal cord. Here respiration is further modified by segmental reflexes from muscle and joint proprioceptors, but signals from these proprioreceptors also ascend to the medulla and even to the cortex.[64]

The action of spinal, pontine, and medullary respiratory groups can be substantially modified by projections from the cortex, hypothalamus, and midbrain. These projections allow voluntary control of breathing as well as help coordinate the respiratory and vasomotor responses to exercise and stress.[7, 24]

The respiratory cycle consists of three phases: (1) inspiration, (2) expiration, and (3) a postinspiratory interval in which both inspiratory and expiratory neurons are inhibited (Fig. 14–2). Inspiration consists of a ramp-like increase in the firing pattern of respiratory neurons that is cut short, by inhibitory signals conveyed over the vagus nerves from lung stretch receptors, by activation of expiratory neurons in the pons and medulla, or by a third type of neuron (postinspiratory) identified by Richter and coworkers in the dorsal medulla that

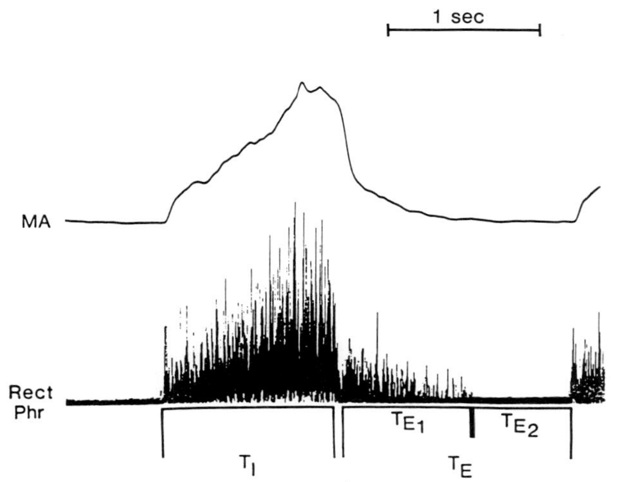

Figure 14–2. Three phases of breathing: T_I = inspiratory phase in which phrenic activity increases; T_{E1} = first phase of expiration (post inspiration) in which after a brief pause phrenic nerve activity declines; T_{E2} = second phase of expiration in which expiratory muscle activity (not shown) may be present. Rect Phr = rectified phrenic nerve activity; MA = the moving average of phrenic nerve activity.

inhibits both inspiration and expiration.[24, 39, 55] After a pause the inspiratory motor neurons fire again, but in a declining fashion, retarding the exit of air from the lung, which possibly improves gas exchange. Following this, expiration under usual conditions continues with air being pushed out of the body by the passive relaxation of the lungs and chest wall. The expiratory muscles are silent electrically. When respiratory drives intensify, the ramp increases in inspiratory activity grow steeper, inspiratory flow into the lungs accelerates, the duration of the postinspiratory phase decreases, and expiratory muscles, such as the abdominal muscles and the internal intercostals, contract more forcibly.[24] One expiratory muscle, the transverse sterni, is active in animals and probably in humans as well, even during quiet breathing.

It is generally believed that the oscillatory breathing sequence is the result of an interaction of a network of neurons (the central pattern generator) and is shaped further by neurons with different time courses of firing (early and late inspiratory, early and late expiratory, and phase spanning) in the DRG, VRG, and PRG.[39] However, the site of the central pattern generator has as yet not been determined. Moreover, pacemaker cells located in slice preparations in different parts of the medulla (both ventral and dorsal) have been identified, but it is still uncertain what role such pacemaker cells play in shaping normal breathing patterns (eupnea) in the intact medulla.[39, 55]

Central and Peripheral Chemoreceptors

The respiratory neurons in the medulla receive information on the level of arterial PO_2 and PCO_2 in the body from the peripheral chemoreceptors (the carotid and aortic bodies).[25, 29] Each are highly vascularized bits of tissue loaded with a variety of amines and neuropeptides.[25, 51, 53] The peripheral chemoreceptors consist of islands of cells (type I and type II) surrounding a blood vessel and supplied by an afferent nerve (Fig. 14–3). The type I cell, which contains granules packed with a variety of neuroactive substances, seems to be the primary chemoreceptive element, with the type II cell serving as a supporting element. Although the same nerve fiber can respond to changes in both arterial oxygen pressure (PaO_2) and arterial carbon dioxide pressure ($PaCO_2$), discharge rates increase linearly with rising PO_2 but hyperbolically with hypoxia. The CO_2 and hypoxic signals affect each other in a multiplicative fashion; the responses to reductions in arterial PO_2 are greater when arterial PCO_2 is higher; and hypercapnic responses are greater when hypoxia is more severe.[51]

The mechanisms underlying the formation of the two signals are also different.[35] The hypoxic signal may be triggered by a change in the ratio of adenosine diphosphate (ADP) to adenosine triphosphate (ATP) (the phosphate potential) or in intracellular levels of calcium produced by hypoxia, which causes the release of one or more neuroactive substances (neurotransmitters) from the type I cells.[25, 53] Acetylcholine and substance P (SP) are two possible neurotransmitters in a rather long list of suggested agents that may be released during hypoxia and excite increased afferent activity.[25, 53] The response to CO_2, in comparison, seems to involve changes in the intracellular hydrogen ion concentration, although extracellular acidosis also increases chemoreceptor output.[51] The response to hypoxia but not to CO_2 can be blocked by a number of agents, such as antimycin, which blocks electron transfer of mitochondria, or oligomycin, which prevents formation of ATP, or by anti-SP, in appropriate concentrations.[53] The response to CO_2, but not hypoxia, is interfered with by carbonic anhydrase inhibitors.[1, 51]

Although the carotid body responds to changes in the arterial tension of O_2, it is relatively unaffected by anemia or by carbon monoxide. The aortic body responds more to changes in O_2 content and may have weaker response to CO_2 than the carotid body.[35] Both the aortic body and carotid body also have a vasopressor action triggered by hypoxia and by systemic hypotension and cause changes in heart rate.[51] The circulatory action of the aortic body seems to be stronger than its respiratory actions, whereas the reverse seems to be true of the carotid body.[37] The action of the peripheral chemoreceptors, but the carotid body in particular, may be modified by efferent nerves from the brain, which inhibit its discharge, and by autonomic nerves from the cervical ganglia, which alter the blood flow through the receptors.[51] A decrease in blood flow stimulates both peripheral chemoreceptors. For example, neuropeptide Y, a vasoconstricting agent, excites the carotid body.[52]

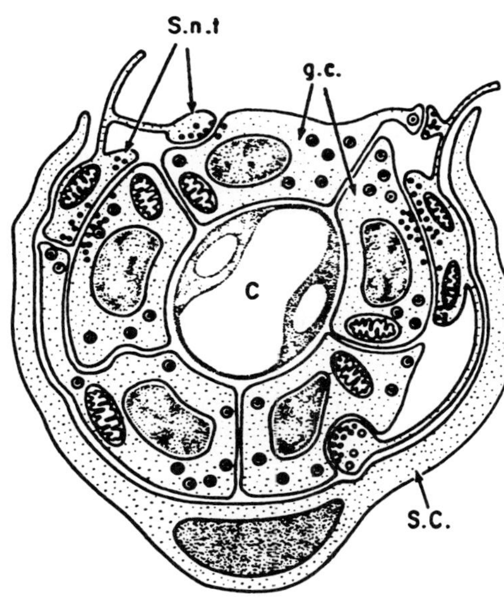

Figure 14–3. Schematic representation of the microscopic structure of the carotid body. S.n.t. = nerve terminals; g.c. = glomerular cells (type I); C = capillaries; S.C. = supporting cells (type II). (Reproduced with permission from Eyzaguirre C, Zapata P. Perspectives in carotid body research. J Appl Physiol 1984; 57:931–957.)

However, a number of agents found in the carotid body seem to have direct stimulatory or inhibitory effects independent of their action on blood vessels. Substance P and acetylcholine, mentioned earlier, stimulate the carotid body as does vasoactive intestinal peptide (VIP), serotonin, epinephrine, and adenosine. Dopamine and the enkephalins diminish carotid body discharge. These agents have similar actions on the aortic body.[25, 53]

Even in carotid body– and aortic body–denervated animals, inhaled CO_2 stimulates respiration. The site of this action continues to be debated, but evidence indicates that important sites are superficially located areas near the ventrolateral medullary surface (VMS).[6, 7, 42, 62] Cooling of the ventrolateral medulla or applying local anesthetics decreases or eliminates breathing or produces apnea and depresses respiratory responses to hypercapnia. Tonically firing cells have been identified in this area.[31, 42, 45] These neurons are excited by a variety of afferent inputs, including signals evoked by limb flexion or extension, stimulation of hypothalamic regions for the defensive reactions evoked by stress, stimulation of midbrain locomotor center, inhaled CO_2, and excitation of peripheral chemoreceptors.[6, 45] These neurons are also tightly interlinked and even intermingled with pressor and depressor vasomotor neurons located in the same area.[42] Interconnections have also been demonstrated with the dorsal respiratory group.[7]

Further studies that have involved focal intramedullary cooling or local injection of anesthetics, amines, and peptides suggest that the main body of chemoreceptive neurons near the VMS are actually located in a superficial portion of the nucleus paragigantocellularis lateralis.[7, 42, 45] Like the cells in the carotid body, these neurons contain a variety of neuroactive agents, including acetylcholine, neurotensin, and SP, all of which have been shown to stimulate breathing when administered to this area.[28, 31, 38] Other inhibitory substances, enkephalins, somatostatin, and gamma-aminobutyric acid (GABA), reduce breathing when the neurons in the VMS are exposed to them.[30, 31] However, the idea that these cells are the only central chemoreceptors has been seriously challenged by later reports concerning cells elsewhere in the brain, in the DRG for example, which also seem to respond to changes in CO_2.[7]

Respiration is depressed by metabolic alkalosis as are responses to hypoxia.[19] This depressive action is believed to take place at central as well as peripheral chemoreceptors. While it was once believed that the VMS cells were primarily responsive to changes in cerebrospinal fluid (CSF) pH or brain extracellular fluid pH, that idea no longer seems tenable. For the same change in pH at the VMS, respiration is more excited by CO_2 increases than by changes in bicarbonate.[38] However, the hypothesis that all the respiratory changes that were elicited from this area were indirect and caused by excitation of vasomotor neurons also seems to be disproved.[38] Although respiratory and vasomotor neurons in the VMS are closely linked, they are not identical.[42, 46]

The compensatory changes in ventilation caused by hypoxia or hypercapnia depend on feedback adjustments in respiratory activity provoked in response to signals from the peripheral and central chemoreceptors (see Fig. 14–4). Ventilation also increases nearly linearly with the increases in carbon dioxide output (V_{CO_2}) and oxygen uptake (V_{O_2}) produced by hypermetabolism, as occurs during exercise.[11, 72] The way in which this feed-forward control occurs remains in doubt, but there are a number of intriguing possibilities.[61, 72] Afferent signals from exercising limbs or projections from locomotor neurons in the brain to medullary respiratory neurons may roughly bring respiratory levels in line with metabolic levels. Finer adjustment in respiratory control could then take place through feedback via chemoreceptors.[61] Neural signals from mechanoreceptors in the joints and muscles of the limbs also help increase breathing during exercise.[45, 64] Motor areas in the cortex for the limbs also send projections to respiratory neurons and stimulate breathing.[64] Chemical inputs from peripheral and central chemoreceptors modify the activity of upper airway muscles and alter upper airway resistance.[23, 30]

It has been shown that the oscillations in P_{CO_2} occur in the blood and at the VMS during the respiratory cycle.[61] The oscillations in the blood and perhaps in the brain grow greater when metabolic rate is increased.[61] The carotid body activity rises as the rate of change of P_{CO_2} increases and as the absolute level of P_{O_2} increases. It could be that the carotid body conveys a metabolically related signal to brain respiratory neurons by its response to the rate of change of P_{CO_2}.

Because exercise increases ventilation even in carotid body–denervated animals, both the neural signals from the limbs and metabolic signals from the brain may play a significant role in the respiratory response.[61, 64, 72]

Reflex and Behavioral Regulation of Breathing

Mechanoreceptors in the lung and chest wall can modify both the level and pattern of breathing, as shown in Figure 14–4.[16, 64]

Receptors in the lung communicate with respiratory neurons in the brain via the vagus nerves.[16] Three types of receptors have been identified: stretch and irritant receptors, which transmit signals over myelinated fibers, and a third receptor type (C or J receptors), which signal over unmyelinated fibers. Stretch and irritant receptors are located in the airways, mainly the larger ones. C-fiber receptors are found mainly in the smaller airways and lung interstitium. All three types of receptors have complex circulatory as well as respiratory effects.

Stretch receptors have been the most extensively studied.[59] They are activated by lung inflation, cut short inspiration but have little effect on the steepness of the inspiratory ramp, and stimulate expiratory activity. Stretch receptors are believed to be excited by the amount of lung expansion, although increasing the rate of lung filling also has some stimulatory action. Stretch receptors are responsible for the Hering-Breuer reflex in animals, in which sufficiently great inflation of the lung produces apnea. In animals also, vagotomy and destruction of the PRGs produce prolonged inspiratory activity (so-called apneustic breathing).[16, 24]

Irritant receptors are excited by lung deflation but also by certain noxious substances in the inspired air and by chemical agents, such as histamine and prostaglandins.[16] The high rates of airflow into the lung can also excite irritant receptors. Irritant receptor stimulation causes coughing, but, when less severe, intensifies breathing, producing tachypnea with diminished tidal volumes. Irritant receptor stimulation may contribute to the rapid shallow breathing observed during asthmatic attacks.[33, 50] Irritant receptor stimulation has a vasopressor effect, whereas stretch receptor stimulation has a vasodepressor effect.[16, 50]

Receptors innervated by C fibers (unmyelinated fibers) are stimulated in many of the same ways as those for irritant receptors and like them often cause rapid, shallow breathing.[16] The rapid breathing, however, is often preceded by a brief interval of apnea. The C fibers can be activated by the injection of capsaicin or diphenylguanidine into the bronchial or pulmonary arteries.[50] Tachykinins such as substance P may be the neurotransmitter used in C-fiber signaling. C-fiber reflexes are believed to be an important contributor to the tachypnea seen with pulmonary edema.[50]

The respiratory muscles contain both tendon organs, which measure force and in general have an inhibitory effect on breathing, and spindles, which monitor muscle fiber length,

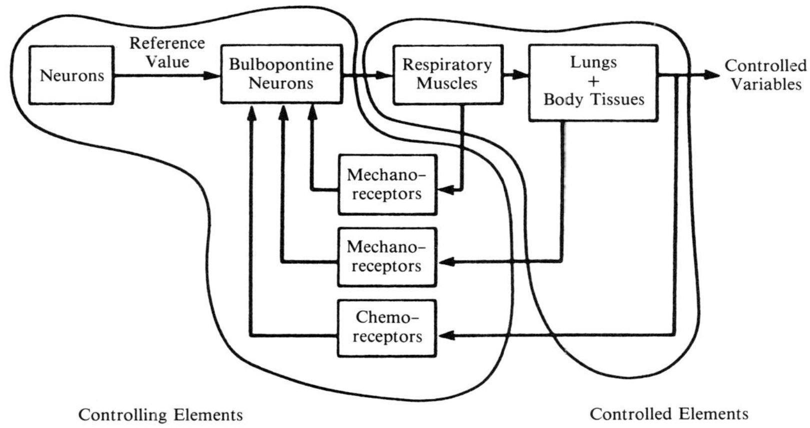

Figure 14–4. Block diagram of respiratory control system. The system can be divided, roughly, into controlling and controlled elements. Neurons located in the medulla provide reference values to premotor neurons also located in the medulla, which drive respiratory muscles, ventilate the lungs, and produce changes in pH, partial pressure of carbon dioxide (Pco_2), and partial pressure of oxygen (Po_2), the controlled variables, in the blood and body tissues. These changes in blood gases and pH act on central and peripheral chemoreceptors. Signals from these receptors are relayed to the bulbopontine neurons. When there are differences between reference values (the desired levels) and actual values, the activity of the bulbopontine neurons is modified and the appropriate ventilation changes are produced. Mechanoreceptors located in the respiratory muscles and the lungs measure the forces and displacements produced by the respiratory neurons and further modify the pattern and level of their discharge. (Reproduced with permission from Longobardo GS, Cherniack NS. Abnormalities in respiratory rhythm. In: Cherniack NS, Widdicombe JG, eds. Handbook of Physiology, vol. 2, part II, section 3. Bethesda: American Physiological Society, 1986, 729–750.)

are excited by muscle stretch, and in general increase breathing.[64] A unique arrangement that permits spindle length to be independently set through gamma efferent fibers allows spindle activity to be excitatory even during inspiration when the main muscle fibers innervated by alpha efferent fibers shorten. While tendon organs and spindles have an important reflex action at the spinal segmental level both in respiration and in the maintenance of posture, their signals reach the cortex and may play a role there in producing the sense of dyspnea.[9, 32, 64]

A number of other reflexes from the joints and from the upper airways affect breathing.[64] For example, negative pressures in the upper airway, as might occur during inhalation when the nose or oropharynx is blocked, lengthen inspiration.[59]

Higher brain centers have major effects on breathing through voluntary acts, such as talking, which alter respiratory patterns, and changes in state between sleep and wakefulness.[14, 49] Although the effects of state changes are discussed more fully in other chapters, in general, sleep has a depressant action on breathing and responses to CO_2 and hypoxia. Sleep can alter responses to reflexes.[69] For example, laryngeal stimulation, which can give rise to coughing during wakefulness, can produce apnea if it occurs while asleep. The pattern of breathing is also altered by sleep. In general, breathing becomes more regular during non-REM sleep but more erratic in REM sleep. Airway resistance tends to rise during sleep.[69]

Changes in mental activity can affect breathing even during wakefulness. Mental arithmetic stimulates breathing, whereas closing the eyes decreases breathing.[14] Tranquilizers, alcohol, and opiates all depress breathing, presumably in large part by their effects on higher brain centers.[60, 63]

Control of Airway Smooth Muscle Tone

Although the tone of airway smooth muscle, and hence airway caliber, largely depends on local effects on the airway, a number of reflexes can affect airway resistance.[34]

The parasympathetic motor nerves that innervate the smooth muscle of the tracheal bronchial tree have a respiratory modulation.[44] As respiration intensifies, so does the constricting effect on the airways. Both hypercapnia and hypoxia can act centrally to constrict airway smooth muscle.[29] In addition, groups of neurons in the ventral medulla have been described that act to increase airway tone independently of effects of breathing, whereas there seem to be other groups which decrease tone.[18]

Stimulation of irritant and C-fiber receptors besides producing breathing changes also narrows airways. Alternatively, excitation of pulmonary stretch receptors dilates the airways.[59]

Responses to Acute Loading of the Respiratory Muscles

Chronic obstructive pulmonary disease interferes with the ability of the thoracic pump to ventilate the lung.[12, 13] In order to study the compensatory mechanisms investigators have devised different experimental methods of acutely interfering with the mechanical function of the thorax and then comparing the responses of healthy individuals with those of patients with COPD.[2] One commonly used intervention requires subjects to breathe through narrow tubes or increased resistances; but other kinds of experimental paradigms have been used, such as forcing subjects to breathe at large lung volumes, against positive pressures, or after some bronchoconstricting agent has been given.[12, 13, 33] Although none of these exactly simulates the effects of COPD, they have permitted a systematic cataloguing of the mechanisms and tactics that the subjects can employ when loads are present for a short time.

Very important in compensation are the properties of the skeletal muscles themselves, which allow the force exerted at a given level of nerve stimulation to increase when muscles are preloaded (lengthened as the expiratory muscles are in the inflated lung) or afterloaded as the respiratory muscles are when airway resistance is increased.[56]

In addition, proprioceptive and pulmonary reflexes can have compensating effects.[64] Spindles in the intercostal muscles increase the drive to the respiratory muscles when tidal volumes achieved are less than expected. Although the diaphragm contains very few spindles, motor output to that muscle is increased through an intercostal-to-diaphragm reflex if the depth of breathing is inadequate. Failure of the lung to expand normally also decreases the inhibition of respiration exerted by pulmonary stretch receptors, and this effect increases the duration of inspiration, so that tidal volume returns toward normal levels.[16] Bronchoconstriction usually excites irritant and unmyelinated receptors, augmenting the motor drive to the respiratory muscles.[16]

Breathing at increased lung volume may reduce the mechanical advantage and produce misalignment of the diaphragm.[56] The abnormal and weakened action of the diaphragm may be partially offset by a redistribution of motor drives to other respiratory muscles. Thus, the abdominal muscles may be made to contract more forcibly, allowing the diaphragm to begin its inspiratory contraction at a longer length and hence in a better mechanical advantage. The accessory muscles of respiration may be activated and drive to the intercostal muscles may increase. It is of interest, though, that a recent study has shown that expiratory muscles use O_2 less efficiently than do inspiratory muscles.[20]

Postinspiratory activity is generally decreased during acute obstruction of the airways, allowing expiration to proceed more rapidly.[13]

The hypoxia and hypercapnia that result from inadequate ventilation also increase both inspiratory and expiratory activity and, in addition, have an excitatory effect on the dilator muscles of the upper airways.[23, 30]

Further compensation is achieved by behavioral mechanisms. It has been shown that an increase in airway resistance in conscious subjects is frequently followed on the next breath by a more forcible contraction of the respiratory muscles.[3, 12, 13] This response is usually eliminated or reduced during sleep and can be reduced even by mild tranquilizing agents.

Effect of Sustained Loading

The responses to mechanical impairment undergo changes with time. Changes occur in the muscles themselves. Fatigue-resistant fibers, for example, increase in chronically loaded respiratory muscles.[58] Changes in muscle strength also occur.[56] Hyperinflated lungs can be produced in animals by the inhalation of elastase or elastase-like enzymes. This resulting permanent hyperinflation leads to diaphragm shortening and reduction in the length of each diaphragm sarcomere.[57] However, with time the number of sarcomeres per diaphragm fiber diminishes and the length of each sarcomere once again increases. Because the force that can be exerted during diaphragm contraction depends on sarcomere and not fiber length, contractile force returns to pre-lung hyperinflation levels.

However, not all the adjustments that occur with time improve the ability of the respiratory system to compensate for loads. Patients with COPD are less able to detect changes in airway resistance than are healthy individuals and respond behaviorally with less force production when acutely obstructed.[2, 12] One group of investigators has attributed this finding to a chronic increase in the release of endorphins, since the response to acute obstruction reverts to normal in patients with COPD when they are given naloxone.[63, 66] It is not certain that this diminution in the response to loads is a consequence just of the obstruction. Older individuals with normal lungs respond to load with less force production than do younger individuals.[12, 13] Some of the subnormal response of COPD patients may be due to their advanced age. Resting levels of cerebral perfusion and brain blood flow in patients with COPD are usually within normal limits. However, the chronic hypoxia that occurs with COPD may diminish cognitive function. Severe hypoxia, in addition, may even diminish ventilation by a central depressive effect.[21]

Responses to Chemical Stimuli in COPD

Ventilatory sensitivity to CO_2 and hypoxia is usually expressed by the relationship between some index of respiratory output and the changes in arterial gas tension.[11, 54] Because respiratory output tends to increase linearly with P_{CO_2}, the slope of the line relating respiratory output, such as ventilation, to P_{CO_2} is used to evaluate and compare hypercapnic responses among patients (Fig. 14–5).

The response to hypoxia is curvilinear (Fig. 14–5), and sensitivity is expressed by relating respiratory output to some function of arterial P_{O_2} such as its reciprocal, log transformation, or percent of oxygen saturation (Sa_{O_2}).[54] All of these derivations linearize the relationship between respiratory output and the hypoxic stimulus.

In patients with COPD the ventilatory responses to hypoxia

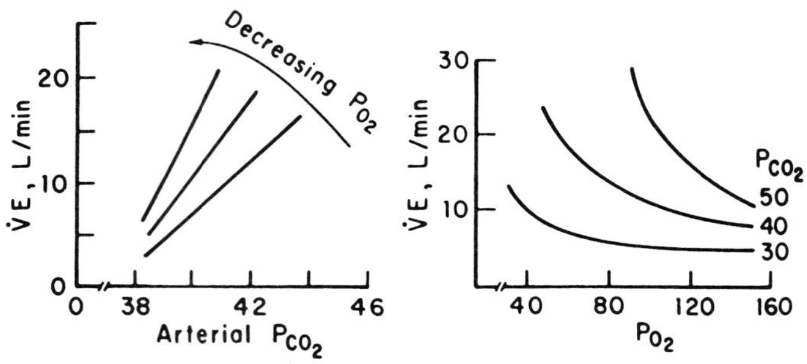

Figure 14–5. Effect of changes in arterial partial pressure of carbon dioxide (P_{CO_2}) and partial pressure of oxygen (P_{O_2}) on ventilation (VE). Decreasing P_{O_2} increases the response to P_{CO_2}, while decreasing P_{O_2} increases the response to hypoxia. (Reproduced with permission from Cherniack NS, Longobardo GS. The chemical control of respiration. Ann Biomed Eng 1981; 9:395–407.)

and hypercapnia tend to be subnormal.[2, 54] This is usually attributed to the mechanical interference with ventilatory function produced by the disease.[2, 54] A similar decrease in ventilatory response is seen in normal subjects made to breathe through severe resistances.[2, 12, 13, 54] Responses in COPD tend to be normal when output is expressed as the force developed with each breath, when ventilation is expressed as a percent of maximal voluntary ventilation, or when electrical activity of the diaphragm is used as an index of the respiratory output.[11, 22]

When healthy subjects are made alkalotic by bicarbonate infusion or by potassium depletion, the respiratory response to CO_2 diminishes.[19] A similar decrease in response occurs in hypercapnic COPD patients who retain bicarbonate so as to restore pH to normal levels.[54] The mechanism for respiratory inhibition is believed to be a decrease in extracellular fluid hydrogen concentration, since acid infusion stimulates breathing.[19] The initial depression of ventilation caused by alkalosis may take place at the carotid body. Subsequently, a variety of mechanisms, which actively readjust bicarbonate levels in the brain extracellular fluid and intracellularly, may contribute to the depression.[19] In COPD, CO_2 retention produces compensatory increases in bicarbonate both in the CSF and in the plasma.[54] The respiratory depression caused by the bicarbonate retention in COPD reduces the ability of the chemoreceptors to compensate for loads.

The response of the carotid body to hypoxia also depends on the level of hydrogen ion.[25, 54] Hence, bicarbonate retention in COPD may also diminish the respiratory response to hypoxia. In addition, it has been observed in animals that reside on mountains and in human high-altitude inhabitants that prolonged exposure to hypoxia decreases and may even abolish the response to hypoxia.[36] A similar decrease in hypoxic response occurs in individuals who are hypoxemic as a result of right-to-left cardiac shunts.[36] Whereas it was once believed that exposure to hypoxia at birth was required for this reduced response to occur, more recently it has been shown that it is better related to the duration of the exposure.[36, 54] However, it seems clear that newborns and children are more susceptible to this effect than are adults. An enlargement and increase in perfusion to the carotid body with prolonged hypoxia may contribute to this depression. It is not clear whether similar changes in the carotid body can occur in COPD.[54] However, some studies suggest that the response to hypoxia is better preserved in COPD than is the response to CO_2.[54] Removal of an excitatory effect of hypoxia explains the rise in P_{CO_2} seen in patients with COPD who are given oxygen.

One might imagine that a reduction in upper airway resistance might be beneficial in patients with COPD, but studies show that laryngeal expiratory resistance is increased.[17] The increase in resistance, although it interferes with lung emptying, may act like pursed-lip breathing to improve gas exchange.

BREATHING PATTERNS IN COPD AND THEIR RELATION TO RESPIRATORY FAILURE

The control system functions sufficiently well in most patients with COPD so that normal blood gas tensions of CO_2 are maintained.[54, 68] Even though there may be a modest degree of hypoxemia, O_2 delivery to the tissues is preserved by an increase in cardiac output, a greater extraction of O_2 from the blood, an increase in red cell mass, or some combination of these three factors. There is a price for this. Respiratory muscle work is greater than normal and the O_2 usage by the muscles is increased. Efferent drive to the muscles is increased, which can produce dyspnea.[15, 64]

In a minority of patients, compensatory mechanisms fail and hypercapnia ensues.[64] Most often, hypercapnia is the consequence of more severe disease.[54, 64] However, it has been clear for many years that some patients with equal degrees of lung dysfunction will retain CO_2 but others will not. The hypercapnic patients can be divided into two groups: those with normal or even increased levels of minute ventilation, who constitute the bulk of the group with COPD respiratory failure; and a smaller group in which levels of minute ventilation are decreased.[64]

Of the patients with greater-than-normal levels of ventilation, those with respiratory failure tend to have smaller tidal volumes (Fig. 14–6).[64] In these patients, respiratory drive and chemosensitivity (assessed using some index of respiratory output other than ventilation) are normal, but patterns of breathing are not. Because tidal volume is low and because COPD is associated with enlargement of the physiologic dead space, alveolar ventilation is less than normal.

There are several factors that might cause this rapid, shallow sort of breathing in patients with COPD.

Many patients with COPD who develop respiratory failure have chronic bronchitis as well, caused by injury to the airway and the lung parenchyma.[5] The bronchitis excites irritant receptors, which in turn produces the rapid, shallow breathing observed.[5] Many patients with hypercapnia, but not all, are cyanotic (blue) and edematous (bloated). These "blue bloaters" characteristically have a chronic cough.

It has been demonstrated that the occurrence of respiratory muscle fatigue depends on forces developed by the respiratory muscles and the time of contraction.[57, 58] Fatigue is said to occur when the product of the force used in each breath (as a percent of maximum inspiratory force) and inspiratory time (as a percent of the total duration of a breath) reaches some limit (about 0.15).[58] As the disease becomes more severe and maximum inspiratory force declines, shallower breathing may be employed at the expense of hypercapnia to avoid respiratory muscle fatigue, which may potentially produce irreversible injury to the muscles.[57, 58]

The ratio of inspiratory force per breath to maximal inspiratory force is also an important determinant of dyspnea.[14] As this ratio increases, dyspnea becomes increasingly intense.[14] In comparison, dyspnea develops much less rapidly when breathing frequency rises. Hence, the rapid, shallow breathing employed by some patients with COPD may be a strategy used to minimize discomfort.

A smaller group of patients with COPD breathe less than normal and develop respiratory failure on that basis. Some have depressed respiratory responses to CO_2 or to hypoxia.[54] This depression may occur because of the injudicious use of tranquilizers, O_2, or diuretics resulting in metabolic alkalosis. But there are other causes. Intermittent nocturnal hypoxia and hypercapnia in patients with COPD and the sleep apnea syndrome may lead to bicarbonate retention or hypoxic depression, or both, and thereby to respiratory failure. Cerebrovascular disease in the elderly patient with COPD may depress central chemoreceptor function.[54]

Some of the patients may have genetically depressed chemosensitivity. Siblings of patients with CO_2 retention have CO_2 sensitivities in the low to subnormal range.[47] Abnormal neurotransmitter function could play a role in causing a reduction in sensitivity, which may be sufficient to allow adequate gas exchange in ordinary circumstances but not when the respiratory system is stressed.

In the extremely rare patient COPD may be sufficiently severe that the additional CO_2 produced by the muscles in ventilating the lungs renders useless attempts to reduce arterial CO_2 by more breathing.[15, 54, 56]

DIAGNOSIS OF CONTROL SYSTEM ABNORMALITIES IN COPD

The diagnosis of abnormalities in chemoreceptor function is difficult in patients with lung disease, particularly in those with COPD. All assessments should begin with a complete evaluation of pulmonary function, including tests of gas exchange and mechanics. Spirometry alone is not enough. The abnormalities in the thoracic pump mechanism caused by the disease may depress the ventilatory response to CO_2, normally more than 1 L/min per mm Hg change in P_{CO_2}, even if the chemoreceptors are normal. However, at least two techniques seem useful in evaluating respiratory control even when lung function is abnormal.

One test, occlusion pressure, uses inspiratory force as a measure of respiratory output (Fig. 14–7), and the other, respiratory muscle electrical activity.[2, 33, 41] In both instances,

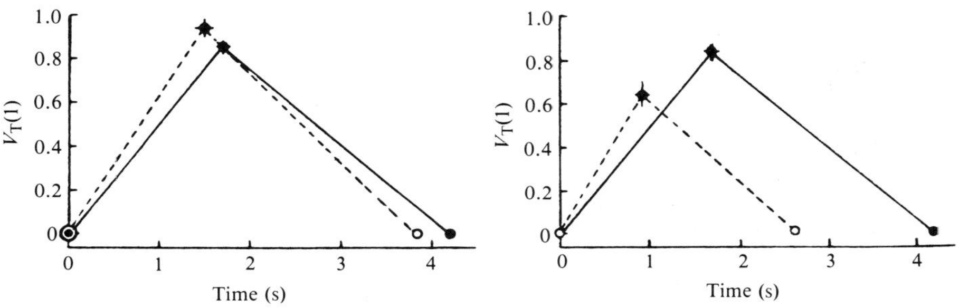

Figure 14–6. Plots of volume against time in single breath. Solid lines show responses of healthy individuals during resting breathing. Dotted lines in left-hand panel show tidal volume in COPD patients with normal levels of carbon dioxide partial pressure (P_{CO_2}). Dotted lines in right-hand panel show tidal volume of COPD patients with elevated P_{CO_2}. Note in the patients with elevated P_{CO_2}, tidal volume is smaller. (Reproduced with permission from Sorli J, Grassino A, Lorange G, Milic-Emili J. Control of breathing in patients with chronic obstructive lung disease. Clin Sci Mol Med 1978; 54:295–304.)

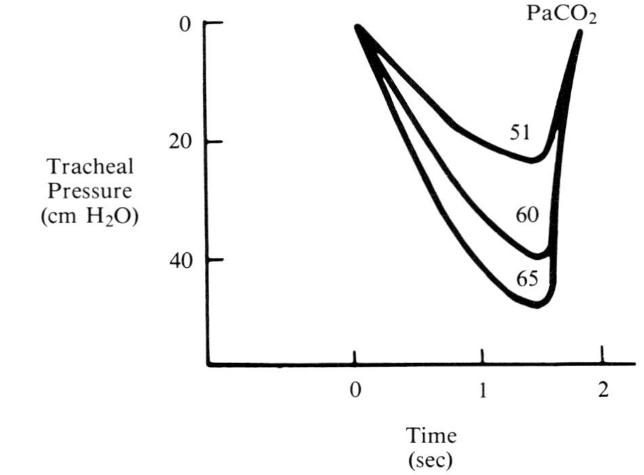

Figure 14–7. Changes in tracheal pressure during inspiratory occlusion in an animal. Note that the occluded pressure becomes greater (more negative) as partial pressure of carbon dioxide (P_{CO_2}) rises. Similar changes in occlusion pressure occur in humans, but behavioral changes are likely to distort all but the first 100 to 150 msec of the pressure curve.

change in chemical drive can be produced by steady state gas inhalation or by rebreathing. In the rebreathing test, after a period of O_2 breathing to produce normal or supernormal levels of arterial P_{O_2}, the patient rebreathes from a bag containing 7% CO_2 in O_2 so that progressive hypercapnia develops.[11] As rebreathing proceeds, the CO_2 in the patient's lungs and in the bag equilibrates; then P_{CO_2} in the end-tidal gas and in the arterial blood rises linearly with the time at the same rate, which depends on the volume of the patient's lung, the bag, the buffering capacity of the patient's body, and the CO_2 production.[54] Intermittently a valve is turned at end expiration so that the subsequent inspiration is occluded and mouth pressure or esophageal pressure is measured. The occlusion is random and lasts 100 to 200 msec to prevent conscious affects from altering breathing efforts. The slope of the change in the occlusion pressure with CO_2 is compared with values obtained in normal individuals in the same laboratory. Ventilation can be measured on unoccluded breaths during the same test.

This procedure has the following advantages: It is rapid and should require no more than 5 to 8 minutes of rebreathing. Since the response is measured while the airway is occluded, increased airway resistance will not depress the results. In addition, the test measures the combined activity of all the respiratory muscles. Occlusion pressure will be affected by changes in functional residual capacity (FRC) though the effects are usually slight.[11] When the FRC is larger, the resting length of inspiratory muscles will be less and occlusion pressure may be less. Some investigators have recommended that the test be performed while the patient is supine to minimize any decrease in FRC that sometimes occurs with CO_2 rebreathing. In addition, the results will also be influenced by muscle strength, though these generally have to be large to have any appreciable effect. Originally the test was believed to measure the isometric force produced by the inspiratory muscles. Later studies, however, indicate that considerable shortening of the muscle can occur even when the airway is occluded through distortion of the thoracic cage so that the forces developed are less than isometric.[71] It is also possible to measure changes in occlusion pressure during progressive hypoxia under isocapnic conditions, which can also be produced by a rebreathing technique.[11]

The responses of individual muscles to stimulation by hypercapnia or hypoxia can be assessed by measurement of muscle electrical activity.[11, 41] It is known that when the electrical discharge of the diaphragm with each breath is integrated using a moving average technique, peak electrical activity is proportional to changes in tidal volume in healthy subjects.[22] Moreover, changes in peak activity in muscles, such as the intercostals, normally parallel changes in the diaphragm. Surface electrodes over the upper abdomen or lower rib cage can measure diaphragm electrical activity during CO_2 rebreathing or during hypoxia. However, there is some risk that the electrical signal will be contaminated by the activity of other muscles. This risk can be diminished by recording diaphragm electrical activity with an electrode inserted in an esophageal catheter and positioned so that it is near the diaphragm.[11]

Both the occlusion pressure and electromyelographic tests of chemosensitivity may be abnormal in patients with hypercapnia and COPD because of elevated bicarbonate levels even if chemoreceptors are adequately functioning.[19] In these patients some clue as to the integrity of chemoreceptor function may be obtained in the following way: patients who retain CO_2 because of poor chemoreceptor responsivity can usually achieve normal arterial P_{CO_2} levels by voluntary hyperventilation. In addition, these patients have excessively high arterial P_{CO_2} levels in relation to the FEV_1. In patients with COPD there tends to be a hyperbolic relationship between FEV_1 and arterial P_{CO_2}. If chemoreceptors are defective or the muscles weak, arterial P_{CO_2} will lie above this curve (Fig. 14–8). The relationship between maximal inspiratory pressure and P_{CO_2} is also hyperbolic. Patients with poor chemoreceptor function will have a disproportionally great P_{CO_2} for their level of maximal inspiratory force.

Sleep studies are important to carry out in hypercapnic patients since sleep apnea, which produces severe hypoxemia, can intensify respiratory failure.[69]

Measurement of chemosensitivity is useful in patients with COPD even if they do not have hypercapnia. Low responsivity may identify patients at special risk for respiratory failure if pulmonary function worsens.

TREATMENT OF RESPIRATORY CONTROL SYSTEM ABNORMALITIES

Although much is being learned about the biochemical mechanisms involved in signal transduction in the carotid body

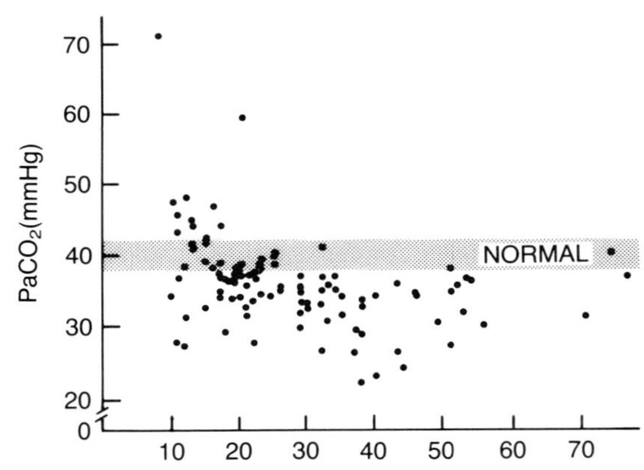

Figure 14–8. Arterial carbon dioxide partial pressure (P_{CO_2}) in an acute asthmatic patient plotted against forced expiratory volume in one second (FEV_1). Note that arterial carbon dioxide pressure (Pa_{CO_2}) rises as FEV_1 decreases in a curvilinear manner. In asthmatic patients changes in Pa_{CO_2} are seen when FEV_1 falls below 15% to 20% of predicted. In patients with COPD, Pa_{CO_2} rises with less decrease in FEV_1, approximately when FEV_1 is 30% of predicted. (Reproduced with permission from McFadden ER, Lyons H. Arterial blood gas tensions in asthma. N Engl J Med 1968; 278:1027.)

and in the brain, no specific measures are available currently that correct defects in respiratory chemoreceptors.

A number of respiratory stimulants have been developed, such as doxapram, which act to excite the carotid body, or nikethamide, a central respiratory stimulant, which can be given intravenously, and have been used experimentally for short periods of time to allow O_2 to be administered with excessive respiratory depression.[54] Intravenous theophylline has a respiratory stimulating action, perhaps because of its antagonism to adenosine, and can be used for the same purpose.[54]

Progesterone is probably the agent most frequently given to stimulate breathing and can be taken orally.[54] Its action is uncertain, although it is believed to be central. It seems to be effective in the patient with primary alveolar hypoventilation but is occasionally helpful in the patient with COPD because it increases the tidal volume.[67]

Acetazolamide, by creating a metabolic acidosis, has been used as a respiratory stimulant in patients with COPD with CO_2 retention and occasionally produces dramatically beneficial results.[67]

Almitrine, like acetazolamide and progesterone, can be given orally.[26] Although it is not available in the United States, it may to some degree improve ventilation and perfusion inequalities but probably improves oxygenation and reduces hypercapnia mainly by its action as a carotid body stimulant. Weight loss or peripheral neuropathy, or both, sometimes occur in individuals taking the drug in doses of more than 100 mg/d.[26]

Treatment of COPD itself is the most efficacious strategy to improve function even in patients with control system abnormalities. Improved respiratory muscle strength and endurance can have especially significant effects. It may also be important to reverse even minor degrees of sleep apnea. Metabolic alkalosis is a respiratory depressant and if present should be corrected.

Administration of O_2 may reverse hypoxic depression, improve respiratory muscle dysfunction, and have some bronchodilating action. Oxygen must be given with care and its effects during both sleep and wakefulness must be evaluated if life-threatening respiratory acidosis and coma are to be avoided.

REFERENCES

1. Ahmad HR, Loeschcke HH, Woidtke HH. Three compartment model for the bicarbonate exchange of the brain extracellular fluid with blood and cells. In: Fitzgerald RS, Gautier H, Lahiri S, eds. The Regulation of Respiration During Sleep and Anesthesia. New York: Plenum, 1978, 195–209.
2. Altose MD, McCauley WC, Kelsen SG, Cherniack NS. Effects of hypercapnia and inspiratory flow-resistive loading on respiratory activity in chronic airway obstruction. J Clin Invest 1977; 59:500–507.
3. Altose MD, Kelsen SG, Cherniack NS. Respiratory responses to change in airflow resistance in conscious man. Respir Physiol 1979; 37:185–200.
4. Aubier MD, Murciano M, Fournier M, et al. Central respiratory drive in acute respiratory failure of patients with chronic obstructive pulmonary disease. Am Rev Respir Dis 1980; 122:191–199.
5. Bellemare F, Grassino A. Force reserve of the diaphragm in patients with chronic obstructive pulmonary disease. J Appl Physiol 1983; 55:8–15.
6. Bledsoe SW, Hornbein TF. Central chemoreceptors and the regulation of their chemical environment. In: Hornbein TF, ed. Regulation of Breathing. New York: Marcel Dekker, 1981, 347–406.
7. Bruce EN, Cherniack NS. Central chemoreceptors. J Appl Physiol 1987; 62:389–402.
8. Campbell AH, Imberger H, Jones BM. Increased upper airway resistance in patients with airway narrowing. Br J Dis Chest 1976; 70:58.
9. Campbell EJM, Howell JBL. The sensation of breathlessness. Br Med Bull 1963; 19:36–40.
10. Cherniack NS, Longobardo GS. Oxygen and carbon dioxide gas stores of the body. Physiol Rev 1970; 50:196–243.
11. Cherniack NS, et al. Conference Report: Workshop on assessment of respiratory control in humans. I. Methods of measurement of ventilatory responses to hypoxia and hypercapnia. Am Rev Respir Dis 1977; 115:117–119.
12. Cherniack NS, Altose MD. Respiratory responses to ventilatory loading. In: Hornbein TF, ed. Regulation of Breathing, II. New York: Marcel Dekker, 1981, 905–964.
13. Cherniack NS, Milic-Emili J. Mechanical aspects of loaded breathing. In: Roussos C, Macklem PT, eds. Thorax. New York: Marcel Dekker, 1985, 751–786.
14. Cherniack NS, Altose MD. Mechanisms of dyspnea. Clin Chest Med 1987; 8(2):207–214.
15. Cherniack RM. The oxygen consumption and efficiency of the respiratory muscles in health and emphysema. J Clin Invest 1959; 38:494–499.
16. Coleridge HM, Coleridge JCG. Reflexes evoked from the tracheobronchial tree and lungs. In: Cherniack NS, Widdicombe JG, eds. Handbook of Physiology; Vol. 2, Part II, Section 3, Control of Breathing. Bethesda: American Physiological Society, 1986, 395–431.
17. Collett PW, Brancatisano A, Engel LA. Changes in the glottic aperture during bronchial asthma. Am Rev Respir Dis 1983; 128:719–723.
18. Connelly JC, McCallister LW, Kaufman MP. Stimulation of the caudal ventrolateral medulla decreases total lung resistance in dogs. J Appl Physiol 1987; 63:912–917.
19. Dempsey JA, Forster HV. Mediation of ventilatory adaptations. Physiol Rev 1982; 62:262–346.
20. Dodd DS, Yarom J, Loring SH, Engel LA. O_2 cost of inspiratory and expiratory resistive breathing in humans. J Appl Physiol 1988; 65:2518–2523.
21. Easton PA, Slykerman LJ, Anthonisen NR. Ventilatory responses to sustained hypoxia in normal adults. J Appl Physiol 1986; 61:906–911.
22. Eldridge FL. Relationship between respiratory nerve and muscle activity and muscle force output. J Appl Physiol 1975; 39:567–574.
23. England SJ, Bartlett D Jr, Knuth SL. Comparison of human vocal cord movements during isocapnic hypoxia and hypercapnia. J Appl Physiol 1982; 53:81–86.
24. Euler, C von. Brain stem mechanisms for generation and control of breathing pattern. In: Cherniack NS, Widdicombe JG, eds. Handbook of Physiology; Vol. 2, Part II, Section 3, Control of Breathing. Bethesda: American Physiological Society, 1986, 1–67.
25. Eyzaguirre C, Zapata P. Perspectives in carotid body research. J Appl Physiol 1984; 57:931–957.
26. Gothe B, Cherniack NS, Bachand RT, et al. Long-term effects of almitrine bimesylate on oxygenation during wakefulness and sleep in chronic obstructive pulmonary disease. Am J Med 1988; 84:436–444.
27. Grassino A, Macklem PT. Respiratory muscle failure and ventilatory failure. Am J Med 1984; 35:625–647.
28. Haxhiu MA, Mitra J, van Lunteren E, et al. Hypoglossal and phrenic responses to cholinergic agents applied to ventral medullary surface. Am J Physiol 1984; 247:R939–R944.
29. Haxhiu MA, Deal EC Jr, Norcia MP, et al. Influence of the ventrolateral medulla on reflex tracheal constriction. J Appl Physiol 1986; 61:791–796.
30. Haxhiu MA, Mitra J, van Lunteren E, et al. Responses of hypoglossal and phrenic nerves to decreased respiratory drive in cats. Respiration 1986; 50:130–138.
31. Haxhiu MA, Deal EC Jr, Trivedi RD, et al. Tracheal and phrenic responses to neurotensin applied to the ventral medulla. Am J Physiol 255 (Reg Int Comp Physiol 24) 1988; R780–786.
32. Homma I, Obata T, Sibuya M, Uchida M. Gate mechanisms in breathlessness caused by chest wall vibration in humans. J Appl Physiol 1984; 56:8–11.
33. Kelsen SG, Fleegler B, Altose MD. The respiratory neuromuscular response to hypoxia, hypercapnia and obstruction to airflow in asthma. Am Rev Respir Dis 1979; 120:517–527.

34. Kim CS, Eldridge MA, Wanner A. Airway responsiveness to inhaled and intravenous carbachol in sheep, effect of airway muscles. J Appl Physiol 1988; 65:2744–2751.
35. Lahiri S, Mokashi A, Mulligan E, Nishino T. Comparison of aortic and carotid chemoreceptor responses to hypercapnia and hypoxia. J Appl Physiol 1981; 51:55–61.
36. Lahiri S, Edelman NH, Cherniack NS, Fishman AP. Role of carotid chemoreflex in respiratory acclimatization to hypoxemia in goat and sheep. Respir Physiol 1981; 46:367–382.
37. Lahiri S, Mulligan E, Nishino T, et al. Relative responses of aortic and carotid body chemoreceptors to carboxy hemoglobinemia. J Appl Physiol 1981; 50:580–586.
38. Loeschcke HH. Respiratory chemosensitivity in the medulla oblongata. Acta Neurobiol Exp 1973; 33(Suppl):97–112.
39. Long S, Duffin J. The neuronal determinants of respiratory rhythm. Prog Neurobiol 1986; 27:101–182.
40. Longobardo GS, Cherniack NS, Damokosh-Giordano A. Possible optimization of respiratory controller sensitivity. Ann Biomed Eng 1980; 8:143–158.
41. Lourenco RV, Miranda JM. Drive and performance of the ventilatory apparatus in chronic obstructive lung disease. N Engl J Med 1968; 279:53–59.
42. McAllen RM. Location of neurons with cardiovascular and respiratory function at the ventral surface of the cat's medulla. Neuroscience 1986; 18:43–49.
43. McFadden ER Jr, Kiser R, DeGroot WJ. Acute bronchial asthma: relation between clinical and physiological manifestations. N Engl J Med 1973; 288:221–225.
44. Mitchell RA, Herbert DA, Baker DG. Inspiratory rhythm in airway smooth muscle tone. J Appl Physiol 1985; 58:911–920.
45. Mitra J, Prabhakar NR, Pantaleo T, et al. Do structures in the region of the nucleus paragigantocellularis integrate and mediate ventilatory drive inputs. Soc Neurosci Abst 1986; 12:304.
46. Mitra J, Prabhakar NR, Overholt J, Cherniack NS. Respiratory and vasomotor effects of excitatory amino acid on ventral medullary surface. Brain Res Bull 1987; 15:681–684.
47. Mountain R, Zwillich C, Weil JV. Hypoventilation in obstructive lung disease, the role of familial factors. N Engl J Med 1978; 298:521–525.
48. Oliven A, Cherniack NS, Deal EC, Kelsen SG. The effects of acute bronchoconstriction on respiratory activity in patients with chronic obstructive pulmonary disease. Am Rev Respir Dis 1985; 131:236–241.
49. Orem J. Inspiratory neurons that are activated when inspiration is inhibited behaviorally. Neurosci Lett 1987; 83:282–286.
50. Paintal AS. Vagal sensory receptors and their reflex effects. Physiol Rev 1973; 53:159–227.
51. Pallot DJ. The mammalian carotid body. Adv Anat Embryol Cell Biol 1987; 102:1–90.
52. Potter EK, McCloskey DI. Excitation of carotid body chemoreceptors by neuropeptide Y. Respir Physiol 1987; 67:357–365.
53. Prabhakar NR, Mitra J, Lagercrantz H, et al. Substance P and hypoxic excitation of the carotid body. In: Henry J, ed. Substance P and Neurokinins. New York: Springer-Verlag, 1987, 84–87.
54. Rebuck AS, Slutsky AS. Control of breathing in diseases of the respiratory tract and lungs. In: Cherniack NS, Widdicombe JG, eds. Handbook of Physiology; Vol 2, Part II, Section 3, Control of Breathing. Bethesda: American Physiological Society, 1986, 771–792.
55. Richter DW. Generation and maintenance of the respiratory rhythm. J Exp Biol 1982; 100:93–108.
56. Rochester DF, Arora NS, Braun NMT, Goldberg SK. The respiratory muscles in chronic obstructive pulmonary diseases. Bull Eur Physiopathol Respir 1979; 18:951–975.
57. Roussos CS, Macklem PT. Diaphragmatic fatigue in man. J Appl Physiol 1977; 43:189–197.
58. Roussos C, Moxham J. Respiratory muscle fatigue. In: Roussos C, Macklem PT, eds. Thorax. New York: Marcel Dekker, 1985, 829–870.
59. Sant'Ambrogio G, Remmers JE. Reflex influences on the respiratory muscles of the chest wall. In: Roussos C, Macklem PT, eds. Thorax. New York: Marcel Dekker, 1985, 531–580.
60. Santiago TV, Edelman NH. Opioids and breathing. J Appl Physiol 1985; 59:1675–1685.
61. Saunders KB. Oscillations of arterial CO_2 tension in a respiratory model: some implications for the control of breathing in exercise. J Theor Biol 1980; 84:163–179.
62. Schlaefke ME. Central chemosensitivity, a respiratory drive. Rev Physiol Biochem Pharmacol 1981; 90:171–244.
63. Scardella AT, Parisi RA, Phair DK, et al. The role of endogenous opioids in the ventilatory response to acute flow resistive loads. Am Rev Respir Dis 1986; 133:26–31.
64. Shannon R. Reflexes from respiratory muscles and costovertebral joints. In: Cherniack NS, Widdicombe JG, eds. Handbook of Physiology; Vol 2, Part 1, Section 3, Control of Breathing. Bethesda: American Physiological Society, 1986, 431–448.
65. Sharp JT, Druz WS, Moisan T, et al. Postural relief of dyspnea in severe chronic obstructive pulmonary disease. Am Rev Respir Dis 1980; 122:201–211.
66. Simon PM, Pope A, Lahive K, et al. Naloxone does not alter response to hypercapnia or resistive loading in chronic obstructive pulmonary disease. Am Rev Respir Dis 1989; 139:134–138.
67. Skatrud JB, Dempsey JA. Relative effectiveness of acetazolamide and medroxyprogesterone acetate in the correction of chronic CO_2 retention. Am Rev Respir Dis 1983; 127:405–412.
68. Sorli J, Grassino A, Lorange G, Milic-Emili J. Control of breathing in patients with chronic obstructive lung disease. Clin Sci Mol Med 1978; 54:295–304.
69. Strohl KP, Cherniack NS, Gothe B. Physiologic basis of therapy for sleep apnea. Am Rev Respir Dis 1986; 134:791–802.
70. Thomson RL, Stocker CL, Ross JC. The efficacy of purse-lips breathing in patients with chronic obstructive pulmonary disease. Am Rev Respir Dis 1966; 93:100–106.
71. van Lunteren E, Arnold JS, Cherniack NS. Vagal influences on parasternal intercostal muscle inspiratory shortening during hypercapnia and airway occlusion. Respir Physiol 1988; 71:201–212.
72. Whipp BJ. Ventilatory control during exercise. Annu Rev Physiol 1984; 45:393–415.

Chapter 15

EFFECTS OF COPD ON BEHAVIORAL CONTROL OF BREATHING

Tatsuya Chonan **Neil S. Cherniack** **Murray D. Altose**

IMPORTANCE OF DYSPNEA AS A SYMPTOM IN PATIENTS WITH COPD

Breathing usually occurs effortlessly without conscious awareness. Dyspnea, or the sense of difficulty in breathing, is one of the major symptoms in patients with COPD and is often their chief complaint. Dyspnea is not a specific symptom of COPD, but almost all patients with COPD have difficulty breathing, which limits activity and impairs quality of life. Many patients who have dyspnea may adopt breathing patterns that minimize its occurrence.[20, 23] When pulmonary dysfunction is mild or moderate, difficulty in breathing may be overlooked by both physicians and the patients themselves unless the patients perform moderate to heavy exercise. However, it becomes obvious as pulmonary function deteriorates further owing to such factors as smoking, aging, and respiratory tract infection, and once it becomes symptomatic, it is difficult to eliminate or reduce unless pulmonary function, respiratory muscle performance, or physical condition is improved.[3, 21]

Dyspnea, in a general sense, results when disease or an experimental intervention, such as the application of resistance to the mouth, impedes the movement of the respiratory muscles and there is perception of effort associated with breathing. Like other sensations, this awareness of increased effort may be associated with qualities such as a sense of unpleasantness. In contrast, difficulty in breathing experienced by habitual runners may not be perceived by them as being unpleasant. Thus, dyspnea can differ both in its intensity and in its quality.

METHODS OF EVALUATING RESPIRATORY SENSATIONS AND DYSPNEA

The ability to detect impediments to breathing has been studied extensively,[7, 14, 15, 52, 81] but it was not until recently that respiratory sensations and dyspnea were assessed directly. In 1970, Bakers and Tenney[6] first applied psychophysical techniques to the quantitative measurement of the intensity of respiratory sensations. Now several scales are used to evaluate the magnitude of respiratory sensations and dyspnea.

In healthy subjects the ability to detect changes in external loads, e.g., resistances, elastances added to a breathing circuit, follows Weber's law, i.e., there is a constant relationship between the just-noticeable change in a load (ΔR) and the basal load (R); hence, $\Delta R/R$ is constant.[52] It is to be expected that the size of the added resistance needed to evoke a change in perception will be greater in patients with COPD than in healthy subjects, because baseline airway resistance is greater in the patients. However, it has been reported that the just-noticeable difference in airflow resistance, even expressed as a percentage of the baseline resistance, is higher in patients than in healthy individuals,[40] which suggests an impairment of the patients' ability to detect added loads.

Magnitude Estimation and Production

Two psychophysical techniques, magnitude estimation and magnitude production, have been established to quantify the sensations produced by respiratory maneuvers. In the magnitude estimation method, the subject is required to assign numbers proportional to the apparent magnitude of the sensations produced by a series of stimuli.[77] Magnitude production is the inverse of the magnitude estimation. The subject is given numerical values and is required to produce the corresponding stimuli.

According to Stevens' power law, there is a power function relationship between the stimulus (ϕ) and the magnitude of sensation (ψ), i.e., $\psi = K \cdot \phi^{\beta}$ where β is the exponent of the power function and K is a constant.[78] It predicts that the ratio of sensation change is proportional to the ratio of stimulus change. This power law has been reported to be obeyed by many sensory modalities, including vision, hearing, pain, and perceived magnitude of added loads,[13, 61, 77] although the exponent is different among the sensory modalities. It has been reported that results obtained with direct ratio scales, such as open magnitude scaling, generally fit Stevens' power law better than do category scales.[79]

Visual Analog Scales

Visual analog scales (VAS) have been used to assess sensory intensity of such sensations as pain and dyspnea.[2, 22, 68, 76] The VAS usually consists of a line 10 to 15 cm in length, the two ends of which are designated by adjectives, such as "none at all" at one end and "most intense imaginable" at the other.[22] These adjectives help the subject rate the sensory intensity consistently over a certain period of time.[1, 76] A major advantage of the VAS is that it allows intersubject comparisons to be made more easily than with open magnitude scales. Although the VAS is basically a category scale, it has been reported to have ratio properties, i.e., there is a fixed proportional relationship between the scale ratings and the perceived sensation.[68]

TABLE 15–1. 10-point Borg Category Scale

0	Nothing at all
0.5	Very, very slight (just noticeable)
1	Very slight
2	Slight
3	Moderate
4	Somewhat severe
5	Severe
6	
7	Very severe
8	
9	Very, very severe (almost maximal)
10	Maximal

Borg Scales

The Borg category scale was originally developed to assess ratings of perceived exertion. It was a 21-grade scale with verbal anchors.[9] The Borg scale was later reconstructed by Borg[10] to increase its linearity with exercise intensity. The scale values of the modified Borg scale range from 6 to 20 where the numbers are intended to denote heart rate ranging from 60 to 200 beats per minute. Descriptive terms ranging from "very, very light" to "very, very hard" were anchored to each of the odd numbers and helped subjects rate their sensory intensity in a relatively absolute fashion. Although this modified scale could be used conveniently to examine direction of changes in perceptual intensity, it lacked ratio properties.

The latest Borg scale, which has a number range from 0 to 10, was developed to reduce category effects and obtain ratio properties (Table 15–1).[11] In using this scale, the subjects are allowed to employ decimals and also to go beyond 10 if necessary.

The Borg scales have been applied to evaluate the intensity of respiratory sensations in dyspnea both in healthy subjects[22, 48] and in patients with COPD.[74] The Borg scales, like visual analog scales, have the advantage that they allow comparison to be made easily among different subjects.

Clinical Dyspnea Ratings

Several clinical scales have been employed to evaluate the sensation of dyspnea. These clinical dyspnea scales focus on when breathlessness occurs during different levels of daily activities. It has been reported that these clinical methods are interrelated and correlate with pulmonary function.[51] Among these, the Medical Research Council (MRC) scale has been used by many investigators and clinicians (Table 15–2).[57]

These clinical methods are convenient in approximately evaluating the impact of dyspnea on the patient's activity, but they may not be sufficiently precise to assess the patient's perceptual experience over time, to investigate the mechanisms of dyspnea, or to assess the effect of treatment. For these purposes, the direct scaling techniques described earlier are more useful.

TABLE 15–2. Modified Medical Research Council Dyspnea Scale

GRADE	
0	Not troubled with breathlessness except with strenuous exercise
1	Troubled by shortness of breath when hurrying on the level or walking up a slight hill
2	Walks slower than people of the same age on the level because of breathlessness or has to stop for breath when walking at own pace on the level
3	Stops for breath after walking about 100 yards or after a few minutes on the level
4	Too breathless to leave the house or breathless when dressing or undressing

Many patients with pulmonary diseases have decreased exercise capacity because of dyspnea on exertion. Therefore, one indirect method of evaluating a patient's dyspnea is to measure his or her exercise capacity. The incremental exercise test on a treadmill or cycle ergometer is used widely to assess exercise performance. The 12-minute walking distance (TMD) test is a simple method to evaluate exercise performance and has been reported to correlate with the maximum oxygen consumption in an incremental exercise test.[55] One problem in using exercise capacity as an index of dyspnea is that exercise performance can be limited by many factors other than the dyspnea, such as leg discomfort, cardiac function, physical conditioning, and motivation.

ATTEMPTS TO SIMULATE AIRWAY OBSTRUCTION AND EVALUATE EFFECTS ON DYSPNEA

Airway obstruction probably plays a central role in the genesis of breathlessness in patients with COPD because the exercise capacity of patients with COPD is limited owing to dyspnea and is correlated with the degree of airway obstruction.[23, 27] Airway obstruction can be simulated in healthy subjects by imposing resistive loads to breathing either externally or internally by the administration of bronchoconstrictive drugs.

External Loads

Burdon and colleagues,[13] using the magnitude estimation method, reported that the perceived magnitude of an externally added inspiratory resistance increased with the size of the load and as the underlying level of ventilatory drive increased. Altose and associates[3] reported that imposition of an external resistive load to inspiration resulted in an increase in the degree of breathlessness at any given level of ventilation during exercise in healthy subjects. Futhermore, they found that the intensity of dyspnea was related to the level of respiratory efferent activity as measured by the mouth occlusion pressure during progressive treadmill exercise both with and without inspiratory resistive loads. This finding is illustrated in Figure 15–1. Expiratory resistive loading as well as inspiratory loading causes dyspnea in proportion to the expiratory motor output.[25]

These findings are consistent with the hypothesis that dyspnea is caused by increased effort in breathing, which is determined by respiratory motor output. The size of the motor command to the respiratory muscles has been postulated to be the major factor responsible for dyspnea.[48] Are there any differences in the intensity of dyspnea between patients with COPD and healthy subjects if the respiratory motor output is the same? Altose[3] observed that the intensity of dyspnea was not different between the two groups at a given occlusion pressure corrected for maximum inspiratory muscle strength.

Bronchoconstriction

Kelsen and colleagues[45] reported that in normal subjects the ventilatory responses to bronchoconstriction were different from those to externally added resistive loads. They also

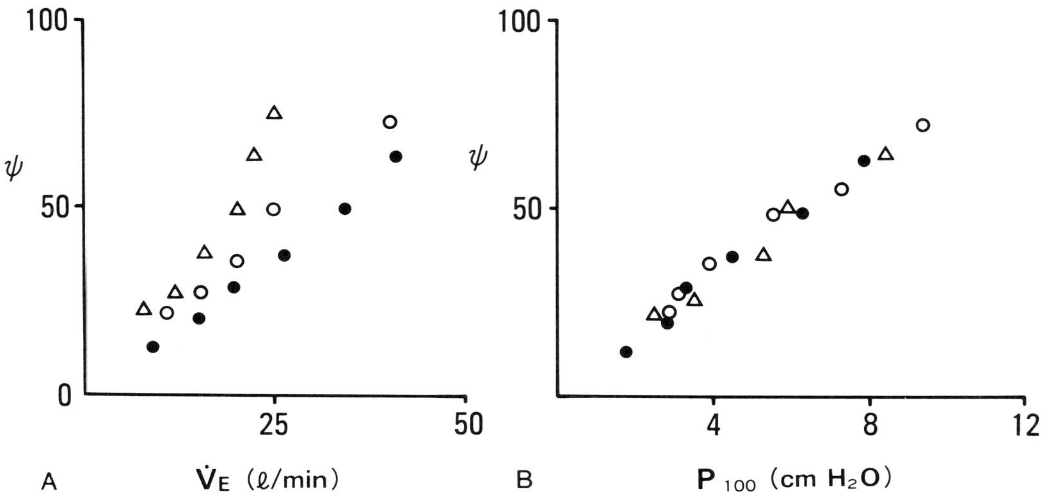

Figure 15–1. Relationship between (*A*) minute ventilation ($\dot{V}_E$) and the intensity of the sensation of difficulty in breathing (ψ), and (*B*) mouth occlusion pressure (P_{100}) and ψ, in a healthy subject during incremental exercise on a bicycle ergometer with and without external inspiratory resistive loads. Closed circles, control data without loads; open circles, data with a small inspiratory resistance (5 cm H_2O/L/seconds); triangles, data with a large inspiratory resistance (55 cm H_2O/L/sec). The intensity of dyspnea was rated using an open magnitude scale. Although the intensity of dyspnea at a given level of ventilation rises with the increase in load, the dyspnea intensity at a given respiratory neuromuscular output measured as P_{100} is unchanged by loading.

observed that the sense of effort was greater with bronchospasm than with external loading, which produced the same level of resistance. These results suggest that, at a given level of resistance to breathe, mechanoreceptors, probably in the airways, which are supplied by the vagus nerves, respond differently depending on the site of increased resistance and contribute to generation of the sensation of dyspnea. Consistent with this hypothesis, Taguchi and colleagues[80] reported that airway anesthesia decreased dyspnea induced by histamine at a given level of airway resistance but did not affect dyspneic sensations during external loading. Kikuchi and associates[46] reported that inhaled prostaglandin E_2 (PGE_2), which is known to stimulate airway irritant receptors and C fibers,[28] increased the magnitude of dyspnea without changing airway resistance and lung volume at a given intensity of exercise in healthy subjects.

Respiratory loads, external or internal, increase the force output of the respiratory muscles needed to achieve a constant level of ventilation and hence increase the sense of effort. Stimulation of airway receptors appears to augment the sensation of dyspnea.

SENSORY EFFECTS OF INCREASED BREATHING

Attempts have been made to stimulate ventilation through various mechanisms and evaluate the effect on perception and dyspnea. One major issue here is whether the intensity and quality of respiratory sensations vary depending on the nature of the stimulus.

Burdon and colleagues[13] reported that perceived magnitude of externally added loads increased with inspiratory muscle force, and at a given level of respiratory motor output was the same during exercise, hypercapnia, and hypoxia.

Stark and colleagues[76] reported that, in healthy subjects, hypercapnia produced by rebreathing caused greater breathlessness in relation to ventilation than did exercise. Chonan and colleagues[24] also compared the sensation of dyspnea during progressive hypercapnia with that during incremental exercise under conditions in which the time course of the increase in ventilation was the same. They found that the intensity of dyspnea grew linearly with increases in ventilation both in hypercapnia and exercise, but the change in dyspnea intensity produced by a given change in ventilation was significantly greater during hypercapnia than during exercise. These investigators also reported that rebreathing produced more dyspnea than did isocapnic voluntary hyperventilation at a given increase in ventilation (Fig. 15–2). These results suggest that dyspnea is accentuated by higher levels of CO_2 even when levels of ventilation are similar. It is not clear why hypercapnia causes greater dyspnea than does an isocapnic increase in ventilation. One explanation would be that dyspnea is modulated by afferent inputs from chemoreceptors.

Respiratory sensations may also be qualitatively different during hypercapnia as opposed to exercise.[76] During exercise, an increase in ventilation closely approximates the greater metabolic demand, and the acid-base status of the arterial blood with moderate exercise is maintained within the normal range, whereas during CO_2 breathing, acidity of the arterial blood increases acutely. Hypercapnia introduces an insatiable demand to breathe, which seems to be sensed as an additional discomfort.

Reported data are inconsistent on whether the intensity of dyspnea is different or not between exercise and isocapnic voluntary hyperventilation (IVH). Altose and associates[4] reported that both exercise and IVH caused a similar intensity of breathlessness at a given level of ventilation or occlusion pressure in healthy subjects. Chonan and colleagues[24] also observed that dyspnea was accentuated with ventilation increases both during exercise and IVH and that the change in the intensity of dyspnea induced by a given increase in ventilation was not significantly different between exercise and IVH.

In comparison, Lane and colleagues[50] reported that in healthy subjects exercise caused a greater increase in breathlessness than did IVH. Freedman and associates[35] also reported that voluntary copying of breathing pattern, which was measured during exercise, diminished or abolished breathlessness in patients with chronic airflow limitation. The differences between the data of the two groups may be explained by differences in the quality of sensations measured. It is possible that the sense of effort was underestimated in the latter group of experiments because in this group the experimenters instructed their subjects to avoid rating their awareness that

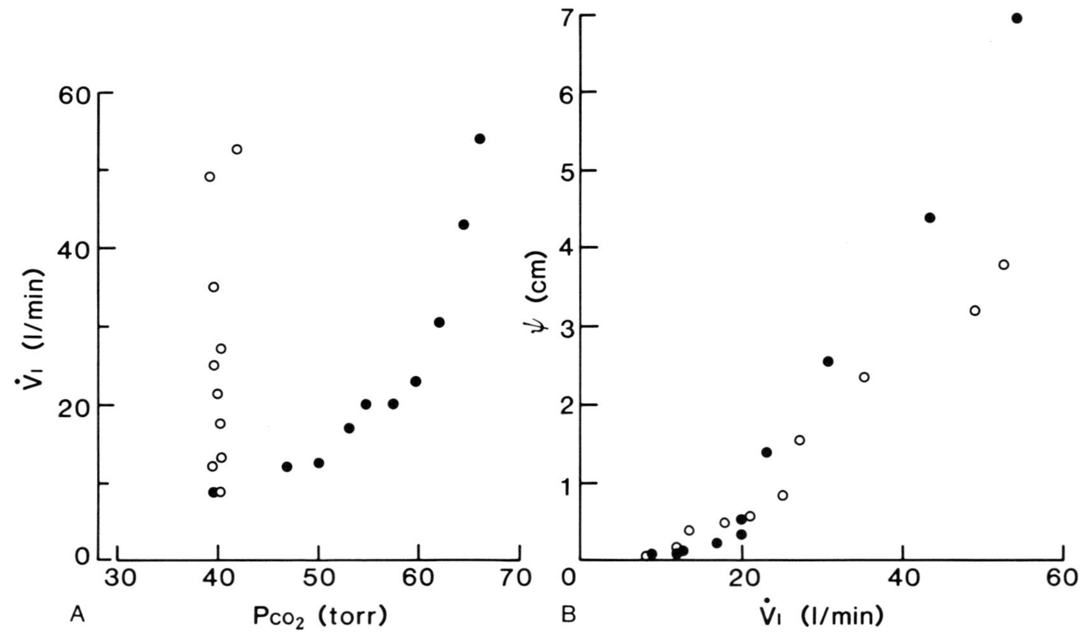

Figure 15–2. ***A,*** **Relationship between end-tidal carbon dioxide partial pressure (P_{CO_2}) and minute ventilation ($\dot{V}_I$) during progressive hypercapnia (closed circle) and during isocapnic voluntary hyperpnea (open circle) in one subject.** ***B,*** **Relationship between minute ventilation and intensity of the sensation of difficulty in breathing (ψ) during progressive hypercapnia (closed circle) and isocapnic voluntary hyperpnea (open circle) in the same subject. The intensity of dyspnea was rated using visual analog scales. The dyspnea intensity at a given level of ventilation is greater during hypercapnia than isocapnic hyperpnea, and the difference in sensory intensity grows with the widening of the difference in carbon dioxide partial pressure (P_{CO_2}) between hypercapnic and isocapnic trials. (Reproduced with permission from Chonan T, et al. J Appl Physiol 1990; 68:2100–2106.)**

breathing had merely increased, whereas in the former group the subjects were instructed to rate their sensation of difficulty in breathing, whether it was distressing or not.

EFFECTS OF RESTRAINING BREATHING

Breath-holding is an extreme example of restrained breathing. Fowler[34] has shown that respiratory distress caused by breath-holding can be relieved temporarily by a short period of rebreathing despite a progressive reduction in arterial oxygen saturation and a rise in alveolar CO_2 tension. It has also been reported that the highest tolerable P_{CO_2} is greater during rebreathing as compared with breath-holding[42, 49] and greater at high compared with low levels of ventilation during voluntarily controlled breathing.[69]

Chonan and colleagues[22] examined the effects of voluntary constraining thoracic displacement during hyperoxic hypercapnia on the sensation of dyspnea. Two types of experiments were carried out in healthy subjects. In the first set of experiments, P_{CO_2} was increased progressively while ventilation was held constant; in the second set of experiments, ventilation was reduced while P_{CO_2} was maintained at a constant level. In both experiments dyspnea was accentuated at a given level of P_{CO_2} when the ventilation was reduced below the spontaneously adopted level. These results suggest that sensory feedback originating from mechanoreceptors in the lung, chest wall, or both, as a result of thoracic displacement decreases dyspnea by acting either on brainstem respiratory neurons or on higher brain centers, or both. The accentuation of dyspnea produced by restraining breathing may be explained by a loss of this inhibitory feedback.

POSSIBLE ORIGIN OF SENSATIONS INVOLVED IN DYSPNEA

Lung and Airway Receptors

Chaudhary and Burki[18, 19] examined the effects of airway anesthesia on the ability to detect added inspiratory resistive or elastic loads in healthy individuals. They reported that airway anesthesia produced by lidocaine inhalation did not significantly change the threshold for load detection or the Weber fraction.

Guz and coworkers[41] reported that bilateral blockade of the vagus and glossopharyngeal nerves with locally injected lidocaine prolonged maximum breath-holding time with alleviation of the associated distress, although the detection of added loads to the airway was unaffected. Davies and colleagues[30] reported an extreme exertional dyspnea that appeared in a patient with unilateral pulmonary venous obstruction. They observed a marked relief of the dyspnea with the alteration of breathing pattern after vagotomy. These data suggest the importance of lung and airway vagal receptors in mediating respiratory sensations. However, among the various airway receptors each type seems to play a different role. Stimulation of pulmonary stretch receptors by lung inflation may have an inhibitory effect on the sensation of dyspnea because a reduction in thoracic displacement intensifies dyspnea, as discussed in the previous section. In comparison, stimulation of irritant receptors or C fibers, or both, appears to augment dyspnea because it is accentuated by inhalation of histamine or PGE_2.[46, 80]

Muscle Receptors

Two types of mechanoreceptors in respiratory muscles that influence respiratory control, muscle spindle endings, which are considered to be length receptors, and tendon organs, which are force receptors,[72] may also affect the occurrence of dyspnea. Mechanoreceptors in respiratory muscles may have important roles in shaping respiratory sensations either by acting on the medullary respiratory neurons or through direct projection to the cerebral cortex. Bolser and coworkers[8] have reported that intercostal tendon organs and not muscle spindle endings have an inhibitory effect on medullary inspiratory activity.

Davenport and colleagues[29] have reported that evoked potentials can be recorded in the somatosensory region of the cortex by inspiratory occlusion in conscious humans. Gandevia and Macefield[39] have observed that microstimulation of intercostal muscles can evoke cortical potentials in conscious humans. These data suggest that nerve fibers from intramuscular receptors project to the cerebral cortex. However, Eisele and associates[32] observed that spinal anesthesia up to T1 did not affect the ability to detect added elastic and resistive loads or the sensation and duration of breath-holding.

Newsom-Davis[59] reported that detection of added inspiratory resistance was impaired in patients with upper spinal cord lesions. Afferents from muscular receptors in the diaphragm may be important in mediating respiratory sensations. Consistent with this idea are the observations that muscle paralysis[16] or phrenic nerve blockade[60] prolong breath-holding duration and eliminate its distressing effects. These reports are not in keeping with the findings that voluntary inhibition of breathing augments the sensation of dyspnea[22] and that unpleasant sensation during breath-holding is relieved by static inspiratory efforts against a closed airway that simply increase muscle tension.[70]

Chest wall vibration stimulates muscle spindle endings and has been used to investigate the mechanisms of dyspnea.[72] Homma and colleagues[43] reported that vibration out of phase with the respiratory cycle of the inspiratory and expiratory intercostal muscles induced breathlessness in healthy individuals. Altose and coworkers[5] reported that in-phase upper chest wall vibration during inspiration and lower chest wall vibration during expiration reduced the dyspnea during constrained breathing but had no effect on dyspnea during hyperpnea, suggesting that chest wall afferents stimulated by vibration play a role in the accentuation of dyspnea during constrained breathing.

Corollary Inputs of Central Motor Command

In limb skeletal muscles it has been reported that humans can distinguish sense of effort from that of tension, which is sensed by peripheral muscle receptors.[53, 54, 71] It has been hypothesized that a sense of effort or perceived motor command is mainly generated centrally by a corollary discharge or efferent copy from motor to sensory centers.[53, 54] For example, perceived heaviness seems to depend on the motor output to the contracting muscles because weights seem heavier when lifted by muscles weakened by paralysis and fatigue.[36, 37]

Campbell and colleagues[17] reported that during curarization load detection ability was not impaired, but the size of inspiratory resistive load was overestimated. Gandevia and coworkers[38] also reported that healthy subjects could distinguish between a sense of motor command and a sense of achieved tension during loaded breathing and that inspiratory loads were overestimated when the respiratory muscles were fatigued. The findings suggest that there is similarity in sensory mechanisms in respiratory and peripheral muscles; in both, the sense of tension and effort are separable, and the size of load is judged through the sense of effort.

Killian and colleagues[48] examined the effects of increased lung volume and hence the weakening of inspiratory muscles on the respiratory sensations during external elastic loading. They found that both sensations of breathlessness and effort became greater, but that the perceived tension was unchanged at a given inspiratory pressure when the lung volume was increased. They have suggested that sensations of breathlessness and effort are psychophysically the same. Sense of effort appears to be one major component of dyspnea and would explain the dyspnea in COPD in which breathing efforts are frequently greater because of the lung disease and secondary impairment of muscle function. Afferent inputs from mechanoreceptors in the airway and respiratory muscles, and from chemoreceptors, may evoke an additional sense of discomfort as discussed.

POSSIBLE EFFECTS OF RESPIRATORY SENSATIONS ON BREATHING

In the previous sections we have described that an increase in breathing produces sense of effort and that restraining breathing augments dyspnea at a constant level of P_{CO_2}. Therefore, it is possible that the level of breathing is controlled not only automatically but also in part behaviorally to minimize respiratory sensations in awake humans. It may also be possible that breathing pattern is adjusted in part to minimize respiratory sensations, because breathing patterns can affect respiratory sensations.[47]

Behavioral control of breathing is well established[12, 31, 33, 34, 47, 58, 63, 65, 66, 73] and can be exerted by cortical action over anatomic pathways separate from those used by medullary neurons.

Killian and coworkers[47] showed that the sense of effort associated with breathing increased as follows:

$$\psi = P^{1.3} \times ti^{0.56}$$

where P = pressure developed at the airway, and ti = inspiratory time. The equation shows that pressure developed at the mouth is the major factor determining sense of effort. Because mouth pressure decreases as tidal volume is reduced, at the same level of minute ventilation, the sense of effort can be minimized by breathing rapidly and shallowly.

Chonan and coworkers[22, 26] examined the effects of voluntary changes in the level and pattern of breathing on the sensation of dyspnea at a constant level of hypercapnia. They found that during steady-state hypercapnia at P_{CO_2} 50 torr dyspnea intensified when ventilation was either voluntarily raised or lowered from the spontaneously adopted level. At a constant level of minute ventilation dyspnea was augmented when the breathing frequency was either voluntarily increased or decreased, with reciprocal changes in tidal volume, from the spontaneously adopted level (Fig. 15–3). These results indicate that dyspnea is intensified when the level or pattern of breathing is voluntarily changed from the spontaneously adopted range. This finding is consistent with the possibility that breathing responses to changes in chemical drive may be regulated in part to minimize sensations of respiratory effort and discomfort.

It has been reported that breathing patterns may be regulated to minimize the work of breathing or force output.[56, 64] Poon[67] has proposed a respiratory control model in which it is hypothesized that ventilation is controlled to minimize a total cost consisting of chemical stimulation and the work of breathing. The hypothetic total cost proposed by Poon could be the sensation of dyspnea.

The need to minimize dyspnea may be particularly important in patients with COPD, and respiratory sensation may be especially important in determining patterns and levels of ventilation.

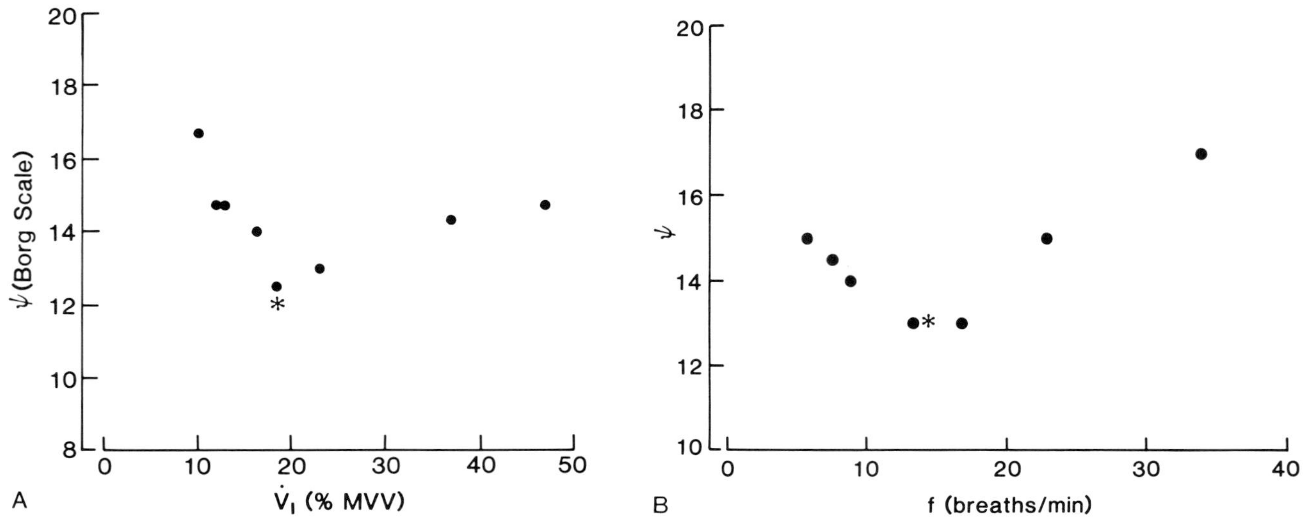

Figure 15–3. ***A,*** **Effects of voluntary changes in minute ventilation ($\dot{V}_I$), expressed as percent of maximum voluntary ventilation (MVV) on the intensity of dyspnea (ψ) in a single subject. Asterisk indicates spontaneous breathing.** ***B,*** **Effects of voluntary changes in breathing frequency (f) on the intensity of dyspnea (ψ) at a constant steady state carbon dioxide partial pressure (P_{CO_2}) of 50 torr, in a single subject. Minute ventilation was maintained at a spontaneous level. Asterisk indicates spontaneous breathing. The intensity of dyspnea was rated using a modified Borg scale. (Reproduced with permission from Chonan T, et al. J Appl Physiol 1990 [in press].)**

Sorli and colleagues,[75] in a study of patients with COPD, showed that hypercapnic patients differed from eucapnic patients by breathing with smaller tidal volumes, and the smaller tidal volumes decreased alveolar ventilation. The difference in tidal volumes spontaneously adopted in the two groups could not be explained by the difference in lung mechanics or by ventilatory responses to CO_2. However, a requirement to minimize dyspnea in the hypercapnic patients could have accounted for the smaller tidal volume.

The role of sensation in the response of patients with COPD to resistive loads was examined by Oliven and coworkers.[62] Patients with COPD were required to breathe on resistive loads for at least 10 minutes. About half of the group studied increased P_{CO_2} levels while on the load whereas the other did not. The exponent for magnitude production of respiratory force was also determined in the same patient group. There was a significant positive correlation between the magnitude of the exponent and the increase in P_{CO_2} while on the load. In addition, tidal volume on the load was inversely related to P_{CO_2} changes. This finding suggests that patients with COPD who were sensitive to changes in respiratory force (high exponent) might have chosen to breathe with smaller tidal volumes when breathing was further impeded by respiratory loading even at the expense of increases in P_{CO_2}. These findings are consistent with the idea that minimization of tidal volume to reduce dyspnea and to maintain P_{CO_2} are important competing priorities in the patients with COPD.

REFERENCES

1. Adams L, Chronos N, Lane R, Guz A. The measurement of breathlessness induced in normal subjects: validity of two scaling techniques. Clin Sci 1985; 69:7–16.
2. Adams L, Lane R, Shea SA, et al. Breathlessness during different forms of ventilatory stimulation: a study of mechanisms in normal subjects and respiratory patients. Clin Sci 1985; 69:663–672.
3. Altose MD. Assessment and management of breathlessness. Chest 1985; 88:77S–83S.
4. Altose MD, Mulholland MB, Hudgel DW. Comparison of the intensity of breathlessness during exercise and voluntary hyperventilation [abstract]. Fed Proc 1986; 45:159.
5. Altose MD, Syed I, Shoos L. Effects of chest wall vibration on the intensity of dyspnea during constrained breathing [abstract]. XXXI International Congress of Physiological Sciences, 1989, 388.
6. Bakers JHCM, Tenney SM. The perception of some sensations associated with breathing. Respir Physiol 1970; 10:85–92.
7. Bennett ED, Jayson MIV, Rubenstein D, Campbell EJM. The ability of man to detect added non-elastic loads to breathing. Clin Sci 1962; 23:155–162.
8. Bolser DC, Lindsey BG, Shannon R. Medullary inspiratory activity: influence of intercostal tendon organs and muscle spindle endings. J Appl Physiol 1987; 62:1046–1056.
9. Borg GAV. Physical Performance and Perceived Exertion. Lund, Sweden: Gleerup, 1962, 1–63.
10. Borg GAV. Perceived exertion as an indicator of somatic stress. Scand J Rehab Med 1970; 2:92–98.
11. Borg GAV. Psychophysical bases of perceived exertion. Med Sci Sports Exer 1982; 14:377–381.
12. Bunn JC, Mead J. Control of ventilation during speech. J Appl Physiol 1971; 31:870–872.
13. Burdon JGW, Killian KJ, Campbell EJM. Effect of ventilatory drive on the perceived magnitude of added loads to breathing. J Appl Physiol 1982; 53:901–907.
14. Burki NK. Effects of added inspiratory loads on load detection thresholds. J Appl Physiol 1981; 50:162–164.
15. Campbell EJM, Freedman S, Smith PS, Taylor ME. The ability of man to detect added elastic loads to breathing. Clin Sci 1961; 20:223–231.
16. Campbell EJM, Godfrey S, Clark TJH, et al. The effect of muscular paralysis induced by tubocurarine on the duration and sensation of breath-holding during hypercapnia. Clin Sci 1969; 36:323–328.
17. Campbell EJM, Gandevia SC, Killian KJ, et al. Changes in the perception of inspiratory resistive loads during partial curarization. J Physiol (Lond) 1980; 309:93–100.
18. Chaudhary BA, Burki NK. Effects of airway anesthesia on the ability to detect added inspiratory resistive loads. Clin Sci Mol Med 1978; 54:621–626.
19. Chaudhary BA, Burki NK. The effects of airway anesthesia on detection of added inspiratory elastic loads. Am Rev Respir Dis 1980; 122:635–639.
20. Cherniack NS. Potential role of optimization and respiratory instability. In: Euler C von, Lagercrantz H, eds. Neurobiology of the Control of Breathing. New York: Raven Press, 1986, 45–50.
21. Cherniack NS. Dyspnea. In: Murray JF, Nadel JA, eds. Textbook of Respiratory Medicine. Philadelphia: WB Saunders Company, 1988, 389–396.
22. Chonan T, Mulholland MB, Cherniack NS, Altose MD. Effects of voluntary constraining of thoracic displacement during hypercapnia. J Appl Physiol 1987; 63:1822–1828.

23. Chonan T, Hida W, Kikuchi Y, et al. Role of CO_2 responsiveness and breathing efficiency in determining exercise capacity of patients with chronic airway obstruction. Am Rev Respir Dis 1988; 138:1488–1493.
24. Chonan T, Mulholland MB, Leitner J, et al. Sensation of dyspnea during hypercapnia, exercise and voluntary hyperventilation. J Appl Physiol 1990; 68:2100–2106.
25. Chonan T, Altose MD, Cherniack NS. Effects of expiratory resistive loading on the sensation of dyspnea. J Appl Physiol 1990; 69:91–95.
26. Chonan T, Mulholland MB, Altose MD, Cherniack NS. Effects of changes in level and pattern of breathing on the sensation of dyspnea. J Appl Physiol 1990 (in press).
27. Clark TJH, Freedman S, Campbell EJM, Winn RR. The ventilatory capacity of patients with chronic airways obstruction. Clin Sci 1969; 36:307–316.
28. Coleridge HM, Coleridge JCG, Ginzel KH, et al. Stimulation of "irritant" receptors and afferent C fibers in the lungs by prostaglandins. Nature 1976; 264:451–453.
29. Davenport PW, Friedman WA, Thompson FJ, Franzen O. Respiratory-related cortical potentials evoked by inspiratory occlusion in humans. J Appl Physiol 1986; 60:1843–1848.
30. Davies SF, McQuaid KR, Iber C, et al. Extreme dyspnea from unilateral pulmonary venous obstruction. Am Rev Respir Dis 1987; 136:184–188.
31. Dudley DL, Pitts-Poarch AR. Psychophysiologic aspects of respiratory control. Clin Chest Med 1980; 1:131–143.
32. Eisele J, Trenchard D, Burki N, Guz A. The effect of chest wall block on respiratory sensation and control in man. Clin Sci 1968; 35:23–33.
33. Euler C von. Some aspects of speech breathing physiology. In: Grillner S, Lindblom B, Lubker J, Persson A, eds. Speech Motor Control. Oxford: Pergamon Press, 1982, 95–103.
34. Fowler WS. Breaking point of breath holding. J Appl Physiol 1954; 6:539–545.
35. Freedman S, Lane R, Guz A. Breathlessness and respiratory mechanics during reflex or voluntary hyperventilation in patients with chronic airflow limitation. Clin Sci 1987; 73:311–318.
36. Gandevia SC, McCloskey DI. Sensation of heaviness. Brain 1977; 100:345–354.
37. Gandevia SC, McCloskey DI. Interpretation of perceived motor commands by reference to afferent signals. J Physiol (Lond) 1978; 283:493–499.
38. Gandevia SC, Killian K, Campbell EJM. The effect of respiratory muscle fatigue on respiratory sensations. Clin Sci 1981; 60:463–466.
39. Gandevia SC, Macefield G. Projection of low-threshold afferents from human intercostal muscles to the cerebral cortex. Respir Physiol 1989; 77:203–214.
40. Gottfried SB, Altose MD, Kelsen SG, Cherniack NS. Perception of changes in airflow resistance in obstructive pulmonary disorders. Am Rev Respir Dis 1981; 124:566–570.
41. Guz A, Noble MIM, Widdicombe JG, et al. The role of vagal and glossopharyngeal afferent nerves in respiratory sensation, control of breathing and arterial pressure regulation in conscious man. Clin Sci 1966; 30:161–170.
42. Hill L, Flack M. The effect of excess of carbon dioxide and of want of oxygen upon the respiration and circulation. J Physiol (Lond) 1908; 37:77–111.
43. Homma I, Obata T, Sibuya M, Uchida M. Gate mechanism in breathlessness caused by chest wall vibration in humans. J Appl Physiol 1984; 56:8–11.
44. Hudgel DW, Kinsman RA. Interaction among behavioral style, ventilatory drive, and load recognition. Am Rev Respir Dis 1983; 128:246–248.
45. Kelsen SG, Prestel TF, Cherniack NS, et al. Comparison of the respiratory responses to external resistive loading and bronchoconstriction. J Clin Invest 1981; 67:1761–1768.
46. Kikuchi Y, Taguchi O, Hida W, et al. Effects of PGE_2 inhalation on dyspnea during exercise [abstract]. XXXI International Congress of Physiological Sciences, 1989, 73.
47. Killian KJ, Bucens DD, Campbell EJM. Effect of breathing patterns on the perceived magnitude of added loads to breathing. J Appl Physiol 1982; 52:578–584.
48. Killian KJ, Gandevia SC, Summers E, Campbell EJM. Effect of increased lung volume on perception of breathlessness, effort, and tension. J Appl Physiol 1984; 57:681–691.
49. Kobayasi S, Sasaki C. Breaking point of breath holding and tolerance time in rebreathing. Jpn J Physiol 1967; 17:43–56.
50. Lane R, Cockcroft A, Guz A. The effect of voluntary isocapnic hyperventilation on breathlessness during exercise in normals [abstract]. Clin Sci 1987; 72:37P.
51. Mahler DA, Rosiello RA, Harver A, et al. Comparison of clinical dyspnea ratings and psychophysical measurements of respiratory sensation in obstructive airway disease. Am Rev Respir Dis 1987; 135:1229–1233.
52. Mahutte CK, Campbell EJM, Killian KJ. Theory of resistive load detection. Respir Physiol 1983; 51:131–139.
53. McCloskey DI, Ebeling P, Goodwin GM. Estimation of weights and tension and apparent involvement of a "sense of effort." Exp Neurol 1974; 42:220–232.
54. McCloskey DI. Kinesthetic sensibility. Physiol Rev 1978; 58:763–820.
55. McGavin CR, Gupta SP, McHardy GJR. Twelve-minute walking test for assessing disability in chronic bronchitis. Br Med J 1976; 1:822–823.
56. Mead J. Control of respiratory frequency. J Appl Physiol 1960; 15:325–336.
57. Medical Research Council Committee on Research into Chronic Bronchitis. Instruction for use on the questionnaire on respiratory symptoms. Devon: WJ Holman, 1966.
58. Mitchell RA, Berger AJ. Neural regulation of respiration. Am Rev Respir Dis 1975; 111:206–224.
59. Newsom-Davis J. Contribution of somatic receptors in the chest wall to detection of the diaphragm in the sensation of holding the breath. Clin Sci 1970; 41:275–283.
60. Noble MIM, Eisele JH, Frankel HL, et al. The role of the diaphragm in the sensation of holding the breath. Clin Sci 1971; 41:275–283.
61. Ohnhaus EE, Adler R. Methodological problems in the measurement of pain: a comparison between the verbal rating scale and visual analogue scale. Pain 1975; 1:379–384.
62. Oliven A, Kelsen SG, Deal EC Jr, Cherniack NS. Respiratory pressure sensation. Relationship to changes in breathing pattern in patients with chronic obstructive lung disease. Am Rev Respir Dis 1985; 132:1214–1218.
63. Orem J. Neural basis of behavioral and state-dependent control of breathing. In: Lydic R, Biebuyck JF, eds. Clinical Physiology of Sleep. Bethesda, MD: Am Physiol Soc, 1988, 79–96.
64. Otis AB, Fenn WO, Rahn H. Mechanics of breathing in man. J Appl Physiol 1950; 2:592–607.
65. Phillipson EA, McClean PA, Sullivan CE, Zamel N. Interaction of metabolic and behavioral respiratory control during hypercapnia and speech. Am Rev Respir Dis 1978; 117:903–909.
66. Plum F. Neurological integration of behavioral and metabolic control of breathing. In: Porter R, ed. Hering-Breuer Centenary Symposium. London: Churchill Livingstone, Inc., 1970, 159–175.
67. Poon CS. Optimal control of ventilation in hypoxia, hypercapnia and exercise. In: Whipp BJ, Wilberg DM, eds. Modelling and Control of Breathing. New York: Elsevier Science Publishing Co., 1983, 189–196.
68. Price DD, McGrath PA, Rafii A, Buckingham B. The validation of visual analogue scales as ratio scale measures for chronic and experimental pain. Pain 1983; 17:45–56.
69. Remmers JE, Brooks JG III, Tenney SM. Effect of controlled ventilation on the tolerable limit of hypercapnia. Respir Physiol 1968; 4:78–90.
70. Rigg JRA, Rebuck AS, Campbell EJM. A study of factors influencing relief of discomfort in breath-holding in normal subjects. Clin Sci Mol Med 1974; 47:193–199.
71. Roland PE, Ladegaard-Pedersen H. A quantitative analysis of sensations of tension and of kinesthesia in man. Brain 1977; 100:671–692.
72. Shannon R. Reflexes from respiratory muscles and costovertebral joints. In: Handbook of Physiology, Sec 3, Vol II, part I. Bethesda MD: Am Physiol Soc, 1986, 431–447.
73. Shea SA, Walter J, Pelley C, et al. The effect of visual and auditory stimuli upon resting ventilation in man. Respir Physiol 1987; 68:345–357.
74. Silverman M, Barry J, Hellerstein H, et al. Variability of the perceived sense of effort in breathing during exercise in patients with chronic obstructive pulmonary disease. Am Rev Respir Dis 1988; 137:206–209.

75. Sorli J, Grassino A, Lorange G, Milic-Emili J. Control of breathing in patients with chronic obstructive lung disease. Clin Sci Mol Med 1978; 54:295–304.
76. Stark RD, Gambles SA, Lewis JA. Methods to assess breathlessness in healthy subjects: a critical evaluation and application to analyse the acute effects of diazepam and promethazine on breathlessness induced by exercise or exposure to raised levels of carbon dioxide. Clin Sci 1981; 61:429–439.
77. Stevens SS. On the psychophysical law. Psychol Rev 1957; 64:153–181.
78. Stevens SS. Neural events and the psychophysical law. Science 1970; 170:1043–1050.
79. Stevens SS. Issues in psychophysical measurement. Psychol Rev 1971; 78:426—450.
80. Taguchi O, Kikuchi Y, Kida W, et al. Effects of airway anesthesia on dyspnea during bronchoconstriction and loaded breathing in normal subjects [abstract]. Am Rev Respir Dis 1989; 139: A322.
81. Wiley RL, Zechman FW Jr. Perception of added airflow resistance in humans. Respir Physiol 1966/67; 2:73–87.

Chapter 16

EFFECTS OF COPD ON THE RESPIRATORY MUSCLES

Dudley F. Rochester

Respiratory muscle dysfunction contributes significantly to the clinical and physiologic manifestations of acute and chronic obstructive pulmonary disease (COPD). In 1862, Waters recognized that patients with emphysema displayed excessive contraction of the inspiratory muscles in the neck, whereas the diaphragm had little or no respiratory action.[258] As a result of the abnormal pattern of respiratory muscle contraction, the respiratory excursion of the rib cage exceeded that of the abdomen. In 1920, Hoover described the physical sign that bears his name, i.e., Hoover's sign, the inspiratory retraction of the lower rib cage in patients with severe emphysema.[117] In 1936, Cournand and associates[61] postulated that respiratory muscle dysfunction contributed to dyspnea, and later work strongly supports this concept.

This chapter begins by outlining the characteristics of COPD that most affect the respiratory muscles, including mechanical, neural, and metabolic aspects of COPD. The respiratory muscle structural and biochemical responses to the COPD environment in animal models and human disease are reviewed. Human respiratory muscle strength and endurance in COPD are compared with respiratory muscle performance in healthy subjects, and similar comparisons are made for healthy and emphysematous animals. The relationships among respiratory muscle fatigue, dyspnea, and hypercapnic respiratory failure are discussed, and a distinction is made between overt and incipient fatigue. Lastly, the chapter outlines treatment of respiratory muscle failure, with particular reference to respiratory muscle rest and restoration of contractility.

The author thanks Ms. Elizabeth Crawford for her expert help in preparation of this manuscript.

HOW COPD AFFECTS THE RESPIRATORY MUSCLES

Mechanical Factors

The hallmarks of obstructive pulmonary disease are increased resistance to airflow and hyperinflation of the lungs. It is important to appreciate that resistance to airflow is elevated in inspiration as well as in expiration[54, 168] and that both inspiratory and expiratory airflow resistance affect the respiratory muscles.

Expiratory airflow limitation causes air trapping and is responsible for most of the hyperinflation. In young, healthy subjects, residual volume (RV) is about 25% of total lung capacity (TLC) and functional residual capacity (FRC) is about 50% of TLC. In older healthy subjects, RV and FRC are about 30% and 55% TLC, respectively. In COPD, typical values for RV and FRC are 70% and 85% of predicted TLC, respectively.[211] Because breathing is performed at FRC, it can be seen that patients with COPD must breathe at a volume that is one and a half to two times normal. Such hyperinflation causes the inspiratory muscles, especially the diaphragm, to be shortened before they contract, thereby putting the inspiratory muscles at a distinct mechanical disadvantage.

The increased inspiratory airflow resistance is partially offset by hyperinflation, but at very high lung volumes static compliance is reduced. As a result of both factors, the effective dynamic compliance during breathing is much lower than normal, and the inspiratory work of breathing is increased.

Gas exchange is severely impaired in COPD, owing to abnormal lung structure and the resultant imbalance of ventilation and perfusion. In consequence, the level of minute ventilation required to maintain arterial carbon dioxide pressure (Pa_{CO_2}) at normal levels may be two to three times normal. Thus, the total work and energy cost of breathing in COPD are greatly elevated.

Work, Pressure-Time Index, and Energy Cost of Breathing

Most of the increase in respiratory work in COPD is work done on the lungs. Currently available techniques do not permit the work done on the chest wall to be measured, but to the extent that the chest wall is distorted from its relaxed configuration, work, or energy, must be expended for this as well.[108] The work done on the lung can be assessed from analyzing pressure across the lung and the volume displacement. Graphs of inspired volume plotted as a function of inspiratory and expiratory pleural pressures show a large increase in the area of the pressure-volume curves. The area of the pressure-volume curve represents the work done on the lung consequent to the high airway resistance and low dynamic compliance. In COPD patients who are well enough to be studied in the laboratory, the work done on the lung is two to five times greater than normal,[53, 96, 168] and about 75% of the increased work is borne by the inspiratory muscles. Similar levels of work occur in acute asthma[164, 165] and in COPD patients with acute respiratory failure.[92]

A second approach to quantifying the burden on the inspiratory muscles was introduced by McGregor and Becklake[168] and refined by Bellemare and Grassino.[28, 29] This is called the inspiratory pressure-time index (PTI). Whereas work represents the product of pressure and volume, i.e., the area under the volume-pressure curve, the PTI represents the product of inspiratory pressure and time (the area under the inspiratory pressure-time curve; see section on Respiratory Muscle Strength and Endurance for details). As in the case of work, PTI is estimated from pleural or transdiaphragmatic pressure and, thus, does not include pressure required to displace and/or deform the chest wall. The PTI gives important information about the force and duration of inspiratory muscle contraction, and is closely correlated with respiratory muscle energy expenditure.[57, 91, 212] In patients with COPD or acute asthma attacks, the PTI may be 10 to 20 times normal.[29, 99, 165]

A third approach to assessing respiratory muscle activity is to calculate the energy cost of breathing. This approach takes into account energy expended in volume displacement of both the lung and the chest wall. It is assessed by measuring total body oxygen consumption ($\dot{V}O_2$) and minute ventilation ($\dot{V}_E$) during quiet breathing and again after $\dot{V}_E$ has been augmented by voluntary hyperventilation, inhalation of CO_2, or breathing through an external dead space.[53, 96] The ratio $\dot{V}O_2/\Delta\dot{V}_E$ is referred to as the oxygen cost of breathing (O_2 cost, ml/L), and the product of O_2 cost and $\dot{V}_E$ represents respiratory muscle oxygen consumption ($RM\dot{V}O_2$). The energy equivalent of 1 ml O_2/minute is 4.81 cal/minute or 0.335 watts.

The oxygen cost of breathing increases as $\dot{V}_E$ increases, because both airflow and tidal volume increase. Analyses of the experimental data of Cherniack and Fritts and colleagues[53, 96] show that the oxygen cost is almost linearly related to $\dot{V}_E$, such that $O_2 \text{ cost} = K'\dot{V}_E$. This relationship holds for healthy subjects and patients with COPD, but the value of K′ is much higher in COPD.[211] Because $RM\dot{V}O_2 = O_2 \text{ cost} \times \dot{V}_E$, it follows that $RM\dot{V}O_2 = K'\dot{V}_E^2$.

Typical values for $\dot{V}_E$ and $RM\dot{V}O_2$ during quiet breathing are shown in the left half of Table 16–1. Note that owing to elevations of O_2 cost and $\dot{V}_E$, $RM\dot{V}O_2$ in COPD may be 10 to 20 times that of healthy subjects.[53, 90, 96, 168] Similar results have been obtained in asthma[94] and in cystic fibrosis.[129] During voluntary hyperventilation sufficient to lower Pa_{CO_2} by about 10 mm Hg, respiratory muscle oxygen consumption was 4 times higher in COPD patients than it was in healthy subjects.[196]

As $\dot{V}_E$ is increased by physical exercise, the oxygen consumed by the respiratory muscles becomes a progressively larger fraction of total oxygen consumption, as much as 40% to 50% in COPD patients at relatively light exercise.[146] The exercise ventilation level in the right half of Table 16–1 is appropriate for a healthy subject who is walking rapidly or performing light work. For COPD patients, this is a very high level of ventilation, as manifest by the extremely high levels of respiratory muscle oxygen consumption. Because they use so much oxygen just to breathe, both patients have much less oxygen left over to support physical activity. Because more oxygen can be extracted from the inspired air in the presence of hypercapnia, patient COPD-B has a higher total oxygen consumption than does patient COPD-A. Thus, patient COPD-A is limited to one third of the normal exercise capacity, whereas COPD-B can perform at two thirds of the normal level. In severe COPD there comes a point where increasing $\dot{V}_E$ no longer supplies the body with more oxygen, because the $RM\dot{V}O_2$ is so high.[211]

The Pattern of Breathing in COPD

Patients with COPD generally have an increased ventilatory drive,[5, 231, 238, 241, 265] and they also tend to exhibit rapid, shallow breathing relative to the normal breathing pattern. These findings are most apparent when breathing is measured from body surface movements, using the technique of respiratory inductance plethysmography to avoid the effects of a mouthpiece on breathing.[95, 215, 222, 252] Both eucapnic and hypercapnic COPD patients have smaller tidal volumes and higher respiratory rates than do healthy subjects.[153, 154, 252] Those COPD patients with hypercapnia, more airflow limitation, or both, have even higher rates and smaller tidal volumes.[125, 153, 154, 197, 238, 241] Patients with hypoxemia alone have increased respiratory rates with normal tidal volumes.[197] When patients with COPD experience increased bronchoconstriction, or when they develop acute respiratory failure, the rapid, shallow breathing pattern is even more pronounced and parallels increases in the neural drive to breathe.[19, 187] Rapid shallow breathing also develops when COPD patients exercise,[98] particularly when they retain CO_2 during exercise.[107]

The rapid, shallow pattern of breathing affects inspiratory muscle performance. It contributes to hyperinflation and to mechanical disadvantage, because the shortened expiratory time prevents the respiratory system from falling back to its relaxation volume.[135, 164] In exacerbation of asthma, there is an increase in tonic electrical activity of inspiratory muscles during expiration, which decreases with administration of bronchodilator.[54, 159] However, the rate at which inspiratory muscle activity declines after the end of inspiration is faster in COPD than in healthy subjects,[159] being related to recruitment of abdominal muscles during expiration.[159]

RIB CAGE AND ABDOMINAL EXCURSIONS. Normally, the rib cage and abdomen move outward smoothly and synchronously with inspiration. In acute, severe asthma, the abdominal excursion was found to be synchronous with respired volume, but the rib cage excursion lagged behind to an extent that was greater in patients with the lowest FEV_1.[116] Conversely, in COPD patients with severe reductions of FEV_1, rib cage motion was in phase with respired volume and the abdomen lagged behind[17] or else actually moved inward with inspiration.[235]

The inward inspiratory motion of the abdomen is associated

TABLE 16–1. Typical Values for Minute Ventilation ($\dot{V}E$), and Respiratory Muscle Oxygen Consumption ($RM\dot{V}O_2$) in a Healthy Subject, a Eucapnic Patient (COPD-A), and a Hypercapnic Patient (COPD-B)

VARIABLE	REST			EXERCISE		
	Normal	COPD-A	COPD-B	Normal	COPD-A	COPD-B
$\dot{V}E$ (L/min)	6	12	8	25	25	25
$RM\dot{V}O_2$ (ml/min)	5	70	35	60	300	300
$RM\dot{V}O_2$ (% total)	2	25	12	6	50	35

with a decrease in abdominal pressure.[106] Inspiratory indrawing of the lower rib cage is attributable to the insertional action of the flattened diaphragm, whereas inspiratory indrawing of the lower sternum may be attributable to the relaxation of the abdominal muscles.[106] Assuming a leaning forward or supine posture caused inspiratory abdominal pressure to become positive and restored normal outward inspiratory abdominal excursion.[76] In COPD, indices of chest-abdomen asynchrony do not necessarily correlate with the severity of airflow limitation.[105] Overall, the phenomenon of chest-abdomen asynchrony reflects increased activity of the rib cage and neck inspiratory muscles,[42] as well as of the abdominal muscles.

Chest-abdomen asynchrony may develop during exercise even if not present at rest, or the breathing pattern worsens from that seen during quiet breathing.[68] However, paradoxical motions do not always occur.[73] That is, recruitment of expiratory muscles in expiration, with early inspiratory relaxation, may only result in an increase in the contribution of the abdominal compartment to ventilation. Such actions lessen the burden on the diaphragm.[73] Some COPD patients have chest-abdomen asynchrony with arm but not leg exercise.[51]

Asynchronous breathing often develops during weaning from mechanical ventilation and tends to be worse in patients whose weaning trials are unsuccessful.[253, 255] In addition, more severe degrees of asynchrony tend to be seen in more disabled patients and in those with respiratory failure.[17, 235] Because chest-abdomen asynchrony can be elicited in healthy subjects by inspiratory resistive loading, it appears to be a response to imposed loads.[221, 254]

Nutritional and Metabolic Abnormalities

It is likely that 30% to 40% of patients with COPD are underweight, and some are severely underweight.[261] Severe weight loss is associated with a significant reduction in diaphragm muscle mass in patients without chronic lung disease as well as those with COPD.[12, 15, 251] Muscle wasting in emphysema results mainly from decreased muscle protein synthesis,[176] but the mechanism for this is unclear. Severe infection also contributes to muscle wasting.[24] Respiratory muscle strength is lower in underweight COPD patients than in normal-weight COPD patients with equivalent degrees of airflow limitation.[192] Underweight patients without chronic lung disease also have severe respiratory muscle weakness.[13]

Patients with COPD exhibit a variety of metabolic abnormalities in all their muscles. Even in the absence of severe blood gas derangement, patients with COPD have low concentrations of ATP in their muscles,[48] and these are lower in respiratory failure.[89, 100, 173] The ATP concentrations improve with treatment of acute respiratory failure.[100] Low levels of phosphagens are accompanied by intracellular acidosis; increases in muscle cell lactate, sodium, chloride, bicarbonate, and water concentrations; and decreases in muscle cell potassium and magnesium concentrations.[88, 173]

Hypophosphatemia occurs in acute respiratory failure and is associated with severe diaphragmatic weakness, which is partly correctible by phosphate infusion.[20] Other causes of respiratory muscle weakness include hypomagnesemia[174] and perhaps steroid-induced myopathy.[171]

Acute blood gas derangements affect respiratory muscle strength and endurance. Hypercapnia induced by CO_2 inhalation reduced transdiaphragmatic pressure in healthy human volunteers by 30% to 50%, when end-tidal P_{CO_2} was about 50 to 60 torr.[128] Acute hypoxemia induced by inhalation of 13% O_2 curtailed inspiratory muscle endurance, thereby predisposing patients to fatigue.[124]

STRUCTURAL ADAPTATIONS TO HYPERINFLATION

Data from Animal Models

Animal models of emphysema have been used to assess the effects of chronic pulmonary hyperinflation on the lung, chest wall, and respiratory muscles. Instillation of pancreatic elastase produces emphysema, which gradually progresses over the animal's lifetime. In emphysematous hamsters, the FRC can range from 2 to 5 times that of healthy hamsters.[84, 85, 190, 250] The TLC increases by 60% to 100% over control.[84, 132, 245, 250] These increases in lung volume are accompanied by slight increases in airway resistance and doubling of lung compliance.[190] The volume-pressure curve of the chest wall is shifted upward such that for a given pleural pressure, chest wall volume is about 25% to 75% higher in emphysematous animals, and linear dimensions at various sites on the rib cage are increased by 10% to 20%.[250]

Muscle Fiber Type and Biochemistry

The alterations in lung volume and chest wall structure affect the respiratory muscles, especially the diaphragm. Kelsen and colleagues[132] described the changes in diaphragm muscle from hamsters that had emphysema for 12 weeks. The weight of the hamster diaphragm and its water content are unaffected. The diaphragm from emphysematous animals is about 30% thicker than that from control animals, and the cross-sectional area of diaphragm muscle fibers also increases by 30% to 40%. The increase is greater in slow-twitch oxidative fibers than in fast-twitch fibers. In contrast, Farkas and Roussos[86] showed that after 24 weeks of emphysema, there is no significant change in slow-twitch oxidative fibers, and the fast-twitch fibers become atrophied, with a 30% reduction in their cross-sectional area. No significant changes were found in internal intercostal muscles, and mild atrophy was found in fast-twitch glycolytic fibers of external intercostal muscles. Exercise training of emphysematous animals prevented atrophy of fast-twitch fibers in the diaphragm but not in the external intercostal muscles. Training produced hypertrophy of slow-twitch diaphragmatic fibers.[86] In a rabbit model of emphysema in which FRC was increased by only 45%, no changes in diaphragm muscle fiber diameter were observed.[69]

The relative distribution of muscle fiber types by number is virtually the same in emphysematous animals as in control animals of the same species.[69, 86, 132] Emphysema enhanced the oxidative capacity of the diaphragm and intercostal muscles. Emphysema also enhanced glycolytic capacity in intercostal muscles but reduced it in the diaphragm.[86] Exercise training had no additional effect on the diaphragm but slightly enhanced glycolytic capacity of intercostal muscles.

MUSCLE FIBER LENGTH. The most pronounced effect of emphysema on the hamster diaphragm is shortening of its muscle fibers. Muscle fibers are composed of individual units called sarcomeres, linked in series. Both Supinski and Kelsen[245] and Farkas and Roussos[85] showed that emphysema causes the costal diaphragm muscle to shorten by 15% to 20% as compared with diaphragm muscle from control animals. About 65% to 80% of this shortening is due to loss of sarcomeres, with the balance due to shortening of the remaining sarcomeres.[84, 85, 132, 245] Both the degree of diaphragm muscle shortening and the loss of sarcomeres from muscle fibers are related to the magnitude of the increase in FRC.[84, 85] We estimated from these data that diaphragm length was 90% normal in animals when FRC was 2.7 times normal, and 74% normal when FRC was 4.6 times its baseline value.[15] No alteration exists in the length of limb muscles in emphysematous hamsters.[245]

FUNCTIONAL SIGNIFICANCE. The functional significance of these structural and biochemical changes is two-fold. The first consideration involves the relation between the resting length of the diaphragm and its force output in response to supramaximal stimulation. Every muscle has an optimal resting length (Lo) at which stimulated force output is maximal. At lengths above or below Lo, force output falls off (Fig. 16–1*A*). When length is expressed as a percentage of Lo, the force-length (length-tension) relationships of diaphragms from healthy and emphysematous animals are virtually identical (Fig. 16–1*A*). However, when length is expressed in absolute units, the maximal force output of the diaphragm from emphysematous hamsters is at an Lo that is 20% shorter than the normal Lo (Fig. 16–1*B*). The circle indicates that acute 20% shortening of the normal diaphragm reduces its force output by 25%. The distance from the circle to the triangle shows the extent to which force output of the diaphragm in emphysema is restored by the process of sarcomere adaptation.

The second consequence is that the diaphragm of emphysematous animals has greater endurance capacity and is more resistant to fatigue. Atrophy of fast-twitch fibers causes the relative area contributed by slow-twitch fibers to increase from 20% in control animals to 32% in emphysematous animals (calculated from data in Farkas and Roussos).[86] The slow-twitch fibers are the most resistant to fatigue, and the increase in the relative area proportion of these fibers may explain the observed increases in the oxidative capacity of the diaphragm.[86]

Emphysema also affects some expiratory abdominal muscles. In emphysematous hamsters, the optimal resting length of the transversus abdominis muscle was 8% shorter than that in control animals, whereas the length of the external oblique muscle was unchanged. This result is contrary to what one would expect from the increases in lung volume and rib cage dimensions,[25] and its functional significance is as yet unclear.

Data from COPD Patients

Owing to diversity in the type, stage, and complications of COPD, it is not surprising that measurements of the dimensions of the diaphragm at necropsy have produced variable results. One would think that some differences could be resolved by relating dimensions of the diaphragm to body weight and either the lung volume or the morphologic extent of emphysema. However, data in support of this hypothesis are relatively scant, particularly with regard to establishing independent effects of lung volume and weight loss.

DIAPHRAGMATIC DIMENSIONS. Diaphragm weight varies linearly with body weight and inversely with the morphologic extent of emphysema.[251] Arora and Rochester[15] found that diaphragm muscle mass varies linearly with body weight, in the same way in patients with COPD and those without chronic lung disease. In both COPD patients and other patients, the ratio of diaphragm muscle mass (DMM) to body weight (BW) was 3.3 to 3.4 g/kg, and in COPD patients DMM = 4.95 BW − 97.4 ($r = 0.89$, $P < 0.001$). This relationship is virtually identical to that in healthy subjects and patients without chronic lung disease. Taking body weight into account, the reported values for diaphragm weight or muscle mass in three separate studies are very much alike.[15, 123, 251] This observation suggests, but by no means proves, that lung volume or the degree of pulmonary hyperinflation has little independent effect on diaphragm muscle mass. If hyperinflation does exert an independent effect, it is most likely mediated by loss of sarcomeres.

Substantial disagreement among investigators exists as to the effect of COPD on the thickness of diaphragm muscle.

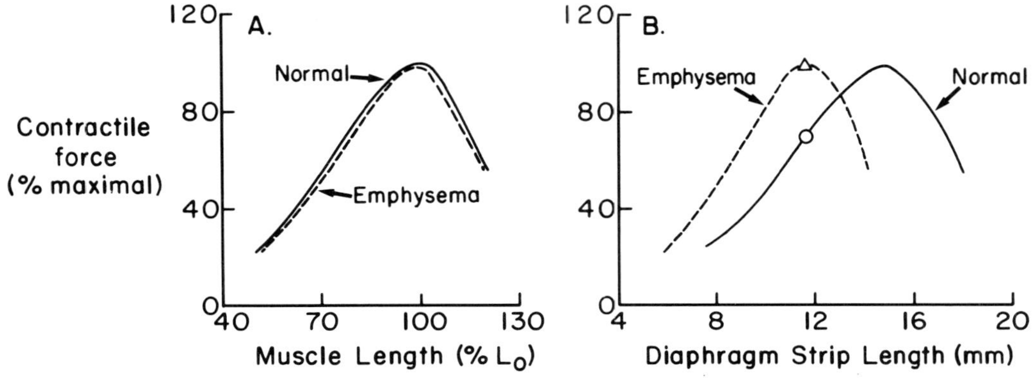

Figure 16–1. Force-length (length-tension) curves for diaphragm muscle strips obtained from healthy hamsters (solid lines) and emphysematous hamsters (dashed lines). Force is expressed as percent of maximal force, which was the same in both groups. *A* shows that when length is expressed as percent of optimal resting length (Lo), the force-length relationship is the same for both sets of diaphragms. *B* shows that maximal force of diaphragms from emphysematous hamsters was reached at a length (Lo) that was 20% shorter than normal. The open circle shows that the force of the normal diaphragm is 75% of maximal when it is acutely shortened to the length that is optimal for the diaphragm in emphysema. The distance from the open circle to the open triangle represents the restoration of force gained by sarcomere adaptation in diaphragms from emphysematous animals. (Adapted from Farkas GA, Roussos C. J Appl Physiol 1982; 53:1263–1272, with permission.)

Thickness also varies with body weight, and in our series the relationship was again similar for patients without and with COPD.[15] In underweight patients with chronic bronchitis, diaphragm muscle thickness was 0.23 cm,[242] which is consistent with our results. However, in normal-weight COPD patients diaphragm muscle thickness averaged 0.50 cm,[123] whereas we would predict a value of 0.30 cm for patients of this weight.[15] This difference could be explained by acute as opposed to chronic changes in lung volume. With chronic hyperinflation, loss of sarcomeres would reduce muscle length, area, and mass, so that thickness should be relatively unaffected. However, acute hyperinflation consequent to immediate pre-mortem events could reduce muscle length and area, while leaving mass unchanged. If these events occurred, diaphragm muscle thickness measured at necropsy would be substantially increased.

Diaphragm and diaphragm muscle surface area are substantially below control values in many patients with emphysema,[45] chronic bronchitis,[242] or mixed forms of COPD.[123] However, in our series of COPD patients, diaphragm muscle surface area and muscle lengths were well within normal limits.[15] When diaphragm area is low, the reduction is entirely due to loss of muscle area, because the area of the central tendon does not change.[45]

The variability of results of diaphragm surface area measurements suggests that lung volume should have an effect on diaphragm muscle length and surface area. That is, the type of sarcomere adaptation seen in the hamster model of emphysema might be expected to occur in human COPD as well. Our study does not support this hypothesis, as we found no relation between diaphragm muscle length and lung volume.[15] However, for the most part, our patients were not severely hyperinflated. Moreover, the degree of hyperinflation in human COPD seldom approaches that seen in hamster emphysema. Data from hamsters indicate that the degree of diaphragmatic shortening is modest in animals with lesser degrees of hyperinflation,[15] and there is much overlap in muscle fiber length and sarcomere counts between healthy and emphysematous animals.[84, 85, 245] Sharp and colleagues[232] showed that in human emphysema the rib cage expands differently in various subjects. Thus, in patients whose hyperinflation is mainly in the upper rib cage, diaphragmatic area may be less affected. Of interest, from analysis of rib angles and the angles made by intercostal muscles with adjacent ribs, it appears that hyperinflation has relatively little effect on the resting length of intercostal muscles.[232]

RESPIRATORY MUSCLE FIBER TYPE AND BIOCHEMISTRY. A number of studies have addressed questions concerning respiratory muscle fiber type and ultrastructure in COPD. The distribution of muscle fiber types by number is the same in COPD as in healthy individuals. Sanchez and colleagues found that there is mild atrophy of both slow- and fast-twitch fibers in the diaphragm but not the intercostal muscles.[225, 226] In the costal portion of the diaphragm and in the internal intercostal muscle the degree of atrophy was greater in patients who had more severe airflow limitation.[48, 119, 226] Some degree of atrophy was found in nonrespiratory as well as respiratory muscles, being more severe in fast-twitch fibers.[119] In addition to atrophy, there were other morphologic abnormalities of intercostal muscles including targeting, fiber splitting, and increased variability in fiber size.[48] Only one study shows diaphragm muscle fiber cross-sectional area in COPD to be increased over that in non-COPD patients.[230] However, without knowing the nutritional status of the patients studied, it is difficult to assess the significance of these results.

The metabolic profile of the diaphragm in COPD patients and in healthy subjects was assessed by measuring activities of oxidative and glycolytic enzymes.[224] Biopsy specimens of diaphragms from COPD patients had slightly less oxidative capacity and significantly less glycolytic activity as compared with control diaphragms, but COPD had no effect on the enzymatic activities of the latissimus dorsi muscle. In healthy subjects, activities of all enzymes were 60% to 120% greater in the diaphragm than in the latissimus dorsi. Thus, in human COPD it appears that the diaphragm is somewhat detrained, partly in relation to weight loss and partly in relation to hyperinflation of the lungs.[224] These results are opposite to those in the hamster diaphragm.[86]

NECK INSPIRATORY MUSCLES. The sternocleidomastoid muscles of patients with COPD are more visible than those of healthy subjects and usually contract with inspiration even during quiet breathing. Using anthropometric techniques, arm muscle circumference, thickness of the triceps skin fold, and thickness of the sternocleidomastoid muscle were assessed in normal-weight and underweight COPD patients and in healthy individuals.[14] The normal-weight COPD patients weighed significantly less than the healthy subjects but their arm muscle circumferences were normal. However, both their triceps skin folds and sternocleidomastoid muscles were about 30% thinner than those in healthy individuals. In the underweight COPD patients all three anthropometric indices were substantially decreased, by 14% for arm muscle circumference and by 45% to 50% for triceps skin fold and sternocleidomastoid muscle thickness.[14]

Because increasing lung volume should shorten and thicken the sternocleidomastoid muscles, and the results of our study were not corrected for muscle length, the degree of sternocleidomastoid muscle atrophy is probably even more pronounced than we indicated. As yet, we are unaware of any data concerning the dimensions of the scalene muscles in either healthy subjects or patients with COPD.

RESPIRATORY MUSCLE STRENGTH AND ENDURANCE

Contractile Properties of Hamster Muscles

The intrinsic contractile properties of respiratory muscles excised from emphysematous hamsters are normal. Diaphragm strips from both normal and emphysematous animals develop maximal tetanic tensions of 1.7 to 2.1 kg/cm^2, and twitch tensions are 25% to 35% of maximal tetanic tension.[84, 85, 245] Contraction and relaxation times and the force-frequency responses are also the same in healthy as in emphysematous animals.[84, 245] The transverse abdominis and external oblique muscles develop somewhat higher peak tetanic tensions and have a somewhat lower ratio of twitch-to-tetanic tension, but these tensions and the contraction and relaxation times are the same in healthy and emphysematous animals.[10, 11]

The diaphragm *in situ* behaves much differently in emphysematous animals than in healthy ones. At lung volumes from normal RV to normal TLC, the transdiaphragmatic pressure (Pdi) generated by the normal diaphragm is greater than that which can be generated by the diaphragm from emphysematous animals.[190] However, at lung volumes above normal TLC, Pdi in emphysematous animals progressively exceeds Pdi in healthy animals (Fig. 16–2). At a lung volume equivalent to FRC in emphysema (triangle), the Pdi response to phrenic nerve stimulation in emphysematous animals is twice that in healthy animals. In the rabbit model of emphysema, the Pdi response to phrenic nerve stimulation is lower than that in control animals when uncorrected for the increase in FRC.[169] However, by taking into account the higher FRC in emphysematous animals, the results confirm those in the hamster model.

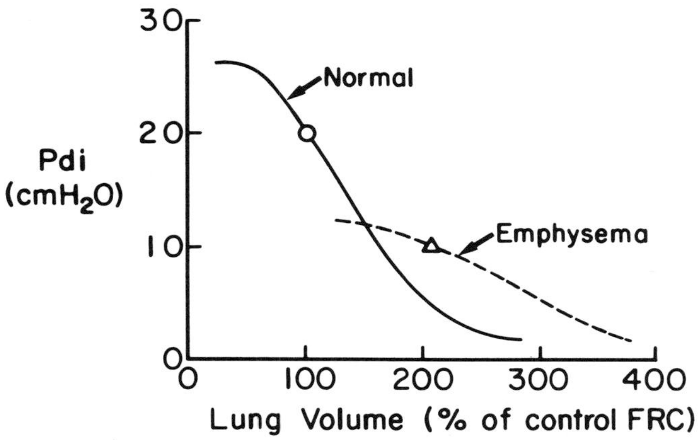

Figure 16–2. Transdiaphragmatic pressure (Pdi) responses to phrenic nerve stimulation in healthy hamsters (solid line) and emphysematous hamsters (dashed line). The circle and the triangle depict the Pdi responses at functional residual capacity (FRC) in the healthy and emphysematous animals, respectively. At lung volumes above 150% of normal FRC, Pdi is greater in animals with emphysema than in control animals. (Modified from the data of Oliven A, et al. J Appl Physiol 1986; 60:225–231.)

These results probably cannot be explained solely by loss of sarcomeres from the diaphragm.[85, 245] Given the complex changes that occur in the thoracic cage and abdominal muscles,[10, 250] it seems likely that there are significant alterations in the linkage among the respiratory muscles and between the muscles and the rib cage, which contribute to the advantage of the *in situ* diaphragm in emphysema.

Respiratory Muscle Strength in Patients with COPD

EVALUATION OF METHODS. Respiratory muscle strength is usually assessed from the maximal pressures that can be generated by maximal voluntary effort. In most cases the inspiratory and expiratory efforts are made against a closed airway. In some cases an inspiratory sniff or an expiratory cough maneuver may be used.[209] Other maneuvers include maximum expulsive efforts with the glottis open, which cause the diaphragm to contract against the abdominal muscles, and a combined inspiratory-expulsive maneuver.[138]

Maximal respiratory pressures are usually measured at the mouth. To record sniff or cough pressures, it is necessary to place a balloon catheter in the esophagus and to record abdominal or transdiaphragmatic pressures (Pdi). It is also necessary to place a catheter in the stomach.

The level of neural drive to respiratory muscles varies according to the type of maneuver. For example, in the Müller maneuver, in which subjects make maximal inspiratory efforts against a closed airway, neural drive to rib cage inspiratory muscles is maximal but the diaphragm is not maximally activated.[115] Gibson and colleagues[101] showed that the pattern of abdominal muscle activity is variable in Müller maneuvers. Diaphragmatic activation and Pdi are maximal in expulsive or combined inspiratory-expulsive maneuvers.[26, 115, 138] However, even with those maneuvers, diaphragmatic activation is incomplete after breathing to exhaustion through a severe inspiratory resistance.[27]

Given the aforementioned considerations, it is quite possible that respiratory muscle strength is underestimated in patients with COPD, especially in the more dyspneic patients. However, the variability of diaphragmatic activation and abdominal muscle activity during Müller maneuvers does not affect the minimum pleural or overall inspiratory muscle pressure.[101, 115] Thus, measurements of maximal inspiratory pressure probably do reflect the maximal available inspiratory muscle strength.

MAXIMAL INSPIRATORY PRESSURES. In 1968, Sharp[236] reported that maximal inspiratory pressures are substantially below normal in patients with COPD. Older, healthy subjects can generate a PI max of -99 ± 21 cm H_2O at residual volume.[37, 40, 67, 101, 160, 175, 185, 191] Data for older, healthy subjects and patients with COPD are shown in Figure 16–3. At the patients' RV, PI max averaged -69 ± 23 cm H_2O, and lung volume was 75% ± 6% predicted TLC. At the patients' FRC, PI max was -58 ± 11 cm H_2O and lung volume was 105% ± 15% predicted TLC. The higher the lung volume at which the maximal inspiratory effort was made, the lower was the resultant PI max. When healthy subjects and COPD patients made the effort from a comparable lung volume, e.g., about 75% of predicted TLC, then PI max values were similar for the two groups.

Transdiaphragmatic pressure (Pdi) behaves in a similar fashion.[29, 76, 101] Data from healthy subjects[209] show that Pdi is about 120 cm H_2O at 60% TLC, 85 cm H_2O at 80% TLC, and 35 cm H_2O at 100% TLC. Values obtained in COPD patients agree well with the normal values at equivalent lung volume. For example, in one series Pdi was 89 ± 36 cm H_2O at a lung volume of approximately 85% predicted TLC,[29] and in another Pdi was 58 ± 45 cm H_2O at a lung volume of $109 \pm 3\%$ predicted TLC.[101]

Rochester and Braun[213] related PI max in patients with COPD to their PE max and to the length of the diaphragm estimated roentgenographically. The patients with COPD had RV values ranging from 30% to 130% predicted TLC, with a mean value of 70 ± 25% predicted TLC. There was significant inverse relationship between PI max and lung volume ($r = 0.42$, $P < 0.02$), but there were stronger correlations between PI max and either PE max or diaphragm length (Fig. 16–4*A* and *B*). The highest correlation was obtained when PI max was expressed as a combined function of diaphragm length and PE max ($R = 0.82$, $P < 0.001$). We interpreted this to indicate that inspiratory muscle strength in COPD is determined not only by the degree of mechanical disadvantage to

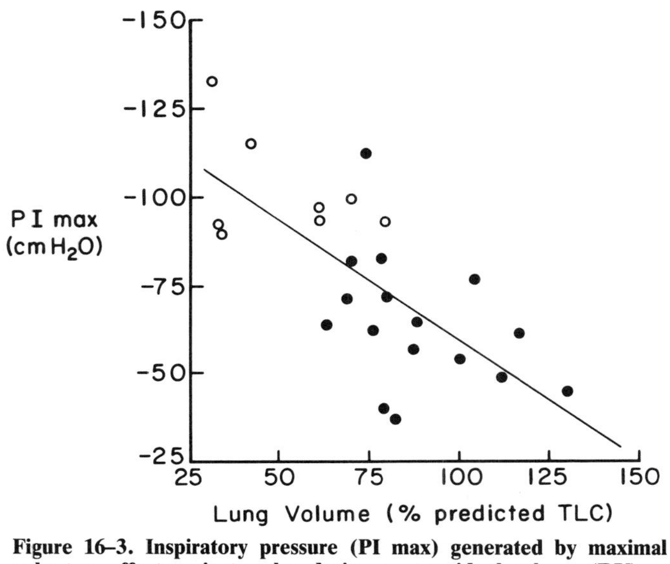

Figure 16–3. Inspiratory pressure (PI max) generated by maximal voluntary effort against a closed airway at residual volume (RV) or functional residual capacity (FRC). PI max is shown as a function of the lung volume at which the inspiratory effort was made. Data points represent mean values for COPD patients (closed circles) and age-matched healthy subjects (open circles). Note that PI max decreases as lung volume increases. The equation of the line is PI max (cm H_2O) = 128 − 0.68 volume (% predicted total lung capacity [TLC]), ($r = -0.69$, $P < 0.001$).

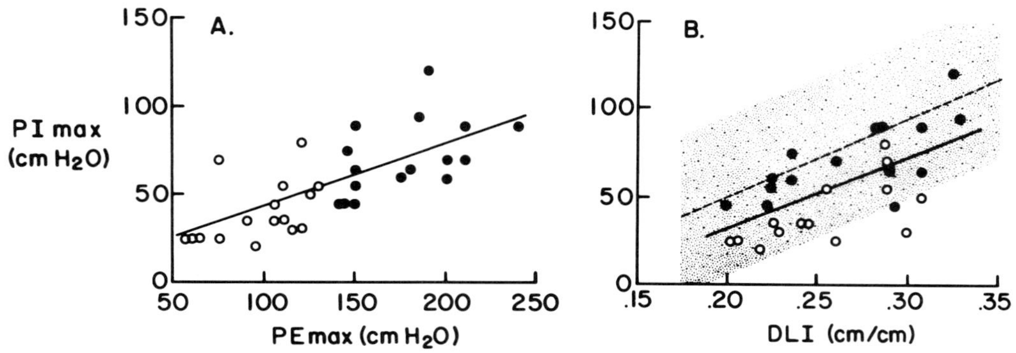

Figure 16–4. Determinants of maximal inspiratory pressure (PI max) in COPD. Each point represents data from a single patient. *A* shows that PI max is higher in patients whose maximal expiratory pressure (PE max) is in the normal range (closed circles) than it is in patients who have expiratory muscle weakness (open circles). *B* shows that PI max is higher in patients whose diaphragm length index at RV is greater. Diaphragm length was measured from chest roentgenograms and normalized to the patient's height to yield a diaphragm length index (DLI). The slope of the relationship between PI max and DLI in COPD patients (solid line) parallels that from healthy subjects (dashed line) who were studied at lung volumes matching the range of RV values in COPD. These results indicate that PI max in COPD is determined both by generalized muscle strength (*A*) and the force-length relationship of the diaphragm (*B*). (Reproduced with permission from Rochester DF, Braun NMT. Am Rev Respir Dis 1985; 132:42–47.)

the diaphragm but also by the presence or absence of generalized muscle weakness.

The contractile force of the sternocleidomastoid muscles has also been measured in healthy subjects and patients with COPD. One technique is based on measuring the force vector directed anteriorly against a transducer that lies against the tendon, which attaches the sternal head of the muscle to the sternum.[263] With contraction the muscle attempts to straighten, and its tendon pushes anteriorly against the transducer. In another technique, the subject is studied while semirecumbent and tries to lift the head against a restraining plate connected to a force transducer.[79] Measured this way, force produced by maximal voluntary sternocleidomastoid contraction was 5.2 kg in normal subjects. In 25 patients with severe respiratory disease, most of whom had COPD, sternocleidomastoid force was 3.1 kg, a reduction of 40% below normal. However, half the patients were in respiratory failure and their PI max and PE max were low, 40 and 75 cm H_2O, respectively. All three measures of respiratory muscle strength improved by about 30% after recovery from respiratory failure but were still well below normal.[79]

MAXIMAL EXPIRATORY PRESSURES. There is no obvious mechanical disadvantage to the expiratory muscles in COPD.

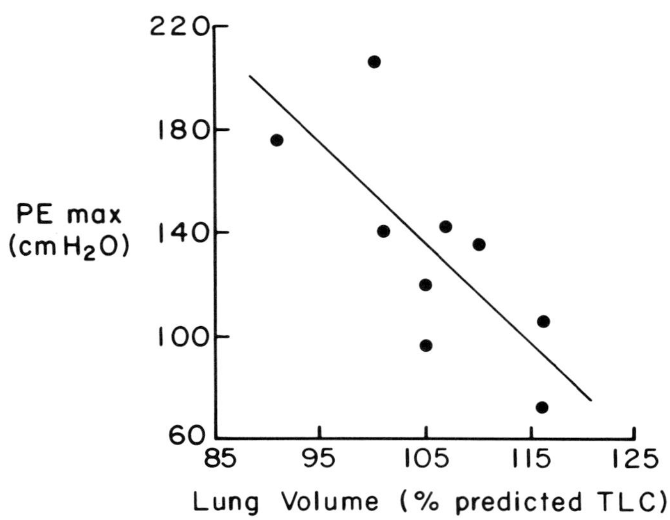

Figure 16–5. Expiratory pressure (PE max) generated by maximal voluntary effort against a closed airway at total lung capacity (TLC). Data points represent mean values for COPD patients. Note that patients with the largest TLCs have the lowest PI max (see text). The equation of the line is PE max (cm H_2O = 539 − 3.84 volume [% predicted TLC]), (r = −0.75, *P* < 0.05).

One might expect them to be overstretched, but there is no evidence for this in human intercostal muscles[232] or in hamster abdominal muscles.[10] The abdominal muscles of emphysematous hamsters have normal force responses to tetanic stimulation,[11] but COPD patients often have low values of PE max.

Based on data from multiple sources,[47, 67, 160, 175, 191, 213] PE max in COPD patients averages 133 ± 43 cm H_2O. This is significantly lower than the value of 167 ± 32 cm H_2O calculated for age-matched healthy subjects.[37, 40, 67, 160, 191] When individual series mean values are plotted as a function of the lung volume at which the maximal expiratory effort was made, it can be seen that there is a significant inverse relationship between PE max and lung volume (Fig. 16–5). The PE max effort was initiated at TLC, but owing to gas compression the final lung volume is lower than TLC. Those patients whose PE max was performed at lung volumes between 91% and 101% predicted TLC had normal values for PE max (175 ± 33 cm H_2O). Patients who made the effort at lung volumes between 105% and 128% predicted TLC had significantly lower values, i.e., 108 ± 26 cm H_2O.

The relationship between PE max and lung volumes in COPD is probably not mediated by the length-tension relationship. Those patients who are more hyperinflated likely are also more flow limited and more dyspneic. They may also be underweight. Thus, their low values of PE max may reflect true muscle weakness, but it is also possible that these patients may not have maximally activated their expiratory muscles, owing to dyspnea.

Asthma and Cystic Fibrosis

Maximal respiratory pressures are usually normal in children or young adults with asthma, cystic fibrosis, or other forms of COPD.[16, 99, 140, 162, 193, 199] The observed values of PI max are often lower than those predicted for healthy individuals at normal RV. However, after correcting for lung volume, PI max values in asthma, cystic fibrosis, and childhood COPD are either normal or greater than normal.[16, 162, 206]

Two exceptions to these results should be noted. Children with cystic fibrosis who are malnourished or whose lungs are exceptionally hyperinflated have lower values of maximal respiratory pressures than well-nourished patients or age-matched controls.[248] Some obese patients with asthma treated with corticosteroids have marked inspiratory muscle weakness not related to lung volume.[171]

COUPLING AMONG INSPIRATORY MUSCLES. The ability to generate inspiratory pressure and volume displacements depends on the nature of the mechanical coupling among various inspiratory muscles and between these muscles and the rib cage. Muscles can be arranged mechanically in parallel or in series, as shown schematically in Figure 16–6. The in-parallel

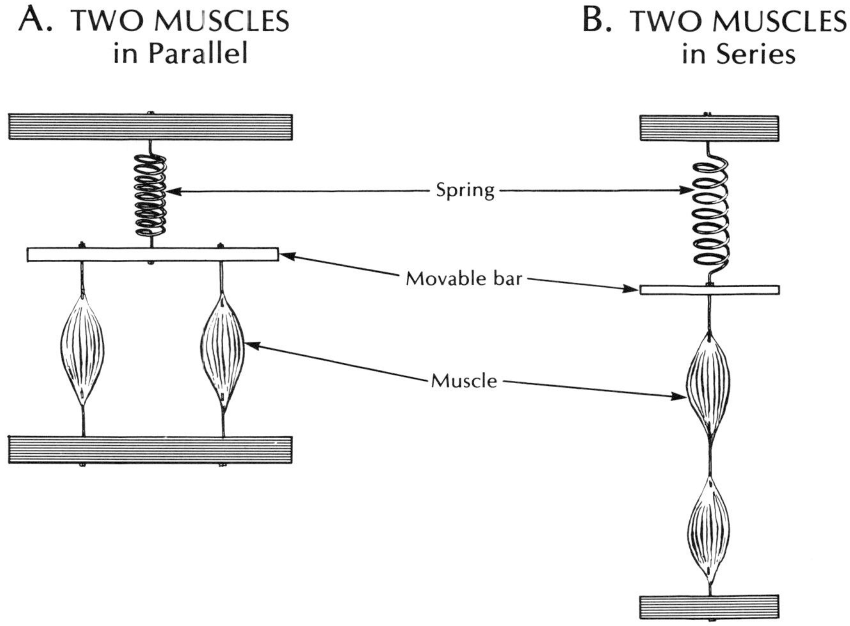

Figure 16–6. Theoretic arrangements of two muscles. The muscles are attached to a fixed block at one end and to a movable bar at the other. The bar is attached to a stretchable spring, which is anchored at the top. The two muscles are equal in size and strength and receive identical neural stimulation. When the muscles are arranged in parallel (*A*), they apply twice as much force to the bar as one muscle alone, but the muscles can shorten and stretch the spring only as much as a single muscle. Conversely, when the muscles are arranged in series (*B*), the two muscles can exert only as much force as a single muscle, but they can stretch the spring twice as far as a single muscle could.

arrangement enhances applied force, whereas the in-series arrangement increases linear displacement.

DeTroyer and colleagues[70] pointed out that the diaphragm consists of two distinct components, which differ with regard to their embryologic origins and their nerve supply. Both parts of the diaphragm cause the dome to descend, thus increasing abdominal pressure and displacing the abdominal wall outward. However, the costal part of the diaphragm also acts to expand the lower rib cage, whereas the crural diaphragm does not.[71] From these observations, Macklem and colleagues[156] developed a scheme to describe coupling among the inspiratory muscles. At normal FRC, the right and left costal diaphragms are arranged in parallel with each other and with the lower inspiratory intercostal muscles (Fig. 16–7*A*). The costal diaphragm is also in parallel with the crural diaphragm. Conversely, the neck inspiratory muscles, such as the scalene and sternomastoid muscles, are mostly in series with the diaphragm (see Fig. 16–7*A*). The in-parallel arrangement favors pressure generation, whereas the in-series arrangement favors volume displacement.

These arrangements by themselves do not account for all the experimental results of stimulating different muscles.[71] It is necessary to add the effects of the inspiratory increase in abdominal pressure.[156] This increase exerts an inflationary effect on the lower rib cage through the zone of apposition of the diaphragm to the lower rib cage, as described by Loring and Mead.[151] Thus, at normal FRC, the upper rib cage and neck inspiratory muscles are mainly responsible for expanding the upper rib cage. The lower intercostal muscles and the costal part of the diaphragm expand the lower rib cage and

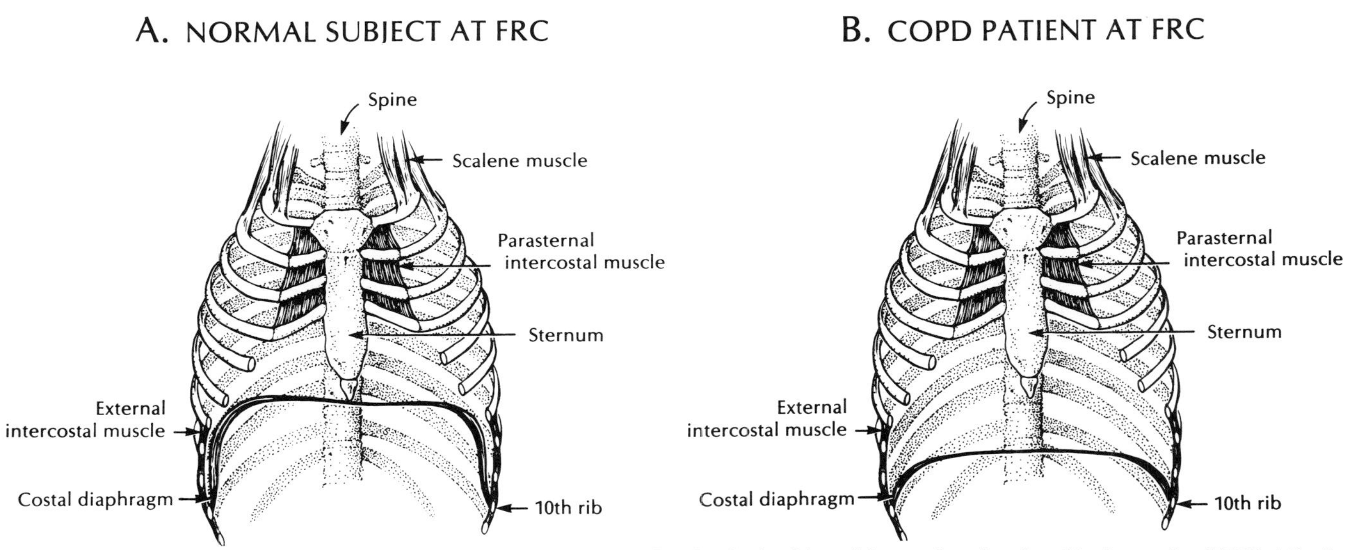

Figure 16–7. Coupling between the diaphragm and the rib cage muscles. In the healthy subject at functional residual capacity (FRC) (*A*), the right and left costal diaphragms are in parallel with each other and with the lower intercostal muscles. In contrast, the scalene and parasternal intercostal muscles and the diaphragm are arranged more in series than in parallel. In the COPD patient at FRC (*B*), hyperinflation of the lung has depressed and shortened the diaphragm so that it is no longer in parallel with lower rib cage muscles or in series with the upper rib cage muscles.

both parts of the diaphragm cause the diaphragm dome to descend. Yet this action, by increasing abdominal pressure, also expands the lower rib cage.

All of these relationships are altered at high lung volumes such as are commonly found in COPD (Fig. 16–7*B*). The two parts of the diaphragm behave more as if they were mechanically in series.[156] The zone of apposition shrinks, and the shortened diaphragm loses its ability to increase abdominal pressure. Thus, the direct and indirect contributions of the diaphragm to expanding the lower rib cage largely disappear. When hyperinflation of the lungs is severe, contraction of the diaphragm actually exerts a deflationary effect on the lower rib cage.[117, 156]

LAPLACE RELATIONSHIP. The dome of the diaphragm is similar to a segment of a sphere. The pressure (P) inside a sphere is related to the tension (T) in the wall of the sphere by the Laplace equation: $P = 2T/R$, where R is the radius of curvature. For the diaphragm, P represents inspiratory transdiaphragmatic pressure and T represents the force of muscle contraction. For a given contractile force (tension), P will decrease if R increases. Thus, when hyperinflation in COPD causes the diaphragm to flatten, its radius of curvature becomes very large, and the conversion of contractile force to inspiratory pressure is severely impaired.

It appears that most of the loss of Pdi as lung volume increases from normal FRC toward normal TLC can be accounted for by the force-length relationship.[134, 210] Therefore, the Laplace relationship probably only affects Pdi at lung volumes higher than normal TLC. Any effect of the Laplace relationship on Pdi would be added to the effects of shortening the resting length of the diaphragm.

MAGNITUDE OF INSPIRATORY MUSCLE SHORTENING. Among the inspiratory muscles, the diaphragm undergoes the greatest degree of shortening as lung volume increases. In normal subjects, the diaphragm shortens by about 40% between RV and TLC.[39] In COPD, the length of the diaphragm at RV, which is the longest the diaphragm can be, is equivalent to the length of the normal diaphragm at 60% to 100% of normal TLC.[213] In contrast, hyperinflation has relatively little effect on the lengths of the parasternal, intercostal, scalene, and sternomastoid muscles.[231, 233]

Thus, the principal cause of impaired ability to generate inspiratory pressure in COPD is shortening of the diaphragm. This affects the muscle directly, through the force-length relationship, but it also has indirect effects mediated through altered coupling of the diaphragm to other inspiratory muscles and the rib cage. With extreme hyperinflation, flattening of the diaphragm increases its radius of curvature, depresses conversion of tension to pressure, and further reduces inspiratory pressure.

One must also keep in mind the effect that diaphragmatic shortening has on inspiratory volume displacement. Owing to its great capacity to shorten and its anatomic arrangement, the normal diaphragm is exceptionally well suited to the task of inspiratory expansion of the lungs. When the diaphragm is shortened to the point so that further shortening can only be minimal, the capacity of the diaphragm to displace volume is lost. Therefore, in COPD the task of inspiratory volume displacement must be borne mainly by the intercostal and neck inspiratory muscles, which are much less suited for this task.

Ventilatory and Respiratory Muscle Endurance

MAXIMAL VOLUNTARY AND SUSTAINABLE VENTILATION

In healthy subjects the maximal voluntary ventilation (MVV) can be sustained for only 15 to 30 seconds. The level of ventilation that can be sustained for longer periods is referred to as the maximal sustainable ventilation (MSV) or maximal sustainable ventilatory capacity (MSVC). This is a measure of ventilatory endurance. Healthy subjects typically can breathe at 80% to 90% of their MVV for 5 minutes and at about 70% of their MVV for 10 to 15 minutes.[209]

In COPD, the MVV is much lower than normal, largely because of the mechanical abnormalities in the lungs and airways. However, in COPD, as in healthy subjects, the MVV is also dependent to some extent on respiratory muscle strength.[2] The MSVC is also severely reduced in COPD, but when expressed as a percentage of MVV, the MSVC is either normal or above normal. That is, patients with COPD can breathe at about 90% of their MVV for 4 to 10 minutes[55, 263] and can sustain about 75% of their MVV for 15 to 30 minutes.[32, 130, 196, 198, 267] In essence, patients with COPD seem to have a ventilatory endurance equivalent to that in well-trained healthy subjects.

Patients with COPD utilize a very high fraction of their MVV during exercise. For example, healthy individuals at maximal exercise breathe at about 65% of their MVV, whereas COPD patients breathe at about 90% of their MVV.[107, 172, 182] At the end of a 12-minute treadmill walk at 4 to 7 kph, ventilation was about 80% of MVV.[263] At a lower intensity of exercise, walking on a treadmill at 1.6 kph for 30 minutes, other COPD patients used about 50% of their MVV.[80] Electromyographic evidence of intercostal muscle fatigue occurred when exercise ventilation was about 40% of MVV.[239] As would be expected, maximal exercise ventilation in COPD is strongly correlated with forced expiratory volume in one second (FEV_1). However, a better prediction of maximal exercise ventilation can be made using both FEV_1 and peak inspiratory flow rate, which is strongly correlated with PI max.[72]

Respiratory Muscle Endurance

Bellemare and Grassino[28] showed that respiratory muscle endurance is related to the force and duration of respiratory muscle contraction. The duration of contraction is defined as the ratio of inspiratory time (Ti) to total breath cycle time (Ttot). The force of contraction is estimated as the mean inspiratory pressure ($\overline{P}$breath) expressed as a fraction of the maximal inspiratory pressure (Pmax). The pressure-time index (PTI) is the product of these two ratios, i.e., $PTI = (Ti/Ttot) \times (\overline{P}breath/Pmax)$. Note that the PTI is dimensionless.

When healthy subjects are made to breathe through external inspiratory resistances, inspiratory muscle or diaphragmatic fatigue occurs when PTI exceeds 0.15.[28] During quiet breathing adult COPD patients have a PTI of 0.05 ± SD 0.04, about three times normal.[29] When their breathing pattern was modified by increasing the tidal volume and Ti/Ttot, the PTI rose to 0.17 and electromyographic evidence of diaphragmatic fatigue developed.[29] Children with COPD also have a PTI close to the fatiguing level, even during quiet breathing.[99]

Pressure-time index is increased in COPD mainly because the ratio of $\overline{P}$breath-to-PI max is increased. The increase in the ratio is substantial because $\overline{P}$breath rises while PI max falls. By and large, the ratio of Ti/Ttot is either normal or even slightly low in COPD.[29, 63, 99]

In adult COPD patients, the pleural PTI was 0.10, and the diaphragmatic PTI was 0.12 at the end of exhausting exercise.[46] Others have found even higher values of diaphragmatic PTI from 0.17 to 0.22, during bicycle ergometer exercise.[63] Analysis of the patterns of respiratory muscle contraction during exercise shows that COPD patients develop higher values of Pdi during the first half of inspiration than during the second half, in contrast to age-matched healthy subjects.[144] Chronic obstructive pulmonary disease patients also exhibit much higher pressure swings attributable to use of inspiratory accessory muscles and to postexpiratory recoil, which is a measure of early inspiratory relaxation of abdominal muscles. Thus, the pattern of breathing used in COPD patients tends to distribute the work of breathing among all the respiratory muscles.

Upper extremity exercise in the form of arm cycling was accompanied by a pattern of respiratory muscle contraction that is similar to that seen in leg bicycle exercise.[63, 64] However, unsupported arm exercise, i.e., moving rings on a pegboard at shoulder level, was associated with higher levels of diaphragmatic PTI and with a shorter endurance time, even though minute ventilation and oxygen consumption were lower with unsupported arm exercise.[64]

Another type of endurance test is based on performing a series of maximal voluntary muscle contractions in which contraction time is one-half to two-thirds total cycle time. To test the respiratory muscles, subjects make maximal inspiratory and expiratory efforts against a closed airway, so as to measure PI max and PE max. Using this test, it has been shown that the ability to sustain maximal voluntary inspiratory or expiratory contractions is somewhat better in young adult asthma patients than in age-matched healthy individuals.[169]

A third type of endurance test is based on inspiratory threshold loading. The load is increased every 2 minutes, and endurance is assessed for the highest load that can be sustained for 2 minutes, as well as from the inspiratory pressures required to support the maximal load. By these criteria, a group of eight COPD patients had much lower inspiratory muscle endurance than age- and sex-matched control subjects.[175] The COPD patients had lower values for PI max, but even when corrected for these differences, their endurance was only 63% of normal.

In summary, ventilatory endurance, expressed as a fraction or a percent of maximal voluntary ventilation, is either normal or better than normal in patients with COPD. However, inspiratory muscle endurance for threshold loads is reduced. Both healthy subjects and COPD patients are prone to develop inspiratory muscle fatigue when their PTI exceeds a value of about 0.15. It seems likely that ventilatory and respiratory muscle endurance are well below normal in acutely ill COPD patients, but data on this point are lacking. Maximal respiratory pressures are extremely low in acute respiratory failure,[3, 203] as are transdiaphragmatic pressure responses to phrenic nerve stimulation.[20–22, 181] At present, it is not known whether respiratory muscle endurance in acute respiratory failure is compromised because the muscles are so weak or whether other factors also play a role.

DYSPNEA, FATIGUE, AND RESPIRATORY FAILURE

The Respiratory Muscles and Dyspnea

The sensation of dyspnea in COPD is related to the force of inspiratory muscle contraction.[163, 184] More specifically, dyspnea is related to the pressure required to inspire a breath ($\overline{\text{P}}$breath), expressed as a fraction of maximal inspiratory pressure (PI max).[185] Thus, a high value of the ratio of $\overline{\text{P}}$breath-to-PI max appears to be as important for the sensation of breathlessness as it is for inspiratory muscle endurance.

The mechanism that relates dyspnea to the ratio of $\overline{\text{P}}$breath-to-PI max is probably the sense of effort required to breathe.[4, 133] The increased sense of effort is closely linked to the increase in the neural drive to breathe.[44] During quiet breathing, patients with COPD evidently adopt a breathing pattern that requires the least sense of effort, because switching to a slower, deeper breathing pattern increases $\overline{\text{P}}$breath-to-PI max and brings on dyspnea.[111] During exercise, dyspnea in COPD patients is a function of multiple variables, including $\overline{\text{P}}$breath-to-PI max, inspiratory duty cycle, respiratory rate, tidal volume, and mean inspiratory flow rate.[141] These variables are related to inspiratory muscle contractile force, duration of contraction, and degree and rate of muscle shortening.

The close relationship between respiratory muscle function and dyspnea in asthma and COPD is highlighted by several observations. In acute asthma attack, dyspnea correlates with hyperinflation and recruitment of the sternocleidomastoid muscles, and during treatment dyspnea subsides when sternocleidomastoid activity ceases, even though the FRC is still well above normal.[167] Abdominal strapping exacerbates dyspnea during exercise, perhaps because the intercostal and neck inspiratory muscles are shortened and receive an increased motor command.[74]

Sharp and colleagues[234] showed that those COPD patients with postural relief of dyspnea are more hyperinflated than are other patients with equivalent expiratory airflow limitations. These patients also have greater increases in sternocleidomastoid electrical activity on standing, along with a less effective diaphragmatic contraction. Postural relief of dyspnea is associated with a reduction in diaphragmatic electrical activity and an increase in inspiratory transdiaphragmatic pressure.[77] Patients with postural relief of dyspnea are able to generate higher values of PI max while in the leaning forward position.[191]

It appears that the sensation of greater respiratory effort during inspiratory resistive loading is mainly related to the increases in motor drive to rib cage and neck inspiratory muscles. When healthy subjects inspired through resistances severe enough to produce electromyographic evidence of diaphragmatic fatigue, the respiratory effort sensation correlated strongly with electrical activation of the parasternal intercostal and sternocleidomastoid muscles but not with electrical activation of the diaphragm.[257]

We have observed extreme dyspnea in COPD patients with pneumothorax whose diaphragms were displaced downward. Downward displacement of the hemidiaphragm by pleural effusion is associated with dyspnea. Thoracentesis relieves the dyspnea when diaphragmatic position is restored to normal.[82]

Yet another link between dyspnea and respiratory muscle activity is provided by the effects of mechanical ventilation. When patients with chronic respiratory failure from COPD or thoracic restrictive diseases were ventilated in an "iron lung" there was prompt cessation of diaphragmatic electrical activity coupled with an immediate loss of dyspnea.[214, 215] Patients who were more dyspneic when supine showed increased electrical activity of the diaphragm on assuming the supine position but obtained prompt relief when the ventilator abolished their inspiratory muscle contraction. Similar observations are routine in intubated patients being weaned from positive-pressure mechanical ventilation. If the weaning trial is unsuccessful, dyspnea and tachypnea ensue.[56] With restoration of full mechanical ventilatory support, spontaneous ventilatory efforts cease and dyspnea is abolished.[161]

Although there are strong associations between dyspnea and inspiratory muscle contractile effort in COPD, it is clear that other causes of dyspnea are not closely related to inspiratory muscle activity. For example, dynamic airway compression is associated with dyspnea in COPD,[186] and dyspnea in acute asthma may be abolished by vagal blockade or anesthesia of the airways.[200] In the clinical setting, dyspnea, which cannot be abolished by mechanical ventilation, suggests the presence of processes such as airway inflammation, pneumonia, pulmonary edema, pulmonary embolism, or pneumothorax. Dyspnea in these processes is most likely mediated by stimulation of afferent fibers in the vagus nerve rather than by excessive inspiratory muscle contraction.

Respiratory Muscle Weakness, Fatigue, and Respiratory Failure

VENTILATORY DRIVE. In 1968, Lourenco and Miranda[152] used the integrated electrical activity of the diaphragm (EMGdi) as an index of central drive to breathe. They found that during inhalation of CO_2 the EMGdi of COPD patients in respiratory failure increased, but the magnitude of increase was far less than in healthy subjects or COPD patients without respiratory failure. This result was interpreted to indicate that there was a secondary depression of the respiratory center. However, the hypercapnic patients also had the most severe mechanical impairment, and it could well be that their diaphragmatic activation was so high prior to CO_2 inhalation that it could not increase further.[113] Altose and colleagues[5] reported that hypercapnic COPD patients had low mouth occlusion pressures ($P_{0.1}$) at rest and in response to CO_2 inhalation, as compared with eucapnic COPD patients and healthy individuals. Both $P_{0.1}$ and EMGdi responses to CO_2 inhalation were higher in eucapnic COPD patients than in healthy subjects.[5, 152]

By way of contrast, other data support the concept that neural drive to breathe is increased in acute respiratory failure, whether neural drive is estimated from the diaphragm EMG[113] or from mouth occlusion pressure.[19, 187] Moreover, in COPD patients with chronic respiratory failure the mouth occlusion pressures are the same as in eucapnic patients.[227, 241] Thus, it is very unlikely that primary depression of the respiratory center is the major cause of hypercapnic respiratory failure in COPD.

RESPIRATORY MUSCLE DYSFUNCTION. There is strong evidence to support the concept that respiratory failure in COPD is related to respiratory muscle dysfunction. Muscle weakness impairs the ability to compensate for added flow-resistive loads[149, 188] and to increase minute ventilation in response to CO_2 inhalation.[112] In acute respiratory failure the transdiaphragmatic pressure responses to phrenic nerve stimulation are extremely low.[20–22, 181] Both acute and chronic respiratory failure are accompanied by asynchronous patterns of respiratory muscle contraction.[17, 103, 235] Chronic hypercapnia is associated with respiratory muscle weakness,[135, 191, 213] and the Pa_{CO_2} is inversely related to PI max when PI max falls below half normal (Fig. 16–8). During trials of weaning COPD patients from mechanical ventilation, patients who were unable to be weaned within 10 hours had lower values of Pdi max and higher ratios of Pdi breath-to-Pdi max compared with patients who weaned successfully.[203]

It is also clear that in COPD only a small departure from quiet breathing is necessary to put the inspiratory muscles into a fatiguing pattern of contraction. This can occur merely by adopting a slower, deeper pattern of breathing,[29, 111] by moderate voluntary hyperventilation,[196] or by physical exercise.[59, 194, 239, 263] Fatiguing patterns of inspiratory muscle contraction also occur in unsuccessful trials of weaning from mechanical ventilation.[56]

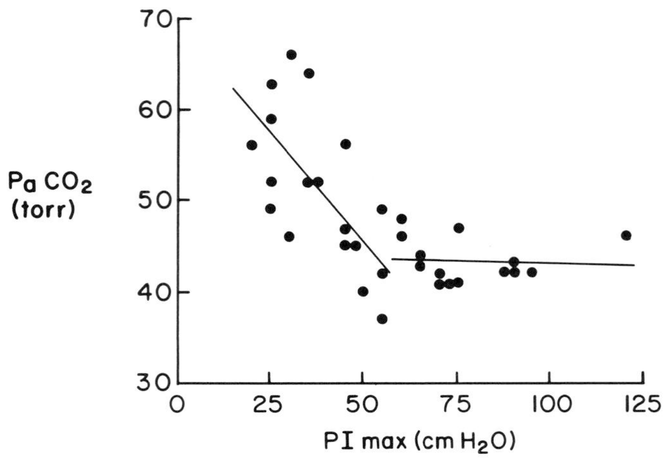

Figure 16–8. Relationship between Pa_{CO_2} and PI max in ambulatory COPD patients. Note that when PI max is less than half normal, there is a significant inverse relationship between Pa_{CO_2} and PI max. The equation of the regression line for 18 COPD patients whose PI max is 20 to 55 cm H_2O is Pa_{CO_2} = 68.4 − 0.464 PI max (r = −0.66, $P < 0.005$). (Reproduced with permission from Rochester DF, Braun NMT. Am Rev Respir Dis 132:42–47, 1985.)

Incipient versus Overt Fatigue

It is important to distinguish between incipient and overt fatigue.[208] Overt fatigue represents inability to carry on with a prescribed task because the workload is too high. Incipient fatigue means that the inspiratory muscles are contracting in a fatiguing pattern. In other words, the muscles will become fatigued if that pattern of contraction persists. The manifestations of incipient and overt fatigue are summarized in Table 16–2. Experiments in healthy subjects show that a diaphragmatic PTI of 0.15 could be sustained for about 90 minutes, and a PTI of 0.25 could be sustained for about 15 minutes before the subject could no longer continue the prescribed pattern of breathing.[28] In this type of experiment, the high-to-low ratio of the EMG power spectrum falls, and the diaphragmatic relaxation rate becomes prolonged soon after the fatiguing pattern of contraction has begun.[81] In addition, there may be a cyclic alteration in the contractions of the diaphragm and other inspiratory muscles.[221] Thus, these phenomena are really indicators of incipient rather than of overt fatigue.

In experiments designed to produce inspiratory muscle fatigue in healthy individuals, the subjects are required to breathe in a fixed pattern. However, when animals are subjected to external flow-resistive loads, or when patients experience respiratory failure, they adopt a rapid, shallow pattern of breathing. This has important implications concerning neural control mechanisms and respiratory muscle function.

When animals are made to inspire through a severe resistance to airflow, their tidal volume falls and their respiratory rate and Pa_{CO_2} rise.[1, 189, 223] The diaphragm may or may not become fatigued, but electrical activation of the diaphragm, which initially rises in response to the load, subsequently

TABLE 16–2. Manifestations of Incipient Versus Overt Inspiratory Muscle Fatigue*

INCIPIENT	OVERT
Fall in high-to-low ratio or centroid frequency of electromyogram (EMG) power spectrum (diaphragm or other inspiratory muscle)	Reduction in Pdi response to phrenic nerve stimulation
Slowing of inspiratory muscle relaxation	Reduction in stimulated force response of sternomastoid muscle
Chest-abdomen asynchrony	Fall in Pdi-to-Edi ratio during spontaneous breathing
Rapid, shallow breathing	

*To qualify as signs of fatigue, these phenomena must have developed as a consequence of breathing with a pressure-time index that lies in the fatigue range.

falls.[189, 223] This suggests that central neural drive is reduced. The tidal volume can be restored to or above control levels by cutting the vagus nerves[1] or by administration of the opioid antagonist naloxone.[229] Naloxone also reverses the fall in the high-to-low ratio of the diaphragm EMG.[201] Thus, the alteration in breathing induced by flow-resistive loads is under neural control with both vagally mediated reflexes and elaboration of endogenous opioids playing a role. One need not invoke overt inspiratory muscle fatigue to explain the load response. Although respiratory muscle fatigue can by itself produce rapid, shallow breathing,[97, 207] this too is probably mediated by neural reflex mechanisms.

Another example of load adaptation is afforded by an experiment in which COPD patients breathed through an external inspiratory and expiratory flow-resistive load.[188] The patients who successfully compensated for the load increased their tidal volume by 13% and their inspiratory time by 37%. The patients who could not compensate reduced their tidal volume by 15%, increased their inspiratory time by only 9%, and experienced a 9-torr elevation in Pa_{CO_2}. The baseline patterns of breathing and airflow limitation were the same in both groups, but PI max was -69 cm H_2O in those who compensated as compared with -49 cm H_2O in those who retained CO_2. The changes in inspiratory time and tidal volume during loaded breathing were directly proportional to PI max. In effect, those who retained CO_2 reduced the rate and extent of inspiratory muscle shortening in response to the load, which would minimize their pressure-time index and energy expenditure.

The ability of COPD patients to compensate for inspiratory loads may depend on endogenous opioids. Naloxone restored load compensation in some patients who lacked this ability[227] but not in others.[237] Naloxone also increases the ventilatory responses to hypoxia and CO_2.[228, 249] When stable COPD patients are breathing quietly without any added hypercapnic, hypoxic, or load stimulus, naloxone has little effect on tidal volume, respiratory rate, or minute ventilation.[227, 228, 249] However, in such patients the mean inspiratory flow rate increases by 30% to 40%.[228, 249] In COPD patients with acute respiratory failure, infusion of naloxone or naltrexone can lower Pa_{CO_2}.[205]

The process of weaning patients from mechanical ventilation represents a clinical experiment that also sheds light on the integrated response of the respiratory system to loading. On switching from fully supported mechanical ventilation to spontaneous breathing, tidal volume falls by about 40% to 50%, and the spontaneous respiratory rate is higher than the ventilator rate.[104, 155, 161, 255] The pattern of respiratory muscle contraction becomes asynchronous, especially when the weaning trial is unsuccessful.[56, 203, 253] The high-to-low ratio of the diaphragm EMG also falls in unsuccessful trials.[56] However, as noted previously, the fall in the EMG high-to-low ratio is a sign of incipient rather than overt fatigue, and the same is probably true for the asynchronous pattern of respiratory muscle contraction.[221, 254]

In summary, respiratory failure in COPD does not necessarily result from overt fatigue of the respiratory muscles. Physical exercise can produce overt fatigue of the sternocleidomastoid muscles, as judged by the fact that the force responses to tetanic electrical stimulation are reduced after exercising.[263] However, this does not affect the patient's ability to perform a 12-minute walk or to increase ventilation during CO_2 rebreathing. Both diaphragmatic and sternomastoid force responses to electrical stimulation are reduced in acute respiratory failure,[20, 79, 181] but these results can be explained by muscle weakness and do not necessarily imply muscle fatigue. The manifestations of acute respiratory failure, such as rapid, shallow asynchronous breathing, are most likely mediated by neural responses to the load. Respiratory muscle weakness and fatigue may well contribute to those neural responses and to the reduction in tidal volume but need not do so.[247] Increased production of endogenous opioids may play a role in modifying the pattern of breathing in acute or chronic respiratory failure, but evidence to support this hypothesis in human COPD is sketchy.

The integrated response of the respiratory system to loads has an impact on respiratory muscle function. Roussos[220] emphasized the concept that a rapid, shallow breathing pattern protects the respiratory muscles from fatigue. A smaller tidal volume is accompanied by less shortening of the inspiratory muscles, with correspondingly less encroachment on the limits of their function set by the force-length and force-velocity relationships. In effect, rapid, shallow breathing lowers the inspiratory PTI and thereby either delays the onset of overt fatigue or prevents it altogether.

TREATMENT OF RESPIRATORY MUSCLE FAILURE

If patients with COPD were able to breathe more freely, they would improve their blood-gas composition and in some cases have a greater capacity for physical exercise. Because the ability to increase minute ventilation depends on the functional capacity of the respiratory muscles, it is of interest to examine treatments that may enhance respiratory muscle strength and endurance. Five types of interventions are summarized in Table 16–3; positive responses to the first three can be expected to occur within a few days, whereas it takes weeks to months to rebuild the contractile apparatus by nutritional repletion and muscle training.

Remove Adverse Influences

The first step in restoring respiratory muscle contractility is to return the muscles to a normal environment insofar as is possible. Multiple metabolic abnormalities that adversely affect the respiratory muscles are often present in critically ill patients.[216] The depressant effects of electrolyte imbalance and deficiency states such as hypokalemia, hypocalcemia, hypophosphatemia, and hypomagnesemia are readily reversed by appropriate replacement therapy. Similarly, the depressant effects of hypoxemia and hypercapnia can be overcome by administration of oxygen and use of mechanical ventilation.

Infection causes the diaphragm to lose muscle mass.[38, 75]

TABLE 16–3. Treatment of Respiratory Muscle Failure

STAGE	THERAPEUTIC PRINCIPLE	TECHNIQUES
Acute	Restore normal environment	Correction of metabolic and blood-gas abnormalities
	Rest respiratory muscles	Intubation and mechanical ventilation and vigorous treatment of underlying lung disease, or both
	Enhance contractility pharmacologically	Aminophylline infusion, mainly for patients not receiving mechanical ventilation
Chronic	Rebuild contractile apparatus	Nutritional repletion
		Inspiratory muscle training

Both infection and endotoxic shock seriously impair diaphragmatic contractility.[38, 120, 121] Indeed, both circulatory and endotoxic shock lead to respiratory failure and arrest.[23, 120] Bronchospasm, airway inflammation, and infection exaggerate pulmonary hyperinflation and thereby put the inspiratory muscles at an even greater mechanical disadvantage. Therefore, it is essential to control infection, stabilize the circulation, and improve airway function as much as possible in order to optimize the environment in which the respiratory muscles have to work.

Respiratory Muscle Rest

The only way to restore contractility to muscles that have become overtly fatigued is to allow them to rest. In patients with COPD, this usually requires some form of mechanical ventilatory support. Conventional positive-pressure ventilation abolishes inspiratory muscle activity, provided it is used in the control mode, with the inspiratory flow rate above 1 L per second.[257] Analysis of currently available data leads to the conclusion that respiratory muscle rest is also beneficial for incipient respiratory muscle fatigue.[208] Part of the benefit may result from relief of dyspnea,[214, 215] which may in turn lead to an increase in neural drive. Circumstantial support for this hypothesis is based on studies in which removing an external inspiratory resistance from animals or providing 1 hour of negative-pressure ventilation to COPD patients led to increases in the high-to-low ratio of the diaphragm EMG power spectrum.[201, 204]

Among 12 reports about the effects of respiratory muscle rest in patients with COPD, five concern short-term application of mechanical ventilatory support, that is, for one half to several hours over one to several days. Negative-pressure ventilation in an iron lung was applied to a group of 8 COPD patients, only 2 of whom were hypercapnic. Although 1-to-1 phase locking of the patient's breathing with the ventilator cycle was readily achieved, the diaphragm EMG remained at 70% or more of the spontaneous breathing value.[219] In contrast, when the iron lung was used for seven chronically hypercapnic COPD patients, diaphragmatic electrical activity was reduced to less than 10% of the spontaneous breathing level.[215] As little as 1 hour of negative-pressure ventilation led to increases in both the EMG high-to-low ratio and maximal transdiaphragmatic pressures of seven patients with severe chronic airflow limitation.[204] In eight COPD patients, five of whom were hypercapnic, 3 to 6 hours of negative pressure ventilation increased respiratory muscle strength by 14%, approximately doubled an index of respiratory muscle endurance, and relieved dyspnea.[65] Moreover, Pa_{CO_2} in the five hypercapnic patients fell by 8 torr. No changes occurred in a control group of seven COPD patients.

Two preliminary communications describe the effects of mechanical positive-pressure ventilation by nose mask.[49, 58] A total of seven COPD patients in acute respiratory failure were studied. All benefited with regard to blood-gas composition, and in four patients recordings of esophageal pressure and diaphragmatic electrical activity documented that inspiratory muscle contractions were almost completely suppressed by mechanical positive-pressure ventilation via nose mask.

The effects of daily intermittent mechanical ventilation, 2 to 12 hours per day for 3 to 26 weeks, are summarized in Table 16–4. These results are from 42 patients, almost all of whom had COPD. Most of them were treated with negative-pressure body ventilators of either the body wrap or cuirass type. The tabulated data were calculated using the mean values from five reports.[41, 87, 143, 202, 266] Overall, daily intermittent negative-pressure ventilation produced significant ($P < 0.001$)

TABLE 16–4. Effects of Prolonged, Daily, Intermittent Mechanical Ventilation (MV) on Pa_{CO_2}, Respiratory Muscle Strength, and Ventilatory or Exercise Endurance in 42 COPD Patients*

VARIABLE	BASELINE VALUE	% CHANGE WITH MV
Pa_{CO_2} (torr)	49 ± 5	-7 ± 10
PI max (cm H_2O)	38 ± 11	29 ± 30
Endurance (%)	100	35 ± 66

*(Values are mean ± SD, calculated from mean values in references 41, 87, 143, 202, 266.)

improvement in inspiratory muscle strength, ventilatory or exercise endurance, and Pa_{CO_2}. However, in individual series the improvement was limited to reduction of dyspnea[202, 266] or to a small increase in ventilatory endurance.[87] In one series the percent increase in exercise endurance was large but the absolute gain was small, and the negative-pressure ventilation group fared no better than a control group treated with rehabilitation alone.[143]

Eight hours of negative-pressure ventilation for only 1 day a week for 4 months brought about improvements in PI max, exercise endurance time, and Pa_{CO_2} similar to the mean values in Table 16–4.[114] In this study most of the improvement had occurred by the end of the first month. Both these patients and those described by Braun and Marino[41] experienced considerable functional improvement as well.

Collectively, both the short- and long-term results of respiratory muscle rest therapy raise a series of as yet unanswered questions. One would expect that the effectiveness of respiratory muscle rest would depend on how well mechanical ventilation suppresses spontaneous inspiratory effort and on how long the treatment is applied. There is so much variability among the reported regimens that it is impossible to assess which is the most effective. It is difficult to suppress inspiratory activity by mechanically ventilating healthy subjects.[215, 218] The same may be true for eucapnic COPD patients,[219] whereas hypercapnic patients may find it easier to relax and let the ventilator do the work.[215] Most patients find it hard to get used to negative-pressure ventilation and often experience several types of distress, including musculoskeletal pain, air swallowing, thermal discomfort, and claustrophobia.[266] Nose mask positive-pressure ventilation might become a suitable alternative. Thus far, negative-pressure ventilation for patients with COPD has not had nearly the success that it has had in patients with kyphoscoliosis or neuromuscular disease.

Pharmacologic Enhancement of Respiratory Muscle Contractility

Aubier and his colleagues have shown that numerous drugs commonly used in the clinical setting can enhance or depress diaphragmatic performance.[18, 21, 22, 179, 180, 256] Effects of drugs on various aspects of diaphragmatic contractility as observed in studies of isolated, perfused diaphragm muscle or in the *in situ* animal diaphragm are summarized in Table 16–5. The effects of methylxanthines and digitalis glycosides are probably mediated through increased intracellular free calcium concentration, resulting either from enhanced release from the sarcoplasmic reticulum or from enhanced influx of extracellular calcium. The beta-adrenergic agonists may have multiple actions, and the anticholinesterases exert their effects at the neuromuscular junction.

EFFECTS IN HEALTHY VOLUNTEERS. Most experience with pharmacologic agents in humans has been with methylxanthines. Aminophylline, which is converted to theophylline in

TABLE 16–5. Actions of Drugs on Isolated, Perfused, or *In Situ* Animal Diaphragm Muscle

CATEGORY	DRUGS	EFFECTS
Methylxanthines	aminophylline theophylline caffeine	Increase force or Pdi Increase endurance Reverse fatigue, depression by CO_2, and acidosis
Beta-adrenergic agonists	isoproterenol terbutaline salbutamol	Reverse fatigue, and depression by CO_2, acidosis, or calcium-channel blocker
Digitalis glycosides	ouabain deslanoside digoxin	Increase force or Pdi Reverse fatigue
Anticholinesterase	neostigmine	Reverse fatigue, depression by CO_2, and acidosis
Beta-adrenergic antagonist	propranolol	Depress Pdi
Calcium-channel blockers	verapamil diltiazem	Depress force

the blood, has been reported to increase transdiaphragmatic pressure (Pdi) responses to spontaneously generated diaphragmatic electrical activity (Edi), with an increase in the Pdi-to-Edi ratio.[18, 244] Aminophylline also increases the twitch Pdi response to stimulation of the phrenic nerves, but enprofylline, a xanthine that does not inhibit adenosine receptors, does not.[180] Caffeine also increases the Pdi-to-Edi ratio[244] and the stimulated force output of the adductor pollicis muscle.[150]

When the diaphragm was fatigued by breathing through a severe inspiratory resistance, aminophylline restored its force response to tetanic stimulation of the phrenic nerves within 30 minutes, whereas without the drug there was no recovery during this time.[18] Caffeine had a similar effect on the adductor pollicis muscle.[150] In addition, caffeine prolonged respiratory muscle endurance time when subjects inspired against threshold loads and reduced the sense of effort during loaded breathing.[246]

In contrast to these positive results, other investigators have found that aminophylline in the usual therapeutic dose has relatively little effect on respiratory muscle function. For example, aminophylline failed to increase the twitch Pdi response to stimulation of one phrenic nerve[177] and did not enhance the tetanic force responses of the sternomastoid or adductor pollicis muscles before or after fatigue.[148, 260] Aminophylline produced a mere 2% increase in unloaded ventilatory endurance.[34] The beta-adrenergic agonist albuterol had no effect on voluntary Pdi max before or after fatigue, nor did the drug prolong endurance time for loaded breathing.[126]

RESULTS IN COPD PATIENTS. In one study of 15 COPD patients, ten received oral aminophylline for 30 days and five received placebo.[179] Prior to treatment, both groups had similar values of Pdi max during voluntary efforts. Moreover, during inspiratory resistive loaded breathing the ratio of $\bar{P}$breath-to-Pmax lay in the fatiguing range, and both groups developed electromyographic evidence of diaphragmatic fatigue. These indicators of incipient fatigue remained unchanged after placebo. However, in the patients treated with aminophylline, Pdi max increased by 16% after 7 days. Because of this, the ratio of $\bar{P}$breath-to-Pmax was lower during loaded breathing, and there was no longer any electromyographic evidence of fatigue. By way of contrast, theophylline had no effect on diaphragmatic contractility in a series of 20 ambulatory COPD patients whose FEV_1 averaged 68% predicted.[93] Specifically, the Pdi generated by maximum voluntary effort against a closed airway was unchanged from control at serum theophylline levels of 5, 12, and 19 mg per liter.

The effects of aminophylline on ventilatory endurance and capacity for physical exercise are also marginal. In six patients with moderate airflow limitation (FEV_1 = 1.8 L), PI max increased by more than 20% after aminophylline, and peak inspiratory flow rate during exercise increased by 8%.[183] There was a 12% increase in maximal oxygen consumption, a 9% increase in maximal work, and a 30-second increase in exercise duration. In patients with greater airflow limitation (FEV_1 = 0.8 L), the sustainable ventilatory capacity increased by 7% after aminophylline, from 39 to 42 L per minute.[34] For 12 COPD patients whose FEV_1 was 1.4 L (40% predicted), sustained-release theophylline reduced dyspnea but did not alter the distance they could walk in 12 minutes.[158] In six patients whose FEV_1 was 30% predicted, aminophylline increased the distance walked in 6 minutes by 6% and increased the ventilatory and mouth pressure responses to CO_2 inhalation by 20%.[60] There were no changes in PI max, PE max, or sensation of dyspnea. In all of these studies, placebo therapy was without effect on any of the variables.

Several studies concerned drugs other than methylxanthines. In one, five COPD patients recovering from acute respiratory failure were given digoxin intravenously.[22] Within 90 minutes, the twitch Pdi response to bilateral phrenic nerve stimulation increased by 20%, but there was no change in cardiac output. A second study concerned the effects of dopamine on diaphragmatic contractility.[21] The drug was infused for 30 minutes, at 10 μg/kg body weight per minute into eight COPD patients who were receiving mechanical ventilation for acute respiratory failure. Cardiac output increased by 40%, and diaphragmatic blood flow increased by 30%. The Pdi twitch response to bilateral phrenic nerve stimulation averaged 5 cm H_2O prior to dopamine and 7 cm H_2O on dopamine ($P < 0.001$). Enhancement of the Pdi twitch response lasted only as long as the infusion and was attributed to the increase in diaphragmatic blood flow. In ten ambulatory COPD patients, oral terbutaline produced a small but statistically insignificant increase in PI max as compared with placebo.[243]

INTERPRETATION AND RECOMMENDATION. Methylxanthines, digitalis glycosides, and beta-adrenergic agonists exert small and inconsistent effects on human respiratory muscles when the drugs are given in nontoxic, therapeutic doses. The effects on muscle strength are at most about 15%. Perhaps the effects on delaying the onset of fatigue or reversing it would be of greater clinical relevance. However, as indicated in the section Dyspnea, Fatigue, and Respiratory Failure, the spontaneous pattern of breathing changes so as to minimize fatigue.

There is at least circumstantial evidence that the best results of pharmacologic intervention would be obtained in the presence of acute or chronic respiratory failure. All of the reports that show minimal or no effects of drugs are either about healthy subjects or COPD patients who are eucapnic. The two studies with the most positive results were in COPD patients who had chronic hypercapnia[179] or who were studied within 48 hours of their admission for acute respiratory failure.[22] In animal studies, aminophylline and neostigmine reversed the depressant effects of hypercapnia.[118] In dogs subjected to severe inspiratory resistive loads, the onset of diaphragmatic fatigue and acute respiratory failure with hypoxemia, hypercapnia, and acidosis was postponed by 4 minutes, a 36% increase in endurance.[256] When aminophylline was given in the recovery period, it, but not oxygen, restored diaphragmatic contractile responses to phrenic nerve stimulation.

Aminophylline has multiple actions, including enhancement of ventilatory drive and bronchodilation. Its toxicity is well recognized, and although side effects produce considerable distress, there is a wide margin of safety before dangerously toxic levels are achieved. The drug is also relatively inexpensive. Therefore, it seems reasonable to give a patient a trial of aminophylline. The end points in clinical practice will have to be simple assessments of endurance, such as walk distance, and subjective evaluation of dyspnea. All studies of aminophylline effects in COPD patients are in agreement on the absence of any meaningful changes in spirometric evaluation of pulmonary function. A similar statement can be made about beta-adrenergic agonists, and these agents are less effective at reversing the depressant effects of hypercapnia. At the present time experience with digoxin is limited. Its therapeutic range is narrow, and its toxicity is potentially dangerous. Therefore, this drug should be used with caution as a treatment for respiratory muscle dysfunction.

Nutritional Repletion

Underweight patients with and without COPD generally have less diaphragm muscle mass.[12, 15, 251] Underweight patients also have lower values of PI max and PE max,[13, 147, 192] although the differences between normal weight and underweight COPD patients are not always statistically significant.[192] Moreover, patients with COPD have a resting energy expenditure that is 15% to 60% higher than in healthy subjects or underweight patients without COPD.[109, 110, 192, 262] Thus, it is of interest to consider the effects of nutritional repletion on respiratory muscle strength and endurance.

Kelly and colleagues[131] showed that the inspiratory muscle strength of critically ill patients correlated with their body cell mass, as estimated from measurement of total body potassium. Of the 29 patients who received parenteral hyperalimentation for several weeks, 21 improved and eight worsened, probably because their underlying disease was not controlled. The 21 who improved had a 37% increase in PI max and a 12% increase in body cell mass.

Nutritional repletion appears to facilitate weaning from mechanical ventilation. Data from 70 patients studied retrospectively show that weaning trials were successful in 89% of the 25 patients given adequate nutritional support, as compared with 48% of 42 patients who did not receive nutritional support.[25, 166] This difference is highly significant ($P < 0.001$). However, the retrospective nature of the studies and lack of information about severity of lung disease and complications that could have influenced the outcome indicate that these results must be interpreted with caution. Regimens that provide an excess of carbohydrate calories can lead to respiratory failure, especially during weaning trials.[62, 66] To prevent this complication, the total caloric intake should not exceed 10% to 20% above the resting energy expenditure.[259]

Ambulatory COPD patients generally tolerate diets containing up to 300 g of carbohydrate quite well. A single meal containing 170 g of carbohydrate and 920 kcal caused CO_2 production to increase by 30% and raised minute ventilation by 14% to 24%.[43, 102] The Pa_{CO_2} was unchanged, even in hypercapnic patients,[102] but the 12-minute walk distance fell by about 5%.[43] Feeding diets containing 125 to 350 g of carbohydrate and 1800 to 2000 calories for 5 days also had small effects.[9] On a low-carbohydrate, high-fat regimen, the CO_2 production was 20% lower than baseline, and 10% lower than on a high-carbohydrate, low-fat regimen. Baseline Pa_{CO_2} averaged 49 torr, and was only 2 torr lower on the 125-g carbohydrate diet. In contrast, dietary composition had a greater effect on COPD patients whose baseline Pa_{CO_2} averaged 57 torr.[137] The baseline carbohydrate intake was about 300 g, and total caloric intake remained at 2000 kcal per day throughout the study. Cutting the daily carbohydrate to 200 g for a week, then to 50 g for a week, led to reductions in Pa_{CO_2} of 6 to 9 torr. The Pa_{CO_2} increased from 51 to 62 torr, and all patients felt subjectively better.

The effects of nutritional repletion on respiratory muscle strength and endurance have been examined in five studies involving 58 ambulatory COPD patients.[78, 110, 136, 147, 262] Their body weights averaged 82% of ideal, their FEV_1 was 34% predicted, and their PI max was -48 cm H_2O. The duration of nutritional supplementation ranged from 2 to 3 weeks[110, 262] to 2 to 3 months.[78, 136, 147]

On average, PI max increased by 6 cm H_2O (13%) for all patients. Statistically insignificant changes of -3 to $+11\%$ were seen when caloric intake exceeded baseline by only 15% to 20%.[136, 147] When caloric intake was set at 40% to 70% above the baseline level, there was a 13% to 43% increase in PI max, averaging 11 cm H_2O.[78, 110, 262] In these studies, the strength and endurance of limb skeletal muscles also improved with nutritional repletion, which amounted to about 50 kcal/kg per day. Efthimiou and colleagues[78] pointed out that when patients resumed their baseline diet, all the gains attained during the period of dietary supplementation were lost.

In summary, it seems clear that nutritional repletion can improve skeletal and respiratory muscle function in ambulatory COPD patients, provided that the level of nutritional supplementation is high enough. The available data indicate that benefits can be attained when caloric intake is increased by 40% to 50% above baseline but not when the increase is 20% or less.

Excessive carbohydrate feeding can be dangerous, especially for patients susceptible to acute respiratory failure. However, when an appropriate total caloric intake is prescribed and the proportion of carbohydrate calories is reduced, these problems are overcome without difficulty. Supplements that are high in fat and low in carbohydrate are effective but expensive. It seems likely that most ambulatory COPD patients can benefit from nutritional repletion when daily caloric intake is adjusted to approximately 50 kcal/kg of baseline body weight, with protein and carbohydrate components of the regimen accounting for about 15% and 45% of the calories, respectively.

Respiratory Muscle Training

TECHNIQUES. Physical exercise training programs can increase maximal voluntary ventilation (MVV) in COPD patients by about 10%.[217] Although Belman and Kendregan[31] reported that physical training is without effect on the maximal sustainable ventilatory capacity (MSVC), a reanalysis of their data indicates that arm or leg cycle ergometer exercise for 6 weeks can in fact increase MSVC by about 10%, which is statistically significant ($P < 0.02$). Training increased the exercise endurance capacity of these COPD patients by about 70%. In patients with cystic fibrosis, exercise training (swimming and canoeing) for 6 weeks increased MSVC by 53%, without affecting MVV or maximal exercise oxygen consumption.[130]

Breathing exercises of the traditional type focus on increasing diaphragmatic and abdominal excursion, synchronization of rib cage and abdominal motion, and relaxation of the neck inspiratory muscles. One study focused on a combination of physical exercise training for 9 weeks in the control patients and the same regimen plus breathing retraining for the last 3 weeks in the test group.[50] Both groups increased their maximal oxygen consumption by about 50% in the first 6 weeks. At the end of 9 weeks the breathing retraining group had increased their maximal oxygen consumption by 50% above the 6-week level, whereas in the control group the increase was only 10%. The pattern of breathing during exercise was also modified by breathing retraining, with a lower respiratory rate and a larger tidal volume.

Some forms of respiratory muscle training augment respiratory muscle strength. Practicing maximal inspiratory and expiratory efforts for several weeks increased PI max by 50% and PE max by 37% in a group of patients with COPD, healed tuberculosis and pneumoconiosis.[142] Diaphragmatic breathing exercises elevated the Pdi recorded at TLC by 30% ($P < 0.05$), whereas abdominal breathing exercises had no significant effect.[122] Daily performance of 10 PE max maneuvers for 1 month, combined with inspiratory resistive training for 30 minutes a day, raised PE max by 41%.[6] However, there were no changes in spirometric test results, blood-gas composition, or 12-minute walk distance.

Training for inspiratory muscle endurance can be carried out in two ways. The first involves daily voluntary hyperventilation, usually at the level of the maximal sustainable ventilatory capacity (MSVC). To prevent lowering the Pa_{CO_2}, the subject may rebreathe through a dead space, but most studies have been carried out using a system that allows for enough supplemental oxygen to prevent hypoxemia while at the same time keeping Pa_{CO_2} constant.

The second type of training regimen involves inspiring against a load. In most cases the load is of the flow-resistive type. The magnitude of the resistance may be fixed or variable. In many applications the resistive load is simply an orifice. By decreasing the caliber of the orifice, the magnitude of the inspiratory effort can be increased. A major problem with flow-resistive devices is that the inspiratory pressure needed to breathe varies greatly with the pattern of breathing.[35] By inspiring slowly, a subject can take in a given tidal volume through a small orifice using a lower inspiratory pressure than would be required for a high inspiratory flow rate through a larger orifice. It is critically important for the subject to use a constant pattern of breathing, and in most studies this variable has not been assessed.

In the other inspiratory loading technique, the applied load is the threshold type. To initiate inspiration, the subject must exert a level of inspiratory pressure that depends on the magnitude of the threshold load. For the remainder of inspiration, inspiratory pressure remains constant and is independent of the inspiratory flow rate. The pattern of breathing is also important with inspiratory threshold loading, because for a given load, a tidal volume may be inspired rapidly or slowly. The magnitude of the inspiratory pressure is the same in either case, but its duration is shorter with a high inspiratory flow rate. Thus, the PTI, which is probably the most important training variable, could change widely from rapid to slow inspiration of a constant tidal volume.

EFFECTS OF MAXIMAL SUSTAINABLE VENTILATORY CAPACITY TRAINING. In four cystic fibrosis patients who trained at their maximal sustainable ventilatory capacity (MSVC) for 25 minutes daily, 5 days a week for 6 weeks, the MSVC increased by 52%, compared with 22% in four healthy control subjects.[130] A similar regimen applied to six COPD patients for a month led to an average 23% improvement in MSVC, with four patients having improvements at 17% to 64%, and two not improving at all.[198] Untrained COPD control subjects had no change in MSVC over a month.

A regimen of 30 minutes of training daily for 6 weeks led to a 31% increase in MSVC, a 19% increase in MSVC normalized to FEV_1, and a 12% increase in MVV.[32] In these ten patients, maximal exercise ventilation also increased by 12%, as did their 12-minute walk distance. Endurance time for submaximal cycle ergometry exercise increased by 54% (leg) and 82% (arm). Levine and colleagues[145] conducted a controlled study in which 15 COPD patients underwent an MSVC training regimen, and 17 patients used intermittent positive-pressure breathing (IPPB) as placebo therapy. The MSVC of the MSVC trainers improved by 41% ($P < 0.001$), whereas in the IPPB group the 18% rise in MSVC was not statistically significant. Yet both groups increased their physical exercise capacity, by 8% for 12-minute walk distance, 15% for stair climbing, and 58% endurance time for a submaximal bicycle legometer test. Both groups also experienced improvement with regard to psychologic status and ability to perform activities of daily living.

EFFECTS OF INSPIRATORY RESISTIVE TRAINING. A group of 11 patients with cystic fibrosis received inspiratory resistive training (IRT) for 15 minutes twice daily, over 4 weeks.[16] One half of the subjects went through a 4-week control period followed by training, and the other half went through the reverse sequence. Training increased PI max by 7 cm H_2O (9%). The highest load the patients could tolerate also increased. Maximal exercise oxygen consumption did not change, but endurance time for submaximal exercise improved by 31%.

When using the IRT device acutely, COPD patients raise their tidal volume but lower their respiratory rate so that minute ventilation falls by about 15%. This results in a small increase in end-tidal P_{CO_2} and a small decrease in arterial oxyhemoglobin saturation.[127] This breathing pattern was not modified by training even though the patients could tolerate a smaller orifice. This finding represents failure to compensate for the load, but it does not necessarily mean that IRT has no benefit on inspiratory muscle strength and endurance.

Three uncontrolled studies involving a total of 20 COPD patients examined the effects of IRT 30 minutes a day for 3 to 8 weeks.[7,127,195] Their FEV_1 was approximately 30% to 35% predicted. After training, nearly all patients were able to tolerate a higher resistive load (smaller orifice), and many experienced less dyspnea. In the study by Pardy and colleagues,[195] patients who developed incipient diaphragmatic fatigue, as manifest by a fall in EMG high-to-low ratio, on cycle ergometer exercise prior to training, did not do so after 8 weeks of IRT. Moreover, their submaximal exercise endurance time and maximal exercise oxygen consumption increased by 88% and 32%, respectively. Results after 8 weeks of IRT were almost always better than after 4 weeks.[7,195]

A large series of COPD patients underwent daily IRT for 3 months.[8] The subset of 51 eucapnic patients whose FEV_1 averaged 0.75 L increased their steady-state exercise time by 65%. The subset of 14 hypercapnic patients whose FEV_1 was 0.55 L doubled their 12-minute walk distance, and their Pa_{CO_2} fell from 56 to 51 torr.

Two studies examined the effects of physical exercise training and IRT. In the first, the protocol involved a 6-week period of adaptation without training, followed by a 6-week period of physical exercise training in the form of climbing stairs 45 minutes per day.[157] In the last 6-week period, physical training was discontinued and IRT for 30 minutes a day was instituted. The ten participating COPD patients, whose FEV_1 was 0.85 L, showed modest improvement during the control adaptation period. With physical exercise training, they increased their maximal oxygen consumption, stair-climbing ability, and 12-minute walk distance by 10%, 11%, and 19%, respectively. However, these indices of exercise performance declined by 6% to 10% during the period of IRT, even though the patients could tolerate a higher resistive load after IRT.

In the second study, over 60 COPD patients underwent a rehabilitation program that involved simultaneous physical exercise training and IRT for 10 weeks.[264] The maximum tolerable steady-state workload increased by 14%. Exercise endurance times while inhaling air and oxygen increased by 57% and 98%, respectively, and the 12-minute walk distance increased by 51% and 72%, respectively. Their PI max improved by 14 cm H_2O, or, 37%. The patients were grouped into four categories based on their FEV_1 values, which ranged from less than 0.6 to greater than 1.8 L. Improvements in exercise performance and PI max were equally distributed among the four groups.

A number of reports compare training with an inspiratory load to sham training, or to training at two levels of load or physical exercise. In all of the studies, the patients had severe, irreversible airway obstruction, with the FEV_1 lying between 25% and 42% predicted. The duration of training, which was completed by all patients, ranged from 1 to 3 months. Exercise endurance time rose by 60% in 12 patients who used IRT for 3 months.[83] After training, these patients were less dyspneic, and their respiratory rates were lower. The 15 patients who sham trained increased exercise endurance time by 22% but had no changes in breathing pattern or dyspnea. A group of six patients who used IRT for 6 weeks had significant improvement in their inspiratory muscle endurance, maximal oxygen consumption, work rate, exercise ventilation, and MVV, whereas four sham-trained patients had no change in exercise performance.[240] A group of nine patients who underwent IRT 30 minutes a day for 4 weeks raised their steady-state exercise endurance time by 65% and their 12-minute walk distance by 13%, whereas 8 patients undergoing physical exercise training had insignificant results in these performance measures.[194]

Training with a single-orifice IRT, which was connected to a feedback device in order to monitor and control the pattern of breathing and inspiratory pressure, was tested at low and high intensity in 17 patients.[33] The respiratory rate was 12.5 per minute, and the duty cycle was 0.44. With this pattern and the selected orifice, the end-tidal CO_2 concentration remained nearly constant. Low-intensity trainees developed a $\overline{P}$breath that was about 12% to 16% of their PI max. High-intensity trainees increased the pressure target throughout the study, so that their $\overline{P}$breath generally reached 50% of their PI max. After training, both groups increased the PI max and $\overline{P}$breath attained during their timed resistive breathing endurance tests, but the elevations were relatively small in the low-intensity group, whereas they averaged 30% in the high-intensity group. Moreover, the high-intensity group also had significant increases of about 15% in their MSVC and peak inspiratory flow rates. Exercise performance after IRT was not tested.

Larson and colleagues[139] assessed the effects of inspiratory threshold loading, 30 minutes daily for 8 weeks, at two different loads. The ten patients who trained with an inspiratory load equal to 30% of their PI max had a 20% increase in their PI max, an 8% rise in their 12-minute walk distance, and an 81% increase in steady-state exercise endurance time. In contrast, the 12 patients whose training loads were 15% of PI max had smaller and statistically insignificant results in their performances.

Three reports compare the results of IRT with sham training in patients who were concomitantly undergoing physical exercise training. In two of these,[36, 170] all 46 patients improved their exercise performance to a modest degree, as judged by maximal workload or stair-climbing ability. However, there were no differences between groups. Both control subjects and trained patients increased their PI max slightly,[170] whereas only the IRT patients were able to tolerate a higher resistive load.[36] In the third study of this type, the seven patients in the IRT group improved their exercise endurance time by 69%, and their sustainable inspiratory pressure, a measure of inspiratory muscle endurance, increased by 59% even though PI max improved only slightly.[52] The six sham-trained patients had no improvement in any of these variables.

Inspiratory muscle training has also been used in acute respiratory failure. Two COPD patients utilized MSVC training to improve their MSVC from 14 to 24 and 22 to 29 L per minute, respectively.[30] Aldrich and colleagues[3] treated 27 patients on mechanical ventilation with IRT for 5 weeks. Prior to training, their ventilatory endurance averaged 6.4 hours. After training, 12 patients whose PI max increased by 15 cm H_2O (38%) were successfully weaned from mechanical ventilation, whereas patients whose PI max increased less than 10% could not be weaned.

SUMMARY AND RECOMMENDATIONS. The results of controlled studies of inspiratory muscle training (IMT) in COPD are summarized in Table 16–6. For the most part, control represents sham training, but in one instance it is physical exercise instead of MSVC training, and in two instances it is a low- instead of a high-intensity load. The data in the table were calculated from published mean values for trained and control groups. Baseline values for each variable were similar in the two groups, averaging 40 ± 15 L/min for MSVC, 5.7 ± 2.4 minutes for steady-state exercise endurance time, −59 ± 8 cm H_2O for PI max, and 783 ± 51 meters for 12-minute walk distance.

Inspiratory resistive load training almost always increases the severity of the resistance that can be tolerated, whereas sham training has no effect on the tolerable resistance level. Inspiratory load training increases PI max by 15% (10 cm H_2O), as compared with 8% (5 cm H_2O) in the control subjects (see Table 16–6). When results of a large, uncontrolled study are added,[264] PI max of 95 patients increased with IMT by 12 cm H_2O or 30% above baseline. However, the baseline value in the uncontrolled study was only 38 cm H_2O, and the training regimen also included physical exercise.

Training increases the MSVC and also increases steady-state exercise endurance time. Adding results of uncontrolled studies to the controlled ones has only small effects on baseline values or on the percent change of either variable with IMT. A relatively large number of patients have had their steady-state exercise time tested in a controlled fashion, so it seems clear that IMT really does improve this variable. However, only a few patients have undergone MSVC training with an appropriate control regimen. Even when uncontrolled studies are added, results are available from only 31 experimental patients and 21 control patients.

In controlled studies, IMT has no significant effect on the distance walked in 12 minutes (see Table 16–6), but when results of two large uncontrolled studies are added,[8, 264] the 12-minute walk distance is elevated by 38%. However, the baseline values range from 125 to over 6000 meters, far outside the range of values in the controlled studies.

The practical value of inspiratory muscle training is not yet established with certainty. Training with resistive or threshold loads does improve inspiratory muscle strength and endurance, but more experiments are needed in which the pattern of breathing and the magnitude of the training load are carefully controlled. The duration of inspiration should probably be 40% to 50% of the total breath time (duty cycle 0.4 to 0.5), and the inspiratory load should probably lie between 30% and 50% of PI max. Thus, the training PTI would lie between 0.12 and 0.25. With 30 minutes of training per day, benefits after 2 months are generally greater than after 1 month. Therefore, it would be worthwhile to explore the effects of a longer period of training earlier on, perhaps 1 hour per day in divided intervals.

In these experiments, there should be a control group that undergoes sham training using an identical pattern of breathing without added load. Patients in the test and control groups should be matched as closely as possible for age, sex, nutri-

TABLE 16–6. Effects of Inspiratory Muscle Training (IMT) Versus a Control Regimen in COPD Patients*

	IMT			CONTROL			
VARIABLE	N	X	SD	N	X	SD	P
PI max†	35	15	10	34	8	5	<0.001
MSVC	29	30	12	30	10	9	<0.001
SSEET	58	72	25	60	24	14	<0.001
12MWD	42	7	6	45	5	3	NS

*Data are calculated from mean values in various published reports, and expressed as percent change from baseline values in each group.
†PI max = maximal inspiratory pressure against closed airway; MSVC = maximal sustainable ventilatory capacity; SSEET = steady-state exercise endurance time; 12MWD = 12-minute walk distance.

tional status, degree of airflow limitation, and extent of hyperinflation. More work is also needed with MSVC training, mainly to enroll adequate numbers of patients, matched as described previously.

In all of these studies, there should also be some attempt to standardize the output variables. Quantitative dyspnea scores, performance on 12-minute walk, and capacity for activities of daily living may have more practical clinical value than performance of steady-state bicycle exercise. If the last is used, the workload should be standardized at approximately two thirds of the maximal workload.

CONCLUSION

Chronic obstructive pulmonary disease places great demands on the respiratory muscles, while at the same time the mechanical, nutritional, and metabolic consequences of the disease make it difficult for the respiratory muscles to perform extra work. Weight loss, muscle wasting, electrolyte imbalance, hypophosphatemia and other deficiency states, infection, and abnormal blood-gas composition are relatively common complications in COPD and respiratory failure.

Even when the respiratory muscles are not particularly affected by metabolic disturbances, they still must work at a mechanical disadvantage. Acute hyperinflation shortens the inspiratory muscles, which reduces their maximal force output. This may be offset by the adaptive process of losing sarcomeres so that remaining sarcomeres are of normal length. However, shortening of the diaphragm means that its capacity to contribute to inspired volume is diminished, even if its maximal force output is restored to normal. Moreover, with acute bronchospasm or bronchitis, the lungs become acutely inflated beyond the baseline level, which negates some of the advantage due to sarcomere adaptation. Alterations in linkages among inspiratory muscles and in the shape of the diaphragm also occur with acute or chronic hyperinflation. These combine to reduce the effective inspiratory pressure even if neural drive increases and sarcomere adaptation occurs.

The pressure developed by maximal voluntary inspiratory effort against a closed airway (PI max) is almost always reduced in COPD. In the absence of generalized muscle weakness, PI max is about 70% of normal. The pressure developed by maximal expiratory effort (PE max) is often normal but tends to be lower in severely hyperinflated patients. When generalized muscle weakness is present, both PI max and PE max are further reduced.

The endurance of the respiratory muscles is variable. Maximal sustainable ventilatory capacity (MSVC), expressed as a fraction of maximal voluntary ventilation (MVV), is generally higher in COPD patients than in healthy individuals. Patients with COPD develop evidence of inspiratory muscle fatigue at the same PTI that fatigues healthy subjects. However, the capacity to sustain added inspiratory pressure loads may be below normal in COPD.

The pattern of breathing in COPD has a major effect on respiratory muscle endurance. By decreasing the tidal volume, the inspiratory muscles are not required to shorten as much, thus reducing the ratio of $\overline{P}$breath-to-Pmax. Increasing the respiratory rate might cause the inspiratory muscles to shorten more rapidly, but available evidence suggests that mean inspiratory flow rates are not raised, except in conditions leading to acute respiratory failure. Thus, rapid, shallow breathing should be considered an adaptive mechanism that tends to minimize dyspnea and the chance for developing overt fatigue of the inspiratory muscles. The disadvantage of this strategy is that small tidal volumes predispose the patient to hypercapnia and hypoxemia.

Respiratory muscle dysfunction in COPD is clearly associated with dyspnea and respiratory failure. These phenomena represent a complex set of interactions between central neural control of breathing and muscle weakness. In some cases, overt respiratory muscle fatigue may occur, but it seems likely that most of the time the inspiratory muscles do not become overtly fatigued. When complications that predispose to acute respiratory failure occur, the inspiratory muscles are often put into a fatiguing pattern of contraction, as manifest by pressure-time indices above the critical level, redistributions of power in the electromyogram from higher to lower frequencies, and asynchronous movements of rib cage and abdomen. However, even when the respiratory muscles are in a fatiguing pattern of contraction, overt fatigue does not occur immediately. When overt fatigue does occur, it probably reflects a combination of inadequate neural drive (central fatigue), impaired function of the nerves or neuromuscular junction (transmission fatigue), and fatigue processes operating at the level of the muscle cell.

Treatment of acute respiratory muscle failure is based on several principles. The burden on the respiratory muscles must be reduced. In some cases it is sufficient to treat bronchospasm, infection, edema, or other factors that increase the work of breathing. At other times, it is necessary to put the respiratory muscles to rest, using some form of mechanical ventilation. Conditions such as hypoxemia, acidosis, electrolyte imbalance, deficiency states, and infection adversely affect the environment of the muscle, and these must be corrected. Pharmacologic enhancement of respiratory muscle contractility may be of value, perhaps mainly in the presence of hypercapnic respiratory failure. Aminophylline (theophylline) appears to be the drug of choice, but clear-cut demonstration of its efficiency remains to be established. In the absence of hypercapnic respiratory failure, the effects of aminophylline and beta-sympathetic agonists appear to be minimal.

For long-term enhancement of respiratory muscle contractility, two approaches are promising. Nutritional repletion increases respiratory muscle strength provided that an adequate level of support can be provided. Taking nutritional supplements often causes patients to reduce their regular diet, and in any case it is often hard for patients to comply with the regimen. More work is needed to define the lowest level of nutritional repletion that would be effective. Because COPD patients have a high resting energy expenditure, they need to sustain the nutritional repletion program indefinitely in order to preserve its benefits.

Inspiratory muscle training can increase strength and endurance, but effects on dyspnea and capacity for physical exercise are less clear cut. Several issues need more careful investigation. The optimal pattern of breathing and the optimal type and magnitude of the training load must be defined. We still need criteria to decide which COPD patients should be trained. Preliminary evidence supports the concept that training may even be of value in acute respiratory failure. For stable, ambulatory patients, training probably improves physical exercise capacity only in those whose exercise capacity is limited by inspiratory muscle fatigue.

Therapeutic modification of the breathing pattern may be helpful in patients who have excessive use of the neck inspiratory and abdominal muscles and lack of coordination between rib cage and abdominal excursions. However, attempts to breathe deeply and slowly can put the respiratory muscles into a fatiguing pattern of contraction.

Despite uncertainty about the value of individual measures, treatment directed at restoring respiratory muscle strength and endurance does appear to facilitate weaning from mechanical ventilation and recovery from respiratory failure. Because the performance of the air pump is more susceptible to therapeutic interventions than function of the lungs, it is important to apply all reasonable measures to enhance respiratory muscle contractility in COPD.

REFERENCES

1. Adams JM, Farkas GA, Rochester DF. Vagal afferents, diaphragm fatigue and inspiratory resistance in the anesthetized dog. J Appl Physiol 1988; 64:2279–2286.
2. Aldrich TK, Arora NS, Rochester DF. The influence of airway obstruction and respiratory muscle strength on maximal voluntary ventilation in lung disease. Am Rev Respir Dis 1982; 126:195–199.
3. Aldrich TK, Karpel JP, Uhrlass RM, et al. Weaning from mechanical ventilation: adjunctive use of inspiratory muscle training. Crit Care Med 1989; 17:143–147.
4. Altose MD. Assessment and management of breathlessness. Chest 1985; 88:775–825.
5. Altose MD, McCauley WC, Kelsen SG, Cherniack NS. Effects of hypercapnia and inspiratory flow-resistive loading on respiratory activity in chronic airways obstruction. J Clin Invest 1977; 59:500–507.
6. Ambrosino N, Paggiaro PL, Roselli MG, Contini V. Failure of resistive breathing training to improve pulmonary function tests in patients with chronic obstructive pulmonary disease. Respiration 1984; 45:455–459.
7. Andersen JB, Dragsted L, Kann T, et al. Resistive breathing training in severe chronic obstructive pulmonary disease: a pilot study. Scand J Respir Dis 1979; 60:151–156.
8. Andersen JB, Falk P. Clinical experience with inspiratory resistive breathing training. Int Rehab Med 1984; 6:183–185.
9. Angelillo VA, Sukhdarsham B, Durfee D, et al. Effects of low and high carbohydrate feedings in ambulatory patients with chronic obstructive pulmonary disease and chronic hypercapnia. Ann Intern Med 1985; 103:883–885.
10. Arnold JS, Thomas AJ, Kelsen SG. Length-tension relationship of abdominal expiratory muscles: effect of emphysema. J Appl Physiol 1987; 62:739–745.
11. Arnold JS, Thomas AJ, Kelsen SG. Contractile properties of expiratory abdominal muscles: effect of elastase-induced emphysema. J Appl Physiol 1987; 62:2314–2319.
12. Arora NS, Rochester DF. Effect of body weight and muscularity on human diaphragm muscle mass, thickness, and area. J Appl Physiol 1982; 52:64–70.
13. Arora NS, Rochester DF. Respiratory muscle strength and maximal voluntary ventilation in undernourished patients. Am Rev Respir Dis 1982; 126:5–8.
14. Arora NS, Rochester DF. Effect of chronic airflow limitation (CAL) on sternocleidomastoid muscle thickness. Chest 1984; 85:58S–59S.
15. Arora NS, Rochester DF. COPD and human diaphragm muscle dimensions. Chest 1987; 91:719–724.
16. Asher MI, Pardy RL, Coates AL, et al. The effects of inspiratory muscle training in patients with cystic fibrosis. Am Rev Respir Dis 1982; 126:855–859.
17. Ashutosh K, Gilbert R, Auchincloss JH Jr, Peppi D. Asynchronous breathing movements in patients with chronic obstructive pulmonary disease. Chest 1975; 67:553–557.
18. Aubier M, DeTroyer A, Sampson M, et al. Aminophylline improves diaphragmatic contractility. N Engl J Med 1981; 305:249–252.
19. Aubier M, Murciano D, Fournier M, et al. Central respiratory drive in acute respiratory failure of patients with chronic obstructive pulmonary disease. Am Rev Respir Dis 1980; 122:191–199.
20. Aubier M, Murciano D, Lecocguic Y, et al. Effect of hypophosphatemia on diaphragmatic contractility in patients with acute respiratory failure. N Engl J Med 1985; 313:420–424.
21. Aubier M, Murciano D, Menu Y, et al. Dopamine effects on diaphragmatic strength during acute respiratory failure in chronic obstructive pulmonary disease. Ann Intern Med 1989; 110:17–23.
22. Aubier M, Murciano D, Viires N, et al. Effects of digoxin on diaphragmatic strength generation in patients with chronic obstructive pulmonary disease during acute respiratory failure. Am Rev Respir Dis 1987; 135:544–548.
23. Aubier M, Trippenbach T, Roussos C. Respiratory muscle fatigue during cardiogenic shock. J Appl Physiol 1981; 51:499–508.
24. Baracos V, Rodemann HP, Dinarello CA, Goldberg AL. Stimulation of muscle protein degradation and prostaglandin E_2 release by leucocyte pyrogen (Interleukin-1). N Engl J Med 1983; 308:553–558.
25. Bassili HR, Deitel M. Effect of nutritional support on weaning patients off mechanical ventilators. JPEN 1981; 5:161–163.
26. Bellemare F, Bigland-Ritchie B. Assessment of human diaphragm strength and activation using phrenic nerve stimulation. Respir Physiol 1984; 58:263–277.
27. Bellemare F, Bigland-Ritchie B. Central components of diaphragmatic fatigue assessed by phrenic nerve stimulation. J Appl Physiol 1987; 62:1307–1316.
28. Bellemare F, Grassino A. Effect of pressure and timing of contraction on human diaphragm fatigue. J Appl Physiol 1982; 53:1190–1195.
29. Bellemare F, Grassino A. Force reserve of the diaphragm in COPD patients. J Appl Physiol 1983; 55:8–15.
30. Belman MJ. Respiratory failure treated by ventilatory muscle training (VMT): a report of two cases. Eur J Respir Dis 1981; 62:391–395.
31. Belman MJ, Kendregan BA. Exercise training fails to increase skeletal muscle enzymes in subjects with chronic obstructive pulmonary disease. Am Rev Respir Dis 1981; 123:256–261.
32. Belman MJ, Mittman C. Ventilatory muscle training improves exercise capacity in chronic obstructive pulmonary disease patients. Am Rev Respir Dis 1980; 121:273–280.
33. Belman MJ, Shadmehr R. Targeted resistive ventilatory muscle training in chronic obstructive pulmonary disease. J Appl Physiol 1988; 65:2726–2735.
34. Belman MJ, Sieck GC, Mazar A. Aminophylline and its influence on ventilatory endurance in humans. Am Rev Respir Dis 1985; 131:226–229.
35. Belman MJ, Thomas SG, Lewis MI. Resistive breathing training in patients with chronic obstructive pulmonary disease. Chest 1986; 9:662–669.
36. Bjerre-Jepsen K, Secher NH, Kok-Jenson A. Inspiratory resistance training in severe chronic obstructive pulmonary disease. Eur J Respir Dis 1981; 61:405–411.
37. Black LF, Hyatt RE. Maximal respiratory pressures: normal values and relationship to age and sex. Am Rev Respir Dis 1969; 99:696–702.
38. Boczkowski J, Dureuil B, Branger C, et al. Effects of sepsis on diaphragmatic function in rats. Am Rev Respir Dis 1988; 138:260–265.
39. Braun NMT, Arora NS, Rochester DF. Force-length relation of the normal human diaphragm. J Appl Physiol 1982; 53:405–412.

40. Braun NMT, Arora NS, Rochester DF. Respiratory muscle and pulmonary function in polymyositis and other proximal myopathies. Thorax 1983; 38:616–623.
41. Braun NMT, Marino WD. Effect of daily intermittent rest of respiratory muscles in patients with severe chronic airflow limitation (CAL). Chest 1984; 85:59S–60S.
42. Brennan NJ, Morris AJR, Green M. Thoracoabdominal mechanics during tidal breathing in normal subjects and in emphysema and fibrosing alveolitis. Thorax 1983; 38:62–66.
43. Brown SE, Nagendran RC, McHugh JW, et al. Effects of a large carbohydrate load on walking performance in chronic air-flow obstruction. Am Rev Respir Dis 1985; 132:960–962.
44. Burki NK. Breathlessness and mouth occlusion pressure in patients with chronic obstruction of the airways. Chest 1979; 76:527–531.
45. Butler C. Diaphragmatic changes in emphysema. Am Rev Respir Dis 1976; 114:155–159.
46. Bye PTP, Esau SA, Levy RD, et al. Ventilatory muscle function during exercise in air and oxygen in patients with chronic air-flow limitation. Am Rev Respir Dis 1985; 132:236–240.
47. Byrd RB, Hyatt RE. Maximal respiratory pressures in chronic obstructive lung disease. Am Rev Respir Dis 1968; 98:848–856.
48. Campbell JA, Hughes RL, Sahgal V, et al. Alterations in intercostal muscle morphology and biochemistry in patients with obstructive lung disease. Am Rev Respir Dis 1980; 122:679–686.
49. Carrey Z, Gottfried SB, Petrof B, Levy RD. Cycling nasal ventilation in respiratory failure [abstract]. Chest 1988; 94:42S.
50. Casciari RJ, Fairshter RD, Harrison A, et al. Effects of breathing retraining in patients with chronic obstructive pulmonary disease. Chest 1981; 79:393–398.
51. Celli BR, Rassulo J, Make BJ. Dyssynchronous breathing during arm but not leg exercise in patients with chronic airflow obstruction. N Engl J Med 1986; 314:1485–1490.
52. Chen H-I, Dukes R, Martin BJ. Inspiratory muscle training in patients with chronic obstructive pulmonary disease. Am Rev Respir Dis 1985; 131:251–255.
53. Cherniack RM. The oxygen consumption and efficiency of the respiratory muscles in health and emphysema. J Clin Invest 1959; 38:494–499.
54. Citterio G, Agostoni E, Del Santo A, Marazzini L. Decay of inspiratory muscle activity in chronic airway obstruction. J Appl Physiol 1981; 51:1388–1397.
55. Clark TJH, Freedman S, Campbell EJM, Winn RR. The ventilatory capacity of patients with chronic airways obstruction. Clin Sci 1969; 36:307–316.
56. Cohen C, Zagelbaum G, Gross D, et al. Clinical manifestations of inspiratory muscle fatigue. Am J Med 1982; 73:308–316.
57. Collett PW, Perry C, Engel LA. Pressure-time product, flow, and oxygen cost of resistive breathing in humans. J Appl Physiol 1985; 58:1263–1272.
58. Conoscenti C, Meduri GU, Menashe P, Nair S. Face mask positive pressure-mechanical ventilation in acute respiratory failure [abstract]. Chest 1988; 94:3S.
59. Cooke NT, Wilson SH, Freedman S. Blood lactate and respiratory muscle fatigue in patients with chronic airways obstruction. Thorax 1983; 38:184–187.
60. Cooper CB, Davidson AC, Cameron IR. Aminophylline, respiratory muscle strength and exercise tolerance in chronic obstructive airway disease. Bull Eur Physiopathol Respir 1987; 23:15–22.
61. Cournand A, Brock HJ, Rappaport I, Richards DW Jr. Disturbance of action of respiratory muscles as a contributing cause of dyspnea. Arch Intern Med 1936; 57:1008–1026.
62. Covelli HD, Black JW, Olsen MS, Beekman J. Respiratory failure precipitated by high carbohydrate loads. Ann Intern Med 1981; 95:579–581.
63. Criner GJ, Celli BR. Ventilatory muscle recruitment in exercise with O_2 in obstructed patients with mild hypoxemia. J Appl Physiol 1987; 63:195–200.
64. Criner GJ, Celli BR. Effect of unsupported arm exercise on ventilatory muscle recruitment in patients with severe chronic obstruction. Am Rev Respir Dis 1988; 138:856–861.
65. Cropp A, Dimarco AF. Effects of intermittent negative pressure ventilation on respiratory muscle function in patients with severe chronic obstructive pulmonary disease. Am Rev Respir Dis 1987; 135:1056–1061.
66. Dark DS, Pingleton SK, Kerby GR. Hypercapnia during weaning. A complication of nutritional support. Chest 1985; 88:141–143.
67. Decramer M, Demedts M, Rochette F, Billiet L. Maximal transrespiratory pressures in obstructive lung disease. Bull Eur Physiopathol Respir 1980; 16:479–490.
68. Delgado HR, Braun SR, Skatrud JB, et al. Chest wall and abdominal motion during exercise in patients with chronic obstructive pulmonary disease. Am Rev Respir Dis 1982; 126:200–205.
69. Delpierre S, Fornaus M, Pelissier JF, Payan MJ. Contractile and histochemical characteristics of the rabbit diaphragm in elastase-induced emphysema. Lung 1985; 163:221–232.
70. DeTroyer A, Sampson M, Sigrist S, Macklem PT. The diaphragm: two muscles. Science 1981; 213:230–238.
71. DeTroyer A, Sampson M, Sigrist S, Macklem PT. Action of costal and crural parts of the diaphragm on the rib cage in dogs. J Appl Physiol 1982; 53:30–39.
72. Dillard TA, Piantadosi S, Rajagopal KR. Prediction of ventilation at maximal exercise in chronic air-flow obstruction. Am Rev Respir Dis 1985; 132:230–235.
73. Dodd DS, Brancatisano TP, Engel LA. Chest wall mechanics during exercise in patients with severe chronic air-flow obstruction. Am Rev Respir Dis 1984; 129:33–38.
74. Dodd DS, Brancatisano TP, Engel LA. Effect of abdominal strapping on chest wall mechanics during exercise in patients with severe chronic air-flow obstruction. Am Rev Respir Dis 1985; 131:816–821.
75. Drew JS, Farkas GA, Pearson RD, Rochester DF. Effects of a chronic wasting infection on skeletal muscle size and contractile properties. J Appl Physiol 1988; 64:460–465.
76. Druz WS, Danon J, Fishman HC, et al. Approaches to assessing respiratory muscle functions in respiratory disease. Am Rev Respir Dis 1979; 119:145–149.
77. Druz WS, Sharp JT. Electrical and mechanical activity of the diaphragm accompanying body position in severe chronic obstructive pulmonary disease. Am Rev Respir Dis 1982; 125:275–280.
78. Efthimiou J, Fleming J, Gomes C, Spiro SG. The effect of supplementary oral nutrition in poorly nourished patients with chronic obstructive pulmonary disease. Am Rev Respir Dis 1988; 137:1075–1082.
79. Efthimiou J, Fleming J, Spiro SG. Sternomastoid muscle function and fatigue in breathless patients with severe respiratory disease. Am Rev Respir Dis 1987; 136:1099–1105.
80. Emmanuel GE, Moreno F. Distribution of ventilation and blood flow during exercise in emphysema. J Appl Physiol 1966; 21:1532–1544.
81. Esau SA, Bellemare F, Grassino A, et al. Changes in relaxation rate with diaphragmatic fatigue in humans. J Appl Physiol 1983; 54:1353–1360.
82. Estenne M, Yernault J-C, DeTroyer A. Mechanism of relief of dyspnea after thoracocentesis in patients with large pleural effusions. Am J Med 1983; 74:813–819.
83. Falk P, Eriksen A-M, Kolliker K, Andersen JB. Relieving dyspnea with an inexpensive and simple method in patients with severe chronic airflow limitation. Eur J Respir Dis 1985; 66:181–186.
84. Farkas GA, Roussos C. Adaptability of the hamster diaphragm to exercise and/or emphysema. J Appl Physiol 1982; 53:1263–1272.
85. Farkas GA, Roussos C. Diaphragm in emphysematous hamsters: sarcomere adaptability. J Appl Physiol 1983; 54:1635–1640.
86. Farkas GA, Roussos C. Histochemical and biochemical correlates of ventilatory muscle fatigue in emphysematous hamsters. J Clin Invest 1984; 74:1214–1220.
87. Feiss G, Levy S, Henson D, Levine S. Effects of a hospital-based outpatient ventilatory muscle rest therapy (VMRT) program in COPD subjects (COPDs) [abstract]. Chest 1988; 94:15S.
88. Fiaccadori E, Del Canale S, Arduini U, et al. Intracellular acid-base and electrolyte metabolism in skeletal muscle of patients with chronic obstructive lung disease and acute respiratory failure. Clin Sci 1986; 71:703–712.
89. Fiaccadori E, Del Canale S, Vitali P, et al. Skeletal muscle energetics, acid-base equilibrium and lactate metabolism in patients with severe hypercapnia and hypoxemia. Chest 1987; 92:883–887.
90. Field S, Kelly SM, Macklem PT. The oxygen cost of breathing

in patients with cardiorespiratory disease. Am Rev Respir Dis 1982; 126:9–13.

91. Field S, Sanci S, Grassino A. Respiratory muscle oxygen consumption estimated by the diaphragm pressure-time index. J Appl Physiol 1984; 57:44–51.
92. Fleury B, Murciano D, Talamo C, et al. Work of breathing in patients with chronic obstructive pulmonary disease in acute respiratory failure. Am Rev Respir Dis 1985; 131:822–827.
93. Foxworth JW, Reisz GR, Knudson SM, et al. Theophylline and diaphragmatic contractility. Investigation of a dose-response relationship. Am Rev Respir Dis 1988; 138:1532–1534.
94. Freedman AR, Lavietes MH. Energy requirements of the respiratory musculature in asthma. Am J Med 1986; 80:215–222.
95. Freedman AR, Mangura BT, Lavietes MH. Minute ventilation in asthma. Enhancement by mouthpiece and depression by oxygen administration. Am Rev Respir Dis 1983; 128:800–805.
96. Fritts HW Jr, Filler J, Fishman AP, Cournand A. The efficiency of ventilation during voluntary hyperpnea: studies in normal subjects and in dyspneic patients with either chronic pulmonary emphysema or obesity. J Clin Invest 1959; 38:1339–1348.
97. Gallagher CG, Im Hof V, Younes M. Effect of inspiratory muscle fatigue on breathing pattern. J Appl Physiol 1985; 59:1152–1158.
98. Gallagher CG, Younes M. Breathing pattern during and after maximal exercise in patients with chronic obstructive lung disease, interstitial lung disease, and cardiac disease, and in normal subjects. Am Rev Respir Dis 1986; 133:581–586.
99. Gaultier C, Boule M, Tournier G, Girard F. Inspiratory force reserve of the respiratory muscles in children with chronic obstructive pulmonary disease. Am Rev Respir Dis 1985; 131:811–815.
100. Gertz I, Hedenstierna G, Hellers G, Wahren J. Muscle metabolism in patients with chronic obstructive lung disease and acute respiratory failure. Clin Sci Molec Med 1977; 52:395–403.
101. Gibson GJ, Clark E, Pride NB. Static transdiaphragmatic pressures in normal subjects and in patients with chronic hyperinflation. Am Rev Respir Dis 1981; 124:685–689.
102. Gieseke T, Gurushanthaiah G, Glauser FL. Effects of carbohydrates on carbon dioxide excretion in patients with airway disease. Chest 1977; 71:55–58.
103. Gilbert R, Ashutosh K, Auchincloss JH Jr, et al. Prospective study of controlled oxygen therapy. Poor prognosis of patients with asynchronous breathing. Chest 1977; 71:456–462.
104. Gilbert R, Auchincloss JH Jr, Peppi D, Ashutosh K. The first few hours off a respirator. Chest 1974; 65:152–157.
105. Gilmartin JJ, Gibson GJ. Abnormalities of chest wall motion in patients with chronic airflow obstruction. Thorax 1984; 39:264–271.
106. Gilmartin JJ, Gibson GJ. Mechanisms of paradoxical rib cage motion in patients with chronic obstructive pulmonary disease. Am Rev Respir Dis 1986; 134:683–687.
107. Gimenez M, Servera E, Candina R, et al. Hypercapnia during maximal exercise in patients with chronic airflow obstruction. Bull Eur Physiopathol Respir 1984; 10:113–119.
108. Godfrey S, Leventhal A, Weintraub Z, et al. Distortion of chest movement by increased airways resistance. Thorax 1972; 27:148–155.
109. Goldstein S, Askanazi J, Weissman C, et al. Energy expenditure in patients with chronic obstructive pulmonary disease. Chest 1987; 91:222–224.
110. Goldstein SA, Thomashow BM, Kvetan V, et al. Nitrogen and energy relationships in malnourished patients with emphysema. Am Rev Respir Dis 1988; 138:636–644.
111. Grassino A, Bellemare F, Laporta D. Diaphragm fatigue and the strategy of breathing in COPD. Chest 1984; 85:51S–54S.
112. Gribbin HR, Gardiner IT, Geinz GR III, et al. Role of impaired inspiratory muscle function in limiting the ventilatory response to carbon dioxide in chronic airflow obstruction. Clin Sci 1983; 64:487–495.
113. Gribbin HR, Pride NB, Bye PTP, et al. Electrical activation of the diaphragm during stimulated breathing in patients with severe chronic airflow limitation and CO_2 retention. Chest 1984; 85:50S–51S.
114. Gutierrez M, Beroiza T, Contreras G, et al. Weekly cuirass ventilation improves blood gases and inspiratory muscle strength in patients with chronic airflow limitation and hypercarbia. Am Rev Respir Dis 1988; 138:617–623.
115. Hershenson MB, Kikuchi Y, Loring SH. Relative strengths of chest wall muscles. J Appl Physiol 1988; 65:852–862.
116. Hillman DR, Prentice L, Finucane KE. The pattern of breathing in acute severe asthma. Am Rev Respir Dis 1986; 133:587–592.
117. Hoover CF. The diagnostic significance of inspiratory movements of the costal margin. Am J Med Sci 1920; 159:633–646.
118. Howell S, Fitzgerald RS, Roussos Ch. Effects of aminophylline, isoproterenol and neostigmine on hypercapnic depression of diaphragmatic contractility. Am Rev Respir Dis 1985; 132:241–247.
119. Hughes RL, Katz H, Sahgal V, et al. Fiber size and energy metabolites in five separate muscles from patients with chronic obstructive lung disease. Respiration 1983; 44:321–328.
120. Hussain SNA, Graham R, Rutledge F, Roussos C. Respiratory muscle energetics during endotoxic shock in dogs. J Appl Physiol 1986; 60:486–493.
121. Hussain SNA, Sinkus G, Roussos C. Respiratory muscle fatigue: a cause of ventilatory failure in septic shock. J Appl Physiol 1985; 58:2033–2049.
122. Ioli F, Donner CF, Fracchia C. Transdiaphragmatic pressure in the assessment of diaphragmatic and abdominal breathing exercise. Bull Eur Physiopathol Respir 1982; 18(Suppl 4): 177–180.
123. Ishikawa S, Hayes JA. Functional morphometry of the diaphragm in patients with chronic obstructive lung disease. Am Rev Respir Dis 1973; 108:135–138.
124. Jardim J, Farkas G, Prefaut C, et al. The failing inspiratory muscles under normoxic and hypoxic conditions. Am Rev Respir Dis 1981; 124:274–279.
125. Javaheri S, Blum J, Kazemi H. Pattern of breathing and carbon dioxide retention in chronic obstructive lung disease. Am J Med 1981; 71:228–234.
126. Javaheri S, Smith JT, Thomas JP, et al. Albuterol has no effect on diaphragmatic fatigue in humans. Am Rev Respir Dis 1988; 137:197–201.
127. Jederlinic P, Muspratt JA, Miller MJ. Inspiratory muscle training in clinical practice. Physiologic conditioning or habituation to suffocation? Chest 1984; 86:870–873.
128. Juan G, Calverly P, Talamo C, et al. Effect of carbon dioxide on diaphragmatic function in human beings. N Engl J Med 1984; 310:874–879.
129. Katsardis CV, Desmond KJ, Coates AL. Measuring the oxygen cost of breathing in normal adults and patients with cystic fibrosis. Respir Physiol 1986; 65:257–266.
130. Keens TG, Krastins IRB, Wannamaker EM, et al. Ventilatory muscle endurance training in normal subjects and patients with cystic fibrosis. Am Rev Respir Dis 1977; 116:853–860.
131. Kelly SM, Rosa A, Field S, et al. Inspiratory muscle strength and body composition in patients receiving total parenteral nutrition therapy. Am Rev Respir Dis 1984; 130:33–37.
132. Kelsen SG, Wolanski T, Supinski GS, Roessman U. The effect of elastase-induced emphysema on diaphragmatic muscle structure in hamsters. Am Rev Respir Dis 1983; 127:330–334.
133. Killian KJ, Jones NL. Respiratory muscles and dyspnea. Clin Chest Med 1988; 9:237–248.
134. Kim MJ, Druz WS, Danon J, et al. Mechanics of the canine diaphragm. J Appl Physiol 1976; 41:369–382.
135. Kimball WR, Leith DE, Robins AG. Dynamic hyperinflation and ventilator dependence in chronic obstructive pulmonary disease. Am Rev Respir Dis 1982; 126:991–995.
136. Knowles JB, Fairbarn MS, Wiggs BJ, et al. Dietary supplementation and respiratory muscle performance in patients with COPD. Chest 1988; 93:977–983.
137. Kwan R, Mir MA. Beneficial effects of dietary carbohydrate restriction in chronic cor pulmonale. Am J Med 1987; 82:751–758.
138. Laporta D, Grassino A. Assessment of transdiaphragmatic pressure in humans. J Appl Physiol 1985; 58:1469–1476.
139. Larson JL, Kim MJ, Sharp JT, Larson DA. Inspiratory muscle training with a pressure threshold breathing device in patients with chronic obstructive pulmonary disease. Am Rev Respir Dis 1988; 138:689–696.
140. Lavietes MH, Grocela JA, Maniatis T, et al. Inspiratory muscle strength in asthma. Chest 1988; 93:1043–1048.
141. Leblanc P, Bowie DM, Summers E, et al. Breathlessness and exercise in patients with cardiorespiratory disease. Am Rev Respir Dis 1986; 133:21–25.
142. Lecoq A, Delhez L, Janssons F, Petil JM. Réentrainement de la

fonction motrice ventilatoire chez des insuffisants respiratoires chroniques. Acta Tuber Pneumol Belg 1970; 61:63–69.
143. Lee H, Criner G, Rassulo J, et al. A controlled study of rehabilitation vs. rehabilitation and respiratory muscle resting with negative external ventilation in patients with severe COPD [abstract]. Am Rev Respir Dis 1986; 133:A168.
144. Levine S, Gillen M, Weiser P, et al. Inspiratory pressure generation-comparison of subjects with COPD and age-matched normals. J Appl Physiol 1988; 65:888–899.
145. Levine S, Weiser P, Gillen J. Evaluation of a ventilatory muscle endurance training program in the rehabilitation of patients with chronic obstructive pulmonary disease. Am Rev Respir Dis 1986; 133:400–406.
146. Levison H, Cherniack RM. Ventilatory cost of exercise in chronic obstructive pulmonary disease. J Appl Physiol 1968; 25:21–27.
147. Lewis MI, Belman MJ, Dorr-Uyemura L. Nutritional supplementation in ambulatory patients with chronic obstructive pulmonary disease. Am Rev Respir Dis 1987; 135:1062–1068.
148. Lewis MI, Belman MJ, Sieck GC. Aminophylline and fatigue of the sternomastoid muscle. Am Rev Respir Dis 1986; 133:672–675.
149. Lopata M, Onal E, Cromydas G. Respiratory load compensation in chronic airway obstruction. J Appl Physiol 1985; 59:1947–1954.
150. Lopes JM, Aubier M, Jardim J, et al. Effect of caffeine on skeletal muscle function before and after fatigue. J Appl Physiol 1983; 54:1303–1305.
151. Loring SH, Mead J. Action of the diaphragm on the rib cage inferred from a force-balance analysis. J Appl Physiol 1982; 53:756–760.
152. Lourenco RV, Miranda JM. Drive and performance of the ventilatory apparatus in chronic obstructive lung disease. N Engl J Med 1968; 279:53–59.
153. Loveridge B, West P, Anthonisen NR, Kryger MH. Breathing patterns in patients with chronic obstructive pulmonary disease. Am Rev Respir Dis 1984; 130:730–733.
154. Loveridge B, West P, Kryger MH, Anthonisen NR. Alteration in breathing pattern with progression of chronic obstructive pulmonary disease. Am Rev Respir Dis 1986; 134:930–934.
155. MacIntyre N. Respiratory function during pressure support ventilation. Chest 1986; 89:677–683.
156. Macklem PT, Macklem DM, DeTroyer A. A model of inspiratory muscle mechanics. J Appl Physiol 1983; 55:547–557.
157. Madsen F, Secher NH, Kay L, et al. Inspiratory resistance versus general physical training in patients with chronic obstructive pulmonary disease. Eur J Respir Dis 1985; 67:167–176.
158. Mahler DA, Matthay RA, Snyder PE, et al. Sustained-release theophylline reduces dyspnea in nonreversible obstructive airway disease. Am Rev Respir Dis 1985; 131:22–25.
159. Marazzini L, Cavestri R, Mastropasqua B, et al. Pressure available for expiration in chronic airway obstruction. Respiration 1983; 44:241–251.
160. Marazzini L, Vezzoli F, Rizzato G. Intrathoracic pressure development in chronic airways obstruction. J Appl Physiol 1974; 37:575–578.
161. Marini JJ, Rodriquez RM, Lamb V. The inspiratory workload of patient-initiated mechanical ventilation. Am Rev Respir Dis 1986; 134:902–909.
162. Marks J, Pasterkamp H, Tal A, Leahy F. Relationships between respiratory muscle strength, nutritional status, and lung volume in cystic fibrosis and asthma. Am Rev Respir Dis 1986; 133:414–417.
163. Marshall R, Stone RW, Christie RV. The relationship of dyspnea to respiratory effort in normal subjects, mitral stenosis and emphysema. Clin Sci 1954; 13:625–631.
164. Martin J, Powell E, Shore S, et al. The role of respiratory muscles in the hyperinflation of bronchial asthma. Am Rev Respir Dis 1980; 121:441–447.
165. Martin JG, Shore SA, Engle LA. Mechanical load and inspiratory muscle action during induced asthma. Am Rev Respir Dis 1983; 128:455–460.
166. Mattar JA, Velasco IT, Esgaib AS, Takaoka F. Parenteral nutrition (PN) as a useful method for weaning patients from mechanical ventilation (MV) [abstract]. JPEN 1978; 2:50.
167. McFadden ER Jr, Kiser R, de Groot WJ. Acute bronchial asthma. Relations between clinical and physiologic manifestations. N Engl J Med 1973; 288:221–225.
168. McGregor M, Becklake MR. The relationship of oxygen cost of breathing to respiratory mechanical work and respiratory force. J Clin Invest 1961; 40:971–980.
169. McKenzie DK, Gandevia SC. Strength and endurance of inspiratory, expiratory and limb muscles in asthma. Am Rev Respir Dis 1986; 134:999–1004.
170. McKeon JL, Turner J, Kelly C, et al. The effect of inspiratory resistive training on exercise capacity in optimally treated patients with severe chronic airflow limitation. Aust NZ J Med 1986; 16:648–652.
171. Melzer E, Souhrada JF. Decrease of respiratory muscle strength and static lung volumes in obese asthmatics. Am Rev Respir Dis 1980; 121:17–22.
172. Mohan-Kumar T, Gimenez M. Maximal ventilation at rest and exercise in patients with chronic pulmonary disease. Respiration 1984; 46:291–302.
173. Moller P, Bergstrom J, Furst P, et al. Energy-rich phosphagens, electrolytes and free amino acids in leg skeletal muscle of patients with chronic obstructive lung disease. Acta Med Scand 1982; 211:187–193.
174. Molloy DW, Dhingra S, Solven F, et al. Hypomagnesemia and respiratory muscle power. Am Rev Respir Dis 1984; 129:497–498.
175. Morrison NJ, Richardson J, Dunn L, Pardy RL. Respiratory muscle performance in normal elderly subjects and patients with COPD. Chest 1989; 95:90–94.
176. Morrison WL, Gibson JNA, Scrimgeour C, Rennie MJ. Muscle wasting in emphysema. Clin Sci 1988; 75:415–420.
177. Moxham J, Miller J, Wiles CM, et al. Effect of aminophylline on the human diaphragm. Thorax 1985; 40:288–292.
178. Muller N, Bryan AC, Zamel N. Tonic inspiratory muscle activity as a cause of hyperinflation in asthma. J Appl Physiol 1981; 50:279–282.
179. Murciano D, Aubier M, Lecocguic Y, Pariente R. Effects of theophylline on diaphragmatic strength and fatigue in patients with chronic obstructive pulmonary disease. N Engl J Med 1984; 311:349–353.
180. Murciano D, Aubier M, Viires N, et al. Effects of theophylline and enprofylline on diaphragmatic contractility. J Appl Physiol 1987; 63:51–57.
181. Murciano D, Lecocguic Y, Aubier M, et al. Assessment of diaphragmatic force in acute respiratory failure in COPD in patients by bilateral phrenic stimulation [abstract]. Am Rev Respir Dis 1985; 131:A329.
182. Nery LE, Wasserman K, Andrews JD, et al. Ventilatory and gas exchange kinetics during exercise in chronic airways obstruction. J Appl Physiol 1982; 53:1594–1602.
183. Nietrzeba RM, Elliott CG, Adams TD, et al. Effects of aminophylline upon the exercise performance of patients with stable chronic airflow obstruction. Bull Eur Physiopathol Respir 1984; 20:361–367.
184. Nisell O. The respiratory work and pressure during exercise, and their relation to dyspnea. Acta Med Scand 1960; 166:113–119.
185. O'Connell JM, Campbell AH. Respiratory mechanics in airways obstruction associated with dyspnea. Thorax 1976; 31:669–676.
186. O'Donnell DE, Sanii R, Anthonisen NR, Younes M. Effect of dynamic airway compression on breathing pattern and respiratory sensation in severe chronic obstructive pulmonary disease. Am Rev Respir Dis 1987; 135:912–918.
187. Oliven A, Cherniack NS, Deal EC, Kelsen SG. The effects of acute bronchoconstriction on respiratory activity in patients with chronic obstructive pulmonary disease. Am Rev Respir Dis 1985; 131:236–241.
188. Oliven A, Kelsen SG, Deal EC, Cherniack NS. Mechanisms underlying CO^2 retention during flow-resistive loading in patients with chronic obstructive pulmonary disease. J Clin Invest 1983; 71:1442–1449.
189. Oliven A, Lohda S, Adams ME, et al. Effect of fatiguing resistive loads on the level and pattern of respiratory activity in awake goats. Respir Physiol 1988; 73:311–324.
190. Oliven A, Supinski GS, Kelsen SG. Functional adaptation of diaphragm to chronic hyperinflation in emphysematous hamsters. J Appl Physiol 1986; 60:225–231.
191. O'Neill S, McCarthy DS. Postural relief of dyspnoea in severe chronic airflow limitation: relationship to respiratory muscle strength. Thorax 1983; 38:595–600.
192. Openbrier DR, Irwin MM, Rogers RM, et al. Nutritional status

and lung function in patients with emphysema and chronic bronchitis. Chest 1983; 83:17–22.
193. Orzalesi MM, Cook CD, Hart MC. Pulmonary function in symptom-free asthmatic patients. Acta Paediatr 1964; 53:401–407.
194. Pardy RL, Rivington RN, Despas PJ, Macklem PT. Inspiratory muscle training compared with physiotherapy in patients with chronic airflow limitation. Am Rev Respir Dis 1981; 123:421–425.
195. Pardy RL, Rivington RN, Despas PJ, Macklem PT. The effects of inspiratory muscle training on exercise performance in chronic airflow limitation. Am Rev Respir Dis 1981; 123:426–433.
196. Pardy RL, Roussos CH. Endurance of hyperventilation in chronic airflow limitation. Chest 1983; 83:744–750.
197. Parot S, Miara B, Milic-Emili J, Gautier H. Hypoxemia, hypercapnia and breathing pattern in patients with chronic obstructive pulmonary disease. Am Rev Respir Dis 1982; 126:882–886.
198. Peress L, McLean P, Woolf CR, Zamel N. Ventilatory muscle training in obstructive lung disease. Bull Eur Physiopathol Respir 1979; 15:91–92.
199. Peress L, Sybrecht G, Macklem PT. The mechanisms of increase in total lung capacity during acute asthma. Am J Med 1976; 61:165–169.
200. Petit JM, Delhez L. Quelques données experimentales recentes concernant l'origine de la dyspnée et la regulation ventilatoire chez le malade asthmatique. Acta Tuberc Pneumonol Belg 1970; 61:169–186.
201. Petrozzino JJ, Scardella AT, Li J K-J, et al. The effect of naloxone on spectral shifts of the diaphragm EMG during inspiratory flow resistive loading [abstract]. FASEB J 1988; 2:A513.
202. Pluto LA, Fahey PJ, Sorenson L, Chandrasekhan AJ. Effect of 8 weeks of intermittent negative pressure ventilation on exercise parameters in patients with severe chronic obstructive lung disease [abstract]. Am Rev Respir Dis 1985; 131:A64.
203. Pourriat JL, Lamberto CH, Hoang PH, et al. Diaphragmatic fatigue and breathing pattern during weaning from mechanical ventilation in COPD patients. Chest 1986; 90:703–707.
204. Rabinovitch B, Pardy RL, Hussain SNA, Macklem PT. The acute effects of rest on ventilatory muscle (VM) function in patients with severe chronic airflow limitation (CAL) [abstract]. The Physiologist 1983; 26:A21.
205. Reents SB, Beck CA Jr. Naloxone and naltrexone. Application in COPD. Chest 1988; 92:217–219.
206. Ries AL, Sosa G, Prewitt L, et al. Restricted pulmonary function in cystic fibrosis. Chest 1988; 94:575–579.
207. Road J, Vahi R, DelRio P, Grassino A. *In vivo* contractile properties of fatigued diaphragm. J Appl Physiol 1987; 63:471–478.
208. Rochester DF. Does respiratory muscle rest relieve fatigue or incipient fatigue [editorial]? Am Rev Respir Dis 1988; 138:516–517.
209. Rochester DF. Tests of respiratory muscle function. Clin Chest Med 1988; 9:249–261.
210. Rochester DF, Arora NS, Braun NMT. Maximum contractile force of human diaphragm muscle, determined *in vivo*. Trans Am Clin Climatol Assoc 1981; 93:200–208.
211. Rochester DF, Arora NS, Braun NMT, Goldberg SK. The respiratory muscles in chronic obstructive pulmonary disease (COPD). Bull Eur Physiopathol Respir 1979; 15:951–975.
212. Rochester DF, Bettini G. Diaphragmatic blood flow and energy expenditure in the dog. Effect of inspiratory airflow resistance and hypercapnia. J Clin Invest 1976; 57:661–672.
213. Rochester DF, Braun NMT. Determinants of maximal inspiratory pressure in chronic obstructive pulmonary disease. Am Rev Respir Dis 1985; 132:42–47.
214. Rochester DF, Braun NMT. The diaphragm and dyspnea. Evidence from inhibiting diaphragmatic activity with respirators. Am Rev Respir Dis 1979; 119:77–80.
215. Rochester DF, Braun NMT, Laine S. Diaphragmatic energy expenditure in chronic respiratory failure: The effect of assisted ventilation with body respirators. Am J Med 1977; 63:223–232.
216. Rochester DF, Esau SA. Critical illness, infection, and the respiratory muscles [editorial]. Am Rev Respir Dis 1988; 138:258–259.
217. Rochester DF, Goldberg SK. Techniques of respiratory physical therapy. Am Rev Respir Dis 1980; 122(5):133–146.
218. Rodenstein DO, Cuttita G, Stanescu DC. Ventilatory and diaphragmatic EMG changes during negative-pressure ventilation in healthy subjects. J Appl Physiol 1988; 64:2272–2278.
219. Rodenstein DO, Stanescu DC, Cuttita G, et al. Ventilatory and diaphragmatic EMG responses to negative-pressure ventilation in airflow obstruction. J Appl Physiol 1988; 65:1621–1626.
220. Roussos C. Ventilatory muscle fatigue governs breathing frequency. Bull Eur Physiopathol Respir 1984; 20:445–451.
221. Roussos C, Fixley M, Gross D, Macklem PT. Fatigue of the inspiratory muscles and their synergic behavior. J Appl Physiol 1979; 46:897–904.
222. Sackner MA, Gonzalez H, Rodriquez M, et al. Assessment of asynchronous and paradoxic motion between rib cage and abdomen in normal subjects and in patients with chronic obstructive pulmonary disease. Am Rev Respir Dis 1984; 130:588–593.
223. Sadoul N, Bazzy AR, Akabas SR, Haddad GG. Ventilatory response to fatiguing and nonfatiguing resistive loads in awake sheep. J Appl Physiol 1985; 59:969–978.
224. Sanchez J, Bastien C, Medrano G, et al. Metabolic enzymatic activities in the diaphragm of normal men and patients with moderate chronic obstructive pulmonary disease. Bull Eur Physiopathol Respir 1984; 20:535–540.
225. Sanchez J, Derenne JP, Debesse B, et al. Typology of the respiratory muscles in normal men and in patients with moderate chronic respiratory diseases. Bull Eur Physiopathol Respir 1982; 18:901–914.
226. Sanchez J, Medrano G, Debesse B, et al. Muscle fiber types in costal and crural diaphragm in normal men and in patients with moderate chronic respiratory disease. Bull Eur Physiopathol Respir 1985; 21:351–356.
227. Santiago TV, Remolina C, Soder V, Edelman NH. Endorphins and the control of breathing: ability of naloxone to restore flow-resistive load compensation in chronic obstructive pulmonary disease. N Engl J Med 1981; 304:1190–1195.
228. Santiago TV, Sheft SA, Khan AU, Edelman NH. Effect of naloxone on the respiratory responses to hypoxia in chronic obstructive pulmonary disease. Am Rev Respir Dis 1984; 130:183–186.
229. Scardella AT, Parisi RA, Phair DK, et al. The role of endogenous opioids in the ventilatory response to acute flow-resistive loads. Am Rev Respir Dis 1986; 133:26–31.
230. Scott KWM, Hoy J. The cross sectional area of diaphragmatic muscle fibers in emphysema, measured by an automated image analysis system. J Pathol 1976; 120:121–128.
231. Sergysels R, van Meerhaeghe A, Scano G, et al. Respiratory drive during exercise in chronic obstructive lung disease. Bull Eur Physiopathol Respir 1981; 17:755–766.
232. Sharp JT, Beard GAT, Sunga M, et al. The rib cage in normal and emphysematous subjects: a roentgenographic approach. J Appl Physiol 1986; 61:2050–2059.
233. Sharp JT, Danon J, Druz WS, et al. Respiratory muscle function in patients with chronic obstructive pulmonary disease: its relationship to disability and to respiratory therapy. Am Rev Respir Dis 1974; 110(suppl):154–167.
234. Sharp JT, Druz WS, Moisan T, et al. Postural relief of dyspnea in severe chronic obstructive pulmonary disease. Am Rev Respir Dis 1980; 122:201–211.
235. Sharp JT, Goldberg NB, Druz WS, et al. Thoracoabdominal motion in chronic obstructive pulmonary disease. Am Rev Respir Dis 1977; 115:47–56.
236. Sharp JT, vanLith P, Nuchprayoon CV, et al. The thorax in chronic obstructive lung disease. Am J Med 1968; 44:39–46.
237. Simon PM, Pope A, Lahive K, et al. Naloxone does not alter response to hypercapnic or resistive loading in chronic obstructive pulmonary disease. Am Rev Respir Dis 1989; 139:134–138.
238. Skatrud JB, Dempsey JA, Bhansali P, Irvin C. Determinants of chronic carbon dioxide retention and its correction in humans. J Clin Invest 1980; 65:813–821.
239. Smidt U, Worth H, Petro W. Ventilatory limitation of exercise in patients with chronic bronchitis and/or emphysema. Bull Eur Physiopathol Respir 1979; 15:95–101.
240. Sonne LJ, Davis JA. Increased exercise performance in patients with severe COPD following inspiratory resistive training. Chest 1982; 81:436–439.
241. Sorli J, Grassino A, Lorange G, Milic-Emili J. Control of breathing in patients with chronic obstructive lung disease. Clin Sci Mol Med 1978; 54:295–304.
242. Steele RH, Heard BE. Size of the diaphragm in chronic bronchitis. Thorax 1973; 28:55–60.

243. Stoller JK, Wiedemann HP, Loke J, et al. Terbutaline and diaphragm function in chronic obstructive pulmonary disease: a double-blind randomized clinical trial. Br J Dis Chest 1988; 82:242–250.
244. Supinski GS, Deal EC Jr, Kelsen SG. Some effects of caffeine and theophylline on diaphragm contractility. Am Rev Respir Dis 1984; 130:429–433.
245. Supinski GS, Kelsen SG. Effect of elastase-induced emphysema on the force-generating ability of the diaphragm. J Clin Invest 1982; 70:978–988.
246. Supinski GS, Levin S, Kelsen SG. Caffeine effect on respiratory muscle endurance and sense of effort during loaded breathing. J Appl Physiol 1986; 60:2040–2047.
247. Swartz MA, Marino PL. Diaphragmatic strength during weaning from mechanical ventilation. Chest 1985; 88:736–739.
248. Szeinberg A, England S, Mindorff C, et al. Maximal inspiratory and expiratory pressures are reduced in hyperinflated, malnourished young adult male patients with cystic fibrosis. Am Rev Respir Dis 1985; 132:766–769.
249. Tabona MVZ, Ambrosino N, Barnes PJ. Endogenous opiates and the control of breathing in normal subjects and patients with chronic airflow obstruction. Thorax 1982; 38:384–389.
250. Thomas AJ, Supinski GS, Kelsen SG. Changes in chest wall structure and elasticity in elastase-induced emphysema. J Appl Physiol 1986; 61:1821–1829.
251. Thurlbeck WM. Diaphragm and body weight in emphysema. Thorax 1978; 33:483–487.
252. Tobin MJ, Chadha TS, Jenouri G, et al. Breathing patterns 2. Diseased subjects. Chest 1983; 84:286–294.
253. Tobin MJ, Guenther SM, Perez W, et al. Konno-Mead analysis of rib cage–abdominal motion during successful and unsuccessful trials of weaning from mechanical ventilation. Am Rev Respir Dis 1987; 135:1320–1328.
254. Tobin MJ, Perez W, Guenther SM, et al. Does rib cage–abdominal paradox signify respiratory muscle fatigue? J Appl Physiol 1987; 63:851–860.
255. Tobin MJ, Perez W, Guenther SM, et al. The pattern of breathing during successful and unsuccessful trials of weaning from mechanical ventilation. Am Rev Respir Dis 1986; 134:1111–1118.
256. Viires N, Aubier M, Murciano D, et al. Effects of aminophylline on diaphragmatic fatigue during acute respiratory failure. Am Rev Respir Dis 1984; 129:396–402.
257. Ward ME, Corbeil C, Gibbons W, et al. Optimization of respiratory muscle relaxation during mechanical ventilation. Anesthesiology 1988; 69:29–35.
258. Waters ATH. Researches on the Nature, Pathology and Treatment of Emphysema of the Lungs and its Relations with other Diseases of the Chest. London: John Churchill, 1862, 56–60.
259. Weissman C, Kemper M, Elwyn DH, et al. The energy expenditure of the mechanically ventilated critically ill patient. An analysis. Chest 1986; 89:254–295.
260. Wiles CM, Moxham J, Newham D, Edwards RHT. Aminophylline and fatigue of adductor pollicis in man. Clin Sci 1983; 64:547–550.
261. Wilson DO, Rogers RM, Hoffman RM. State of the art: nutrition and chronic lung disease. Am Rev Respir Dis 1985; 132:1347–1365.
262. Wilson DO, Rogers RM, Sanders MH, et al. Nutritional intervention in malnourished patients with emphysema. Am Rev Respir Dis 1986; 134:672–677.
263. Wilson SH, Cooke NT, Moxham J, Spiro SG. Sternomastoid muscle function and fatigue in normal subjects and in patients with chronic obstructive pulmonary disease. Am Rev Respir Dis 1984; 129:460–464.
264. Zack MB, Palange AV. Oxygen supplemented exercise of ventilatory and nonventilatory muscles in pulmonary rehabilitation. Chest 1985; 88:669–675.
265. Zackon H, Despas PJ, Anthonisen NR. Occlusion pressure responses in asthma and chronic obstructive pulmonary disease. Am Rev Respir Dis 1976; 114:917–927.
266. Zibrak JD, Hill NS, Federman EC, et al. Evaluation of intermittent long-term negative pressure ventilation in patients with severe chronic obstructive pulmonary disease. Am Rev Respir Dis 1988; 138:1515–1518.
267. Zocche GP, Fritts HW Jr, Cournand A. Fraction of maximum breathing capacity available for prolonged hyperventilation. J Appl Physiol 1960; 15:1073–1075.

Chapter 17

NEUROMUSCULAR PHYSIOLOGY OF COUGH AND OTHER RESPIRATORY TRACT REFLEXES

Erik van Lunteren Thomas E. Dick

Cough is an important mechanism for defending the respiratory system. Patients with an impaired ability to cough due to neuromuscular disorders, e.g., the muscular dystrophies or spinal cord injuries, or in whom airway mechanics or respiratory muscle fatigue prevents adequate expiratory flow rates, e.g., some patients with severe obstructive abnormalities, are at increased risk for developing serious pulmonary infections and respiratory failure with attendant morbidity and mortality. Coughing also provides a clue to the pathology of the respiratory tract and is elicited by acute and chronic infections, bronchoconstriction, structural abnormalities such as benign and malignant tumors, and a variety of inhaled airway irritants.

Descriptions of coughing have identified four phases in this complex act: inspiration, compression, expulsion, and termination (Fig. 17–1).[1, 7, 21, 35, 36, 37, 69] A cough is initiated with the inspiratory phase, during which lung volume is variably increased. To the extent that the lung and thorax expand, inspiratory and expiratory airflow profiles become mechanically more advantageous. Increases in the precontractile lengths of the expiratory muscles allow greater expiratory forces to be generated during the subsequent phases. In a variant of cough, the expiration reflex, the expiratory phases are not preceded by an increment in lung volume. The inspiratory phase is followed by the compressive phase, characterized by intrathoracic and intra-abdominal pressures becoming markedly positive while the glottis is closed. The build-up of positive pressures in the thorax and abdomen during the compressive phase of coughs allows expiratory flow to start abruptly during the expulsive phase. Loss of the compressive phase, as occurs in intubated or tracheostomized patients, reduces but does not totally abolish the mechanical efficacy and efficiency of coughs. The expulsive phase is initiated by opening of the larynx, with the driving force for the high rates of expiratory airflow being provided by the expiratory muscles of the abdomen and thorax. Abdominal and thoracic pressures continue to increase during the early portion of the expulsive phase and subside as lung volume diminishes. Finally, the cough is terminated by relaxation of the expiratory muscles. Several compressive and expulsive phases may occur sequentially with or without intervening inspiratory phases.

This chapter focuses on lung and airway receptors (afferents) responsible for initiating cough, central projections of these afferents, and activity of the respiratory muscles during coughing. The effects of cough on the clearance of lung and airway secretions and the clinical relevance of cough in patients with chronic obstructive pulmonary disease are discussed elsewhere.

PULMONARY AND AIRWAY RECEPTORS (AFFERENTS) AND THEIR CENTRAL PROJECTIONS

Receptors that induce cough are located mainly in the airway epithelium, concentrated at the larynx and at points where the tracheobronchial tree branches.[30, 35, 65] Mechano-, thermo-, chemo-, and irritant-sensitive receptors have been identified within the airways,[8, 9, 65–68] and stimuli acting on a variety of receptors may induce cough[7] as well as other respiratory and cardiovascular reflexes. Sensory receptors have been categorized by different schemes, which leads to confusion in the nomenclature.[9, 67] In addition to being classified according to these effective stimuli, receptors have been identified on the basis of their morphology, location, activated nerve, and elicited response. Briefly, the morphology of airway and pulmonary receptors appears to be similar to other general sensory receptors of the body, with the exception of special sensory receptors subserving olfaction and taste. Receptors are either encapsulated or free-nerve endings located in the airway epithelium.[46, 68] The airway has afferent innervation from three cranial nerves and from sympathetic nerves (Fig. 17–2): (1) the vagus nerve (cranial nerve X) innervates the bronchial tree and lung parenchyma, (2) the internal branch of the superior laryngeal nerve (arising from cranial nerve X) innervates the larynx, (3) the glossopharyngeal nerve (cranial nerve IX) innervates the pharyngeal wall, and (4) the trigeminal nerve (cranial nerve V) innervates nasal passages. Inhaled substances elicit reflexes depending on the specific afferent nerve stimulated as well as on the intensity of the stimulus.[68] Afferents coursing with the sympathetic nerves innervate the airways having endings in the epithelial cell layer.

The *vagus nerve* innervates extra- and intrathoracic trachea, bronchi, and lung parenchyma. Myelinated fibers innervate rapidly and slowly adapting receptors.[33] Morphologic studies of rapidly adapting receptors have shown that the myelinated nerves branch in the subepithelium and terminate in fine, unmyelinated, varicose arborizations between epithelial cells.[16] Unlike rapidly adapting receptors that are located in the epithelium, slowly adapting receptors are located in the smooth muscle of the airways.[16] Unmyelinated fibers terminate as free nerve endings in the bronchi ("C" fibers)[8] and innervate "J" receptors, which are named for their juxtacapillary location in the lung parenchyma.[44, 45, 47]

Cell bodies of vagal afferents are located in the nodose ganglion and their axons project centrally to the nucleus of the solitary tract (NTS). The feline NTS has been divided into subnuclei based on its cytoarchitectonics.[23] Only the ventrolateral subnucleus contains cells that are depolarized during inspiration, whether or not the lungs inflate. Medial, dorsal, and commissural subnuclei contain cells that discharge in relationship to lung volume. Central sensory projections to specific subnuclei have been investigated using anatomic and electrophysiologic methods. Anatomic experiments have shown that axons project differentially based on receptive field, and physiologic experiments have shown differential projection patterns based on receptor type. Injections of a retrograde tracer in the extrathoracic trachea have revealed vagal afferent collaterals predominantly in the ventrolateral NTS with moderate labeling in the dorsal, dorsolateral, medial, and interstitial nuclei.[23, 24] Injections in the intrathoracic trachea revealed predominantly the dorsolateral NTS with moderate labeling in the dorsal commissural and ventrolateral nuclei, and injections in the bronchi revealed predominantly the ventrolateral NTS with moderate labeling in the interstitial and intermediate subnuclei of the NTS.[23, 24] In electrophysiologic experiments, afferents arising from rapidly adapting receptors were found to terminate predominantly in the ipsilateral commissural and medial NTS,[12, 27, 29] whereas afferents from slowly adapting receptors were found to terminate predominantly in the medial and ventrolateral NTS.[4, 25, 26] Afferents from unmyelinated C fibers have not been mapped. However, J receptors, which are innervated by unmyelinated afferents, project mainly to the ventrolateral and dorsolateral subnuclei of the NTS, with moderate projection to the commissural subnucleus.[23]

The *internal branch of the superior laryngeal nerve* contains the sensory innervation from the larynx. Afferent fibers from irritant receptors are myelinated; have an irregular discharge, which is indicative of rapidly adapting receptors; and induce cough. Unmyelinated nerve fibers elicit cough also; selective stimulation of C-fiber endings by capsaicin can cause cough.[30]

In addition to irritant receptors, the superior laryngeal nerve contains afferent fibers that have regular, repetitive activity related to respiratory events. Three types of receptors have been identified and these may have a role in regulating respiration.[2, 3] These receptors are (1) pressure receptors, (2) "drive" receptors that respond to laryngeal movement, and (3) cold or flow receptors.[51, 52]

Cell bodies for the internal branch of the superior laryngeal nerve are located in the nodose ganglion. Axons project into the medulla and terminate preferentially in the interstitial nucleus and to a lesser extent in the dorsolateral, ventrolateral, and commissural subnuclei.[24]

The *glossopharyngeal nerve* is a mixed, i.e., both motor and sensory function, nerve with fibers innervating mechano-, thermo-, and irritant-sensitive receptors in the pharynx. Fillenz and Widdicombe,[16] in one of the few histologic studies examining the morphology of airway receptors, have described fine nerve terminals of myelinated glossopharyngeal afferents within the epipharynx. These terminals are in the epithelium

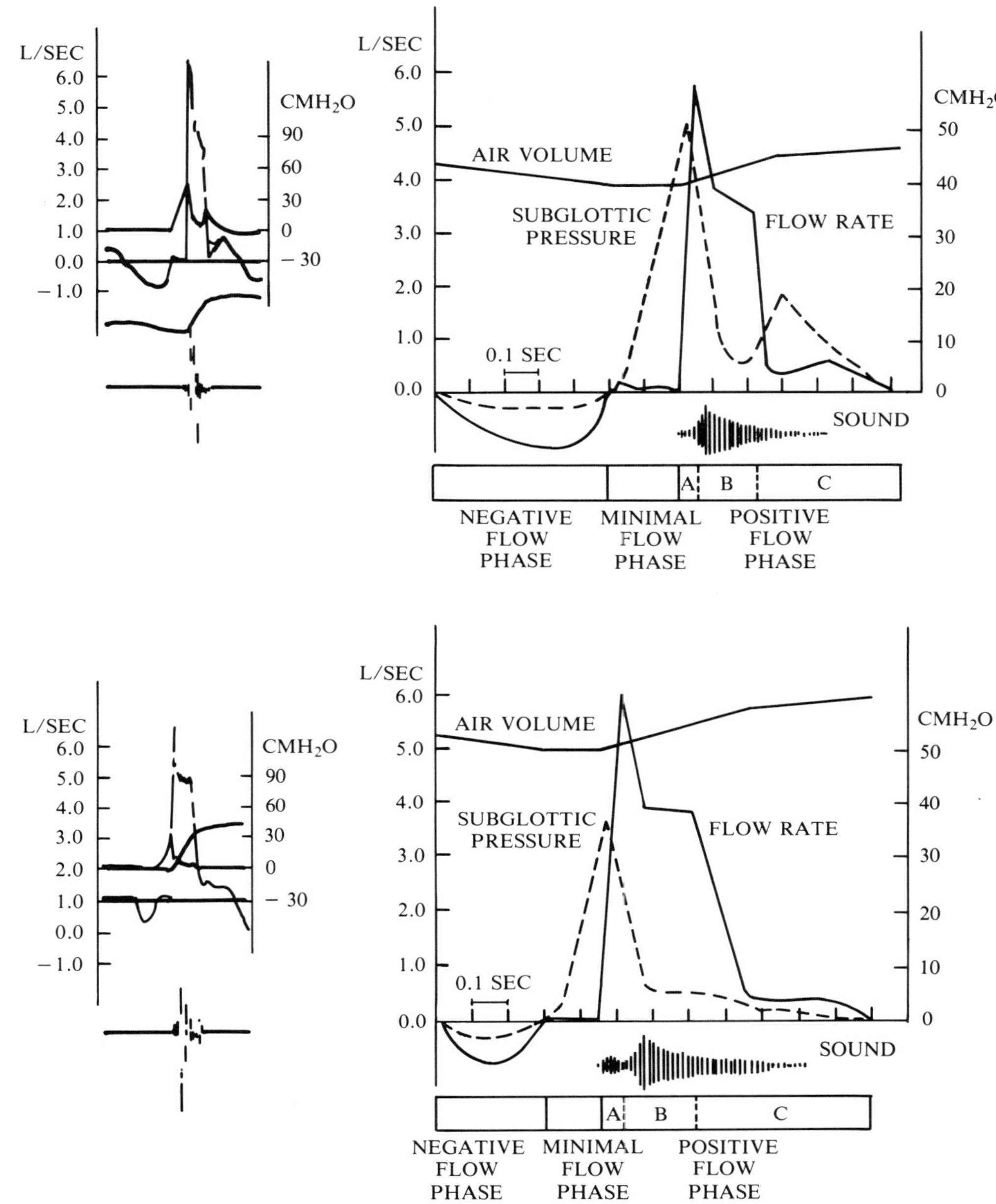

Figure 17–1. Illustration of the inspiratory (negative flow), compressive (minimal flow), and expulsive (positive flow) phases of two coughs recorded in humans. Traces indicate flow at the airway opening (flow rate), spirometric volume change (air volume), subglottic pressure, and sound level. Recordings on left are diagrammed on right. The positive flow phase is divided into increasing *(A)*, constant *(B)*, and decreasing *(C)* parts. (Reproduced with permission from Vanagihara N, Von Leden H, Werner-Kukuk E. Acta Otolaryngol 1966; 61:495–510.)

under a layer of squamous cells. Unmyelinated afferents are located also in the pharyngeal region.

Cell bodies for glossopharyngeal afferents are located in the petrosal ganglion. Axons project centrally into the medulla and terminate in the NTS. The projection pattern appears similar to vagal afferents.

The *trigeminal nerve* is an afferent nerve that divides into three main branches. Two of these, the ophthalmic and maxillary, supply the nasal mucosa. The majority of nerve fibers are unmyelinated, terminating as free nerve endings within the epithelium. The cell bodies of these fibers are located in the trigeminal, i.e., semilunar, ganglion, and projecting fibers enter the brainstem in the lateral pons where the nerve divides into a short ascending branch and a long descending branch.

Axons in the short branch terminate in the principal sensory nucleus of V and in the mesencephalic nucleus of V. The principal sensory nucleus of V is located in the lateral pons just rostral to the point of entry of the trigeminal nucleus. Somatotopic organization is retained in the sensory nucleus such that fibers of the ophthalmic branch terminate ventrally below those in the maxillary branch.[32] Cells of the principal sensory nucleus have spontaneous activity and respond to pressure stimuli with little adaptation and with large receptive fields.[64] The mesencephalic nucleus of V receives sensory information only from the mandibular branch of the trigeminal nerve.

Axons in the long branch from the spinal tract of V descend posterolaterally, i.e., near the spinothalamic tract, to the upper cervical segments. These fibers terminate in the spinal nucleus of V. The three branches of the trigeminal nerve retain their somatotopic organization within the spinal tract, with the ophthalmic branch being the most anterior and with the maxillary branch situated in the middle. This organization is retained for the length of the tract and within the paratrigeminal nucleus.[54] Cells throughout the spinal tract of V respond to touch of the nasal epithelium, supporting extensive termination of afferents along the length of the nucleus.

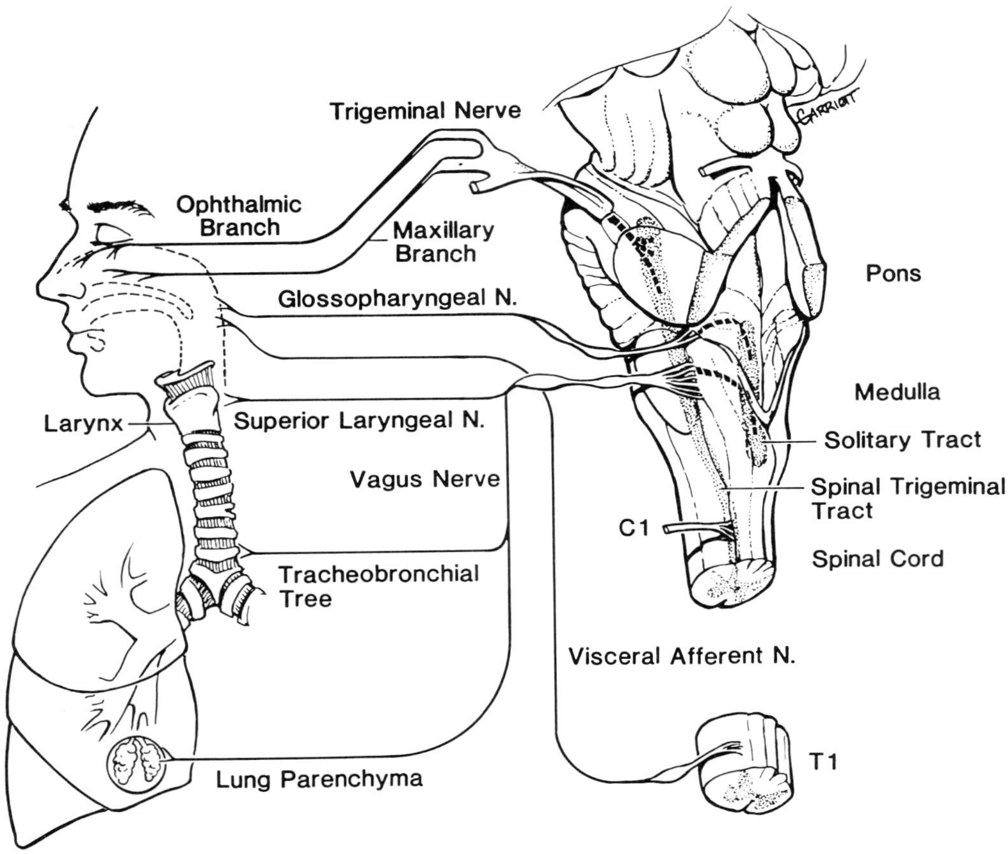

Figure 17–2. Diagrammatic illustration of afferent innervation of the airways and lung parenchyma. Please see text for details. Briefly, the nasal mucosa has afferent innervation by the ophthalmic and maxillary branches of the trigeminal nerve (cranial nerve V); the pharyngeal region by the glossopharyngeal nerve (cranial nerve IX); and the larynx, tracheobronchial tree, and lung parenchyma by the vagus nerve (cranial nerve X). These afferent nerves project to the pons and medulla. In addition, the airway is innervated by sympathetic afferent nerves, which project to the thoracic spinal cord.

Projections to and from the trigeminal sensory nuclei have been studied using ortho- and retrograde tracers.[42, 48] These nuclei receive projections from the neighboring reticular formation and from other brainstem nuclei, as well as from trigeminal afferents, and send extensive projections to the thalamus. The trigeminal nuclei also project to the ipsilateral parabrachial nuceli and to other medullary nuclei, especially the facial nucleus. The parabrachial nucleus has been associated with many visceral functions and with respiration.

AIRWAY AND PULMONARY AFFERENTS AND CONTROL OF BREATHING

Stimulation of pulmonary and airway receptors elicits a variety of responses depending on the intensity of stimulation and the distribution of receptors stimulated.[65] Teleologically, the purpose of these reflexes is interpreted to defend the airway and to prevent damage to pulmonary tissue.

Activation of other specific receptors in the tracheobronchial tree can elicit different responses. For example, stimulation of free nerve endings innervated by nonmyelinated C-fiber afferents results in rapid, shallow breathing; stimulation of rapidly adapting irritant receptors innervated by myelinated afferents elicits coughing; and stimulation of slowly adapting, stretch receptors also innervated by myelinated fibers elicits the Hering-Breuer reflex inhibiting inspiration and facilitating expiration.

Mechanical and chemical irritations of the laryngeal and tracheal airway elicit coughing. Rapidly adapting receptors have been identified at these zones from which coughing can be elicited. This correlation leads to the speculation that rapidly adapting receptors are the irritant receptors that underlie the cough reflex.

Stimulation of the nasopharyngeal region elicits either an aspiration or a sneeze reflex. Aspirations are intense inspiratory efforts that may be mediated through the cells in the ventrolateral subnucleus of the solitary tract.[59] Stimulation of the glossopharyngeal nerve activates NTS neurons.[5] In addition, extensive lesions of the NTS block the response to glossopharyngeal stimulation.[38]

Stimulation of the nasal mucosa can elicit an apnea or a sniff. The apnea is an aspect of the diving reflex elicited by wetting the face of a mammal or bird and is mediated through trigeminal afferents. Sniffing is a more complex response and may be one of those reflexes mediated by a combination of stimulated afferents. In particular, receptors supplied by the trigeminal nerve are important but signals from olfactory receptors also contribute.[59]

The state of arousal has a strong influence in determining the effectiveness of a stimulus in producing coughing. In awake and sleeping dogs, Sullivan and colleagues[56, 57] assessed the respiratory effects of mechanical stimulation of the larynx and tracheobronchial tree. Airway stimulation during wakefulness was very effective in producing coughing. In contrast, during both slow-wave sleep and rapid eye movement sleep, single coughs rarely occurred and a fully developed cough response never occurred in the absence of arousal. Jamal and colleagues[22] assessed cough responses to inhaled aerosols of citric acid in healthy human subjects during wakefulness and both slow-wave and rapid eye movement sleep. The concentration of citric acid required to elicit coughing was significantly higher during sleep than during wakefulness but was not significantly different for the two types of sleep. Cough was always associated with arousal, but no information was given regarding the temporal relationship between cough and arousal. Power and coworkers[49] recorded cough frequency during wakefulness and sleep in ten subjects with severe chronic bronchitis and emphysema who complained of nocturnal cough. Each patient had a mean of approximately 15 bouts of coughing per night, with each bout lasting on average 4 seconds. The majority of coughs (85%) occurred during electroencephalographically confirmed wakefulness and not during true sleep. Of coughs during sleep, none took place during stages three and four, and only one patient coughed during rapid eye movement sleep. Only once did cough during sleep lead to arousal.

RESPIRATORY MUSCLE USE DURING COUGHING

Inspired lung volume during coughing is highly variable and ranges from a fraction of to several times eupneic tidal volume.[6, 19, 20, 31, 34, 43, 50, 56, 57, 69] Studies in which patients were instructed to cough voluntarily suggest a large degree of volitional control over inspired volume.[20, 34, 50, 69] In comparison, during a vigorous nonvolitional series of coughs in awake animals one or more of the expiratory efforts are typically preceded by a large increase in thoracic volume.[56, 57] In anesthetized humans and animals most studies of cough report an augmentation of inspiratory volume relative to tidal volume.[6, 31, 43] The augmentation of inspired volume may improve the mechanical efficiency of the subsequent expiratory phase by increasing the diameter of the tracheobronchial tree, increasing the recoil of the lung, and optimizing the precontractile lengths of the expiratory muscles.

Many muscles contribute to thoracic expansion during breathing. During resting breathing the most important are the costal and crural diaphragms and the parasternal intercostal muscles, with the interosseous intercostal muscles at different interspaces, as well as the scalene muscles, which play lesser roles. When breathing is stimulated chemically, (e.g., by hypoxia or hypercapnia), metabolically (e.g., by exercise), or mechanically (e.g., by bronchoconstriction), the activation of these muscles increases, although not necessarily proportionately. In addition, muscles minimally active or not previously active, such as the lower interosseous intercostal and the sternocleidomastoid muscles, are recruited.

Several studies have confirmed that electromyographic activity of the costal diaphragm and electroneurographic activity of the phrenic nerve increase during the inspiratory phase of coughing relative to that during resting breathing.[6, 59, 61, 70] Tomori and Widdicombe[59] found in spontaneously breathing anesthetized cats that during coughing the spike frequency recorded simultaneously from multiple motor units of the phrenic nerve increased three- to four-fold relative to values during breathing, whereas in artificially ventilated animals single or pauci-fiber motor unit discharge frequency increased from a baseline of 4 to 5 impulses per second during breathing to 7 to 9 impulses per second during the inspiratory phase of coughs. These data indicate that the discharge frequency of phrenic motor units already active increases, and that in addition new motor units are recruited, findings which were confirmed by Yanaura and coworkers[70] in anesthetized dogs. In the last study, the mean amplitude of phrenic spike potentials was greater during coughing than during breathing, and hence the newly recruited motor units were larger than those active during breathing. In anesthetized dogs the value for the autocorrelation coefficient of the phrenic electroneurogram was lower during coughing than during breathing.[70] In spontaneously breathing anesthetized cats, the peak electrical activity of the costal and crural diaphragms and the parasternal intercostal muscles was found to increase two- to five-fold during coughing, compared with that during breathing, with the activity of both the crural diaphragm and the parasternal intercostal increasing proportionately more than the activity of the costal diaphragm.[61] This pattern of differential muscle recruitment did not appear to vary from the pattern of muscle activation in response to hypercapnia, suggesting similarities between breathing and coughing during inspiration, unlike during expiration, as discussed subsequently.

Traditionally, expiration of breathing is considered to be a passive process, with the rate and degree of emptying of the lungs determined solely by the resistive and compliance characteristics of the chest wall, airways, and lung parenchyma. Later evidence indicates that expiration is an active process, with airflow being retarded by continued activation of the diaphragm and other inspiratory muscles during the early phase of expiration (post-inspiratory inspiratory activity) and augmented by contraction of expiratory muscles of the thorax and abdomen during the later phases of expiration. Muscles that may increase expiratory airflow include the triangularis sterni, the internal interosseous, the pectoralis muscles of the chest wall, and the transverse, rectus, and internal and external oblique muscles of the abdomen. The degree to which expiration is actively regulated is variable among species and is influenced by posture and respiratory drive. In contrast to breathing, in which active control of expiration plays a modulatory as opposed to a primary role, vigorous recruitment of expiratory muscles is an essential component of coughing and sneezing.

Several studies have quantified electrical activity of expiratory muscles during coughing, and all agree that the abdominal, intercostal, and triangularis sterni muscles are activated to levels exceeding values during stimulated breathing (Fig. 17–3).[6, 11, 14, 18, 41, 55, 59, 62] Floyd and Silver[18] recorded abdominal muscle activity in humans using surface electrodes placed slightly lateral to the midline, which records rectus abdominis activity, and over the lateral abdominal wall of the upper abdomen, which they believed recorded predominantly external oblique muscle activity, and lower abdomen, which they believed recorded predominantly external oblique activity. During coughing upper and lower abdominal muscle activity was vigorous, whereas rectus abdominis activity was minimal. Strohl and colleagues[55] also recorded abdominal muscle activity in humans from electrodes placed in similar locations, although

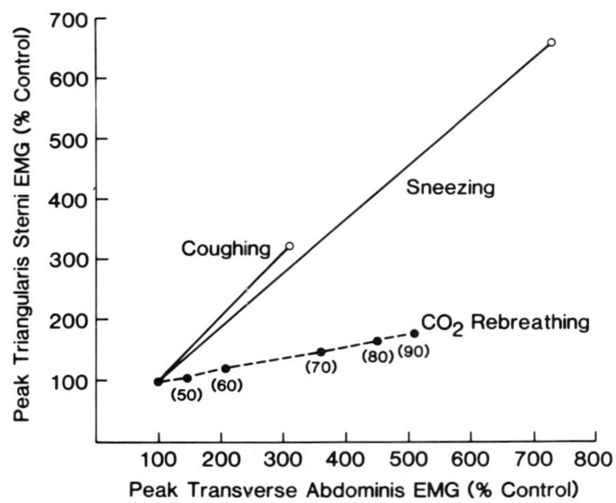

Figure 17–3. Peak electromyographic (EMG) activity recorded from two expiratory muscles, the transverse abdominis and the triangularis sterni, as a percent of values found during quiet oxygen breathing in anesthetized dogs. Mean values are illustrated for coughing and sneezing and compared with values for breathing during progressive hyperoxic hypercapnia. CO_2 rebreathing; numbers indicate values for end-tidal carbon dioxide partial pressure (P_{CO_2}) in mm Hg. (Reproduced with permission from van Lunteren E, Haxhiu MA, Cherniack NS, Arnold JS. J Appl Physiol 1988; 65:2440-2445.)

based on sonographic evidence they did not believe upper and lower abdominal muscle recordings were specific for the external and internal oblique muscles, respectively. The same study confirmed the greater activation of upper and lower lateral abdominal muscles, compared with the rectus abdominis muscle during coughing.

DeTroyer and colleagues[14] found that in humans the triangularis sterni, an expiratory rib cage muscle, was active during coughing. Regarding animal studies, in anesthetized cats the rectus abdominis is activated during coughing,[6, 41, 59] although the degree of rectus activation has not been directly compared with that of other abdominal muscles. In anesthetized, artificially ventilated animals, Tomori and Widdicombe[59] found that rectus abdominis single- or pauci-fiber motor unit firing frequency increased from less than 0.5 impulses per second during breathing to 6 to 8 impulses per second during fictive coughs. In anesthetized dogs, both the triangularis sterni and the transverse abdominis are electrically active during resting breathing, and the peak activity of both muscles increases approximately three-fold during coughing and six- to seven-fold during sneezing (Fig. 17–3).[62] Furthermore, electrical activity of the expiratory muscles reaches a peak within 50 to 200 milliseconds or sooner after cough onset, in contrast to during breathing when peak values of electromyographic activity occur much later into expiration. The pattern of recruitment of different muscles during coughing may not be identical to during breathing. For example, in anesthetized animals during progressive hypercapnia, increases in transverse abdominis electrical activity as a percent of control values during resting breathing exceed those of the triangularis sterni, whereas during coughing the relative recruitment of the two muscles is much more similar.[62]

Electromyographic and mechanical evidence shows that the inspiratory muscles remain active during the early expiratory portion of coughs.[10, 39, 40, 59, 61, 70] These agonist-antagonist interactions between inspiratory and expiratory muscles of the thorax in humans are of a smaller magnitude during coughing than during forced vital capacity maneuvers, as assessed from measurements of esophageal and gastric pressure.[39, 40] In anesthetized cats, direct recordings of diaphragm and phrenic nerve electrical activity show obvious persistence of activation of inspiratory muscles during the early expiratory phase of coughing.[59, 61] Tomori and Widdicombe[59] found that the intensity of diaphragm activity during early expiration of coughs exceeded that during inspiration of coughs. However, the activation was relatively short-lived, lasting in the order of 0.1 to 0.2 seconds and ceasing prior to the attainment of peak-positive intrapleural pressure. In a later study on anesthetized cats, the duration of activity during early expiration of coughs averaged 0.17 seconds for the costal diaphragm, 0.25 seconds for the crural diaphragm, and 0.31 seconds for the parasternal intercostal muscles, values that were similar to the duration of early expiratory activity during breathing.[61] These data indicate that agonist-antagonist relations are not limited to the diaphragm, but that they are present for the rib cage muscles as well. The persistent activation of inspiratory muscles during expiration is believed to optimize the timing of pressure distributions between the abdomen and thorax during the compressive phase of coughs. In addition, it may maintain the expiratory muscles at longer lengths until the onset of the expulsive phase and, hence, optimize their force of contraction by retaining favorable positions on their length-tension relationships.

During breathing, many dilator muscles located at the nasal, pharyngeal, and laryngeal portions of the upper airways are rhythmically active in phase with inspiration. The resulting dilation of the upper airway reduces total respiratory resistance and prevents airway occlusion due to gravitational forces. During expiration, airflow profiles may be modified by reciprocal activity of dilating and constricting muscles of the larynx and to a lesser extent more proximal portions of the upper airways.

The activity of upper airway muscles during coughing is inferred mainly from descriptions of vocal cord and supraglottic movements, because of the paucity of direct electromyographic recordings.[15, 17, 58, 63, 69] In humans, recordings of laryngeal and supraglottic movements indicate that during inspiration of coughs the vocal cords initially open. This is then followed by a rapid and firm closure of the cords during the compressive phase and a reopening of the glottis during the expulsive phase.[63] The glottic closure during the compressive phase is longer lasting than that during phonation and is reinforced by adduction of the ventricular folds and by covering of the laryngeal inlet by the epiglottis. During the expulsive phase, high-frequency, low-amplitude vocal cord vibrations are superimposed on the overall abduction. These vibrations start at the onset of abduction and cease prior to attainment of maximal glottic dilation. Lower frequency vibrations of the aryepiglottic fold and epiglottis occur as well, but these are of shorter duration. The overall cycle of glottic dilation, narrowing, and dilation during the first three phases of coughing are the direct consequence of laryngeal muscle contraction,[17, 63] whereas the superimposed vibrations during the expulsive phase are believed to represent aerodynamic phenomena related to the flow profiles during coughing.[63] Faaborg-Anderson[15] recorded electromyograms from laryngeal adductors (cricothyroid, vocal, and arytenoid muscles), and a laryngeal abductor (posterior cricoarytenoid muscle), using intramuscular electrodes in human subjects with normal vocal cord function and in patients with vocal cord paresis. During coughing the adductors were maximally active prior to the onset of sound production, with tapering of activity thereafter (Fig. 17–4). The interval between the onset of adductor activity and the onset of sound production was greater during coughing with a range of 0.12 to 1.09 seconds, than during vocalization, with a range of 0.10 to 0.34 seconds. Furthermore, the peak electrical activity of the laryngeal adductors was greater during coughing than either resting breathing or vocalization. Regarding the posterior cricoarytenoid muscle, its activity pattern was reciprocal to that of the laryngeal adductors, with a period of inhibition starting 0.35 seconds and ending 0.08 seconds prior to sound production.

Coughing also requires activation of other striated muscles of the upper airways. During coughing, in contrast to sneezing, expiratory airflow primarily traverses the oral passageways. This requires appropriate movement of the soft palate to close the nasopharynx, and, in addition, the muscles responsible for

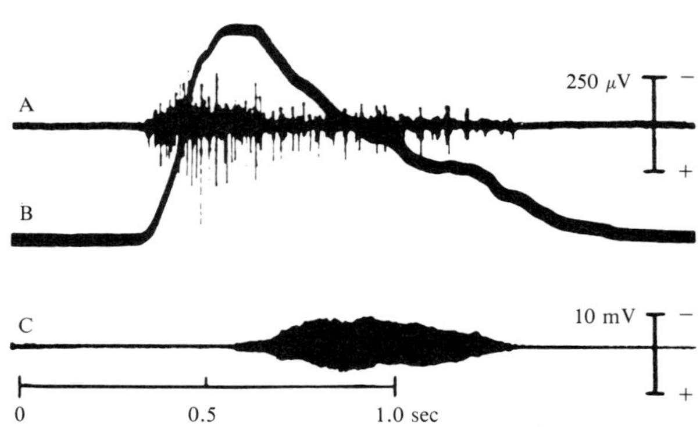

Figure 17–4. Laryngeal abductor muscle activity during cough in humans. Traces indicate the electromyogram recorded from the left vocal muscle *(A)*, mean amplitude of the vocal muscle electromyogram *(B)*, and microphone recording of sound *(C)*. (Reproduced with permission from Faaborg-Andersen K. Acta Physiol Scand 1957; 41:1–148.)

lowering the jaw and opening the mouth need to be recruited. In anesthetized cats, the genioglossus muscle is activated when coughing is produced by mechanically stimulating the larynx or tracheobronchial tree, although this response appears to be in part a consequence of the mucosal stimulation and not totally an integral part of the cough response.[58]

CONCLUSIONS

Cough is a complex component of the respiratory defensive system involving multiple respiratory and neuromuscular structures. Receptors and afferent nerves subserving cough are located both in the tracheobronchial tree and the upper airways. A large number of stimuli are capable of initiating defensive reflexes, with the resultant response determined by location and type of receptor stimulated. Central neuronal groups located especially in the NTS but also elsewhere in the medulla receive input from the peripheral receptors and via interneurons produce activation of the medullary and spinal motoneurons, comprising the efferent limb of the defensive reflexes. The identity of the medullary and pontine structures involved in respiratory rhythmicity have been largely identified, and it appears that these areas participate in but are not totally responsible for generation of the more complex defensive rhythms. Efferent nerves involved in respiratory defensive reflexes supply inspiratory and expiratory muscles of the thorax, abdomen, and neck, and the dilator and constrictor muscles of the upper airways. Coordination between muscle groups results in single or repetitive cycles of a four-phased motor output consisting of inspiration, compression, expulsion, and termination. Optimization of the inspiratory and compressive phases maximizes the mechanical efficiency of the subsequent expulsive phase and hence potentiates the removal of secretions and exogenous substances from the lungs.

REFERENCES

1. Banner AS. Cough: physiology, evaluation, and treatment. Lung 1986; 164:79–92.
2. Bartlett D Jr, Remmers JE, Gautier H. Laryngeal regulation of respiratory airflow. Respir Physiol 1973; 18:194–204.
3. Bartlett D Jr. Regulation of respiratory movements by afferents from the upper airways. Presented at Central Neural Production of Periodic Respiratory Movements International Symposium, April 14–18, 1982, Lake Bluff, IL.
4. Berger AJ, Averill DB. Projection of single pulmonary stretch receptors to solitary tract region. J Neurophysiol 1983; 49:819–830.
5. Berger AJ. Dorsal respiratory group neurons in the medulla of cat: spinal projections, responses to lung inflation and superior laryngeal nerve stimulation. Brain Res 1977; 135:231–254.
6. Boushey HA, Richardson PS, Widdicombe JG. Reflex effects of laryngeal irritation on the pattern of breathing and total lung resistance. J Physiol 1972; 224:501–513.
7. Bucher K. Pathophysiology and pharmacology of cough. Pharmacol Rev 1958; 10:43–58.
8. Coleridge HM, Coleridge JCG. Reflexes evoked from tracheobronchial tree and lungs. In: Geiger SR, ed. Handbook of Physiology, section 3, The Respiratory System, Fishman AP, ed. vol II, Control of Breathing, part 1, Cherniack NS, Widdicombe JG, eds. Bethesda, MD: American Physiological Society, 1986, 395–429.
9. Coleridge JCG, Coleridge HM. Afferent vagal C fibre innervation of the lungs and airways and its functional significance. Rev Physiol Biochem Pharmacol 1984; 99:1–110.
10. Coryllos PN. Action of the diaphragm in cough. Experimental and clinical study on the human. Am J Med Sci 1937; 194:523–535.
11. Cox ID, Wallis PJW, Apps MCP, et al. An electromyographic method of objectively assessing cough intensity and use of the method to assess effects of codeine on the dose-response curve to citric acid. Br J Clin Pharmacol 1984; 18:377–382.
12. Davies RO, Kubin L. Projection of pulmonary rapidly adapting receptors to the medulla of the cat: an antidromic mapping study. J Physiol 1986; 373:63–86.
13. Davies RO, Kubin L, Pack AI. Pulmonary stretch receptor relay neurones of the cat: location and contralateral medullary projections. J Physiol 1987; 383:571–585.
14. De Troyer A, Ninane V, Gilmartin JJ, Lemerre C, Estenne M. Triangularis sterni muscle use in supine humans. J Appl Physiol 1987; 62:919–925.
15. Faaborg-Anderson K. Electromyographic investigation of intrinsic laryngeal muscles in humans. Acta Physiol Scand 1957; 41:1–148.
16. Fillenz M, Widdicombe JG. Receptors of the lungs and airway. In: Neil E, ed. Enteroceptor, Volume III, section 1, Handbook of Sensory Physiology, Autrum H, Jung R, Loewenstein WR, MacKay DM, Teuber HL (eds). New York: Springer-Verlag, 1972, 81–112.
17. Floersheim GL. Über die rolle der glottis beim husten. Helv Physiol Pharmacol Acta 1959; 17:153–165.
18. Floyd WF, Silver PHS. Electromyographic study of patterns of activity of the anterior abdominal wall muscles in man. J Anat 1950; 84:132–145.
19. Hanácek J, Davies A, Widdicombe JG. Influence of lung stretch receptors on the cough reflex in rabbits. Respiration 1984; 45:161–168.
20. Harris RS, Lawson TV. The relative mechanical effectiveness and efficiency of successive voluntary coughs in healthy young adults. Clin Sci 1968; 34:569–577.
21. Irwin RS, Rosen MJ, Braman SS. Cough. A comprehensive review. Arch Intern Med 1977; 137:1186–1191.
22. Jamal K, McMahon G, Edgel G, Fleetham JA. Cough and arousal responses to inhaled citric acid in sleeping humans. Am Rev Respir Dis 1983; 127:A237.
23. Kalia M, Mesulam M-M. Brain stem projections of sensory and motor components of the vagus complex in the cat: II. Laryngeal tracheobronchial, pulmonary, cardiac, and gastrointestinal branches. J Comp Neurol 1980; 193:467–508.
24. Kalia M, Mesulam M-M. Brain stem projections of sensory and motor components of the vagus complex in the cat: the cervical vagus and nodose ganglion. J Comp Neurol 1980; 193:435–465.
25. Kalia M, Richter D. Morphology of physiologically identified slowly adapting lung stretch receptor afferents stained with intra-axonal horseradish peroxidase in the nucleus of the tractus solitarius of the cat. II. An ultrastructural analysis. J Comp Neurol 1985; 241:521–535.
26. Kalia M, Richter D. Morphology of physiologically identified slowly adapting lung stretch receptor afferents stained with intra-axonal horseradish peroxidase in the nucleus of the tractus solitarius of the cat. I. A light microscopic analysis. J Comp Neurol 1985; 241:503–520.
27. Kalia M, Richter D. Rapidly adapting pulmonary receptor afferents: I. Arborization in the nucleus of the tractus solitarius. J Comp Neurol 1988; 274:560–573.
28. No reference.
29. Kalia M, Richter D. Rapidly adapting pulmonary receptor afferents: II. Fine structure and synaptic organization of central terminal processes in the nucleus of the tractus solitarius. J Comp Neurol 1988; 274:574–594.
30. Karlsson J-A, Sant'Ambrogio G, Widdicombe J. Afferent neural pathways in cough and reflex bronchoconstriction. J Appl Physiol 1988; 65:1007–1023.
31. Kasé Y, Wakita Y, Kito G, Miyata T, Yuizone T, Kataoka M. Centrally-induced coughs in the cat. Life Sci 1970; 9:49–59.
32. Kerr FWL. The divisional organization of afferent fibres of the trigeminal nerve. Brain 1963; 86:721–732.
33. Knowlton GC, Larrabee MG. A unitary analysis of pulmonary volume receptors. Am J Physiol 1946; 147:100–114.
34. Knudson RJ, Mead J, Knudson DE. Contribution of airway collapse to supramaximal expiratory flows. J Appl Physiol 1974; 36:653–667.
35. Korpáš J, Tomori Z. Cough and other respiratory reflexes. In: Herzog H, ed. Progress in Respiration Research, vol 12, New York: S. Karger, 1979.
36. Leith DE. Cough. In: Lenfant C, ed. Lung Biology in Health and Disease, Respiratory Defense Mechanisms, vol 5, Brain JD,

Proctor DF, Reid LM, eds. New York: Marcel Dekker Inc., 1977, 545–592.
37. Leith DE, Butler JP, Sneedon SL, Brain JD. Cough. In: Geiger SR, ed. Handbook of Physiology, section 3, The Respiratory System, Fishman AP, ed. vol III, Mechanics of Breathing, Macklem PT, Mead J, eds. Bethesda, MD: American Physiological Society, 1986, 315–336.
38. McCrimmon DR, Speck DF, Feldman JL. Role of the ventrolateral region of the nucleus of the tractus solitarius in processing respiratory afferent input from vagus and superior laryngeal nerves. Exp Brain Res 1987; 67:449–459.
39. Mellissinos CG, Bruce E, Leith DE. Factors affecting pleural pressure during cough in normal man. Clin Res 1976; 24:643A.
40. Mellissinos CG, Leith DE, Brody JS, et al. Thoracoabdominal mechanics in spontaneous cough. Am Rev Respir Dis 1978; 117:372.
41. Mori M, Sakai Y. Re-examination of centrally-induced cough in cats using a micro-stimulation technique. Jpn J Pharmacol 1972; 22:635–643.
42. Nasution ID, Shigenaga Y. Ascending and descending internuclear projections within the trigeminal sensory nuclear complex. Brain Res 1987; 425:234–247.
43. Nishino T, Hiraga K, Mizuguchi T, Honda Y. Respiratory reflex responses to stimulation of tracheal mucosa in enflurane-anesthetized humans. J Appl Physiol 1988; 65:1069–1074.
44. Paintal AS. Impulses in vagal afferent fibres from specific pulmonary deflation receptors. The response of these receptors to phenyl diguanide, potato starch, 5-hydroxytryptamine and nicotine, and their role in respiratory and cardiovascular reflexes. Q J Exp Physiol 1955; 40:89–111.
45. Paintal AS. Mechanism of stimulation of type J pulmonary receptors. J Physiol 1969; 203:511–32.
46. Paintal AS. Cardiovascular receptors. In: Neil E, ed. Enteroceptors. volume III, section 1, Handbook of Sensory Physiology, Autrum H, Jung R, Loewenstein WR, MacKay DM, Teuber HL, eds. New York: Springer-Verlag, 1972, 1–45.
47. Paintal AS. The location and excitation of pulmonary deflation receptors by chemical substances. Q J Exp Physiol 1957; 42:56–71.
48. Panneton WM, Burton H. Projections from the paratrigeminal nucleus and the medullary and spinal dorsal horns to the peribrachial area in the cat. Neuroscience 1985; 3:779–797.
49. Power JT, Stewart IC, Connaughton JJ, Brash HM, Shapiro CM, Flenley DC, Douglas NJ. Nocturnal cough in patients with chronic bronchitis and emphysema. Am Rev Respir Dis 1984; 130:999–1001.
50. Ross BB, Gramiak R, Rahn H. Physical dynamics of the cough mechanism. J Appl Physiol 1955; 8:264–268.
51. Sant'Ambrogio G. Information arising from the tracheobronchial tree of mammals. Physiol Rev 1982; 62:531–569.
52. Sant'Ambrogio G, Mathew OP, Fisher JT, Sant'Ambrogio FB. Laryngeal receptors responding to transmural pressure, airflow and local muscle activity. Respir Physiol 1983; 54:317–330.
53. Sant'Ambrogio G, Mathew OP, Sant'Ambrogio FB, Fisher JT. Laryngeal cold receptors. Respir Physiol 1985; 59:35–44.
54. Shigenaga Y, Okamoto T, Nishimori T, et al. Oral and facial representation in the trigeminal principal and rostral spinal nuclei of the cat. J Comp Neurol 1986; 244:1–18.
55. Strohl KP, Mead J, Banzett RB, et al. Regional differences in abdominal muscle activity during various maneuvers in humans. J Appl Physiol 1981; 51:1471–1476.
56. Sullivan CE, Kozar LF, Murphy E, Phillipson EA. Arousal, ventilatory, and airway responses to bronchopulmonary stimulation in sleeping dogs. J Appl Physiol 1979; 47:17–25.
57. Sullivan CE, Murphy E, Kozar LF, Phillipson EA. Waking and ventilatory responses to laryngeal stimulation in sleeping dogs. J Appl Physiol 1978; 45:681–689.
58. Tatar M, Webber SE, Widdicombe JG. Lung C-fibre receptor activation and defensive reflexes in anaesthetized cats. J Physiol 1988; 402:411–420.
59. Tomori Z, Widdicombe JG. Muscular, bronchomotor and cardiovascular reflexes elicited by mechanical stimulation of the respiratory tract. J Physiol 1969; 200:25–49.
60. van Lunteren E, Strohl KP. Striated respiratory muscles of the upper airways. In: Mathew OP, Sant'Ambrogio G, eds. Respiratory Function of the Upper Airway, New York: Marcel Dekker Inc., 1988, 87–123.
61. van Lunteren E, Daniels R, Deal EC Jr, Haxhiu MA. Role of costal and crural diaphragm and parasternal intercostals during coughing in cats. J Appl Physiol 1989; 66:135–141.
62. van Lunteren E, Haxhiu MA, Cherniack NS, Arnold JS. Role of triangularis sterni during coughing and sneezing in dogs. J Appl Physiol 1988; 65:2440–2445.
63. von Leden H, Isshiki N. An analysis of cough at the level of the larynx. Arch Otol 1965; 81:616–625.
64. Wall PD, Taub A. Four aspects of trigeminal nucleus and a paradox. J Neurophysiol 1962; 25:110–126.
65. Widdicombe JG. Nasal and pharyngeal reflexes. Protective and respiratory functions. In: Lenfant C, ed. Lung Biology in Health and Disease, Respiratory Function of the Upper Airway, vol 35, Mathew OP, Sant'Ambrogio G, eds. New York: Marcel Dekker Inc., 1988, 233–258.
66. Widdicombe JG. Sensory innervation of the lungs and airways. In: Cervero F, Morrison JFB, eds. Progress in Brain Research, The Netherlands: Elsevier Science Publishing Co., 1986, 49–64.
67. Widdicombe JG. Respiratory reflexes and defense. In: Lenfant C, ed. Lung Biology in Health and Disease, Respiratory Defense Mechanisms, vol 5, Brain JD, Proctor DF, Reid LM, eds. New York: Marcel Dekker Inc., 1977, 593–630.
68. Widdicombe JG. Reflexes from the upper respiratory tract. In: Geiger SR ed. Handbook of Physiology, section 3: The Respiratory System, Fishman AP, ed. volume II: Control of Breathing, part 1, Cherniack NS, Widdicombe JG, eds. Bethesda, MD: American Physiological Society, 1986, 363–394.
69. Yanagihara N, von Leden H, Werner-Kukuk E. The physical parameters of cough: the larynx in a normal single cough. Acta Otolaryngol 1966; 61:495–510.
70. Yanaura S, Kamei J, Goto K, et al. Analysis of efferent discharges of the phrenic nerve during the cough reflex. Jpn J Pharmacol 1982; 32:795–801.

Section IV

SYSTEMIC EFFECTS OF CHRONIC OBSTRUCTIVE PULMONARY DISEASE

Chapter 18

COPD AND THE PERIPHERAL CIRCULATION

Robert A. Wise

The goal of this chapter is to describe the ways in which chronic obstructive lung disease affects the peripheral circulation and left ventricle. Fundamental principles of the mechanics of the peripheral circulation and the performance of the left ventricle are discussed as a basis for understanding their interactions with respiratory events. This section addresses the ways in which obstructive lung disease in its chronic state and during acute exacerbations may influence systemic venous return to the right side of the heart, and how chronic obstructive lung disease may influence the function of the left ventricle.

SYSTEMIC VENOUS RETURN

Cardiac output must be increased under conditions of either greater oxygen utilization, e.g., exercise, or reduced oxygen content of the blood, e.g., hypoxemia. Total steady state cardiac output is determined by the total amount of blood which can return from the peripheral circulation to the heart, as well as by the ability of the heart to pump the blood into the peripheral circulation. The ways in which respiratory mechanics interact with the peripheral circulation have been analyzed in detail elsewhere.[1–6] Respiratory mechanical events that interfere with the delivery of blood back to the heart from the periphery or that interfere with the ability of the heart to eject blood into the peripheral circulation lead to a reduction in cardiac output.

To understand the determinants of systemic venous return, four important concepts are presented subsequently: mean systemic pressure, resistance to venous return, backpressure to venous return, and collapsibility of the veins.

Mean Systemic Pressure

No matter how complicated the mechanical properties of the peripheral circulation in terms of parallel and series compliances and resistances, it can be demonstrated that an equivalent steady-state circuit can be formulated consisting of a single arterial resistance, a venous compliance, and a venous resistance.[7] The pressure in the equivalent compliant region is termed the mean systemic pressure, not to be confused with systemic arterial pressure. The mean systemic pressure can be defined as the peripheral circulatory pressure that is independent of the flow through the circuit. When the flow through the circuit is zero, the pressure at all points along the circuit will be equal to the mean systemic pressure.[8] If both ends of the circuit are connected to an active pump, i.e., the heart, then the increase in flow will be accompanied by an increase in pressure at all locations upstream from the compliance, and a decrease in pressure at all locations downstream from the compliance. The mean systemic pressure in the compliant region, then, is independent of flow through the circuit and, thus, independent of the function of the heart.

The mean systemic pressure depends only on the pressure-volume characteristics of the circulation and the volume of blood in the peripheral circulation. The mean systemic pressure can be considered the static recoil pressure of the peripheral circulation, which tends to return blood to the heart. Although the exact locus of this pressure has not been measured, it is thought to exist in the small veins, which are the seat of the major vascular compliance of the peripheral circulation (Fig. 18–1).

In experimental animals, mean systemic pressure can be readily measured by momentarily stopping the circulation and measuring the equilibration pressure. Alternatively, the mean systemic pressure can be measured by raising the right atrial pressure to cause a reduction in systemic venous return, and extrapolating to the value of right atrial pressure at which flow equals zero. The mean systemic pressure is normally approximately 7 mm Hg. It is decreased in hypovolemia or peripheral vascular collapse and is increased in volume loading or adrenergic stimulation.[12, 13]

Resistance to Venous Return

The resistance to systemic venous return is not to be confused with systemic or peripheral vascular resistance. The resistance to blood flow returning to the right side of the heart from the peripheral circulation can be described by the pressure gradient from any point in the peripheral circulation to the right atrial pressure divided by the blood flow between those two points. It is common clinical practice to measure the gradient between aortic pressure and right atrial pressure and divide this pressure gradient by total cardiac output, thereby calculating systemic vascular resistance. Although it is not easily performed clinically, it is of great conceptual importance to understand the meaning of the resistance to venous return. This is measured using the pressure gradient between the pressure at the static locus, i.e., the mean systemic pressure, and the right atrium. It can be measured experimen-

The author gratefully acknowledges the helpful discussions with Dr. Solbert Permutt and Dr. James Robotham and the excellent secretarial assistance of Ms. Brenda Jordan.

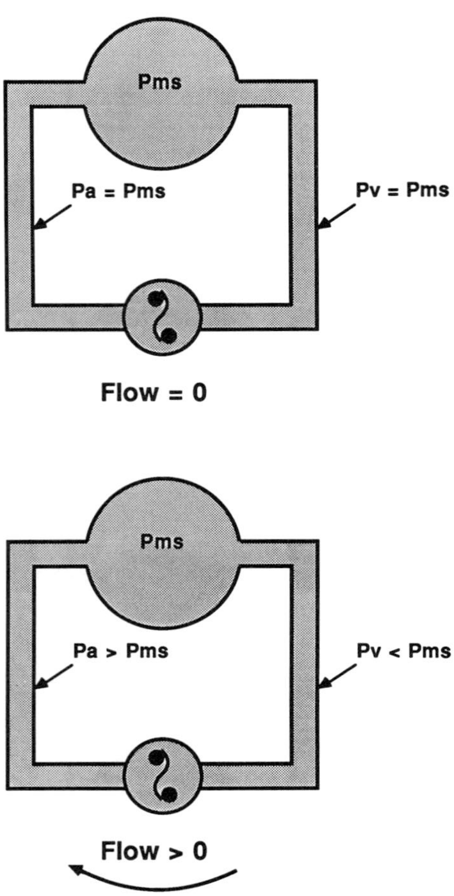

Figure 18–1. The steady state flow characteristics of the peripheral circulation can be grouped into a single equivalent circuit, which consists of an arterial conduit with resistance but no compliance, a peripheral compliance with no resistance, and a venous resistance with no compliance. This circuit is attached to a rotary pump, which represents the heart.

When the pump is turned off *(upper panel)*, the pressures everywhere in the circuit are equal to mean systemic pressure (Pms). This pressure is determined by the volume of blood in the circuit and the pressure volume characteristics of the compliance.

When the pump is activated *(lower panel)*, the pressures on the venous side of the circuit fall, and the pressures on the arterial side of the circuit rise. The pressures in the compliant portion of the circuit, however, do not change.

When there is flow through the circuit, the volume of blood returning to the pump, the "venous return," is determined by the pressure gradient between the mean systemic pressure in the compliant region and the inflow end of the pump, the "right atrial" pressure. Viewed from this perspective, the total flow through the circuit can be considered to be determined in part by the ability of the pump to lower the inflow pressure with respect to the mean systemic pressure.

tally in animals by elevating right atrial pressure (e.g., by pericardial tamponade or by obstruction of the tricuspid valve) at constant blood volume and thus constant mean systemic pressure. The resistance to venous return is calculated by dividing the change in right atrial pressure by the change in cardiac output.[7, 9]

Backpressure to Venous Return

The backpressure to venous return is the right atrial pressure, which is determined by the diastolic volume of the right side of the heart, its pressure-volume characteristics, and the surrounding pressures in the pericardial and pleural spaces.[10] If the systemic blood-volume and vascular pressure-volume characteristics are unaltered, then an elevation of right atrial pressure leads to a reduction in systemic venous return. An acute elevation of right atrial pressure such as can occur with a Valsalva maneuver, chest compression, pericardial tamponade, or right-sided heart failure (e.g., acute pulmonary embolism) frequently leads to a sufficient reduction in cardiac output to cause syncope. If there were no reflex changes, an elevation of right atrial pressure to the level of mean systemic pressure of only 7 mm Hg would lead to a cessation of all systemic venous return. After a period of time, however, sympathetic reflex responses tend to restore the cardiac output through reduction in compliance or unstressed volume of the peripheral circulation.[11, 12] In addition, there may be redistribution of blood from the central circulation to the peripheral circulation or redistribution of blood flow from slowly draining beds, such as the splanchnic circulation, to more quickly draining beds, such as the muscle.[11–14]

Collapse of the Vena Cava

Although elevation of right atrial pressure is very effective in reducing systemic venous return, lowering of right atrial pressure below about −2 mm Hg does not increase systemic venous return above a maximal venous return, owing to collapse of the vena cava and flow limitation in the systemic veins.[15, 16] Similar to the determinants of maximal expiratory airflow in the lungs, the maximal systemic venous return is dependent on the elastic recoil pressure of the peripheral circulation (i.e., mean systemic pressure), the resistance to flow upstream to the site of collapse (i.e., resistance to venous return), and the collapsibility characteristics of the conduit (i.e., the vena cava).[17, 18] Therefore, when the right atrial pressure is reduced markedly below atmospheric pressure, such as occurs with deep or obstructed inspiration, systemic venous return cannot increase above the flow-limiting amount. Only an increase in the elastic recoil pressure of the peripheral venous circulation, such as by volume loading or by sympathetic tone, or a decrease in the resistance to venous return, such as by redistribution of blood flow away from slowly draining regions, can significantly raise maximum systemic venous return under these circumstances.

How Chronic Obstructive Lung Disease Affects Systemic Venous Return

Chronic obstructive lung disease can change the determinants of systemic venous return through altered mechanical characteristics of either the heart or the lungs.

EFFECTS OF PLEURAL PRESSURE ON SYSTEMIC VENOUS RETURN

It is a common incorrect clinical intuition that acute exacerbations of airway obstruction that are due to expiratory airflow obstruction cause an elevation of pleural pressure. Several studies have confirmed the opposite: acute episodes of bronchospasm lead to very negative pleural pressure swings during inspiration, accompanied by modest elevations of pleural pressure during expiration.[19–21] The inspiratory pleural pressure is reduced to about −30 cm H_2O while the expiratory pleural pressure is increased to only −2 to +4 cm H_2O.[21] Breathing at high lung volumes, while preventing airway collapse, increases the work of breathing and leads to the large negative pleural pressure swings. With exercise, however, some patients with chronic obstructive lung disease adopt a breathing strategy with very positive pleural pressure swings during expiration, using forced expiration to prevent hyperinflation.[22] Although the negative swings in pleural pressure have little effect on systemic venous return because of the flow limitation of the venae cavae, the positive swings cyclically decrease systemic venous return, and this can lead to an exaggeration of respiratory variation in arterial blood pressure or *pulsus paradoxus*.[23, 24] Pulsus paradoxus is present in two-thirds of patients with severe chronic obstructive lung disease and is correlated with the degree of airflow obstruction.[25]

EFFECT OF COR PULMONALE ON SYSTEMIC VENOUS RETURN

Chronic hypoxemia in advanced chronic obstructive pulmonary disease leads to pulmonary hypertension and cor pulmonale.[26] The dilatation and hypertropy of the right side of the heart leads to elevation of right atrial pressure, manifested by the physical finding of elevated jugular venous pressure. Cardiac output is sustained by the retention of fluid, which leads to elevated peripheral venous pressures, manifested by the physical finding of peripheral edema. In the setting of increased right atrial pressures due to cardiac dilatation from pulmonary hypertension, elevation of mean systemic pressure is necessary to maintain a gradient for systemic venous return. For this reason, in the setting of cor pulmonale, dehydration or overuse of diuretics can be particularly dangerous, leading to reduced cardiac output. When right atrial pressure is elevated in the setting of low cardiac output, intravenous fluid administration is often necessary to sustain adequate cardiac output, if it can be delivered without causing pulmonary vascular congestion and lung edema. Elevated jugular venous pressure, in the setting of a reduced cardiac output, can be an indication for volume administration, not diuresis. In the acutely ill patient, monitoring of left ventricular filling pressures may be necessary to prevent pulmonary vascular engorgement and pulmonary edema.

EFFECT OF HYPOXEMIA ON SYSTEMIC VENOUS RETURN

Although chronic hypoxemia may lead to a decrease in cardiac output through right-sided heart failure, acute hypoxemia generally leads to an increase in cardiac output. Although this is partially mediated by an increase in myocardial contractility from catecholamine release, animal experiments suggest that important peripheral circulatory effects also occur. A redistribution of blood flow and blood volume from the high capacitance splanchnic regions occurs, to the lower capacitance cardiac, cerebral, and muscle regions, which leads to an improved gradient for venous return and a reduction in the resistance to venous return. These effects are mediated not only by sympathetic nervous system stimulation but by increased circulating levels of peptide hormones.[27–33]

EFFECTS OF LUNG INFLATION ON SYSTEMIC VENOUS RETURN

Lung hyperinflation occurs in chronic obstructive lung disease as a consequence of the reduced elastic recoil pressure of the lung and the presence of associated bronchospasm. The effect of lung hyperinflation on systemic venous return in this disorder remains to be fully understood, but there is evidence that increases in lung volume may directly impede systemic venous return through compression of the vena cava or heart. When the lungs are hyperinflated with positive pressure ventilation, there is direct compression of the heart by the expanding and less deformable lung.[34] It remains to be seen if this phenomenon can actually lead to an increase in right atrial pressure relative to atmospheric pressure with spontaneous inspiration. Kussmaul's sign (inspiratory elevation of venous pressure) can be observed on occasion in acute right-sided heart failure, and compression of the heart may be the mechanism for Kussmaul's sign.

Lung inflation can also indirectly compress the heart through the linkage of the diaphragm with the pericardium. When the diaphragm is contracted, tension is developed in the pericardiophrenic ligaments, which increases pericardial pressure.[35] This could also lead to a paradoxical inspiratory decrease in systemic venous return.

Normally, inspiration leads to an increase in systemic venous return due to the fall in right atrial pressure. When the lungs are markedly hyperinflated in advanced chronic obstructive lung disease, some patients exhibit paradoxical reduction or cessation of systemic venous return from the inferior vena cava during inspiration.[36] It is postulated that the inflated lungs can directly compress the vena cava leading to distortion and reduction in venous return.[37, 38] Some cases have been reported in which resection of giant bullae have been thought to improve cardiac exercise limitation by removing this compression of the vena cava. In most cases, however, inspiration leads to normal augmentation of systemic venous return.[39]

EFFECTS OF ABDOMINAL PRESSURE ON VENOUS RETURN

During exercise of hyperventilation, some individuals with chronic obstructive lung disease actively expire, leading to an increase in abdominal pressure.[22] Although this effect has not been studied in humans with chronic obstructive lung disease, the effect of increases in abdominal pressure on systemic venous return have shown conflicting and confusing results. Some studies have shown increases in systemic venous return, whereas others have shown decreases in systemic venous return associated with increases in abdominal pressure.[40–47]

Studies in animals have shown that these conflicting results can be explained by considering the intravascular volume status.[41, 43, 48] When the intravascular volume is low, an increase in abdominal pressure causes collapse of the vena cava and obstructs blood flow from the lower extremities. This leads to a fall in systemic venous return from the inferior vena cava. When the intravascular volume is high, an increase in abdominal pressure raises the gradient for systemic venous return from the abdominal compartment and causes a net increase in inferior vena caval blood flow. The effects of abdominal pressure on systemic venous return can be considered analogous to the effects of alveolar pressure on pulmonary venous return.[49] When alveolar pressure is high relative to pulmonary venous pressure (zone II), pulmonary venous return falls with an increase in alveolar pressure. When alveolar pressure is low relative to pulmonary venous pressure (zone III), pulmonary venous return rises with an increase in alveolar pressure.

Thus, increases in expiratory abdominal pressure during vigorous ventilation in patients with chronic obstructive lung disease could either assist or inhibit cardiac output depending on intravascular volume status. If venous pressure is high, then cardiac output would be aided. If venous pressure is low, cardiac output would be reduced.

LEFT VENTRICULAR FUNCTION

A large body of experimental evidence has emphasized that the function of the left ventricle can be characterized as a time-varying elastance.[50, 51] During the course of ventricular ejection, the ventricle follows a reproducible path through a family of approximately linear pressure-volume lines that intersect at the unstressed volume of the ventricle (Vo). The degree of maximum stiffening of the ventricle (Emax), the slope of the end-systolic pressure-volume curve, is an excellent indicator of the contractile state of the left ventricle and is independent of changes in preload or afterload (Fig. 18–2).

The effect of an increase in afterload on the left ventricle is determined by the Emax slope. If Emax is high, i.e., the ventricle has good contractility and is very stiff at end-systole, then an increase in end-systolic transmural ventricular pressure would have little effect on end-systolic volume. Stroke volume would be little impaired. Alternatively, if Emax is low, i.e., the ventricle has poor contractility and is very compliant at end-systole, then an increase in end-systolic transmural pressure would cause a large increase in end-systolic volume, leading to a large reduction in stroke volume.

Although the measurement of Emax in humans is difficult because it requires the accurate measurement of ventricular volume at several end-systolic pressures with constant contractile state, it provides the basis for contemporary measures of ventricular functional assessment. Because the pleural pressure surrounding the heart is an important determinant of the transmural ventricular pressure, the effect of changes in pleural pressure on the end-systolic volume and stroke volume depend on the contractile state of the ventricle.

Effects of Pleural Pressure on Left Ventricular Performance

A large body of work in investigating the effect of pleural pressure on left ventricular performance has been done.[52–59] This is an important consideration because of the alterations in pleural pressure swings that are present in chronic obstructive lung disease. Large negative pleural pressure swings during inspiration are countered by slightly positive pleural pressure swings during expiration. These pleural pressure swings are exaggerated during periods of acute bronchospasm or during exercise hyperventilation.[19–22]

The stress on the left ventricle during ejection is determined by its radius of curvature and the transmural pressure across the wall of the ventricle. Usually, left ventricular wall stress is considered to be dominated by the pressure on the inside of

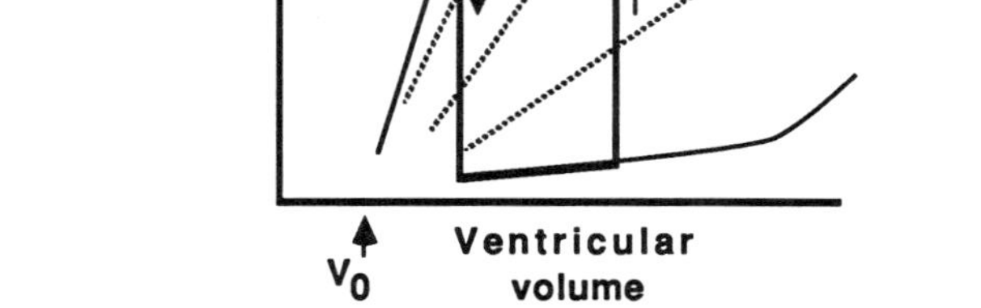

Figure 18–2. The pressure-volume relationships of the left ventricle change throughout the course of systole as indicated by the dotted lines, which intersect at Vo. The maximum stiffening of the ventricle occurs at near the end of systole. The slope of this line (Emax) is a good indicator of the contractility of the ventricle. The steeper the line, the lower the end-systolic volume for a particular end-systolic transmural ventricular pressure.

The systolic pressure-volume loop of the ventricle is superimposed on the pressure-volume lines and represents the cycle of diastolic filling, isovolumic contraction, ejection, and isovolumic relaxation.

the ventricle, which is equal to aortic pressure in the absence of aortic valve stenosis. A negative pressure on the exterior surface of the ventricle will also increase wall stress. A major determinant of the stress placed on the left ventricle is the aortic pressure relative to pleural pressure, or the aortic transmural pressure. With normal cardiac contractility and normal ventilatory mechanics, pleural pressure is only a minor determinant of steady-state left ventricular performance. When ventricular contractility is depressed, or when pleural pressure swings are exaggerated, there can be significant effects of negative pleural pressure on cardiac performance, manifest by an exaggerated inspiratory fall in stroke volume, pulsus paradoxus, or an elevation of left ventricular filling pressure. The severity of an asthma attack can be assessed by determining the degree of respiratory variation in systolic pressure, an indirect measure of the magnitude of pleural pressure fluctuation.[60–64] It has been speculated that the sustained stress of exaggerated pleural pressure swings could lead to the unexplained left ventricular hypertrophy that has been reported to occur in patients with chronic obstructive lung disease, described subsequently. In cases of acute respiratory failure with concomitant left ventricular failure, the load imposed by the negative pleural pressure of spontaneous ventilation may contribute to the development of pulmonary edema during weaning from positive pressure ventilation.[65] This adverse effect of respiratory stresses on the heart may, in part, account for the poor prognosis of a patient with chronic obstructive lung disease who sustains acute myocardial infarction.[66]

Effect of Right Ventricular Distention on Left Ventricular Performance

Chronic obstructive lung disease leads to destruction of the pulmonary vascular bed and hypoxemia, which results in pulmonary hypertension and right ventricular distention. This distention of the right ventricle can have important effects on left ventricular function by decreasing diastolic compliance of the left ventricle.[67–75] This phenomenon is known as ventricular interdependence and is mediated by the pericardial constraints[76] or alterations in the geometry of the ventricle, due to leftward septal shift.[77, 78] Thus, distention of the right ventricle leads to an increase in left ventricular filling pressure, which exacerbates pulmonary vascular congestion and pulmonary edema. Convincing evidence exists that acute increases in right ventricular volume, which occur with spontaneous inspiration, can inhibit diastolic filling of the left ventricle and contribute to respiratory variation in stroke volume.[79, 80]

It remains unsettled whether distention of the right ventricle affects systolic function of the left ventricle. Some studies show an improvement[73, 76, 81] in left ventricular ejection and some show a worsening.[59, 74, 75] These conflicting results are consistent with the interpretation that a moderate amount of right ventricular distention serves to stiffen the septal wall of the left ventricle, prevent deformation of the ventricle, and improve ejection. In contrast, excessive degrees of distention deform the septum convex toward the left ventricle. This distortion of the septal left ventricular wall could lead to a geometric inability of the contracting left ventricle to decrease its volume or could potentially impede the left ventricular outflow tract.[82]

Effect of Lung Distention on Left Ventricular Performance

Just as the hyperinflated lungs in chronic obstructive lung disease patients may mechanically impede systemic venous return, the hyperinflated lungs can impede filling of the left side of the heart through direct compression. Animal studies have demonstrated that when the lungs are hyperinflated, the distribution of pleural surface pressure is not uniform throughout the thorax. Pleural pressure is higher where the lungs directly contact the heart.[83-87] Thus, lung hyperinflation may contribute to poor pulmonary venous return or otherwise unexplained elevation of left ventricular filling pressures.

Hypoxemia and Left Ventricular Function

Hypoxemia is a frequent complication of advanced or decompensated chronic obstructive lung disease and may occur at severe levels during sleep in otherwise normoxic patients with chronic obstructive lung disease.[88]

The effect of acute hypoxic hypoxemia on the myocardium is an increase in wall thickness and a decrease in diastolic compliance, which is only partly attributed to greater coronary blood flow causing myocardial tumescence.[89, 90] Hypoxemia leads to increased levels of sympathetic and vagal tone, with a doubling of coronary sinus catecholamine levels and either an increase or no change in ventricular contractility.[91, 92] The variable effects of hypoxemia on myocardial contractility may reflect that the hypoxic myocardium is resistant to the positive inotropic effects of catecholamines, as well as other inotropic drugs, such as methylxanthines and ouabain.[93, 94]

Hypercapnia and Left Ventricular Function

Hypercapnia, which results from alveolar hypoventilation, either in chronic or acute respiratory failure, can reduce cardiac contractility at very high levels.[92] The effect of extremely high levels of hypercapnia is to induce bradycardia and impaired ventricular function to a degree that can mimic a cardiogenic shock syndrome. This is thought to be the result of disordered intramyocardial calcium flux, which can be overcome by catecholamine or calcium infusion.[95]

Abnormal Left Ventricular Function in Chronic Obstructive Lung Disease

Patients with advanced chronic obstructive lung disease frequently manifest dyspnea, orthopnea, jugular venous distention, ankle edema, and rales in the absence of pulmonary vascular congestion. It, therefore, has been an area of considerable clinical interest and controversy—how best to determine which patients with chronic obstructive lung disease have left ventricular dysfunction, and if this is a primary manifestation of chronic obstructive lung disease or the result of other known causes of left ventricular failure. Few areas of clinical research have been pursued with more vigor or with more conflicting findings.

LEFT VENTRICULAR HYPERTROPHY

Autopsy series as early as 1936 found that 59% of obstructive lung disease patients had pathologic thickening of the left ventricle.[96] Many other studies have confirmed a high prevalence of left ventricular thickening in autopsied cases with chronic obstructive lung disease, with prevalence ranging from 24% to 90%.[97-102] Electrocardiographic evidence of left ventricular hypertrophy has been found in 18% of patients with chronic obstructive lung disease.[103] The largest and most thorough autopsy study was performed by Murphy and colleagues.[104] Of 72 autopsied cases, 28% had left ventricular hypertrophy determined by chamber weights, a more accurate method than measuring wall thickness. Of these cases, half involved conditions that could account for left ventricular hypertrophy, but these investigators could not rule out hypertension in the other cases. Murphy's group concluded that if left ventricular hypertrophy did occur as a consequence of obstructive lung disease, it is an uncommon finding. In some cases, however, they did attribute left ventricular hypertrophy to concomitant coronary artery disease, itself a controversial association.

Left ventricular fibrosis has been reported to occur in patients with cor pulmonale, but careful pathologic studies have shown that this does not occur in the absence of coronary artery disease or myocardial infarction.[105] Exercise-induced hypoxemia may predispose the patient to the development of myocardial infarction, however, because reversible thallium perfusion defects have been shown with exercise in hypoxemic patients with chronic obstructive lung disease, even with angiographically normal coronary arteries.[106]

LEFT VENTRICULAR FUNCTION

Over the past two decades, many studies have been performed to determine whether chronic obstructive lung disease, either by itself or as a consequence of cor pulmonale, leads to dysfunction of the left ventricle. The results of these studies are more consistent than the interpretations of investigators who conclude that unexplained left ventricular dysfunction is either a common or an uncommon finding.[107, 108] These studies are summarized in Table 18–1.[109-131, 144, 145] The prevalence of unexplained left ventricular dysfunction appears to be most closely related to the methodology used and to the diligence of seeking out occult coronary artery disease, alcoholism, or valvular heart disease. Kachel[132] reviewed the literature available prior to 1978, and his conclusions, which follow, remain valid at present:

1. A significant percentage of patients with chronic obstructive pulmonary disease have coronary artery disease, which may depress left ventricular function. Even excluding patients with angina or electrocardiographic patterns of infarction still leaves some with silent disease.
2. The majority of patients with chronic pulmonary disease have normal left ventricular function once other known causes of impairment are excluded. This is so in spite of a clinical picture that often indicates the contrary.
3. There does seem to be a group of patients who have some left ventricular impairment, as demonstrated by sophisticated means. This impairment occurs in the absence of hypertension, coronary disease, alcoholism, or valvular disease. The demonstrated abnormalities have not been clinically significant, although their natural history is totally unknown. Whether these abnormalities are, in fact, related to the pulmonary disease or some other unsuspected variable is also unknown.
4. If left ventricular failure secondary to chronic obstructive pulmonary disease occurs, it is uncommon.

As more sophisticated noninvasive cardiovascular techniques are developed to establish the presence of ventricular dysfunction and coronary artery disease, it appears that most of the cases of left ventricular dysfunction that occur in chronic obstructive lung disease patients are associated with other causes, coronary artery disease and alcoholic cardiomyopathy in particular. No convincing evidence supports the notion of a primary pulmonary cardiomyopathy. Rather, it should be emphasized that the stresses placed on the left ventricle by chronic obstructive lung disease, right ventricular distention, negative pleural pressures, and hypoxemia all have adverse effects on the left side of the heart that are exaggerated with

TABLE 18–1. Studies of Left Ventricular Function in Patients with COPD

AUTHOR	REF NO.	YEAR	NUMBER SUBJECTS	METHOD OF ANALYSIS	NUMBER ABN LVF	NUMBER OTHER CAUSE	NUMBER UNEXPLAINED	COMMENTS
Williams	109	1968	16	Cath/Methoxamine	—	—	—	Normal response to afterload in 16 subjects.
Lockhart	112	1969	86	Cath/Exercise	30	—	—	Abnormal PCW in 30 of 86 pts not due to increased pleural pressure or gradient between PCW and LA.
Davies	113	1970	12	Cath	0	—	0	12 subjects with normal hemodynamics.
Baum	114	1971	15	Cath/Angiotensin	14	2	12	14 of 15 COPD subjects had abnormal response to angiotensin load.
Khaja	115	1971		Cath/Exercise				Normal LVEDP at rest and exercise in COPD patients.
Burrows	116	1972	17	Cath/Exercise	2	—	—	Only two of 17 subjects had abnormal LV function.
Frank	117	1973	11	Cath, CBF	—	—	—	Increased LVESV and reduced LVEF in COPD patients compared to younger controls.
Hooper	118	1974	28	STI	15	—	—	All 15 COPD subjects had abnormal systolic time intervals.
Steele	119	1975	120	Nucl Probe	48	20/20	—	Although 48 of 120 subjects had abnormal LVEF, coronary artery disease usually was present.
Unger	120	1975	28	Cath, STI, Echo	7	—	—	7 of 28 had abnormal PCW at rest or exercise, but STI were unreliable.
Kline	121	1977	20	Echo, Cath, GERV	3	0	3	3 of 20 subjects had unexplained LV dysfunction.
Matthay	123	1978	15	Nucl Probe/ Aminophylline	5	—	—	5 of 15 subjects had abnormal LV function improved by aminophylline in two.
Matthay	122	1976	23	Cath, Nucl Probe/ Dextran	4	4	0	Normal baseline function and response to Dextran infusion in all except four of 23 patients with concomitant CAD.
Matthay	124	1978	10	Nucl Probe/ Methoxamine	0	—	0	Normal response to afterload with methoxamine in all subjects.
Rao	111	1978	8	Cath/Clinical Exam	8	0	8	Case series of clinically diagnosed LV failure in eight COPD patients.
Christianson	125	1979	19	Cineangiography	3	2	1	Quantitative cineangiography was normal in 16 of 19 subjects. Two of three abnormal subjects had proven CAD.
Matthay	126	1980	30	FPRV/Exercise	6	—	6	6 of 30 COPD patients did not show normal increase in LVEF with exercise.
Slutsky	127	1980	37	FPRV	16	8	8	Early ejection indices were abnormal in 16 of 37 subjects. Eight of 16 had other causes.
Louridas	130	1981	64	STI/Exercise	13	13	0	STI were always abnormal at rest or exercise in COPD.
Slutsky	127	1981	20	Cath/FPRV/ Exercise	14	8	6	Associated fall in EF with rise in PAP.
Hooper	128	1982	14	FPRV	7	—	—	15% increase in LVEF with Terbutaline.
Mathur	148	1985	15	Cath/Exercise/GERV/ Digoxin	4	—	—	Digoxin normalized LV function in all 4 cases.
Seibold	129	1986	27	GERV/Echo/ Exercise	5	5	0	Attributed all dysfunction/dyskinesia to CAD.
Bratel	141	1988	11	Cath/Felodipine	—	—	—	14% increase in LVEF with calcium channel blocker.
Mols	131	1988	10	Cath/GERV/ Salbutamol	—	—	—	Decrease in LVESV with salbutamol.

KEY

ABN	= Abnormal	LVEDP	= Left ventricular end-diastolic pressure
CAD	= Coronary artery disease	LVEF	= Left ventricular ejection fraction
Cath	= Intracardiac catheterization	LVF	= Left ventricular function
CBF	= Coronary blood flow	LVESV	= Left ventricular end-systolic volume
COPD	= Chronic obstructive pulmonary disease	Nucl Probe	= First pass nuclear scintillation counter
Echo	= Echocardiography	PAP	= Pulmonary artery pressure
FPRV	= First-pass radioventriculography	PCW	= Pulmonary capillary wedge pressure
GERV	= Gated equilibrium radioventriculography	REF	= Reference number
LA	= Left atrium	STI	= Systolic time intervals

an impaired myocardium. Mild degrees of pulmonary vascular congestion can be of greater clinical consequence in the presence of pulmonary decompensation.

It is often difficult to determine whether patients with chronic obstructive lung disease suffer from left ventricular failure. Physical examination is often not helpful or is misleading. The overall body of evidence does support the practice that left ventricular dysfunction can be accurately diagnosed in stable patients with noninvasive radionuclide studies and two-dimensional echocardiography. Unfortunately, about one third of the studies are not of satisfactory quality for evaluation. When indicated, pulmonary capillary wedge pressures are generally accurate reflections of left atrial pressure, although occasional discrepancies do occur, particularly if the catheter is wedged in a zone I or zone II region of the lung. Systolic time intervals are not reliable indices of abnormal left ventricular function in severe obstructive lung disease.[121]

It is possible that there is an increased association of coronary artery disease with chronic obstructive lung disease. Tobacco cigarette smoking is a primary risk factor for both disorders. Also, abnormalities of pulmonary function are strong risk factors for cardiac mortality.[133, 134] Alcoholism is a cause of cardiomyopathy that can be overlooked. Although the causal relationship of alcohol abuse to development of chronic obstructive lung disease is controversial, there are associations of alcohol use with cigarette consumption.[135, 136] Thus, it must be considered a plausible hypothesis that chronic obstructive lung disease itself represents a major risk factor for coronary artery disease either by common pathogenetic mechanisms or by individual susceptibility.[137–139]

EFFECT OF CARDIOACTIVE DRUGS ON LEFT VENTRICULAR FUNCTION IN CHRONIC OBSTRUCTIVE LUNG DISEASE

Several studies have examined whether the left ventricle (LV) responds normally to vasodilators or positive inotropic agents. It has been demonstrated that patients with chronic obstructive lung disease do show improved LV function acutely when treated with vasodilators, including alpha-adrenergic blockade,[140] calcium-channel blockers,[141] and nitrates.[142] Positive inotropic agents, which have been shown to improve left ventricular function in chronic obstructive lung disease, include beta agonists,[140, 141, 145] aminophylline,[93, 146] and digitalis.[147, 148]

The treatment of patients with combined coronary artery disease and chronic obstructive lung disease is often particularly frustrating. The use of nitrates for the treatment of coronary artery disease or the use of hydralazine for afterload reduction in patients with congestive heart failure is associated with an increase in alveolar-arterial gradient for oxygen. In chronic lung disease patients these drugs can occasionally cause frank hypoxemia. This is thought to be the consequence of reversal of local hypoxic vasoconstriction and worsening of ventilation-perfusion matching. Utilizing beta-blockade for treatment of coronary artery disease has the potential for exacerbation of bronchospasm in susceptible individuals, which at times is life-threatening. The employment of aminophylline and beta-agonists for bronchospasm can increase heart rate and myocardial oxygen consumption, causing an exacerbation of angina. Management of such patients requires the judicious use of selective agents, careful titration of dosage, and close monitoring of respiratory and cardiac function.

ARRHYTHMIAS

Arrhythmias are common in patients with chronic obstructive pulmonary disease, occurring in 85% to 90% of those having prolonged electrocardiographic monitoring.[149, 150] Factors that have been associated with arrhythmias in chronic obstructive lung disease have included hypoxemia,[151] hypercarbia,[152] alkalosis,[153] hypokalemia,[154] and drugs, including digitalis glycosides, theophylline, beta-adrenergic agonists, fluorocarbon inhaler propellants;[155] and alcohol-induced sleep apnea.[156]

Ambulatory electrocardiographic monitoring in hypoxemic patients has shown that one third of such patients have more than 25 ventricular premature beats per hour, and that nearly one in four have episodes of nonsustained ventricular tachycardia within a 24-hour period. Runs of supraventricular tachycardia occurred in about two thirds of the patients. Risk factors for complicated ventricular arrhythmias included male gender, hypercarbia, and peripheral edema. Despite the occurrence of these rather ominous rhythm disturbances, mortality was not predicted in this patient population when the presence of coexisting coronary artery disease was taken into account.[157] Sinus tachycardia is the only cardiac rhythm disturbance that is predictive of survival in stable patients with chronic obstructive lung disease.[158] It is, therefore, probably not indicated to treat ventricular arrhythmias in patients with chronic obstructive pulmonary disease in a chronic stable state if they are asymptomatic and do not have coronary artery disease.[159]

In contrast to the lack of prognostic significance of ventricular arrhythmias in ambulatory patients, hospitalized patients with acute respiratory failure are at greater risk for death if complex ventricular arrhythmias are present. One study showed a 70% in-hospital mortality in this group of patients.[160] Similar high mortality rates are present in patients who manifest multifocal atrial tachycardia.[161] It is reasonable, therefore, to treat acutely ill patients with chronic obstructive lung disease for both ventricular and atrial arrhythmias with particular attention to maintenance of satisfactory arterial blood oxygenation and acid-base balance, and avoidance of drug toxicity.

Drugs Affecting the Heart Rhythm

BETA-AGONISTS. Inhaled as well as oral beta-agonists can induce both supraventricular and ventricular arrhythmias, although the frequency with which this is of clinical importance is not well established.[162–165] Patients at risk appear to be those who are older, who are treated with higher doses for longer periods of time, or who may have combined treatment with other drugs, such as diuretics or xanthine derivatives.[166, 167] Prolonged use of beta agonists causes more ventricular arrhythmias because the mechanism by which beta agonists induce serious arrhythmias is not only through direct sympathetic stimulation of the heart. Prolonged use of beta agonists can induce hypokalemia and hypomagnesemia, which put patients at risk for serious heart rhythm disturbances.[168–170] It is believed that the mechanism for hypomagnesemia is renal wasting.[171] The mechanism for hypokalemia is believed to be a consequence of the effect of beta agonists on membrane-bound $Na+/K+$ ATPase, which allows shifts of potassium into muscles.[172]

THEOPHYLLINE. Theophylline has well-established potential for exacerbating atrial as well as ventricular arrhythmias.[173] At therapeutic concentrations, theophylline decreases atrioventricular conduction time and decreases sinus node recovery time.[174] These are mediated, in part, by increased catecholamine levels as well as by the direct effect of the drug. In particular, multifocal atrial tachycardia, which portends a very poor prognosis in a chronic obstructive lung disease patient with acute respiratory failure, has been closely associated with the use of theophylline.[175–177] In susceptible individuals, this arrhythmia can occur with normal therapeutic concentrations of theophylline and in the absence of acute respiratory failure. Verapamil is the drug of choice for treatment of this rhythm disturbance.[176, 178–180]

CONCLUSIONS

An understanding of the principles by which mechanical stresses of respiration interact with the heart and peripheral circulation is useful in the management of acutely ill patients with chronic obstructive lung disease. Derangements of arterial blood gas values, acid-base balance, and the adverse effects of bronchodilator agents all can have important effects on cardiac function and rhythm. The coexistence of myocardial disease with chronic obstructive lung disease is a common and particularly challenging combination requiring an understanding of the pathophysiologic interrelations of the two disorders. Treatment of the lung disease can worsen the heart disease, and treatment of the heart disease can worsen the lung disease. Minimal, judicious therapy with careful monitoring of heart and lung function is often the best course.

REFERENCES

1. Permutt S, Wise RA. Control of cardiac output through coupling of heart and blood vessels. In: Yin FCP, ed. Ventricular/Vascular Coupling. New York: Springer-Verlag, 1987.
2. Permutt S, Wise RA. Mechanical interaction of respiration and circulation. In: Macklem PT, ed. Handbook of Physiology: The Respiratory System III. Rockville, MD: American Physiological Society, 1985.
3. Wise RA, Robotham JL, Summer WR. Effects of spontaneous ventilation on the circulation. Lung 1981; 159:175–186.
4. Permutt S, Wise RA, Sylvester JT. Interaction between the circulatory and ventilatory pumps. In: Roussos C, Macklem PT, eds. The Thorax (part B). New York: Marcel Dekker, 1985, 701–736.
5. Robotham JL. Hemodynamic events: a physiological approach. In: Montenegro HD, ed. Chronic Obstructive Pulmonary Disease. New York: Churchill Livingstone, 1984, 183–217.
6. Wise RA. Effect of alterations of pleural pressure on cardiac output. South Med J 1985; 78:423–428.
7. Sylvester JT, Goldberg HS, Permutt S. The role of the vasculature in the regulation of cardiac output. Clin Chest Med 1983; 4:111–126.
8. Guyton AC, Polizo D, Armstrong GG Jr. Mean circulatory filling pressure measured immediately after cessation of heart pumping. Am J Physiol 1954; 179:261–267.
9. Permutt S, Caldini P. Regulation of cardiac output by the circuit: venous return. In: Baan J, Noordergraff A, Raines J, eds. Cardiovascular System Dynamics. Cambridge, MA: The MIT Press, 1978, 465–479.
10. Janicki JS, Shroff SG, Weber KT. Influence of extracardiac forces on the cardiopulmonary unit. In: Yin FCP, ed. Ventricular/Vascular Coupling; Clinical, Physiological, and Engineering Aspects. New York: Springer-Verlag, 1987.
11. Brunner MJ, Shoukas AA, MacAnespie CL. The effect of the carotid sinus baroreceptor reflex on blood flow and volume redistribution in the total systemic vascular bed of the dog. Circ Res 1981; 48:74–285.
12. Caldini P, Permutt S, Wadell JA, Riley RL. Effect of epinephrine on pressure, flow, and volume relationships in the systemic circulation of dogs. Circ Res 1974; 34:606–623.
13. Mitzner W, Goldberg H. Effects of epinephrine on resistive and compliant properties of the canine vasculature. J Appl Physiol 1975; 39:272–280.
14. Mitzner W, Goldberg H, Lichtenstein S. Effect of thoracic blood volume changes on steady state cardiac output. Circ Res 1976; 38:255–261.
15. Guyton AC, Adkins LH. Quantitative aspects of the collapse factor in relation to venous return. Am J Physiol 1954; 177:523–527.
16. Holt JP. The collapse factor in the measurement of venous pressure: the flow of fluid through collapsible tubes. Am J Physiol 1941; 134:292–299.
17. Pride NB, Permutt S, Riley RL, Bromberger-Barnea B. Determinants of maximal expiratory flow from the lungs. J Appl Physiol 1967; 23:646–662.
18. Mead J, Turner JM, Macklem PT, Little JB. Significance of the relationship between lung recoil and maximum expiratory flow. J Appl Physiol 1967; 22:95–108.
19. Permutt S. Some physiological aspects of asthma. Ciba Foundation Symposium. Identification of Asthma. London: Churchill Livingstone, 1971, 63.
20. Stalcup SA, Mellins RB. Mechanical forces producing pulmonary edema in acute asthma. N Engl J Med 1977; 297:592–596.
21. Even P, Sors H, Safran D, Reynaud P. Interaction between ventilation and circulation in bronchial asthma and pulmonary emphysema. In: Cumming G, Bonsignore G, eds. Pulmonary Circulation in Health and Disease. New York: Plenum Press, 1980, 279–296.
22. Potter WA, Olafsson S, Hyatt RE. Ventilatory mechanics and expiratory flow limitation during exercise in patients with obstructive lung disease. J Clin Invest 1971; 50:910.
23. Natarajan TK, Wise RA, Karam M, et al. Immediate effect of expiratory loading on left ventricular stroke volume. Circulation 1987; 75:139–145.
24. Ruskin J, Bache RJ, Rembert JC, Greenfield JC Jr. Pressure flow studies in man: effect of respiration on left ventricular stroke volume. Circulation 1973; 48:79–85.
25. Bilgi C, Jones RL, Sproule BJ. Relation between pulses paradoxus and pulmonary function in patients with chronic airways obstruction. Can Med Assoc J 1977; 117:1389–1392.
26. Burrows B. Arterial oxygenation and pulmonary hemodynamics in patients with chronic airways obstruction. Am Rev Respir Dis 1974; 110:64–70.
27. Rose CE Jr, Godine RL Jr, Rose KY, et al. Role of arginine vasopressin and angiotensin II in cardiovascular responses to combined acute hypoxemia and hypercapnic acidosis in conscious dogs. J Clin Invest 1984; 74:321–331.
28. Grisoni ER, Brown-Armstrong E, Kalhan SC. Vasoactive intestinal polypeptide potentiates the hypoxemia-induced decrease in splanchnic circulation in the rat. J Pediatr Surg 1988; 23:1193–1197.
29. Phillips BA, McConnell JW, Smith MD. The effects of hypoxemia on cardiac output. A dose-response curve. Chest 1988; 93:471–475.
30. Rose CE Jr, Althaus JA, Kaiser DL, et al. Acute hypoxemia and hypercapnia: increase in plasma catecholamines in conscious dogs. Am J Physiol 1983; 245:H924–H929.
31. Nesarajah MS, Matalon S, Krasney JA, Farhi LE. Cardiac output and regional oxygen transport in the acutely hypoxic conscious sheep. Respir Physiol 1983; 53:161–172.
32. Borgia JF, Horvath SM. Effects of acute prolonged hypoxia on cardiovascular dynamics in dogs. J Appl Physiol 1977; 43:784–789.
33. Ffoulkes-Crabbe DJ, Creighton RE, Volgyesi GA, et al. The effect of splenectomy on circulatory adjustments to hypoxaemia in the anaesthetized dog. Br J Anaesth 1976; 48:639–641.
34. Butler J. The heart is in good hands. Circulation 1983; 67:1163–1168.
35. Dock W. Inspiratory traction on the pericardium. Arch Intern Med 1961; 108:81–84.
36. Nakhjavan FK, Palmer WH, McGregor M. Influence of respiration on venous return in pulmonary emphysema. Circulation 1966; 33:8–16.
37. Wise RA, Taylor WR, Bromberger-Barnea B, Permutt S. Effect of positive end-expiratory pressure (PEEP) on determinants of venous return. Fed Proc 1980; 39:270.
38. Fessler H, Brower R, Wise R, et al. Effects of abdominal pressure and elastance on venous return during positive end-expiratory pressure. Fed Proc 1989; 3:A1182.
39. Natori H, Tamaki S, Kira S. Ultrasonic evaluation of ventilatory effect on inferior vena caval configuration. Am Rev Respir Dis 1979; 129:421–427.
40. Diamant M, Benumof JL, Saidman LJ. Hemodynamics of increased intra-abdominal pressure: interaction with hypovolemia and halothane anesthesia. Anesthesiology. 1978; 48:23–27.
41. Kashtan J, Green JF, Parsons G. Hemodynamic effects of increased abdominal pressure. J Surg Res 1981; 30:249.

42. Doppman JR, Robinson RM, Rockoff SD, et al. Mechanism of obstruction on the infradiaphragmatic portion of the inferior vena cava in the presence of increased intra-abdominal pressure. Invest Radiol 1986; 1:37–53.
43. Lloyd TC. Effect of inspiration on inferior vena caval blood flow in dogs. J Appl Physiol 1983; 55:1701–1706.
44. Kelman GR, Swapp GH, Smith I, et al. Cardiac output and arterial blood gas tension during laparoscopy. Br J Anaesth 1972; 44:1155–1161.
45. Richardson JD, Trinkle JK. Hemodynamic and respiratory alterations with increased intra-abdominal pressure. J Surg Res 1976; 20:401–404.
46. Lynch FP, Tomoshige O, Scully JM, et al. Cardiovascular effects of increased intra-abdominal pressure in newborn piglets. J Pediatr Surg 1974; 9:621–626.
47. Masey SA, Koehler RC, Rock JR, et al. Effect of abdominal distension on central and regional hemodynamics in neonatal lambs. Pediatr Res 1985; 19:1244–1249.
48. Wise RA, Robotham JL. Determinants of inferior vena cava blood flow with changes in abdominal pressure. Am Rev Respir Dis 1987; 135:A115.
49. Brower R, Wise RA, Hassapoyannes C, et al. Effect of lung inflation on lung blood volume and pulmonary venous flow. J Appl Physiol 1985; 58:954–963.
50. Sagawa K, Suga H, Shoukas A, Bakalar KM. End-systolic pressure-volume ratio: a new index of contractility. Am J Cardiol 1977; 40:748–753.
51. Kono A, Maughan WL, Sunagawa K, et al. The use of left ventricular end-ejection pressure and peak pressure in the estimation of the end-systolic pressure-volume relationship. Circulation 1984; 70:1057–1065.
52. Summer W, Permutt S, Sagawa K, et al. Effects of spontaneous respiration on canine left ventricular function. Circ Res 1979; 45:719–728.
53. Buda AS, Pinsky MR, Ingles NB, Alderman E. Effect of intrathoracic pressure on left ventricular performance. N Engl J Med 1979; 301:453–459.
54. Karam M, Wise RA, Natarajan TK, et al. Mechanism of decreased left ventricular stroke volume during inspiration in man. Circulation 1984; 69:866–873.
55. Scharf SM, Brown R, Saunders N, Green LH. Effects of normal and loaded spontaneous inspiration on cardiovascular function. J Appl Physiol 1979; 47:582–590.
56. Scharf SM, Brown R, Tow DE, Parisi AF. Cardiac effects of increased lung volume and decreased pleural pressure in man. J Appl Physiol 1979; 47:257–262.
57. Wead WB, Norton JF. Effects of intrapleural pressure changes on canine left ventricular function. J Appl Physiol 1981; 50:1027–1035.
58. Schrijen F, Ehrlich W, Permutt S. Cardiovascular changes in conscious dogs during spontaneous deep breaths. Pflugers Arch 1975; 355:205–215.
59. Robotham JL, Mitzner W. A model of the effects of respiration on left ventricular performance. J Appl Physiol 1979; 46:411–418.
60. Martin J, Jardim J, Sampson M, Engel LE. Factors influencing pulsus paradoxus in asthma. Chest 1981; 80:543–549.
61. Rebuck AS, Pengelly LD. Development of pulsus paradoxus in the presence of airways obstruction. N Engl J Med 1973; 288:66–69.
62. Shim C, Williams MH Jr. Pulsus paradoxus in asthma. Lancet 1978; i:530–531.
63. Pulsus paradoxus in the bedside assessment of patients with bronchial asthma. S Afr Med J 1976; 50:1210–1203.
64. Gluck JC, Busto R, Marks MB. Pulsus paradoxus in childhood asthma—its prognostic value. Ann Allergy 1977; 38:405–407.
65. Lemaire F, Teboul JL, Cinotti L, et al. Acute left ventricular dysfunction during unsuccessful weaning from mechanical ventilation. Anesthesiology 1988; 69:171–179.
66. Henning H, Gilpin EA, Covell JW, et al. Prognosis after acute myocardial infarction: a multivariate analysis of mortality and survival. Circulation 1979; 59:1124–1136.
67. Bemis CE, Serur JR, Borkenhagen D, Sonnenblick EH. Influence of right ventricular filling on left ventricular pressure and dimension. Circ Res 1974; 34:498.
68. Bove AA, Santamore WP. Ventricular interdependence. Prog Cardiovasc Dis 1981; 23:365–388.
69. Santamore WP, Lynch PR, Heckman JL. Left ventricular effects on right ventricular developed pressure. J Appl Physiol 1976; 41:925–930.
70. Santamore WP, Lynch PR, Heckman JL, et al. Myocardial interaction between the ventricles. J Appl Physiol 1976; 41:362–368.
71. Santamore WP, Lynch PR, Meier GD. Myocardial interaction between the ventricles. J Appl Physiol 1976; 41:362–368.
72. Janicki JS, Weber KT. Factors influencing the diastolic pressure-volume relation of the cardiac ventricles. Fed Proc 1980; 39:133–140.
73. Maughan WL, Kallman CH, Shoukas A. The effect of right ventricular filling on the pressure-volume relationship of ejecting canine left ventricle. Circ Res 1981; 49:382–388.
74. Elzinga G, Van Grondell R, Westerhof N, Van den Bos GC. Ventricular interference. Am J Physiol 1974; 226:941–947.
75. Moulopoulos SD, Sarcas A, Stamatelopoulos S, Arealis E. Left ventricular performance during bypass or distention of the right ventricle. Circ Res 1965; 17:484–491.
76. Janicki JS, Weber KT. The pericardium and ventricular interaction, distensibility and function. Am J Physiol 1980; 238:H494–H503.
77. Stool EW, Mullins CB, Leshin SJ, Mitchell JH. Dimensional changes of the left ventricle during acute pulmonary arterial hypertension in dogs. Am J Cardiol 1974; 33:868–875.
78. Alderman EL, Glantz SA. Acute hemodynamic intervention with the diastolic pressure-volume curve in man. Circulation 1976; 54:662–671.
79. Brinker JA, Weiss JL, Lappe DC, et al. Leftward septal displacement during right ventricular loading in man. Circulation 1980; 61:626–633.
80. Robotham JL, Stuart RS, Borkon AM, et al. Effects of changes in left ventricular loading and pleural pressure on mitral flow. J Appl Physiol 1988; 65:1662–1675.
81. Langille BL, Jones DR. Mechanical interaction between the ventricles during systole. Can J Physiol 1977; 55:373–382.
82. Weber KT, Janicki JS, Shroff SG, Likoff MJ. The cardiopulmonary unit: the body's gas transport system. Clin Chest Med 1983; 4:101–110.
83. Lloyd TC Jr. Respiratory system compliance as seen from the cardiac fossa. J Appl Physiol 1982; 53:56–62.
84. Wallis T, Robotham J, Compean R, Kindred MK. Mechanical heart-lung interaction with positive end-expiratory pressure. J Appl Physiol 1983; 54:1039–1047.
85. Brookhart JM, Boyd TE. Local differences in intrathoracic pressure and their relation to cardiac filling pressure in the dog. Am J Physiol 1947; 148:434–444.
86. Culver BH, Marini JJ, Butler J. Lung volume and pleural pressure effects on ventricular function. J Appl Physiol 1981; 50:630–635.
87. Wise RA, Robotham JL, Bromberger-Barnea B, Permutt S. Effect of PEEP on left ventricular function in right-heart bypassed dogs. J Appl Physiol 1981; 51:541–546.
88. Fletcher EC, Levin DC. Cardiopulmonary hemodynamics during sleep in subjects with chronic obstructive pulmonary disease; The effect of short- and long-term oxygen. Chest 1984; 85:6–14.
89. Scharf SM, Permutt S, Bromberger-Barnea B. Effects of hypoxic and CO hypoxia on isolated hearts. J Appl Physiol 1975; 39:752–758.
90. Wyman RM, Farhi ER, Bing OH, et al. Comparative effects of hypoxia and ischemia in the isolated, blood-perfused dog heart: evaluation of left ventricular diastolic chamber distensibility and wall thickness. Circ Res 1989; 64:121–128.
91. Krause PC, Inoue H, Zipes DP. Electrophysiologic alterations produced by hypoxia in the canine heart. Am Heart J 1989; 117:550–561.
92. Beierholm EA, Grantham RN, O'Keefe DD, et al. Effects of acid-base changes, hypoxia, and catecholamines on ventricular performance. Am J Physiol 1975; 228:1555–1561.
93. Gomez A, Eng J, Mink SN. Aminophylline has little positive inotropic effect and a slightly negative diastolic effect on the left ventricle during hypoxic conditions in dogs. Am Rev Respir Dis 1988; 137:1296–1303.
94. Cunningham MJ, Apstein CS, Weinberg EO, Lorell BH. Deleterious effect of ouabain on myocardial function during hypoxia. Am J Physiol 1989; 256:H681–H687.
95. Steinhart CR, Permutt S, Gurtner GH, Traystman RJ. Beta-

adrenergic activity and cardiovascular response to severe respiratory acidosis. Am J Physiol 1983; 244:H46–H54.
96. Kountz WB, Alexander HL, Prinzmetal M. The heart in emphysema. Am Heart J 1936; 11:163–172.
97. Spain DM, Handler BJ. Chronic cor pulmonale. Arch Intern Med 1946; 77:37–65.
98. Walzer I, Frost TT. Cor pulmonale. Dis Chest 1954; 26:192–198.
99. Spatt SD, Grayzel DM. Cor pulmonale: observations on forty-two autopsied patients. Am J Med 1948; 5:252–255.
100. Scott RW, Garvin CF. Cor pulmonale: observations in fifty autopsy cases. Am Heart J 1941; 22:56–63.
101. Michelson N. Bilateral ventricular hypertrophy due to chronic pulmonary disease. Dis Chest 1960; 38:435–486.
102. Fluck DC, Chandrasekar RG, Gardner RV. Left ventricular hypertrophy in chronic bronchitis. Br Heart J 1986; 28:92–97.
103. Millard FJC. The electrocardiogram in chronic lung disease. Br Heart J 1967; 29:43–50.
104. Murphy ML, Adamson J, Hutcheson F. Left ventricular hypertrophy in patients with chronic bronchitis and emphysema. Ann Intern Med 1974; 81:307–313.
105. Murphy ML, de Soyza N, Thenabadu PN. Quantitation of fibrosis of the heart in chronic obstructive pulmonary disease with and without cor pulmonale. Chest 1983; 84:535–538.
106. Mehrotra PP, Weaver YJ, Higginbotham EA. Myocardial perfusion defect on thallium-201 imaging in patients with chronic obstructive pulmonary disease. J Am Coll Cardiol 1983; 2:233–239.
107. Hooper GH, Whitcomb ME. Systolic time intervals in chronic obstructive pulmonary disease. Circulation 1974; 50:1205–1209.
108. Frank MJ, Weisse AB, Moschos CB, Levinson GE. Left ventricular function, metabolism, and blood flow in chronic cor pulmonale. Circulation 1973; 47:798–806.
109. Williams JF, Childress RH, Boyd DL, et al. Left ventricular function in patients with chronic obstructive pulmonary disease. J Clin Invest 1968; 47:1143–1153.
110. Jezek V, Schrijen F. Left ventricular function in chronic obstructive pulmonary disease with and without cardiac failure. Clin Sci Mol Med 1973; 45:267–279.
111. Rao BS, Cohn KE, Eldridge FL, Hancock EW. Left ventricular failure secondary to chronic pulmonary disease. Am J Med 1968; 45:229–241.
112. Lockhart A, Tzareva M, Nader F, et al. Elevated pulmonary artery wedge pressure at rest and during exercise in chronic bronchitis: fact or fancy. Clin Sci 1969; 37:503–517.
113. Davies H, Overy HR. Left ventricular function in cor pulmonale. Chest 1970; 58:8–14.
114. Baum GL, Schwartz A, Llamas R, et al. Left ventricular function in chronic obstructive lung disease. N Engl J Med 1971; 285:361–365.
115. Khaja F, Parker JO. Right and left ventricular performance in chronic obstructive lung disease. Am Heart J 1971; 82:319–327.
116. Burrows B, Kettel LJ, Niden AH, et al. Patterns of cardiovascular dysfunction in chronic obstructive lung disease. N Engl J Med 1972; 286:912–918.
117. Frank MJ, Weisse AB, Moschos CB, et al. Left ventricular function, metabolism, and blood flow in chronic cor pulmonale. Circulation 1973; 47:798–806.
118. Hooper RG, Whitcomb ME. Systolic time intervals in chronic obstructive pulmonary disease. Circulation 1974; 50:1205–1209.
119. Steele P, Ellis JH, Van Dyke D, et al. Left ventricular ejection fraction in severe chronic obstructive airways disease. Am J Med 1975; 59:21–28.
120. Unger K, Shaw D, Karliner JS, et al. Evaluation of left ventricular performance in acutely ill patients wth chronic obstructive lung disease. Chest 1975; 68:135–142.
121. Kline LE, Crawford MH, MacDonald WJ Jr, et al. Noninvasive assessment of left ventricular performance in patients with chronic obstructive pulmonary disease. Chest 1977; 72:558–564.
122. Matthay RA, Ellis JH Jr, Steele PP. Effect of dextran loading on left ventricular performance in chronic obstructive pulmonary disease. Am Heart J 1976; 92:730–736.
123. Matthay RA, Berger HJ, Loke J, et al. Effects of aminophylline upon right and left ventricular performance in chronic obstructive pulmonary disease: noninvasive assessment by radionuclide angiocardiography. Am J Med 1978; 65:903–910.
124. Matthay RA, Ellis JH Jr, Steele PP. Methoxamine-induced increase in afterload. Effect on left ventricular performance in chronic obstructive pulmonary disease. Am Rev Respir Dis 1978; 117:871–877.
125. Christianson LC, Shah A, Fisher VJ. Quantitative left ventricular cineangiography in patients with chronic obstructive pulmonary disease. Am J Med 1979; 66:399–404.
126. Matthay RA, Berger HJ, Davies RA, et al. Right and left ventricular exercise performance in chronic obstructive pulmonary disease: radionuclide assessment. Ann Intern Med 1980; 93:234–239.
127. Slutsky R, Hooper W, Ackerman W, et al. Evaluation of left ventricular function in chronic pulmonary disease by exercise gated equilibrium radionuclide angiography. Am Heart J 1981; 101:414–420.
128. Hooper WW, Slutsky RA, Kocienski DE, et al. Right and left ventricular response to subcutaneous terbutaline in patients with chronic obstructive pulmonary disease: radionuclide angiographic assessment of cardiac size and function. Am Heart J 1982; 104:1027–1032.
129. Seibold H, Roth U, Lippert R, et al. Left heart function in chronic obstructive lung disease. Klin Wochenschr 1986; 64:433–441.
130. Louridas G, Patakas D, Christaki R, Stavropoulos C. Systolic time intervals in chronic obstructive pulmonary disease. Cardiology 1981; 68:30–41.
131. Mols P, Ham H, Naeije N, et al. How does salbutamol improve the ventricular performance in patients with chronic obstructive pulmonary disease? J Cardiovasc Pharmacol 1988; 12:127–133.
132. Kachel RG. Left ventricular function in chronic obstructive pulmonary disease. Chest 1978; 74:286–290.
133. Beaty TH, Cohen BH, Newill CA, et al. Impaired pulmonary function as a risk factor for mortality. Am J Epidemiol 1982; 116:102–113.
134. Schroll M. Smoking habits in the Glostrup population of men and women, born in 1914. Implications for health, evaluated from ten-year mortality, incidence of cardiovascular manifestations and pulmonary function, 1964–1974. Acta Med Scand 1980; 208:245–256.
135. Lebowitz MD. Respiratory symptoms and disease related to alcohol consumption. Am Rev Respir Dis 1981; 123:16–19.
136. Cohen BH, Celentano DD, Chase GA, et al. Alcohol consumption and airway obstruction. Am Rev Respir Dis 1980; 121:205–215.
137. Marcus EB, Curb JD, MacLean CJ, et al. Pulmonary function as a predictor of coronary heart disease. Am J Epidemiol 1989; 129:97–104.
138. Bhargava RL, Woolf CR. Relationships between ischemic heart disease and chronic diffuse pulmonary disease. Chest 1970; 59:254–261.
139. Sobol BJ, Herbert WH, Emergal C. The high incidence of pulmonary functional abnormalities in patients with coronary artery disease. Chest 1974; 65:148–151.
140. Gould L, Zahir M, DeMartino A, Gomprecht R. Haemodynamic effects of phentolamine in chronic obstructive pulmonary disease. Br Heart J 1971; 33:445–450.
141. Bratel T, Hedenstierne G, Lundquist H, et al. Cardiac function and central haemodynamics in severe chronic obstructive lung disease; Acute and long-term effects of felodipine. Eur J Respir Dis 1988; 1:262–268.
142. Morrison D, Caldwell J, Lakshminaryan S, et al. The acute effects of low flow oxygen and isosorbide dinitrate on left and right ventricular ejection fractions in chronic obstructive pulmonary disease. J Am Coll Cardiol 1983; 2:652–660.
143. Hooper WW, Slutsky RA, Kocienski DE, et al. Right and left ventricular response to subcutaneous terbutaline in patients with chronic obstructive pulmonary disease: radionuclide angiographic assessment of cardiac size and function. Am Heart J 1982; 104:1027–1032.
144. Brent BN, Mahler D, Berger HJ, et al. Augmentation of right ventricular performance in chronic obstructive pulmonary disease by terbutaline: a combined radionuclide and hemodynamic study. Am J Cardiol 1982; 50:313–319.
145. Sunderrajan EV, Byron WA, McKenzie WN, et al. The effect of terbutaline on cardiac function in patients with stable chronic obstructive lung disease. JAMA 1983; 250:2151–2156.
146. Matthay RA, Berger HJ, Loke J, et al. Effects of aminophylline upon right and left ventricular performance in chronic obstructive

pulmonary disease: noninvasive asssessment by radionuclide angiocardiography. Am J Med 1978; 65:903–910.
147. Mathur PN, Fowles P, Pugsley SO, et al. Effect of digoxin on right ventricular function in severe chronic airflow obstruction. A controlled clinical trial. Ann Intern Med 1981; 95:283–288.
148. Mathur PN, Fowles AC, Pugsley SO, et al. Effect of long-term administration of digoxin on exercise performance in chronic airflow obstruction. Eur J Respir Dis 1985; 66:273–283.
149. Kleiger RE, Senior RM. Long-term electrocardiographic monitoring of ambulatory patients with chronic airway obstruction. Chest 1974; 65:482–487.
150. Holford FD, Mithoefer JC. Cardiac arrhythmias in hospitalized patients with chronic obstructive pulmonary disease. Am Rev Respir Dis 1973; 108:879–885.
151. Tirlapur VG, Mir MA. Nocturnal hypoxemia and associated electrocardiographic changes in patients with chronic obstructive airways disease. N Engl J Med 1982; 306:125–130.
152. Rogers RM, Spear JF, Moore EN, et al. Vulnerability of canine ventricle to fibrillation during hypoxia and respiratory acidosis. Chest 1973; 63:986–994.
153. Ayres SM, Grace WJ. Inappropriate ventilation and hypoxemia as causes of cardiac arrhythmias—the control of arrhythmias without antiarrhythmic drugs. Am J Med 1969; 46:495–505.
154. Levine PA, Klein MD. Mechanisms of arrhythmias in chronic obstructive lung disease. Geriatrics 1976; 31:47–56.
155. Webb-Johnson DC. When drug therapy for lung disease affects the heart. Geriatrics 1976; 31:79–87.
156. Dolly FR, Block AJ. Increased ventricular ectopy and sleep apnea following ethanol ingestion in COPD patients. Chest 1983; 83:469–472.
157. Shih HT, Webb CR, Conway WA, et al. Frequency and significance of cardiac arrhythmias in chronic obstructive lung disease. Chest 1988; 94:44–48.
158. Burrows B, Earle RH. Course and prognosis of chronic obstructive lung disease—a prospective study of 200 patients. N Engl J Med 1969; 280:387–404.
159. Pratt CM. Asymptomatic ventricular arrhythmias in patients with obstructive lung disease. Should they be treated [editorial]? Chest 1988; 94:2–4.
160. Hudson LD, Kurt TL, Petty TL, Genton E. Arrhythmias associated with acute respiratory failure in patients with chronic airway obstruction. Chest 1973; 63:661–665.
161. Shine K, Kastor JA, Yurchak PM. Multifocal atrial tachycardia—clinical and electrocardiographic features in 32 patients. N Engl J Med 1968; 279:344–349.
162. Assael R, Martt JM, Okeson GC. Frequency of isoproterenol hydrochloride-induced cardiac arrhythmia in 19 patients with chronic obstructive pulmonary disease: a prospective study. Am Rev Respir Dis 1975; 111:743–747.
163. Eidelman DH, Sami MH, McGregor M, Cosio MG. Combination of theophylline and salbutamol for arrhythmias in severe COPD. Chest 1987; 91:808–812.
164. Conradson TB, Eklundh G, Olofsson B, et al. Cardiac arrhythmias in patients with mild-to-moderate obstructive lung disease. Comparison of beta-agonist therapy alone and in combination with a xanthine derivative, enprofylline or theophylline. Chest 1985; 88:537–542.
165. Montenegro HD, Chester EH, Jones PK. Cardiac arrhythmias during routine tests of pulmonary function in patients with chronic obstruction of airways. Chest 1978; 73:133–139.
166. Higgins RM, Cookson WOCM, Lane DG, et al. Cardiac arrhythmias caused by nebulised beta-agonist therapy. Lancet 1987; ii:863–864.
167. Sears MR, Rea HH, Fenwick J, et al. 75 deaths in asthmatics prescribed home nebulisers. Br Med J 1987; 294:477–480.
168. Lipworth BJ, McDevitt DG, Struthers AD. Prior treatment with diuretic augments the hypokalemic and electrocardiographic effects of inhaled albuterol. Am J Med 1989; 86:653–657.
169. Lipworth BJ, Clark RA, Dhillon DP, et al. Metabolic effects of cumulative doses of salbutamol from a metered-dose inhaler in bronchial asthma. Br J Clin Pharmacol 1988; 25:667P–668P.
170. Whyte KF, Reid C, Addis GJ, et al. Salbutamol induced hypokalemia: the effect of theophylline alone and in combination with adrenaline. Br J Clin Pharmacol 1988; 25:571–578.
171. Bos WJW, Postma DS, Van Doormeal JJ. Magnesuric and calciuric effects of terbutaline in man. Clin Sci 1988; 74:595–597.
172. Whyte KF, Addis GJ, Whitesmith R, Reid JL. The mechanism of salbutamol induced hypokalemia. Br J Clin Pharmacol 1987; 23:65–71.
173. Patel AK, Skatrud JB, Thomsen JH. Cardiac arrhythmias due to oral aminophylline in patients with chronic obstructive pulmonary disease. Chest 1981; 80:661–665.
174. Eiriksson CE Jr., Writer SL, Vestal RE. Theophylline-induced alterations in cardiac electrophysiology in patients with chronic obstructive pulmonary disease. Am Rev Respir Dis 1987; 1335: 322–326.
175. Levine JH, Michael JR, Guarnieri T. Multifocal atrial tachycardia: a toxic effect of theophylline. Lancet 1985; i:12–14.
176. Marchlinski RE, Miller JM. Atrial arrhythmias exacerbated by theophylline. Response to verapamil and evidence for triggered activity in man. Chest 1985; 88:931–934.
177. Biggs FD, Lefrak SS, Kleiger RE, et al. Disturbances of rhythm in chronic lung disease. Heart Lung 1977; 6:256–261.
178. Levine JH, Michael JR, Guarnieri T. Treatment of multifocal atrial tachycardia with verapamil. N Engl J Med 1985; 312:21–25.
179. Salerno DM, Anderson B, Sharkey PJ, Iber C. Intravenous verapamil for treatment of multifocal atrial tachycardia with and without calcium pretreatment. Ann Intern Med 1987; 107:623–628.
180. Hazard PB, Burnett CR. Verapamil in multifocal atrial tachycardia. Hemodynamic and respiratory changes. Chest 1987; 91:68–70.

Chapter 19

BRAIN BLOOD FLOW

Norman H. Edelman

PHYSIOLOGY OF REGULATION OF BRAIN BLOOD FLOW

A review of the regulation of brain blood flow as it relates to respiratory control may be found in Santiago and Edelman.[10]

Pressure-Flow Relationships

In humans virtually all the arterial input into the circulation of the brain is from the circle of Willis, which is fed by the internal carotid and basilar arteries. The venous drainage is principally through the cavernous sinuses into the internal jugular veins. The unique arrangement of the cerebrospinal fluid (CSF) system protects this circulation from abrupt variations in hemodynamic driving pressure due to sudden changes in the position of the head relative to the heart. Thus, under most circumstances, the effective driving pressure for brain perfusion is the difference between arterial and CSF pressures. This effect is relevant to chronic obstructive pulmonary disease (COPD) in circumstances associated with increased intracranial pressure, such as intense cough or acute hypercapnia.

The brain manifests a high degree of pressure-flow autoregulation under physiologic conditions. By this is meant that blood flow remains relatively constant over a wide range of driving pressures. However, the phenomenon is both variable and fragile. For example, the lower limit of autoregulation may be a blood pressure of 70 mm Hg during hemorrhagic hypotension and as low as 40 mm Hg during drug-induced hypotension. In the acute setting, the upper limit is generally found to be 150 mm Hg. Important to this discussion is the fact that in a variety of experimental settings acute hypoxia has been shown to obliterate or deteriorate pressure-flow autoregulation and render brain blood flow a more nearly passive function of perfusion pressure.

As in other vascular beds resistance to brain blood flow has an important component related to blood viscosity, principally as determined by blood hematocrit value. In COPD accompanied by respiratory insufficiency, the hematocrit level may play a critical role in setting brain perfusion (see subsequent discussion).

Hypoxia

Arterial hypoxemia has been shown to produce significant increases of brain blood flow in humans. Whereas some studies demonstrate a threshold value of O_2 tension in arterial blood of 50 mm Hg, others demonstrate an inverse relationship between brain blood flow and $Pa{O_2}$. What seems to remain constant over a wide range and in a variety of circumstances is the product of O_2 content in arterial blood and brain blood flow, i.e., O_2 delivery to the brain. The relationship seems to hold for anemia, although a role for decreased viscosity of blood is accepted, and carboxyhemoglobinemia. It seems likely that O_2 availability to tissues rather than the product of brain blood flow and O_2 content per se is closer to the true controlling variable. This finding is well demonstrated in the study of Wade and colleagues[14] in which they showed that, despite greater blood viscosity, patients with polycythemia due to hemoglobin with a high affinity for O_2 (oxygen half-saturation pressure of hemoglobin, P_{50} = 13 mm Hg) had a greater than normal brain blood flow.

The distribution of brain blood flow response to acute hypoxia is not uniform. Relatively greater flow is provided to the brainstem than the cortex. This flow is likely to be related to nonuniform distribution of neural effects on the brain vasculature (see subsequent discussion) rather than to inherent differences in the responsiveness of vessels in various regions of the brain to hypoxia.[7] The protective role of such a distribution for basic respiratory and circulatory control mechanisms is clear.

As arterial blood CO_2 tension has a powerful influence on brain blood flow, the brain vasculature dilation caused by hypoxia can be readily reversed by hypocapnia, which may result from accompanying hyperventilation. Although not studied, it thus seems quite unlikely that the hypoxia and hypocapnia that accompany moderately severe asthma result in increased brain perfusion. Decreased perfusion is actually more likely.

The effects of prolonged hypoxia on brain blood flow are difficult to discern from studies of disease states because of the complicating influences of compensatory mechanisms such as polycythemia. Detailed studies have been done by Krasney and associates[5] in sheep exposed to simulated high altitude. These studies show a relatively rapid return to near prehypoxic values for global and regional brain blood flow within 24 to 48 hours. The time course of the phenomenon seems to parallel that of ventilatory acclimatization to high altitude. The implication is that the key variable for both phenomena is the improving tissue oxygenation within the brain.

Hypercapnia

Carbon dioxide tension in arterial blood is a powerful regulator of brain blood flow. The control is bidirectional—hypocapnia is vasoconstricting and hypercapnia is vasodilating. Although widely different values have been reported, it seems likely that the gain of the system is about 2 cc/minute/100 gm/mm Hg. An acute change in arterial $P{CO_2}$ of just 1 mm Hg may change brain blood flow by 5%. The mechanism that relates brain blood flow to arterial P_{CO_2} seems strongly linked to brain metabolic rate. Thus, anesthesia, hypothermia, and certain forms of brain trauma reduce the brain metabolic rate and the brain blood flow response to CO_2 in parallel.

Prolonged hypercapnia results in an attenuation of the effect of P_{CO_2} on brain blood flow. The elegant studies of Fencl and coworkers[4] suggest that the key determinant of brain blood flow over the full spectrum of acid-base variations is the hydrogen ion concentration $[H^+]$ in brain interstitial fluid. Thus, brain blood flow declines as the metabolic compensation for acute respiratory acidosis progresses. These studies also suggested that a single variable, i.e., interstitial $[H^+]$, determined both brain blood flow and ventilatory changes in response to acid base alterations.

Metabolic Rate

Both globally and regionally, brain blood flow and metabolic rate are tightly linked. Unlike other organs, the metabolic rate for the whole brain varies little under physiologic conditions. Thus, brain blood flow differs little under such diverse conditions as sleep and exercise. However, on a regional basis, the situation is quite different. Stimulation of specific neuronal pathways results in abrupt and sometimes pronounced increases in blood flow to the relevant neuronal pools, presumably reflecting metabolic events within cells or shifting ionic gradients (notably K^+) across cell membranes.

Neural Control

There is no longer any doubt that the blood supply to the brain is under neural control. Both adrenergic and cholinergic systems have been demonstrated, with the former better documented than the latter and likely to play the more important role. The neural effects that are exerted on arteries and arterioles are generally larger than those invoked in metabolic control. Another generalization of importance is that adrenergic nerve terminals are more abundant in the anterior (forebrain) than in the posterior (hindbrain) circulations. Thus, activation of the adrenergic nervous system, such as during acute hypoxia, is likely to redistribute brain blood flow in a manner that favors perfusion of the hindbrain.

Metabolic control of brain blood flow tends to counterbalance neural effects except at certain extremes. That is, neurally mediated vasoconstriction of larger vessels will result in a greater metabolically generated signal in the region of small vessels, thereby minimizing the effect on tissue perfusion. This balancing is least likely to be operative under extreme conditions. For example, the vasoconstrictor effect of adrenergic activation is most readily demonstrated in a vascular bed that has been near maximally dilated by hypercapnia. In theory at least, this effect would render the hypoxic, hypercapnic patient more sensitive to neurally mediated variations in brain blood flow.

BRAIN BLOOD FLOW DURING SLEEP

Just as the control of breathing has been found to be profoundly influenced by sleep so has the control of the cerebral vasculature been found to be state related in a significant way. During slow-wave sleep, despite a slight (about 10%) reduction in whole brain metabolic rate, brain blood flow is increased. The increase parallels the increase in Pa_{CO_2} and can be related to it, i.e., the increase per mm Hg increase in Pa_{CO_2} is the same as that in awake subjects given CO_2 to breathe.

During rapid eye movement (REM) sleep the situation is quite different. When brain blood flow is monitored continuously it is found to be quite irregular, with surges that parallel periods of intense REM. These surges are not related to increases in brain oxidative metabolism and, as a consequence, result in a transient decline in calculated brain tissue or measured brain venous P_{CO_2}.[8, 11] We[8] have postulated that this phenomenon occurs in the region of the central chemoreceptor and plays a role in the generation of the reduced neural output to the diaphragm, which is characteristic of the intense REM phase of REM sleep. Because as many as half the patients with emphysema may have weakened diaphragms (the only major pump muscle of breathing activated during phasic REM sleep), this phenomenon is of potentially great importance in that disease.

BRAIN BLOOD FLOW IN PATIENTS WITH COPD

Normative data are difficult to obtain for various reasons. Techniques for measuring brain blood flow vary substantially as do the normal values associated with each technique and in fact with each laboratory. Although it is clear that age adjustments (decrease in flow with increase in age) must be made, the magnitude is unclear. The influence of concomitant diffuse cerebrovascular disease is difficult to discern.

Nevertheless, some generalizations may be made from limited clinical studies and studies in healthy subjects. It would appear that acid-base state is a key determinant of brain blood flow. Either a normal P_{CO_2} value or normal arterial pH (pHa) value in the presence of an elevated Pa_{CO_2} is associated with normal values for brain blood flow. Hypercapnia resulting in uncompensated or not fully compensated respiratory acidosis is associated with increased values for brain blood flow.[9, 13] Although more difficult to assess, moderate chronic hypoxia, i.e., Pa_{O_2} not below 55 mm Hg, seems to have little effect on brain blood flow in patients with COPD. One possible exception may be found in a comparison of patients with primary polycythemia to those with polycythemia secondary to chronic lung disease. Despite similar hematocrit values, the patients with polycythemia secondary to chronic lung disease had higher values for cerebral blood flow, although they were not found to have acidosis.[12]

The most attention has been paid to the role of secondary polycythemia.[1, 6, 9, 12, 15, 16] Of five studies that inferred effects of hematocrit levels, four involved venesection and one compared blood flow among subjects with elevated and normal hematocrit levels (Table 19–1). All agree that a significant inverse relationship exists between brain blood flow and hematocrit value. Following venesection, the magnitude of the increase in flow paralleled the magnitude of the decrease in hematocrit level, although the relationship varied considerably.

The greatest increase in flow is described in a work designed to compartmentalize brain blood flow.[16] In that study, a reduction of hematocrit value from 60 to 44% resulted in a rise in supratentorial flow of 78%. In no study did Pa_{CO_2} increase following venesection, but it did decrease in two.[15, 16] Thus, the effect of relieving secondary polycythemia upon brain blood flow may have been underestimated. The effect on O_2 delivery to the brain was variable. In one study, the greater flow more than compensated for the lesser oxygen-carrying capacity of the blood,[6] whereas in two other studies it did not.[12, 15] Cerebral function was assessed by questionnaire related to symptoms in three studies (e.g., headache, "full-

TABLE 19–1. Effect of Hematocrit Value on Brain Blood Flow and Cerebral Function in COPD

STUDY	HCT	Δ HCT	Δ BBF (%)	Δ PSYCH	Δ O_2 DEL
Menon et al.[6]	51.5	–	+27	+	+
Wade et al.[15]	61.3	−11.8	+21	+	–
York et al.[16]	59.6	−15.7	+57	+	Not determined
Semple et al.[12]	61.4	−13.0	+16	–	–
Bornstein et al.[1]	53.5	− 5.4	+ 9	+	Not determined

HCT = hematocrit; BBF = brain blood flow; PSYCH = psychologic function; O_2 DEL = product of O_2 content in arterial blood and brain blood flow; Δ = change following venesection except in the study of Menon and colleagues in which it refers to a comparison between groups with elevated and normal hematocrit values.

ness" in the head, and lethargy or hypersomnolence) and by formal psychometric testing in two. Four of the five studies reported improvement in cerebral function[2, 6, 15, 16]; one did not.[12] Improvement in cerebral function was variably related to improvement in brain blood flow and poorly or not at all related to change in the product of brain blood flow and O_2 content of arterial blood. Thus, it would appear that the majority of patients with significant secondary polycythemia (hematocrit level above 50%) due to COPD are likely to experience improved cerebral function following venesection. The procedure is to be recommended for this purpose and for protection against thrombosis.

EFFECT OF THEOPHYLLINE ON BRAIN BLOOD FLOW

Theophylline is widely used to treat chronic airways obstructive disease. Its beneficial effects have been ascribed to its action as a bronchodilator, a respiratory stimulant, and an enhancer of skeletal muscle endurance. However, the risk-benefit ratio has been questioned for certain subsets of patients because of significant toxic effects including those on the central nervous system. Further studies raise the possibility that some toxic effects may be mediated by a substantial decrease in brain blood flow. Recommended therapeutic dosages (loading dose of 6 mg/kg followed by 0.5 mg/kg/hr) caused 20% to 30% reductions in brain blood flow in normal volunteers and in patients with "moderately severe" COPD. At least some subjects hyperventilated, but the decrease in P_{CO_2} could not account for the decrease in brain blood flow.[2, 3]

The mechanism of this effect is unclear. Theophylline in therapeutic doses is known to antagonize the actions of adenosine, a potent vasodilator that is higher in concentration in the hypoxic brain. However, the data available do not allow an assessment as to whether the effect was greater in more hypoxic patients. In addition, in healthy subjects given an hypoxic gas mixture to breathe, the effect of aminophylline infusion on brain blood flow did not increase.[3]

Whether or not the central nervous system side effects of theophylline are related to its restriction of brain blood flow is a matter of conjecture at the moment. However, a potential 20% to 30% decline in brain blood flow in an already hypoxic, hypercapnic patient is certainly a cause for concern on theoretic grounds.

REFERENCES

1. Bornstein R, Menon D, York E, et al. Effects of venesection on cerebral function in chronic lung disease. Le Journal Canadien des Sciences Neurologique 1980; 7:293–296.
2. Bowton DL, Alford PT, McLees BD, et al. The effect of aminophylline on cerebal blood flow in patients with chronic obstructive pulmonary disease. Chest 1987; 91:874–877.
3. Bowton DL, Haddon WS, Prough DS, et al. Theophylline effect on the cerebral blood flow response to hypoxemia. Chest 1988; 94:371–375.
4. Fencl V, Vale JR, Broch JA. Respiration and cerebral blood flow in metabolic acidosis and alkalosis in humans. J Appl Physiol 1969; 27:67–76.
5. Krasney JA, McDonald BW, Matalon S. Regional circulatory responses to 96 hours of hypoxia in conscious sheep. Respir Physiol 1984; 57:73–88.
6. Menon D, York EL, Bornstein RA, et al. Optimal hematocrit and blood viscosity in secondary polycythemia as determined from cerebral blood flow. Clin Invest Med 1981; 4:117–121.
7. Neubauer JA, Edelman NH. Nonuniform brain blood flow response to hypoxia in unanesthetized cats. J Appl Physiol 1984; 57:1803–1808.
8. Parisi RA, Neubauer JA, Frank MM, et al. Linkage between brain blood flow and respiratory drive during rapid eye movement (REM) sleep. J Appl Physiol 1988; 64:1457–1465.
9. Patakas D, Sproule B, Jones D, et al. Cerebral blood flow, oxygen, carbon dioxide tensions, and blood bicarbonate in controlling drive and timing in patients with chronic obstructive pulmonary diseases. Respiration 1984; 46:45–51.
10. Santiago TV, Edelman NH. Brain blood flow and control of breathing. In: Handbook of Physiology, section 3: The Respiratory System, Fishman AP (ed), vol II. Control of Breathing, Part 1, Cherniack NS, Widdicombe JG (eds). Bethesda: American Physiological Society, 1986, 163–179.
11. Santiago TV, Neubauer JA, Edelman NH. Correlation between ventilation and brain blood flow during hypoxic sleep. J Appl Physiol 1986; 60:295–298.
12. Semple Pd'A, Lowe GDO, Patterson J, et al. Comparison of cerebral blood flow after venesection of bronchitic secondary polycythaemic and primary polycythaemic patients. Scott Med J 1983; 28:332–337.
13. Skinhoj E. CBF adaptation in man to chronic hypo- and hypercapnia and its relation to CSF pH. Scand J Clin Lab Invest 1968; 102 (Suppl 8A).
14. Wade JP, DuBoulay GH, Marshall J, et al. Cerebral blood flow, haematocrit and viscosity in subjects with a high oxygen affinity haemoglobin variant. Acta Neurol Scand 1980; 61:210–215.
15. Wade JPH, Pearson TC, Russell RWR, Wetherley-Mein G. Cerebral blood flow and blood viscosity in patients with polycythaemia secondary to hypoxic lung disease. Br Med J 1981; 283:689–692.
16. York EL, Jones RL, Menon D, Sproule BJ. Effects of secondary polycythemia on cerebral blood flow in chronic obstructive pulmonary disease. Am Rev Respir Dis 1980; 121:813–818.

Chapter 20

ACID-BASE DISORDERS IN CHRONIC OBSTRUCTIVE PULMONARY DISEASE

Philip L. Schiffman

COMMON PRESENTATIONS

Compensated respiratory acidosis is seen commonly in chronic bronchitis and emphysema of the bronchitic type. Mild chronic hypoventilation produces respiratory acidosis. Metabolic compensation is mediated via renal retention of bicarbonate ions, almost normalizing the pH. Progressive worsening of airway obstruction over time may lead to further increases in arterial carbon dioxide pressure (Pa_{CO_2}) with subsequent further secondary compensatory metabolic alkalosis.[9] When a patient so affected experiences acute exacerbations of disease, measurements of arterial blood gas values may show severe respiratory acidosis that is partially compensated. Thus, the presence of an elevated bicarbonate level in a patient who presents with hypercapnic ventilatory failure indicates underlying chronic hypercapnia.

Respiratory alkalosis is the most common acid-base disorder seen during acute asthmatic attacks.[13, 15] Although hypoxemia is almost uniformly present owing to ventilation-perfusion mismatching, hypocapnia is mostly present owing to stimulation of stretch receptors in the chest, which causes a sensation of dyspnea and heightened ventilatory drive. Despite the increased work of breathing, the muscles of ventilation are commonly overdriven early in bronchospastic episodes unless the degree of airway obstruction is extremely severe. Thus, even a normal Pa_{CO_2} (eucapnic hypoxemia) is an ominous sign of impending ventilatory failure, and hypercapnia is a finding that should never be ignored.

Respiratory alkalosis is also the most common finding in chronic bronchitis, but eucapnia and hypercapnia occur more frequently and earlier than in asthma and denote the presence of severe airways obstruction.[12] Patients who present with subacute exacerbations of asthma frequently exhibit non–anion gap metabolic acidosis. In one study, 45% of patients who presented at an emergency room with severe asthmatic attacks were found to have metabolic acidosis not secondary to lactic acid. In most of the patients, the asthma attacks had been present at least 2 days. It is likely that prolonged respiratory alkalosis in the early stages of the attacks stimulated a significant bicarbonate diuresis by the kidney in an attempt to maintain a normal blood pH.[16] Similarly, patients with chronic stable asymptomatic asthma, chronic bronchitis, and emphysema frequently present with compensated respiratory alkalosis.[6]

Acute respiratory alkalosis and respiratory acidosis may have clinical effects. Respiratory alkalosis may cause secondary bronchoconstriction[13] and also produce systemic vasoconstriction and decreased cerebral blood flow. Other complications of respiratory alkalosis include increased neuroexcitability, which may lead to heightened dyspnea, cardiac arrhythmia, seizures, and other neurologic manifestations. Acute respiratory acidosis can give rise to cardiovascular, gastrointestinal (GI), renal, and cerebral complications, including narcosis, bicarbonate retention, headache, dyspnea, and arrhythmias.

EXOGENOUS FACTORS

Acid-base disturbances in patients with chronic obstructive pulmonary disease may be produced by exogenous factors as listed in Table 20–1. In general, factors decreasing ventilatory drive or weakening respiratory muscles cause respiratory acidosis, whereas respiratory stimulants may give rise to respiratory alkalosis. Some agents listed as causing metabolic acidosis and metabolic alkalosis are either directly acidic (ammonium chloride) or alkalotic (bicarbonate). Others produce their effects by promoting loss of acid (nasogastric suction, loop diuretics) or loss of alkali (outdated tetracycline, amphotericin B, acetazolamide) by the kidneys or GI tract. Some agents act on a metabolic pathway resulting in the formation of an organic acid (phenformin, methanol, ethylene glycol). Patients with severe airway obstruction may be more prone to respiratory acidosis from the effects of sedating drugs than other patients. Inappropriate oxygen administration may cause respiratory acidosis in patients. This effect was once thought solely to be secondary to depression of respiratory drive, but further studies suggest that an increase in the dead space-tidal volume ratio (V_D/V_T) is another important factor.[4, 18]

Several of the agents in Table 20–1 may be responsible for more than one type of acid-base derangement. Aspirin (in children) and paraldehyde cause metabolic acidosis. However, they act also as respiratory stimulants. This effect can be greater than the metabolic acidosis aspirin and paraldehyde produce, resulting in respiratory alkalosis.

Banked red blood cells preserved in citric acid—trisodium citrate—dextrose solution (ACD) are acidic; thus, massive transfusions may cause metabolic acidosis. As the ACD is metabolized, a metabolic alkalosis state may develop.[14] Note that corticosteroids are listed in Table 20–1 as causing metabolic alkalosis—a mineralocorticoid effect.

OTHER FACTORS

The earliest studies on blood gas chemistry and acid-base balance in patients with chronic obstructive pulmonary disease

TABLE 20–1. Exogenous Factors Leading to Acid-Base Disturbances

METABOLIC ACIDOSIS	METABOLIC ALKALOSIS	RESPIRATORY ACIDOSIS	RESPIRATORY ALKALOSIS
Acetazolamide	Corticosteroids	Sedating drugs	Progesterone
Spironolactone	Loop diuretics	Barbiturates	Nicotine
Ammonium chloride	Bicarbonate therapy	Benzodiazepines	Theophylline
Theophylline	Massive blood transfusion (late)	Narcotics	Epinephrine
Phenformin	Nasogastric suction	Anesthetics	Aspirin (in adults)
Diarrhea (cathartics)		Paralyzing agents	Paraldehyde
Starvation		Curare	
Ileostomy loss		Succinyl choline	
Ethylene glycol		Organophosphates	
Ethanol		Oxygen	
Methanol			
Aspirin (in children)			
Cholestyramine			
Amphotericin B			
Tetracycline (outdated)			
Paraldehyde			
Isoniazid			
Massive blood transfusion (early)			

(COPD) focused on the resting awake state. It is now known that sleep, exercise, and dietary intake may contribute to acid-base abnormalities.

During sleep, patients with COPD may develop oxygen desaturation secondary to hypoventilation. When arterial blood gas measurements have been obtained,[5, 11] concomitant rises in Pa_{CO_2} have been confirmed. Sleep apnea is not necessary for this phenomenon to occur,[5] and patients who are hypercapnic when awake appear to have greater risk of hypoventilation than those who are eucapnic.[17]

During aerobic exercise, healthy subjects are able to match minute ventilation to increasing CO_2 production, resulting in eucapnia. At increasing work levels, exercise becomes anaerobic and metabolic acidosis develops. In patients with chronic airflow obstruction, CO_2 retention and respiratory acidosis may occur during exercise. The inappropriately low minute ventilation during exercise that causes this respiratory acidosis is not due to reduced respiratory drive but rather is due to mechanical derangements limiting ventilation and to an increase in V_D/V_T.[10, 19] Reduced muscle levels of ATP and phosphocreatine and intracellular acidosis with increased muscle levels of lactate have been shown to occur in patients with severe hypercapnia and hypoxemia and suggest that the muscles may be metabolizing anaerobically.[8]

The composition of the diet affects metabolism and CO_2 production. Diets in which carbohydrate content makes up a high percent of total calories will produce a relatively high respiratory quotient and correspondingly greater CO_2 production. When a patient is unable to match minute ventilation to CO_2 production, respiratory acidosis and even respiratory failure may develop.[7] In ambulatory, chronically hypercapnic patients with COPD, diets with low carbohydrate content produced lower arterial Pa_{CO_2} than did diets with higher carbohydrate content.[2]

Various reports show that some asthmatic patients during severe attacks of bronchospasm may develop metabolic acidosis (lactic acidosis).[1, 3] This finding is at odds with previous studies in which lactic acidosis was not reported.[12, 13, 15, 16] Increased lactic acid production may arise from overworked respiratory muscles, from hypoperfusion of skeletal muscle and liver, or from both.[1, 3] An alternative theory is that the lactic acidosis may be linked to treatment with β-adrenergic medications that were not given as treatment in the previous studies.[1]

REFERENCES

1. Alberts WM, Williams JH, Ramsdell JW. Metabolic acidosis as a presenting feature in acute asthma. Ann Allergy 1986; 57:107–109.
2. Angelillo VA, Bedi S, Durfee D, et al. Effects of low and high carbohydrate feedings in ambulatory patients with chronic obstructive pulmonary disease and chronic hypercapnia. Ann Intern Med 1985; 103:883–885.
3. Appel D, Rubenstein R, Schrager K, Williams MH. Lactic acidosis in severe asthma. Am J Med 1983; 73:580–584.
4. Aubier M, Murciano D, Milic-Emili J, et al. Effects of the administration of O_2 on ventilation and blood gases in patients with chronic obstructive pulmonary disease during acute respiratory failure. Am Rev Respir Dis 1980; 122:747–754.
5. Catterall JR, Douglas NJ, Calverley PMA, et al. Transient hypoxemia during sleep in chronic obstructive pulmonary disease is not a sleep apnea syndrome. Am Rev Respir Dis 1983; 128:24–29.
6. Cochrane GM, Prior JG, Wolff CB. Chronic stable asthma and the normal arterial pressure of carbon dioxide in hypoxia. Br Med J 1980; 281:705–710.
7. Covelli HD, Black JW, Olsen MS, Beekman JF. Respiratory failure precipitated by high carbohydrate loads. Ann Intern Med 1981; 95:579–581.
8. Fiaccadori E, Del Canale S, Vitali P. Skeletal muscle energetics, acid-base equilibrium and lactate metabolism in patients with severe hypercapnia and hypoxemia. Chest 1987; 92:883–887.
9. Filley GF. Acid regulation and CO_2 retention. Chest 1970; 58 (Supp 2):417–422.
10. Gimenez M, Servera E, Candina R, et al. Hypercapnia during maximum exercise in patients with chronic airflow obstruction. Bull Eur Physiopathol Respir 1984; 20:113–119.
11. Guilleminault C, Cummiskey J, Motta J. Chronic obstructive airflow disease and sleep studies. Am Rev Respir Dis 1980; 122:397–406.
12. Hodgkin JE, Balchum OJ, Kass I, et al. Chronic obstructive airway diseases. Current concepts in diagnosis and comprehensive care. JAMA 1975; 232:1243–1260.
13. Hypoxemia and hypocapnia in asthma. N Engl J Med 1968; 278:1068.
14. Litwin MS, Smith LL, Moore FD. Metabolic alkalosis following massive transfusion. Surgery 1959; 45:805–813.
15. McFadden ER, Lyons HA. Arterial-blood gas tension in asthma. N Engl J Med 1968; 278:1027–1032.
16. Okrent DG, Tessler S, Twersky RA, Tashkin DP. Metabolic acidosis not due to lactic acidosis in patients with severe acute asthma. Crit Care Med 1987; 15:1098–1101.
17. Perez-Padilla R, Conway W, Roth T, et al. Hypercapnia and

sleep O_2 desaturation in chronic obstructive pulmonary disease. Sleep 1987; 10:216–223.

18. Sassoon CSH, Hassell KT, Mahutte CK. Hyperoxic-induced hypercapnia in stable chronic obstructive pulmonary disease. Am Rev Respir Dis 1987; 135:907–911.

19. Van Meerhaeghe A, Sergysels R. Control of breathing during exercise in patients with chronic airflow limitation with or without hypercapnia. Chest 1983; 84:565–570.

Chapter 21

FLUID RETENTION ASSOCIATED WITH PULMONARY INSUFFICIENCY AND RESPIRATORY FAILURE

Kaye H. Kilburn

Fluid retention may develop in patients with lung disease and occurs more frequently in patients with chronic bronchitis and emphysema during respiratory failure. In a prospective study of 176 episodes of respiratory failure, fluid retention was observed in 22% of patients with chronic obstructive pulmonary disease (COPD).[2] In 39 episodes, patients lost 16 to 65 lb (7.3 to 29.5 kg) during recovery from respiratory failure (Fig. 21–1).[25] The arterial oxygen pressures (Pa_{O_2}) of these patients were less than 55 torr, and in 33 the arterial carbon dioxide pressure (Pa_{CO_2}) was greater than 50 torr. Visible or palpable edema is not unusual, and massive fluid retention occurs when alveolar hypoventilation is combined with obesity, i.e., Pickwickian syndrome, as in Figure 21–2. Some of these patients so affected have cardiac problems, but all patients with fluid retention have impaired ability to excrete water even during recovery. This problem has been verified by giving water loads of 20 ml/kg orally or intravenously and measuring urine volume during 4 hours. Thus, both impaired cardiac and renal functions seem to be mechanisms of fluid retention in pulmonary patients.

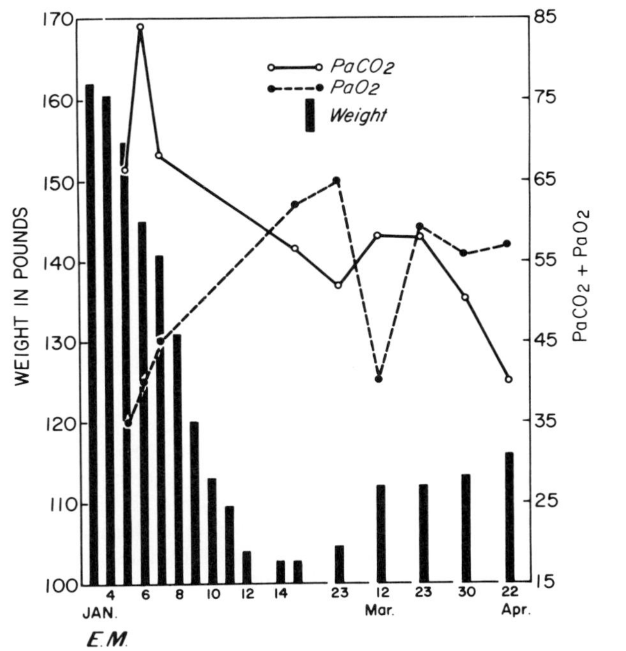

Figure 21–1. A 46-year-old patient with chronic bronchitis and emphysema had anasarca, which was refractory to a combination of bed rest, digitalis, and diuretics. Initial Pa_{O_2} was 35 torr and Pa_{CO_2} was 67 torr. Treatment with oxygen and intermittent assisted ventilation produced a diuresis of 59 lbs. in 6 days. (Reproduced with permission from Kilburn KH, Dowell AR. Arch Intern Med 1971; 127:754–762.)

HISTORICAL BACKGROUND

In the early 1950s, Flint in Sheffield[20] and Wood in London[41] observed that 10% to 25% of patients with congestive heart failure (CHF) admitted to hospitals in Britain had chronic lung disease as the underlying cause. In Sheffield City Hospital in 1952, fully 40% of the episodes of CHF in men and 8.5% of CHF in women were classified as caused by cor pulmonale. These observations were underscored further in the 1950s, 1960s, and 1970s,[11, 12, 18, 19, 23, 27, 39] pointing to an interplay between cardiac failure and pulmonary failure. Wood estimated that chronic cor pulmonale was responsible for between 5% and 10% of all instances of organic heart disease.[41] Kellaway, in 1959,[23] studied the features of 18 patients in Edinburgh and found of 334 consecutive patients admitted with CHF that 25 had histories of chronic lung disease. In 15, this was considered the sole etiologic factor in cardiac failure. Those patients showing right ventricular strain by electrocardiography were least likely to survive. The most satisfactory treatment was oxygen, which increased survival. Kellaway

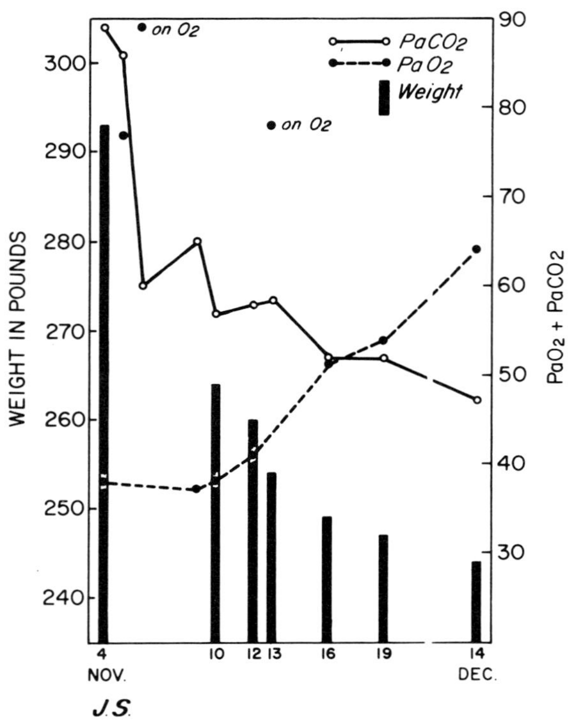

Figure 21–2. A 42-year-old male with chronic bronchitis and obesity was admitted with respiratory failure and edema. Pa_{O_2} was 37 torr and Pa_{CO_2} was 88 torr. During 12 days of treatment with oxygen and assisted ventilation he lost 46 lbs. (Reproduced with permission from Kilburn KH, Dowell AR. Arch Intern Med 1971; 127:754–762.)

predicted the reductions in renal plasma flow and glomerular filtration rate found later by others.[12, 19, 27]

Turning the question around, Wade and Bishop observed, in 1962,[38] that despite physiologic studies, no prevalent information was available concerning the status of the heart and pulmonary circulation in patients with emphysema, chronic bronchitis, or chronic obstructive pulmonary disease. Notwithstanding intense interest in cor pulmonale over the years, this situation remains true today.

HYPERCAPNIA AND FLUID RETENTION

Hypercapnia can affect both circulatory and renal functions; acute hypercapnia can affect cardiac work. The acute effects of breathing 10% CO_2 and of exercise on the pulmonary circulation have been compared in normal subjects and in patients with hypercapnic respiratory failure during recovery. Although both stimuli raised cardiac output equally, hypercapnia in both groups raised pulmonary vascular resistance significantly when compared during exercise.[24] Also, infusion of bicarbonate during CO_2 breathing did not reduce the pulmonary vascular resistance.

In 1960, Campbell,[11] in reviewing edema in patients with lung disease, observed that edema was rarely present when the Pa_{CO_2} was normal. When edema was present, Pa_{CO_2} was almost always raised, although edema did not occur in all patients with CO_2 retention. Campbell suggested that the greater absorption of bicarbonate bound base, known to occur experimentally in dogs, could expand extracellular fluid in the lungs and elsewhere, increasing nonelastic pulmonary resistance and decreasing compliance. However, a decade earlier, Fishman and colleagues[19] had shown in dogs, Davies and Kilpatrick had inferred clinically,[12] and Lewis and colleagues[27] had shown in humans, that hypoxia, hypercapnia, or both reduced renal plasma flow and glomerular filtration rate. By 1964, two additional studies indicated that renal function was affected by hypoxia. One showed that as arterial oxygenation was reduced the kidneys enlarged and became cyanotic and autonomic control of the renal vessels was lost in dogs.[3] The other study showed that glomerular lesions, consisting of dilatation of capillaries, increased capillary loops, hypercellularity of mesangium, and deposition of granulofibrillar material, developed with hypoxia. In addition, a prominent juxtaglomerular apparatus was seen in the kidneys of individuals who had died of cyanotic congenital heart disease and primary pulmonary hypertension.[36] These findings suggested that abnormalities in renal function may be even more important than abnormal cardiac function in edema production.

CARDIAC MECHANISMS

Some patients with pulmonary impairment, coronary artery disease, and borderline ventricular function develop heart failure or decreased cardiac output during hypoxia and retain fluid. Left ventricular failure may occur in conjunction with respiratory failure.[14, 30] Left ventricular hypertrophy in individuals with chronic bronchitis has been documented by measuring cardiac wall thickness of hearts obtained at autopsy.[21] The causes of this finding remain controversial. In another study, normal left ventricular function was found in patients with chronic obstructive pulmonary disease.[40] The clinical comparability of patients in these different studies is uncertain because groups vary as to history of angina, electrocardiographic changes of left ventricular stress or hypertrophy, and heart size as determined on the chest radiograph. Systemic hypertension is uncommon and seldom contributes to heart failure in these patients.

Obesity, associated with alveolar hypoventilation and chronic phlegm production, is sometimes accompanied by edema, hypoxemia, and hypercapnia. Although the incidence of fluid retention is unknown, these patients are younger than the usual patients with COPD and have smoked less. They have frequently been edematous for weeks or months before hospitalization often despite administration of diuretics, salt restriction, and digitalis.[25]

Pulmonary emboli in the presence of obstructive pulmonary disease are frequently overlooked. Yet embolic episodes may imitate or even cause airway obstruction. It is difficult to know the extent of small or microscopic emboli in a pulmonary arterial tree that has suffered frequently from the destruction of lung parenchyma and the accompanying loss of vascular bed. Other patients with edema who are bedridden or sedentary suffer venous thrombosis and pulmonary embolization. Clearly, emboli further reduce the already restricted pulmonary vascular bed and elevate the output impedance for the right side of the heart.

A decrease in effective arterial blood volume can cause salt and water retention leading to the development of edema. It is observed when heart failure decreases cardiac output or when chronic hepatic cirrhosis with hypoalbuminemia decreases plasma oncotic pressure. Edema occurred in experimental animals when large arteriovenous fistulae were created.[9] The decline in "effective arterial blood volume" triggers renal vascular constriction causing a redistribution of renal blood flow, decreased renal blood flow, increased filtration fraction, and increased proximal tubular reabsorption of sodium and water. Glomerular filtration rate is decreased, while renin output is increased. Higher levels of aldosterone acting on the distal renal tubule promote sodium absorption. The usual rise in central venous pressure in heart failure increases capillary pressure transudation and thus increases interstitial fluid. The interaction of greater plasma volume and greater vascular transudation from renal retention of salt and water enhances the increase in interstitial volume, producing edema. A reduction in atrial natriuretic hormone[15] and an elevation in antidiuretic hormone may also contribute to edema formation.

These processes probably account for fluid retention in patients with COPD with low cardiac output, i.e., heart failure. However, it is difficult to make a case for a decrease in "effective arterial blood volume" in most patients with COPD who have normal cardiac outputs and normal systemic blood pressures. Little data indicate renal vasoconstriction or higher vasopressin levels in patients with COPD with fluid retention.[18] Mean central venous pressure is not usually elevated in patients with COPD, although exaggerated fluctuations in venous pressures may occur with breathing. Thus, the mechanisms that account for fluid retention in low output heart failure, arteriovenous fistula, or hypoalbuminemic edema states[35] are probably not operative in most edematous patients with respiratory failure from airway obstruction.

CARDIAC OUTPUT IN CHRONIC AIRWAY OBSTRUCTION

In 1962, Wade and Bishop[38] studied over 200 patients with chronic airways obstruction, most of whom had emphysema but some had chronic bronchitis only. These workers found normal cardiac indices by the Fick method, although stroke volumes were decreased because of high cardiac rates. No apparent relationship was observed among the cardiac index and the oxygen saturation of arterial blood or the cardiac index and the right atrial mean pressure. Patients who had retained fluid, i.e., had "congestive failure," had the same distribution of cardiac indices as the normal subjects and those with emphysema without congestive failure. Wade and Bishop found that elevated cardiac output (high output failure) was unusual and that low output was exceptional. Thus, these patients retained salt and water without a reduction in cardiac output or cardiac congestive failure.

RENAL MECHANISMS

Impaired renal function may be even more important than cardiac abnormalities as a cause of salt and water retention and edema in patients with severe respiratory insufficiency.[6, 24, 26, 35] Major factors are thought to be increased renal vascular resistance, decreased renal plasma flow, and increased filtration fraction, which reduces peritubular hydrostatic pressure and glomerular filtration rate. It is not clear whether the increase in renal vascular resistance or the decrease in renal blood flow is primary. Additionally, as mentioned, renal bicarbonate reabsorption that helps compensate for respiratory acidosis contributes to edema formation.[31] The reabsorption of filtered bicarbonate and regeneration of new bicarbonate occur in the proximal tubular cells where hydrogen ion, formed by splitting water into hydrogen and hydroxyl ions, is secreted into the tubular lumen. The hydroxyl ion catalyzed by carbonic anhydrase combines with CO_2 to form HCO_3, which diffuses across the cell membrane and enters the extracellular bicarbonate pool. The hydrogen ion secreted into the lumen combines with filtered bicarbonate, forming H_2CO_3. This is dehydrated further along in the proximal tubule to form CO_2. The CO_2 diffuses from the lumen to the peritubular blood so that the filtered bicarbonate ion is reclaimed. Secreted hydrogen ions continue to combine with nonbicarbonate buffers to be excreted in the urine. Bicarbonate, the original product formed in the tubular cell, enters the peritubular blood and thus a bicarbonate ion is regenerated. The secretion of the hydrogen ion into the tubular lumen is frequently accompanied by a transfer of sodium from the lumen into the cell where it freely moves into the peritubular blood. This effect seems to explain the sodium retention that accompanies bicarbonate retention and enhances water retention.[11]

For additional detail, the reader may wish to refer to Smith[37] or Pitts.[28] A clear explanation of state of the art concerning edema and sodium retention is provided by Levy and Seely.[26]

PATHOPHYSIOLOGY OF INCREASED RENAL SODIUM RETENTION IN PATIENTS WITH RESPIRATORY FAILURE

The possible mechanisms for increased renal sodium retention include (1) abnormal volume receptors that respond inadequately to expansion of blood volume, in the brain, the left atrium, the great vessels, or the kidney itself; (2) a disturbance in the normal ratio of plasma volume to available vascular capacity; (3) a plasma volume contraction because of unusual space partition; (4) a reduction in renal perfusion because of either a reduction in cardiac output or a decrease in peripheral vascular resistance; and (5) a direct intrarenal vascular readjustment, i.e., a change in the fraction of sodium reabsorbed by the renal tubules.

Cardiac failure, as postulated by Berns and Schrier,[6] has three effects: (1) greater venous pressure; (2) greater left atrial pressure; and (3) less effective arterial filling, which can alter renal function. The first of these effects raises renal venous pressure; the second raises renal vascular resistance; and the third promotes tubular sodium reabsorption by diminishing renal blood flow. Aldosterone levels may rise because hepatic congestion reduces its degradation or because renal hypoprofusion and activation of the juxtaglomerular receptor raises renin and angiotensin-II levels and thereby stimulates aldosterone.

Decreased renal perfusion is an important final pathway in edema formation and leads to a reduction in effective renal plasma flow and a less marked reduction in glomerular filtration rate, elevating the filtration fraction. The kidney, which is sensitive to a reduction in perfusion, adaptively retains sodium to restore its blood flow. However, in patients with respiratory failure, edema usually occurs with a normal or an elevated cardiac output and in all probability with increased renal blood flow rather than decreased.

Respiratory failure in COPD is more common in the older individual. Renal function decreases in subjects older than 50 years. Davies and Shock[13] studied renal plasma flow and glomerular filtration rate using classic techniques with constant infusion of iodopyracet (Diodrast) and inulin in subjects between 20 and 89 years of age. Inulin and iodopyracet clearance and iodopyracet transfer maximum were lower in subjects older than 60 years. In fact, both renal plasma flow and glomerular filtration rate are significantly reduced after 50 years of age and are reduced to about half the maximal values by 80 to 89 years of age.

RENAL EFFECTS OF RESPIRATORY FAILURE

The hypoxia and hypercapnia that occur in respiratory failure can have direct effects, which can produce fluid retention. In fact, some sources fail to even mention this possibil-

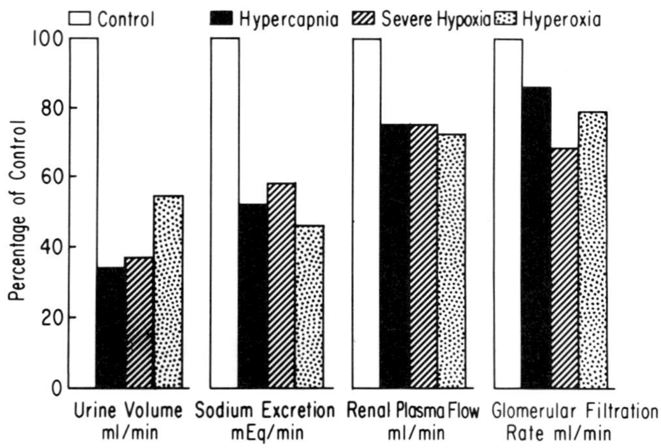

Figure 21–3. Urine flow shown in bars decreased as arterial blood oxygen decreased. During subsequent hyperoxia, induced by administration of 40% oxygen, urine flow initially doubled and then fell as Pa_{O_2} exceeded 148 torr. (Reproduced with permission from Kilburn KH, Dowell AR. Arch Intern Med 1971; 127:754–762.)

ity.[9, 10, 42] Similarly, some textbooks of renal disease have also overlooked possible direct effects of hypoxia and hypercapnia on the kidney.[8, 22, 33]

An early study (1960) of 23 patients with chronic bronchitis after they had developed congestive failure showed that renal plasma flows were reduced but glomerular filtration rates remained normal as CO_2 tensions rose and O_2 saturation fell. These effects resulted in elevated filtration fractions that persisted after recovery.[29] Another study compared eight COPD patients with edema with ten COPD patients without edema.[1] Renal blood flow varied with cardiac output, was lowest in patients with edema, but was reduced significantly in all patients. Cardiac output was inversely related to pulmonary artery pressure. Positive correlations were found between Pa_{CO_2}, tubular reabsorption of bicarbonate, and reduced excretion of both sodium and water.[1]

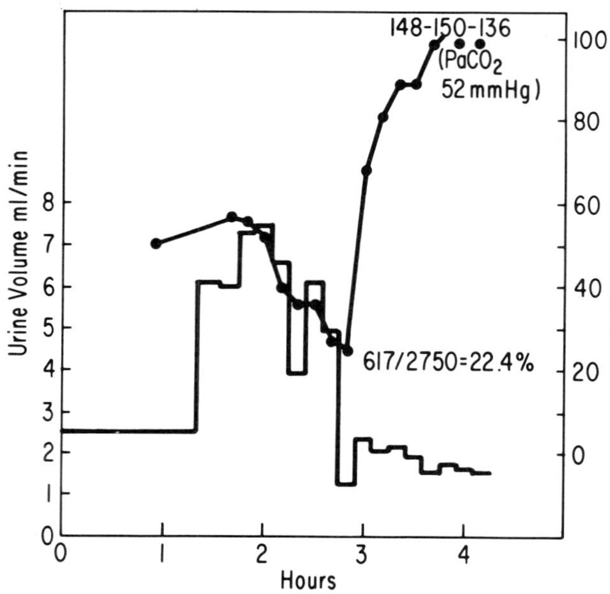

Figure 21–4. Hypercapnia, severe hypoxia, and hyperoxia reduced urine volume, sodium excretion, renal plasma flow, and glomerular filtration rate in three groups of patients studied during their recovery from respiratory failure, which was accompanied by edema. (Reproduced with permission from Kilburn KH, Dowell AR. Arch Intern Med 1971; 127:754–762.)

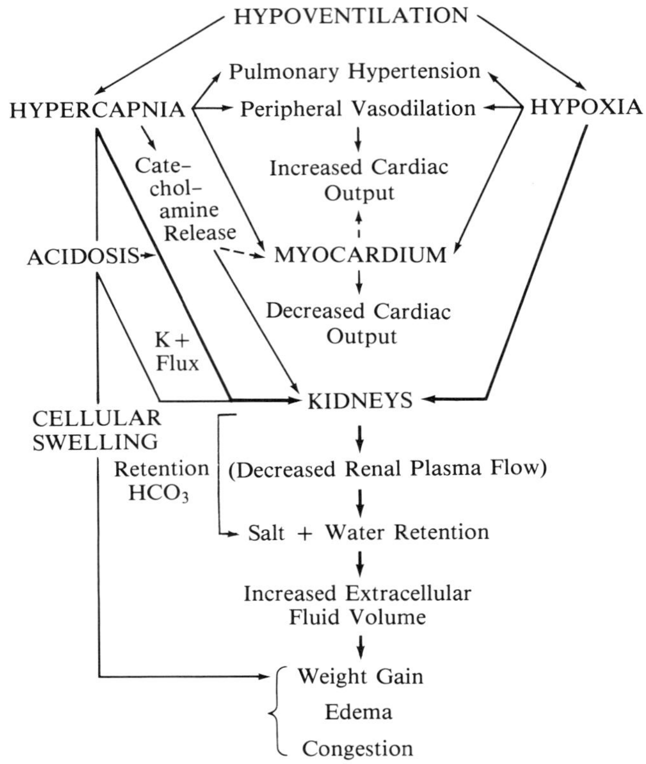

Figure 21–5. The renal effects of hypercapnia and hypoxia appear to play a pivotal role in fluid retention and edema in patients with respiratory failure due to chronic bronchitis with or without emphysema. Hypercapnia acidosis appears to act synergistically with hypoxemia to activate the renin-angiotensin system and diminish renal plasma flow. (Reproduced with permission from Kilburn KH, Dowell AR. Arch Intern Med 1971; 127:754–762.)

Additional clues came from studies of water loading in 20 patients with obstructive airway disease who had hypercapnia but not edema. When given 20 ml of water/kg body weight orally, they excreted only 51% of the administered load compared with 106% in 13 controls. Sodium output was only 0.073 mEq/minute in the patients compared with 0.237 mEq/minute in the controls.[39] The glomerular filtration rate of patients was 77 ml/minute compared with 117 ml/minute in the controls; water clearance was 2.1 and osmolar clearance 2.0 as compared with 7.4 and 4.5, respectively, in the controls. The most striking difference between patients and controls was the greater Pa_{CO_2} of 61.2 torr in the patients, which correlated inversely with the percentage of the water load excreted. Although White and Woodings speculated that increased vasopressin activity might be responsible for the abnormal water excretion, this possibility was ruled out in other studies.

Normal vasopressin levels were found in patients with elevated Pa_{CO_2} by Farber and colleagues,[18] who demonstrated impaired excretion of a water load and decreased effective renal plasma flow with normal glomerular filtration rates. In their study, ten hypercapnic patients were unable to have a normal solute diuresis or a maximal water diuresis. The investigators attributed this finding to a reduced sodium excretion that was 15 mEq in 4 hours (0.06 mEq/minute) in the hypercapnic patients, half as much as in the eucapnic subjects (0.14 mEq/minute). Total solute excretion was 114 mOsm in patients compared with 172 mOsm in eucapnic subjects. in contrast, plasma vasopressin levels were in the normal range (1.9 ± 0.7 pg/ml) in the hypercapnic patients and were suppressed appropriately with water loading. The hypercapnic patients had slightly lower baseline vasopressin levels (1.1 ± 0.2 pg/ml), which also were suppressed appropriately. Decreased water output and 4-hour sodium excretions were correlated significantly.

A study of water loading in 17 patients during convalescence from 26 episodes of respiratory failure due to airways obstruction also showed impaired excretion.[25] Thus, in only three of 26 episodes was 70% or more of a 20 ml/kg water load excreted in 4 hours.[14] Studies repeated in three patients during recovery showed marked improvement with greater oxygenation and reduction in Pa_{CO_2}, from 10% to 20% excretion of the water load to 50% to 90% excretion. However, there were too few observations to permit correlations with Pa_{CO_2} or Pa_{O_2}.

A study of 41 subjects with diffuse obstructive pulmonary emphysema (cardiac status unspecified) showed a 20% increase in total exchangeable sodium, using ^{24}Na dilution, and a 30% decrease in total body exchangeable potassium, ^{42}K. The extracellular fluid was increased from 163 ml/kg to 233 ml/kg.[4] Retained sodium and Pa_{CO_2} had a correlation coefficient of 0.41, which was significant.

EFFECTS OF HYPOXIA

The effects of acute hypoxia on renal function were studied in nine normal subjects who breathed 14% oxygen to reduce arterial Pa_{O_2} to approximately 50 torr. Renal plasma flow did not decrease during hypoxemic periods but rather increased slightly, and sodium and chloride excretion and urine flow increased.[5]

The effects of hypoxia on kidney function were studied in two groups of patients with cor pulmonale secondary to emphysema and chronic bronchitis, using classic renal clearance techniques. Four patients who remained in heart failure at the time of study were compared with nine who had been in heart failure but had recovered.[19] Those in heart failure had higher filtration fractions, lower glomerular filtration rates, and much lower renal plasma flows measured by para-aminohippurate (PAH) than did those who had recovered. An increased filtration fraction was found. The renal plasma flow varied inversely with the changes in Pa_{O_2}, and sodium excretion was correlated with renal plasma flow. Thus, when hypoxemia was varied by administering oxygen or low oxygen mixtures, renal plasma flow varied inversely with Pa_{O_2} as did sodium excretion. Relief of hypoxemia depressed renal plasma flow, whereas increasing hypoxemia produced a higher renal plasma flow. The levels of hypoxia used had no effect on the excretion of PAH.

Renal clearances in 14 patients during recovery from respiratory failure showed the expected reductions in glomerular filtration rate and renal plasma flow during control periods breathing air,[25] as in Figure 21–3. Breathing a low oxygen gas mixture that reduced Pa_{O_2} from 54 to 30 torr and Pa_{CO_2} from 55 to 47 torr for 2 to 3 hours, reduced average urine flow from 6.3 to 2.3 ml/minute and water clearance from 2.8 to 1.2 ml/minute as renal plasma flow fell from 293 to 219 ml/minute and glomerular filtration rate from 81 to 56 ml/minute. Although the filtration fraction dropped only slightly, sodium excretion fell from 0.19 mEq/minute to 0.11 mEq/minute.

Breathing oxygen raised Pa_{O_2} from 49 to 160 torr and raised Pa_{CO_2} from 55 to 59 torr, reduced urine volume from 6.1 to 3.3 ml/minute, reduced water clearance from 2.9 to 1.0 ml/minute, reduced renal plasma flow from 291 to 211 ml/minute, and reduced glomerular filtration rate from 77 to 61 ml/minute.[14] Sodium excretion fell from 0.26 to 0.12 mEq/minute during 2 to 3 hours of hyperoxia.

Breathing 5% CO_2 raised Pa_{CO_2} from 58 to 75 torr, decreased urine volume from 6.1 to 2.0 ml/minute, water clearance from 2.4 to 0.1 ml/minute, renal plasma flow from 337 to 253 ml/minute, glomerular filtration rate from 97 to 83 ml/minute, and sodium excretion from 0.20 to 0.09 mEq/minute.[14]

Viewed together, these studies on convalescent patients suggest that hypercapnia, severe hypoxemia, and hyperoxia to a mean of 162 torr each interferes with sodium and water excretion and decreases renal plasma flow. When the urine flow as a percent of maximal output is plotted against changes in Pa_{O_2}, it rises as hypoxia becomes more severe (to 30 to 50 torr) and then plummets, in individual patients, with further hypoxia as seen in Figure 21–4.

Similar experiments on conscious dogs measured plasma renin activity and angiotensin II concentrations during hypoxia, hypercapnia, and combined hypercapnia and hypoxia. Hypoxemia or hypercapnia alone stimulated the renin-angiotensin system moderately. Hypoxemia and hypercapnic acidosis were synergistic, strongly activating the renin-angiotensin system. Angiotensin II blockade, using 1-sarcosine-8-alanine-angiotensin II, during acute hypoxemia and hypercapnic acidosis decreased renal plasma flow.[34]

No strong evidence implicates atrial-derived peptide or natriuretic factor in edema in patients with chronic obstructive lung disease.[15] Dintenfass and Read have suggested a novel hypothesis that decreased deformation of red blood cells in increased aggregation alters distribution of red blood cells to critical capillary beds and leads to edema.[16]

Thus, it appears that patients with hypoxic and hypercapnic respiratory failure from airway obstructive disease due to emphysema, chronic bronchitis, or both, as shown in Figure 21–5, manifest impaired renal function with reduced renal plasma flow and smaller decreases in glomerular filtration. Salt and water are retained with little or no elevation of the vasopressin levels but, probably, with considerable stimulation of the renin-angiotensin system. When hypercapnia exceeds a level of approximately 60 torr in the arterial blood and hypoxia falls below 40 torr, further salt and water are retained.[7] In addition, it appears that hyperoxia may inhibit renal plasma flow at least temporarily.[17] Further observations in patients during therapeutic administration of oxygen are needed to determine whether this inhibition can have adverse effects on the excretion of sodium and water.[32]

REFERENCES

1. Aber GM, Bayley TJ, Bishop JM. Inter-relationships between renal and cardiac function and respiratory gas exchange in obstructive airways disease. Clin Sci 1963; 25:159–170.
2. Asmundsson T, Kilburn KH. Survival of acute respiratory failure. Ann Intern Med 1969; 70:471–485.
3. Axelrod DR, Pitts RF. Effects of hypoxia on renal tubular function. J Appl Physiol 1952; 4:593–601.
4. Baum GL, Dick MM, Blum A, et al. Total body exchangeable potassium and sodium and extracellular fluid in chronic pulmonary insufficiency. Am Heart J 1959; 58:53–58.
5. Berger EY, Gladston M, Horwitz SA. The effect of anoxic anoxia on the human kidney. J Clin Invest 1949; 28:648–652.
6. Berns AS, Schrier RW. The kidney in heart failure. In: Suki WN, Eknoyan G, eds. The Kidney in Systemic Disease, 2nd ed. New York: John Wiley & Sons, 1981.
7. Black DAK, Stanbury SW. Renal insufficiency in terminal respiratory failure. Br Med J 1958; 1:872–873.
8. Black DAK, Jones NF. Renal Disease, 4th ed. Oxford: Blackwell Scientific, 1979.
9. Braunwald E. Edema. In: Petersdorf RG, Adams RD, Braunwald E, et al., eds. Harrison's Principles of Internal Medicine, 10th ed. New York: McGraw-Hill, 1983.
10. Braunwald E. Heart Disease, A Textbook of Cardiovascular Medicine, 3rd ed. Philadelphia: WB Saunders Company, 1988.
11. Campbell JM, Short DS. The cause of oedema in "cor pulmonale." Lancet 1960; i:1184–1186.

12. Davies CE, Kilpatrick JA. Renal circulation in "low-output" and high-output" heart failure. Clin Sci 1951; 10:53–63.
13. Davies DF, Shock NW. Age changes in glomerular filtration rate, effective renal plasma flow, and tubular excretory capacity in adult males. J Clin Invest 1950; 29:496–507.
14. Davies H, Overy HR. Left ventricular function in cor pulmonale. Chest 1970; 58:8–14.
15. de Bold AJ. Atrial natriuretic factor: a hormone produced by the heart. Science 1985; 230:767–770.
16. Dintenfass L, Read J. Pathogenesis of heart failure in acute-on-chronic respiratory failure. Lancet 1968; i:570–572.
17. Editorial. Renal function in respiratory failure. JAMA 1971; 216:131–132.
18. Farber MO, Bright TP, Strawbridge RA, et al. Impaired water handling in chronic obstructive lung disease. J Lab Clin Med 1975; 85:41–49.
19. Fishman AP, Maxwell MH, Crowder Ch, Morales P. Kidney function in cor pulmonale: particular consideration of changes in renal hemodynamics and sodium excretion during variation in level of oxygenation. Circulation 1951; 3:703–721.
20. Flint FJ. Cor pulmonale incidence and aetiology in an industrial city. Lancet 1954; ii:51–58.
21. Fluck DC, Chandrasekar RG, Gardner FV. Left ventricular hypertrophy in chronic bronchitis. Br Heart J 1966; 28:92–97.
22. Hamburger J, Crosnier J, Grunfeld JP. Nephrology. New York: John Wiley & Sons, 1979.
23. Kellaway G. Acute anoxic cardiac failure in pulmonary heart disease. Lancet 1954; ii:768–773.
24. Kilburn KH, Asmundsson T, Britt RC, Cardon R. Effects of breathing 10 per cent carbon dioxide on the pulmonary circulation of human subjects. Circulation 1969; 39:639–653.
25. Kilburn KH, Dowell AR. Renal function in respiratory failure. Arch Intern Med 1971; 127:754–762.
26. Levy M, Seely JF. Pathophysiology of edema formation. In: Brenner BM, Rector FC Jr, eds. The Kidney. Philadelphia: WB Saunders Company, 1981.
27. Lewis SC Jr, Samuels AJ, Daines MC, et al. Cardiovascular-renal adjustments in cor pulmonale. Am J Med 1951; 10:765.
28. Pitts RF. Physiology of the Kidney and Body Fluids. Chicago: Yearbook Medical Publishers, 1963.
29. Platts MM, Hammond JDS, Stuart-Harris CH. A study of cor pulmonale in patients with chronic bronchitis. Quart J Med 1960; 29:559–574.
30. Rao BS, Cohn KE, Eldridge FL, Hancock EW. Left ventricular failure secondary to chronic pulmonary disease. Am J Med 1968; 45:229–241.
31. Rector FC Jr. Structure and transport along the nephron: Hydrogen ion transport along the nephron. In: Robinson RR, ed. Nephrology, vol. I. New York: Springer-Verlag, 1984.
32. Richens JM, Howard P. Editorial review—Oedema in cor pulmonale. Clin Sci 1982; 62:255–259.
33. Rose BA. Pathophysiology of Renal Disease. New York: McGraw-Hill, 1981.
34. Rose CE Jr, Kimmel DP, Godine RL Jr, et al. Synergistic effects of acute hypoxemia and hypercapnic acidosis in conscious dogs: Renal dysfunction and activation of the renin-angiotensin system. Cir Res 1983; 53:202–213.
35. Skorecki KL, Brenner BM. Body fluid homeostasis in congestive heart failure and cirrhosis with ascites. Am J Med 1982; 72:323–338.
36. Spear GS. The glomerulus in cyanotic congenital heart disease and primary pulmonary hypertension: a review. Nephron 1964; 1:238–248.
37. Smith HW. Principles of Renal Physiology. New York: Oxford University Press, 1956.
38. Wade OL, Bishop JM. Cardiac Output and Regional Blood Flow. Philadelphia: FA Davis Company, 1962.
39. White RJ, Woodings DF. Impaired water handling in chronic obstructive airways disease. Br Med J 1971; 2:561–563.
40. Williams JF Jr, Childress RH, Boyd DL, et al. Left ventricular function in patients with chronic obstructive pulmonary disease. J Clin Invest 1968; 47:1143–1153.
41. Wood PO. Diseases of the Heart and Circulation. Philadelphia: JB Lippincott Company, 3rd ed., 1968.
42. Wyngaarden JB, Smith LH Jr. Cecil Textbook of Medicine, 18th ed. Philadelphia: WB Saunders Company, 1988.

Chapter 22

EFFECTS OF COPD ON SLEEP

Melvin Lopata

Along with the multitude of studies that have defined the nature and extent of primary sleep disorders that result in impaired breathing, there has been increased recognition of sleep-induced respiratory dysfunction in primary pulmonary disorders, mainly chronic obstructive pulmonary disease (COPD). This chapter reviews the effects of COPD on nocturnal (sleep-related) respiration, the marked impairment of ventilation and gas exchange that occurs during sleep in some patients with COPD, its causes, consequences, and treatment. In addition, this chapter focuses on the relationship between COPD and the primary sleep-induced breathing disorder, sleep apnea. Considering that patients with COPD predominate any practice of pulmonology, awareness of the relatively new insights in sleep-induced respiratory dysfunction in these patients is of great importance.

SLEEP AND RESPIRATION IN HEALTHY INDIVIDUALS

Sleep has a primary effect on respiratory control that can result in significant alterations of respiratory drive and respiratory mechanics. These sleep-related changes in respiration have little functional influence on ventilation and gas exchange in healthy adults but can have profound impact on patients with respiratory disease.

The act of falling asleep, the mechanisms of which are unknown, is essentially the loss of the waking state with diminished cerebral activity due to inhibition of the pontine reticular activating system.[63] This lack of wakefulness stimulation, along with decreased metabolic rate and the specific effects of active sleep, especially rapid eye movement (REM) sleep, influences respiratory control and, thereby, ventilation. To understand the effects of sleep on respiration from a physiologic as well as a functional point of view, it is necessary to separate the roles of nonrapid eye movement (NREM) and REM sleep.

The state of NREM sleep has four stages, reflecting the electroencephalographic and behavioral changes as sleep progresses from sleep onset to deep sleep. Changes in respiration during NREM sleep are dependent on sleep stage with the effects of light sleep (stages I and II) being different from slow-wave (stages III and IV) sleep. Light sleep is somewhat unstable, characterized by sleep interspersed with brief arousals or wakenings.[69] This unsteady sleep is associated with unstable respiration that waxes and wanes with the alternation of wakefulness and sleep, respectively, and results in the periodic breathing characteristic of sleep onset.[11, 92] Hypopnea and apnea can occur during this period, which is usually short-lived, until stable stage II sleep is reached.[11, 92] The prevalence of periodic breathing of sleep onset is not known, but it probably increases with age and there may be individual determinants to its occurrence.[6, 92]

Once stable stage II or slow-wave sleep is attained, breathing becomes quite regular.[11, 55, 92] However, ventilatory control continues to be impaired so that responses to CO_2 and hypoxic chemostimulation are reduced when compared with those occurring in the state of wakefulness.[5, 11, 28, 29, 43] As a result, ventilation decreases as well, mostly owing to reduction in tidal volume, and arterial carbon dioxide pressure ($Paco_2$) increases approximately 3 to 4 torr.[11, 12, 44, 55]

The most apparent change in respiratory mechanics associated with NREM sleep pertains to the upper airway. Pharyngeal resistance increases more than twice that during waking, probably owing to a decrease in activity of the upper airway dilating muscles, which have a respiratory function to maintain integrity and patency of the upper airway during inspiration.[50, 74] In contrast, during NREM sleep respiratory muscle activity either does not change (diaphragm)[60, 89] or is increased (inspiratory intercostals and diaphragm).[60, 83, 91]

Rapid eye movement sleep is inherently an unsteady state characterized by bursts of phasic eye movements (rems) and skeletal muscle twitching, along with loss of tone of the postural muscles.[3] During REM sleep, breathing is also unsteady or irregular.[92] In contrast to the relatively regular irregularity, i.e., periodic breathing at sleep onset, respiration during REM sleep is usually irregularly irregular with sudden changes, especially shallow, rapid respirations, associated with bursts of rems,[11, 89] though periodic breathing can occur as well.[92] Apneas may also result at this time.[55]

Responses to chemostimulation during REM sleep are variable, depending on the presence or absence of phasic activity, the presence of phasic activity being associated with diminished responsiveness.[5, 11, 28, 29] Similarly, ventilation is decreased during bursts of rems.[26] As in NREM sleep, upper airway muscle activity is diminished, especially with rems, and pharyngeal resistance increases in REM sleep as well.[50] In contrast to NREM sleep, inspiratory intercostal muscle activity is inhibited during REM sleep, resulting in diminished rib cage displacements or even in paradoxical chest wall movement (abdomen out and rib cage in) during inspiration and a decrease in functional residual capacity.[64, 83, 89] As a result of impaired ventilation and respiratory mechanics, not only is there a small elevation in $Paco_2$, but there may be a relatively greater reduction in partial pressure of oxygen (Po_2) due to impaired gas exchange.[26, 64] Thus, REM sleep represents a precarious period for respiration, which can become critical in patients with pulmonary disease.

COPD AND SLEEP

The effects of sleep on ventilation and oxygenation in patients with COPD have been the subject of investigation for over 2 decades. Although nocturnal oxygen desaturation is now well recognized in patients with severe chronic airways obstruction, the role of sleep-related hypoxemia in the pathogenesis of some of the sequelae of COPD and its therapeutic implications are not clear at this time.

Oxygen Desaturation During Sleep

Although early studies demonstrated that arterial oxygen tension or saturation decreased and CO_2 tension increased in patients with COPD during sleep,[17, 54, 57, 70, 74, 88] the reported degree of blood gas worsening was variable and not even considered by some investigators to be greater than normal.[54, 57, 70] Not until continuous monitoring of arterial oxygen saturation (Sao_2) was possible did the extent of sleep-induced impairment of oxygenation become known.[27, 39] From the works of Flick and Block and Douglas and colleagues,[27, 39] it was clearly demonstrated in these patients that oxygen desaturation during sleep could be severe and prolonged and that REM sleep was the state typically associated with such desaturation (Fig. 22–1).

Although almost all patients studied and reported have severe airways obstruction, i.e., $FEV_1 < 1$ L, the degree of nocturnal hypoxemia as well as CO_2 retention was quite variable.[2, 17, 23, 27, 39, 41, 54, 57, 70, 74, 88, 95] The decrease in Sao_2 and Pao_2 can vary from 4% to 70% and 5 to 35 mm Hg, respectively, whereas the increase in $Paco_2$ can range from 5 to 15 mm Hg.[17, 27, 39, 54, 57] Three distinct patterns of oxygen desaturation related to different sleep stages and incurring different degrees and duration of hypoxemia have been recognized (see Fig. 22–1). The first occurs at sleep onset and is evident by a mild to moderate decrease of the waking baseline oxygen saturation, or tension, which persists throughout sleep.[39, 54] Superimposed on this baseline shift are two types of episodic desaturations: one, referred to as sleep-disordered breathing,[95] occurs in stages I and II NREM sleep and REM sleep and is associated with the periodic breathing evident in these sleep states.[11, 92] This disordered breathing is manifest as periodic hypopneas or apneas, often due to upper airway obstruction, hence similar to the disordered breathing of sleep apnea (Fig. 22–2).[67] The degree of associated desaturation is usually mild to moderate and of relatively brief duration (< 30 seconds).[2, 95] The second pattern of episodic desaturation occurs essentially during REM sleep and may account for over 50% of the transient desaturations and usually the great majority of severe desaturations.[95] These desaturations are usually associated with some decrease in respiratory effort evident by decreased chest wall or pleural pressure excursions (Fig. 22–3).[2, 27, 49, 52, 95] There also may be no obvious change in the ventilatory pattern.[95] These episodes of desaturation can be the most severe and prolonged, lasting from 5 to over 30 minutes.[2, 27, 95]

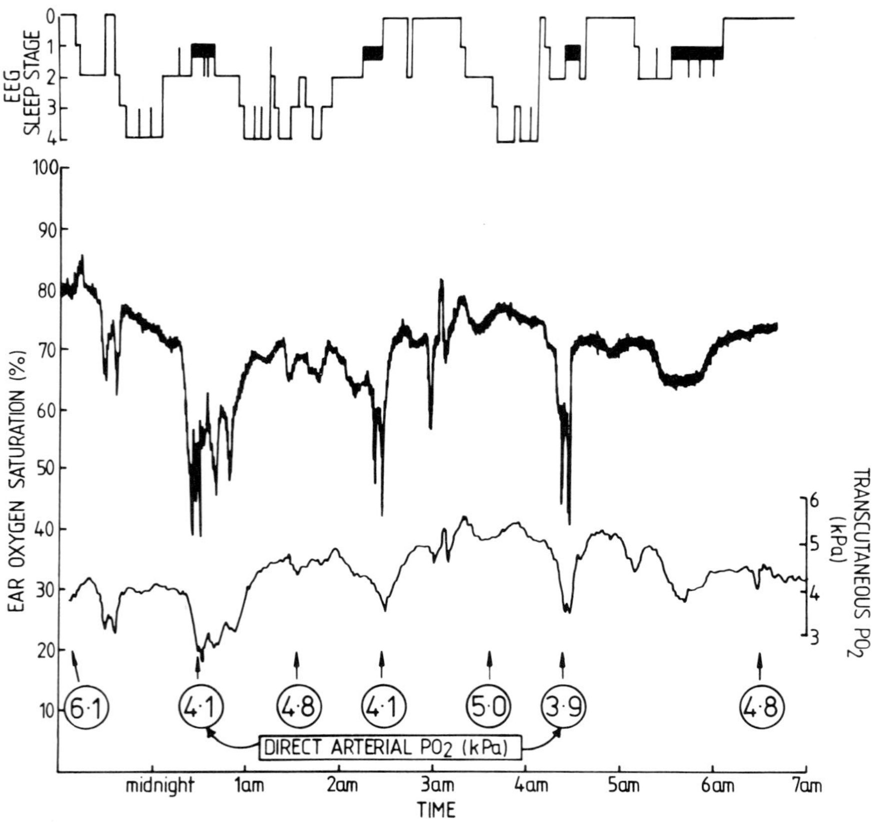

Figure 22–1. Continuous oxygen saturation, transcutaneous Po_2, and sleep state (closed bars = rapid eye movement [REM] sleep) during the night in a patient with severe airways obstruction and daytime hypoxemia and hypercapnia, i.e., a "blue bloater" breathing room air. Note drop in baseline saturation at sleep onset and episodic desaturation, the most severe being in REM (1 pka = 7.5 mm Hg). (Reproduced with permission from Flenley DC. Clin Chest Med 1985; 6:651–661.)

Epidemiology of Oxygen Desaturation

What is the prevalence of sleep-associated hypoxemia in patients with COPD and which patients are at risk for developing significant oxygen desaturation during sleep? True epidemiologic studies have not been done to answer the first question. Studies reporting on sleep effects in COPD usually included relatively few patients who were selected for their severe airways obstruction.[2, 17, 23, 27, 33, 39, 41, 54, 57, 70, 81, 88, 95] Most, if not all, patients in this group experience nocturnal decreases in Pao_2 and, depending on the baseline Pao_2, many show oxygen desaturation. However, the degree of desaturation is quite variable and one would hope to be able to select those patients who are at risk for severe deterioration of blood gases during sleep.

Patients classified as "blue bloaters" have been shown to be at risk for severe nocturnal desaturation. These patients have severe hypoxemia, hypercapnia, and cor pulmonale and are often obese as opposed to the thin, mildly hypoxemic, normocapneic "pink puffers." The former group has been shown to manifest severe and prolonged oxygen desaturation during sleep, compared with the mild impairment of oxygenation seen in the latter.[2, 16, 23, 27, 41, 81] The degree of airways obstruction does not distinguish between those patients who do or do not experience desaturation.[27, 54, 57, 70, 88]

The most apparent reason for the susceptibility of the blue bloater to nocturnal desaturation is the presence of a low waking Pao_2 and thereby a low baseline oxygen saturation. By being on the steep part of the oxygen dissociation curve, changes in Pao_2 can result in profound changes in saturation and could explain the differences between the blue bloater and pink puffer.[81] Thus, the true risk factor may be the waking

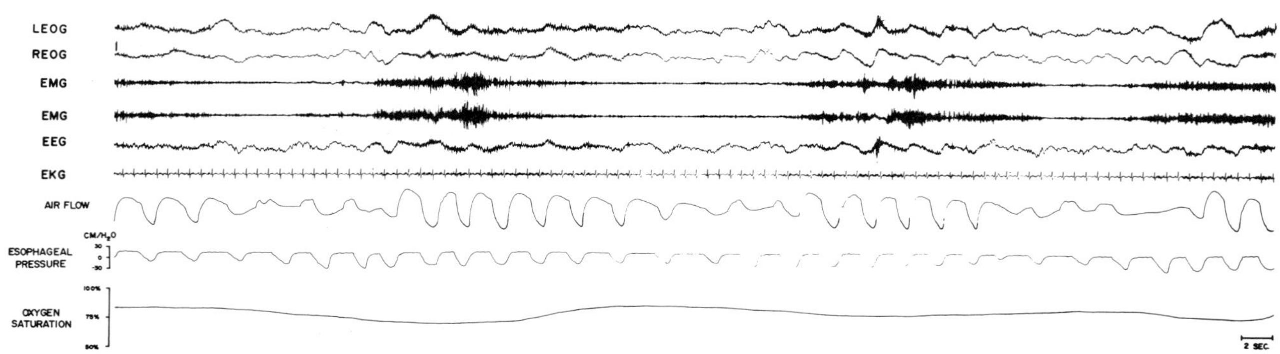

Figure 22–2. Continuous recording of left and right electro-oculogram (LEOG and REOG), submental electromyocardiogram (EMG), electroencephalogram (EEG), and electrocardiogram (EKG), airflow, esophageal pressure, and oxygen saturation in a patient with chronic obstructive pulmonary disease (COPD) during nonrapid eye movement (NREM) sleep. Note periodicity of breathing pattern with intermittent hypopneas associated with increasing pleural pressures during the hypopnea and desaturation ending in arousal. (Reproduced with permission from Arand DL, McGinty DJ, Littner MR. Chest 1981; 80:183–190.)

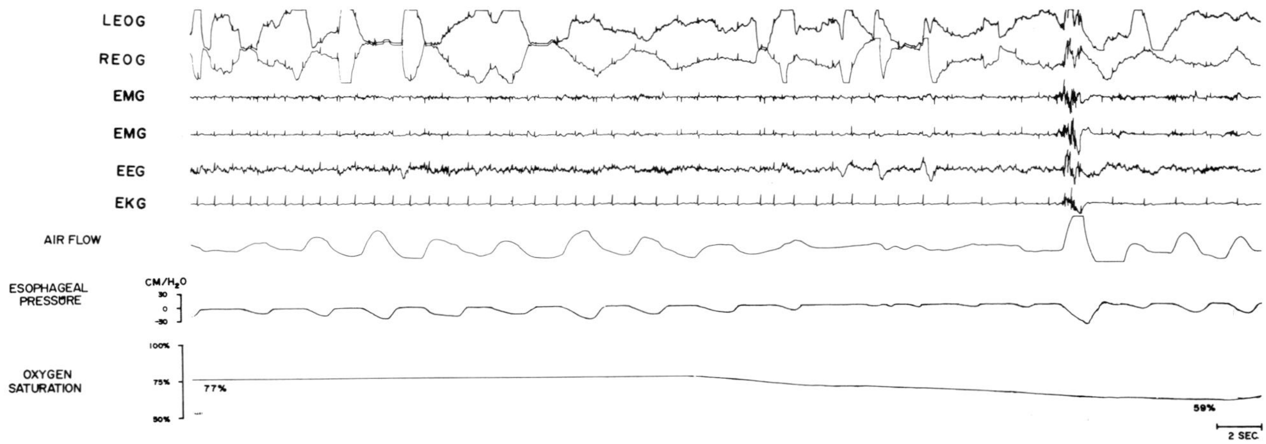

Figure 22–3. Similar recording depicting prolonged desaturation associated with decreased pleural pressure during rapid eye movement (REM) sleep. (Reproduced with permission from Arand DL, McGinty DJ, Littner MR. Chest 1981; 80:183–190.)

Pa_{O_2} or saturation. Baseline Pa_{O_2} above 60 torr and saturation above 90%, as in the pink puffer, would not be associated with nocturnal deterioration of oxygenation, whereas lesser values would be a harbinger of sleep-induced hypoxia. Indeed, a number of studies have shown a significant relationship between the degree of nocturnal hypoxemia or desaturation and the baseline or waking Pa_{O_2} or Sa_{O_2},[21, 32, 33, 54, 70, 81, 84] such that the lower the baseline value the greater the nocturnal deterioration. Daytime hypoxemia has been found to account for three fourths of the variation in nocturnal hypoxemia.[81] Thus, waking Pa_{O_2} is probably the best predictor of nocturnal desaturation, but patients with reasonable Pa_{O_2} above 60 torr can experience significant desaturation.[2, 23, 95] However, one study has shown that the great majority of such patients do not develop severe nocturnal hypoxia.[37]

A somewhat ill-defined predictor of nocturnal desaturation in these patients is the so-called level of chemosensitivity or their responsiveness to CO_2 and hypoxic stimulation. A number of studies have shown a negative correlation between the ventilatory or occlusion pressure response to CO_2, or hypoxia, and the degree of nocturnal desaturation in sleeping patients with severe COPD,[32, 43, 84] although one study failed to confirm these findings.[21] In addition, it has also been shown that such responses to chemical stimulation were significantly lower in patients who experienced desaturation at night compared with those who did not.[58] Thus, the less a given patient is able to increase respiratory drive in response to hypoxia and hypercapnia, the greater the likelihood of desaturating during sleep. Whether ventilation or occlusion pressure responses in these patients actually reflect central drive or the state of respiratory mechanics and muscle function is not clear, but the tests appear to serve as a marker of risk for sleep-induced desaturation. More importantly, the results of these studies may provide some insight into the mechanisms of nocturnal desaturation to be discussed subsequently.[32, 43, 58, 84]

Sequelae of Nocturnal Oxygen Desaturation

The impairment of oxygenation during sleep must result in physiologic dysfunction due to tissue hypoxia. The effects of sleep-induced oxygen desaturation on pulmonary artery pressure, myocardial function, sleep behavior, and sleep architecture have been studied in COPD patients who exhibit nocturnal hypoxemia.

PULMONARY VASCULAR EFFECTS. Episodes of oxygen desaturation, whether associated with hypopneas and apneas or REM, uniformly result in increased pulmonary artery pressure (PAP) (Fig. 22–4).[7, 17, 27, 36] Although most of the patients studied have waking pulmonary hypertension, which worsens during sleep,[17, 36, 95] patients with normal baseline pulmonary pressures also can show increases in PAP associated with oxygen desaturation.[7] The degree of PAP elevation is inversely proportional to the degree of desaturation. The mechanism mediating the pulmonary hypertension is likely pulmonary vasoconstriction induced by hypoxia or possibly acidosis secondary to acute hypoventilation occurring with the desaturation episode.[7, 36] The fact that pulmonary vascular resistance increases with the PAP elevation[36] and that oxygen administration, which eliminates the desaturations, eliminates the increase in PAP during sleep supports the role of hypoxia as the main culprit (see Fig. 22–4).[7, 36] Based on our understanding of the relationship between hypoxia and pulmonary hypertension[1] and the known effects on pulmonary pressure of sleep-induced hypoxemia in the sleep apnea syndrome,[18, 86] the occurrence of sleep-related pulmonary hypertension in COPD is certainly not unexpected. However, the importance of this process relates to the premise that episodes of transient elevation of PAP during sleep can lead to sustained pulmonary hypertension.[65, 72] This contention implicates sleep-related desaturation in the natural history and daytime morbidity of COPD, and presupposes the use of nocturnal oxygen therapy to prevent hypoxemia and its pulmonary vascular sequelae.

MYOCARDIAL EFFECTS. Interestingly, left ventricular function apparently is not impaired during the desaturation episodes because pulmonary capillary wedge pressure is not elevated during these periods[7, 36]; however, it has been calculated that during sleep in those patients who desaturate, there is an increased demand for myocardial blood flow equivalent to that of maximal exercise.

Patients with severe COPD are at risk for sudden death, presumably because of arrhythmias,[13, 24, 47] likely occurring during sleep.[51, 80] At least three studies have documented electrocardiographic changes and multiple arrhythmias at night in these patients,[40, 77, 87] though sleep was not documented electroencephalographically in two.[40, 87] Premature ventricular contractions, often frequent and multifocal, unsustained ventricular tachycardia, and idioventricular rhythm have been shown to occur during sleep,[40, 77, 87] especially at the nadir of a severe episode of desaturation.[77]

Electrocardiographic (ECG) abnormalities, such as ST-T depression, right bundle branch block, and prolonged QT interval have also been associated with sleep.[87] The patients at greatest risk are those who experience desaturation the most

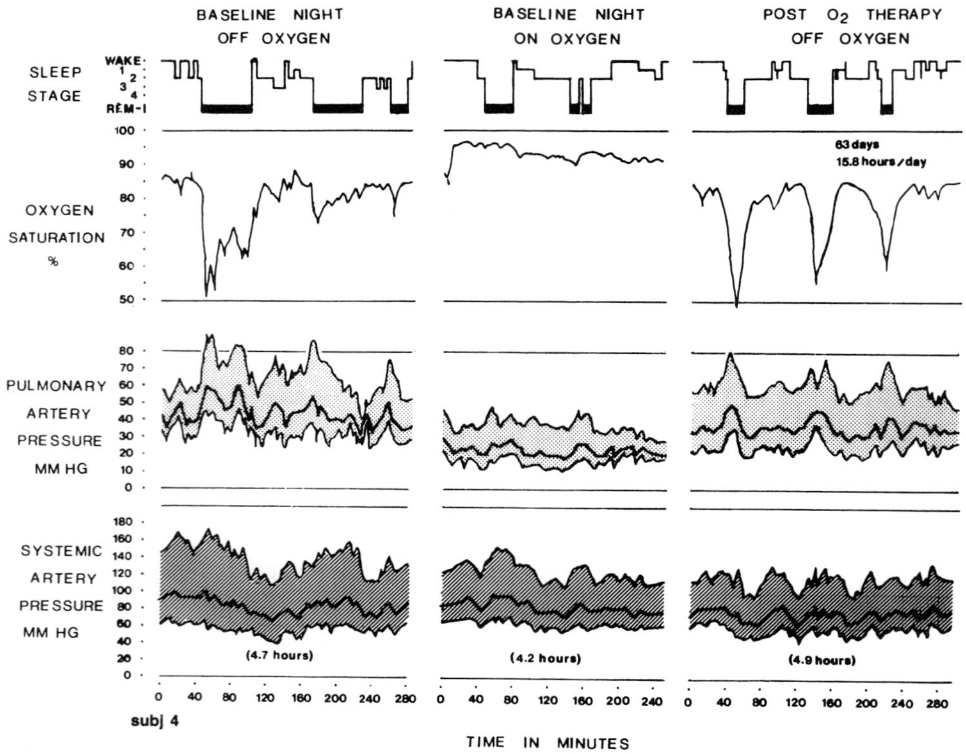

Figure 22–4. Continuous nocturnal recording of sleep stage, oxygen saturation, and pulmonary artery pressure in a patient with severe chronic obstructive pulmonary disease (COPD) breathing room air (left), while breathing oxygen (center), and while breathing room air after 2 months of therapy with continuous (>15 hours per day) oxygen therapy. At baseline, severe desaturations occur associated with marked increase in pulmonary artery pressure (PAP); oxygen therapy eliminates the desaturations along with the increased pulmonary pressures, but returning to room air after chronic oxygen therapy results in the same sequelae as during the baseline study. (Reproduced with permission from Fletcher EC, Levin DC. Chest 1984; 85:6–14.)

during sleep,[77] those with low baseline Pa_{O_2} or Sa_{O_2}, i.e., the so-called "blue bloaters."[87] Elimination of nocturnal desaturation with oxygen decreases the amount of premature ventricular contractions (PVCs) and may eliminate the occurrence of arrhythmias, such as ventricular tachycardia and idioventricular rhythm, as well as the described ECG abnormalities.[40, 87] The potential efficacy of oxygen to reduce the risk of sleep-induced arrhythmia and sudden death implies the benefits of nocturnal oxygen therapy.

SLEEP BEHAVIOR EFFECTS. Sleep is disturbed in patients with severe COPD.[17, 95] When sought, complaints are common, including sleeping difficulty with repeated awakenings and daytime somnolence.[2, 21] Monitoring sleep architecture confirms disturbed sleep, and findings from multiple studies are fairly consistent. Generally, total sleep time is decreased and there may be an increase in sleep latency.[14, 17] The decreased time in sleep is due to multiple arousals resulting in more time spent in wakening.[10, 14, 17, 21, 53, 57] The effects of this fractionated sleep on specific sleep states are not clear. Although there is some evidence for reduction in REM and slow wave sleep,[33, 57, 95] the changes in these sleep states are quite variable and may not be different from those of a healthy population of the same age. Though the number of arousals has been shown to be related to the severity of oxygen desaturation, i.e., patients with the lowest Sa_{O_2} had the greatest number of arousals or awakenings,[21] only half of arousals are associated with episodes of desaturation, and there is no relationship between the number of arousals and the number of desaturation episodes per hour of sleep.[10, 21] In addition, one study has shown that pink puffers with less severe daytime hypoxemia and nocturnal desaturation had more disturbed sleep than blue bloaters.[14] These data certainly indicate that poor oxygenation is not the sole cause of arousal and disturbed sleep, that other factors, such as nocturnal dyspnea, retained secretions, and cough must be important as well. The multifactorial mechanisms for causing sleep disruption are supported by the variable effects of nocturnal oxygen on this pattern of disturbed sleep. Preventing desaturation by administering oxygen via a nasal cannula has not been shown to improve sleep dramatically, although there are reports of improved sleep efficiency with oxygen administration.[53, 57] Other studies have shown no improvement[14, 33] or only an insignificant trend toward improvement.[42]

The importance of disturbed sleep in the clinical context of COPD is not clear. Certainly this sleep abnormality is not associated with marked or disabling symptoms such as those seen in patients with sleep apnea.[21] But it is possible that sleep disruption, like nocturnal pulmonary hypertension, may have a significant bearing on the morbidity and course of COPD. Nocturnal exacerbation of hypoxemia and hypercapnia over a prolonged period of time could lead to diminished responsiveness to chemical stimuli as observed in patients with chronic hypoxia or intermittent hypercapnia.[30, 76, 93] More pertinent, sleep disruption could result in diminished chemosensitivity and ventilatory performance.[20, 68, 94] This resultant disturbance in respiratory control could impair load compensation and contribute to the development of daytime hypoventilation in COPD as has been proposed for patients with obesity-hypoventilation.[59] However, at present no data exist to support the role of nocturnal sleep disruption, along with hypoxia and acidosis, in the development of CO_2 retention in COPD.

Mechanisms of Oxygen Desaturation

The mechanisms of sleep-induced hypoxemia in COPD must be understood in the context of the three patterns of oxygen desaturation. The decrease in baseline Sa_{O_2} at sleep onset, the desaturation associated with periodic breathing during mostly light NREM sleep, and the prolonged REM desaturations are all abnormalities based on disease-exaggerated sleep state and stage effects on respiratory control, ventilation, and respiratory mechanics. The sleep-induced hypoventilation at sleep onset, resulting in minimal changes in Pa_{O_2} in healthy individuals, results in significant desaturation in hypoxemic patients on the steep part of their O_2-dissociation curve. Middle-aged to elderly men with COPD, especially if plagued by the common afflictions of obesity and snoring, experience periodic breathing and associated apneas and hypopneas during early sleep as do their nonsmoking counterparts, and, even without meeting criteria for sleep apnea, will experience significant desaturation due to their abnormal baseline blood gases. Patients with COPD may have true sleep apnea, which will be discussed subsequently. The striking effect of REM sleep on respiratory function and chest wall mechanics in healthy individuals becomes profound in patients with COPD and results in oxygen desaturation that is far more severe than that occurring in the other stages.

The mechanism of REM-induced blood gas abnormalities has been studied in a number of laboratories and is reasonably well understood. Both hypoventilation and gas exchange abnormalities have been implicated as the cause of hypoxemia. Hypoventilation, as denoted by an increase in Pa_{CO_2}, does occur[15, 17, 39, 54, 57] and is associated with decreased ventilation[15, 35, 49] and respiratory effort as indicated by decreased chest wall displacement and inspiratory pressure generation.[2, 15, 49, 52] The decrease in ventilation is mainly due to tidal volume reduction,[15, 49] and thoracic displacement is diminished more than that of the abdomen.[49, 52] The cause of this impaired ventilation is in large part due to REM-induced inhibition of intercostal/accessory muscles whose activity is necessary to compensate for impaired diaphragmatic function in patients with chronic airways obstruction.[39, 51] A decrease, or loss, of phasic and tonic inspiratory intercostal/accessory activity as well as expiratory activity results in chest wall distortion and reduced functional residual capacity.[16, 52, 64] Both hypoventilation and impaired gas exchange result, though the relative contribution of both of these pathophysiologic components to REM-induced hypoxemia is not really known.[31, 48] A number of studies have determined that the alveolar-arterial oxygen gradient (A-aO_2D) is increased during REM desaturations, implying $\dot{V}/\dot{Q}$ mismatching,[16, 39, 54, 57] but accurate calculation of the gradient depends on a stable respiratory quotient, which probably does not occur in the nonsteady state of REM sleep.[15] However, the increase in venous admixture that occurs with REM desaturation indicates that impaired gas exchange does indeed occur,[35] as would be expected in conditions in which FRC fell below closing volume.[31, 48]

The rise in Pa_{CO_2} indicative of hypoventilation, which occurs during these episodes, is rather modest compared with the fall in Pa_{O_2}, likely due to the large body stores of CO_2 compared with those of oxygen.[15] Though this hypoventilation is probably mostly due to REM inhibition of postural muscles, which include the intercostal/accessory muscles, the detection of diminished diaphragmatic electromyocardiogram (EMG) and decreased oxygen utilization during REM desaturations suggest that a more global component of hypoventilation also occurs.[35, 49]

However, centrally mediated impairment of respiratory drive does not appear to contribute greatly to REM hypoventilation, because almitrine, not approved for use in the U.S., and progesterone (peripheral and central respiratory stimulants, respectively) when tested in patients with COPD, result in less overall nocturnal desaturation due to increase in waking Pa_{O_2} but do not really eliminate or alter the nocturnal episodes that cause desaturation.[19, 22, 25, 61, 71, 79, 85] Interestingly, COPD patients who have undergone carotid body resection with resultant loss of hypoxic drive are reported to have disordered sleep and nocturnal desaturation no different from a comparable group of patients who have not undergone this resection.[90]

In this context it should be recalled that data exist indicating that patients with low responses to chemostimulation are particularly at risk for nocturnal oxygen desaturation[32, 43, 84] and would seem to conflict with the contention that central hypoventilation does not contribute greatly to REM desaturation. However, these studies tested waking responsiveness and thus reflected waking function, either of respiratory mechanics or control, which determines waking blood gas levels. The resulting baseline Pa_{O_2} markedly influences nocturnal gas tensions and the severity of sleep-induced desaturations but does not necessarily contribute to the basic mechanism of the desaturations.

COPD and Sleep Apnea

The majority of sleep-induced desaturation episodes in patients with severe COPD are not associated with apneas.[16, 33] Obstructive apneas and hypopneas can occur, especially in light sleep, but are a minor component of the nocturnal respiratory disorder of these patients and not a major factor in the occurrence of significant desaturations.[16, 33, 81] However, most patients with severe COPD are middle-aged to elderly males, a group that is also at risk for sleep apnea.[6] The relatively high prevalence of obesity further increases the probability of sleep apnea in this population.[62] These epidemiologic factors probably account for the fact that some (usually small) degree of apneas and hypopneas occurs during sleep in these patients, but the mere presence of obstructive episodes does not make a diagnosis of sleep apnea unless the number of events is sufficient to at least satisfy conventional criteria.[4, 46] However, it must be apparent that there are patients with COPD who have a significant degree of sleep apnea; thus the two diseases, COPD and obstructive sleep apnea (OSA), can coexist or, as has been stated previously, overlap.[34, 38, 45]

The importance of recognizing patients with this overlap is due to the probable additive effects of both disease processes on sleep-induced blood gas impairment and on daytime respiratory dysfunction as well. The presence of airways obstruction in patients with predominant OSA probably contributes to the morbidity of sleep apnea by being a determinant in the development of hypercapnia and pulmonary hypertension.[8, 9, 56] Besides adding to the nocturnal oxygen desaturation, airways obstruction adds to the mechanical load imposed by obesity in a disease process in which load compensation is impaired,[59] thereby contributing to the development of CO_2 retention with worsening daytime hypoxemia and, secondarily, pulmonary hypertension. On the other hand, the presence of OSA in patients with airways obstruction can contribute to or independently result in hypercapneic respiratory failure and cor pulmonale that may be attributable to the COPD because the presence of OSA is overlooked or its importance to the clinical picture is not understood. Such recognition of OSA can be crucial to proper patient management because OSA can be treated and its sequelae of cardiorespiratory failure are reversible with treatment,[38, 45, 82] but this is not the case with COPD. Patients with COPD who may have OSA demonstrate the typical features of the latter disease, e.g., obesity, daytime somnolence, snoring, and morning headaches.

One should be especially cognizant of the COPD patient with CO_2 retention who does not have the severe degree of airways obstruction that is typically associated with hypercapnia in such a patient.[73] An FEV_1 of greater than 1 to 1.3 L in such a clinical context should arouse suspicion of disease in addition to COPD and warrants consideration of the presence of OSA and an appropriate workup. The treatment of OSA with tracheostomy or nasal continuous positive airway pressure (CPAP) should ameliorate or even completely reverse the hypercapnia and cor pulmonale.[38, 45, 82] This remarkable therapeutic benefit should not be missed by failing to consider the diagnosis of OSA in certain patients with COPD.

Therapy of Sleep Desaturation

It is not clear whether there is, or more appropriately, should be, specific treatment for sleep-associated oxygen desaturation in COPD. Certainly nocturnal desaturation can be prevented by administering oxygen, which can also prevent nocturnal exacerbation of pulmonary hypertension, arrhythmias, and may improve sleep quality.[7, 14, 33, 36, 42, 53, 57] As noted, intermittent, yet chronic, pulmonary hypertension and sleep disruption have been proposed to contribute to the sequelae of COPD by leading to sustained pulmonary hypertension or by contributing to the development of CO_2 retention. However, even if this contention were true no evidence exists that treatment with nocturnal oxygen would prevent the sequelae or alter the natural course of the disease. In this regard the inability of 12-hour nocturnal oxygen administration to improve survival in patients with severe COPD certainly does not support nocturnal oxygenation only[66]; however, since the Nocturnal Oxygen Therapy Trial study did not investigate sleep behavior, the results do not definitively negate such use of oxygen.

The consideration of nocturnal oxygen in patients who demonstrate sleep-induced hypoxemia is rather moot because the majority of patients who significantly desaturate are severely hypoxemic and generally already meet the criteria for continuous oxygen therapy.[66] The real consideration for nocturnal therapy is in those patients whose waking Pa_{O_2} is above 60 torr. About a quarter of these patients will experience REM desaturation, but usually not to a severe degree, and there is no way to predict who is at risk.[37]

Screening such patients with routine polysomnography or monitoring nocturnal oxygen saturation would overwhelm sleep laboratories and certainly not justify the expense. Even if a relatively normoxic patient were found to have severe desaturation, nocturnal oxygen cannot be easily justified because its efficacy and cost-effectiveness are not known. A sleep study may be warranted in patients with a Pa_{O_2} of > 60 torr if they have sleep-related complaints or pulmonary hypertension or hypercapnia. If REM desaturations are present, nocturnal or continuous oxygen may be warranted. Therapy with oxygen should result in amelioration of the sleep complaint or the pulmonary vasculature and blood gas abnormalities to justify its long-term use. However, it is also quite likely that patients with these clinical features may have OSA. Certainly proving or disproving the efficacy of nocturnal oxygen in this clinical context requires extensive longitudinal studies that are yet to be performed.

Another therapeutic approach to prevent nocturnal oxygen desaturation is using drugs that stimulate ventilation. Both almitrine and progesterone have been studied and generally found to improve nocturnal oxygenation without affecting the REM events that cause the desaturations.[19, 22, 25, 61, 71, 79, 85] This improvement is due to the ability of these drugs to increase waking Pa_{O_2}.[19, 22, 25, 61, 71, 79] As with oxygen therapy, which is more effective than drugs in improving oxygenation, the efficacy and cost-effectiveness of drug therapy is not known and their routine use cannot be justified at this time.

REFERENCES

1. Abraham AS, Kay JM, Cole RB, Pincock AC. Hemodynamic and pathologic study of the effect of chronic hypoxia and subsequent recovery on the heart and pulmonary vasculature of the rat. Cardiovasc Res 1971; 5:95–102.
2. Arand DL, McGinty DJ, Littner MR. Respiratory patterns associated with hemoglobin desaturation during sleep in chronic obstructive pulmonary disease. Chest 1981; 80:183–190.
3. Aseunsky E, Kleetman N. Regularly occurring periods of eye mobility and concomitant phenomena during sleep. Science 1953; 118:273–274.
4. Berry DTR, Webb WB, Block AJ. Sleep apnea syndrome: a critical review of the apnea index as a diagnostic criterion. Chest 1984; 86:529–531.
5. Berthon-Jones M, Sullivan CE. Ventilatory and arousal responses to hypoxia in sleeping humans. Am Rev Respir Dis 1982; 125:632–639.
6. Block AJ, Wynne JW, Baysen PG. Sleep disordered breathing and nocturnal oxygen desaturation in normal subjects: a strong male performance. N Engl J Med 1979; 300:513–517.
7. Boysen PG, Block AJ, Wynne JW, et al. Nocturnal pulmonary hypertension in patients with chronic obstructive pulmonary disease. Chest 1979; 76:536–542.
8. Bradley TD, Rutherford R, Lue F, et al. Role of diffuse airway obstruction in the hypercapnia of obstructive sleep apnea. Am Rev Respir Dis 1986: 134:920–924.
9. Bradley TD, Rutherford R, Grossman RF, et al. Role of daytime hypoxemia in the pathogenesis of right heart failure in the obstructive sleep apnea syndrome. Am Rev Respir Dis 1985; 131:835–839.
10. Brezinova V, Catterall JR, Douglas NJ, et al. Night sleep of patients with chronic ventilatory failure and age matched controls: number and duration of the EEG episodes of intervening wakefulness and drowsiness. Sleep 1982; 5:123–130.
11. Bulow K. Respiration and wakefulness in man. Acta Physiol Scand 1963; 59:1–110.
12. Bulow K, Ingvar D. Respiration and state of wakefulness in normals, studied by spirography, capnography and EEG. Acta Physiol Scand 1961; 51:230–236.
13. Burrows B, Earle RH. Course and prognosis of chronic obstructive lung disease. N Engl J Med 1969; 280:397–404.
14. Calverley PMA, Brezinova V, Douglas NJ, et al. The effect of oxygenation on sleep quality in chronic bronchitis and emphysema. Am Rev Respir Dis 1982; 126:206–210.
15. Catterall JR, Calverley PMA, MacNee W, et al. Mechanism of transient nocturnal hypoxemia in hypoxic chronic bronchitis and emphysema. J Appl Physiol 1985; 59:1698–1703.
16. Catterall JR, Douglas NJ, Calverley PMA, et al. Transient hypoxemia during sleep in chronic obstructive pulmonary disease is not a sleep apnea syndrome. Am Rev Respir Dis 1983; 128:24–29.
17. Coccagna G, Lugaresi E. Arterial blood gases and pulmonary and systemic arterial pressure during sleep in chronic obstructive pulmonary disease. Sleep 1978; 1:117–124.
18. Coccagna G, Mantovani M, Brignani F, et al. Continuous recording of the pulmonary and systemic arterial pressure during sleep in syndromes of hypersomnia with periodic breathing. Bull Physiopathol Respir 1972; 8:1159–1172.
19. Connaughton JJ, Douglas NJ, Morgan AD, et al. Almitrine improves oxygenation when both awake and asleep in patients with hypoxia and carbon dioxide retention caused by chronic bronchitis and emphysema. Am Rev Respir Dis 1985; 132:206–210.
20. Cooper, KR, Phillips BA. Effect of short term sleep loss on breathing. J Appl Physiol 1982; 53:855–858.
21. Cormick W, Olson L, Hensley JM, Saunders NA. Nocturnal hypoxaemia and quality of sleep in patients with chronic obstructive lung diseases. Thorax 1986; 41:846–854.
22. Daskalopoulou E, Patakas D, Tsara V, et al. Almitrine effect on nocturnal hypoxaemia in patients with chronic obstructive pulmonary disease (COPD). Bull Clin Respir Physiol 1987; 23(Suppl):185s–190s.
23. DeMarco FJ, Wynne JW, Block AJ. Oxygen desaturation during sleep as a determinant of the "blue and bloated" syndrome. Chest 1981; 79:621–625.
24. Diener CV, Burrows B. Further observations on the course and prognosis of chronic obstructive lung disease. Am Rev Respir Dis 1975; 111:719–724.
25. Dolly FR, Block AJ. Medroxyprogesterone acetate and COPD: Effect on breathing and oxygenation in sleeping and awake patients. Chest 1983; 84:394–398.
26. Douglas NJ. Control of breathing during sleep. Clin Sci 1984; 67:465–471.
27. Douglas NJ, Calverley PMA, Leggett RJE, Brash HM. Transient hypoxemia during sleep in chronic bronchitis and emphysema. Lancet 1979; i:1–4.

28. Douglas NJ, White DP, Weil JV. Hypercapnic ventilatory responses in sleeping adults. Am Rev Respir Dis 1982; 126:758–762.
29. Douglas NJ, White DP, Weil JV, et al. Hypoxic ventilatory responses decrease during sleep in normal men. Am Rev Respir Dis 1982; 125:286–289.
30. Edelman HN, Lahiri S, Braudo L. The blunted ventilatory response to hypoxia in cyanotic congenital heart disease. N Engl J Med 1970; 282:405–411.
31. Findley LJ, Ries AL, Lisi GM, Wagner PD. Hypoxemia during apnea in normal subjects: mechanisms and impact of lung volume. J Appl Physiol 1983; 55:1777–1783.
32. Fleetham JA, Mezon B, West P. Chemical control of ventilation and sleep arterial oxygen desaturation in patients with COPD. Am Rev Respir Dis 1980; 122:583–589.
33. Fleetham J, Mezon B, West P, et al. Sleep, arousals, and oxygen desaturation in chronic obstructive pulmonary disease. Am Rev Respir Dis 1982; 126:429–433.
34. Flenley DC. Sleep in chronic obstructive lung disease. Clin Chest Med 1985; 6:651–661.
35. Fletcher EC, Gray BA, Levin DC. Nonapneic mechanisms of arterial oxygen desaturation during rapid-eye-movement sleep. J Appl Physiol 1983; 54:632–639.
36. Fletcher EC, Levin DC. Cardiopulmonary hemodynamics during sleep in subjects with chronic obstructive pulmonary disease. The effect of short and long-term oxygen. Chest 1984; 85:6–14.
37. Fletcher EC, Miller J, Divine GW, et al. Nocturnal oxyhemoglobin desaturation in COPD patients with arterial oxygen tensions above 60 mm Hg. Chest 1987; 92:604–608.
38. Fletcher EC, Schaaf JW, Miller J, Fletcher JG. Long-term cardiopulmonary sequelae in patients with sleep apnea and chronic lung disease. Am Rev Respir Dis 1987; 135:525–533.
39. Flick MR, Block AJ. Continuous *in vivo* monitoring of arterial oxygenation in chronic obstructive lung disease. Ann Intern Med 1977; 36:725–730.
40. Flick MR, Block AJ. Nocturnal vs. diurnal cardiac arrhythmias in patients with chronic obstructive pulmonary disease. Chest 1979; 75:8–11.
41. Gimeno F, van Veenen R, Steenhuis EJ. Ear oximetry studies during sleep in patients with severe chronic obstructive pulmonary disease in a stable state. Ann Allergy 1986; 56:142–144.
42. Goldstein RS, Ramcharan V, Bowes G, et al. Effect of supplemental nocturnal oxygen on gas exchange in patients with severe obstructive lung disease. N Engl J Med 1984; 310:425–429.
43. Gothe B. Effect of chemosensitivity on arterial O_2-saturation during sleep [abstract]. Am Rev Respir Dis 1979; 119:119.
44. Gothe B, Altose MD, Goldman MD, Cherniack NS. Effect of quiet sleep on resting and CO_2-stimulated breathing in humans. J Appl Physiol 1981; 50:724–730.
45. Guilleminault C, Cummiskey J, Motta J. Chronic obstructive airflow disease and sleep studies. Am Rev Respir Dis 1980; 122:397–406.
46. Guilleminault C, van den Heod J, Mitler M. Clinical overview of the sleep apnea syndrome. In: Guilleminault C, Dement W, eds. Sleep Apnea Syndromes. New York: Alan R. Liss, 1978, 1–12.
47. Holford FD, Mithoefer JC. Cardiac arrhythmias in hospitalized patients with COPD. Am Rev Respir Dis 1973; 108:879–895.
48. Hudgel DW, Devadatta P. Decrease in functional residual capacity during sleep in normal humans. J Appl Physiol 1984; 57:1319–1322.
49. Hudgel DW, Martin RJ, Capehart M, et al. Contribution of hypoventilation to sleep oxygen desaturation in chronic obstructive pulmonary disease. J Appl Physiol 1983; 55:669–677.
50. Hudgel DW, Martin RJ, Johnson B, Hill P. Mechanics of the respiratory system and breathing pattern during sleep in normal humans. J Appl Physiol 1984; 56:133–137.
51. Hudson LD, Kurt TL, Petty TL, Genton E. Arrhythmias associated with acute respiratory failure in patients with chronic airway obstruction. Chest 1973; 63:661–665.
52. Johnson MW, Remmers JE. Accessory muscle activity during sleep in chronic obstructive pulmonary disease. J Appl Physiol 1984; 57:1011–1017.
53. Kearley R, Wynne JW, Block AJ, et al. The effect of low flow oxygen on sleep-disordered breathing and oxygen desaturation. A study of patients with chronic obstructive lung disease. Chest 1980; 78:682–685.
54. Koo KW, Sax DS, Snider GL. Arterial blood gases and pH during sleep in chronic obstructive pulmonary disease. Am J Med 1975; 58:663–670.
55. Krieger J, Turlot JC, Mangin P, Kurtz D. Breathing during sleep in normal young and elderly subjects. Hypopneas, apneas and correlated factors. Sleep 1983; 6:108–120.
56. Leech JA, Önal EO, Baer P, Lopata M. Determinants of hypercapnia in occlusive sleep apnea syndrome. Chest 1987; 92:807–813.
57. Leitch AG, Clancy LJ, Leggett RJE, et al. Arterial blood gas tensions, hydrogen ion, and electroencephalogram during sleep in patients with chronic ventilatory failure. Thorax 1976; 31:730–735.
58. Littner MR, McGinty DJ, Arand DL. Determinants of oxygen desaturation in the course of ventilation during sleep in chronic obstructive pulmonary disease. Am Rev Respir Dis 1980; 122:849–857.
59. Lopata M, Önal E. Mass loading, sleep apnea, and the pathogenesis of obesity hypoventilation. Am Rev Respir Dis 1982; 126:640–645.
60. Lopes JM, Tabachnik E, Muller NL, et al. Total airway resistance and respiratory muscle activity during sleep. J Appl Physiol 1983; 54:773–777.
61. Marrone O, Milone F, Coppola P, et al. Effects of almitrine bismesylate on nocturnal hypoxemia in patients with chronic bronchitis and obesity. Eur J Respir Dis 1986; 69(Suppl 146):641–648.
62. Prevalence of overweight in selected states—behavioral risk factor surveillance, 1986. MMWR 1988; 37:9–11.
63. Morcizzi G, Magvun HW. Brainstem reticular formation and activation of the EEG. Electroencephalogr Clin Neurophysiol 1949; 1:445–479.
64. Muller NL, Francis PW, Gurwitz D, et al. Mechanism of hemoglobin desaturation during rapid-eye–movement sleep in normal subjects and in patients with cystic fibrosis. Am Rev Respir Dis 1980; 121:463–469.
65. Nattie EE, Bartlett D, Johnson K. Pulmonary hypertension and right ventricular hypertrophy caused by intermittent hypoxia and hypercapnia in the rat. Am Rev Respir Dis 1978; 118:653–658.
66. Nocturnal Oxygen Therapy Trial Group: Continuous or nocturnal oxygen therapy in hypoxemic chronic obstructive lung disease. Ann Intern Med 1980; 93:391–398.
67. Önal E, Lopata M. Periodic breathing and the pathogenesis of occlusive sleep apneas. Am Rev Respir Dis 1982; 126:676–680.
68. Phillips BA, Cooper KR, Burke TV. The effect of sleep loss on breathing in chronic obstructive pulmonary disease. Chest 1987; 91:29–32.
69. Phillipson EA. Control of breathing during sleep. Am Rev Respir Dis 1978; 118:909–939.
70. Pierce AK, Jarrett CE, Werkle G, Miller WF. Respiratory function during sleep in patients with chronic obstructive lung disease. J Clin Invest 1966; 45:631–636.
71. Racineux JL, Meslier N, Hubert P. The effect of long-term almitrine therapy on sleep hypoxaemia in patients with chronic airways obstruction. Bull Clin Respir Physiol 1987; 23 (Suppl):183s.
72. Ressl J, Urbanova D, Widimsky J, et al. Reversibility of pulmonary hypertension and right ventricular hypertrophy induced by intermittent high altitude hypoxia in rats. Respiration 1974; 31:38–46.
73. Rhoads GG, Brody JS. Idiopathic alveolar hypoventilation: clinical spectrum. Ann Intern Med 1969; 71:271–278.
74. Robin ED. Some interrelations between sleep and disease. Ann Intern Med 1958; 102:669–675.
75. Sauertienal EK, Harper RM. The human tongue during sleep: electromyographic activity of the genioglossus muscle. Exp Neurol 1976; 51:160–170.
76. Schafer KE. Adaptation to breath-hold diving. In: Rahn H, Yokoyama T, eds. Physiology of Breath-hold Diving and the AMA of Japan. Washington, DC: National Academy of Sciences–National Research Council, 1965 (Publication no. 1341:237–252).
77. Shepard JW, Garrison MW, Grither DA, et al. Relationship of ventricular ectopy to nocturnal oxygen desaturation in patients with chronic obstructive pulmonary disease. Am J Med 1985; 78:28–34.
78. Shepard JW, Schweitzer PK, Keller CA, et al. Myocardial stress—exercise versus sleep in patients with COPD. Chest 1984; 86:366–374.

79. Skatrud JB, Dempsey JA, Iber C, Berssenbrugge A. Correction of CO_2 retention during sleep in patients with chronic obstructive pulmonary diseases. Am Rev Respir Dis 1981; 124:260–268.
80. Smolensky M, Halberg F, Sargent F II. Chronobiology of the life sequence. In: Itoh S, Ogata K, Hoshimure H, eds. Advances in Climatic Physiology. Tokyo: Igaku Shoin Ltd., 1972, 281–318.
81. Stradling JR, Lane DJ. Nocturnal hypoxaemia in chronic obstructive pulmonary disease. Clin Sci 1983; 64:213–222.
82. Sullivan CE, Berthon-Jones M, Issa FG. Reversal of obstructive sleep apnea by continuous positive airway pressure applied through the nares. Lancet 1981; i:862–865.
83. Tabachnik E, Muller NL, Bryan C, Levison H. Changes in ventilation and chest wall mechanics during sleep in normal adolescents. J Appl Physiol 1987; 51:557–564.
84. Tatsumi K, Kimura H, Kunitomo F, et al. Sleep arterial oxygen desaturation and chemical control of breathing during wakefulness in COPD. Chest 1986: 90:68–73.
85. Tatsumi K, Kimura H, Kunitomo F, et al. Effect of chlormadinone acetate on sleep arterial oxygen desaturation in patients with chronic obstructive pulmonary disease. Chest 1987; 91:688–692.
86. Tilkian AG, Guilleminault C, Schroeder JS, et al. Hemodynamics in sleep induced apnea. Ann Intern Med 1976; 85:714–719.
87. Tirlapur VG, Mir MA. Nocturnal hypoxemia and associated electrocardiographic changes in patients with chronic obstructive airways disease. N Engl J Med 1982; 306:125–130.
88. Trask CH, Cree EM. Oximeter studies on patients with chronic obstructive emphysema, awake and during sleep. N Engl J Med 1962; 266:639–642.
89. Tusiewicz K, Moldafsky H, Brian SC, Bryan AC. Mechanics of the rib cage and diaphragm during sleep. J Appl Physiol 1977; 43:600–602.
90. Vermeire P, de Backer W, van Maele R, et al. Cartoid body resection in patients with severe chronic airflow limitation. Bull Clin Respir Physiol 1987; 23(Suppl): 165s–166s.
91. Warner G, Skatrud JB, Dempsey JA. Effect of hypoxia-induced periodic breathing on upper airway obstruction during sleep. J Appl Physiol 1987; 62:2201–2211.
92. Webb P. Periodic breathing during sleep. J Appl Physiol 1974; 37:899–909.
93. Weil JV, Byrne-Quinn E, Sodal IE, et al. Acquired alteration of chemoreceptor function in chronically hypoxic man at high altitude. J Clin Invest 1971; 50:186–195.
94. White DP, Douglas NJ, Pickett CK, et al. Sleep deprivation and the control of ventilation. Am Rev Respir Dis 1983; 128:984–986.
95. Wynne JW, Block AJ, Hemenway J, et al. Disordered breathing and oxygen desaturation during sleep in patients with chronic obstructive lung disease (COLD). Am J Med 1979; 66:573–579.

Chapter 23

LIMITATION OF EXERCISE IN CHRONIC AIRWAY OBSTRUCTION

Norman L. Jones Kieran J. Killian

Dynamic exercise requires the repetitive shortening of skeletal muscle fibers, in response to motoneuron activation under central neurologic control. The action potential releases calcium, which becomes bound to troponin, leading to fiber shortening and hydrolysis of ATP, with liberation of energy. For exercise to continue for more than a few seconds, ATP has to be reformed from creatine phosphate and other metabolic pathways that lead to the production of lactate or require the delivery of oxygen through central cardiorespiratory and peripheral cardiovascular adaptations. Acid-base control is required to limit the increase in intracellular H^+ ion concentration to prevent the metabolic pathways from becoming inhibited.

Although limitation of exercise capacity is often ascribed to limitation of the oxygen delivery mechanisms, it is clear from this simple description of the processes involved that many mechanisms may contribute, from the cerebral cortex down. Thus, with greater exercise intensity a point is reached where the subject is unable to continue. This point is not necessarily the point where oxygen transport has reached its capacity. For these reasons a broader approach is required to identify the causes of exercise limitation, both in healthy individuals and those with cardiorespiratory disorders. The approach that we use, to assess the factors that contribute to exercise intolerance in patients with chronic airflow obstruction, is one that identifies the subjective limitations experienced by the patients and attempts to quantify the factors that contribute to these limitations. The approach extends also into the clinical assessment of patients and provides a contrast to the methods usually applied to disability evaluation.

Patients with chronic airflow limitation present to their physicians with limitations in their ability to perform and sustain functional activities, such as walking, dressing, climbing stairs, or specific activities unique to their employment. During the clinical interview the limitation is most often related to the discomfort associated with the act of breathing. The quality of this sensation of dyspnea or breathlessness varies in description, but its severity is usually identified from the intensity of activity associated with discomfort. Thus, if discomfort occurs at a level of activity where it is unexpected, breathlessness is considered present. Breathlessness is most severe if it occurs at rest and is considered normal or physiologic if it occurs at high-intensity exercise. This approach was formalized in the grading system first proposed by the British Medical Research Council[1] and later adopted by the American Thoracic Society.[2] A questionnaire identifies if breathlessness is experienced in walking activities, e.g., up hills (grade 1), at an ordinary pace on the level (grade 2), at a slow pace (grade 3), and at rest (grade 4).

Less commonly than dyspnea, exercise is limited by subjective fatigue—a sensation that an excessive amount of muscular effort is required in tasks previously performed with much less effort. Of course, the aforementioned description is inadequate to include the entire range of symptoms that leads a patient with airflow limitation to seek medical advice, but it does apply to a majority of patients with moderate to severe airflow limitation.

After symptoms are identified, most physicians direct their examinations and investigations toward heart or lung disorders. Often, examination findings may be inconclusive, and frequently the clinical problem becomes the distinction between heart and lung disease. Further history, clinical examination, and laboratory investigations center on identifying and specifying the disease process. The general assumption inherent in this approach is that the degree of organ impairment is reasonably and closely related to the disability experienced (reduced capacity to perform functional activities) and the severity of symptoms experienced in everyday life (handicap).[3] Thus, the model may be represented in the following scheme:

Organ Impairment → Disability → Handicap

Also inherent in this approach is a tacit assumption that the degree of handicap and disability is more or less directly related to the degree of functional organ impairment. Once a diagnosis is established, the therapeutic approach is largely centered on correcting organ impairment to eliminate disability and handicap. Improvement in organ capacity is assumed to result in comparable improvements in disability and handicap. Thus, the usual train of events is that the patient presents with symptoms and reduced functional performance; the physician identifies a specific disease; accepted and validated modes of therapy are applied; and disability and handicap are eliminated or minimized. When the handicap and symptoms are greater than expected, or do not respond to conventional treatment, a psychogenic cause often is considered or the patient suspected of a compensation neurosis.

The procedure as described may caricature the diagnostic approach to disabled patients with chronic airflow limitation, but it serves to set the scene for a critical analysis of the relationships among organ impairment, disability, and handicap.

ORGAN IMPAIRMENT AND DISABILITY IN CHRONIC AIRFLOW LIMITATION

If we select a representative population of patients with chronic airflow limitation we can ascertain to what extent the aforementioned relationships are true. The selection of a representative population may be impossible, because of the uncertainty regarding the consequences of specific pathologic features, but at least we may identify the presence of airflow limitation, quantify its severity, and measure functional capacity in the same patients. Patients with functional performances out of keeping with airflow limitations may have structural changes in the lungs or a variety of pathophysiologic abnormalities, which may be identified, corrected, or ameliorated.

In such a representative population a close relationship exists between exercise capacity and severity of airflow limitation (Fig. 23–1), as reflected in the forced expiratory volume in 1 second (FEV_1). Although several studies have demonstrated a decline in exercise capacity with declining FEV_1,[4] Figure 23–1 illustrates a wide range of exercise capacity in patients with comparable severity of airflow limitation. If reduction in ventilatory capacity were the dominant single factor in limiting performance, such a wide range in responses would not be expected. Adding a measurement of the capacity to exchange gas, such as the carbon monoxide transfer capacity (D_{CO}), explains some of the range effect, but its contribution is small.[4,5] Resting measurements of FEV_1 and D_{CO} do not predict exercise capacity with any precision.

Because dyspnea is the main complaint of patients who find their exercise capacity to be limited as part of their airflow obstruction, it is helpful to consider what is known of the factors that underlie this symptom.

DYSPNEA IN AIRFLOW LIMITATION

Discomfort experienced during breathing is generally assumed to limit exercise in patients with chronic airflow limi-

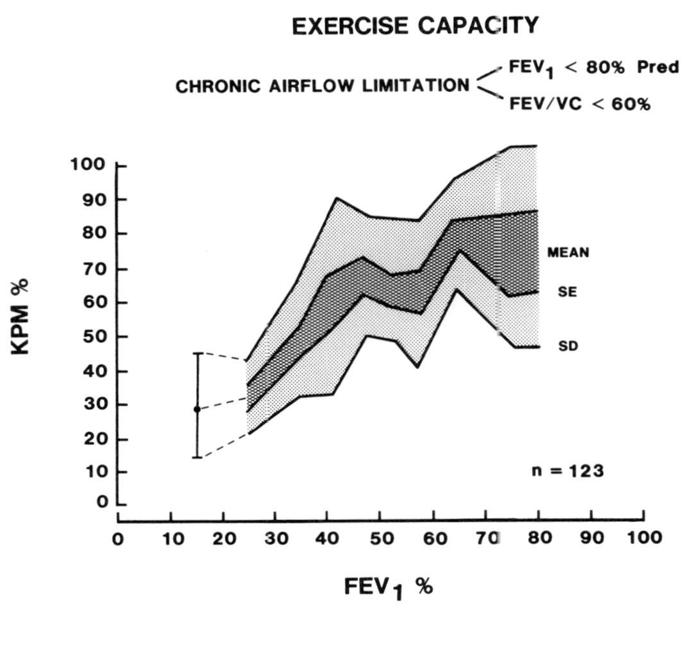

Figure 23–1. Relationship between forced expiratory volume in one second (FEV_1), expressed as % predicted and the maximum power output % predicted in 123 patients with chronic airflow obstruction. FEV/VC = forced expiratory volume/vital capacity; KPM = kilopond meters.

tation. To what extent can be determined by asking patients what prevented them from continuing in an incremental or endurance exercise study in the laboratory. Patients readily identify specific limiting symptoms in exercise tests, including breathlessness, leg fatigue, and less commonly in respiratory patients chest pain and a variety of other complaints. Although most patients with severe airflow limitation are restricted by breathlessness, about one third are restricted by leg fatigue, either alone or combined with dyspnea.

Rather than confining our examination of breathlessness to its severity at maximum exercise, we may also study the relationship between breathlessness and exercise by asking patients to grade the intensity of breathing discomfort at each incremental step during an exercise test continued to maximum performance (Fig. 23–2). Breathlessness is increased in patients when compared with that of healthy subjects, but at maximum exercise the intensity of breathlessness is similar in healthy subjects and patients with airflow limitation. Breathlessness is not unique to airflow limitation but is present in healthy subjects, although at a much higher absolute exercise intensity. The basis for this analysis was provided by studies in which dyspnea was quantified, using established and validated psychophysical methods.[6–8] The application of these methods to studies of exercise and loaded breathing in healthy subjects and patients with respiratory disorders has increased our understanding by allowing a quantitative analysis of the factors contributing to limiting symptoms.

Mechanisms Contributing to Dyspnea

Dyspnea is the dominant symptom at maximum exercise in most patients with chronic airflow obstruction and in many healthy subjects. Several studies have demonstrated a close relationship between the intensity of the sensation and the pressure generated by inspiratory muscles as a proportion of their capacity to generate this pressure.[9–12] The capacity to generate pressure itself is a function of the static strength and the contractile properties of the inspiratory muscles as expressed in the length-tension and force-velocity characteristics. In this analysis, tension and force are reflected by maximum esophageal pressures, length is reflected by volume changes, and velocity by inspiratory airflow. To utilize these indirect measurements to indicate the basic properties of respiratory muscle may require a stretch of the imagination for neuromuscular physiologists but they have been successful for clinical physiologists[7, 11] in a number of studies that have quantified dyspnea in healthy subjects and in patients with airflow obstruction. These studies have yielded quantitative information on the relationship between the intensity of dyspnea, in terms of additional tension generated by respiratory muscles, and the reduced capacity to generate tension.

Ventilation During Exercise

The increase in ventilation that occurs in exercise is closely correlated with the increase in metabolic demands, expressed in terms of CO_2 output. For a given intensity of total body dynamic exercise, or O_2 intake, CO_2 output is influenced by a number of factors. The dietary history related to exercise exerts a strong effect by modulating the balance between fats and carbohydrates as fuel sources. On the one hand, if subjects fast for 24 hours, fat is the predominant fuel source for exercise and CO_2 output is relatively low. On the other hand, exercise taken shortly following a meal, when elevations in plasma insulin concentrations effectively inhibit the mobilization of free fatty acids,[13] is accompanied by high CO_2 output. Conditions associated with lactate production are also associated with increases in CO_2 output through their effects on acid-base variables. Subjects who are poorly conditioned accumulate lactate at relatively low exercise levels, associated with increased CO_2 output. Similarly, patients with cardiac impairment or severe arterial O_2 desaturation are exposed to poor O_2 delivery to exercising tissues, with elevations in lactate production and CO_2 output.[14] In contrast, trained individuals exhibit low CO_2 output during exercise, due not only to less lactate accumulation than untrained individuals but also to a greater use of fat as an aerobic fuel.[15, 16]

The efficiency of the lung as a gas exchanger also influences the ventilation at a given power output. An increase in deadspace ventilation due to areas in the lung with a high ventilation perfusion ($\dot{V}/\dot{Q}$) ratio is associated with an increase in total ventilation ($\dot{V}_E$). Conditions associated with

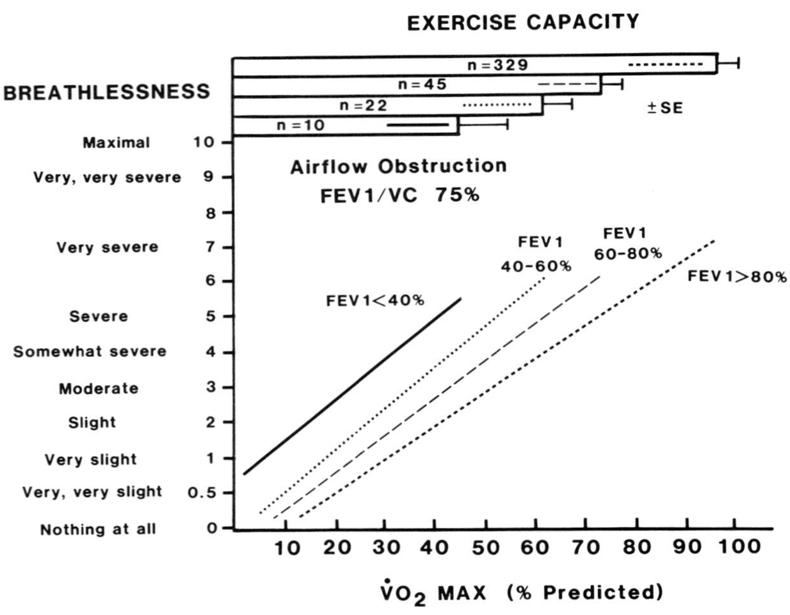

Figure 23–2. Dyspnea during exercise (Borg scale) in groups of patients with differing airflow obstruction. $\dot{V}O_2$ MAX = maximum oxygen consumption. (Reproduced with permission from Killian KJ. Chest 1985; 88:845–905.)

hypoxia are also accompanied by elevations in ventilation during exercise through the effects of hypoxemia on respiratory control mechanisms.[17, 18]

Respiratory Muscle Tension

Increases in ventilation during exercise are accompanied by increases in tension generated by the respiratory muscles, as defined by the mechanical characteristics of the lung. These may be expressed in terms of the pressures that are required to overcome elastic and resistive components. Pressure (Prs) generated against the elastance of the lung is a function of volume, and against resistance a function of flow, as expressed in the following equation:[19]

$$Prs = (V \times E) + (\dot{V} \times R) + (\ddot{V} \times I)$$

The intrathoracic pressures generated during exercise have been measured in healthy subjects.[20–22] Pressures recorded at zero flow at the end of inspiration and expiration represent the pressures generated to achieve changes in volume (V), against the elastance (E) of the respiratory system. Pressures generated during active inspiratory and expiratory flow ($\dot{V}$), insofar as they deviate from these static characteristics, represent the pressures required to overcome flow resistance (R). Accelerative forces ($\ddot{V}$) against inertial impedance are assumed to be insignificant. During exercise, elevations in inspiratory pressure occur gradually, but once tidal volume exceeds 50% of the vital capacity the change in pressure gradually increases (Fig. 23–3). End-expiratory pressure shows little change until high levels of exercise when an increase is observed, representing a reduction in the end-expiratory lung volume.[23] This may be considered an adaptive response, in that a reduction in end-inspiratory volume minimizes end-inspiratory volume and thus the end-inspiratory pressure.

The contributions of elastance and resistance to both the pressure generated by respiratory muscles and the sense of effort in breathing have been obtained by studies in which breathing has been "loaded" by the imposition of graded resistances and elastances during inspiration.[9, 12] These studies have shown that the sense of effort rises with increased pressure generation by the respiratory muscles, but also that the forces may be modified considerably by changes in the pattern of breathing. Thus, with an elastic load, inspiratory pressures may be minimized by the adoption of a smaller tidal volume and greater frequency of breathing. Similarly, when a resistive load is imposed, inspiratory airflow may be slowed, and the time spent in inspiration is relatively lengthened (an increase in the duty cycle, T_i/T_{tot}).

Studies of loaded breathing have also allowed measurement of the oxygen cost. These studies have shown that the maximum oxygen consumption of the respiratory muscles is 100 to 300 ml/minute.[9] This increase in metabolic demands theoretically may contribute to a limitation of maximal oxygen intake, but as the oxygen uptake ($\dot{V}O_2$) of respiratory muscles will seldom exceed 10% of the total body $\dot{V}O_2$ max, this effect is a small one in healthy subjects. However, in patients whose maximal oxygen uptake is severely restricted, the greater oxygen cost of breathing imposed by increases in respiratory impedance may well contribute to reductions in exercise capacity.

Capacity of Respiratory Muscles to Generate Pressure

In the healthy population a wide range in respiratory muscle strength is found, as measured by maximal inspiratory and expiratory pressures against an occluded airway (MIP, MEP). This variation may be as much as five-fold, between 60 cm H_2O and 300 cm H_2O for MIP.[24] Studies of loaded breathing in healthy subjects have shown that the intensity of respiratory effort for a given development of pressure is related to the respiratory muscle strength; subjects with weak respiratory muscle strength indicate a higher sense of effort for a given pressure generated than subjects with higher respiratory muscle strength.[9, 11] Differences among subjects are minimized when the sense of effort is related to the pressure generated. This value is expressed as a percentage of the maximum pressure-generating capacity.[12]

In addition to the effect of static muscle strength, the dynamic characteristics of respiratory muscle influence the functional capacity under varying operational conditions. These characteristics are classically defined in terms of the length-tension and force-velocity characteristics of muscle.[25]

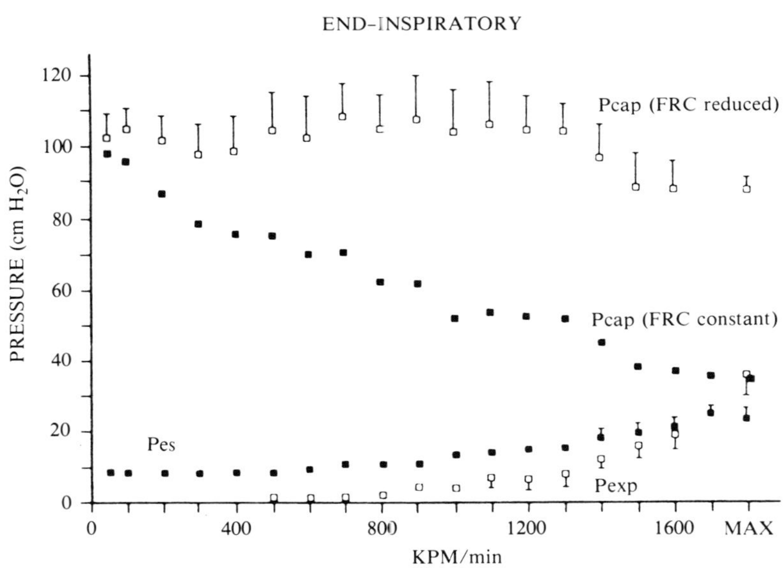

Figure 23–3. Peak inspiratory and expiratory pressures during exercise in normal subjects, showing concomitant reduction in inspiratory capacity. FRC = functional residual capacity. (Reproduced with permission from Leblanc P, Summers E, Inman MD, et al. J Appl Physiol 1988; 64:2482–2489.)

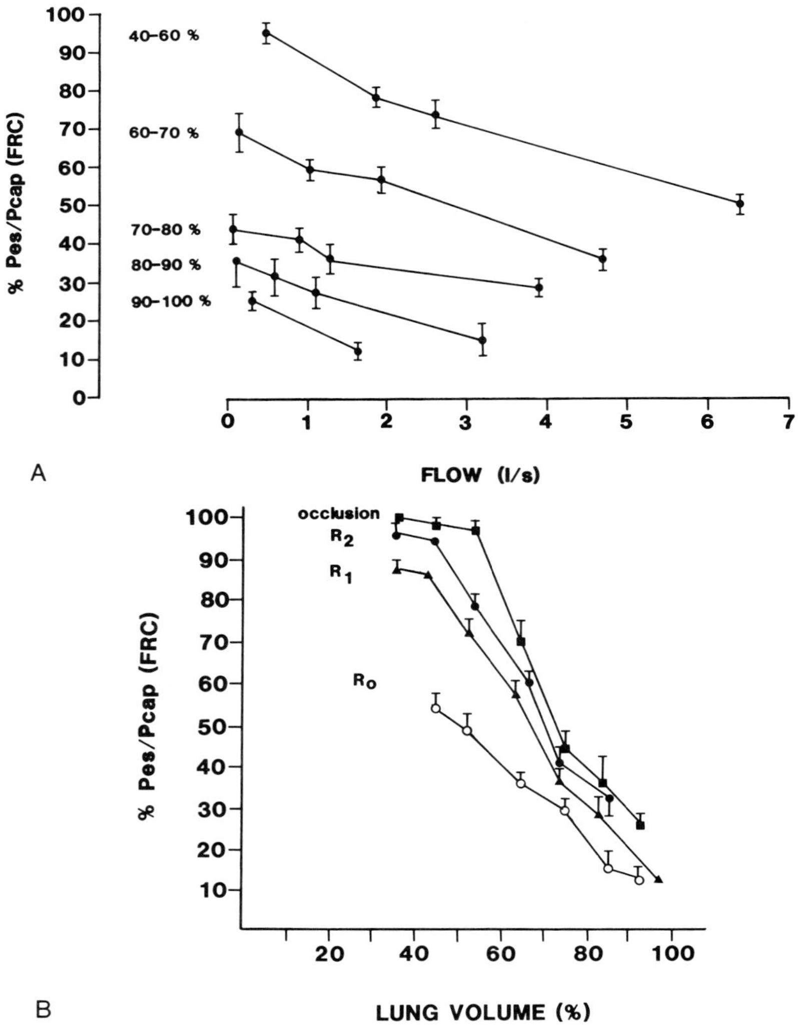

Figure 23–4. Effect of inspiratory flow *(A)* and end-expiratory lung volume *(B)* to generate maximum inspiratory pressure in healthy subjects. (Reproduced with permission from Leblanc P, Summers E, Inman MD, et al. J Appl Physiol 1988; 64:2482–2489.)

Capacity falls as the muscle becomes shorter and as it contracts faster. In applying these classic muscle characteristics to respiratory muscle, changes in volume are used as indications of changes in respiratory muscle length, and changes in inspiratory flow are used as indications of changes in respiratory muscle velocity of contraction. However imperfect, these conventions have allowed the changes in respiratory muscle capacity to be functionally defined in terms of the operating characteristics of the respiratory muscles. Thus, Leblanc and colleagues[21] applied a similar approach to the early work of Agostoni and Fenn[26] in the context of ventilation during exercise. They showed that tension-generating capacity of respiratory muscles declined linearly by 1.7% for each 1% of total lung capacity (TLC) increase in volume above functional residual capacity and by 5% for each 1 L/second increase in inspiratory flow (Fig. 23–4). These investigators also established the interaction between these two effects. When these findings were applied to studies of loaded breathing during exercise, the sense of respiratory effort was found to be closely related to the pressure generated by the respiratory muscles as a percentage of the pressure-generating capacity, corrected for the effects of end-inspiratory volume and peak inspiratory flow. El Manshawi and coworkers[12] derived an equation to express the increase in respiratory effort with rising esophageal pressure (Prs), inspiratory flow ($\dot{V}_i$), T_i/T_{tot}, and frequency (f_b):

$$\text{Breathlessness} = 0.11\ \text{Prs} + 0.61\ \dot{V}_i + 1.99\ T_i/T_{tot} + 0.04\ f_b - 2.6$$

where breathlessness was scored in arbitrary units from 0 to 10 by the Borg scale as shown in Figure 23–2.[6] This equation was derived from studies of imposed resistive loads to breathing and indicates the influence of the peak esophageal pressure and the effect of the velocity of respiratory muscle contraction, the duration of that contraction, and the frequency of breathing.

In addition to quantifying the factors that contributed to the sense of effort in breathing, the results of a number of studies in healthy subjects during exercise suggest that the pattern of breathing adopted by a given subject may serve to optimize the sense of effort by minimizing the tension generated in respiratory muscles and by maintaining the tension-generating capacity.

Respiratory Muscle Fatigue

The maximum force generating capacity of respiratory muscles, just as in skeletal muscles, as well as being influenced by isometric strength and force-velocity and length-tension characteristics, may change with the duration of activity. For any skeletal muscle the relationship between power and length of time for which it may be sustained is represented as a curve that declines exponentially as described in the following general equation:[27]

$$W = E + S/t$$

This equation states that below a threshold (E), power (W) may be maintained indefinitely. Above the threshold, fatigue will occur after a duration (t) that is influenced by the power output and the muscle's maximum strength (S). In this context fatigue is defined as failure to maintain a given power.[28] Thus, when considering the capacity to generate power above the threshold, time should enter the determination. It may be appreciated that the definition of capacity becomes very complex if we are to allow for all the relevant factors (strength, velocity, extent of contraction, frequency of contraction, duty cycle, and duration of exercise). In cycling exercise the extent of contraction may be kept constant, allowing the effects of velocity and time to be defined. Such studies have shown that peak power is a function of velocity. Thus, maximum power is developed at high velocities; however, the decline in power with time is less at the lower velocities of contraction.[29]

In the case of respiratory muscles the length of time for which a given ventilation may be sustained can be given with a fair degree of precision. The threshold is usually defined as the ventilation that can be maintained for 15 minutes—the maximum sustained ventilatory capacity.[30] The form of the curve is similar to that of skeletal muscle in showing a hyperbolic decline from the classic 15-second maximum breathing capacity to a threshold value that is about 60% of the maximum. Bellemare and Grassino[31] extended these findings by introducing the concept of the tension-time integral, obtained by multiplying the pressure generated by the respiratory muscles expressed as a proportion of maximum by the duty cycle (T_i/T_{tot}). Thus, if pressure is 0.5 of maximum and T_i/T_{tot} is 0.4, the tension-time integral is 0.2. These investigators showed that when the tension-time integral for the diaphragm exceeded 0.15, electromyographic signs of muscle failure would be found if the pattern of breathing continued long enough. This index includes the pressure as a proportion of maximum and the duration of contraction, but Bellemare and Grassino indicated that the effects of velocity and extent of contraction should also be kept in mind in relation to fatigue development.

The identificiation of fatigue in respiratory muscle is not as clear-cut as in skeletal muscle, making it difficult to identify whether respiratory muscle fatigue limits exercise. For this reason a number of indirect measures of fatigue have been suggested. Electromyographic changes associated with the development of fatigue in skeletal muscle may be identified as an increase in amplitude of the lower frequency component (20 to 50 Hz), a decrease in amplitude of the high frequency component (150 to 350 Hz), and a decrease in ratio of the high to low frequency. Such changes using esophageal or chest electrodes may be identified.[32] Also, the occurrence of paradoxical movement of the abdomen and rib cage during breathing has been advocated as an indication of respiratory muscle fatigue. However, it has been argued that neither the electromyographic changes[33] nor the presence of paradoxical movement[34] is necessarily an indicator of muscle fatigue.

When the respiratory muscles respond to a given load in the fatigued state, the sense of effort is greater than in controlled conditions.[35] It seems likely that during exercise the intensity of dyspnea that occurs as muscle tension approaches its maximum capacity will lead to the subject stopping or reducing exercise before actual respiratory failure occurs.

DYSPNEA DURING EXERCISE IN PATIENTS WITH AIRFLOW LIMITATION

On this background we may examine the factors that contribute to the sense of respiratory effort during exercise in patients with chronic airflow obstruction.

Ventilation During Exercise

In patients with chronic airflow obstruction the total ventilation generally is within the normal range or elevated in relation to the power output or oxygen intake. Although alveolar underventilation frequently occurs, it is seldom sufficiently severe as to lead to a reduction in the total ventilatory response to exercise, as it is almost invariably accompanied by a high physiologic deadspace in % of tidal volume (V_D/V_T ratio).[36] Because the capacity to increase ventilation is severely limited, any factor tending to increase ventilation at a given exercise level will contribute to a reduction in the total exercise capacity, often to a marked degree. For example, oxygen uptake at a given power output in a patient with severe airflow obstruction is increased on average by about 200 ml/minute above that in a normal subject at comparable loads.[4] Because this value is similar to the maximal increase in oxygen uptake shown in a healthy subject during loaded breathing,[9] it seems likely that these greater metabolic costs are due to the greater tension developed by the respiratory muscles in overcoming the impedance to breathing.

Elevations in CO_2 output can occur following a meal or a glucose infusion and are accompanied by elevations in ventilation. If ventilatory capacity is severely limited, a reduction in exercise capacity results.[37] An increase in CO_2 output also accompanies the increase in oxygen intake at a given level of exercise, which accompanies the greater O_2 cost of breathing. Lactate production in a patient with chronic airflow obstruction is unusual,[38] mainly because the maximum power output achieved by such a patient is too low to require muscle glycolysis. However, in less disabled subjects, who are capable of achieving relatively high exercise levels, or in subjects who become severely hypoxemic or who have an impaired cardiac output response to exercise, lactate production may contribute to a rise in CO_2 output and ventilation.

It might be thought that hypoxemia leads to increases in ventilation by stimulating chemoreceptors. However, falls in arterial O_2 saturation in patients with chronic airflow limitation are the consequence of impaired ventilatory capacity, respiratory control and gas exchange, and thus have little independent effect on increasing ventilation. Studies in patients have shown correlations among arterial O_2 desaturation in exercise and reduction in FEV_1 (severity of airflow obstruction), reduction in D_{CO} (severity of gas exchange impairment), and intensity of exercise (O_2 demands).[36]

The efficiency of the lungs in terms of gas exchange is very frequently impaired in a patient with chronic airflow obstruction.[39] Marked inhomogeneity in the distribution of ventilation and perfusion leads to areas with a high ventilation-perfusion ratio, which act as dead space, and areas with a low ventilation-perfusion ratio, which act as venous admixture and contribute to arterial O_2 desaturation. A high V_D/V_T leads to a high ventilation for a given carbon dioxide output (V_{CO_2}) and thus contributes to dyspnea. In some patients, this effect is lessened by alveolar underventilation with a higher arterial partial pressure CO_2 (P_{CO_2}), by as much as 20 torr during exercise.[36] Thus, hypoventilation acts to reduce the sensation of dyspnea but at the uncertain expense of a rise in P_{CO_2}.

Impedance to Breathing

In patients with chronic airflow obstruction the dominant impedance is resistive. Indeed, in patients with emphysema the elastic components to impedance may actually be reduced, owing to the fall in elastic recoil. Airflow resistance is worse during expiration than inspiration in most patients. In patients with severe reductions in elastic recoil, the limitation of expiratory airflow at low lung volumes may become extreme (Fig. 23–5).

As mentioned previously, ventilatory capacity is conventionally assessed by expiratory flow measurements, such as the FEV_1. Several studies have shown correlations between FEV_1 and maximum ventilation during exercise,[4] suggesting that expiratory flow limitation leads to impaired ventilatory capacity and to limited exercise capability. Armstrong and coworkers[40] suggested that the FEV_1 may be utilized in conjunction with submaximal exercise ventilation to predict maximum exercise capacity. The data in these studies, while showing significant correlations, indicate a large residual variance. This variance may be understood when one considers that (1) maximum ventilation during exercise depends as much on inspiratory as on expiratory flow and that (2) inspiratory flow is extremely variable in patients with a given reduction in FEV_1. For example, in patients with emphysema FEV_1 may be very low, whereas during inspiration airflow resistance may be normal. In these patients, the limitation of expiratory flow leads to a prolongation of expiratory time, in turn placing a heavy responsibility on the increases in inspiratory flow and thus on decreases in inspiratory time in order to achieve a given tidal volume and total ventilation. T_i/T_{tot} may be less than 0.2, and relatively high levels of ventilation are obtained if the respiratory muscles are of normal strength and inspiratory resistance is low.

By comparison, in patients with severe chronic bronchitis reductions in inspiratory flow may be due to reductions in airway caliber (see Fig. 23–5). This effect limits the extent to which T_i/T_{tot} may be reduced. Ventilation during exercise in such patients may be very limited.

Increases in inspiratory flow may also be limited in patients with weak respiratory muscles (Fig. 23–5) or in patients with respiratory muscle strength compromised by gross increases in functional residual capacity (see Fig. 23–5). If the pattern of breathing in terms of tidal volume and inspiratory and expiratory flow is considered in the context of the flow-volume loop, the adopted pattern of breathing may usually be explained. Also, changes in end-expiratory lung volume may be understood. Patients with airflow obstruction seldom are able to reduce end-expiratory lung volume, owing to the extreme decline in airflow at low lung volumes. Thus, the adaptation that is available to healthy subjects in heavy exercise is not available to these patients. Some patients with airflow obstruction increase inspiratory lung volume, but this strategy is seldom observed in patients with poor inspiratory flow, because of elevations in inspiratory resistance, respiratory muscle weakness, or very high functional residual capacity (FRC).[41] This finding is presumably obtained because the gains in expiratory flow achieved by a gain in end-inspiratory lung volume are offset by the accompanying reduction in inspiratory flow capacity.

Factors Tending to Reduce Respiratory Muscle Capacity in Chronic Airflow Obstruction

The strength of the respiratory muscles is compromised by both static and dynamic factors in patients with chronic airflow obstruction. Hyperinflation, associated with increases in FRC, may be marked. As this condition is associated with shortening of the inspiratory muscles, they are unable to generate a normal maximum inspiratory pressure. To this effect may be added other factors that tend to weaken respiratory muscle, such as prolonged inactivity, steroid administration, and chronic hypoxemia. These effects may be quantified by determination of maximum inspiratory pressure, corrected for the volume at which it is measured. Reductions in maximum inspiratory pressure may be shown to contribute to dyspnea during exercise, independently of reductions in FEV_1.[42] Thus, both the degree of obstruction and respiratory muscle weakness contribute to dyspnea (Fig. 23–6). During exercise the increase in end-inspiratory volume associated with greater tidal volume serves to weaken muscles further. However, the most important factor tending to weaken respiratory muscles in a dynamic sense is the increase in the velocity of inspiratory muscle contraction required to reduce inspiratory time and raise inspiratory flow. Because of the dominant effect of expiratory airflow slowing, the inspiratory muscles have to contract at a much faster velocity than those in healthy subjects at comparable work loads. In addition to requiring greater muscle forces, as previously pointed out, these changes are associated with progressive functional weakening of the inspiratory muscles.

These factors were quantified by Leblanc and colleagues,[42]

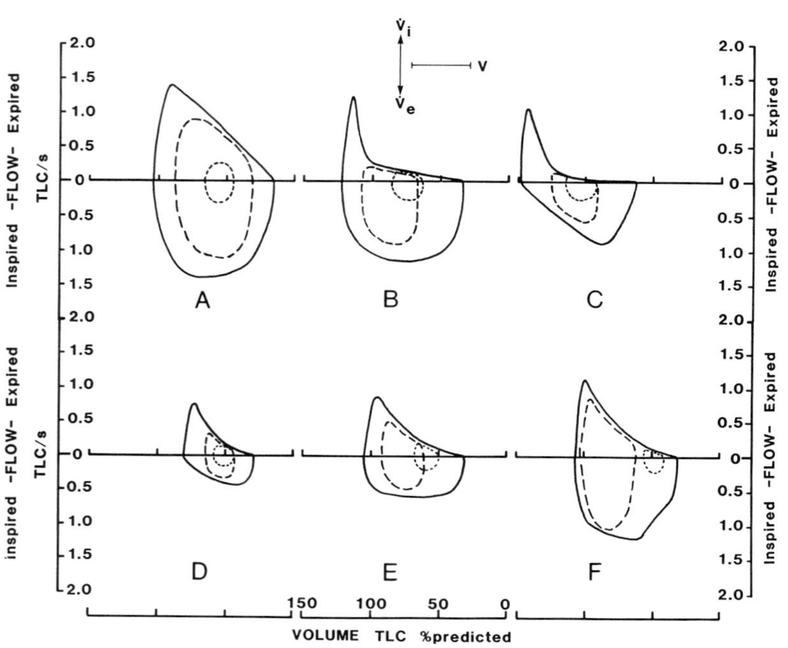

Figure 23–5. Pattern of flow: volume loop in normal subject (A) and patients with airflow obstruction (B–F), showing maximum resting loop (—), quiet breathing at rest (.....) and in maximum exercise (----).
A. Increase in tidal volume (V_T), inspiratory ($\dot{V}_i$) and expiratory ($\dot{V}_e$) flows in normal subject.
B. Patient with severe expiratory flow reduction, but normal inspiratory flow and respiratory muscle strength.
C. Severe obstruction with increase in FRC reducing strength and leading to marked reduction in $\dot{V}_i$ at higher lung volumes.
D. Inspiratory and expiratory obstruction with normal strength.
E. Inspiratory muscle weakness.
F. Less severe obstruction than B and C, normal strength, showing marked increase in end-expiratory volume with exercise.

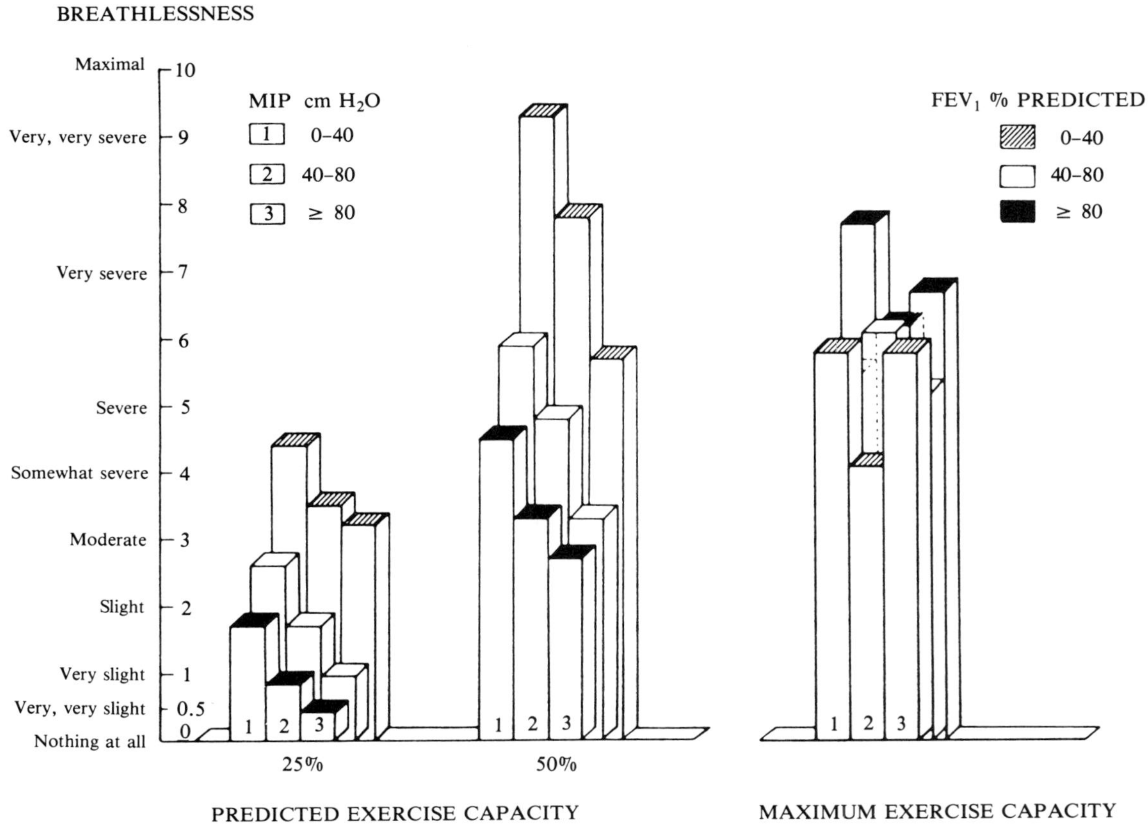

Figure 23–6. Diagram to show the contribution of reduction in FEV_1 and of maximum inspiratory pressure (MIP) on dyspnea in patients with airflow obstruction. (Reproduced with permission from Killian KJ. Chest 1985; 88:845–905.)

who measured esophageal pressures in patients with respiratory disorders and showed that the sense of effort in breathing was related to the pressure generated as a proportion of maximum static capacity (Ppl/MIP), the inspiratory flow rate ($\dot{V}_i$), the tidal volume expressed as a proportion of vital capacity (VT/VC), breathing frequency (f_b), and duty cycle (T_i/T_{tot}) in the following equation:

$$\text{Borg Rating} = 3.0\ \text{Ppl/MIP} + 1.2\ \dot{V}_i + 4.5\ (V_T/V_C) + 0.13\ f_b + 5.6\ T_i/T_{tot} - 6.2$$

where the Borg rating scale is in arbitrary units, i.e., 0 to 10, as in Figure 23–2.[6]

Although in a number of studies the sensation of dyspnea was related to the indices of respiratory muscle forces and the capacity to meet them, some later studies cast doubt on this simple interpretation. Lane and coworkers,[43] in a small number of subjects, found that changes in arterial O_2 saturation influenced dyspnea independently of the mechanical accompaniments. The same investigating group found that different intensities of breathlessness occurred when the subjects voluntarily copied patterns of breathing first used in CO_2 breathing and exercise studies.

Respiratory Muscle Fatigue

As previously pointed out, there is no doubt that combinations of respiratory loading and exercise can lead to situations in which the forces required exceed the capacity to meet them. In healthy subjects, this situation is associated with an extreme sense of dyspnea together with an elevation in P_{CO_2} and a fall in arterial O_2 saturation.[9] Although elevations of P_{CO_2} and falls in arterial O_2 saturation occur during exercise in patients with chronic airflow obstruction, these changes should not be construed as indicating respiratory failure. The individual tolerance to both changes is extremely variable in patients with chronic airflow obstruction. Furthermore, in some patients such changes may be "accepted" as part of the price paid to reduce ventilation and sense of dyspnea.

The McGill group has shown that changes in the electromyographic frequency spectrum consistent with diaphragm fatigue occur in patients with chronic airflow obstruction during exercise.[32, 44] However, Levine and colleagues[45] did not find such changes in exercising patients who were generating large pressures. Furthermore, Gallagher and coworkers,[46] in finding similar breathing patterns during recovery as were found in exercise, reasoned that respiratory muscle fatigue was unlikely to have occurred. A 1970 study by Raimondi and associates[47] approached the same situation by determining if exercise duration could be prolonged by helium-oxygen breathing. Because duration and ventilation were unaffected, these investigators also concluded that the onset of fatigue was not responsible for exercise limitation. Although respiratory muscle fatigue as a factor limiting exercise seems unlikely, little doubt exists that the forces generated by patients during exercise are high and that the capacity to meet these demands is reduced by a number of dynamic factors, including the time exercise is maintained. The sensation of dyspnea thereby increases with both the intensity and the duration of exercise and ultimately leads to the patient stopping or reducing exertion.

A primary objective in the management of patients is an

increase in exercise tolerance. Theoretically, in a given patient, the options might include reductions in respiratory impedance (bronchodilation), reductions in ventilation (endurance training, O_2 therapy), gains in respiratory muscle strength and endurance (xanthines, ventilatory muscle training), and changes in the pattern of force deployment (education). Such strategies may be chosen on the basis of exercise studies. There is little point, for example, in instituting training of the respiratory muscles, if their strength is normal and dyspnea is solely due to severe airflow obstruction. The topic of training is briefly reviewed next.

Other Factors That May Limit Exercise in Airflow Obstruction

Dyspnea is not the only symptom to limit exercise. Many patients, while they experience severe dyspnea, indicate that they are unable to continue exercising because of severe leg muscle effort. In a large series of patients with chronic airflow obstruction, Killian found that 30% were limited by leg fatigue, 26% by dyspnea, and 44% by a combination of the two sensations (unpublished, 1988).

Reductions in patients' activity in everyday life are usual accompaniments to chronic airflow limitation and may be expected to lead to impaired skeletal muscle function. The most extreme example or model for these effects is limb immobilization, which over a period of 4 to 6 weeks is accompanied by marked reductions in (1) muscle strength, (2) muscle fiber cross-sectional area,[48] (3) energy stores, and (4) metabolic enzyme activities.[49] Bed rest for a similar period, even in otherwise fit individuals, is accompanied by reductions in maximal O_2 uptake and by impaired cardiovascular control.[50] Differences between active and sedentary individuals in muscle strength and oxidative enzyme activities are also well known. Such effects are particularly marked in elderly individuals.[51] Few studies have been carried out in patients with disability due to heart or pulmonary disorders. Jones and McCartney[52] measured maximal quadriceps isokinetic power in patients who were recovering from myocardial infarction. During a 12-week observation period, maximal power fell in patients who were inactive and rose in those who were active and entered into a rehabilitation program. Although we are unaware of published data, our own experience suggests that many patients who are seriously disabled by chronic respiratory disorders have weak quadriceps muscles that contribute to poor exercise performance. In 50 patients in whom FEV_1 was less than 60% predicted, we measured maximal isometric strength of the quadriceps muscles and related the findings to maximal exercise performance. In patients in whom exercise capacity was in the normal range, isometric strength was also normal; in patients in whom exercise capacity was 60% to 80% predicted, strength was also normal. However, in patients with severe reduction in exercise capacity to below 60%, strength was reduced to 55% of the mean of the other two groups. Apart from inactivity, steroid-induced myopathy and diuretic therapy may account for weakness in some patients, and theoretically hypoxemia and hypercapnia may also impair muscle function.

Among other factors that contribute to exercise intolerance in patients with chronic airflow obstruction, coexisting coronary artery disease or leg atherosclerosis is usually not difficult to identify. Whether heart failure constitutes a limitation to exercise has been debated.[53] As a patient with "right heart failure" usually is hypoxemic and hypercapnic and has a low ventilatory capacity, it usually is difficult to separate individual effects. Patients with right-sided heart failure associated with idiopathic hypoventilation may have virtually normal exercise capacity, making it unlikely that heart failure per se limits the ability to exercise.

THE PLACE OF EXERCISE IN THE MANAGEMENT OF CHRONIC AIRFLOW OBSTRUCTION

A number of ways in which exercise capacity might be increased in patients are known. These include overall endurance exercise and exercise specifically designed to improve the strength and endurance of the respiratory muscles.

Respiratory Muscle Training

In patients who are unable to generate adequate ventilatory pressures, owing to respiratory muscle weakness, or whose muscles fatigue rapidly, specific training of the muscles should increase maximum ventilation and power in exercise, reduce dyspnea, and improve quality of life. The principles of training regimens have been reviewed by Pardy and Leith[30] and are not detailed here. Training methods have included isocapnic hyperventilation, resistive breathing, and threshold inspiratory loading. All three methods are successful in raising the maximal sustained ventilatory capacity and respiratory muscle strength.[54] Other studies have suggested that regimens that incorporate prescribed flow rates and tidal volumes during training may be more effective than those with unprescribed training.[55] Although ventilatory capacity and endurance may be improved by as much as 50% by these means, the associated effects in exercise tolerance and activities in everyday life are not as consistent. Keens and colleagues,[56] in adult patients with cystic fibrosis, and Belman and Mittman,[57] in adults with chronic airflow limitation, found improvements in exercise capacity following respiratory muscle training. However, Levine and colleagues[45] compared outcome measures in a control group who received intermittent positive pressure breathing and did not find a significant benefit of respiratory muscle training in terms of exercise tolerance or activities of daily living.

It is generally considered that endurance exercise training is unlikely to benefit patients with chronic airflow limitation because they are unable to exercise at an intensity sufficient to elicit a training response. This type of training in healthy subjects and patients with coronary artery disease improves exercise capacity and reduces heart rate and blood pressure during exercise. Associated with these changes is a reduction in lactate accumulation in blood and in CO_2 output. Theoretically, the associated reduction in ventilation and dyspnea would be of great value to patients who are limited by dyspnea. However, such benefits are likely to be limited to patients who accumulate lactate during exercise, prior to training. In most patients, exercise is limited at an intensity that is not associated with lactate production. Also, theoretically, the elevation in ventilation that occurs during training exercise may be associated with improvements in respiratory muscle strength, if the respiratory muscles are weak in the first place. Chester and colleagues,[58] among others, have demonstrated a reduced ventilation following training in 21 patients with moderately severe airway obstruction. An increase in sustained ventilatory capacity has been a feature of several other training studies.[56, 59]

Studies of training, both whole body endurance and respiratory muscle, have shown variable effects in patients with chronic airflow limitation.[54] The reasons for the variable responses have not been systematically investigated. In part, they may be due to the experimental design, as several have

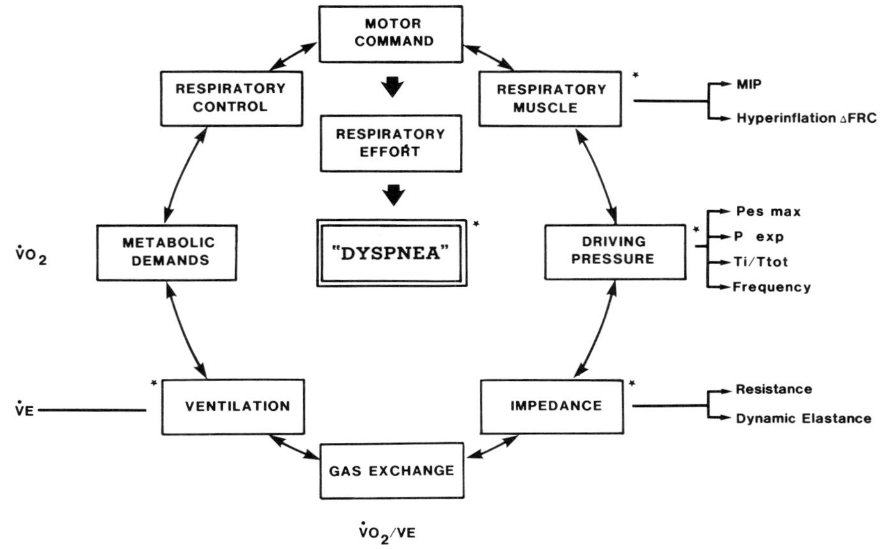

Figure 23–7. Scheme to show the multiple factors that contribute to dyspnea in exercise. (MIP = maximum inspiratory pressure; FRC = functional residual capacity; Ti/Ttot = duty cycle; $\dot{V}E$ = ventilation; $\dot{V}O_2$ = oxygen intake.)

not included a control group. In some studies, appropriate outcome measures may not have been used. More important, however, may be a poor identification of the objectives of training. By clarifying the mechanisms that underlie limiting symptoms, treatment measures may be specifically tailored to an individual. On the one hand, if respiratory muscle weakness is identified, respiratory muscle training is likely to help. On the other hand, a patient who shows increased CO_2 output and ventilation during exercise may be helped more by a general exercise program. In such a program it may prove difficult to prescribe an appropriate exercise intensity using the guidelines developed for cardiac patients. In respiratory patients, the usual aerobic program in which exercise is maintained for a prolonged time may be associated with an unacceptable intensity of dyspnea. In such patients, improvements in muscle function may be achieved by high intensity muscle forces sustained for only short periods but repeated frequently. This type of exercise has proved helpful in cardiac patients.[60]

CONCLUSIONS

Our understanding of the factors that reduce exercise capacity and handicap patients with chronic airflow obstruction and our approach to their therapeutic management have been placed on a sounder basis by a systematic study of the factors that contribute to limiting systems. By quantifying the intensity of the symptoms in relation to the reductions in exercise capacity, the relative roles of the ventilatory demands of exercise, the effects of gas exchange disturbances, the changes in the mechanical characteristics of the respiratory system, and the weakness of respiratory muscles may all be assessed (Fig. 23–7). Each of these unit processes may play a unique role in a given patient and thus allow us to manage this patient on a more logical basis.

REFERENCES

1. Medical Research Council. Standardized questionnaire on respiratory symptoms. Br Med J 1960; 2:1665–1668.
2. Renzetti A. Evaluation of impairment/disability secondary to respiratory disorders. Am Rev Respir Dis 1986; 133:1205.
3. World Health Organization. International Classification of Impairment, Disabilities and Handicaps. Geneva: WHO, 1980.
4. Jones NL, Jones G, Edwards RHT. Exercise tolerance in chronic airway obstruction. Am Rev Respir Dis 1971; 103:477–491.
5. Johnson RL, Taylor HF, Degraff AC. Functional significance of a low pulmonary diffusing capacity for carbon monoxide. J Clin Invest 1965; 44:789–800.
6. Borg GAV. Psychophysical bases of perceived exertion. Med Sci Sports Exercise 1982; 14:377–381.
7. Killian KJ. The objective measurement of breathlessness. Chest 1985; 88:84S–90S.
8. Mahler DA, Weinberg DH, Wells CK, Feinstein AR. The measurement of dyspnea. Chest 1984; 85:751–758.
9. Jones GL, Killian KJ, Summers E, Jones NL. Inspiratory muscle forces and endurance in maximal resistive loading. J Appl Physiol 1985; 58:1608–1615.
10. Killian KJ, Jones NL. The use of exercise testing and other methods in the investigation of dyspnea. Clin Chest Med 1984; 5:99–108.
11. Killian KJ, Campbell EJM. Dyspnea and exercise. Ann Rev Physiol 1983; 45:465–479.
12. El-Manshawi A, Killian KJ, Summers E, Jones NL. Breathlessness during exercise with and without resistive loading. J Appl Physiol 1986; 61:896–905.
13. Molé PA. Exercise metabolism. In: Exercise Medicine: Physiologic Principles and Clinical Application. Orlando: Academic Press 1983, 43–88.
14. Weber KT, Wilson JR, Janicki JS, Likoff ML. Exercise testing in the evaluation of the patient with chronic cardiac failure. Am Rev Respir Dis 1984; 129(Suppl):S60–S62.
15. Henriksson J. Training-induced adaptation of skeletal muscle and metabolism during submaximal exercise. J Physiol (Lond) 1977; 270:661–675.
16. Taylor R, Jones NL. The reduction by training of CO_2 output during exercise. Eur J Cardiol 1979; 9:53–62.
17. Hughes RL, Clode M, Edwards RHT, et al. Effect of inspired O_2 on cardiopulmonary and metabolic responses to exercise in man. J Appl Physiol 1968; 24:336–347.
18. Vidruk EH, Dempsey JA. Peripheral and central nervous system mechanisms controlling exercise-induced breathing patterns. Exercise Sport Sci Rev 1980; 8:129–147.
19. Otis AB. The work of breathing. Physiol Rev 1954; 34:449–458.
20. Grimby G, Saltin B, Wilhelmsen L. Pulmonary flow-volume and pressure-volume relationship during submaximal and maximal exercise in young well-trained men. Bull Physiopath Resp 1971; 7:157–168.
21. Leblanc P, Summers E, Inman MD, et al. Inspiratory muscles during exercise: a problem of supply and demand. J Appl Physiol 1988; 64:2482–2489.
22. Stubbing DG, Pengelly LD, Morse JLC, Jones NL. Pulmonary mechanics during exercise in normal males. J Appl Physiol 1980; 49:506–510.
23. Inman MD, Campbell EJM, Killian KJ. The effect of expiratory

muscle activity on human ventilation during exercise. J Appl Physiol (In press).
24. De Troyer A, Yernault J. Inspiratory muscle force in normal subjects and patients with interstitial lung disease. Thorax 1980; 35:92–100.
25. Edgerton VR, Roy RR, Gregor RJ, Rugg S. Morphological basis of skeletal muscle power output. In: Jones NL, McCartney N, McComas AJ, eds. Human Muscle Power. Champaign, Ill: Human Kinetics, 1986, 43–58.
26. Agostoni E, Fenn WO. Abdominal and thoracic pressures at different lung volumes. J Appl Physiol 1960; 15:1087–1092.
27. Wilkie DG. Muscle function: a historical view. In: Jones NL, McCartney N, McComas AJ, eds. Human Muscle Power. Champaign, Ill: Human Kinetics, 1986, 3–14.
28. Edwards RHT. Human muscle function and fatigue. In: Human Muscle Fatigue: Physiological Mechanisms. Ciba Foundation Symposium 1981; 82:1–18.
29. McCartney N, Obminski G, Heigenhauser GJF. Torque-velocity relationship in isokinetic cycling exercise. J Appl Physiol 1985; 58:1459–1462.
30. Pardy RL, Leith DE. Ventilatory muscle training. In: Roussos C, Macklem PT, eds. The Thorax. New York: Marcel Dekker, 1985, 1353–1372.
31. Bellemare F, Grassino A. Effect of pressure and timing of contraction on human diaphragm fatigue. J Appl Physiol 1982; 53:1190–1195.
32. Roussos C, Macklem PT. The respiratory muscles. N Engl J Med 1982; 307:786–798.
33. Bazzy AR, Korten JB, Haddad GG. Increase in electromyogram low-frequency power in nonfatigued contracting skeletal muscle. J Appl Physiol 1986; 61:1012–1017.
34. Tobin MJ, Perez W, Guenther SM, et al. Does rib cage abdominal paradox signify respiratory muscle fatigue? J Appl Physiol 1987; 63:851–860.
35. Gandevia SC, Killian KJ, Campbell EJM. The effect of respiratory muscle fatigue on respiratory sensations. Clin Sci 1981; 60:463–466.
36. Jones NL. Pulmonary gas exchange during exercise in patients with chronic airflow obstruction. Clin Sci 1966; 31:39–50.
37. Brown SE, Nagendran RC, McHugh JW, et al. Effects of a large carbohydrate load on walking performance in chronic air-flow obstruction. Am Rev Respir Dis 1985; 132:960–962.
38. Daly JJ, Duff RS, Jackson E, Turino GM. Effect of exercise on arterial lactate, pyruvate and excess lactate in chronic bronchitis. Br J Dis Chest 1967; 61:193–197.
39. Jones NL, Berman LB. Gas exchange in chronic air-flow obstruction. Am Rev Respir Dis 1984; 129:S81–S83.
40. Armstrong BW, Workman JN, Holcombe HH, Roemmich WR. Clinicophysiologic evaluation of physical working capacity in persons with pulmonary disease. Am Rev Respir Dis 1966; 93:90–99.
41. Stubbing DG, Pengelly LD, Morse JLC, Jones NL. Pulmonary mechanics during exercise in subjects with chronic airflow obstruction. J Appl Physiol 1980; 49:511–515.
42. Leblanc P, Bowie DM, Summers E, et al. Breathlessness and exercise in patients with respiratory disease. Am Rev Respir Dis 1986; 133:21–25.
43. Lane R, Cockroft A, Adams L, Guz A. Arterial oxygen saturation and breathlessness in patients with chronic obstructive airways disease. Clin Sci 1987; 72:693–698.
44. Bye PTB, Esau SA, Levy RD, et al. Ventilatory function during exercise in air and oxygen in patients with chronic air-flow limitation. Am Rev Respir Dis 1985; 132:236–240.
45. Levine S, Weiser P, Gillen J. Evaluation of a ventilatory muscle endurance training program in the rehabilitation of patients with chronic obstructive pulmonary disease. Am Rev Respir Dis 1986; 133:400–406.
46. Gallagher CG, Younes MK. Breathing pattern during and following exercise in patients with chronic obstructive lung disease, interstitial lung disease and cardiac disease and in normal subjects. Am Rev Respir Dis 1986; 133:581–586.
47. Raimondi AC, Edwards RHT, Denison DM, et al. Exercise tolerance breathing a low density gas mixture, 35% oxygen and air in patients with chronic obstructive bronchitis. Clin Sci 1970; 39:675–685.
48. Sargeant AJ, Davies CTM, Edwards RHT, et al. Functional and structural changes after disuse of human muscle. Clin Sci Molec Med 1977; 52:337–342.
49. MacDougall JD, Ward GR, Sale DG, Sutton JR. Biochemical adaptation of human skeletal muscle to heavy resistance training and immobilization. J Appl Physiol 1977; 43:700–703.
50. Saltin B, Blomqvist G, Mitchell JH, et al. Response to exercise after bed rest and after training. A longitudinal study of adaptive changes in oxygen transport and body composition. Circulation 1968; 37/38 (Suppl 7):1–78.
51. Aniansson A, Grimby G, Hedberg M, Krotkiewski M. Muscle morphology, enzyme activity and muscle strength in elderly men and women. Clin Physiol 1981; 1:73–86.
52. Jones NL, McCartney N. Influence of muscle power on aerobic performance and the effects of training. Acta Med Scand 1986; 711(suppl):115–122.
53. Matthay RA, Berger HJ, Davies RA, et al. Right ventricular exercise performance in chronic obstructive pulmonary disease: radionuclide assessment. Ann Int Med 1980; 93:234–239.
54. Pardy RL, Rivington RN, Despas PJ, Macklem PT. The effects of inspiratory muscle training on exercise performance in chronic airflow limitation. Am Rev Respir Dis 1981; 123:426–433.
55. Clanton TL, Dixon GF, Drake J, Gadek JE. Effects of breathing pattern on inspiratory muscle endurance in humans. J Appl Physiol 1985; 59:1834–1841.
56. Keens TG, Krastins TRB, Wannamaker EM, et al. Ventilatory muscle endurance training in normal subjects and patients with cystic fibrosis. Am Rev Respir Dis 1977; 116:853–860.
57. Belman MJ, Mittman C. Ventilatory muscle training improves exercise capacity in chronic obstructive lung disease patients. Am Rev Respir Dis 1980; 121:273–280.
58. Chester EH, Belman MJ, Behler RC, et al. Multidisciplinary treatment of chronic pulmonary insufficiency. 3. The effect of physical training on cardiopulmonary performance in patients with chronic obstructive pulmonary disease. Chest 1979; 72:695–702.
59. Orenstein DM, Franklin BA, Doershuk CF, et al. Exercise conditioning and cardiorespiratory fitness in cystic fibrosis. Chest 1981; 80:392–398.
60. Kelemen MH, Stewart KJ, Gillian RE, et al. Circuit weight training in cardiac patients. J Am Coll Cardiol 1986; 1:38–42.

Chapter 24

HEMATOLOGIC MANIFESTATIONS OF COPD

Clement Cahan **Kingman P. Strohl**

This chapter describes the hematologic manifestations of COPD, emphasizing new developments in the understanding of normal erythropoietic function and responses relevant to COPD and its sequelae, the foremost of which is hypoxemia. This chapter also reviews the clinical assessment of erythropoietic abnormalities that may be present in the patient with COPD.

THE NORMAL RESPONSE TO HYPOXEMIA

Information concerning erythropoietic responses to hypoxemia is derived from two large studies on high altitude natives. In 1945, Hurtado and colleagues[32] reported observations on Andean natives of South American Indian extraction. They found a correlation among hematocrit value, hemoglobin level, red blood cell volume, and arterial oxygen saturation at high altitude. A graphic presentation of some of these data can be seen in Figure 24–1. This figure indicates the mean hemoglobin and arterial oxygen saturation measured in natives living at different altitudes and suggests an inverse relationship between the degree of arterial oxygen saturation and the level of hemoglobin in circulating blood. In a selected group of subjects, Hurtado and colleagues[32] also reported on red blood cell mass in relation to altitude. Whereas the degree of increase varied according to the method used, a greater red blood cell mass, as compared with that at sea level, was found at both altitudes of 12,240 ft and 14,900 ft. This report by Hurtado and colleagues[32] is one most often cited as indicating that the normal response to hypoxia is an elevation in red blood cell mass and a graded increase in hematocrit value.

Weil and colleagues[63] reported values for red blood cell mass, hematocrit, and hemoglobin in healthy Caucasians living at high altitudes. All subjects were in good health by clinical history and physical examination, chest roentgenogram, and pulmonary function studies. Iron deficiency was excluded by serum measurements. Data from these subjects at sea level, 1600 m, and 3100 m showed a direct relationship between red blood cell mass and oxygen saturation, as shown in Figure 24–2. Red blood cell mass, expressed as % of predicted normal in order to normalize for body size, was inversely correlated with arterial oxygen saturation. As reviewed by Stradling,[58] the relationship between red blood cell mass and arterial oxygen saturation might depend on reaching a certain threshold of hypoxemia, with no significant rise until Sa_{O_2} falls below 92%, and a linear relationship with O_2 saturation below this level. These observations by Weil and colleagues[63] did not extend to arterial oxygen saturations less than 83%. Nevertheless, this database on healthy individuals is relevant to North American and, possibly, European populations, with which COPD patients who have significant alterations in gas exchange can be compared.

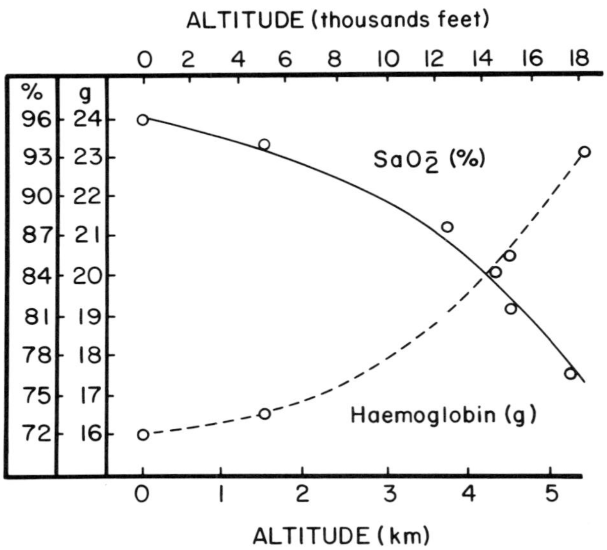

Figure 24–1. Correlation between concentration of hemoglobin in peripheral blood and % arterial oxygen saturation (Sa_{O_2}) at various altitudes. (Reproduced with permission from Hurtado A, Merino C, Delgado E. Arch Intern Med 1945; 75:284.)

PHYSIOLOGIC INFLUENCES ON ERYTHROPOIETIC RESPONSES TO HYPOXEMIA

The factors that influence the erythropoietic response to hypoxemia are presented schematically in Figure 24–3.

THE CHEMISTRY OF OXYGEN BINDING BY HEMOGLOBIN. The relationship between the arterial oxygen pressure (Pa_{O_2}) and the oxygen-carrying capacity of hemoglobin is described by the oxyhemoglobin dissociation curve. The characteristics of the curve are explained by the structure of the hemoglobin molecule.

Hemoglobin is a tetramer consisting of two nonidentical polypeptide chains. Hemoglobin A, which comprises 97% of all adult hemoglobin, has two alpha and two beta chains. An iron-containing prosthetic heme group is attached to each

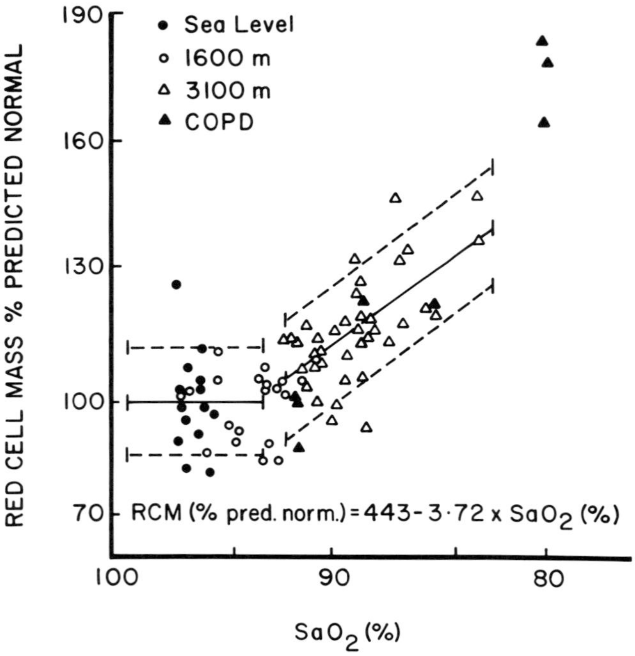

Figure 24–2. Red cell mass (RCM)/Sao_2 relationship using % predicted normal RCM. Regression of 3100-meter data analyzed separately. Broken lines represent 95% confidence limits on individual estimates. Also included are nine patients with COPD. (Adapted from Weil JV, et al. J Clin Invest 1968; 47:1627–1639.)

chain. The T (taut) quaternary structure is constrained by salt chains between the different subunits and is associated with a low affinity for oxygen. These salt links are absent from the R (relaxed) form, which has a high affinity for oxygen. Upon oxygenation the iron atom moves into the plane of the heme. This motion cleaves some of the salt links, resulting in a transition from T to R forms (Fig. 24–4). The binding of oxygen to one heme subunit will facilitate the binding of oxygen to the other heme subunits. This translates into a sigmoidal shape for the oxyhemoglobin dissociation curve.[2, 3, 45–47]

The oxygen affinity of hemoglobin is usually expressed in terms of oxygen tension at which 50% of the hemoglobin is saturated (P_{50}). At sea level, in healthy subjects, this value is 26 to 28 mm Hg. When oxygen affinity is increased the O_2 dissociation curve is shifted to the left so that Sao_2 increases at any given Pao_2 and the P_{50} decreases. Conversely, when oxygen affinity is decreased and the dissociation curve is shifted to the right, P_{50} increases.

Various factors (pH, temperature, $Paco_2$) influence the oxyhemoglobin dissociation curve. The most potent of these is the organic phosphate 2,3 diphosphoglycerate (2,3 DPG). This intermediate product of glycolysis binds to positively charged groups of the hemoglobin beta chains and introduces additional salt links between the two beta chains of hemoglobin. The taut (T) quaternary form of hemoglobin is stabilized, and oxygen affinity decreased.[3, 45–57] The sigmoidal form of the oxygen hemoglobin dissociation curve is preserved but shifted to the right, which facilitates oxygen release to the tissue.[5, 34, 36]

The second mechanism by which 2,3 DPG influences O_2 affinity is through a reduction in intraerythrocytic pH by the acidity of the DPG molecule itself. The increased presence of hydrogen ions favors the formation of salt bridges by protonation of the terminal histidine residues of the beta subunits. Formation of the salt units forces oxygen out of the tetramer and results in a transition from the R to the T hemoglobin form. Functionally, acidosis acts to shift the curve to the right.

Levels of 2,3 DPG are raised in a variety of clinical situations in which oxygen delivery or supply is impaired. These conditions include cardiac failure, anemia, and arterial oxygen desaturation from lung disease or high altitude. The mechanism of 2,3 DPG response has been explained in the following manner. When oxygen supply falls, deoxyhemoglobin accumulates and binds larger amounts of 2,3 DPG and hydrogen ions (H^+). The reduction in free DPG within the cell, along with the increase in cellular pH, stimulates glycolysis and thereby DPG synthesis. The *in vivo* rise in DPG has a half time of about 4 to 8 hours, a relatively rapid response mechanism, acting within hours to improve available oxygen.

SLEEP AND WAKEFULNESS. The level of Pao_2 is not constant over a 24-hour period. Alveolar ventilation decreases during nonrapid eye movement (NREM) sleep in healthy subjects. Sleep results in an elevation in arterial carbon dioxide ranging from 2 to 8 mm Hg with a reciprocal reduction in Pao_2 of 3 to 10 mm Hg.[18, 48] These changes occur despite the fact that

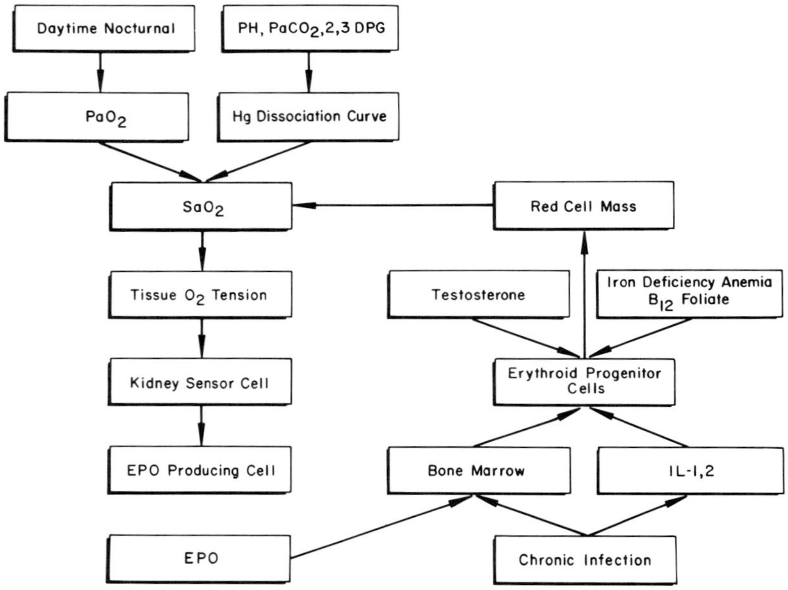

Figure 24–3. Factors that influence the erythropoietic response to hypoxemia. (EPO = erythropoietin; DPG = diphosphoglycerate; $Paco_2$ = arterial carbon dioxide pressure; Pao_2 = arterial oxygen pressure; PH = pulmonary hypertension; IL-1,2 = interleukin-1, interleukin-2.)

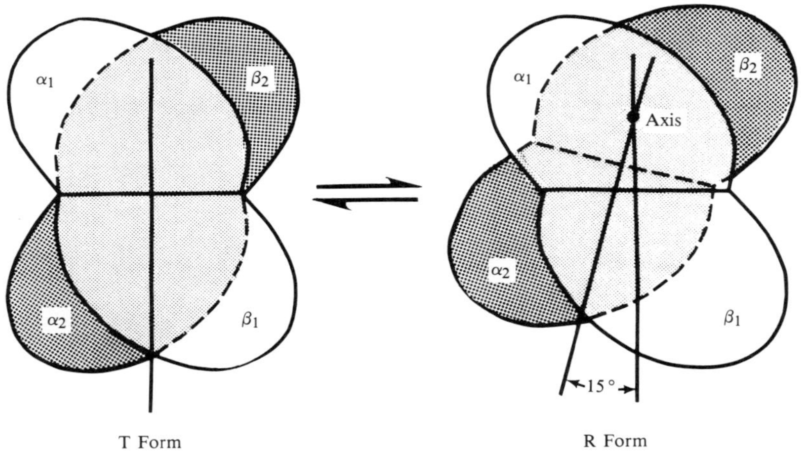

Figure 24–4. Oxygenation results in rupture of salt bonds and a transition of the T form to the R form of hemoglobin. This occurs with a 15° rotation of one pair of subunits relative to the other pair. In this diagram, the α_1/β_1 pair is unshaded and held fixed, and the shaded pair is shown to rotate and shift. (Reproduced with permission from Murray RK, Granner DK, Mays PA. Harper's Biochemistry, 21st edition, Norwalk, CT: Appelton and Lange, 1988.)

oxygen consumption has been reported to decrease on the order of 10% during sleep. Because the Pao_2 of healthy subjects is sufficiently high, with sleep Sao_2 generally decreases by less than 2%. Arterial oxygen pressure values in REM sleep are not as well documented. In most healthy subjects, Pao_2 is at the same level or slightly lower than NREM values. In some healthy individuals, however, both a sustained decrease in Sao_2 and further transient decreases in conjunction with REM-related hypoventilation may be seen.[17, 18, 42, 66] It is not known whether these sleep-related changes in oxygen tension and saturation significantly affect erythropoietic function in healthy subjects.

NUTRITIONAL FACTORS. A deficiency of vitamin B_{12} or folate results in impaired DNA synthesis leading to disturbances in cell division in the hematopoietic tissue. Additionally, exogenous iron is needed in hemoglobin synthesis, and iron deficiency results in decreased production of red blood cells.

ERYTHROPOIETIN. Erythropoietin is an acidic glycoprotein with a molecular mass of 39,000 daltons, produced mainly in the kidney. An auxiliary site of production appears to be the liver, which is the source of approximately 15% of the total circulating erythropoietin. Erythropoietin stimulates bone marrow production of red blood cells by inducing the proliferation and differentiation of committed erythroid progenitor cells.[6, 33] Erythropoietin also accelerates the release of reticulocytes from the bone marrow into the circulation. Both the rapidity of release of erythrocytes and the rate of red blood cell formation is closely related to the plasma concentration of erythropoietin.[33] The stimulus for erythropoietin production is believed to be a decrease in oxygen tissue tension in a sensor cell in the kidney. The mechanisms that regulate the production of erythropoietin itself are not clearly understood.

TESTOSTERONE. The difference in the hematocrit value between men and women is thought to result from the positive effect of testosterone on erythrocytosis. Testosterone increases red blood cell production presumably by increased erythropoietin production. In males, within 20 days after castration there is a 10% decrease in red blood cell mass. Conversely, administration of androgen to women increases red blood cell mass. On the average, hemoglobin level increases by 4.3 g/dl and hematocrit value by 11% in women. Hemoglobin increases by 1.1 g/dl in men treated by pharmacologic doses of testosterone.[16, 35] The presence of renal tissue is not an absolute requirement for stimulation of erythropoietin by androgens.[19, 55] This observation indicates that extrarenal sources of erythropoietin are physiologically important in the maintenance of red blood cell mass.

INFECTION. Chronic inflammatory states and infections are associated with impaired hematopoiesis. The features of the anemia of chronic disease include a low serum iron concentration and low total iron binding capacity. The plasma-iron turnover is elevated and the incorporation of radioactive iron into red blood cells ranges from normal to elevated. In addition, slight hemolysis may occur as the red blood cell half-life is often mildly shortened.

Chronic and acute infections may also be associated with increased secretion of interleukin (IL-1), a 13,000 to 16,000 molecular weight substance derived from monocytes and macrophages. Schooley and coworkers[52] showed that highly purified preparations of IL-1 antagonize the capacity of erythropoietin to stimulate the proliferation of mouse spleen and bone marrow erythroid processor cells in culture. This suppression was produced by both cloned murine IL-1 and purified and cloned human IL-1 and IL-2. Other macrophage products, such as tumor necrosis factor (TNF), were shown to inhibit erythroid progenitor cells *in vitro* and in the *in vivo* model of nude mice with transplanted Chinese hamster ovarian cells expressing the human TNF gene.[34] The effect of IL-1 and TNF on the bone marrow cells of COPD patients may help identify and characterize subgroups of COPD patients with a blunted, hematopoietic response.

CARBON MONOXIDE. Carbon monoxide interferes with oxygen binding in two ways. Carbon monoxide, like oxygen, binds to iron in heme; however, the affinity of hemoglobin for carbon monoxide is about 200 times that for oxygen. In high concentration, carbon monoxide may occupy the iron of all the hemes of the hemoglobin tetramer and result in a molecule that does not bind to oxygen. Hence, carbon monoxide results in a reduction in oxygen content. In low concentrations, carbon monoxide will bind only to some of the available iron sites. This effect changes the affinity of the remaining sites for oxygen and results in a shift of the oxyhemoglobin dissociation curve to the left,[2, 45, 46] thereby impairing oxygen release to tissues.

STUDIES OF HEMATOPOIESIS IN COPD

Most reviews of respiratory and hematologic disorders list polycythemia as a complication of patients with moderate to severe COPD; however, in clinical practice, polycythemia is not usually encountered in these patients. In the literature, several trends have emerged that continue to support this discrepancy between theory and practice. Heterogeneity of response in COPD patients compared with healthy subjects may be seen in Table 24–1.

Weil and colleagues[63] found that, whereas a correlation

TABLE 24–1. Hematopoietic Response of COPD Patients to Hypoxia

STUDY	NO OF PT	Sa_{O_2} RANGE OR MEAN ± S.D.	RBC	Hg	Hct	RCM	RCV	PV	RCT	BM ERYTHROID COMPONENT	CORRELATION OF RCM/Hg/Hct/ TO Sa_{O_2}	COMMENT FOR CORRELATION TO Sa_{O_2}
Wilson 1951[65]	69	70% to 90%	N	N	—	—	—	N	—	N	Low negative r = −0.32 (OCC versus Sa_{O_2})	Oxygen-carrying capacity (OCC) of blood was used as measure of its hemoglobin content. High altitude data show increased retic counts, increased bone marrow erythroid component, and increased Hg, Hct, and red blood cell volume with higher altitudes.
Hammarsten 1957[28]	16	85 ± 7	N	N	I	—	I	—	—	—	r = −0.166 (Hg versus Sa_{O_2})	
Freedman 1963[22]	8	55% to 83%	—	N to I	—	N to I	—	—		—	No correlation	
Vannier 1963[60]	18	73% to 96%	—	N	N	—	I	I		—		1. RCV was increased but less than that in high altitude residents with comparable Sa_{O_2} (Hurtado[32]) 2. RCV measured by Cr^{51}
Ayvazian 1969[1]	18	84% to 97%	—	N	N	—	—	—	—	—	No correlation	47 (59%) of patients had Hg and Hct values below those reported in high altitude Andean residents (Hurtado). RCM decreased versus expected RCM calculated from Andean altitude data (Tura[51]).
Gallo 1964[24]	80	63% to 95%	N	N	N (13 pt)	N (13 pt)	—	N	—	—	No correlation	
Lerzman 1962[40]	25	Pa_{O_2} 28–79 HG	—	— only	N to I	—	—	—	—	—	Moderate inverse correlation between Hct and Pa_{O_2} r = −0.564 and higher correlation with RCM r = 0.775	1. Patients were mainly COPD, seven obese, two CHD. 2. Correlation between Hct and RCM comparable to Andean altitude data (Hurtado[32]).
Shaw & Simpson 1961[56]	33	Sa_{O_2} 85	N	N	N	—	I	I	—	—	RCV negatively correlated to Sa_{O_2}, r = −0.59	RCV measured by Cr^{51}. No difference between r of healthy subjects at altitude and patients in this group.

Murray 1964[44]	17	71–92				I	I	—	—	—	No correlation between RCV and SaO_2	Only 11 patients were COPD; others had interstitial lung disease and CHD. Only in six patients was RCV appropriately elevated to the degree of hypoxemia. Two with mild hypoxia had elevated RCV.
Chan 1969[13]	30	—	—	—	—	—	—	—	—	—	High negative correlation between Hg and SaO_2; $r = -0.85$ and higher correlation between RCM and SaO_2, $r = -0.91$	Patients were coal miners. PFTs showed obstruction.
Weil 1968[60]	9	80–93	—	—	—	I	N to I	—	—	—	High negative correlation $r = -0.96$	Relationship between RCM and SaO_2 in 13 normal individuals at altitude, $r = -0.75$. Steeper increase in RCM in COPD with decrease in SaO_2 versus healthy subjects at altitude.
Harrison 1973[30]	19	86.2 ± 1.8	—	—	—	—	I	N	—	—	Correlation of RCV to SaO_2 moderately negative, $r = -0.486$	When compared with Weil,[63] the RC response to hypoxia in patients seems higher than in healthy subjects, but SaO_2 in patients were not really comparable to that in healthy subjects because patients desaturated more.
Cocking & Darke 1972[14]	45	87 ± 1.2	—	N	N	—	N	—	—	—	Correlation between RCV and SaO_2 moderately negative, $r = -0.66$	Compared with high altitude data there was a subnormal response because RCV SaO_2 regression lines were more shallow than those in healthy subjects at high altitude.

N = normal
I = increased
RBC = red blood cells
Hg = hemoglobin
Hct = hematocrit
RCM = red cell mass
RCV = red cell volume
PV = plasma volume
RCT = reticulocytes
SaO_2 = arterial oxygen saturation
BM = bone marrow
OCC = oxygen-carrying capacity
CHD = congestive heart failure
PFT = pulmonary function tests

between hematocrit value and oxygenation in COPD patients appears to be similar to that found in healthy subjects at different altitudes, the variation around the mean appeared much larger in the patient population. Although the number of observations is too small to confirm this hypothesis, it does support the clinical impression that frank polycythemia and anemia are both uncommon manifestations of stable patients with COPD. The greater variability seen in patients probably arises from factors, such as acidosis, nutrition, or infection, that could blunt erythropoiesis and result in attenuated hematocrit response to hypoxemia.

A number of studies exist that address whether COPD or one of its manifestations could result in changes in plasma volume, which could in turn affect hematocrit levels.[31, 56, 63] But review of these studies suggests that the presence or absence in clinical signs or treatment of fluid overload (congestive heart failure or cor pulmonale) significantly affects the relationship between oxygenation and plasma volume. The literature gives the impression that plasma volume is reduced in patients with COPD compared with healthy subjects at altitude matched for oxygenation. However, few studies statistically indicate significant differences possibly because the number of subjects in each study is insufficient to detect a difference, if present. One way around this problem would be to group studies; however, this approach is hampered because there are few common methodologic criteria on which to justify compilation of values from all these studies.

No studies are available that have systematically examined COPD patients for abnormalities in white blood cell production or function, independent of the effects of acute infection, drug side effect, idiosyncratic reaction, or other complicating illnesses. We assume that clinically significant abnormalities in white blood cell production or peripheral white blood cell function are unusual or not recognized in this patient population.

By far, the majority of studies of hematopoiesis in patients with COPD have been on red blood cell production and function. We have the impression that although there are COPD patients with increased red blood cell production, red blood cell mass, and hematocrit values appropriate to hypoxic exposure, a significant number of these patients have blunted responses and a smaller group have excessive responses. A paucity of studies is available of patients with high hematocrit values. A relatively greater frequency of studies of patients are done for factors that are associated with anemia. The following sections review these areas as well as discuss other factors potentially contributing to the variability in hematopoietic responses in patients with COPD.

FACTORS THAT INFLUENCE THE ERYTHROPOIETIC RESPONSE TO HYPOXEMIA IN COPD

2,3 DPG. Patients with CO_2 retention and acidosis have low levels of 2,3 DPG.[9, 43] This response results in a shift of the oxygen dissociation curve to the right, decreasing Sa_{O_2} at any given Pa_{O_2}. The key element in this counterproductive response appears to be respiratory acidosis. When red blood cell pH decreases, 6-phosphofructokinase activity is decreased, glycolysis is impaired, and 2,3 DPG concentration falls. This response leads to decreased oxygen availability in the peripheral tissues.

CARBOXYHEMOGLOBIN AND SMOKING. Carboxyhemoglobin levels vary among COPD patients according to their smoking habits and change according to the hematopoietic response. Sagone and Balcerzak[50] described five patients in whom smoking appeared to be the only cause of a raised red blood cell mass. Smith and Landaw[57] studied a larger group of 22 smokers with elevated blood carboxyhemoglobin levels of 11.6% and found red blood cell mass elevations in 14 of 18 patients, in which red blood cell mass was measured. The red blood cell mass decreased in all five patients who were able to stop smoking or to reduce it considerably. Similarly, Calverley and associates,[10] in patients with cor pulmonale, found red blood cell mass higher at any given level of Pa_{O_2} in 30 smokers than in 17 nonsmokers. Furthermore, in 12 of these patients, given long-term oxygen therapy, continued smoking prevented the expected fall in red blood cell mass. Foster and colleagues[23] reported similar findings in a study of the effect of supplemental oxygen on hematocrit value in a group of 11 hypoxic (Pa_{O_2}<61 mm Hg) polycythemic COPD patients. Five nonsmokers with a mean carboxyhemoglobin level of 2% to 8% showed a good response to therapy with supplemental oxyen, leading to a decrease in hematocrit value from 57% to 48%. Six smokers with a mean carboxyhemoglobin level of 13% exhibited only a partial response. In spite of similar values of arterial oxygen saturation, the smokers presumably had higher hematocrit levels before and after therapy because of superimposed desaturation due to carboxyhemoglobin.

NOCTURNAL HYPOXEMIA. Studies using intermittent sampling of arterial blood gases during sleep have suggested that hypoxemia can be aggravated during sleep in patients with COPD.[38, 39] This phenomenon was more clearly established following the introduction of ear oximetry. In 1979, two independent groups found that recurrent transient hypoxemia during sleep was frequent in patients with COPD and was particularly marked in those characterized as "blue bloaters."[11, 17, 66] These episodes of hypoxemia are more frequent during the REM phase of sleep in COPD patients as well as in healthy subjects.[12, 17, 20, 21] Many COPD patients are hypoxemic even when awake, so that the arterial Pa_{O_2}/Sa_{O_2} relationship is on the steep part of the oxyhemoglobin dissociation curve. As a result, prominent drops in saturation occur as ventilation and Pa_{O_2} decrease during sleep. In addition, some patients with COPD may have sleep apnea syndrome. The traits of snoring, altered sleep behavior, and excessive daytime sleepiness are clues to the presence of a sleep apnea syndrome independent of COPD.

A study by Wedzicha and coworkers[62] supports this concept of the importance of sleep-related oxygenation. Two groups of COPD patients (ten polycythemic and ten nonpolycythemic) were matched for severity of daytime hypoxemia by the measurement of arterial blood gases. Nocturnal Sa_{O_2} was recorded between 12 a.m. and 6 a.m. with an ear oximeter. The polycythemic group showed greater nocturnal arterial oxygen desaturation than the nonpolycthemic group. Consequently, a group of patients with COPD that seems to be homogeneous with respect to Sa_{O_2} while awake may have heterogeneous 24-hour profiles of oxygenation.

IRON DEFICIENCY. A number of studies of COPD patients report a below normal mean corpuscular hemoglobin concentration (MCHC).[24, 60] Wilson[65] measured serum iron (SI) levels in eight patients and found values of 102 ± 26 μg/100 ml (mean ± S.D.) that were lower than those of the control group (122 ± 38 μg/100 ml). He attributed this finding to chronic infection. In contrast, Hammarsten[28] found serum iron level to be elevated, 129 ± 12.2 μg/100 ml in COPD patients versus 89.4 ± 7.5 μg/100 ml in healthy subjects, and all 18 patients studied by Vannier[60] had a serum iron level that was in the normal range. Measurements of total iron binding capacity (TIBC) allow more complete conclusions. Shaw[56] reported that in 33 hypoxic patients serum iron level was abnormally low (86.3 ± 27.4 μg/100 ml versus 110.4 ± 50.5 μg/100 ml) and TIBC tended to be elevated (mean 378, range 248 to 500 μg/100 ml versus 315 and 249 to 378 μg/100 ml in healthy subjects). Consequently, iron deficiency could be diagnosed in a minority of patients. Furthermore, in many of these studies examinations of the blood smear revealed only minimally hypochromic red blood cells and no marked variation in size and shape of these cells, as opposed to the microcytosis characteristically seen in iron deficiency anemia.

Cocking and Darke[14] found iron deficiency in six of 45 patients with COPD. In this study, red blood cell morphology was normal, but these patients had a low serum iron concentration (mean ± S.D.) of 44.5 ± 10.43 μg/100 ml and high TIBC (438.8 ± 47.11 μg/100 ml) with a saturation ratio less than 16%. Iron deficiency was not associated with clinical evidence of excessive fecal blood loss. Only one of the six patients was considered to consume less than 12 mg of iron per 24 hours—the minimum daily requirement. Six other patients were found by history to have an iron-deficient diet; however, their red blood cell indices and morphology were normal as were their serum iron and TIBC. Although not determined in this study, iron deficiency could have resulted from specific malabsorption of iron or from clinically inapparent hemolytic anemia.

Hence, most studies show that simple iron deficiency is present in a minority of COPD patients, but, when present, may not be associated with fecal blood loss. Factors that may predispose patients to chronic anemia that would further impair tissue oxygen delivery, such as liver dysfunction and alcohol intake commonly occurring in this group, have not been systematically examined.

INFECTION. Wilson and colleagues[65] were among the first investigators to suggest that some patients with COPD had inappropriately low hematocrit values for their degree of hypoxemia and that their responses could be explained by an anemia associated with chronic disease. These workers suggested a connection between chronic bronchitis or chronic lower respiratory tract infections and hematologic findings in patients with stable COPD. Later studies have shown that between 20% and 80% of COPD patients exhibit one or more of the characteristic levels of serum iron, total iron binding capacity, and red blood cell survival commonly found in patients with chronic nonrespiratory inflammatory disease.[1, 40, 51, 56, 60] The variable incidence of hematologic findings consistent with anemia of chronic disease probably arises from small sample sizes and differences in patient selection.

Acute infections may also alter hematopoietic responses in patients with COPD. Unlike other series that studied only stable patients, nine of 15 patients in the series by Tura[51] had evidence of acute infection, e.g., fever, increase in sputum production, and radiographic changes. The degree of erythrocytosis in this group as measured by red blood cell volume was considered to be inappropriately low for the degree of hypoxemia. Mean serum iron level and TIBC were normal and did not suggest either chronic blood loss or infection. However, a moderate decrease in mean red blood cell lifespan and a decrease in incorporation of exogenously given Fe^{59} into red blood cells was noted. The investigators concluded that acute infection could result in decreased red blood cell survival and possibly reduced erythropoiesis. Hence, erythrocytosis in patients with COPD can therefore be affected by both acute and chronic infection.

HORMONES AND ERYTHROPOIETIC FUNCTION: ERYTHROPOIETIN. Gallo and coworkers[24] measured serum erythropoietic activity in 13 COPD patients. Levels were determined in a bioassay of the percent of Fe^{59} uptake in rat bone marrow progenitor cells. The mean value of 17 determinations performed in the 13 COPD patients was 9.5 ± 26% (mean ± S.D.) versus 8.2 ± 1.5% in healthy subjects. In only five of 13 patients was the level of induced erythropoietic activity more than 2 standard deviations (S.D.) above the mean control value. A small but significant negative correlation was found between red blood cell mass and erythropoietin (EPO) levels ($r = -0.5$, $P<0.05$).

Later studies of EPO levels used a radioimmunoassay (RIA) technique.[15] Koefler and Goldwasser[37] reported the serum level of RIA-measured EPO in 26 healthy individuals to be (mean ± S.D.) 14.9 ± 4.2 μ/ml. In the same report, EPO levels in seven patients with lung disease were 80 ± 99 μ/ml. The large S.D. in this group was due to several patients with very high EPO levels. Mean hematocrit value in the group of patients with lung disease was 55% versus 41% in healthy individuals.

More detailed studies were reported by Miller and colleagues.[41] These investigators found immunoreactive serum EPO levels in 48 healthy volunteers ages 20 to 60 to be 18.5 ± 5 μ/ml (mean ± S.D.). Levels of the hormone were also measured sequentially every 4 hours over a 24-hour period in 17 additional healthy volunteers, and no diurnal variation was apparent. Erythropoietin levels were measured also in the 28 patients with stable COPD. The mean EPO level was within the normal range (19.6 ± 1.2 μ/ml); however, in six patients, levels were clearly elevated (up to three times) beyond the normal range. Diurnal variation of EPO levels was measured in 15 COPD patients. In contrast to the findings in healthy subjects, COPD patients exhibited a diurnal variation of EPO levels with peak levels occurring at midnight. These findings were found both in smokers and nonsmokers and no explanation was offered to account for the diurnal rhythm. In this study, direct correlation was shown between hemoglobin levels and the serum EPO level ($r = 0.57$, $P<0.01$). No correlation was found among EPO level and the Po_2, O_2 content, O_2 saturation, pH, $Paco_2$, hematocrit value, and red blood cell mass. However, most of these patients had only mild daytime hypoxemia and little evidence for an increase in red blood cell mass.

Guidet and coworkers[26] reported on EPO levels in 21 patients with severe but stable COPD. Patients had been on supplemental oxygen for at least 1 week but for less than 6 months. Twelve patients were polycythemic (hematocrit value, 52% ± 7; red blood cell mass, 66 ± 7 ml/kg) and nine were nonpolycythemic. Hypoxia was severe in both groups, with a mean Pao_2 of 47 mm Hg. Daytime serum levels of EPO were measured and were found to be elevated in 85% of all patients; however, there was no significant difference between nonpolycythemic and polycythemic groups. This study also evaluated the response of bone marrow isolated from the patient to exogenous EPO. In the absence of exogenous EPO, none of the subjects exhibited spontaneous colonies of medullary erythroid progenitors, thus confirming that polycythemia was not the result of a primary disorder of the bone marrow. After injection of one unit of exogenous EPO, the number of new colonies of erythroid burst-forming units was similar in both polycythemic and nonpolycythemic groups. Apparently, the absence of adaptive polycythemia in the nonpolycythemic group with severe hypoxia was not related to a lack of sensitive erythroid progenitors.

Wedzicha and coworkers[62] studied two selected groups of ten COPD patients: ten with compensatory polycythemia and ten without (with mean red blood cell mass ± 1 S.D. of 24.7 ± 4.2 ml/kg and 47.8 ± 7.5 ml/kg, respectively). Although the two groups were matched for severity of daytime hypoxemia, the polycythemic patients showed greater nocturnal arterial oxygen desaturation than the nonpolycythemic group. Differences in erythropoietin levels were present. However, RIA-measured EPO in both groups were within the same range, although in five of the polycythemia patients, occasional higher levels were present. More studies on larger groups of patients may be necessary to correlate polycythemia, nocturnal desaturation, and EPO levels.

TESTOSTERONE. Depression of urinary 17-ketosteroids has been demonstrated in residents of high altitudes. This finding is interpreted to suggest that testicular endocrine activity is reduced during hypoxic conditions. In a group of 19 hypoxic

COPD patients, Semple and colleagues[54] observed that testosterone levels were decreased in 13 and within the low normal range in the other patients. There was a strong correlation between the degree of testosterone reduction and the degree of hypoxemia ($r = 0.72$) and a slightly less strong correlation between the level of hypercapnia and the degree of testosterone reduction ($r = 0.66$). A decrease in testosterone levels would reduce the bone marrow response to hypoxia, and variable testosterone levels in COPD patients would partially explain the variable erythropoietic response to hypoxemia in COPD patients.

CLINICAL ASSESSMENT OF ERYTHROPOIETIC ABNORMALITIES IN COPD

POLYCYTHEMIA. Other etiologies should be excluded before one can presume that polycythemia is secondary to hypoxemia induced by lung disease. Generally, elevation of red blood cell mass may result either from increased proliferation of erythroid progenitors due to a primary intrinsic cellular defect epitomized by polycythemia rubra vera or from altered erythropoietic regulatory activity. The secondary polycythemia results from either physiologically appropriate signals to compensate for inadequate tissue oxygenation or from inappropriate stimulation of erythropoiesis. The different etiologies of polycythemia are summarized in Table 24–2, and a checklist of the possible workup of polycythemia is presented in Table 24–3.

Because low EPO levels in the presence of an elevated red blood cell mass are characteristic of primary polycythemia, the measurement of EPO levels has replaced other criteria for the diagnosis of polycythemia vera. Secondary polycythemia is caused in many cases by a secondary release or potentiation of EPO effect. In most cases, increased EPO is present and part of a compensatory effect to minimize compromised oxygen tissue delivery. At some high altitudes oxygen availability is decreased. We would expect COPD patients to be more polycythemic if they live at high altitudes. Another condition that may compromise oxygen tissue delivery is a state of increased hemoglobin affinity. This is a result of point mutations that produce single amino acid substitutions that stabilize oxyhemoglobin (e.g., hemoglobins Chesapeake and Yakima) or lead to altered binding of 2,3 DPG (e.g., hemoglobin Little Rock). Rare instances of a high oxygen affinity hemoglobinopathy should be excluded by hemoglobin electrophoresis and complete oxyhemoglobin dissociation curve. Carboxyhemoglobin levels should be measured in COPD patients because many patients continue to smoke.

TABLE 24–2. Classification of Polycythemia

PRIMARY AUTONOMOUS ERYTHROPOIESIS: POLYCYTHEMIA RUBRA VERA SECONDARY
Physiologically appropriate (decreased tissue oxygenation)
High altitude
Chronic lung disease or alveolar hypoventilation
Cardiovascular right-to-left shunt
High oxygen affinity hemoglobinopathy
Congenitally decreased erythrocyte 2,3-diphosphoglycerate
Carboxyhemoglobinemia
Histiotoxic (for example, cobalt)
PHYSIOLOGICALLY INAPPROPRIATE (NORMAL TISSUE OXYGENATION)
Tumors producing erythropoietin or other erythropoietic substances
Renal cell carcinoma
Cerebellar hemangioblastoma
Hypotony
Uterine leiomyoma
Ovarian carcinoma
Pheochromocytoma
Renal disease
Cysts
Hydronephrosis
Bartter syndrome
Transplantation
Adrenocortical hypersecretion
Relative polycythemia (Gaisböck syndrome, spurious or stress erythrocytosis)

Modified from Golde DW, Hocking WG, Koeffler HP, Adamson JW. Ann Intern Med 1981; 95:71–87.

TABLE 24–3. Evaluation of COPD Patients with Polycythemia

HISTORY
Smoking history
Use of steroids and nonsteroidal anti-inflammatory drugs (NSAIDS)
History suggestive of gastrointestinal blood loss (heartburn, epigastric pain)
Detailed nutritional history
Familial history of polycythemia
Hematuria
PHYSICAL EXAMINATION
Plethora, cyanosis, clubbing, hepato- and splenomegaly
Left and right heart failure, heart murmurs, chest bruits, pedal edema
Abdomen, for renal masses and bruits
Neurologic examination
LABORATORY STUDIES
Chest roentgenogram
Arterial blood gases
24-hour oximetry (if inadequate, complete sleep study)
Carboxyhemoglobin level
Red blood cell mass
Erythropoietin, carboxyhemoglobin levels
Hemoglobin electrophoresis (complete oxyhemoglobin dissociation curve if available)
Abdominal, especially renal ultrasound
Computed axial tomography of the head if history and physical examination suggest a central nervous system mass
White blood cell and platelet count
Serum iron, total iron-binding capacity (TIBC), folate, B_{12} levels

The existence of right-to-left cardiac or systemic shunts results in systemic hypoxemia or selective renal hypoxia. Some systemic shunts, like those occurring in patients with cirrhosis of the liver, are caused by pulmonary arteriovenous shunts or direct right-to-left communications between pulmonary veins. Echocardiography of the heart and cineangiography may be necessary to exclude cardiac and renal shunts. Physiologically inappropriate secondary erythrocythemia occurs in two situations: autonomous secretion of erythroid stimulating substances by certain neoplasms, for example, erythropoietin or adrenal corticosteroids, and local renal ischemia, produced by renal mass lesions, hydronephrosis, or renal vascular lesions, or after renal transplantation. Regional ischemia is detected by a presumed renal oxygen sensor and leads to increased EPO secretion and polycythemia.

Considerable evidence indicates that ectopic EPO secretion occurs in some tumors.[29] Circumstantial evidence suggests that the production of other EPO substances, such as steroids, by some tumors leads to erythrocytosis.[59, 61] The tumors most frequently associated with erythrocythemia are renal cell carcinomas, which with other renal tumors account for more than a third of all reported cases.[29] Hepatoma, cerebellar hemangioblastoma, uterus leiomyoma, and adrenal carcinoma also have been associated with polycythemia.[59] Detailed physical diagnosis and, if appropriate, head computed tomography (CT) and magnetic resonance imaging, as well as abdominal

CT or ultrasound, may be necessary to exclude these tumors as causes of secondary polycythemia.

ANEMIA. In the pre-oxygen therapy era, the common practice of recurrent and frequent phlebotomy increased blood loss in COPD patients and resulted in iron deficiency anemia. In our experience, COPD patients are usually not anemic. If anemia is present, blood loss should be suspected. COPD patients may be more prone to gastrointestinal bleeding due to peptic ulcers since they, like all patients with chronic disease, have increased use of nonsteroidal anti-inflammatory agents. Potential nutritional deficiencies should be eliminated by taking a history. However, evidence exists for an iron deficiency anemia of unknown cause and of mild severity in this population.[14]

REFERENCES

1. Ayvazian LF, Richardson DE, Silber R. Erythrokinetic studies during antimicrobial therapy in pulmonary emphysema. Am Rev Respir Dis 1969; 100:305–313.
2. Baldwin J, Chothia C. Hemoglobin: the structural changes related to ligand binding and its allosteric mechanism. J Mol Biol 1979; 129:175–220.
3. Bauer C. On the respiratory function of hemoglobin. Rev Physiol Biochem-Pharmacol 1974; 70:1–29.
4. Beall CM, Strohl KP, Brittenham G. Reappraisal of Andean high altitude erythrocytosis from a Himalayan perspective. Semin Respir Med 1983; 5:195–201.
5. Benesch R, Benesch RE. Intracellular organic phosphates as regulators of oxygen release by hemoglobin. Nature 1969; 221:618–622.
6. Beru N, McDonald J, LaCombe C, Goldwasser E. Expression of the erythropoietin gene. Mol Cell Biol 1986; 6:2571–2575.
7. Beru N, Goldwasser E. The regulation of heme biosynthesis during erythropoietin-induced erythroid differentiation. J Biol Chem 1985; 260:9251–9257.
8. Bondurant M, Koury M. Anemia induces accumulation of erythropoietin mRNA in the kidney and liver. Mol Cell Biol 1986; 6:2731–2733.
9. Brewer J, Eaton J. Erythrocyte metabolism: interaction with oxygen transport. Science 1971; 171:1205.
10. Calverley PM, Leggett RJ, McElderry L, Flenley DC. Cigarette smoking and secondary polycythemia in hypoxic cor pulmonale. Am Rev Respir Dis 1982; 125:507–510.
11. Catterall JR, Douglas NJ, Calverley PM, et al. Transient hypoxemia during sleep in chronic obstructive pulmonary disease is not a sleep apnea syndrome. Am Rev Respir Dis 1983; 128:24–29.
12. Catterall JR, Calverley PM, Macnee W, et al. The mechanism of transient nocturnal hypoxemia in hypoxic chronic bronchitis and emphysema. J Appl Physiol 1985; 59:1698–1703.
13. Chan BW. Polycythemia in coal miners with chronic lung disease. Br Med J 1969; 10:349–350.
14. Cocking JB, Darke CS. Blood volume studies in chronic obstructive nonspecific lung disease. Thorax 1972; 27:44–51.
15. Cotes PM, Dore CJ, LiuYin JA, et al. Determination of serum immunoreactive erythropoietin in the investigation of erythrocytosis. N Engl J Med 1986; 315:283–287.
16. Cunningham GR, Silverman VE. Thornby: the potential for an androgen male contraceptive. J Clin Endocrinol Metab 1979; 49:520–526.
17. Douglas NJ, Calverley PM, Leggett RJ, et al. Transient hypoxemia during sleep in chronic bronchitis and emphysema. Lancet 1979; i:1–4.
18. Douglas NJ, White DP, Pichet CK, et al. Respiration during sleep in normal man. Thorax 1982; 37:840–844.
19. Evans, RP, Amerson AB. Androgens and erythropoiesis. J Clin Pharmacol 1974; 14:94–101.
20. Fleetham J, West P, Mezon B, et al. Sleep, arousals, and oxygen desaturation in chronic obstructive pulmonary disease. The effect of oxygen therapy. Am Rev Respir Dis 1982; 125:429–433.
21. Flick MR, Block AJ. Continuous *in vivo* monitoring of arterial oxygenation in chronic obstructive lung disease. Ann Intern Med 1977; 86:725–730.
22. Freedman BJ, Penington DG. Erythrocytosis in emphysema. Br J Haematol 1963; 9:425–430.
23. Foster LJ, Corrigan K, Goldman AL. Effectiveness of oxygen therapy in hypoxic polycythemic smokers. Chest 1978; 73:572–576.
24. Gallo RC, Fraimow W, Cathcart RT, Erslev AJ. Erythropoietic response in chronic pulmonary disease. Arch Intern Med 1964; 113:559–567.
25. Golde DW, Hocking WG, Koeffler HP, Adamson JW. Polycythemia: Mechanisms and management. Ann Intern Med 1981; 95:71–87.
26. Guidet B, Offenstadt G, Boffa G, et al. Polycythemia in chronic obstructive pulmonary disease. Chest 1987; 92:867.
27. Guilleminault C, Cummiskey J, Motta J. Chronic obstructive air flow disease and sleep studies. Am Rev Respir Dis 1980; 122:397–406.
28. Hammarsten JF, Whitcomb WH, Johnson PC, Lowell JR. The hematologic adaptation of patients with hypoxia due to pulmonary emphysema. Am Rev Tuberc 1958; 78:391–398.
29. Hammond D, Winnick S. Paraneoplastic erythrocytosis and ectopic erythropoietins. Ann NY Acad Sci 1974; 230:219–227.
30. Harrison BD. Polycythemia in a selected group of patients with chronic airway obstruction. Clin Sci 1973; 44:563–570.
31. Hume R. Blood volume changes in chronic bronchitis and emphysema. Br J Haematol 1968; 15:131–139.
32. Hurtado A, Merino C, Delgado E. Influence of anoxemia on the hemopoietic activity. Arch Intern Med 1945; 75:284.
33. Jelkman W. Renal erythropoietin: properties and production. Rev Physiol Biochem Pharmacol 1986; 104:139.
34. Johnson RA, Waddelow TA, Oliff A, Roodman GD. Tumor necrosis factor is an inhibitor of erythropoiesis *in vivo*. Clin Res 1988; 36(3):412A.
35. Kenedy BJ, Gilbertson AS. Increased erythropoiesis induced by androgenic hormone therapy. N Engl J Med 1957; 256:719–726.
36. Kilmartin JV, Rossi-Bernardi L. Interaction of hemoglobin with hydrogen ions, carbon dioxide, and organic phosphates. Physiol Rev 1973; 53:836–890.
37. Koeffler HP, Goldwasser E. Erythropoietin radioimmunoassay in evaluating patients with polycythemia. Am Coll Phys 1981; 94:44–47.
38. Koo KW, Sax DS, Snider GL. Arterial blood gases and pH during sleep in chronic obstructive pulmonary disease. Am J Med 1975; 58:663–670.
39. Leitch AG, Clancy LJ, Leggett RJE, et al. Arterial blood gas tensions, hydrogen ion and electroencephalogram during sleep in patients with chronic ventilatory failure. Thorax 1976; 31:730–735.
40. Lertzman M, Israels LG, Cherniack RM. Erythropoiesis and ferrokinetics in chronic respiratory disease. Ann Intern Med 1962; 56:821–833.
41. Miller ME, Garcia JF, Cohen RA, et al. Diurnal levels of immunoreactive erythropoietin in normal subjects and subjects with chronic lung disease. Br J Haematol 1981; 49:189–200.
42. Miller NL, Francis PW, Gururty D, et al. Mechanism of hemoglobin desaturation during REM sleep in normal subjects and in patients with cystic fibrosis. Am Rev Respir Dis 1980; 121:463–469.
43. Mulhausen R. The affinity of hemoglobin for oxygen [editorial]. Circulation 1970; 42:195.
44. Murray JF. Arterial studies in primary and secondary polycythemic disorders. Am Rev Respir Dis 1965; 92:435–449.
45. Perutz MF. Hemoglobin structure and respiratory transport. Sci Am 1978; 239:92–125.
46. Perutz MF. Regulation of oxygen affinity of hemoglobin: influence of structure of the globin on the heme iron. Ann Rev Biochem 1979; 48:327–386.
47. Perutz MF. Stereochemistry of cooperative effects of hemoglobin. Nature 1970; 228:726–739.
48. Robin EO, Whaley RD, Crump CC, et al. Alveolar gas tensions, pulmonary ventilation and blood pH during physiological sleep in normal subjects. J Clin Invest 1958; 37:981–989.
49. Rorth M. Hypoxia, red cell oxygen affinity and erythropoietin production. Clin Hematol 1974; 3:595–607.
50. Sagone A, Balcerzak SP. Smoking as a cause of erythrocytosis. Ann Intern Med 1975; 82:512–515.
51. Tura S, Pollycove M, Gelpi AP. Erythrocyte and iron-kinetics in patients with chronic pulmonary emphysema. J Nucl Med 1962; 3:110–127.

52. Schooley JC, Kullgreen B, Allison AC. Inhibition by interleukin 1 of the action of erythropoietin on erythroid predecessors and its possible role in the pathogenesis of hypoplastic anemias. Br J Hematol 1987; 67:11–17.
53. Schuster S, Wilson J, Erslev A, Caro J. Physiologic regulation and tissue localization of renal erythropoietin messenger RNA. Blood 1987; 70:316–318.
54. Semple PD'A, Beastall GH, Watson WS, Hume R. Serum testosterone depression associated with hypoxia in respiratory failure. Clin Sci 1980; 58:105–106.
55. Shahide NT. Androgens and erythropoiesis. N Engl J Med 1973; 289:72–80.
56. Shaw DB, Simpson T. Polycythemia in emphysema. Q J Med 1961; 30:135–150.
57. Smith JR, Landaw SA. Smoker's polycythemia. N Engl J Med 1978; 298:6–10.
58. Stradling JR, Lane DJ. Development of secondary polycythemia in chronic airway obstruction. Thorax 1981; 36:321–325.
59. Thorling EB. Paraneoplastic erythrocytosis and inappropriate erythropoietin production: a review. Scand J Hematol 1972; 17:1–166.
60. Vannier T, Mauricio MB, Dulfano J, et al. Emphysema, hypoxia and the polycythemic response. N Engl J Med 1963; 269:176–178.
61. Waldmann TA, Rosse WF, Swarm RL. The erythropoiesis-stimulation factors produced by tumor. Ann NY Acad Sci 1968; 149:509–515.
62. Wedzicha JA, Cotes PM, Empey DW, et al. Serum immunoreactive erythropoietin in hypoxic lung disease with and without polycythemia. Clin Sci 1985; 69:413–422.
63. Weil JV, Jamieson G, Brown DW, et al. The red cell mass-arterial oxygen relationship in normal man. Application to patients with chronic obstructive airway disease. J Clin Invest 1968; 47:1627–1639.
64. Wennesland R, Brown E, Hopper J, et al. Red cell plasma and blood volume in healthy men measured by radiochromium (Cr^{51}) cell tagging and hematocrit: influence of age, somatotype and habits of physical activity on the variance after regression of volumes to height and weight combined. J Clin Invest 1959; 38:1065–1077.
65. Wilson RH, Borden CW, Ebert RV. Adaptation to anoxia in chronic pulmonary emphysema. Arch Intern Med 1951; 88:581–590.
66. Wynne JW, Block AJ, Hemingway J, et al. Disordered breathing and oxygen desaturation during sleep in patients with chronic obstructive lung disease (COLD). Am J Med 1979; 56:573–579.

Chapter 25

SODIUM AND WATER METABOLISM IN COPD

Mark O. Farber **Felice Manfredi**

Edema and hyponatremia are disturbances that are seen commonly in the advanced stages of chronic obstructive pulmonary disease (COPD). Their presence often complicates therapy, owing to the interacting side effects of electrolyte imbalances, diuretics, and digitalis.

The magnitude of the problem is great, although the exact incidence of significant clinical alterations in sodium and water balance in COPD is not well documented. In 350 COPD patients with chronic respiratory failure (CRF) admitted to our intensive care unit during a 5-year period for an acute infectious exacerbation of the disease, edema was noted in approximately 50% (unpublished observations). The frequency of edema remains high through the terminal years of the illness; about one half of the COPD patients followed in our pulmonary clinic for chronic respiratory failure requiring long-term oxygen supplementation are believed to require some form of diuretic therapy for control of excessive body sodium accumulation. Other centers seem to have had similar experiences.

Hyponatremia, i.e., plasma sodium less than 130 mEq/L, presents less of a clinical problem in these patients, except perhaps during episodes of acute respiratory failure.[17] Hyponatremia occurs in approximately 25% of patients with advanced COPD, almost all of whom are edematous.[15]

The major points pertinent to the incidence of edema and hyponatremia in COPD are as follows: (1) edema occurs only in the late stages of the disease, when significant chronic hypercapnia (chronic respiratory failure) is present; (2) edema is more common and more conspicuous when CRF is complicated by episodes of acute respiratory failure; (3) the pattern of hyponatremia parallels that of edema, but with a lower frequency.

PRACTICAL IMPLICATIONS

The previous comments on the frequency distribution of edema and hyponatremia in the progressive course of COPD assume greater import when viewed in the context of their prognostic implications and the therapeutic dilemmas that they may create for the clinician.

"Cor pulmonale" has been clearly defined for over 3 decades as a physiologic disturbance, i.e., right ventricular hypertrophy secondary to lung disease.[8] Yet, this term is frequently used to describe a syndrome of systemic venous hypertension, congested liver, and peripheral edema. It becomes apparent in the course of the discussion on pathogenesis that cor pulmonale is simply associated with but is not the cause of edema formation. Regardless of the meaning assigned to the term, it is clear that cor pulmonale indicates significant hypoxemia and, in the case of COPD, significant hypercapnia. The mean 4-year mortality of all patients with COPD is increased and undoubtedly varies with the severity of the lung disease. With cor pulmonale, read significant hypoxemia and hypercapnia, the 4-year mortality of this subpopulation rises dramatically.[24, 36, 42]

The physician faced with managing an edematous COPD patient is likely to prescribe (1) a restricted sodium diet; (2) a thiazide or a loop diuretic; and (3) a digitalis preparation. Sodium restriction is both appropriate and safe, because the patient certainly has an excess of body sodium. Diuretics are not very rational therapeutic choices since they do not treat any of the underlying physiologic abnormalities, as becomes apparent from the discussion of current views on pathogenesis. In addition, they often complicate matters by producing a hypochloremic, hypokalemic alkalosis resulting in compensatory hypoventilation and by increasing the potential for hyponatremia.[29] Digitalis preparations are unnecessary because global cardiac function is intact and has been shown to be unaffected by these agents. Further, the combination of hypoxemia, hypokalemia, and digitalis therapy is a triad likely to precipitate arrhythmias. If patients also receive beta agonists for bronchospasm, arrhythmias will occur more often.[29]

The distinction between the edematous state of respiratory origin and that of cardiac origin may be a fine one. Chronic obstructive pulmonary disease and heart disease often coexist, because they share the same target population. Dyspnea, orthopnea, cyanosis, and cardiomegaly with gallop sounds are common in both. Electrocardiographic findings may not be helpful. In acutely ill patients, in whom the distinction is most critical, the presence of cold, clammy extremities (expression of a low output state) and pleural effusion (expression of increased pulmonary venous pressure) may help resolve the issue, as these findings are the hallmark of heart failure and are not seen in decompensated COPD patients. Of the laboratory procedures, aside from the proper interpretation of arterial blood gas values, measurement of cardiac function parameters, such as left ventricular wall motion and ejection fraction, can be useful.

Hyponatremia has not been shown to affect prognosis but its presence, too, poses some management difficulties. Water restriction is often mandated, which is pathophysiologically sound, but may impair clearance of bronchial secretions. Profound hyponatremia may become an indication for hypertonic saline infusion, an obviously risky maneuver in patients who are edematous and therefore sodium overloaded. The combination of marked edema and profound hyponatremia in COPD patients in acute respiratory failure may present almost insurmountable therapeutic dilemmas even to the well-trained pulmonary intensivist.

PREVIOUS CONCEPTS

Traditionally, edema in COPD was believed to arise from cor pulmonale and right heart failure with systemic venous hypertension. This condition, in turn, was believed to cause leakage of sodium-rich fluid into interstitial tissues, lead to a reduction in cardiac output, or both, because pulmonary vascular resistance is elevated with consequent decrease in renal blood flow. The sequence of pulmonary hypertension→ right ventricular failure→ venous engorgement→ edema seemed to explain the pathogenesis of right heart failure.[4] The hyponatremia associated with COPD, in the past, was largely ignored. If mentioned, it was (1) left unexplained; (2) ascribed to "sick cell syndrome" or a "reset osmostat"[3]; (3) assumed to have, if associated with edema, the same pathogenesis as that proposed for the hyponatremia seen in other edematous states, i.e., "dilutional," from excessive water intake in the presence of impaired free water excretion[18]; and (4) attributed, loosely, to "salt wasting."[2]

MODERN CONCEPTS

In a now classic paper, Campbell and Short[7] pointed out that edema from lung disease is virtually always associated with an elevated level of arterial carbon dioxide pressure ($Pa{CO_2}$). The following observations have been made that support this idea. In patients with stable, hypercapneic COPD and mild or moderate hypoxemia, effective renal plasma flow (ERPF) is diminished and total body sodium is increased, with or without clinical evidence of edema.[2, 15] Also, the greater the level of CO_2 retention, the greater the decrease in renal perfusion, which is caused by an increase in renal vascular resistance. Diminished capacity to excrete sodium and water is correlated with the reduction in effective renal plasma flow in COPD patients. As the disease progresses, often with worsening CO_2 retention and hypoxemia, renal function declines further and edema develops.[15]

Hormonal perturbations occur along with the changes in renal function. Plasma catecholamine levels, an index of renal sympathetic tone, are elevated early in the course of the disease in association with hypercapnia.[21, 35] Later, when edema is present the renin-angiotensin-aldosterone system is activated.[15, 33, 37] About 40% or more of edematous COPD patients will exhibit secondary hyperaldosteronism with increased plasma levels of renin, angiotensin II, and aldosterone.[15]

A significant proportion of patients with advanced COPD demonstrate hyponatremia. All patients with hyponatremia have inappropriately elevated arginine vasopressin (AVP), an antidiuretic hormone, for the level of plasma osmolality.[15, 17, 43] The elevation of AVP seems to be the cause of the hyponatremia. These patients also demonstrate an exaggerated AVP response to infusion of hypertonic saline.[15, 16]

In the past 3 years, atrial natriuretic hormone (ANH) level has also been shown to be elevated late in the course of COPD.[1, 5, 30] Its potential role in producing hyponatremia is discussed subsequently.

For convenience, three stages of COPD can be described: stage I = normocapnia and mild hypoxemia; stage II = hypercapnia and moderate hypoxemia; and stage III = hypercapnia and moderate to severe hypoxemia. The profile of renal functional and hormonal changes in the course of COPD are illustrated in Table 25–1. Chronic obstructive pulmonary disease patients with normocapnia and mild hypoxemia display normal age-adjusted renal functional parameters and normal hormonal levels.[12, 13] Note the earlier onset of renal functional derangements as compared with onset of hormonal abnormalities later in the course of the disease, when edema and hyponatremia become evident. Significant correlations between the various renal and hormonal parameters are shown in Table 25–2.

CHANGES IN SALT AND H_2O BALANCE WITH DISEASE PROGRESSION

It is clear that patients with advanced lung disease do not have low cardiac output state or heart failure in the usual sense. Many investigations have documented normal to elevated cardiac output in such patients and in most instances right atrial and systemic venous pressures are minimally, if at

TABLE 25–1. Profile of Renal and Hormonal Function in the Three Stages of COPD

	Stage I	Stage II	Stage III
Edema	–	±	+ + +†
Hyponatremia	–	–	+†
GFR	N	±N	↓†
ERPF	N	↓↓*	↓↓↓†
FF	N	↑*	↑↑†
H_2O Excretion	N	↓↓*	↓↓↓†
Na^+ Excretion	N	↓↓*	↓↓*
Catecholamines	N	↑*	↑↑†
PRA	N	±↑	↑↑†
PA	N	±↑	↑↑†
AVP	N	±N	↑†
ANH	N	±N	↑†

*Statistically different from Stage I ($P < 0.05$)
†Statistically different from Stage II ($P < 0.05$)
GFR = glomerular filtration rate; ERPF = effective renal plasma flow; FF = filtration fraction; PRA = plasma renin activity; PA = plasma aldosterone; AVP = arginine vasopressin; ANH = atrial natriuretic hormone.

all, elevated.[10, 20, 21, 26, 35] As the disease worsens and $Paco_2$ rises, cellular pH falls. The kidney responds by increasing the rate of tubular sodium-hydrogen ion (and other cations) exchange as fractional bicarbonate reabsorption increases over the entire nephron.[25] Often, a net increase in sodium reabsorption is likely due to the avid sparing of bicarbonate.

Associated with hypercapnia and intracellular acidosis, stimulation of sympathetic tone increases and the plasma level of norepinephrine increases.[21, 35] Greater renal sympathetic tone enhances tubular sodium reabsorption by diminishing effective renal plasma flow and possibly inducing a redistribution in renal blood flow.[11] When effective renal plasma flow declines, filtration fraction (FF) increases since glomerular filtration rate (GFR) is stable. A concomitant, mandatory increase in peritubular oncotic pressure and in tubular sodium reabsorption also occurs. Impairment of renal sodium and water excretion becomes measurable. Typically, patients with COPD, hypercapnia, and mild hypoxemia are unable to normally excrete a sodium or a water load.[12, 13] Once renal perfusion declines sufficiently so that GRF begins to fall, stimulation of the renin-angiotensin-aldosterone axis occurs, producing a state of "secondary hyperaldosteronism"—late in the course of the disease, as we have seen—which further increases sodium retention. The continued declining ability to excrete sodium and the progressive diminution of renal perfusion, perhaps exacerbated by increasing hypoxemia, invariably lead to edema formation. This pathogenetic scheme is illustrated in Figure 25–1.

TABLE 25–2. Correlations in COPD ($P < 0.05$)

Inverse
$Paco_2$ versus ERPF
ERPF versus FF
$Paco_2$ versus % H_2O excretion
$Paco_2$ versus Na^+ excretion
PRA versus Na^+ excretion
PA versus Na^+ excretion
AVP versus free H_2O clearance
Direct
ERPF versus % H_2O excretion
ERPF versus Na^+ excretion
Na^+ excretion versus % H_2O excretion
PRA versus PA

AVP = arginine vasopressin; ERPF = effective renal plasma flow; FF = filtration fraction; PA = plasma aldosterone; $Paco_2$ = arterial carbon dioxide pressure; PRA = plasma renin activity.

Arginine vasopressin (AVP) elevation then occurs, the *conditio sine qua non* for hyponatremia, although the mechanism of the AVP elevation is unclear. Two main possibilities are available, both invoking nonosmotic stimuli.

Experimental evidence exists that increases in angiotensin II stimulate AVP directly, but this notion is hotly debated.[40] Indirect support for this concept can be derived from a clinical study[16] in which angiotensin-converting enzyme inhibition normalized the slope of the plasma AVP/plasma osmolality line in hypercapneic COPD. Presumably, the resultant reduction in angiotensin II was responsible for correcting the abnormal AVP/Posm relationship (see Fig. 25–1). Another possibility is that advanced hypercapneic COPD with edema leads to a decreased effective circulating blood volume, as postulated in decompensated cirrhosis and congestive heart failure. Low circulating volume stimulates baroreceptors, resulting in the nonosmotic release of AVP.[40]

Measurements of effective circulating volume, defined as the discrepancy between the circulating arterial blood volume and the vascular capacity of the circulation, are not available on COPD patients. Regardless of the mechanism of AVP stimulation, it is clear that hyponatremia in COPD patients is the expression of inappropriate antidiuretic hormone secretion.[15, 17, 43] However, not all patients with elevated AVP levels have hyponatremia. Not uncommonly, some of these patients with plasma AVP levels inappropriately high for plasma osmolality have plasma sodium levels within the normal range. It is well known that plasma sodium may be normal in patients with inappropriate AVP secretion unless water intake is excessive.[15, 38]

POTENTIAL ROLE OF HYPOXEMIA

Hypoxemia may contribute to sodium and water retention in patients with COPD. Studies of acute cases have shown that the removal of supplemental oxygen in hypercapneic COPD patients, which allowed Pao_2 to fall from 80 to 39 mm Hg without a significant $Paco_2$ change, diminished the patients' ability to excrete a sodium load.[35] In contrast, acute hypoxemia of similar degree in normocapneic individuals had no measurable effect. In patients considered for home oxygen therapy, 1 week of oxygen supplementation resulted in significant

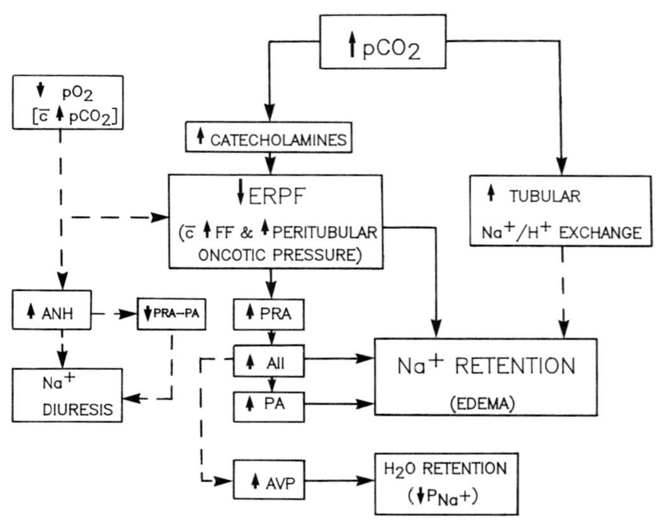

Figure 25–1. Proposed pathogenesis of Na^+ and H_2O retention in COPD. Solid lines indicate established pathways: broken lines indicate nonproven pathways. ANH = atrial natriuretic hormone; ERPF = effective renal plasma flow.

natriuresis.[14] Edematous patients with acute respiratory failure secondary to COPD who experienced diuresis with oxygen therapy if there was no change in Pa_{CO_2} except when plasma renin activity (PRA) and plasma aldosterone (PA) level were extremely high.[17] Animal studies lend support to these clinical investigations.[39]

In hypoxemic, nonhypercapneic patients, sodium and water metabolism is usually normal. No pertinent experimental data exist on the functional renal/hormonal behavior in individuals suffering from chronic hypoxemia alone. Clinical experience teaches us that patients with interstitial lung diseases, with levels of hypoxemia comparable with those of COPD patients but without concomitant hypercapnia, rarely develop edema or hyponatremia. Typically, in the far-advanced stage of the illness, edema may appear in conjunction with a low cardiac output state caused perhaps by myocardial fibrosis in combination with severe hypoxemia.

ATRIAL NATRIURETIC HORMONE

It is logical to assume that atrial natriuretic hormone (ANH) should offset the sodium-retaining propensity evoked by low renal perfusion and high aldosterone secretion. The structure of this hormone and, to some extent, its function, have been defined within the span of a few years.[27] In animal studies, small (1 to 2 mm Hg) increases in atrial pressure stimulate ANH release from the atrium,[22] promote prompt natriuresis and diuresis, lower plasma renin activity and plasma aldosterone levels, and may inhibit AVP release.[31] Atrial natriuretic hormone has been shown to be markedly elevated in patients with left-sided congestive heart failure[6, 34] and to be either normal or elevated in patients with ascites and cirrhosis.[19, 41] Atrial natriuretic hormone has also been shown to be elevated in patients with advanced COPD who are usually edematous[1, 5, 28, 30] but not to the levels seen in left-sided congestive failure.[6, 34] Preliminary studies have demonstrated that the increased ANH level in COPD patients correlates inversely with the Pa_{O_2} level, presumably because of the effect of low oxygen pressure on atrial pressure/volume characteristics.[9]

At present, the precise role of ANH in COPD remains to be elucidated. A study has shown that the normal suppressing effect of ANH on aldosterone is not demonstrable in edematous COPD patients, perhaps because this suppressing potential is overriden by the stimulatory effect of decreased renal perfusion on the renin-aldosterone axis.[30] It may be that in these patients, as proposed for patients with congestive heart failure, the primary function of the ANH system is in acute conditions, where it contributes to reducing the central venous and pulmonary volumes. Conversely, the primary function of the opposing hormonal system, the renin-angiotensin-aldosterone axis, is in chronic conditions, where it contributes to the support of the arterial volume.[23] The interrelationships between these two systems are quite complex; much more work remains to be done before a clear picture will begin to emerge.

THERAPEUTIC IMPLICATIONS

Treatment begins with optimizing ventilatory function and restoring arterial blood gas tensions toward normal. As edema progresses and becomes a clinical problem, its control is often attempted through the use of potent diuretics, such as furosemide, but this can exacerbate existing hypochloremia and hypokalemia from renal compensation if hypercapnia results. Sometimes an alkalosis is created that may cause overt hypoventilation.

Relatively little use has been made in COPD patients of angiotensin-converting enzyme (ACE) inhibitors. In congestive heart failure, these drugs are known to enhance sodium excretion as angiotensin-II and aldosterone generation are blocked while effective renal plasma flow increases.[32] We have seen that in acute studies in COPD patients, ACE inhibition promotes sodium excretion because tubular sodium reabsorption is diminished at constant levels of effective renal plasma flow.[35] It seems logical at present that ACE inhibition should supplement O_2 administration in treating the edema of COPD. In addition, we have indicated that angiotensin II may stimulate AVP secretion. Angiotensin-converting enzyme inhibition could then play an important role in the treatment of hyponatremia in these patients because it prevents angiotensin-II generation. This approach might be used in place of forms of therapy, such as water restriction (likely to result in inspissated bronchial secretions), or hypertonic saline infusion (likely to result in volume overload). Our personal experience indicates that ACE inhibitors are generally well tolerated in COPD patients and often yield the desired effect without any electrolyte complications. Furthermore, this class of "vasodilator" drugs could have a long-term salutary effect on the pulmonary vasculature.

Digitalis preparations should not be used routinely in the management of COPD patients. They promote arrhythmias in patients already on arrhythmogenic drugs (bronchodilators) who also tend to be hypoxemic and hypokalemic, thus increasing the risk with no measurable benefit because cardiac output does not change.

DIRECTIONS FOR FUTURE RESEARCH

Much progress has been made in the past decade toward the understanding of the complex pathophysiologic interplays leading to sodium and water disturbances in COPD patients, but many important questions remain unanswered. Investigations on patients, utilizing rigid experimental designs, are needed to provide applicable answers, notwithstanding the inherent difficulties of such studies.

The many questions that should be addressed include the following:

1. Is the beneficial effect of correcting hypoxemia on the sodium-retaining state mediated via enhancement of renal hemodynamics?
2. Can this favorable oxygen effect be magnified by chronic inhibition of angiotensin converting enzyme?
3. Can depressed renal plasma flow be improved with alpha-adrenergic blockade?
4. Is the syndrome of inappropriate antidiuretic hormone release ameliorated by correcting hypoxemia, by blocking angiotensin, or both?
5. Does the kinin-prostaglandin system participate in the underlying pathophysiology in edematous hyponatremic COPD patients as it does in cirrhotic edematous, hyponatremic patients? Both conditions share the pathophysiologic combination of normal, high cardiac output, low renal perfusion, and stimulation of the sympathetic and the renin-angiotensin-aldosterone axes.

SUMMARY

In the advanced stages of COPD many patients develop sodium retention and edema. When this occurs, prognosis becomes poorer and management more difficult, particularly during acute exacerbations with respiratory failure, because current treatment for edema often entails significant side effects, such as arrhythmias from digitalis and metabolic alkalosis and hypoventilation from diuretics. Sodium retention in these patients is not due to heart failure in the usual sense, because cardiac output is normal. In a long-term attempt to elucidate the pathophysiologic mechanisms at play in the sodium and water retention seen in advanced COPD, we and others have made the following observations over the years.

Patients with COPD generally fall into three groups: (1) normocapneic, mild hypoxemia; (2) hypercapneic, moderate hypoxemia; and (3) hypercapneic, moderate-severe hypoxemia. Most of the last group demonstrate edema, often with concurrent hyponatremia.

Hypercapnia stimulates a cascade of events: increased tubular sodium reabsorption as part of compensation for chronic hypercapnia and stimulation of renal sympathetic tone, which decreases effective renal plasma flow (ERPF), further exacerbating sodium retention. Thus, almost all patients with hypercapnia, even without edema, show significant defects in sodium and water excretory ability. As renal perfusion falls further and glomerular filtration also begins to fall, the renin-angiotensin-aldosterone axis is stimulated and clinical edema usually becomes evident. Antidiuretic hormone is often stimulated at this time, through increased baroreceptor firing or through angiotensin II leading to defective water excretion and hyponatremia. Significant inverse correlations can be demonstrated between the level of Pa_{CO_2} and ERPF, Pa_{CO_2} and sodium excretion, Pa_{CO_2} and water excretion, and plasma AVP levels and free water clearance. Significant positive correlations exist between ERPF and sodium and water excretion, sodium excretion and water excretion, and PRA and PA.

The role of hypoxemia as an independent variable in the previous scheme has yet to be fully clarified. It appears that hypoxemia, when superimposed on hypercapnia, worsens the hypercapnia-induced renal and hormonal perturbations in COPD patients. Atrial natriuretic hormone, which should promote sodium excretion, has begun to be examined in COPD. The hormone is elevated, especially late in the disease when edema and hypoxemia are prevalent, but its importance in the underlying pathophysiology remains obscure. The long-term effect of oxygen administration and of therapy with ACE inhibitors as well as the role of the kinin-prostaglandin system, if any, are also areas ripe for future investigations.

REFERENCES

1. Adnot S, Chabrier PE, Andrivet P, et al. Atrial natriuretic peptide concentrations and pulmonary hemodynamics in patients with pulmonary artery hypertension. Am Rev Respir Dis 1987; 136:951–956.
2. Bauer FK, Telfer N, Herbst HH, et al. Hyponatremia and increased exchangeable sodium in chronic obstructive lung disease. Am J Med Sci 1965; 250:245–253.
3. Bell NH, Schedl HP, Bartter FC. An explanation for abnormal water retention and hypoosmolality in congestive heart failure. Am J Med 1964; 36:351–360.
4. Braunwald E. Edema. In: Braunwald E, Isselbacher KJ, Petersdorf RG, et al., eds. Harrison's Principles of Internal Medicine. 11th Edition. New York: McGraw-Hill Book Company, 1987, 149–151.
5. Burghuber OC, Hartter E, Punzengruber CH, et al. Human atrial natriuretic peptide secretion in patients with pulmonary hypertension. Chest 1988; 93:31–37.
6. Burnett JC Jr, Kao PC, Hu DC, et al. Atrial natriuretic peptide elevation in congestive heart failure in the human. Science 1986; 231:1145–1147.
7. Campbell EJM, Short DS. The cause of oedema in "cor pulmonale." Lancet 1960: i:1184–1186.
8. Campbell RHA, Brand HL, Cox JR, Howard P. Body weight and body water in chronic cor pulmonale. Clin Sci Mol Med 1975; 49:323–335.
9. Davidson AC, Winter RJD, Treacher DF, et al. Increased atrial natriuretic factor in chronically hypoxaemic patients with pulmonary hypertension. Am Rev Respir Dis 1988; 137:105.
10. Dexter L, Whittenberger JL, Gorlin R, et al. The effect of chronic pulmonary disease (cor pulmonale and hypoxia) on the dynamics of the circulation in man. Trans Assoc Am Physician 1951; 64:226–236.
11. DiBona GF. Catecholamines and neuroadrenergic control of renal function. In: Dunn MJ, ed. Renal Endocrinology. Baltimore: Williams & Wilkins, 1983, 323–366.
12. Farber MO, Bright TP, Strawbridge RA, et al. Impaired water handling in chronic obstructive lung disease. J Lab Clin Med 1975; 85:41–49.
13. Farber MO, Kiblawi SO, Strawbridge RA, et al. Studies of plasma vasopressin and the renin-angiotensin-aldosterone system in chronic obstructive lung disease. J Lab Clin Med 1977; 90:373–380.
14. Mannix ET, Dowdeswell IRG, Carlone S, et al. The effect of oxygen on sodium excretion in hypoxemic patients with chronic obstructive lung disease. Chest 1990; 97:840–844.
15. Farber MO, Roberts LR, Weinberger MH, et al. Abnormalities of sodium and H_2O handling in chronic obstructive lung disease. Arch Intern Med 1982; 142:1326–1330.
16. Farber MO, Weinberger MH, Robertson GL, Fineberg NS. The effects of angiotensin converting enzyme inhibition on sodium handling in patients with advanced chronic obstructive lung disease. Am Rev Respir Dis 1987; 136:862–866.
17. Farber MO, Weinberger MH, Robertson GL, et al. Hormonal abnormalities affecting sodium and water balance in acute respiratory failure due to chronic obstructive lung disease. Chest 1984; 85:49–54.
18. Fishman AP. The kidney and acid-base disorders in obstructive pulmonary disease of the airways. In: Fishman AP, ed. Pulmonary Diseases and Disorders. New York: McGraw-Hill Book Company, 1980, 556–557.
19. Gerbes AL, Arendt RM, Ritter D, et al. Plasma atrial natriuretic factor in patients with cirrhosis. N Engl J Med 1985; 313: 1609–1610.
20. Harvey RM, Ferrer MI, Richards DW Jr, Cournand A. Influence of chronic pulmonary disease on the heart and circulation. Am J Med 1951; 10:719–738.
21. Henriksen JH, Christensen NJ, Kok-Jensen A, Christiansen I. Increased plasma noradrenaline concentration in patients with chronic obstructive lung disease: relation to haemodynamics and blood gases. Scand J Clin Lab Invest 1980; 40:419–427.
22. Lang RE, Tholken H, Ganten D, et al. Atrial natriuretic factor—a circulating hormone stimulated by volume loading. Nature 1985; 314:264–266.
23. Laragh JH. The endocrine control of blood volume, blood pressure and sodium balance: atrial hormone and renin system—interactions. J Hypertens 1986; 4(suppl 2):S143–S156.
24. Mitchell RS, Webb WC, Filley GF. Chronic obstructive bronchopulmonary disease, III. Factors influencing prognosis. Am Rev Respir Dis 1964; 89:878–896.
25. Molony DA, Jacobson HR. Respiratory acid-base disorders. In: Kokko JP, Tannen RL, eds. Fluids and Electrolytes. Philadelphia: W.B. Saunders Company, 1986, 305–381.
26. Mounsey JPD, Ritzmann LW, Selverstone NJ, et al. Circulatory changes in severe pulmonary emphysema. Br Heart J 1952; 14:153–172.
27. Needleman P, Adams SP, Cole BR, et al. Atriopeptins as cardiac hormones. Hypertension 1985; 7:469–482.
28. Neilly JB, Doyle J, Stevenson RD. Atrial natriuretic peptide levels in decompensated and treated cor pulmonale. Am Rev Respir Dis 1988; 137:187.
29. Owens GR, Rogers RM. Managing respiratory failure in chronic airflow obstruction. J Respir Dis 1982; 3:24–37.
30. Carlone S, Palange P, Mannix ET, et al. Atrial natriuretic peptide, renin, and aldosterone in obstructive lung disease and heart failure. Am J Med Sci 1989; 296:243–248.
31. Palluk R, Gaida W, Hoefke W. Atrial natriuretic factor. Life Sci 1985; 36:1415–1425.
32. Proceedings of a Symposium. Experience, progress, and clinical perspectives on angiotensin converting enzyme inhibition. Am J Med 1988; 84(suppl 4A):1–46.
33. Raff H, Levy SA. Renin-angiotensin II-aldosterone and ACTH-cortisol control during acute hypoxemia and exercise in patients

with chronic obstructive pulmonary disease. Am Rev Respir Dis 1986; 133:396–399.
34. Raine AEG, Erne P, Burgisser E, et al. Atrial natriuretic peptide and atrial pressure in patients with congestive heart failure. N Engl J Med 1986; 315:533–537.
35. Reihman DA, Farber MO, Weinberger MH, et al. Effect of hypoxemia on sodium and water excretion in chronic obstructive lung disease. Am J Med 1985; 78:87–94.
36. Renzetti AD, McClement JH, Litt BD. The Veterans Administration cooperative study of pulmonary function. III. Mortality in relation to respiratory function in chronic obstructive pulmonary disease. Am J Med 1966; 41:115–129.
37. Richens JM, Howard P. Oedema in cor pulmonale. Clin Sci 1982; 62:255–259.
38. Robertson GL. Diseases of the posterior pituitary. In: Felig P, Baxter J, Broadus AE, et al., eds. Endocrinology and Metabolism. New York: McGraw-Hill Book Company, 1981, 251–277.
39. Rose CE Jr, Kimmel DP, Godine RL Jr, et al. Synergistic effects of acute hypoxemia and hypercapnic acidosis in conscious dogs. Renal dysfunction and activation of the renin-angiotensin system. Circ Res 1983; 53:202–213.
40. Schrier RW, Bichet DG. Osmotic and nonosmotic control of vasopressin release and the pathogenesis of impaired water excretion in adrenal, thyroid, and edematous disorders. J Lab Clin Med 1981; 98:1–15.
41. Shenker Y, Sider RS, Ostafin EA, Grekin RJ. Plasma levels of immunoreactive atrial natriuretic factor in healthy subjects and in patients with edema. J Clin Invest 1985; 76:1684–1687.
42. Stevens PM, Terplan M, Knowles JH. Prognosis for cor pulmonale. N Engl J Med 1963; 269:1289–1291.
43. Szatalowicz VL, Goldberg JP, Anderson RJ. Plasma antidiuretic hormone in acute respiratory failure. Am J Med 1982; 72:583–587.

Section V

EPIDEMIOLOGY AND NATURAL HISTORY OF CHRONIC OBSTRUCTIVE PULMONARY DISEASE

Chapter 26

THE EPIDEMIOLOGY OF COPD

Susan Redline

The epidemiology of chronic obstructive pulmonary disease (COPD) is the study of the population distribution and determinants of a disease that is characterized by mucous hypersecretion or airflow obstruction, or both, that is not completely reversible spontaneously or following medication administration. This chapter reviews the tools by which the epidemiology of COPD is assessed and the application of these tools in assessments of the prevalence of COPD, the relationship of COPD to hypothesized risk factors, the degree to which prevalence of airflow obstruction relates to longitudinal decline in lung function (and the degree to which this differs in populations exposed to different risk factors), and the morbidity and mortality that may be attributable to COPD.

TOOLS

Evaluations of the distribution and natural history of COPD have utilized tools that measure symptoms, exposures, and lung function in large numbers of subjects. Although chest radiography and measurement of static lung volumes and gas exchange have been employed in some epidemiologic studies, most population-based studies have relied on less costly and less complicated assessments of airflow and symptoms. Extensive experience with questionnaires and spirometry has allowed standardization of their applications and elucidation of their validity, reliability, and utility. Biologic and atmospheric measurements of environmental exposures have been popularized as means of more precisely characterizing risk and minimizing information bias. Further, development of sophisticated statistical methods has allowed assessments of exposures with variable or relatively small effects and influences of confounders and interactions among several variables.

Questionnaires

Standardized respiratory symptom questionnaires have been developed by the British Medical Research Council and the American Thoracic Society. These questionnaires attempt characterization and some quantification of occurrences of cough, phlegm, wheezing, breathlessness, chest illnesses, and exposure to cigarette smoking. Samet[1] has reviewed the validity and reliablity of respiratory symptom questionnaires. Assessment of phlegm production with questionnnaires has been validated with measurement of daily expectoration.[2] Validation and establishment of the consistency of responses for other respiratory symptoms, such as wheeze and breathlessness, for which measurement of physiologic correlates is more difficult, however, has been more limited. Only a modest relationship appears to exist between airway hyper-responsiveness measured with bronchoprovocation challenge testing and wheeze symptoms determined with questionnaires in population-based studies.[3, 4] The degree to which differences in responses to challenge tests and wheeze/asthma questions relate to limited specificity and sensitivity of the questionnaire rather than to imprecision and variability in the measurement of selected physiologic responses has not been defined. Similarly, limitations in measuring dyspnea, a symptom based on a number of physiologic and psychologic determinants, limits interpretation of the measured correlations between questionnaire assessment of breathlessness and selected ventilatory parameters. Standardized respiratory questionnaires do not yet attempt to identify specifically the entity "chronic obstructive lung disease." International comparisons of respiratory diseases are limited further by difficulties translating English questionnaires to other languages. For example, the terms "usually," employed to assess chronicity of symptoms, and "wheeze," a commonly employed indicator of airway hyper-reactivity, may be translated into a number of different words, each with different connotations. Despite these limitations, however, questionnaires have provided valuable information regarding the relation of respiratory health to air pollution;[5] active[2, 6–8] and passive[9] smoking; occupational exposures;[10] and genetic factors.[11]

Pulmonary Function

Measurement of forced expiratory volume in 1 second (FEV_1), forced vital capacity (FVC), and the FEV_1 to FVC ratio with spirometry standardly is employed to assess the degree of ventilatory impairment in subjects representing different risk groups. These measures can be obtained easily with portable equipment that can be used in various field settings, including the workplace and home. The FEV_1 and FVC values are highly reproducible (within-individual coefficient of variations are usually $< 5\%$), correlate with clinically and pathologically documented disease,[12, 13] and predict longitudinal decline in lung function[2, 14] as well as mortality.[15, 16] Guidelines for test performance and measurement have been published by The Epidemiology Standardization Project of the American Thoracic Society.[17]

More complicated tests of lung function that have been used in epidemiologic studies include assessments of small airway function with the single breath N_2 test and density dependence of airflow; gas exchange and the integrity of the pulmonary vascular bed with diffusing capacity of carbon monoxide; and airway responsiveness with bronchoprovocation tests and bronchodilator responses. The utility of these tests in epidemiologic studies relates to their ability to provide reliable information concerning "risk" or prognosis not available from spirometry alone.

The single breath N_2 test, which provides data on closing volume (CV/VC%), closing capacity (CC/TLC%), and the slope of the alveolar plateau (ΔN_2/L), is sensitive to the effects of active smoking;[18–20] i.e., measurements derived from this test are frequently abnormal in smokers and improve with smoking cessation. This indicates the sensitivity of these tests in detecting small airway inflammation in smokers. Single breath N_2 variables have been found to correlate moderately strongly with FEV_1 in most,[21–23] but not in all, population studies.[24] To date, however, there is little evidence that this test is sufficiently sensitive and specific for use in the early identification of subgroups of smokers at risk for developing significant irreversible airflow obstruction. A longitudinal study of 734 subjects from two Portland cohorts demonstrated that an abnormal single breath N_2 test preceded the development of an abnormal FEV_1 in 87% of 82 smokers.[21] However, the predictive value of an abnormal test was higher for subjects from the older and more physically impaired cohort than in a more general working-class population. Additionally, a small percentage of subjects (8.5%) with an abnormal FEV_1 had a normal N_2 test. The population utility of this test appears to be limited by its complexity, and the as yet limited evidence suggests a significant ability to predict subsequent development of disease. Further elucidation of the contribution of airway inflammation to the development of irreversible obstructive ventilatory impairment may clarify the role of this test in population studies.

Assessment of the density dependence of airflow, measured with performance of maximal forced maneuvers while the subject breathes air and a helium-oxygen gas mixture, also has been proposed as a means of identifying a subject with small airway disease early in its course. However, the theoretic basis for this has been challenged with the demonstration of "normalization" of low-density gas flow rates in instances wherein large airway obstruction accompanies small airway disease.[25, 26] Further, a population-based study of childhood risk factors for lung disease has demonstrated that determination of density dependence contributed little epidemiologic information over that provided by routinely measured spirometric parameters.[26]

Assessments of airway reversibility and airway hyper-responsiveness have played central roles in many epidemiologic studies. Bronchoprovocation testing has been employed to assess the effects of seasonal[27] and occupational exposures on lung function.[28, 29] It has been hypothesized that characterization of airway hyper-reactivity and reversibility may help identify unique subsets of the population with different susceptibilities to developing severe chronic airflow obstruction. Thus, measures of nonspecific airway hyper-reactivity also have been studied as indices of susceptibility to respiratory irritants or allergens. Accordingly, bronchoprovocation testing has been used to explore the "Dutch hypothesis" (discussed subsequently), which proposes that susceptibility to cigarette smoking may relate to an atopic predisposition partially manifest by airway hyper-responsiveness. In contrast, bronchodilator responses provide information about the presence of fixed versus reversible airflow obstruction. As discussed subsequently, a number of studies of diverse populations suggest that heightened degrees of nonspecific airway reactivity are associated with adverse pulmonary outcomes. However, the relation between airway reversibility (bronchodilator responses) and FEV_1 decline is less clear and appears to vary in studies of different populations. One plausible explanation for apparent differences in risk associated with different degrees of reversibility relates to potentially effective intervention with bronchodilator medication in some of these studies. Comparisons between studies, however, also potentially are limited by differences in the age distribution and disease severity in different populations. Interpretation of data on pulmonary function change following challenge testing also may require consideration of a number of methodologic issues that include adjustment for measurement and biologic variablility in responses;[3, 4] interpretation of data derived from subjects with different levels of baseline function; and "censorship" of data from subjects with very low levels of pulmonary function ($FEV_1 < 65\%$ to 70% of predicted) in whom challenge testing may not be possible. Further understanding of the implications of these limitations may help resolve the role of airway reactivity in the natural history of COPD.

Assessment of Environmental Exposures

Questionnaire data often are used to characterize relevant environmental exposures. Exposure to cigarette smoke is assessed by self-report of current and previous smoking habits, enabling characterization of subjects as "current," "former," and "never" smokers, and estimation of total lifetime exposure in terms of "pack-years." Occupational exposures may be assessed with self-report of dust or fume exposure or with employment history (industry, occupation, or job title). However, there may be variable degrees of information misclassification with self-report, which may be random or nonrandom, as may occur with differential reporting of dust exposure in subjects with respiratory disease. More precise quantification of exposure history may be achieved with measurement of biologic markers of exposure and with physical measurements made using area and personal sampling methods.

Objective assessments of tobacco exposure include measurement of levels of serum thiocyanate, exhaled carbon monoxide, and urinary and salivary cotinine. The last, a nicotine metabolite with a longer serum half-life than nicotine (10 to 40 hours versus 2 hours),[30] appears to be a specific marker of tobacco exposure that is sensitive to involuntary (passive) sidestream tobacco smoke exposure, increases with exposure to increasing numbers of active smokers,[31] and differentiates active from passive exposure.[32] Use of this biologic marker has been important in quantifying the extent of passive smoke exposure in the population. Further, cotinine measurement may be particularly useful for pursuing hypotheses that require precise quantification of tobacco exposure, especially in circumstances where reporting bias is likely. However, the number of cotinine measurements that optimally should be obtained has not been defined and probably will vary according to specific study objectives.

Review of the various area and sampling procedures is beyond the scope of this chapter. These methods can be used to characterize the size and composition of particulates in outdoor and indoor air due to occupational or other environmental sources. Appropriate filters and strategically placed personal samplers can also provide refined estimates of personal exposures to respirable dust for individuals with different activities. The interested reader is referred to Dodgson[33] for further information.

Statistical Methods

Cross-sectional studies have provided important information about the associations of several risk factors, such as active smoking and certain occupational exposures to COPD. Cross-sectional studies of respiratory disease, often less costly, quicker, and simpler to conduct than longitudinal studies, however, may have limited precision in detecting effects of exposures that are small relative to the variability in annual differences in FEV_1 (standard deviation of Δ FEV_1 25–47 ml/year).[34, 35] Cross-sectional studies also provide limited information regarding the temporal, and thus etiologic, association between potential risk factors and COPD. For example, cross-sectional associations between airway hyper-responsiveness and reduced FEV_1 level in smokers may be observed if airway hyper-responsiveness had operated as a risk factor for COPD and caused FEV_1 reductions. Alternatively, measurement of airway hyper-reactivity may be a consequence of lower pulmonary function level. Cross-sectional studies also provide limited assessment of risk factors that may differentially influence subjects born in different birth cohorts ("cohort effects") and are particularly sensitive to "survivor biases" (discussed subsequently).

Longitudinal studies attempt to characterize the effects of exposures that operate during the period of observation, allowing determination of temporal sequence and quantification of effects of exposures of smaller influence. Longitudinal follow-up of lung function in population and occupational-based samples have facilitated elucidation of the role of various risk factors in the development of COPD, as well as furthered our understanding of the natural history of the disorder. Such studies, discussed subsequently, have enabled quantification of the magnitude of decline in lung function for various risk groups and have established the influence of exposures, such as passive smoking during childhood, that may lower FEV_1 growth by relatively small degrees (1% to 5%).[35] However, a number of biases and statistical complexities may arise in longitudinal analyses, which, if inadequately addressed, may seriously limit the findings of such studies. Potential methodologic problems include: (1) *survey biases*, wherein technical differences in data collection among surveys may cause estimates of FEV_1 to vary by +30 to −37 ml per survey;[36] (2) *learning effects*, wherein initial pulmonary function values are depressed by subject inexperience with spirometry; and (3) *survivor biases*, wherein selective loss to follow-up occurs with the dropout or death of subjects whose course differs from those in the larger cohort. Survey biases usually limit the precision of longitudinal estimates; survivor biases and learning effects usually cause systematic underestimation of longitudinal decline in pulmonary function.

Other issues, especially pertinent to longitudinal respiratory data, include adjustment for the nonlinear effects of aging;[37] "regression of data to the mean" (i.e., random measurement differences may cause very low pulmonary function levels on given surveys to appear higher on subsequent surveys, and vice versa); and the "horse-racing effect." The last term refers to the observation that the horse that leads a race at any given point arrives there by running the fastest. This expression was coined to describe an association between pulmonary function *level* and *rate of decline*, i.e., during longitudinal observation, mean level of pulmonary function is correlated with rate of decline.[2] Statistical adjustment for auto or serial correlations has been addressed with the development of random effects[38] and autoregressive statistical models.[39] Further understanding of the uses of nonparametric models also promises to enhance descriptions of nonlinear growth and decline in lung function that occur over a lifetime.[40, 41]

PREVALENCE, MORBIDITY, AND MORTALITY

Prevalence estimates for chronic bronchitis and obstructive lung disease in the U.S. are based (1) on responses to systematic surveys of self-reported disease in large population samples, as provided by the National Health Interview Surveys, National Center for Health Statistics (NCHS); (2) on data for number of office visits provided by the National Ambulatory Medical Care Survey (NCHF) and number of hospital discharges for COPD and allied conditions (NCHS); and (3) on responses to respiratory symptom questionnaires and spirometry in large population samples studied as part of specific research protocols, as in the Harvard Six Cities Study and the Tecumseh, Michigan health study.

In 1986, approximately 11.4 and 2 million Americans were estimated to have chronic bronchitis and emphysema, respectively.[42] More than 17 million office visits were attributed to COPD and allied conditions,[43] and more than 13%, or almost 2 million hospitalizations, resulted from COPD.[43] A prevalence of chronic bronchitis, airflow obstruction, or both, of 14% and 8% was found in adult males and females, respectively, in Tecumseh, Michigan.[6] Prevalence values for specific respiratory symptoms in subjects participating in the Harvard Six Cities Study are provided in Table 26–1. Prevalence is higher in men than in women and is higher in those with lower levels of FEV_1. Hospitalization rates for COPD also appear greater for men than for women.[45] Prevalence rates are strongly influenced by smoking exposure; approximately 3.5% to 6% of nonsmokers versus 15% to 34% of smokers report symptoms of chronic bronchitis.[6, 46] Increasing age also is strongly associated with an increasing prevalence of COPD and increasing numbers of hospitalizations for treatment of COPD (Fig. 26–1).[48]

However, prevalence data may be limited by potential reporting biases and differential use of medical facilities by population subgroups, as is sometimes observed with the apparent greater use of health services by women than men; by difficulty identifying specific disease entities with symptom questionnaires and spirometry; and by the frequent occurrence of overlapping disease entities in given subjects.

The fifth leading cause of death (or 3.6% of all deaths) in the U.S. in 1986 was attributed to COPD and allied conditions. Of these deaths, 95% occurred in subjects older than 55 years of age.[43] Among middle-aged and older subjects, mortality patterns vary by gender (196/100,000 and 81/100,000 for men and women 55 to 84 years of age, respectively) and appear to be changing over time. In both the U.S. and Canada, mortality rates have been increasing for men older than 75 years of age and women older than 55 years of age;[49, 50] appear to be relatively stable for men between 65 and 74 years of age; and may be declining for men less than 65 years of age. Mortality patterns largely reflect (although lag by 20 to 30 years) changes in smoking exposures for cohorts of different ages. Accordingly, relatively high mortality rates among older men[51] can be explained by the heavy exposure to smoking that occurred in men born between 1910 and 1940. The increased mortality observed in middle-aged women can be associated with increased smoking exposure. However, precise determination of COPD mortality is limited by frequent misclassification found on the death certificate.[52] For example, COPD may be absent on the death certificate in 80% of instances in which review of clinical records suggested this diagnosis. Reliance on the death certificate, where COPD also more often is cited as a contributing factor than cause of death, likely may underestimate the impact of COPD on overall health and longevity.[49, 52, 53]

International variability in COPD mortality is an area of great interest. Chronic obstructive pulmonary disease mortality ranges from the relatively low levels observed in Japan (73/100,000) to the four-fold higher levels reported in Romania (433/100,0000).[43] International differences in mortality rates may be explained by national differences in smoking habits (perhaps including type of cigarette smoked); differences in diagnosis and reporting of disease and cause of death; differences in the impact of deaths attributable to other causes (competing risks); differences in genetic susceptibility; and the operation of other environmental influences on respiratory

TABLE 26–1. Number of Subjects Reporting Respiratory Symptoms by Level of Pulmonary Function*

	LEVEL OF FEV_1				
	Best	Good	Fair	Poor	No Test
Men					
Number	922	923	923	921	120
Chronic cough	63 (6.8)	92 (10.0)	129 (14.0)	235 (25.5)	17 (14.2)
Chronic phlegm	73 (7.9)	97 (10.5)	124 (13.4)	233 (25.3)	18 (15.0)
M.D. asthma	5 (0.5)	6 (0.7)	16 (1.7)	40 (4.3)	0 (0.0)
Persistent wheeze	22 (2.4)	39 (4.2)	66 (7.2)	152 (16.5)	12 (10.0)
Women					
Number	1112	1114	1114	1108	170
Chronic cough	49 (4.4)	80 (7.2)	84 (7.5)	155 (14.0)	19 (11.2)
Chronic phlegm	34 (3.1)	62 (5.6)	78 (7.0)	118 (10.6)	17 (10.0)
M.D. asthma	15 (1.3)	10 (0.9)	17 (1.5)	65 (5.9)	4 (2.4)
Persistent wheeze	23 (2.1)	31 (2.8)	36 (3.2)	103 (9.3)	8 (4.7)

*Percentages shown in parentheses.
Reproduced with permission from Speizer FE, Fay ME, Ferris BG Jr. Am Rev Respir Dis 1989; 140(Suppl):541–555.

health. The last may be particularly important in developing nations where childhood respiratory infections and poor indoor ventilation and wood burning may adversely affect respiratory health. In particular, the findings of an usually high prevalence of chronic respiratory disease in nonsmoking African women[54] and death rates as high as 800/100,000 for cor pulmonale in China (personal communication, Bumgarner JR, The World Bank) suggest the potential emergence in the Third World of significant public health problems associated with a variety of respiratory risk factors.

NATURAL HISTORY OF COPD

British and Dutch Hypotheses

Approximately 50% of smokers develop chronic bronchitis; however, only 15% of smokers develop disabling airflow obstruction.[46] This observation has led to intensive investigation of the natural history of COPD, including assessment of the relation between mucous hypersecretion and airflow obstruction and the basis for susceptibility to COPD. Two important hypotheses that have influenced such investigation have become known as the "British" and the "Dutch" hypotheses.

The British hypothesis emphasizes the role of irritants and respiratory infections in COPD. Accordingly, exposure to a variety of inhaled irritants was hypothesized as leading to simple bronchitis. Subsequent mucous hypersecretion would then lead to airway obstruction and predispose to infections and inflammatory destruction of airways and parenchyma, ultimately resulting in irreversible airflow obstruction. This theory initially was advanced in Great Britain at a time of increasing industrial pollution and tobacco smoking and when chronic bronchitis and COPD were emerging as significant public health problems (the death rate for COPD in 1969 in Great Britain was 600/100,000).[55]

In contrast, the Dutch hypothesis emphasizes the role of hypersensitivity in modulating the response of the airways to irritant exposure. In this theory, susceptibility was proposed as relating largely to host characteristics associated with allergy, and partially manifest by wheezing. Infection was considered a secondary phenomenon resulting from impaired airway function.

These hypotheses have been pursued in a variety of ways. The role of mucous hypersecretion, as a marker of airway infection and an independent predictor of FEV_1 decline and COPD mortality, was examined in several British studies[2, 16] and in a French study.[56] A study of 1000 British middle-aged civil servants followed for 8 years demonstrated associations between reduced levels of pulmonary function with both mucous hypersecretion and with more rapid rates of decline in FEV_1. However, phlegm production, assessed by self-report and confirmed with measurement of sputum expectoration, did not prove to be an independent predictor of FEV_1 decline

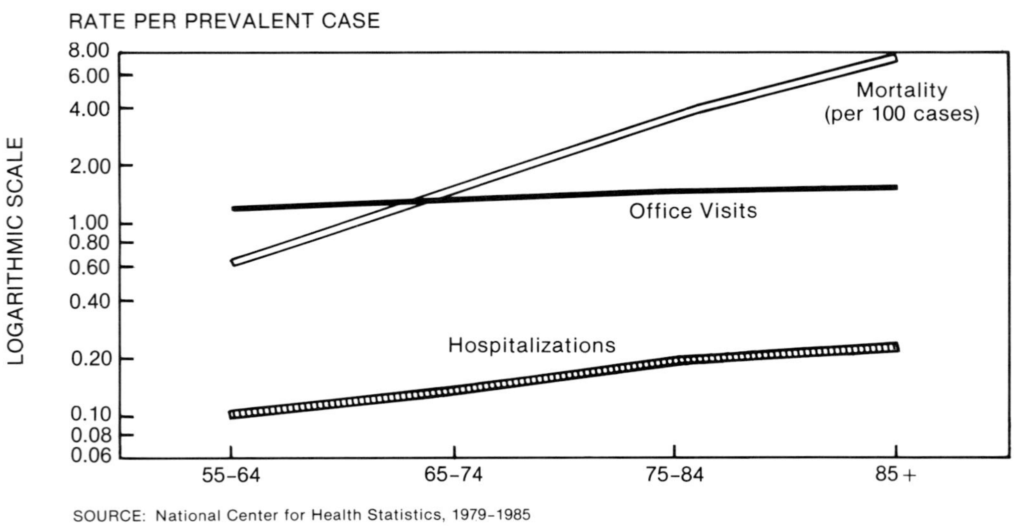

Figure 26–1. Age-related morbidity and mortality in U.S. males, 1979–1985. (Reproduced with permission from Feinleib M, Rosenberg HM, Collins JG, et al. Am Rev Respir Dis 1989; 140: S9–S18.)

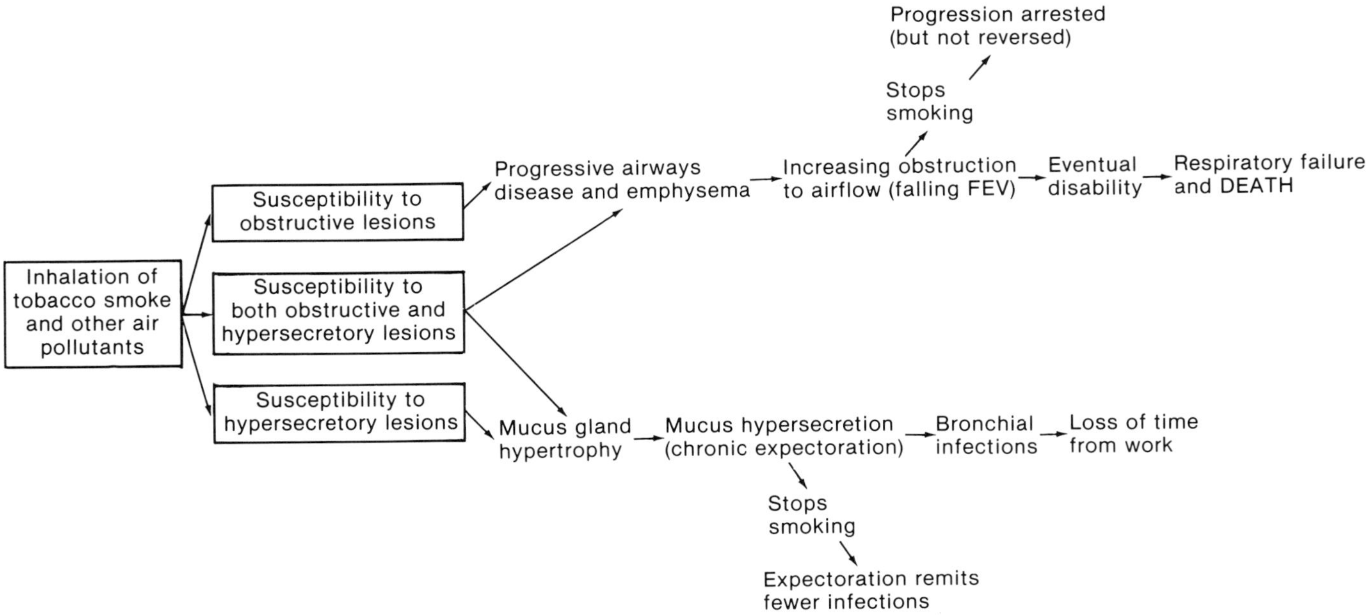

Figure 26–2. Interrelationships between mucous hypersecretion, chronic airflow obstruction, and cigarette smoking/irritant exposure. Mucus hypersecretion and airflow obstruction are independent manifestations of responses to irritant exposures. (Reproduced with permission from Fletcher C, Peto R, Tinker C, Speizer FE. The Natural History of Chronic Bronchitis and Emphysema. An Eight Year Study of Early Chronic Obstructive Lung Disease in Working Men in London. Oxford: Oxford University Press, 1976.)

after adjustment for FEV_1 level. Further, the most rapid decliners did not report mucus hypersecretion. No association was demonstrated between mucous hypersecretion and COPD mortality,[16] which was interpreted as further evidence against a direct association between mucous hypersecretion and susceptibility to airflow obstruction. Rather, it was postulated that mucous hypersecretion and airflow obstruction are independent manifestations of reactions to cigarette smoke exposure and that mucous hypersecretion is not necessary for the development of disabling airflow obstruction (Fig. 26–2). However, the concept of mucous hypersecretion as an "innocent bystander" was challenged with the demonstration of a strong association between phlegm production and overall mortality in a 22-year study of 1474 Parisian factory workers (age- and FEV_1/h^3-adjusted relative risk 20.3 for mucus hypersecretion).[56] The last finding suggests that, in certain instances, information misclassification of COPD on death certificates may cause determination of specific "COPD" mortality to be less useful than examination of "overall" mortality.

The role of atopy and airway hyper-responsiveness in COPD has been and continues to be explored in a number of populations. Eosinophilia and elevated IgE levels have been associated with greater degrees of ventilatory impairment in several population studies.[57–60] However, this relationship may be largely restricted to nonsmokers,[57, 59, 60] a group Burrows has described as having "chronic asthmatic bronchitis." This group may consist of a large proportion of females with a high prevalence of childhood respiratory illnesses. These patients may differ from the more typical patients with COPD associated with smoking exposure. Although mean FEV_1 in this group may be as low as 51%, longitudinal decline does not appear to be substantially increased. Establishment of an independent relationship between atopy and ventilatory impairment in smokers appears to be limited by the potential confounding relationships between elevated eosinophil numbers/IgE levels with active smoking[57, 59] as well as with nonspecific airway hyper-responsiveness,[62] both of which independently predict FEV_1 decline. Further, prospectively collected data on all of these risk factors will be necessary to sort out the role of atopy, including potential interactions between atopy and smoking in COPD.

Tests of airway reactivity may provide information about the relationship of pulmonary "hypersensitivity" and COPD. Augmented responsiveness, measured with bronchodilator[62, 63] or bronchoconstrictor responses,[62, 64, 65] have been demonstrated to predict rapid rates of decline in lung function. In general, bronchodilator and bronchoconstrictor responses are correlated.[66, 67] However, two studies of patients with COPD have suggested that increased reversibility, unlike airway hyperreactivity, is not a risk factor for FEV_1 decline. Large degrees of airway reversibility have been found to predict more favorable outcomes in a small population identified through a Netherlands chest clinic and followed for as long as 21 years[64] and in participants in the intermittent positive pressure breathing (IPPB) trial who had severe airflow obstruction.[68]

Thus, it is not clear whether airway reversibility is a risk factor for COPD in all populations. Airway hyper-responsiveness, however, has been associated fairly consistently with ventilatory impairment determined both cross-sectionally and longitudinally. The degree to which this supports the Dutch hypothesis has not been resolved. Associations between nonspecific airway hyper-responsiveness and ventilatory impairment may be based on mechanisms other than allergy, such as nonallergic airway inflammation. Also, airway reactivity may artifactually appear elevated in subjects with reduced airway caliber because of differential pulmonary deposition of aerosolized bronchoconstrictors onto proximal airways that contribute substantially to total airway resistance[69] or because of measurement of disproportionately large increases in airflow resistance in response to small absolute changes in airway caliber in smaller airways. Prospective studies, wherein airway hyperresponsiveness is measured prior to the development of airflow obstruction, are necessary to determine whether the aforementioned associations are based on etiologic mechanisms.

MODELS OF LONGITUDINAL DECLINE

The concept that susceptibility to COPD can be understood by defining the patterns of age-related decline in lung function and by identifying subjects or groups of subjects in whom longitudinal decline exceeds the usually observed pattern was proposed by Fletcher and colleagues[2] in their 8-year prospective study of pulmonary function in 800 London transit workers. Data from this landmark study suggested that FEV_1 declines at a rate of 36 ml/year in nonsmoking men between the ages of 30 and 59 years. This rate is increased to an average of 44 to 55 ml/year in smokers; however, the "susceptible" smoker may demonstrate losses two-fold greater than this (70–120 ml/year), such that a level of FEV_1 associated with morbidity and mortality is reached in mid or later life (Fig. 26–3). These observations stimulated a great deal of work aimed at further understanding this "natural history" and the basis for individual susceptibility. Data from subsequent larger studies of several populations have confirmed with rather remarkable consistency these initially proposed estimates of FEV_1 decline (Table 26–2) with few modifications.[40, 41, 70, 71]

The concept that age- and size-adjusted levels of pulmonary function (expresed as percentiles relative to the population distribution) remain constant over time in individual nonsmokers, a phenomenon known as "tracking," was furthered by Dockery and colleagues.[73] These investigators provide data that suggest that the pulmonary function levels of adults, as well as of children, "track" over time (Fig. 26–4);[73, 74] i.e., subjects who have low levels of lung function during early childhood also have low levels in late childhood, early adulthood, and late adulthood. Thus, it was proposed that "susceptibility" may result from either an acceleration of rate of decline in lung function during adulthood (i.e., crossing population percentiles) or low childhood and early adulthood levels (genetically or environmentally related) that predispose an individual to the premature development of ventilatory limitation (see Fig. 26–3).

Study of larger numbers of men, women, and children has allowed assessment of nonlinear effects of aging on lung growth and decline. For example, subjects between 35 and 40 years may lose FEV_1 at only one half the rate of subjects greater than 70 years (18 versus 35 ml/year, respectively).[34] Of potentially great importance is work by Tager and colleagues[40] that explores longitudinal change in lung function during early adulthood in detail with nonparametric statistical techniques. This work suggests that pulmonary function in early adulthood is characterized by a "plateau" of relatively stable FEV_1 level. In this model, susceptibility may relate to length of this plateau, i.e., the susceptible smoker experiences a shorter plateau (FEV_1 begins to decline as much as 10 to 15 years earlier than observed in asymptomatic nonsmokers). These observations, if confirmed in other populations, suggest the potential importance of risk factors acting in childhood and early adulthood, the potential utility of screening for susceptibility during this time, and the potential efficacy of interventions aimed at the young adult.

RELATION TO RISK FACTORS

Epidemiologic studies have shed light on the role of smoking, occupational exposures, familial factors, childhood illnesses, and air pollution in COPD. Each of the major risk factors for COPD are discussed in detail in other chapters. A brief discussion of a few representative epidemiologic studies is provided next.

Smoking

Longitudinal studies have not only allowed smoking exposure to be identified as the most significant risk factor associated with susceptibility but have also allowed quantification of this risk and elucidation of the degree to which risk is modified by smoking cessation. There appears to be a reversible and a cumulative irreversible effect on FEV_1. Current smoking increases the age-related loss of FEV_1 by 20%, i.e., for each pack-year of smoking, approximately a 9 ml and a 6 ml additional loss occurs in FEV_1 for men and women, respectively.[70] Expressed alternatively, a one pack per day smoker experiences on average a 1% decrease in his or her predicted level of FEV_1 for each 5 years he or she smokes.[74] Smoking cessation is important in order to reduce respiratory symptoms as well as to reduce additional annual loss in FEV_1. Some recovery also is possible, i.e., following smoking cessation, FEV_1 is increased on average 200 ml in men and 128 ml in women.[70] Further, FEV_1 recovery appears greatest in those who quit smoking at younger ages.[34] Respiratory symptom prevalence may be reduced by one half with smoking cessation (52% to 18% in men and 42% to 19% in women). These last observations suggest that smoking cessation may result in partial resolution of airway inflammation and that the earlier one quits, the better off one is.

The efficacy of antismoking campaigns is suggested by the drop in cigarette sales by 1.8% per year between 1982 and 1986 and by a reduction in smoking prevalence from approximately 53% to 30% in men and 40% to 24% in women.[51] This decrease has been greatest among professionals; however, large segments of the population remain in which smoking is a particular problem.

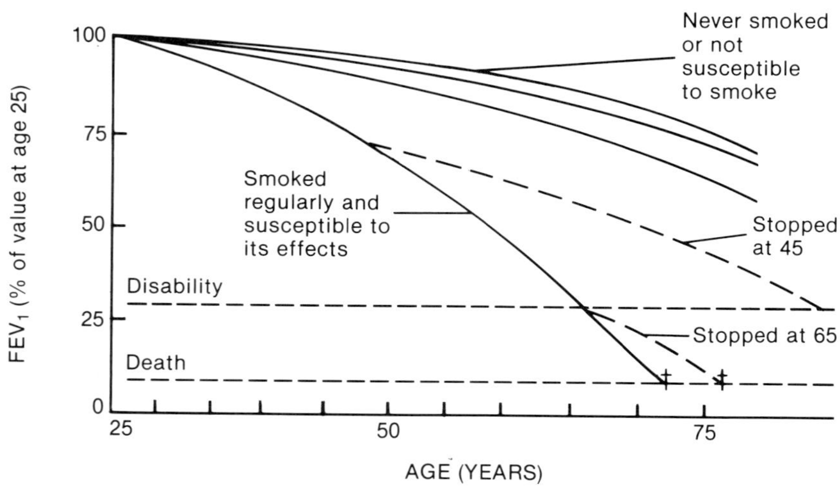

Figure 26–3. Model of longitudinal decline in FEV_1. Cigarette smoking may lead to critically low levels of FEV_1 by causing an accelerated rate of decline in FEV_1 in a susceptible subject. With smoking cessation, rate of decline may decrease to values found in never smokers. This may delay the onset of significant morbidity and mortality.

TABLE 26–2. Longitudinal Estimates of Age-related Change in FEV_1 and Influence of Smoking*

STUDY	FEV_1 (ml/year)			
	Males		Females	
	Nonsmokers	*Smokers*	*Nonsmokers*	*Smokers*
Fletcher et al.[2] 800 London men 30–59 years old 1960–1969	−36	−44 to −55	—	—
Dockery et al.[70] 8842 adults 6 US cities 25–74 years old	−35	−42*	−28	−32
Sherrill et al.[41] Tucson cohort (n = 1705) 20–70 years old	−20	−38	−15	−24
Tager et al.[40] E. Boston cohort (n = 1894) 1975–1985	−35	−40	−30	−35

*Smoking one pack per day

Smoking is more prevalent in blacks than whites (41% and 32% for black versus white men) and in lower socioeconomic classes (40% and 27% for blue versus white collar workers).[51] Also worrisome are the stable or increasing rates of smoking among female adolescents, e.g., young females are twice as likely to be smokers than older males.[70] These observations underscore the need for more effective smoking intervention programs aimed at these segments of the population.

Familial Factors

The nature by which specific host characteristics predispose the smoker to COPD is largely unknown. However, a great deal of evidence suggests that familial factors increase susceptibility to COPD. The familial aggregation of pulmonary function level, as well as of respiratory disease, has been demonstrated in numerous family and twin studies. Asthma or bronchitis may be 25% to 40% higher in subjects with family members who have respiratory diseases.[75–81] Levels of ventilatory function are also highly similar among family members, e.g., sibship correlations range from 0.17 to 0.66.[78, 79, 81] Familial similarities in respiratory disease may suggest the operation of common environmental exposures on family members, such as exposures to active and passive smoking, respiratory infections, or indoor or outdoor air pollution. However, a study of lung function among the members of monozygotic and dizygotic twin families suggests that familial similarities in lung function persist after adjustment for common environmental exposures.[79]

The previous observations suggest the importance of genetic, or possibly prenatal influences, in affecting lung function in later life. However, the basis of genetic susceptibility has not been defined. Clearly, $alpha_1$-antiprotease deficiency predisposes to the premature development of emphysema. However, risk appears to be largely restricted to subjects homozygous for the Z allele, who have deficient and defective antiprotease activities.[82] This risk factor can account only for a small fraction of COPD cases; further, the demonstration that some subjects who both smoke and have antiprotease deficiency have "normal" levels of lung function suggests that disease expression is influenced by, as of yet, undefined environmental or biologic factors.[83] The degree to which familial susceptibility relates to

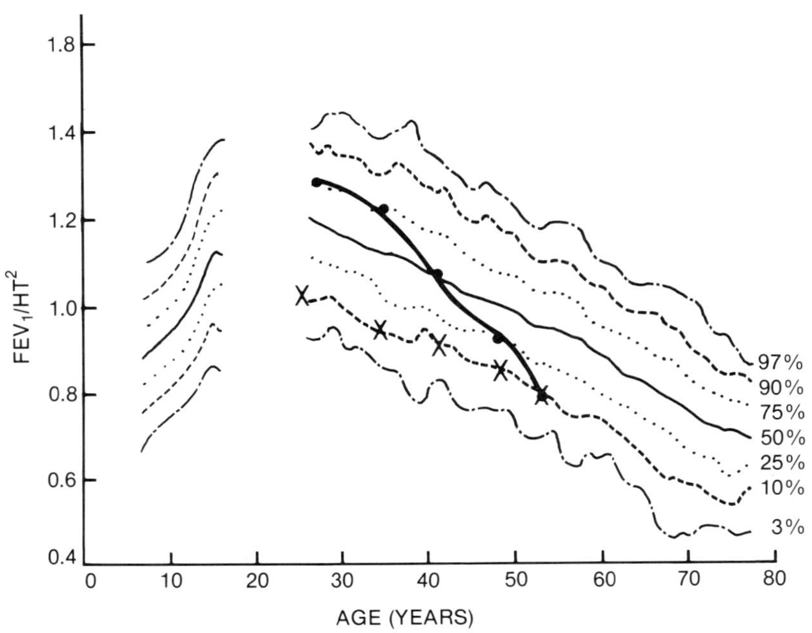

Figure 26–4. Percentiles of height-adjusted FEV_1 by age. Children as well as adults tend to "track" in given percentiles during periods of growth and decline. "Susceptibility," resulting in low FEV_1 levels, may occur if one begins adulthood with low function and continues to track in a given low percentile (X's), or if one begins life with an average level of FEV_1 and then demonstrates an accelerated rate of decline, crossing percentiles (circles). A third concept (not shown) is that age of onset of decline may be earlier in susceptible subjects. (Modified from Dockery DW, Speizer FE, Ferris BG Jr, et al. Am Rev Respir Dis 1988; 137:286–292.)

genetic factors that predispose an individual to allergy, airway responsiveness, airway inflammation, protease-antiprotease imbalance, and so forth, or to environmental factors, such as exposures to respiratory illnesses and environmental allergens or irritants remains to be defined.

Occupational Exposures

An increased prevalence of chronic bronchitis has been demonstrated in numerous studies of dust- and fume-exposed workers.[84–88] Becklake,[89, 90] reviewing data from a number of studies of occupational cohorts (coal, kaolin, potash, copper, and gold workers), has estimated that bronchitis is two to four times more common in dust-exposed than nonexposed workers. Differences between exposed and nonexposed workers are greatest among nonsmokers (two- to five-fold higher). Population-based work also demonstrates an increased prevalence of respiratory symptoms in subjects reporting occupational dust exposure.[10, 91] Chronic phlegm production was estimated to be increased by 40% in exposed subjects. The biologic plausibility of this observation was enhanced with the demonstration of a dose-response relationship between respiratory symptom prevalence and years of dust exposure.[10]

Effects due to dust exposure, in general, appear to be additive to effects due to cigarette smoking.[10, 85, 92] Average levels of ventilatory function also are generally lower in exposed than in nonexposed subjects[93–96] and prevalence of a reduced FEV_1/FVC ratio < 60% may be increased by 68% among dust-exposed subjects.[10] Studies of the relation of occupational dust exposure to respiratory illnesses may be limited by potential biased reporting of symptoms, confounded by the often more significant smoking exposures or lower socioeconomic class of exposed workers, and potential selection bias, wherein symptomatic workers leave the work force (a "health worker" effect). Although many of these concerns have been addressed with adjustment for smoking effects, restriction of analyses to nonsmokers, and examinination of "ex-workers," the degree to which occupational dust exposure increases the risk of COPD in the population is still uncertain. However, given the potentially large proportion of dust-exposed persons in the population (approximately 45% to 50% of male participants in the Tucson and in the Six Cities studies reported occupational exposure to dust or fumes[10, 91]), the attributable risk related to dust exposure may be substantial.

SUMMARY

Patterns of longitudinal decline in middle-aged men have been described in detail and appear to be largely similar to those described in the early 1970s by Fletcher and colleagues.[2] Although the concept of identifying the "rapid decliner," i.e., the subject in whom pulmonary function declines at an accelerated rate, has been very useful in studies of susceptibility, a paucity of knowledge remains about host factors that predispose such subjects to decline at more rapid rates or to cross percentiles. Exposures to environmental irritants may significantly increase the risk of bronchitis and cause some degree of ventilatory limitation. Such exposures may be particularly important in the Third World, where COPD mortality appears to be increasing at inexplicably high rates. Studies that have examined lung growth and decline in subjects of all ages suggest that risk may be increased by factors associated with lower levels of lung function in early adulthood that occur because of reduced lung growth during childhood or because of earlier onset of decline in adulthood (shortening the "plateau"). Childhood respiratory illnesses, passive smoke exposure, and prenatal smoke exposure are a number of factors that continue to be investigated. Identification of biologic and cellular markers that can be used to characterize host responses to common environmental exposures undoubtedly will be important in furthering our understanding of susceptibility to the disease.

REFERENCES

1. Samet JM. A historical and epidemiologic perspective on respiratory symptom questionnaires. Am J Epidemiol 1978; 108:435–446.
2. Fletcher C, Peto R, Tinker C, Speizer FE. The Natural History of Chronic Bronchitis and Emphysema. An Eight Year Study of Early Chronic Obstructive Lung Disease in Working Men in London. Oxford: Oxford University Press, 1976.
3. Redline S, Tager IB, Speizer FE, et al. Longitudinal variability in airway responsiveness in a population-based sample of children and young adults. Am Rev Respir Dis 1989; 140:172–178.
4. Sears MR, Jones DT, Holdaway MD, et al. Prevalence of bronchial reactivity to inhaled methacholine in New Zealand children. Thorax 1986; 41:283–289.
5. Dockery DW, Speizer FE, Stram DO, et al. Effects of inhaled particles on respiratory health of children. Am Rev Respir Dis 1989; 139:587–594.
6. Higgins MW, Keller JB, Metzner HL. Smoking, socioeconomic status and chronic respiratory disease. Am Rev Respir Dis 1977; 116:403–410.
7. Ferris BG Jr, Chen H, Puleo S, Murphy RL. Chronic nonspecific respiratory disease in Berlin, New Hampshire, 1967–1973. A further follow-up study. Am Rev Respir Dis 1976; 113:475–486.
8. Speizer FE, Tager IB. Epidemiology of chronic mucous hypersecretion and obstructive airways disease. Epidemiologic Reviews 1973; 1:124–142.
9. Tager IB, Weiss ST, Munoz A, et al. Longitudinal study of the effects of maternal smoking on pulmonary function in children. N Engl J Med 1983; 309:699–703.
10. Korn RJ, Dockery DW, Speizer FE, et al. Occupational exposures and chronic respiratory symptoms. A population-based study. Am Rev Respir Dis 1987; 136:298–304.
11. Redline S, Tishler PV, Lewitter FI, et al. Assessment of genetic and nongenetic influences on pulmonary function: a twin study. Am Rev Respir Dis 1987; 135:217–222.
12. Cosio M, Ghezzo H, Hogg JC, et al. The relationships between structural changes in small airways and pulmonary function tests. N Engl J Med 1978; 298:1277–1281.
13. Wright JL, Lawson LM, Pare PD, et al. Morphology of the peripheral airways in current smokers and ex-smokers. Am Rev Respir Dis 1983; 127:474–477.
14. Burrows B, Knudson RJ, Camilli AE, et al. The "horse-racing effect" and predicting decline in forced expiratory volume in one second from screening spirometry. Am Rev Respir Dis 1987; 135:788–793.
15. Eisen EA, Dockery DW, Speizer FE, et al. The association between health status and the performance of excessively variable spirometry tests in a population-based study in six U.S. cities. Am Rev Respir Dis 1987; 136:1371–1376.
16. Peto R, Speizer FE, Cochran AL. The relation in adults of airflow obstruction, but not mucous hypersecretion, to mortality from chronic lung disease. Am Rev Respir Dis 1983; 128:491–500.
17. American Thoracic Society. Snowbird workshop on standardization of spirometry. Am Rev Respir Dis 1979; 119:831–838.
18. McCarthy DS, Spencer R, Greene R, Milic-Emili J. Measurement of "closing volume" as a simple and sensitive test for early detection of small airway disease. Am J Med 1972; 52:747–753.
19. Buist AS, Sexton GJ, Nagy JM, Ross BB. The effect of smoking cessation and modification on lung function. Am Rev Respir Dis 1976; 114:115–122.
20. Bake B, Oxhoj H, Sixt R, Wilhelmsen L. Ventilatory lung function following two years of tobacco abstinence. Scand J Respir Dis 1977; 58:311–318.
21. Buist AS, Vollmer WM, Johnson LR, McCamant LE. Does the

single breath N_2 test identify the smoker who will develop chronic airflow limitation? Am Rev Respir Dis 1988; 137:293–301.
22. Tattersall SF, Benson MK, Hunter D, et al. The use of tests of peripheral lung function for predicting future disability from airflow obstruction in middle-aged smokers. Am Rev Respir Dis 1978; 118:1035–1050.
23. Nemery B, Moavero NE, Brasseur L, Stanescu DC. Significance of small airway tests in middle-aged smokers. Am Rev Respir Dis 1981; 124:232–238.
24. Fletcher CM. An 8-year follow-up of FEV and respiratory symptoms in middle-aged men. Scand J Respir Dis 1976; 57:318–319.
25. Castile RG, Pederson OF, Drazen JM, Ingram RH. Density dependence of maximal flow in dogs with central and peripheral obstruction. J Appl Physiol 1983; 55:717–725.
26. Redline S, Tager IB, Castile RG, et al. Assessment of the usefulness of helium-oxygen maximal expiratory flow curves in epidemiologic studies of lung disease in children. Am Rev Respir Dis 1987; 136:834–840.
27. Stanescu DC, Frans A. Bronchial asthma without increased airway reactivity. Eur J Respir Dis 1982; 63:5–12.
28. Hensley MJ, Schittiano R, Saunders NA, et al. Seasonal variation in nonspecific bronchial reactivity: a study of wheat workers with a history of wheat associated asthma. Thorax 1988; 43:103–107.
29. Chan-Yeung M, Vedal S, Kus J, et al. Symptoms, pulmonary function and bronchial hyperreactivity in western red cedar workers compared to those in office workers. Am Rev Respir Dis 1984; 130:1038–1041.
30. Kyerematen GA, Damiano MD, Dvorchik BH, Vesell ES. Smoking-induced changes in nicotine disposition: application of a new HPLC assay for nicotine and its metabolites. Clin Pharmacol Ther 1982; 32:69–80.
31. Coultas DB, Howard CA, Peake GT, et al. Salivary cotinine levels and involuntary tobacco smoke exposure in children and adults in New Mexico. Am Rev Respir Dis 1987; 136:305–309.
32. Samet JM, Marbury MC, Spengler JD. Health effects and indoor air pollution. Part I. Am Rev Respir Dis 1987; 136:1486–1508.
33. Dodgson J. The measurement of dusts and fumes. In: Morgan WKC, Seaton, A, eds. Occupational Lung Diseases, 2nd ed. Philadelphia: W.B. Saunders Company, 1984, 212–236.
34. Camilli AE, Burrows B, Knudson RJ, et al. Longitudinal changes in forced expiratory volume in one second in adults. Effects of smoking and smoking cessation. Am Rev Respir Dis 1987; 135:794–799.
35. Burrows B, Lebowitz MD, Camilli A, Knudson RJ. Longitudinal changes in forced expiratory volume in one second in adults. Methodologic considerations and findings in healthy nonsmokers. Am Rev Respir Dis 1986; 133:974–980.
36. Glindmeyer HW, Engr D, Jones RN, et al. Useful and extraneous variability in longitudinal assessment of lung function. Chest 1987; 92:877–882.
37. Louis TA, Robins J, Dockery DW, et al. Explaining discrepancies between longitudinal and cross-sectional models. J Chron Dis 1986; 39:831–839.
38. Laird NM, Ware JH. Random-effects models for longitudinal data. Biometrics 1982; 38:963–974.
39. Rosner B, Munoz A, Tager IB, et al. The use of an autoregressive model for the analysis of longitudinal data in epidemiologic studies. Stat in Med 1985; 4:457.
40. Tager IB, Segal M, Speizer FE, Weiss ST. The natural history of forced expiratory volumes. Effect of cigarette smoking and respiratory symptoms. Am Rev Respir Dis 1988; 138:837.
41. Sherrill DL, Camilli A, Lebowitz MD. On the temporal relationships between lung function and somatic growth. Am Rev Respir Dis 1989; 140:638–644.
42. National Center for Health Statistics. Current Estimates from the National Health Interview Survey, United States, 1986. Vital and Health Statistics, Series 10, No.164. DHHS (PHS) 897–1592.
43. Higgins MW, Thom T. Incidence, prevalence, and mortality: intra- and intercountry differences. In: Hensley MJ, Saunders NA, eds. Clinical Epidemiology of Chronic Obstructive Pulmonary Disease. New York: Marcel Dekker Inc., 1989, 23–39.
44. Speizer FE, Fay ME, Dockery DW, Ferris BG Jr. Chronic obstructive disease mortality in six U.S. cities. Am Rev Respir Dis 1989; 140(suppl):S49–S55.
45. National Center for Health Statistics. Detailed Diagnosis and Procedures for Patients Discharged from Short-Stay Hospitals, United States, Vital and Health Statistics, 1986.
46. United States Department of Health and Human Services. The Health Consequences of Smoking. Chronic Obstructive Lung Disease. 1984. Washington, DC, U.S. Government Printing Office.
47. Tager IB, Speizer FE. Risk estimates for chronic bronchitis in smokers: A study of male-female differences. Am Rev Respir Dis 1976; 113:619–625.
48. Higgins MW, Keller JB, Landis JR, et al. Risk of chronic obstructive lung disease. Collaborative assessment of the validity of the Tecumseh Index of Risk. Am Rev Respir Dis 1984; 130:380–385.
49. Feinleib M, Rosenberg HM, Collins JG, et al. Trends in COPD morbidity and mortality in the United States. Am Rev Respir Dis 1989; 140(suppl):S9–S18.
50. Higgins MW, Keller JB. Trends in COPD morbidity and mortality in Tecumseh, Michigan. Am Rev Respir Dis 1989; 140 (suppl):S42–S48.
51. Davis RM, Novotny TE. Changes in risk factors. The epidemiology of cigarette smoking and its impact on chronic obstructive pulmonary disease. Am Rev Respir Dis 1989; 140(suppl):S82–S84.
52. Higgins MW. Chronic airways disease in the United States. Trends and determinants. Chest 1989; 96(suppl):328S–334S.
53. Gittelsohn A, Senning J. Studies on the reliability of vital and health records. I. Comparison of cause of death and hospital record diagnoses. Am J Public Health 1979; 69:680–689.
54. Chaulet P. Asthma and chronic bronchitis in Africa; Evidence from epidemiologic studies. Chest 1989; 96(suppl):334S–339S.
55. Holland WW. Chronic airways disease in the United Kingdom. Chest 1989; 96(suppl):318S–321S.
56. Annesi I, Kauffmann F. Is respiratory mucous hypersecretion really an innocent disorder? A 22-year mortality study of 1061 working men. Am Rev Respir Dis 1986; 134:688–693.
57. Burrows B, Hassan FM, Barbee RA, et al. Epidemiological observations on eosinophilia and its relation to respiratory disorders. Am Rev Respir Dis 1980; 122:709–719.
58. Burrows B, Bloom JW, Traver GA, Cline MG. The course and prognosis of different forms of chronic airways obstruction in a sample from the general population. N Engl J Med 1987; 317:1309–1314.
59. Kauffman F, Neukirch F, Korobaeff M, et al. Eosinophils, smoking, and lung function. An epidemiologic survey among 912 working men. Am Rev Respir Dis 1986; 143:1172–1175.
60. Orie NGM, Sluiter HJ, deVries K, et al. The host factor in bronchitis. In: Orie NGM, Sluiter HJ, eds. Bronchitis. Proceedings of the International Symposium on Bronchitis at Gronigen, The Netherlands. Assen: van Gorcum, 1970, 43–59.
61. Taylor RG, Joyce H, Gross E, et al. Bronchial reactivity to inhaled histamine and annual rate of decline in FEV_1 in male smokers and ex-smokers. Thorax 1985; 40:9–16.
62. Barter CE, Campbell AH. Relationship of constitutional factors and cigarette smoking to decrease in 1-second forced expiratory volume. Am Rev Respir Dis 1976; 113:305–314.
63. Kanner RE. The relation between airways responsiveness and chronic airflow obstruction. Chest 1984; 86:54–57.
64. Postma DS, deVries K, Koeter GH, Sluiter HJ. Independent influence of reversibility of air-flow obstruction and nonspecific hyperreactivity on the long-term course of lung function in chronic air-flow obstruction. Am Rev Respir Dis 1986; 134: 276–280.
65. Pham QT, Mur JM, Chau N, et al. Prognostic value of acetylcholine challenge test: a prospective study. Br J Indust Med 1984; 41:267–271.
66. Redline S, Weiss ST, Tager IB, Speizer FE. Airway reversibility following nonspecific bronchoconstriction in a population-based sample of children. Am Rev Respir Dis 1988; 137(suppl):249S.
67. Bahous J, Cartier A, Ouitmet G, et al. Nonallergic bronchial hyperexcitability in chronic bronchitis. Am Rev Respir Dis 1984; 129:216–220.
68. Anthonisen NR, Wright EC, IPPB Trial Group. Bronchodilator response in chronic obstructive pulmonary disease. Am Rev Respir Dis 1986; 133:814–819.
69. Dolovich MB, Shanchis J, Rossman C, Newhouse MT. Aerosol penetrance: A sensitive index of peripheral airways obstruction. J Appl Physiol 1976; 4:468–471.
70. Dockery DW, Speizer FE, Ferris BG Jr, et al. Cumulative and reversible effects of lifetime smoking on simple tests of lung function in adults. Am Rev Respir Dis 1988; 137:286–292.

71. Beaty TH, Menkes HA, Cohen BH, Newill CA. Risk factors associated with longitudinal change in lung function. Am Rev Respir Dis 1984; 129:660–667.
72. Dockery DW, Ware JH, Ferris BG Jr, et al. Distribution of forced expiratory volume in one second and forced vital capacity in healthy, white, adult never-smokers in six U.S. cities. Am Rev Respir Dis 1985; 131:511–520.
73. Dockery DW, Berkey CS, Ware JH, et al. Distribution of forced vital capacity and forced expiratory volume in one second in children 6 to 11 years of age. Am Rev Respir Dis 1983; 128: 405–412.
74. Burrows B, Knudson RJ, Cline M, Lebowitz MD. A reexamination of risk factors for ventilatory impairment. Am Rev Respir Dis 1988; 138:829–836.
75. Tager IB, Rosner B, Tishler PV, et al. Household aggregation of pulmonary function and chronic bronchitis. Am Rev Respir Dis 1976; 114:485–492.
76. Lewitter FI, Tager IB, McGue M, et al. Genetic and environmental determinants of level of pulmonary function. Am J Epidemiol 1984; 120:518–529.
77. Kueppers F, Miller RD, Gordan H, et al. Familial prevalence of chronic obstructive pulmonary disease in a matched pair study. Am J Med 1977; 63:336–342.
78. Redline S, Tishler PV, Lewitter FI, et al. Assessment of genetic and nongenetic influences on pulmonary function. A twin study. Am Rev Respir Dis 1987; 135:217–222.
79. Redline S, Tishler PV, Rosner B, et al. Genotypic and phenotypic similarities in pulmonary function among family members of adult monozygotic and dizygotic twins. Am J Epidemiol 1989; 129:827–836.
80. Hubert HB, Fabsitz RR, Feinleib M, et al. Genetics and environmental influences on pulmonary function. Am Rev Respir Dis 1982; 125:409–415.
81. Astemborski JA, Beaty TH, Cohen BH. Variance components analysis of forced expiration in families. Am J Med Genet 1985; 21:741–753.
82. Bruce RM, Cohen BH, Diamond EL, et al. Collaborative study to assess risk of lung disease in PiMZ phenotype subjects. Am Rev Respir Dis 1984; 130:386–390.
83. Silverman E, Pierce JA, Province MA, et al. Variability in pulmonary function in alpha$_1$-antitrypsin deficiency: Clinical correlates. Ann Intern Med 1989; 111:982–991.
84. Marine WM, Gurr D, Jacobsen M. Clinically important respiratory effects of dust exposure and smoking in British coal miners. Am Rev Respir Dis 1988; 137:106–112.
85. Manfreda J, Sidwall G, Maini K, et al. Respiratory abnormalities in employees of the hard rock mining industry. Am Rev Respir Dis 1982; 126:629–639.
86. Graham BL, Dosman JA, Cotton DJ, et al. Pulmonary function and respiratory symptoms in potash workers. J Occup Med 1984; 26:209–214.
87. Gamble JF, Fellner W, Dimeao MJ. An epidemiologic study of a group of talc workers. Am Rev Respir Dis 1979; 119:741–753.
88. Clark TC, Harrington VA, Asta J, et al. Respiratory effects of exposure to dust in taconite mining and processing. Am Rev Respir Dis 1980; 121:959–966.
89. Becklake MR. Chronic airflow limitation: its relationship to work in dusty occupations. Chest 1985; 88:608–617.
90. Becklake MR. Occupational exposures: evidence for a causal association with chronic obstructive pulmonary disease. Am Rev Respir Dis 1989; 140(suppl):S85–S91.
91. Lebowitz MD. Occupational exposure in relation to symptomatology and lung function in a community population. Environ Res 1977; 14:59–67.
92. Lowe CR, Khosla T. Chronic bronchitis in ex-coal miners working in the steel industry. Br J Ind Med 1972; 29:45–49.
93. Love RG, Miller BG. Longitudinal study of lung function in coal miners. Thorax 1982; 37:193–197.
94. Beck GJ, Maunder LR, Schacter EN. Cotton dust and smoking effects on lung function in cotton textile workers. Am J Epidemiol 1984; 119:33–43.
95. Kauffmann F, Drouet D, Lellouch J, Brille D. Twelve years of spirometric changes among Paris area workers. Br J Ind Med 1982; 39:221–232.
96. Pham QT, Mastrangelo B, Chau N, Haluska J. Five year longitudinal comparison of respiratory symptoms and function in steel workers and unexposed workers. Bull Eur Physiopathol Respir 1979; 15:469–480.

Chapter 27

THE ROLE OF IMMUNE ABNORMALITIES AND INFLAMMATION IN CAUSING AND PERPETUATING COPD

Elizabeth A. Rich

The interrelationships between the immune and inflammatory systems and diseases of the lung, such as chronic obstructive pulmonary disease (COPD), may be considered in three main categories. First, immune functions may directly predispose a patient to the development of COPD. Such an *a priori* role of the immune system occurs in the genetic disorder alpha$_1$-antitrypsin (α1-AT) deficiency, which is associated with emphysema, or in the immunoglobulin deficiencies that often lead to bronchiectasis. Second, disturbances in immune functions and abnormal local and systemic concentrations of immunologic and inflammatory mediators such as immunoglobulins and complement are found in association with various forms of COPD and likely to be important in the perpetuation of the disease process, but the relationships between cause and effect are not at all clear. Third, changes in functions of immunocompetent cells may secondarily aggravate COPD as, for example, when smoking alters alveolar macrophages and neutrophils leading to release from these cells of products injurious to the lung. Overlap inevitably occurs among these three mechanisms by which immune abnormalities participate in the pathogenesis of COPD. This chapter focuses primarily on the first two of these categories. T lymphocytes involved in specific cell-mediated immunity; immunoglobulins in humoral immunity; and macrophages, neutrophils, and complement, which participate in nonspecific immune defenses and inflammation, are considered in turn as regards their possible roles in the pathogenesis of emphysema, bronchitis, bronchiectasis, and cystic fibrosis.

SYSTEMIC AND LOCAL PULMONARY IMMUNE AND INFLAMMATORY RESPONSES

The aspects of the immune system that have been investigated in COPD include, in large part, systemic abnormalities of the cell-mediated and humoral arms of immunity and of nonspecific inflammation. Much less is known about the role of local immunity or inflammation in COPD so that extrapolation of systemic findings to events occurring in the lung should be guarded. A brief review of general systemic and pulmonary immunity and inflammatory responses seems in order before embarking on specific assessment of immunity in COPD.

The major constituents of cell-mediated and humoral immunity and inflammation are depicted in Figure 27–1. Methods of evaluation of immune and inflammatory processes are summarized in Table 27–1.

Systemic cell-mediated responses to infectious agents or other nonself-antigenic substances involve uptake and presentation of the antigen to T lymphocytes by accessory cells (largely macrophages and dendritic cells) expressing HLA-DR determinants on their surface. Activation of T lymphocytes sensitized to a particular antigen then leads to propagation of a variety of T lymphocytes, including specific memory cells for this antigen; T cells producing lymphokines, such as interferon-gamma, a key mediator in the cellular immune response; helper T lymphocytes involved in activating B cells; suppressor T lymphocytes, which are key cells in regulating the cell-mediated and humoral systems; and cytotoxic T lymphocytes important in destroying tumors and virally infected tissues.

Systemic cell-mediated responses are most easily and commonly measured in humans in two ways. Delayed occurrence of induration at a skin test site following intradermal injection of antigens, such as purified protein derivative (PPD) of *Mycobacterium tuberculosis,* is a measure of T-lymphocyte memory cells. These cells express lymphokines and undergo proliferation in response to the specific antigen, a series of events that initiate the typical delayed-type hypersensitivity (DTH) reaction. The other common measure of cell-mediated immunity is an *in vitro* assessment of T-lymphocyte activation by specific antigens or nonspecific mitogens such as phytohemagglutinin and concanavalin A, which are polyclonal stimulants. T-lymphocyte activation *in vitro* is often measured as incorporation of ^{3}H-thymidine into deoxyribonucleic acid (DNA) in response to an *in vitro* stimulus and is an assay of DNA synthesis or blastogenesis.

Systemic humoral immunity involves activation of B lymphocytes by specific antigens. This specific activation requires helper T lymphocytes for optimal B cell responses to most antigens and once initiated is modulated by suppressor T lymphocytes, which inhibit the humoral response. Activated B lymphocytes are precursors of plasma cells, which produce the various classes of humors or antibodies known as immunoglobulin (Ig) molecules. There are several classes of Ig, each with distinctive functions. IgM fixes complement and thus is important in lysis and opsonization of bacteria and other foreign particles. IgG exists in a series of subclasses

This work was supported in part by NIH Grant HL–25830 and HL–01829 from the Public Health Service.

The author would like to thank Dr. Jerrold J. Ellner for his thoughtful and thorough critique, Dr. R. U. Sorensen for his helpful comments, and Trudy Sansbury for her efficient preparation of this manuscript.

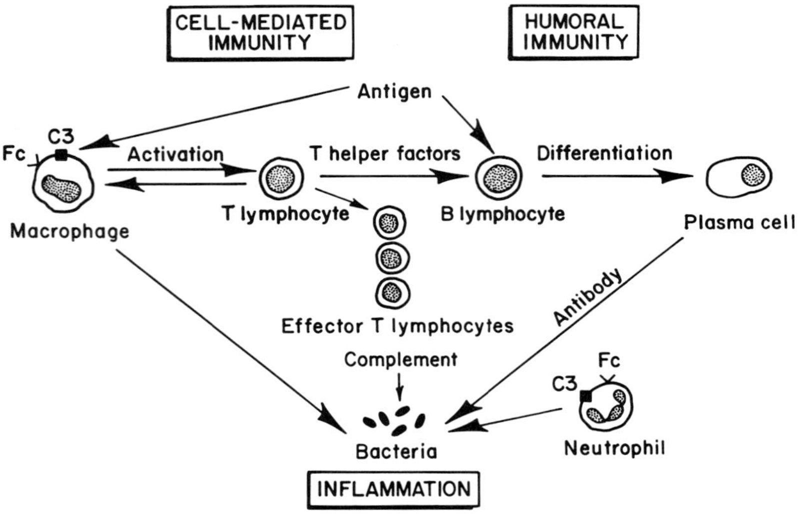

Figure 27–1. Constituents of cell-mediated and humoral immunity and inflammation. Antigen is taken up by antigen-presenting cells, such as macrophages, and presented to T lymphocytes. T lymphocytes are thereby activated to further differentiate into effector T lymphocytes participating in cell-mediated immunity (memory, cytotoxic, regulatory, lymphokine-producing). Activated T lymphocytes also further activate macrophages through release of factors such as interferon gamma. B lymphocytes may respond directly to antigens, and T-helper lymphocytes release factors that stimulate proliferation and then differentiation of B lymphocytes into plasma cells, producing the specific antibodies of humoral immunity. Bacteria can be killed directly by macrophages or neutrophils and by complement, but opsonization of bacteria by antibody or by complement enhances uptake and killing of the organism through Fc or C3 receptors, respectively, on macrophages and neutrophils, which are the major cellular constituents of inflammation.

(IgG1, IgG2, IgG3, IgG4). Both IgG1 and IgG3 can fix complement and are the most efficient IgG subclasses in binding to Fc receptors, which are present on phagocytes. These subclasses, therefore, have a major role in opsonizing microbes, facilitating ingestion by phagocytes. Further details on IgG subclasses are discussed subsequently. IgE molecules are principally responsible for immediate-type allergic reactions, such as those that occur in asthma, and may have a role in immunity to multicellular parasites. The function of IgD is not known. IgA antibodies are the major immunoglobulins on mucosal surfaces, such as the airways where they inhibit adherence of viruses and bacteria to the mucosal surface. IgA in the blood is not functional. Systemic humoral immunity is assessed by measurements of total immunoglobulin levels and of specific classes and subclasses of immunoglobulins in the serum. Specific humoral responses can be measured by assessing antibody levels against organisms or antigens to which the individual is likely to have been exposed, e.g., isohemagglutinins, rubella, and polio virus, or by first immunizing with antigens, e.g., tetanus and diphtheria toxoid, and measuring increments in specific immunoglobulin levels in the blood.

Inflammation is generally considered a localized, nonspecific cellular response to microorganisms or to inert foreign particles. The complement system and the phagocytic/bactericidal activities of macrophages and neutrophils are major examples of networks of inflammation that can be measured in the peripheral blood, providing some insight into mechanisms of localized inflammation. Chemiluminescence (light produced by chemical action) occurs when macrophages and neutrophils are activated. The complement system consists of a large number of plasma and cell membrane–bound proteins, which are activated sequentially by either antibody-coated targets, such as microorganisms, or more traditional immune (antigen-antibody) complexes. These activators stimulate the classic complement pathway. The alternative complement pathway is activated directly by bacterial polysaccharides. The activated C3b complement fragment binds to bacteria helping their attachment to phagocytes (macrophages and neutrophils) through the C3b complement receptors on the cell surface. Activated complement also directly damages certain bacteria and viruses and induces influx of macrophages and neutrophils through chemotactically active fragments of complement proteins (C3a, C5a, C567). Activation and thus consumption of complement can be inferred by measuring levels of specific complement components, such as C3 or C5, or by measuring total hemolytic complement (CH50) levels in the blood. Measurements also may demonstrate depressed levels of complement in disorders of complement synthesis, some of which are hereditary.

Macrophages and neutrophils phagocytose and kill bacteria directly. These cells also express surface Fc and C3b receptors to which the Fc portion of IgG and C3b fragment of complement bind, respectively. Attachment of immunoglobulin or complement-opsonized targets to the appropriate receptors enables these phagocytic cells to ingest and kill opsonized bacteria and viruses efficiently. Antibody also can coat cells infected by virus and expressing viral determinants on the cell surface. This process facilitates destruction by phagocytes (antibody-dependent cellular cytotoxicity).

Phagocytosis and bactericidal activity can be assessed by isolation of monocytes or neutrophils from the blood and then by measuring uptake and killing of radiolabeled bacteria or phagocytosis of inert particles. Chemiluminescence can be measured by mixing the macrophages or neutrophils with an activating stimulus, such as zymosan particles. When these particles are phagocytosed and chemicals such as luminol are

TABLE 27–1. Immune and Inflammatory Processes and Methods of Evaluation

IMMUNE AND INFLAMMATORY PROCESSES	METHODS OF EVALUATION
Cell-mediated immunity	Elicitation of delayed type hypersensitivity by skin testing
	Incorporation of ^{3}H-thymidine into DNA by blood or bronchoalveolar lavage T lymphocytes in response to an *in vitro* antigenic or mitogenic stimulus
Humoral immunity	Levels of total classes and subclasses of immunoglobulin in serum or bronchoalveolar lavage
	Levels of specific antibodies to antigens to which an individual previously has been exposed
	Immunization with antigens and measurement of increments in specific immunoglobulin levels
Inflammation	Levels of specific complement components or total hemolytic complement (CH50)
	Phagocytosis and killing by macrophages and neutrophils from the blood or bronchoalveolar lavage using inert particles or radiolabeled bacteria
	Chemiluminescence by macrophages or neutrophils measured as emission of light after phagocytosis

added, activation by oxygen radicals, for example, causes light generation. The changes in emitted light are then measured in a liquid scintillation counter. Macrophages not only serve as effector cells for phagocytosis and bactericidal activity but also are immunoregulatory cells in processing antigens for T lymphocytes. Macrophages can also regulate cell-mediated immunity by suppressing T lymphocyte responses, particularly in certain chronic infections.

All of the previously described immune and inflammatory activities can be assessed in the peripheral blood but caution must be taken in interpreting these findings in diseases such as COPD. Unfortunately, little is known about the role or even the association of local immune and inflammatory responses in the pathogenesis of COPD. Where data exist, however, such local responses are discussed in this chapter. The reader is referred to more extensive reviews for further information.[6–8, 34, 44, 97, 98, 102, 135]

Inhaled substances can cause local immune or inflammatory responses to occur in three different compartments of the lung. The first is the luminal surface of the bronchoalveolar tree. Although inhaled pathogens, particularly those > 5 to 10μ in size are cleared by the mucociliary ladder, pathogens not as large are retained on the mucosal surface of the smaller bronchi and the epithelial surface of the alveoli. Alveolar macrophages residing on the epithelial surface of alveoli and composing approximately 90% of the total population of bronchoalveolar cells obtained by bronchoalveolar lavage are quite capable of phagocytosis and of killing bacteria. Alveolar macrophages can also take up certain bacterial products and present them to T lymphocytes, thus activating a cell-mediated immune response; however, these cells are particularly adept at inhibiting immune responses, at least *in vitro*. Manifestation of such a suppressive activity may be critical in avoiding excessive and possibly injurious immune responses to inhaled substances. Alveolar T lymphocytes are more difficult to study than alveolar macrophages because they constitute only 6% to 10% of the total number of luminal cells. Some evidence indicates that they are hyporesponsive to mitogens. Currently little is known about the functions of alveolar macrophages or T lymphocytes in COPD. Assessment of the role of these cells in the primary pathogenesis of COPD is complicated by the fact that smoking, which is common in many of the patients, is associated with direct changes in the functions of bronchoalveolar cells, such as immunoregulatory activities and release of inflammatory mediators.

Immunoglobulins, IgA in the upper airways and IgG and IgA in the lower airways and alveoli, also are present on the luminal surface of the bronchoalveolar tree. Secretory IgA is the major immunoglobulin in the upper airways and is of critical importance in the lung's defense against bacteria and viruses. Secretory IgA protects the lung by inhibiting viruses from infecting epithelial cells and by decreasing adherence of certain bacteria to mucosal surfaces. IgA also coats particles and bacteria and in combination with complement and lysozyme promotes phagocytosis. Various components of complement, especially C3, C4, and factor B, are also present on the airway surface but the precise functions of complement in this location are uncertain.

Another compartment where inhaled substances might stimulate immunologic or inflammatory activity is the submucosal region, where lymphoid tissue is distributed along the tracheobronchial tree from Waldeyer's ring to the terminal bronchioles. Submucosal bronchus-associated lymphoid tissue (BALT), as described by Bienenstock and associates,[6] consists mainly of isolated cellular aggregates of one or two follicles containing lymphocytes and plasma cells lying immediately below the epithelium. These cells secrete predominantly IgA antibodies and some IgG. IgA is transported by epithelial cells into the bronchial lumen. During passage through the epithelial cells, IgA acquires a glycoprotein called secretory piece, which confers resistance of the IgA dimer to proteolytic enzymes. The role of macrophages as immunoregulatory or effector cells in the submucosal region of the airways is not known.

Yet another immunologic compartment in the lung is a complex and extensive network of lymphatic channels draining the submucosal lymphoid aggregates. The network resides in connective tissue sheets surrounding bronchioles and blood vessels forming the interlobular septa and ultimately drains into hilar lymph nodes. As suggested by Macklin,[67] the lymphatic system of the tracheobronchial tree may serve as a "sump" for trapping and removing inhaled particles.

ALPHA$_1$-ANTITRYPSIN DEFICIENCY

Primary immune perturbations probably do not predispose to the form of emphysema that is associated with smoking. Smoking has marked effects on blood and alveolar phagocytes and lymphocytes so that it is not clear whether the immune abnormalities in smokers with emphysema are primary or secondary to smoking. Identification of immune abnormalities before the development of emphysema is thwarted by the fact that there are, as yet, no early biologic markers to detect individuals who will develop the disease. Immune system abnormalities may be implicated in the predisposition to and perpetuation of emphysema caused by the inherited disease alpha$_1$-antitrypsin (α1-AT) deficiency. Table 27–2 indicates changes in the immune system reported in α1-AT deficiency.

Mild α1-AT deficiency and phenotypes such as PiMS and PiMZ are associated with certain autoimmune disorders, such as rheumatoid arthritis, systemic lupus erythematosus, and uveitis.[18] There is evidence *in vivo* of lymphocyte hyperresponsiveness in α1-AT deficiency (see Table 27–2). In a study by Breit and colleagues,[15] the delayed-type hypersensitivity (DTH) response in subjects with α1-AT deficiency of the PiZZ phenotype was accelerated. Eight hours after intradermal injection of various antigens, two thirds of the α1-AT deficient subjects who would manifest DTH at 48 hours already were positive, whereas only one of the 20 control subjects was positive at 8 hours. Despite the accelerated responses observed, no difference between the α1–AT-deficient and control groups in the magnitude of positive responses could be detected, perhaps reflecting intact regulatory mechanisms in α1-AT deficiency.

Breit and coworkers[15] also found that lymphocytes (from either healthy or α1–AT-deficient subjects) stimulated *in vitro* with the mitogen phytohemagglutinin showed significantly increased blastogenic responses, as measured by incorporation of ^{3}H-thymidine, when serum from PiZZ α1–AT-deficient subjects was added to cultures. The serum-mediated enhancement of lymphocyte responses was demonstrated to be due to the depressed levels of α1-AT, because addition of highly purified α1-AT resulted in decreases in the PHA response.[17] Similar but less marked effects of α1-AT were observed when another mitogen, concanavalin A, but not pokeweed mitogen, was used as the stimulus. The inhibitory effect of α1-AT on lymphocyte responses was observed to plateau once the protein reached the normal physiologic range (2 to 4 mg/ml). These studies suggest, therefore, that reduced α1-AT levels, as occur in α1–AT-deficient subjects, may result in lymphocyte activation. The mechanism of action of α1-AT on lymphocyte blastogenic responses is not entirely clear. It appears, however, that α1-AT directly inhibits adherent accessory cells, possibly through blocking a membrane-bound serine esterase on monocytes, and has no direct effect on proliferating T cells.[17]

Alpha$_1$-antitrypsin also inhibits the cytotoxic reactions of

TABLE 27–2. Immunologic Activities and Levels in Emphysema Associated with Alpha$_1$-Antitrypsin (α1-AT) Deficiency

COMPARTMENT	IMMUNOLOGIC ACTIVITIES OR LEVELS
Systemic (as obtained from blood or serum)	
T lymphocytes	Accelerated DTH
	Serum-mediated enhancement of responses to mitogens
	Lymphocytes from patients with α1-AT deficiency can kill hepatocytes (not known if these cells kill lung cells)
	α1-AT inhibits T lymphocyte-mediated cytotoxicity and natural killer cell activity directly
B lymphocytes	Ig levels normal
Complement	C3, C5, and factor B increased
Macrophages	α1-AT inhibits accessory cell function
	Chemiluminescence increased
Neutrophils	Chemiluminescence increased
Local	
T lymphocytes	Not known
B lymphocytes	Not known
Complement	Not known
Macrophages, neutrophils	Major role in production of injurious enzymes, particularly neutrophil elastase, which are normally inhibited by α1-AT and are thus unimpeded in α1-AT deficiency

lymphocytes, including antibody-dependent cell-mediated cytotoxicity,[1,96] T lymphocyte-mediated cytotoxicity,[1] and natural killer cell activity.[1,61] It is not known whether α1-AT directly interferes with the cytotoxic cell or modulates target cell binding or destruction. Killing of autologous hepatocytes by peripheral blood lymphocytes from patients with α1-AT deficiency is increased as compared with that which occurs in controls (patients with other forms of chronic liver disease).[80] Killing of lung cells by lymphocytes from subjects with α1-AT deficiency has not been assessed. These studies are provocative, however, since it is possible that deficiency of α1-AT may lead to destruction of lung tissue by uncontrolled activity of cytotoxic lymphocytes.

Serum immunoglobulin levels are normal in α1-AT deficiency[15] and disturbances in antibody activities have not been described. Therefore, abnormalities in systemic humoral immunity cannot be implicated in the predisposition of subjects with α1-AT deficiency to emphysema. There is an increase in some components of complement (C3, C5, factor B, and PH50) but not others (C4 or CH50).[15] Although no direct inhibition of functional complement activity using CH50 and PH50 assays (total hemolytic and total alternative pathway–derived hemolytic complement activity, respectively) by purified α1-AT has been demonstrated,[15] α1-AT was shown to bind directly to C3 and inhibit C3-mediated phagocytosis,[15] suggesting that the observed increase in C3 in patients with α1-AT deficiency may be a direct consequence of the deficiency and not an epiphenomenon.

Studies of macrophages and neutrophils indicate that other nonspecific inflammatory responses in α1-AT deficiency also may be activated. Zymosan-induced chemiluminescence of blood monocytes and neutrophils was enhanced in the presence of α1-AT-deficient sera compared with sera from healthy subjects,[15] but purified α1-AT did not inhibit the chemiluminescence.[16] Since chemiluminescence is dependent on the alternative pathway of complement, and since sera from patients with α1-AT deficiency have elevations of factor B of this pathway as well as of PH50, it has been suggested that the effect of α1-AT–deficient sera on chemiluminescence may be due to these complement components.[18] Alpha$_1$-antitrypsin also reduced chemokinesis of monocytes and neutrophils.[61] Further, monocytes and neutrophils are major producers of such neutral proteases as elastase, collagenases, cathepsin G, and plasminogen activator, which are believed to be of primary importance in tissue destruction in inflammatory diseases, such as emphysema. Since α1-AT inhibits these enzymes, it is likely that in α1-AT deficiency decreased inhibition of these enzymes results in tissue injury.

To summarize, in subjects with α1-AT deficiency, the *in vivo* accelerated DTH response, the *in vitro* serum-mediated enhancement of T-lymphocyte activation, and the increased activity of cytotoxic lymphocytes suggest that uncontrolled immune reactivity may predispose to the lung damage in α1-AT deficiency. The activated monocytes, neutrophils, alternative pathway of complement, and the decreased inhibition of proteases released from phagocytes in α1-AT deficiency together suggest that unimpeded inflammatory responses in this disease directly induce the lung injury leading to emphysema.

CHRONIC BRONCHITIS AND EMPHYSEMA, OR "COPD"

It is difficult to assess the primary role of the immune system in the pathogenesis of chronic bronchitis independently of the direct effects of smoking and infection on immune cells. Unlike emphysema related to α1-AT deficiency, there is no single genetic prototype predisposing the patient to the most common adult form of chronic bronchitis, which is associated with smoking, recurrent infections, cough, obstruction to airflow, hypoxia, and tendency to develop right-sided heart failure. Several inherited immunoglobulin deficiencies exist that are associated with both chronic bronchitis and bronchiectasis, but the clinical characteristics of these diseases differ from the chronic bronchitis of smokers. The general conclusions drawn regarding the functions of the immune system in this disease are summarized in Table 27–3. Because many studies of immune responses in COPD have grouped patients with chronic bronchitis and emphysema, this section focuses on those studies and, when possible, on those studies which address chronic bronchitis alone.

Systemic cell-mediated immunity as assessed by DTH responses has been studied in chronic bronchitis. One study found diminished skin test reactivity to recall antigens in some patients with chronic bronchitis,[145] whereas another found DTH responses comparable between patients with COPD and healthy subjects.[100] Little is known about the role of lymphocytes localized to the lung in the pathogenesis of chronic bronchitis. Clancy and coworkers[28] isolated BALT tissue from surgically resected human bronchial tissue. When the lymphoid cells were challenged *in vitro* with several recall antigens, blastogenic responses occurred. This single study provides an estimate of reactivity of BALT lymphocytes from healthy subjects. Puci and colleagues[95] further characterized the mu-

TABLE 27–3. Immunologic Activities and Levels in Chronic Bronchitis/Emphysema or "COPD"

COMPARTMENT	IMMUNOLOGIC ACTIVITIES OR LEVELS
Systemic (as obtained from blood or serum)	
T lymphocytes	DTH increased or decreased (controversial)
B lymphocytes	
IgA	No relation of serum IgA levels to COPD
IgG, IgM	Normal levels
IgE	Increased levels
IgD	Possibly increased levels
Complement	C3, C4 decreased
Macrophages, neutrophils	Not known
Local	
T lymphocytes	Not known
B lymphocytes	
IgA	Number of IgA (especially IgA1) positive cells in lung necropsy tissues increased IgA levels in saliva and sputum normal
IgG	Increased precipitating IgG to infectious agents in sputum
IgD	Nasal IgD increased
IgE, IgM	Not known
Complement	Not known
Macrophages, neutrophils	Probably major role in production of injurious enzymes and oxygen radicals activated by smoking and infection

cosal cell populations from bronchi of patients with a variety of bronchial disorders, including chronic bronchitis, bronchiectasis, bronchiolitis, carcinoma of the bronchus, and pneumonia. T and B lymphocytes and phagocytic cells were identified. Analysis of T lymphocyte subsets revealed the presence of T lymphocytes capable of binding to the Fc fragment of IgG (Tγ cells), IgM (Tμ), and IgA (Tα). Interestingly, fewer Tα cells were found in acutely inflamed tissues (e.g., bronchiolitis, pneumonia, and abscess) than in chronically inflamed mucosa (e.g., chronic bronchitis, bronchiectasis, and carcinoma of the bronchus). The function of Tα cells is unknown but a possible circuit involving Tα cells and IgA secretion may contribute to local immunoregulation by T lymphocytes. It was suggested by Puci and colleagues[95] that the expanded population of Tα cells in chronically as compared with acutely inflamed mucosa may reflect important differences in the establishment of adaptive control mechanisms regulating lymphocyte proliferation. Whether these or other regulatory mechanisms are hyperresponsive or are in any way dysregulated in those individuals who will develop chronic bronchitis remains to be elucidated.

Lymphocytes lining the epithelial side of the respiratory tract can be retrieved from bronchoalveolar lavage fluid. These cells may or may not, however, reflect those in the mucosal milieu. Cell populations of healthy human subjects, obtained by the lavage procedure, consist largely of macrophages, approximately 6% to 10% lymphocytes and rare granulocytes.[63] The proportion of lymphocytes that are T lymphocytes and B lymphocytes is similar in bronchoalveolar lavage and blood, with T lymphocytes predominating in both. Daniele and colleagues[35] found that the blastogenic responses of bronchoalveolar lymphocytes from healthy nonsmokers to various mitogens were less than that of blood lymphocytes. The responses of bronchoalveolar lymphocytes from healthy smokers to phytohemagglutinin and concanavalin A were significantly less than the responses of lung lymphocytes from healthy nonsmokers.[36] Alveolar macrophages were not responsible for the inhibitory effects in this particular study. Nevertheless, alveolar macrophages inhibit blood lymphocyte responses to a variety of antigens and mitogens,[38, 72, 99, 133, 143] and this suppressive effect is greater with alveolar macrophages from smokers, as compared with nonsmokers.[99] These studies of alveolar lymphocyte responses in healthy individuals and in smokers, and the possible role of alveolar macrophages in regulating these responses, provide a framework for future studies of the role of lymphocyte and macrophage responses in the development of COPD. As yet, however, we know little of the role of luminal, submucosal, or lymphatic lymphocytes and macrophages in COPD.

The contradictory studies of DTH skin test reactions in COPD and the findings of hyporesponsive lung lymphocyte responses and increased immunosuppressive activities of alveolar macrophages in smokers do not themselves support an important role for lymphocytes in chronic bronchitis or emphysema. The generalized hyporesponsiveness of lymphocytes in smokers coupled with the fact that purified α1-AT decreases responsiveness of lymphocytes to mitogens suggests rather that well-regulated T lymphocyte responses may protect against the development of COPD in non α1-AT–deficient subjects.

The role of immunoglobulins in chronic bronchitis has also been examined. IgA deficiency is part of a well-known clinical syndrome associated with bronchitis and recurrent pneumonia in some individuals and is discussed in the next section. Surprisingly, serum IgA levels were found to be increased in COPD patients without acute infection,[84] and the total number of IgA positive cells in specimens of lung tissue from necropsy in those with chronic bronchitis and bronchiectasis was greater than that in control subjects.[21] The IgA1 subset, which is more resistant to proteolysis than IgA2, was also increased in the lungs of subjects with bronchial disease and more so in chronic bronchitis than bronchiectasis.[21] Webb and Condemi[140] described a family study in which COPD was associated with selective IgA deficiency. Zinneman and colleagues,[147] however, measured secretory IgA concentrations in the serum, saliva, and sputum of 91 patients with COPD and found no relationship of IgA concentration to the presence of disease or to its extent. Thus, although bronchitis is often found in patients with IgA deficiency, IgA deficiency does not seem to be a factor in the genesis of COPD in most instances.

Both systemic and local precipitating antibodies (presumably IgG) to a variety of infectious agents have been described in COPD patients. Serum IgG and IgM levels were not significantly increased in COPD patients not acutely infected.[77] IgE-mediated type I hypersensitivity has long been associated with asthma. Pauwels[91] found that total serum levels of IgE were increased in healthy people with a familial history of nonallergic chronic bronchitis, which was termed chronic nonspecific lung disease. The IgE levels were even higher in the patients with chronic nonspecific lung disease. Thus, IgE may predispose an individual through unknown mechanisms to development of chronic bronchitis as well as asthma. Miller and associates[77] found significantly higher levels of serum IgD and nasal IgD and IgM expressed as percentages of total protein in subjects with COPD.[77] These investigators also found that low IgD was more common in healthy control subjects, suggesting that low IgD protects against the development of COPD.[77] A follow-up study with a smaller number of patients did not, however, confirm this initial finding.[86]

Miller and colleagues[78] found significantly lower serum levels of C3 and C4 in COPD patients than in healthy subjects matched for age, sex, occupation, and smoking history.[78] Among the patients there also was a significant correlation among chronic cough and sputum production and low C3 and C4 levels. The more bronchitic subjects tended to have the lowest C3 and C4 values. The mechanisms that account for the low complement values in these patients are speculative. Neutralization of certain viruses may be accomplished through the alternative pathway, and both the alternative and classic pathways are involved in the bactericidal activities of serum. Therefore, activation of complement during periods of infection in patients with COPD may result in periods of low complement levels. Miller and colleagues,[128] however, found no significant correlation between low C3 and C4 levels and the frequency or severity of past respiratory infections. *In vitro* studies have demonstrated that leukocyte lysosomal elastase degrades C3. It is possible, therefore, that the increased levels of active elastase in COPD may be responsible for the lower C3 levels observed in this study by Miller,[78] and even more importantly they might be most relevant for local complement levels. This decrease in complement, in turn, might interfere with local defense mechanisms against infectious agents.

Macrophages and neutrophils are considered to be pivotal in the pathogenesis of smoking-induced emphysema because they release a variety of substances that are toxic to the lung, such as proteases and oxygen radicals.[13, 75] These activities of macrophages and neutrophils are presumably secondary responses to smoking, infection, or both. Cigarette smoke, for example, is believed to oxidize α1-AT. This oxidation induces a functional deficit of the enzyme inhibitor, allowing unimpeded injury to the lung by enzymes such as elastase produced by neutrophils and macrophages.[25] Infection also induces lung damage not only by a direct effect of the microorganisms but by attracting inflammatory cells, such as macrophages and neutrophils, which release proteolytic enzymes and oxygen radicals upon phagocytosis of microbes.

In summary, the role of the immune system in general in predisposing an individual to chronic bronchitis is poorly understood. More is known about T lymphocyte responses in the bronchoalveolar regions of healthy nonsmoking and smoking subjects than about COPD patients. Lung lymphocytes from healthy smokers appear to be hyporesponsive to stimuli. Lymphocytes may play a protective role in COPD. IgA deficiency predisposes to bronchitis but chronic bronchitis or COPD is not associated with IgA deficiency. IgD and IgE may be increased in COPD, suggesting that these immunoglobulins may predispose an individual to COPD but through unknown mechanisms. The complement components, C3 and C4, are decreased in COPD and more so in chronic bronchitis. The low complement levels are not related to smoking history or to infections, suggesting a direct association between complement levels and COPD. Most importantly, inflammatory cells, such as macrophages and neutrophils, which are activated secondarily by smoking or by infection, release products that may directly injure the lung.

BRONCHIECTASIS ASSOCIATED WITH IMMUNOGLOBULIN DEFICIENCIES

Most cases of bronchiectasis are caused by conditions such as infections that lead to collapse or fibrosis of the lung with compensatory stretching and dilation of the bronchial walls.[125] Primary immunoglobulin deficiencies with the attendant recurrent infections are uncommon and account for a small fraction of the cases of bronchiectasis, bronchitis, or sinusitis. In general, immunoglobulin deficiencies are believed to produce bronchiectasis as a result of recurrent infections rather than through a direct effect of the immunologic abnormality on the bronchial tree. Other primary immunologic deficiencies, such as T lymphocyte defects and phagocytic disorders, are associated most commonly with pneumonia and other systemic infections. Less is known about the association of these disorders with bronchiectasis.

Secondarily acquired immune deficiencies usually do not lead to bronchiectasis, perhaps because the offending agent, such as chemotherapy, is eliminated or because the primary disease is fatal, allowing insufficient time for chronic lung damage to occur (e.g., AIDS). Since the lung injury induced by infection or smoking is mediated in part by immune and inflammatory cells, it is perhaps not surprising that immunoincompetence as manifested by immunoglobulin deficiency is not commonly associated with severe lung injury except in those cases of longstanding primary immunoglobulin deficiency. The association of excesses of immunoglobulins and immune complexes with bronchiectasis are considered in the next section.

The clinical hallmark of primary immunoglobulin deficiencies is increased susceptibility to infections, usually beginning early in life. Respiratory, skin, central nervous system, and gastrointestinal infections are the most common. In the lung, the determinants of the progression of recurrent pneumonias or acute bronchitis to bronchiectasis, chronic bronchitis, or both are not well understood. Multiple factors, however, must be involved, including type and severity of the immunoincompetence, age of onset and duration of symptoms, genetic factors, early treatment of infections, and concomitant disorders. The various types of primary immunoglobulin deficiencies and their immunologic characteristics and pulmonary involvement are summarized in Table 27–4. It is not the intent of this section to review these diseases, which are reviewed elsewhere in full,[20, 66, 103, 104] but rather to focus on bronchiectasis as related to primary immunoglobulin abnormalities affecting the lung.

The clinically most severe of the antibody deficiencies is X-linked agammaglobulinemia, first described by Bruton in 1952.[19] The case report by Bruton was that of an 8-year-old male with a 4-year history of recurrent pneumococcal pneumonia and sepsis and unexplained absence of serum gamma globulin (without nephrosis, malnutrition, or other abnormalities of serum proteins). The institution of gamma globulin resulted in no further episodes of sepsis for the 14 months reported. No sequelae of the pneumonia or immune deficiency in the form of bronchiectasis, chronic bronchitis, or pulmonary insufficiency were reported. It was later learned that X-linked agammaglobulinemia is characterized immunologically by complete absence of circulating B lymphocytes and panhypogammaglobulinemia. The defect is assumed to be in B-cell maturation, because pre-B cells in the bone marrow are normal. In the first several years following this initial report of agammaglobulinemia and susceptibility to bacterial pneumonia, a flurry of case reports appeared in the literature. Good and Mazzitello[51] summarized the literature in 1956 and particularly noted that all the patients had recurrent bacterial pneumonias and that the prevalence of bronchiectasis as a complication of congenital agammaglobulinemia was four of the 24 cases reported. In other series the prevalence of bronchiectasis was as high as 67%.[138] Pulmonary infections in X-linked agammaglobulinemia are usually caused by pyogenic bacterial organisms, such as pneumococci, other streptococci, and *Haemophilus influenzae*. Rarely, *Pneumocystis carinii* may

TABLE 27–4. Pulmonary Involvement in Primary Immunoglobulin Deficiencies

DISEASE (REFERENCES)	IMMUNOLOGIC CHARACTERISTICS	PULMONARY INVOLVEMENT
X-linked agammaglobulinemia (Bruton's)[19, 20, 66, 103, 104]	Circulating B cells absent or very low Pre-B cells in marrow normal Panhypogammaglobulinemia Defect likely in B cell maturation	Recurrent pyogenic bacterial pneumonias Chronic sinusitis common Bronchiectasis 17% to 67%
Common variable immunodeficiency (acquired agammaglobulinemia)[20, 51, 53, 62, 66, 103, 104]	B cells present but cannot be stimulated to differentiate into immunoglobulin-producing plasma cells Panhypogammaglobulinemia	Recurrent pyogenic bacterial pneumonias Chronic sinusitis common Bronchiectasis 21% to 67%
Selective immunoglobulin deficiencies		
Single deficiencies of IgG subclass[5, 136]	Deficiencies of IgG2 IgG3 IgG4	Recurrrent pneumonias Bronchiectasis common
Deficiency of more than one IgG subclass[88, 113, 144]	Deficiencies of IgG1, IgG2 and IgG4 IgG1, IgG2 and IgG3 IgG1 and IgG2 IgG2 and IgG3 IgG2 and IgG4	Pneumonia common Bronchiectasis or chronic bronchitis common
Deficiency of IgA[2, 3, 27, 30, 48, 56, 65]	Deficiency of IgA	Upper respiratory tract infections 0% to 36% Bronchiectasis rare
Deficiency of IgA and of IgG subclasses[10, 89]	Deficiencies of IgG2 and IgA IgG3 and IgA	Frequent upper and lower respiratory tract infections Bronchiectasis and COPD common
Deficiency of IgA and IgE[94]	Deficiency of IgA and IgE	Respiratory tract infections rare Bronchiectasis rare

be the cause of the presenting pneumonia or of the recurrent pneumonia despite normal T lymphocyte function in agammaglobulinemia.[108] Patients also may succumb to progressive enteroviral infection despite gammaglobulin replacement.[76] An autosomal recessive agammaglobulinemia also has been described as occurring in female patients that is otherwise indistinguishable from X-linked agammaglobulinemia, but this entity is rare.[58]

In contrast to X-linked agammaglobulinemia, common variable immunodeficiency (CVI), also known as acquired agammaglobulinemia, has an equal sex distribution and occurs later in life (range 7 to 67 years of age).[20, 62, 66, 103, 104, 146] B cells are present in CVI, unlike the X-linked form, but are not functional because they cannot be stimulated to differentiate into immunoglobulin-producing plasma cells. Thus, in CVI, hypogammaglobulinemia or agammaglobulinemia is observed, but lymph nodes and tonsils paradoxically may be enlarged with an increase in B-dependent areas. Serum levels of Ig are low but may not be absent, and the various classes of Ig may not be involved equally. Like congenital agammaglobulinemia, CVI is characterized by recurrent bacterial infections with pyogenic organisms. Bacterial pneumonia occurs in most of the patients, and chronic sinusitis is common. Interestingly, bacteremia and nonpulmonary infections are less common than in X-linked agammaglobulinemia, perhaps because residual antibodies may be present. The reported prevalence of bronchiectasis is 21% to 67%.[51, 53, 62, 138, 146]

The treatment for both congenital and acquired hypogammaglobulinemia includes antibiotics for acute infection and pooled human immune serum globulin for prevention of bacterial infections. Intravenous administration of immune serum globulin is replacing the intramuscular route, because the intravenous route is at least as effective in prevention of infections, and physiologic antibody levels can be achieved and maintained. Furthermore, administration to patients requiring large amounts or having bleeding disorders is facilitated by the intravenous route.[2, 32, 50, 93, 101, 122] The beneficial effect of replacement therapy with serum globulin by either route in reducing the incidence of acute infections is well documented.[2, 4, 32, 50, 64, 92, 101, 122]

Prevention of infection through immunoglobulin replacement therapy will in turn inhibit the development or progression of bronchiectasis. In a study performed before intravenous preparations of serum globulin were available, South and coworkers[124] reported, however, that in 19 of 20 patients with hypogammaglobulinemia (both congenital and acquired) respiratory tract infections progressed despite immunoglobulin therapy.[124] Bjorkander and colleagues[9] found, in contrast, that even with the prophylactic use of intramuscular injections of immunoglobulin, a statistically significant difference was found between the inadequately treated patients ($FEV_1 = 62\%$ of predicted normal, $n = 12$) and the adequately treated patients ($FEV_1 = 82\%$, $n = 12$), $P < 0.05$.

Roifman and colleagues[101] reported the effect of intravenous serum globulin in seven patients with both congenital and acquired hypogammaglobulinemia. All seven patients had radiographic evidence for bronchiectasis. After 6 to 12 months of treatment with intravenous serum globulin, there was a significant decrease in patients with acute infections requiring hospitalization. Cough was markedly reduced in all the patients, but radiographic improvement was noted in only two. Concurrently, there was a 10% to 25% improvement in pulmonary function tests. Watts and colleagues[139] found that 19 reported patients receiving adequate intravenous immunoglobulin therapy maintained stable pulmonary function tests for the 6.9 years of their follow-up study. Interestingly, however, despite improvement or stabilization, physiologic evidence of obstructive lung disease was still apparent in the majority of patients in the studies of both Roifman and Watts. These findings establish, therefore, that with significant reduction in acute infections by immunoglobulin prophylaxis, obstructive lung disease either will be improved or will not be progressive, but that obstructive lung disease once established is irreversible.

A variety of selective immunoglobulin deficiencies has been associated with recurrent pneumonias and bronchiectasis of a severity comparable to that in X-linked agammaglobulinemia or CVI. Rothbach[105] described a patient with recurrent pulmonary infection and right middle lobe bronchiectasis with normal levels of total immunoglobulin and normal levels of IgG, A, M, and E. The patient failed to develop serum antibody responses to specific antigens, e.g., diphtheria, tetanus, pneumococcus, *in vivo*. It is possible therefore that this patient had a selective deficiency in one or more immunoglobulin subclasses or a defect in regulation of antibody formation by other cells, such as T lymphocytes. An isolated deficiency of the immunoglobulin subclass IgG4 was found in three of the first seven subjects with "idiopathic" bronchiectasis, studied by Beck and Heiner.[5] Additionally, four of 29 subjects with recurrent or chronic pulmonary infections had isolated IgG4 deficiency.[5] Three of the same four patients with persistent pulmonary infections who underwent bronchography also had bronchiectasis. IgG4 constitutes only 4% of total IgG and does not fix complement when bound to antigen. Although IgG4 is not detected in all healthy individuals[81] and the function of IgG4 is not clear, this study of Beck and Heiner suggests that IgG4 may play a unique role in pulmonary host defense.

Umetsu and associates[136] described 20 children with recurrent sinopulmonary infections and normal serum IgG levels who had selective deficiency of either IgG2 or IgG3, or both.[136] Because the IgG antibody response to polysaccharide antigens resides predominantly within the IgG2 subclass, serum antibody levels to the capsular polysaccharide of *Haemophilus influenzae* were measured. The antibody levels were low both before and after immunization in the patients with IgG2 deficiency, but the antibody response to a booster of diphtheria toxoid which, because it is a protein, should reside with IgG1 and IgG3, was normal.

Immunodeficiency states involving two or more IgG subclasses also have been described.[88, 113, 144] These patients have recurrent pneumonias and either bronchiectasis or chronic bronchitis. Importantly, a deficiency of either one, two, or three IgG subclasses may be associated with pneumonia, bronchiectasis, and chronic bronchitis even when total serum levels of IgG are normal. Therefore, specific subclasses of IgG should be measured in patients with recurrent bacterial pneumonia without underlying pulmonary anatomic defects and with no other cause of immunodeficiency even if total levels of IgG are normal.

Faulk and colleagues[43] reported an infant with recurrent *Pseudomonas* pneumonia and isolated serum IgM deficiency. Isolated IgM deficiency, however, is rare and has not been reported to be associated with bronchiectasis. Isolated IgD deficiency also has not been found to be associated with bronchiectasis.

IgA is the immunoglobulin that is most frequently deficient. In the general population the frequency of IgA deficiency, defined as $< 10-40$ μg/ml, is 1:310 to 1:3040 depending on the series.[65] The clinical significance of selective IgA deficiency, however, remains controversial. Koistinen[65] found no differences in the clinical history of IgA-deficient and control subjects in a cohort of 64,588 persons. Several other smaller studies also have found IgA deficiency to be present without any signs of disease.[3, 30, 48, 56] In contrast, other studies demonstrate that IgA deficiency is associated with a variety of disorders, including recurrent respiratory tract infections,[2] malabsorption,[49, 109] autoimmune disease,[2] and ataxia telangiectasis.[124] Although a patient with recurrent pneumonias and bronchiectasis in association with selective IgA deficiency has been described,[27] the respiratory infections in IgA deficiency are almost always mild to moderate, involving the upper respiratory tract, and rarely result in abnormalities of pulmonary function.[2]

Because secretory IgA is the major immunoglobulin component of pulmonary as well as other secretions and plays a pivotal role in resistance to pulmonary infections,[73, 115, 134] it is difficult to understand why deficiency of IgA rarely leads to severe pulmonary infection or the chronic sequela of bronchiectasis. When studied, both serum and salivary IgA have been absent in IgA-deficient individuals.[2] One patient has been described, however, who had normal serum levels of IgA but decreased salivary and jejunal IgA; this patient had persistent diarrhea but no pulmonary problems.[127]

Another possible explanation for the discrepancy between the known importance of IgA in lung defense and the paucity of severe pulmonary abnormalities in IgA-deficient subjects is that other immunoglobulins compensate for the deficiency. In support of this possibility, two large series have shown that total serum IgG was significantly increased in IgA-deficient subjects.[2, 65] Other studies demonstrate that the deficient subjects contain compensatory IgM and a low molecular weight IgM, which may have a biologic function in protection.[14, 126]

Several case reports have described IgA deficiency and bronchiectasis in association with diseases, such as sarcoidosis,[107] hemosiderosis,[85] and alpha$_1$-antitrypsin deficiency,[87] suggesting that coexistent abnormalities may influence the evolution of bronchiectasis in individuals with IgA deficiency. Perhaps even more enlightening is the clear association of IgA deficiency with sinopulmonary infections and bronchiectasis with IgG subclass deficiency. Oxelius and colleagues[89] first described coexisting IgG2 deficiency in diseased but not in healthy IgA-deficient subjects.[89] Björkander and colleagues[10] clearly demonstrated that low levels of either IgG2 or IgG3 in IgA-deficient patients were correlated significantly with abnormalities of lung function as determined by spirometry, lung volumes, the single-breath nitrogen test, and static recoil pressures. In addition to providing evidence for a causal relation between low levels of IgG subclasses and deterioration in lung function, these studies suggest that patients with combined IgA and IgG subclass deficiencies might benefit from immunoglobulin prophylaxis. IgA deficiency alone, however, should not be treated with immunoglobulin prophylaxis even if patients are symptomatic, because anaphylaxis may occur due to sensitization of the individual against IgA, even though only trace amounts of IgA are present in the immunoglobulin preparation. IgA deficiency also has been noted in a patient with IgE deficiency and chronic sinopulmonary disease.[23] Polmar and colleagues,[94] however, found that 11 out of 25 individuals with IgA deficiency also had IgE deficiency, and all 11 were asymptomatic. In contrast, a high prevalence (71%) of respiratory tract disease was found in the IgA-deficient subjects who were not IgE deficient.[94] It appears, therefore, that IgE may either be directly pathogenetic in respiratory tract disease or at least its presence may be a marker for other unknown immunologic abnormalities in IgA deficiency.

BRONCHIECTASIS ASSOCIATED WITH IMMUNOGLOBULIN AND IMMUNE COMPLEX EXCESSES

Activation of the immune system may directly participate in the lung injury of bronchiectasis. Certainly the lung damage induced by smoking and infection secondary to immunoglobulin deficiency is mediated in part by products of immune and inflammatory cells. The central bronchiectasis characteristic of allergic bronchopulmonary aspergillosis is thought to be due to tissue damage caused by local deposition of antigen-antibody complexes and complement fixation, and precipitating antibodies to antigens of *Aspergillus fumigatus* are present in patients' sera.[110] Furthermore, precipitating antibodies to *Haemophilus influenzae* and other bacteria are present in other types of bronchiectasis, suggesting that antigens of bacterial or viral origin may lead to the formation of immune complexes that mediate lung damage.[22, 29] Hilton and coworkers[54] found excess anticomplementary activity in the sera of patients with bronchiectasis and further found evidence to suggest the presence of immune complexes of the IgG type in the sera of such patients.[55] Other findings included selective immunoglobulin excesses of IgA, IgG, or IgM, or all three; a high prevalence of autoantibodies (rheumatoid factor 52%, antinuclear antibody 10%); and an association of autoimmune disorders with bronchiectasis.[55] Together these studies lend some credence to the notion that the immune system may cause or perpetuate the lung damage of bronchiectasis.

CYSTIC FIBROSIS

In patients with cystic fibrosis lung damage develops because of chronic pulmonary infection and the ensuing inflammatory response, which leads to the development of fibrosis and COPD. The immune and inflammatory systems in cystic fibrosis are, for the most part, intact apart from responses to *Pseudomonas,* the principal pathogen infecting the lungs of patients with cystic fibrosis. Studies of the immune and inflammatory systems in cystic fibrosis have focused on three areas: (1) characterization of the immune and inflammatory system in the basal state and with progression of lung damage; (2) determination of cellular responses to agents other than *Pseudomonas;* and (3) examination of cellular responses to *Pseudomonas* in particular. These three categories of studies are summarized in Table 27–5.

Although patients with cystic fibrosis are almost invariably infected with some microorganism, some general information has accrued concerning the characteristics of T lymphocytes, the humoral system, immune complexes, and phagocytes. Lymphocytes from individuals with cystic fibrosis do not have abnormalities in chloride metabolism like those that occur in sweat gland cells,[11] but the release of arachidonic acid by lymphocytes from patients with cystic fibrosis is not inhibited by dexamethasone or fetal calf serum as it is in normal lymphocytes.[24] Intact lymphocytes from patients with cystic fibrosis also produce significantly less adenosine 3′, 5′ cyclic adenosine monophosphate (cAMP) in response to the beta-adrenergic agent isoproterenol than do lymphocytes from healthy subjects, although the basal cAMP content and the response to prostaglandin E_1 are normal.[37] Lymphocytes from obligate cystic fibrosis heterozygotes have a reduced cAMP response to isoproterenol as well. Although the implications of these findings for lymphocyte-mediated immunity are not clear, it can be concluded that lymphocytes from patients with cystic fibrosis may express genetically determined functional abnormalities in specific pathways of activation, which may prove ultimately to have a subtle yet significant impact on immune function.

Humoral immunity in cystic fibrosis was examined directly in a series of studies by Matthews and coworkers[71] and Wheeler and coworkers.[141] These investigators performed a large study of 400 patients with cystic fibrosis to examine various aspects of the immune system.[31] In spite of previous reports of hypergammaglobulinemia in cystic fibrosis,[52, 114] these investigators found that 22% of patients under 10 years of age with cystic fibrosis had hypogammaglobulinemia principally attributable to decreases in IgG and to a lesser extent IgA.[71] Only 1% to 2% of the patients over 10 years of age had hypogammaglobulinemia. In contrast, 25% of the patients who were 10 to 20 years of age and 50% who were over 20 years of age were hypergammaglobulinemic. The decrease in immunoglobulin levels was not related to abnormal production or to increased catabolism of immunoglobulin. The patients who were hypogammaglobulinemic had significantly better lung function as demonstrated by arterial blood gases, number of hospitalizations for infections, and chest radiograms. It is intriguing that mortality in the patients with hypogammaglobulinemia at the beginning of the study was significantly less than that for those patients who were hypergammaglobulinemic (3% as compared with 65%).[141] None of the patients who remained hypogammaglobulinemic during the 5-year study period died. Thus,

TABLE 27–5. Immunologic Activities and Levels in Cystic Fibrosis

CATEGORY OF STUDY	CHARACTERISTICS OF CELLS AND IMMUNOLOGIC ACTIVITIES OR LEVELS
Characteristics (not in the context of responses to specific stimuli)	
Lymphocytes	Chloride metabolism normal
	Decreased production of cAMP in response to isoproterenol; normal basal levels of cAMP
Humoral immunity	Association between hypogammaglobulinemia and decreased mortality
Immune complexes	Enhanced clearance of IgA-sensitized erythrocytes
	28% to 100% of patients with elevated circulating immune complexes; may be deposited in airways
Neutrophils	Exceedingly high number obtained by bronchoalveolar lavage
	Lung and airway neutrophils and their proteases likely injurious to the lung
Macrophages	Macrophages obtained by bronchoalveolar lavage ultrastructurally normal
	Decrease in percentage of lavage macrophages as disease progresses, although total number may increase
Cellular Responses to Agents Other than *Pseudomonas*	
Cellular immunity	Number T lymphocytes normal
	Proliferative response to mitogens normal
	DTH preserved
Humoral immunity	Response to parenteral tetanus toxoid normal
Neutrophils, macrophages	Normal or enhanced phagocytosis of *Candida albicans*
Cellular Responses to *Pseudomonas*	
Cellular immunity	Decreased blastogenic responses of T lymphocytes to *Pseudomonas*
Humoral immunity	Antibodies to *Pseudomonas* and its secreted products found in high concentrations in serum and sputum
	Both serum and alveolar lining material contain IgG antibodies that interfere with phagocytosis of *Pseudomonas*
Immune complexes	*Pseudomonas*-specific immune complexes implicated in pathogenesis of lung injury
Neutrophils, macrophages from bronchoalveolar lavage	Decreased phagocytosis of *Pseudomonas,* particularly in the presence of serum from patients with cystic fibrosis

although it is not known whether hypergammaglobulinemia is a cause or an effect of the progressive lung damage in cystic fibrosis, an association clearly exists between hypogammaglobulinemia and decreased mortality.

Deposition of immune complexes is known to cause tissue damage, and several investigators have searched for evidence that immune complexes could contribute to the progressive lung disease in cystic fibrosis. A necrotizing cutaneous venulitis consisting of painful, palpable purpuric lesions on the lower extremities appears to be an extrapulmonary manifestation of immune complex deposition in a few patients with cystic fibrosis, usually those with advanced pulmonary disease.[123] Immune-complex mediated renal disease, however, is not a feature of cystic fibrosis. Clearance by the reticuloendothelial system of immune complexes, as measured by clearance of IgG-sensitized autologous erythrocytes, is decreased in classic immune complex disorders such as systemic lupus erythematosus.[47] Recently, Mantzouranis and colleagues[68] demonstrated that patients with cystic fibrosis as well as those with COPD without cystic fibrosis, unlike those with lupus, have enhanced reticuloendothelial clearance functions. Nevertheless, circulating immune complexes have been demonstrated in a large proportion (28% to 100%) of patients with cystic fibrosis.[39, 57, 82] Associations have been noted between presence of circulating immune complexes, severity of pulmonary function tests,[57] and increased mortality.[39] Serum IgG antibodies, which, as noted, are increased in many patients with cystic fibrosis, especially those with more advanced pulmonary disease, can enter the lungs of patients by passive transudation.[112] IgG and fibrin complexes are also deposited in the airways of patients with cystic fibrosis, and immune complexes have been found in the sputum.[74] Thus, although cystic fibrosis is not primarily an immune complex disorder per se, the evidence that circulating immune complexes and serum IgG are increased in some patients and that immune complexes have been noted in the airways and sputum lends some support to the possibility that airway deposition of immune complexes may be involved in the progressive lung injury.

The predominant types of inflammatory cells in the lumen of bronchoalveolar regions of patients with cystic fibrosis are neutrophils and macrophages. Neutrophils, along with their proteases, are likely to be involved in the progressive lung destruction occurring in patients with cystic fibrosis.[121] The role of macrophages in the pathogenesis of cystic fibrosis is less clear. Macrophages composed 40% to 90% of the total bronchoalveolar cells in patients with cystic fibrosis in fair clinical condition and <1% in patients in poor clinical condition.[131] Most of the other cells were neutrophils. The macrophages ultrastructurally appeared to be normal but unlike neutrophils were not heavily engaged in phagocytosis. In another study macrophages comprised 16% of the total number of bronchoalveolar cells from 15 patients with Schwachman scores ranging from 65 to 90 (mild to moderately poor clinical condition).[26] Thus, the fraction of cells from bronchoalveolar regions that are macrophages is low and decreases as disease progresses. Although the percent of bronchoalveolar macrophages is low in cystic fibrosis, a huge number of bronchoalveolar cells are present in cystic fibrosis compared with healthy subjects. The absolute number of macrophages in the bronchial lumen is therefore exceedingly high. Because these macrophages appear to be capable of responding normally to stimuli, at least for phagocytosis, as described subsequently, it is likely that other activities of macrophages, such as release of inflammatory mediators, are normal or increased. Because many macrophages and even more neutrophils are present, excessive levels of secretory products of these cells could participate in the pathogenesis of the lung disease in cystic fibrosis.

In general, systemic cell-mediated immunity in patients with cystic fibrosis is intact. The number of T lymphocytes, proliferative responses to mitogens, such as phytohemagglutinin and DTH, are preserved.[142] The humoral response to parenteral immunization with tetanus toxoid also is normal.[71] Neutrophils and macrophages obtained by bronchoalveolar lavage from patients with cystic fibrosis also have shown normal or enhanced phagocytosis of microorganisms, such as *Candida albicans*.[26]

The majority of studies of the immune and inflammatory systems in cystic fibrosis have focused on cellular responses to *Pseudomonas*. *Pseudomonas,* especially the mucoid colonial form of *Pseudomonas aeruginosa,* is the dominant pathogen in 70% to 90% of patients with cystic fibrosis. The role of cellular immunity in protection against infection by *Pseudomonas* in humans has not been explored fully. In experimental animals, however, cell-mediated immunity appears to limit *Pseudomonas* infection through both intra- and extracellular killing mechanisms.[69, 92] It is possible, therefore, that defects in activation of cell-mediated immunity in cystic fibrosis are associated with ineffectual killing of *Pseudomonas*. In support of such a possibility, Sorensen and colleagues,[117–119] Van Geffel and colleagues,[137] and Parmely and colleagues[90] have established that patients with cystic fibrosis develop a selective unresponsiveness of blood lymphocytes to killed *P. aeruginosa* and soluble antigens of *Pseudomonas,* particularly as pulmonary disease progresses. Mechanisms of the acquired unresponsiveness to *P. aeruginosa* have not been established, but the unresponsiveness is not caused by serum factors or activated macrophages.

The possibility of compartmentalization to the lung of *P. aeruginosa*-reactive lymphocytes has not been excluded. Furthermore, although the systemic defect in lymphocyte responses to *Pseudomonas* may be associated with defective killing of *Pseudomonas* in the lung, excessive activation of cell-mediated immunity and its mediators, such as cytokines, could lead to local inflammatory reactions injurious to the lung if not properly regulated. Killed *P. aeruginosa* and several exoproducts of *Pseudomonas,* including proteases and phenazine pigments, have been shown to either stimulate or inhibit lymphocyte blastogenesis, depending on the concentration in cell culture assays.[90, 106, 117, 120, 129]

Is the humoral response to *Pseudomonas* protective or deleterious to the patient with cystic fibrosis? Antibodies to both the *Pseudomonas* microbe and to a variety of its secreted products, including elastase and alkaline protease, exist in high concentrations in the serum and sputum of patients with cystic fibrosis.[40, 59, 60] Some evidence exists that these antibodies are produced in response to the mucoid exopolysaccharide of *Pseudomonas*. The lipopolysaccharide is also likely to elicit an antibody response.[33] Large numbers of IgG- and IgA-producing cells are found in the bronchial mucosa of patients with cystic fibrosis.[70] Thus, B lymphocytes generally appear to function normally in response to *Pseudomonas* and other microbes, and anti-*Pseudomonas* antibodies abound. Nevertheless, lung infection with *Pseudomonas* is not eliminated.

Döring and Høiby[41] have demonstrated that as antibodies to secretory products of *Pseudomonas* rise, clinical deterioration in lung function occurs, possibly due to increased bacterial load. The serum of patients with cystic fibrosis with *Pseudomonas* infection, however, contains a factor or factors that are capable of killing *Pseudomonas,*[132] as well as factors that selectively inhibit both phagocytosis and killing of *Pseudomonas* by alveolar macrophages from healthy subjects and patients with cystic fibrosis.[12, 130] Sputum from 18 of 19 patients with cystic fibrosis chronically infected with *Pseudomonas* contained inhibitory factors interfering with the bactericidal activity of serum against the bacteria.[111]

Characterization of the inhibitory moieties for phagocytosis and killing of *Pseudomonas* in the serum and sputum of patients with cystic fibrosis is incomplete. It is possible that the inhibitory activity is a function of the prozone phenomenon, in which high concentrations of functioning antibodies inhibit phagocytosis.[83] It may be, in part, caused by a *Pseudomonas*-specific bactericidal blocking antibody.[45, 46, 132] Fick and colleagues[45] have demonstrated that serum from patients with cystic fibrosis contains IgG antibodies that inhibit phagocytosis and killing of *Pseudomonas* by impairing the attachment of specific antibodies to alveolar macrophages. Further studies show that the alveolar lining material of patients with cystic fibrosis contains an aberrant IgG with the antigenic determinants of the Fab fragment of IgG.[46] This aberrant IgG severely altered the ability of alveolar macrophages from healthy subjects to phagocytose and kill *Pseudomonas*. Moss and coworkers[83] measured total IgG levels and levels of IgG subclass responses to *Pseudomonas* lipopolysaccharide in patients with cystic fibrosis who were or were not colonized with *Pseudomonas*. The patients who were not colonized had lower IgG2 and higher IgG4 subclass antibody responses, whereas the colonized patients had elevated levels of all four IgG subclasses (IgG1–4). Serum levels of IgG4 subclass to *Pseudomonas* lipopolysaccharide correlated inversely with phagocytosis by macrophages, suggesting that this isotype might block uptake of *Pseudomonas* by macrophages. Thus, *in vitro* studies show evidence for local and systemic blocking antibodies, preventing uptake and killing of *Pseudomonas* and an increase in *Pseudomonas*-specific IgG subclasses in the serum. Further studies are needed to decipher where intervention into the humoral response might be therapeutic. Evidence indicates, however, that the effect of blocking antibodies that inhibit phagocytosis and killing of *Pseudomonas* outweighs the protective effect of antibodies that might enhance opsonization of this infectious agent.

Pseudomonas-specific immune complexes may participate in the pathogenesis of lung injury in cystic fibrosis. It is known that proteases of *Pseudomonas* cleave and inactivate elastase secreted by polymorphonuclear leukocytes. Circulating antibodies to proteases of *Pseudomonas* increase over time in many patients with cystic fibrosis. Thus, Döring and associates[42] have suggested that immune complexes containing *Pseudomonas* proteases may be involved in the later stages of lung damage in cystic fibrosis by not allowing free enzymes of *Pseudomonas* to inactivate neutrophil elastase and by continuously stimulating the secretion of proteases by leukocytes.[42] Further studies focusing on deposition of immune complexes in the lung itself will be necessary to elucidate first the presence of immune complexes, particularly involving antigens of *Pseudomonas* in the airways, and second, to determine whether these immune complexes are a cause or an effect of the disease.

Both neutrophils and macrophages obtained by bronchoalveolar lavage from patients with cystic fibrosis have shown decreased phagocytosis of *P. aeruginosa*.[26, 116] In another study, however, phagocytosis of *P. aeruginosa* by alveolar macrophages from patients with cystic fibrosis was found to be equivalent to that of control cells in the presence of normal serum, but specifically inhibited in the presence of serum from patients with cystic fibrosis.[130] Characterization of the inhibitory factor in serum is incomplete.

In summary, in cystic fibrosis certain cellular components of the immune system, such as lymphocytes, are intrinsically normal in some but not all respects. Furthermore, immune responses to agents other than *Pseudomonas* appear to be intact. Nevertheless, a large body of experimental evidence suggests that the immune system is involved in the pathogenesis of the lung injury in this disease through a myriad of humoral and cell-mediated as well as nonspecific inflammatory responses, in particular those directed at the major pathogen *P. aeruginosa*.

IMPLICATIONS OF IMMUNE AND INFLAMMATORY ABNORMALITIES IN COPD

A wide variety of immune and inflammatory abnormalities have been described in COPD, some of which may be important in the pathogenesis of the various forms of this disease. If a cause and effect relationship can be established, attempts to thwart or correct the immune abnormalities should be beneficial in controlling the development of COPD. In general, therapy to be effective must be introduced before the development of irreversible lung disease. The cause may be a specific deficiency, such as α1-AT deficiency, in which α1-AT replacement therapy shows particular promise in containing the progression of lung injury or an immunoglobulin deficiency in which replacement of Ig has prevented infection and further development of bronchiectasis and actually improved pulmonary function. The cause of the immune abnormality in COPD also may be secondary to other factors, such as smoking or infection, the control of which is clearly of paramount importance in preventing lung damage. As described in this chapter, numerous descriptions of abnormalities of the immune and inflammatory systems exist that are associated with COPD and that may or may not be secondary to other factors, such as infection or smoking. These abnormalities, although not as well understood, may be critical in the pathogenesis of COPD. It will be important in these instances to decipher the precise cause of the abnormality and its relevance to disease progression so that specific therapeutic approaches can be devised. A particularly wide gap in the understanding of the role of immune and inflammatory abnormalities in the pathogenesis of COPD is due to the paucity of data concerning the immune response in the lung itself. Efforts in this area should provide a rational approach to specific and perhaps local intervention into the vicious cycle of immune and inflammatory abnormalities leading to COPD. Even when the cause of the lung disease is unknown or irreversible, e.g., cystic fibrosis, understanding of the immune response in disease progression may suggest new avenues to retard the disease process.

REFERENCES

1. Ades EW, Hinson A, Chapuis-Cellier C, Arnaud P. Modulation of the immune response by plasma protease inhibitors. I. Alpha$_2$-macroglobulin and alpha$_1$-antitrypsin inhibit natural killing and antibody-dependent cell-mediated cytotoxicity. Scand J Immunol 1982; 15:109–113.
2. Ammann AJ, Ashman RF, Buckley RH, et al. Use of intravenous γ-globulin in antibody immunodeficiency: results of a multicenter controlled trial. Clin Immunol Immunopathol 1982; 22:60–67.
3. Bachmann R. Studies on the serum gamma-A-globulin level. III. The frequency of A-gamma-A-globulinemia. Scand J Clin Lab Invest 1965; 17:316–320.
4. Barandun S, Riva G, Spengler GA. Immunologic deficiency: diagnosis, forms and current treatment. Birth Defects 1968; 6:40–48.
5. Beck CS, Heiner DC. Selective immunoglobulin G_4 deficiency and recurrent infections of the respiratory tract. Am Rev Respir Dis 1981; 124:94–96.
6. Bienenstock J, Johnston N, Perey DYE. Bronchial lymphoid tissue. I. Morphologic characteristics. Lab Invest 1973; 28:686–692.
7. Bienenstock J, McDermott MR, Befus AD. The significance of bronchus-associated lymphoid tissue. Bull Eur Physiopath Respir 1982; 18:153–177.
8. Bienenstock J. Immunology of the Lung and Upper Respiratory Tract. New York: McGraw-Hill, 1984, 1–414.
9. Björkander J, Bake B, Hanson LÅ. Primary hypogammaglobulinaemia: impaired lung function and body growth with delayed

diagnosis and inadequate treatment. Eur J Respir Dis 1984; 65:529–536.
10. Björkander J, Bake B, Oxelius V-A, Hanson LÅ. Impaired lung function in patients with IgA deficiency and low levels of IgG2 or IgG3. N Engl J Med 1985; 313:720–724.
11. Boucher RC, Ross DW, Knowles MR, et al. Cl^- permeabilities in red blood cells and peripheral blood lymphocytes from cystic fibrosis and control subjects. Pediatr Res 1984; 18:1336–1339.
12. Boxerbaum B, Kagumba M, Matthews LW. Selective inhibition of phagocytic activity of rabbit alveolar macrophages by cystic fibrosis serum. Am Rev Respir Dis 1973; 108:777–783.
13. Brain JD. Pulmonary macrophages. When do they prevent and when do they cause COPD? Chest 1980; 77(suppl):264–265.
14. Brandtzaeg P. Human secretory immunoglobulins. II. Salivary secretions from individuals with selectively excessive or defective synthesis of serum immunoglobulins. Clin Exp Immunol 1971; 8:69–85.
15. Breit SN, Robinson JP, Luckhurst E, et al. Immunoregulation by $alpha_1$ antitrypsin. J Clin Lab Immunol 1982; 7:127–131.
16. Breit SN, Robinson JP, Penny R. The effect of $alpha_1$ antitrypsin on phagocyte function. J Clin Lab Immunol 1983; 10:147–149.
17. Breit SN, Luckhurst E, Penny R. The effect of $alpha_1$ antitrypsin on the proliferative response of human peripheral blood lymphocytes. J Immunol 1983; 130:681–688.
18. Breit SN, Wakefield D, Robinson JP, et al. Review. The role of $alpha_1$-antitrypsin deficiency in the pathogenesis of immune disorders. Clin Immunol Immunopathol 1985; 35:363–380.
19. Bruton, OC. Agammaglobulinemia. Pediatrics 1952; 9:722–728.
20. Buckley RH. Primary immunodeficiency diseases. In: Wyngaarden JB, Smith LH Jr, eds. Cecil Textbook of Medicine (16th ed). Philadelphia: WB Saunders Company, 1982, 1789–1796.
21. Burnett D, Crocker J, Stockley RA. Cells containing IgA subclasses in bronchi of subjects with and without chronic obstructive lung disease. J Clin Pathol 1987; 40:1217–1220.
22. Burns MW. Precipitins to Klebsiella and other enterobacteria in the serum of patients with chronic respiratory disorders. Lancet 1968; i:383–385.
23. Cain WA, Ammann AJ, Hong R, et al. IgE deficiency associated with chronic sinopulmonary infection [abstract]. J Clin Invest 1969; 48:12a.
24. Carlstedt-Duke J, Brönnegård M, Strandvik B. Pathological regulation of arachidonic acid release in cystic fibrosis: the putative basic defect. Proc Natl Acad Sci USA 1986; 83:9202–9206.
25. Carp H, Miller F, Hoidal JR, Janoff A. Potential mechanism of emphysema: $alpha_1$-proteinase inhibitor recovered from lungs of cigarette smokers contains oxidized methionine and has decreased elastase inhibitory capacity. Proc Natl Acad Sci USA 1982; 79:2041–2045.
26. Cassino RJJ, Sordelli DO, Macri CN, et al. Pulmonary nonspecific defense mechanisms in cystic fibrosis. I. Phagocytic capacity of alveolar macrophages and neutrophils. Pediatr Res 1980; 14:1212–1215.
27. Chipps BE, Talamo RC, Winkelstein JA. IgA deficiency, recurrent pneumonias, and bronchiectasis. Chest 1978; 73:519–526.
28. Clancy RL, Pucci A, Jelihovsky T, Bye P. Immunologic "memory" for microbial antigens in lymphocytes obtained from human bronchial mucosa. Am Rev Respir Dis 1978; 117:513–518.
29. Clarke CW. Precipitating antibody to antigens of *Pseudomonas aeruginosa* in chronic obstructive lung disease. Clin Allerg 1977; 7:527–537.
30. Collins-Williams C, Kokubu HL, Lamenza C, et al. Incidence of isolated deficiency of IgA in the serum of Canadian children. Ann Allerg 1972; 30:11–23.
31. Colten HR. Cystic fibrosis: immunologic considerations. In: Daniele RP, ed. Immunology and Immunologic Diseases of the Lung. Cambridge, MA: Blackwell Scientific Publications, 1988, 553–559.
32. Cunningham-Rundles C, Siegal FP, Smithwick EM, et al. Efficacy of intravenous immunoglobulin in primary humoral immunodeficiency disease. Ann Intern Med 1984; 101:435–439.
33. Daley L, Pier GB, Liporace JD, Eardley DD. Polyclonal B cell stimulation and interleukin 1 induction by the mucoid exopolysaccharide of *Pseudomonas aeruginosa* associated with cystic fibrosis. J Immunol 1985; 134:3089–3093.
34. Daniele RP, ed. Immunology and Immunologic Diseases of the Lung. Cambridge, MA: Blackwell Scientific Publications, 1988; 1–183.
35. Daniele RP, Altose MD, Rowlands DT Jr. Immunocompetent cells from the lower respiratory tract of normal human lungs. J Clin Invest 1975; 56:986–995.
36. Daniele RP, Dauber JH, Altose MD, et al. Lymphocyte studies in asymptomatic cigarette smokers. Am Rev Respir Dis 1977; 116:997–1005.
37. Davis PB, Dieckman L, Boat TF, et al. Beta adrenergic receptors in lymphocytes and granulocytes from patients with cystic fibrosis. J Clin Invest 1983; 71:1787–1795.
38. DeSchazo RD, Banks DE, Diem JE, et al. Bronchoalveolar lavage cell-lymphocyte interactions in normal nonsmokers and smokers. Am Rev Respir Dis 1983; 127:545–548.
39. Disis ML, McDonald TL, Colombo JL, et al. Circulating immune complexes in cystic fibrosis and their correlation to clinical parameters. Pediatr Res 1986; 20:385–390.
40. Döring G, Obernesser H-J, Botzenhart K, et al. Proteases of *Pseudomonas aeruginosa* in patients with cystic fibrosis. J Infect Dis 1983; 147:744–750.
41. Döring G, Høiby N. Longitudinal study of immune response to *Pseudomonas aeruginosa* antigens in cystic fibrosis. Infect Immun 1983; 42:197–201.
42. Döring G, Goldstein W, Röll A, et al. Role of *Pseudomonas aeruginosa* exoenzymes in lung infections of patients with cystic fibrosis. Infect Immun 1985; 49:557–562.
43. Faulk WP, Kiyasu WS, Cooper MD, Fudenberg HH. Deficiency of IgM. Pediatrics 1971; 47:399–404.
44. Fels AO, Cohn ZA. The alveolar macrophage. J Appl Physiol 1986; 60:353–369.
45. Fick RB Jr, Naegel GP, Matthay RA, Reynolds HY. Cystic fibrosis *Pseudomonas* opsonins. Inhibitory nature in an *in vitro* phagocytic assay. J Clin Invest 1981;68:899–914.
46. Fick RB Jr, Naegel GP, Squier SU, et al. Proteins of the cystic fibrosis respiratory tract. Fragmented immunoglobulin G opsonic antibody causing defective opsonophagocytosis. J Clin Invest 1984; 74:236–248.
47. Frank MM, Hamburger MI, Lawley TJ, et al. Defective reticuloendothelial system Fc-receptor function in systemic lupus erythematosus. N Engl J Med 1979; 300:518–523.
48. Frommel D, Moullec J, Lambin P, Fine JM. Selective serum IgA deficiency. Frequency among 15,200 French blood donors. Vox Sang 1973; 25:513–518.
49. Gelzayd EA, McCleery JL, Melnyk CS, Kraft SC. Intestinal malabsorption and immunoglobulin deficiency. Arch Intern Med 1971; 127:141–147.
50. Gitlin D, Janeway CA. Agammaglobulinemia, congenital, acquired and transient forms. Prog Hematol 1956; 1:318–329.
51. Good RA, Mazzitello WF. Chest disease in patients with agammaglobulinemia. Dis Chest 1956; 29:9–35.
52. Green MN, Kulczycki LL, Shwachman H. Serum protein paper electrophoresis in patients with cystic fibrosis. Am J Dis Child 1960; 100:365–372.
53. Hermans PE, Diaz-Buxo JA, Stobo JD. Idiopathic late-onset immunoglobulin deficiency. Clinical observations in 50 patients. Am J Med 1976; 61:221–237.
54. Hilton AM, Doyle L. Immunological abnormalities in bronchiectasis with chronic bronchial suppuration. Br J Dis Chest 1978; 72:207–216.
55. Hilton AM, Moore M, Howat JMT, Kimber I. Characterization of circulating immune complexes in bronchiectasis by gel filtration. Clin Allerg 1979; 9:65–74.
56. Hobbs JR. Immune imbalance in dysgammaglobulinemia type IV. Lancet 1968; i:110–114.
57. Hodson ME, Beldon I, Batten JC. Circulating immune complexes in patients with cystic fibrosis in relation to clinical features. Clin Allerg 1985; 15:363–370.
58. Hoffman T, Winchester R, Schulkind M, et al. Hypoimmunoglobulinemia with normal T cell function in female siblings. Clin Immunol Immunopathol 1977; 7:364–371.
59. Høiby N, Axelsen NH. Identification and quantitation of precipitins against *Pseudomonas aeruginosa* in patients with cystic fibrosis by means of crossed immunoelectrophoresis with intermediate gel. Acta Pathol Microbiol Scand (section B) 1973; 81:298–308.
60. Høiby N, Jacobsen L, Jørgensen BA, et al. *Pseudomonas aeruginosa* infection in cystic fibrosis. Acta Paediatr Scand 1974; 63:843–848.
61. Hudig D, Haverty T, Fulcher C, et al. Inhibition of human

natural cytotoxicity by macromolecular antiproteases. J Immunol 1981; 126:1569–1574.
62. Hughes WS, Cerda JJ, Holtzapple P, Brooks FP. Primary hypogammaglobulinemia and malabsorption. Ann Intern Med 1971; 74:903–910.
63. Hunninghake GW, Gadek JE, Kawanami O, et al. Inflammatory and immune processes in the human lung in health and disease: evaluation by bronchoalveolar lavage. Am J Pathol 1979; 97:149–206.
64. Janeway CA, Rosen FS. The gamma globulins. IV. Therapeutic uses of gamma globulin. N Engl J Med 1966; 275:826–831.
65. Koistinen J. Selective IgA deficiency in blood donors. Vox Sang 1975; 29:192–202.
66. Krol RC. Immune deficiency states and recurrent respiratory tract infections. In: Daniele RP, ed. Immunology and Immunologic Diseases of the Lung. Cambridge, MA: Blackwell Scientific Publications, 1988, 563–579.
67. Macklin CC. Pulmonary sumps, dust accumulations, alveolar fluid and lymph vessels. Acta Anat 1955; 23:1–33.
68. Mantzouranis EC, Rosen FS, Colten HR. Reticuloendothelial clearance in cystic fibrosis and other inflammatory lung diseases. N Engl J Med 1988; 319:338–343.
69. Markham RB, Pier GB, Goellner JJ, Mizel SB. *In vitro* T cell-mediated killing of *Pseudomonas aeruginosa*. II. The role of macrophages and T cell subsets in T cell killing. J Immunol 1985; 134:4112–4117.
70. Martinez-Tello FJ, Braun DG, Blanc WA. Immunoglobulin production in bronchial mucosa and bronchial lymph nodes, particularly in cystic fibrosis of the pancreas. J Immunol 1968; 101:989–1003.
71. Matthews WJ Jr, Williams M, Oliphint B, et al. Hypogammaglobulinemia in patients with cystic fibrosis. N Engl J Med 1980; 302:245–249.
72. McCombs CC, Michalski JP, Westerfield BT, Light RW. Human alveolar macrophages suppress the proliferative response of peripheral blood lymphocytes. Chest 1982; 82:266–271.
73. McDermott MR, Befus AD, Bienenstock J. The structural basis for immunity in the respiratory tract. Int Rev Exp Pathol 1982; 23:47–112.
74. McFarlane H, Holzel A, Brenchley P, et al. Immune complexes in cystic fibrosis. Br Med J 1975; 1:423–428.
75. McLeod R, Mack DG, McLeod EG, et al. Alveolar macrophage function and inflammatory stimuli in smokers with and without obstructive lung disease. Am Rev Respir Dis 1985; 131:377–384.
76. Mease PJ, Ochs HD, Wedgwood RJ. Successful treatment of Echovirus meningoencephalitis and myositis-fasciitis with intravenous immune globulin therapy in a patient with X-linked agammaglobulinemia. N Engl J Med 1981; 304:1278–1281.
77. Miller RD, Gleich GJ, Offord KP, Dunnette SL. Immunoglobulin concentrations in serum and nasal secretions in chronic obstructive pulmonary disease. Am Rev Respir Dis 1979; 119:229–238.
78. Miller RD, Kueppers F, Offord KP. Serum concentrations of C3 and C4 of the complement system in patients with chronic obstructive pulmonary disease. J Lab Clin Med 1980; 95:266–271.
79. Mod A, Fust G, Gergely J, et al. Alpha$_1$-antitrypsin-induced inhibition of complement-dependent phagocytosis. Immunobiology 1981; 158:338–346.
80. Mondelli M, Mieli-Vergani G, Eddleston ALWF, et al. Lymphocyte cytotoxicity to autologous hepatocytes in alpha$_1$-antitrypsin deficiency. Gut 1984; 25:1044–1049.
81. Morell A, Skvaril F, Barandun S. Serum concentrations of IgG subclasses. Clin Immunobiol 1976; 3:37–56.
82. Moss RB, Lewiston NJ. Immune complexes and humoral response to *Pseudomonas aeruginosa* in cystic fibrosis. Am Rev Respir Dis 1980; 121:23–29.
83. Moss RB, Hsu Y-P, Sullivan MM, Lewiston NJ. Altered antibody isotype in cystic fibrosis: possible role in opsonic deficiency. Pediatr Res 1986; 20:453–459.
84. Nash DR. Serum immunoglobulin abnormalities in patients with respiratory tract disease. Ann Clin Res 1979; 11:49–52.
85. Nomura S, Kanoh T. Association of idiopathic pulmonary haemosiderosis with IgA monoclonal gammopathy. Thorax 1987; 42:696–697.
86. Offord KP, Gleich GJ, Barbee RA, et al. Serum IgD in subjects with and without chronic obstructive pulmonary disease. Am Rev Respir Dis 1982; 126:118–120.
87. Østergaard PA. Combined IgA and alpha$_1$-antitrypsin deficiency in a boy with severe respiratory tract infections and asthma. Eur J Pediatr 1982; 138:83–85.
88. Oxelius V-A. Chronic infections in a family with hereditary deficiency of IgG2 and IgG4. Clin Exp Immunol 1974; 17:19–27.
89. Oxelius V-A, Laurell A-B, Lindquist B, et al. IgG subclasses in selective IgA deficiency. Importance of IgG2-IgA deficiency. N Engl J Med 1981; 304:1476–1477.
90. Parmely MJ, Iglewski BH, Horvat RT. Identification of the principal T lymphocyte-stimulating antigens of *Pseudomonas aeruginosa*. J Exp Med 1984; 160:1338–1349.
91. Pauwels R, Van Der Straeten M. Total serum IgE levels in normals and patients with chronic nonspecific lung diseases. Allergy 1978; 33:254–260.
92. Pier GB, Markham RB. Induction in mice of cell-mediated immunity to *Pseudomonas aeruginosa* by high molecular weight polysaccharide and vinblastine. J Immunol 1982; 128:2121–2125.
93. Pirofsky B. Intravenous immune globulin therapy in hypogammaglobulinemia. A review. Am J Med 1984; 76(3A):53–60.
94. Polmar SH, Waldmann TA, Balestra ST, et al. Immunoglobulin E in immunologic deficiency diseases. I. Relation of IgE and IgA to respiratory tract disease in isolated IgE deficiency, IgA deficiency and ataxia telangiectasia. J Clin Invest 1972; 51:326–330.
95. Puci A, Clancy R, Jackson G. Quantitation of T-lymphocyte subsets in human bronchus mucosa. Am Rev Respir Dis 1982; 126:364–366.
96. Redelman D, Hudig D. The mechanism of cell-mediated cytotoxicity. I. Killing by murine T lymphocytes requires cell surface thiols and activated proteases. J Immunol 1980; 124:870–878.
97. Reynolds HY. The importance of lymphocytes in pulmonary health and disease. Lung 1978; 155:225–242.
98. Reynolds HY. Lung inflammation: normal host defense or a complication of some diseases? Annu Rev Med 1987; 38:295–323.
99. Rich EA, Tweardy DJ, Fujiwara H, Ellner JJ. Spectrum of immunoregulatory functions and properties of human alveolar macrophages. Am Rev Respir Dis 1987; 136:258–265.
100. Ritts RE, Miller RD, LeDuc PV, Offord KP. Phagocytosis and cutaneous delayed hypersensitivity in patients with chronic obstructive pulmonary disease. Chest 1976; 69:474–478.
101. Roifman CM, Lederman HM, Lavi S, et al. Benefit of intravenous IgG replacement in hypogammaglobulinemic patients with chronic sinopulmonary disease. Am J Med 1985; 79:171–174.
102. Romain PL, Schlossman SF. Human T lymphocyte subsets: functional heterogeneity and surface recognition structures. J Clin Invest 1984; 74:1559–1565.
103. Rosen FS, Cooper MD, Wedgwood RJP. The primary immunodeficiencies (first of two parts). N Engl J Med 1984; 311:235–242.
104. Rosen FS, Cooper MD, Wedgwood RJP. The primary immunodeficiencies (second of two parts). N Engl J Med 1984; 311:300–310.
105. Rothbach C, Nagel J, Rabin B, Fireman P. Antibody deficiency with normal immunoglobulins. J Pediatr 1979; 94:250–253.
106. Rubin H, Sorensen RU, Chase PA, Klinger JD. Suppression of *in vitro* lymphocyte DNA synthesis by killed *Pseudomonas aeruginosa*. Infect Immun 1983; 39:630–637.
107. Rubinstein I, Baum GL. Selective IgA deficiency associated with recurrent sinopulmonary infections in sarcoidosis. Eur J Respir Dis 1984; 65:550–552.
108. Saulsbury FT, Bernstein MT, Winkelstein JA. *Pneumocystis carinii* pneumonia as the presenting infection in congenital hypogammaglobulinemia. J Pediatr 1979; 95:559–561.
109. Savilahti E, Pelkonen P, Visakorpi JK. IgA deficiency in children. A clinical study with special reference to intestinal findings. Arch Dis Child 1971; 46:665–670.
110. Scadding JG. The bronchi in allergic aspergillosis. Scand J Respir Dis 1967; 48:372–377.
111. Schiller NL, Millard RL. *Pseudomonas*-infected cystic fibrosis patient sputum inhibits the bactericidal activity of normal human serum. Pediatr Res 1983; 17:747–752.
112. Schiøtz PO, Clemmensen I, Høiby N. Immunoglobulins and albumin in sputum from patients with cystic fibrosis. Acta Pathol Microbiol Scand, section C 1980; 88:275–280.
113. Schur PH, Borel H, Gelfand EW, et al. Selective gamma-G

globulin deficiencies in patients with recurrent pyogenic infections. N Engl J Med 1970; 283:631–634.
114. Schwartz RH. Serum immunoglobulin levels in cystic fibrosis. Am J Dis Child 1966; 111:408–411.
115. Scott GH, Sydiskis RJ. Responses of mice immunized with influenza virus by aerosol and parenteral routes. Infect Immun 1976; 13:696–703.
116. Sordelli DO, Cassino RJJ, Macri CN, et al. Phagocytosis of *Candida albicans* by alveolar macrophages from patients with cystic fibrosis. Clin Immunol Immunopathol 1982; 22:153–158.
117. Sorensen RU, Stern RC, Polmar SH. Cellular immunity to bacteria: impairment of *in vitro* lymphocyte responses to *Pseudomonas aeruginosa* in cystic fibrosis patients. Infect Immun 1977; 18:735–740.
118. Sorensen RU, Stern RC, Polmar SH. Lymphocyte responsiveness to *Pseudomonas aeruginosa* in cystic fibrosis: relationship to status of pulmonary disease in sibling pairs. J Pediatr 1978; 93:201–205.
119. Sorensen RU, Stern RC, Chase P, Polmar SH. Defective cellular immunity to gram-negative bacteria in cystic fibrosis patients. Infect Immun 1979; 23:398–402.
120. Sorensen RU, Klinger JD, Cash HA, et al. *In vitro* inhibition of lymphocyte proliferation by *Pseudomonas aeruginosa* phenazine pigments. Infect Immun 1983; 41:321–330.
121. Sorensen RU. Immune responses to pseudomonas and other bacteria in cystic fibrosis patients. In: Shapira E, Wilson GB, eds. Immunological Aspects of Cystic Fibrosis. Boca Raton, FL: CRC Press, 1984, 101–123.
122. Sorensen RU, Polmar SH. Immunoglobulin replacement therapy. Ann Clin Res 1987; 19:293–304.
123. Soter NA, Mihm MC Jr, Colten HR. Cutaneous necrotizing venulitis in patients with cystic fibrosis. J Pediatr 1979; 95:197–201.
124. South MA, Cooper MD, Wollheim FA, Good RA. The IgA system. II. The clinical significance of IgA deficiency: studies in patients with agammaglobulinemia and ataxia-telangiectasia. Am J Med 1968; 44:168–177.
125. Spencer H. Diseases of the bronchial tree. In: Spencer H, ed. Pathology of the Lung. New York: Pergamon Press, Inc, 1977, 130–149.
126. Stobo JD, Tomasi TB Jr. A low molecular weight immunoglobulin antigenically related to 19 S IgM. J Clin Invest 1967; 46:1329–1337.
127. Strober W, Krakauer R, Klaeveman HL, et al. Secretory component deficiency. A disorder of the IgA immune system. N Engl J Med 1976; 294:351–356.
128. Taylor JC, Crawford IP, Hugli TE. Limited degradation of the third component (C3) of human complement by human leukocyte elastase (HLE): partial characterization of C3 fragments. Biochemistry 1977; 16:3390–3396.
129. Theander TG, Kharazmi A, Pedersen BK, et al. Inhibition of human lymphocyte proliferation and cleavage of interleukin–2 by *Pseudomonas aeruginosa* proteases. Infect Immun 1988; 56:1673–1677.
130. Thomassen MJ, Boxerbaum B, Demko CA, et al. Inhibitory effect of cystic fibrosis serum on *Pseudomonas* phagocytosis by rabbit and human alveolar macrophages. Pediatr Res 1979; 13:1085–1088.
131. Thomassen MJ, Demko CA, Wood RE, et al. Ultrastructure and function of alveolar macrophages from cystic fibrosis patients. Pediatr Res 1980; 14:715–721.
132. Thomassen MJ, Demko CA. Serum bactericidal effect on *Pseudomonas aeruginosa* isolates from cystic fibrosis patients. Infect Immun 1981; 33:512–518.
133. Toews GB, Vial WC, Dunn MM, et al. The accessory cell function of human alveolar macrophages in specific T cell proliferation. J Immunol 1984; 132:181–186.
134. Tomasi TB, Bienenstock J. Secretory immunoglobulins. Advances Immunol 1968; 9:1–96.
135. Tomasi TB Jr. Mechanisms of immune regulation at mucosal surfaces. Rev Infect Dis 1983; 5:S784–S792.
136. Umetsu DT, Ambrosino DM, Quinti I, et al. Recurrent sinopulmonary infection and impaired antibody response to bacterial capsular polysaccharide antigen in children with selective IgG-subclass deficiency. N Engl J Med 1985; 313:1247–1251.
137. Van Geffel R, Hubert E, Josse M. Study of the relation between the clinical pulmonary condition of children with cystic fibrosis and the lymphoblastic response to the antigen *Pseudomonas aeruginosa*. Ann Immunol 1982; 133D:293–303.
138. Waldmann TA, Laster L. Abnormalities of albumin metabolism in patients with hypogammaglobulinemia. J Clin Invest 1964; 43:1025–1035.
139. Watts WJ, Watts MB, Dai W, et al. Respiratory dysfunction in patients with common variable hypogammaglobulinemia. Am Rev Respir Dis 1986; 134:699–703.
140. Webb DR, Condemi JJ. Selective immunoglobulin A deficiency and chronic obstructive lung disease. A family study. Ann Intern Med 1974; 80:618–621.
141. Wheeler WB, Williams M, Matthews WJ Jr, Colten HR. Progression of cystic fibrosis lung disease as a function of serum immunoglobulin G levels: a five year longitudinal study. J Pediatr 1984; 104:695–699.
142. Wilson GB. Cell-mediated immunity in cystic fibrosis. In: Shapiro E, Wilson GB, eds. Immunological Aspects of Cystic Fibrosis. Boca Raton, FL: CRC Press, 1984:57–58.
143. Yeager H Jr, Sweeney JA, Herscowitz HB, et al. Modulation of mitogen-induced proliferation of autologous peripheral blood lymphocytes by human alveolar macrophages. Infect Immun 1982; 38:260–266.
144. Yount WJ, Hong R, Seligmann M, et al. Imbalances of gamma globulin subgroups and gene defects in patients with primary hypogammaglobulinemia. J Clin Invest 1970; 49:1957–1966.
145. Zembala M, Adamek-Guzik T, Mytar B, Szczeklik A. Immunologic status of patients with recurrent chest infections. Lung 1978; 155:39–53.
146. Zinneman HH, Hall WH, Heller BI. Acquired agammaglobulinemia: report of three cases. JAMA 1954; 156:1390–1393.
147. Zinneman HH, Niewoehner DE, Goodsell MG. Chronic obstructive pulmonary disease and secretory IgA. Minnesota Med 1980; 63:247–249.

Chapter 28

THE RELATIONSHIP OF SMOKING TO COPD

Jonathan M. Samet

At present, most cases of COPD in the United States and in other developed countries are caused by cigarette smoking. The presence of emphysema at autopsy and the clinical syndrome of chronic bronchitis, however, were recognized long before smoking cigarettes was a widespread form of tobacco use.[47, 56, 57] Through the mid-1900s, theories on the etiology of emphysema emphasized physical stresses and aging.[11] In fact, a comprehensive review of emphysema by Christie,[11] published in 1944, did not mention cigarette smoking.

In the 1950s, increasing morbidity and mortality from chronic respiratory conditions prompted clinical and epidemiologic investigations of the etiology of chronic bronchitis and related disorders. At that time, the most widely advanced hypothesis on the causes of COPD linked progressive lung damage to recurrent respiratory infection.[55] This was based on the finding of a history of chronic sputum production and recurrent chest infection in most COPD patients. Air pollution and occupational exposures were also considered to be potential risk factors.[20]

Epidemiologic investigations, however, largely carried out in the United Kingdom, soon indicated the predominant role of cigarette smoking in causing COPD[56, 57] For example, in 1953, Oswald and coworkers[42] reported on the characteristics of 300 patients with chronic cough, sputum, and dyspnea and on those of 300 controls. Nine per cent of patients had never smoked, whereas 21% of the controls had never smoked. Population surveys demonstrated increased symptom prevalence and lower levels of ventilatory function in smokers compared with nonsmokers.[56, 57]

By 1964, the evidence was sufficiently compelling to support the conclusion by the Advisory Committee to the Surgeon General that "Cigarette smoking is the most important of the causes of chronic bronchitis in the United States, and increases the risk of dying from chronic bronchitis and emphysema."[62] The report stopped short, however, of establishing a causal relationship between cigarette smoking and emphysema. The data cited to support these conclusions were drawn from seven prospective studies of mortality in relation to cigarette smoking and from a dozen surveys of respiratory morbidity; only one prospective study on lung function had been reported at the time.

By the early 1970s, cigarette smoking was labeled as a cause of COPD in the Surgeon General's report on smoking.[63] In the comprehensive 1979 report of the Surgeon General on smoking and health, which covered all health effects of smoking, the conclusions of the 1964 report were greatly strengthened.[64] Increased morbidity and mortality from chronic bronchitis and emphysema were documented in cigarette smokers compared with nonsmokers. Additionally, autopsy evidence confirmed that the lungs of smokers were widely damaged, and the protease-antiprotease hypothesis provided a framework for understanding the mechanisms by which cigarette smoke causes emphysema.

The 1984 Surgeon General's report focused on COPD.[65] The overall conclusion was that "Cigarette smoking is the major cause of chronic obstructive lung disease in the United States for both men and women. The contribution of cigarette smoking to chronic obstructive lung disease morbidity and mortality far outweighs all other factors." In contrast to the more limited data in the 1964 report,[62] the 1984 report[65] reviewed numerous cross-sectional and longitudinal studies of morbidity and mortality. The longitudinal studies described the evolution of the cigarette-related decline in lung function that leads to sufficient impairment to result in a clinical diagnosis of COPD. The role of cigarette smoking in causing COPD was further supported by a new understanding of the mechanisms whereby tobacco smoke injures the lung.

CIGARETTE SMOKING

Demographics

The widespread smoking of cigarettes during the 20th century has resulted in the present epidemic of cigarette-related diseases, including COPD. Until the early part of this century, cigarette smoking was a relatively uncommon form of tobacco consumption; chewing tobacco and pipe tobacco accounted for most of the tobacco consumption.[62] Cigarette smoking, however, increased rapidly among males from approximately the time of World War I (Fig. 28–1).[24, 66] Among women, the prevalence of cigarette smoking increased later, beginning at about World War II (Fig. 28–2).[24, 66] From 1900 to 1960, per capita cigarette consumption for persons 15 years of age and older in the United States rose from 49 to 3888 per year.[62] By the 1960s cigarette smoking began to decline among men and women.[24] In 1986, 27% of adults in the United States reported themselves as current cigarette smokers.[60]

The prevalence of cigarette smoking varies with region, educational level, occupation, and race. At present, the prevalence of smoking is highest in the Southeast.[61] A strong correlation of cigarette smoking with educational level has been demonstrated; in both men and women the proportion of cigarette smokers increases with decreasing level of educational attainment.[66] Males with blue-collar jobs are more often smokers than males with white-collar jobs.[66] Cigarette smoking has also become more common among blacks than among whites.[60]

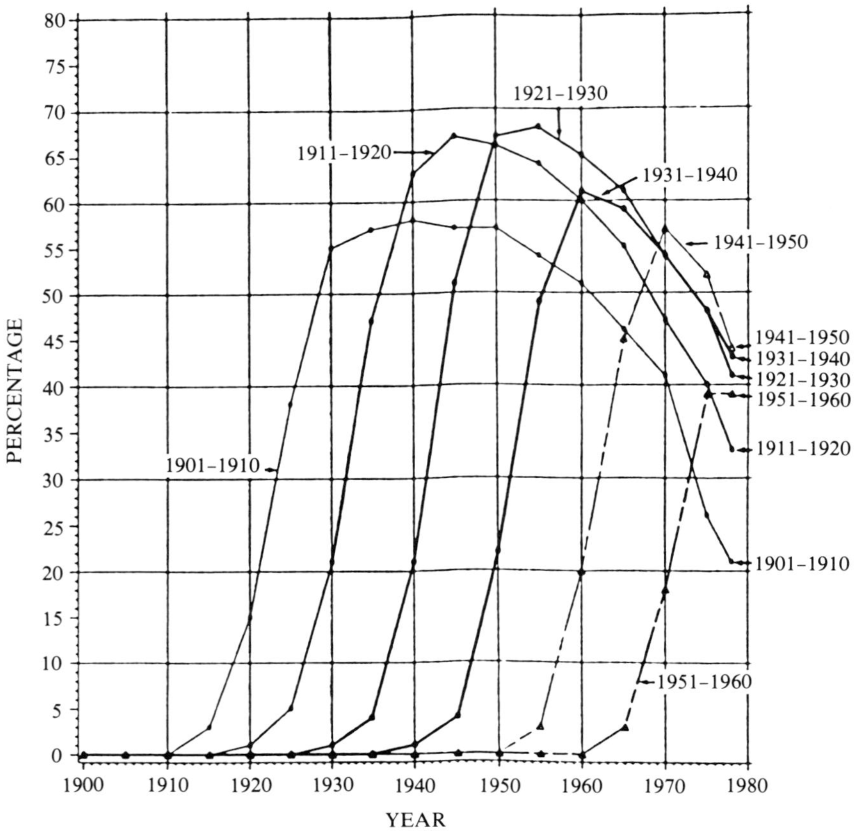

Figure 28–1. Prevalence of cigarette smoking among U.S. men by birth cohort, 1900–1980, based on the National Health Interview Survey.

Cigarette Smoke Composition and Toxicology

The smoke inhaled by a smoker during active smoking is referred to as mainstream smoke; sidestream smoke is released from the smoldering end of the cigarette. Cigarettes are crudely characterized by the yield of tar and nicotine when smoked under standard conditions with a machine.[67] Tar refers to the material, primarily particulate, that is deposited onto a filter during smoking by the machine.[67] The tar yield, however, does not provide an accurate measure of the potential effect of toxic components on the respiratory tract of the smoker.[65]

Mainstream tobacco smoke is a complex aerosol with many toxic and carcinogenic components (Table 28–1).[64, 67] The particle concentration of undiluted mainstream smoke is about 5×10^9 particles/ml, with a median particle diameter of about 0.4 μ. The particles contain a number of toxic constituents, including nicotine and other alkaloids, nitrosamines, aromatic amines, alkanes and alkenes, benzenes and naphthalenes, polynuclear aromatic hydrocarbons, metals, agricultural chemicals, and other organic compounds. The gas phase contains many of the same organic substances in their volatile forms and the toxic gases carbon monoxide, nitrogen oxides, ammonia, and hydrogen cyanide. Estimates of the percentage of smoke particles deposited in the respiratory tract during active smoking range from 47% to 98%.[67] Epithelial surfaces of the

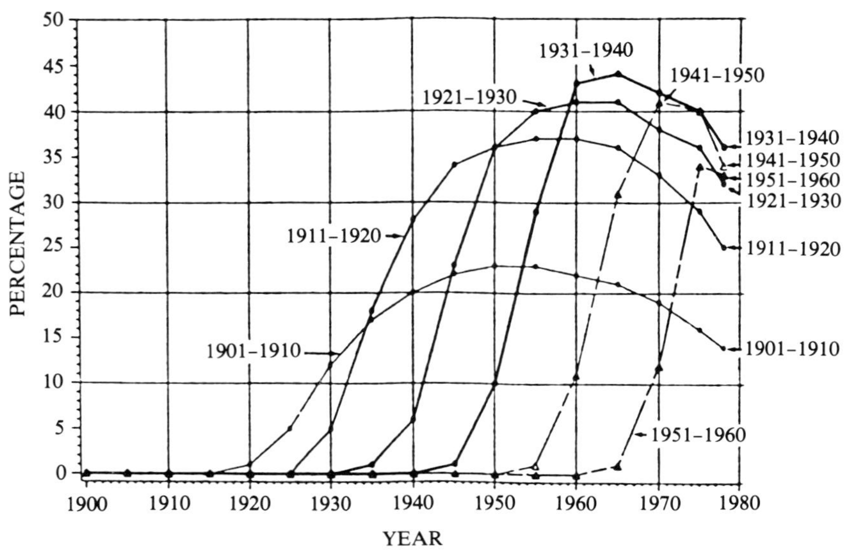

Figure 28–2. Prevalence of cigarette smoking among U.S. women by birth cohort, 1900–1980, based on the National Health Interview Survey.

TABLE 28–1. Some Toxic and Carcinogenic Agents in Cigarette Smoke*

AGENT	BIOLOGIC ACTIVITY
Nitrogen oxides	Toxic
Carbon monoxide	Toxic
Nitrosamines	Carcinogenic
Formaldehyde	Toxic, carcinogenic
Acrolein	Toxic
Hydrogen cyanide	Toxic
Nicotine	Toxic, addicting
Aromatic amines	Carcinogenic
Polynuclear aromatic hydrocarbons	Carcinogenic
Radioactive compounds	Carcinogenic
Metals	Toxic
Benzenes	Carcinogenic

*Based on material from the U.S. Public Health Service. Smoking and health. A report of the Surgeon General. Washington, DC, U.S. Government Printing Office, 1979, DHEW Publ. (PHS) 79-50066.

respiratory tract absorb the soluble components of these particles.

Cigarette smoke has diverse effects on the structure and function of the lung (Table 28–2). Cigarette smoking reduces the efficacy of host defense mechanisms; mucociliary clearance slows and the time for the clearance of particles from the alveoli lengthens.[65] Alveolar macrophage numbers increase and their functional ability can be adversely affected. Local and systemic immune function are also altered by cigarette smoking. Mucus production increases, as do the number of inflammatory cells in the airways and alveoli. The structural changes of greatest physiologic importance in the lungs of smokers are emphysema and small airway changes, including inflammation, fibrosis, increased muscle mass, and narrowing.[65] The pathogenetic mechanisms by which cigarette smoke damages the lung to produce these changes are discussed elsewhere in this volume.

EPIDEMIOLOGIC CONSIDERATIONS

The clinical diagnosis of COPD in older patients is generally made on the basis of sufficient chronic airflow obstruction to result in dyspnea and limitation of exercise capacity. In cigarette smokers, however, clinically evident COPD usually results from a sustained loss of ventilatory function beyond that associated with aging alone, and the disease does not usually develop abruptly. The evolution of lung function changes in cigarette smokers has been partially described in several prospective reports.[10, 19, 65] Although a cohort of cigarette smokers was not followed across their entire life span to observe the entire natural history of COPD, the results of these studies provide a conceptual model for considering the development of the disease.

TABLE 28–2. Effects of Cigarette Smoking on Lung Structure and Function*

LUNG STRUCTURE/ FUNCTION	EFFECTS
Lung defenses	Slowed mucociliary clearance, altered pattern of particle deposition, increased numbers of alveolar macrophages, altered macrophage functioning, altered antigen processing and antibody response.
Large airways	Mucous gland hypertrophy and hyperplasia, epithelial dysplasia, metaplasia, and neoplasia.
Small airways	Inflammation, increased muscle mass, fibrosis, narrowing, and increased number of goblet cells.
Alveoli	Increased numbers of neutrophils and macrophages, emphysema.

*Based on material from U.S. Public Health Service. The health consequences of smoking. Chronic obstructive lung disease: A report of the Surgeon General. Rockville, MD, U.S. Government Printing Office, 1984, DHHS Publ. (PHS) 84-50205.

Ventilatory function, as expressed by the forced expiratory volume in 1 second (FEV_1), increases during childhood and peaks during early adulthood (Fig. 28–3). From the peak level, ventilatory function declines with increasing age. In cigarette smokers who develop COPD a similar loss of function takes place, but at a more rapid rate than in nonsmokers and in smokers who do not develop disease. COPD is likely to be diagnosed when continued excessive loss of ventilatory function results in sufficient impairment to cause dyspnea and limitation of activity.

This conceptual model (Fig. 28–3) suggests three different indexes of COPD-related morbidity: (1) physician-diagnosed disease, which tends to identify persons with the greatest loss of function; (2) reduced ventilatory function, as measured by spirometry; and (3) excessive rate of loss of ventilatory function, which signals the advent of the process that eventually results in COPD. Mortality rates for COPD provide another indication of the burden of COPD in a population, as do studies on morphologic changes in the lungs of smokers. In this section evidence of the relationship of each of these parameters to cigarette smoking is reviewed.

When interpreting information on the occurrence of physician-diagnosed COPD, consideration must be given to the factors influencing the application of a diagnostic label to a particular patient. In a given population, the incidence and prevalence of physician-diagnosed disease reflect not only the size of the affected group, but patterns of medical care access and usage and the diagnostic practices of physicians. For example, in Tucson, Dodge and colleagues[15] found that labeling patients as having chronic bronchitis, asthma, or emphysema by community physicians varied with the age and sex of

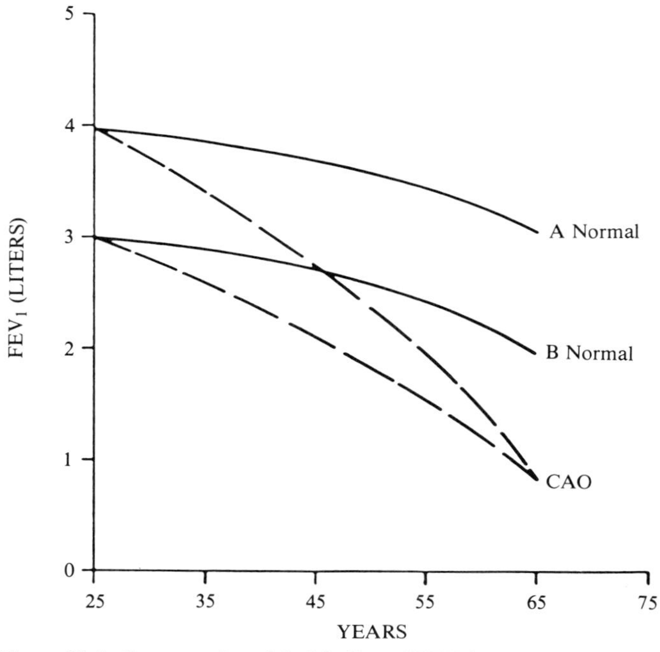

Figure 28–3. Conceptual model of decline of FEV_1 in persons achieving full lung growth (*A*) and not achieving full lung growth (*B*). Excessive decline results in the development of chronic air flow obstruction (CAO). (Reproduced with permission from Samet JM, Tager IB, Speizer FE. Am Rev Respir Dis 1983; 127:508–523.)

TABLE 28–3. Prevalence of Chronic Airflow Obstruction in Selected U.S. Populations*

LOCATION/YEAR	SOURCE OF DATA (Ref. No.)	POPULATION SIZE	INDEX	PREVALENCE (per 100)	
Tecumseh, MI, 1978–1979	65, 27	4930	FEV_1 <65% predicted, and FEV_1:FVC <80%	Men	3.7
				Women	2.2
Glenwood Springs, CO, 1967	35	609	FEV_1:FVC <60%	Men	13.2
				Women	1.5
East Boston, MA, 1973–1974	59	1770	FEV_1 <65% predicted	Men	5.6
				Women	3.4
Six U.S. cities, 1974–1977	18	7909	FEV_1:FVC ≤60%	Men	5.0
				Women	1.9
Burbank and Lancaster, CA, 1973–1974	13	3465 and 4509, respectively	FEV_1 <50% predicted	Age (years)	
				Lancaster	
				18–59	0.8
				60	6.5
				Burbank	
				18–59	1.0
				60	6.2

*Based on material from U.S. Public Health Service. The health consequences of smoking. Chronic obstructive lung disease: A report of the Surgeon General. Rockville, MD, U.S. Government Printing Office, 1984, DHHS Publ. (PHS) 84-50205.

TABLE 28–4. Relationship Between Cigarette Smoking and FEV_1 Level in Selected U.S. Adult Populations

LOCATION/YEAR	SOURCE OF DATA (Ref. No.)	POPULATION	FINDINGS		
Tecumseh, MI, 1959–1960	26	5140 men and women, 16 to 79 years of age	Age-adjusted mean FEV_1 (liters)		
				Men	Women
			Nonsmokers	3.32	2.34
			Ex-smokers	3.31	2.34
			Current smokers	3.12	2.28
Berlin, NH, 1967	17	848 men and women, 30 to 80 years of age	By multiple regression, in men and women, FEV_1 drops by 0.01 liters for each cigarette smoked per day		
Tucson, AZ, 1972–1973	8	2369 men and women, above 14 years of age	By multiple regression analysis, FEV_1 drops by 0.31 and 0.24% of predicted value per pack-year of smoking in men and women, respectively		
East Boston, MA, 1973–1974	58	633 men and women, above 15 years of age	By multiple regression, in men and women, significant reduction of FEV_1 score with increasing lifetime consumption, and in smokers compared with nonsmokers		
Six U.S. cities, 1974–1977	18	8480 men and women, 25 to 74 years of age	Mean residual FEV_1 (liters), after correction for height and age		
			Lifetime Packs	Men	Women
			None	0.25	0.06
			<3000	0.21	0.04
			3000–8999	0.01	−0.05
			9000–17,999	−0.19	−0.20
			≥18,000	−0.45	−0.28
Various California cities, 1973–1975	13, 46	Approximately 8000 men and women, 18 years or older	Prevalence (%) of FEV_1 below 75% predicted, age and sex-adjusted		
			Age group	Never smoked	Current smoker
			18–59 years old		
			Burbank	6.6	12.5
			Lancaster	3.4	6.6
			Long Beach	5.3	10.0
			≥ 60 years old		
			Burbank	15.9	23.5
			Lancaster	13.4	21.7

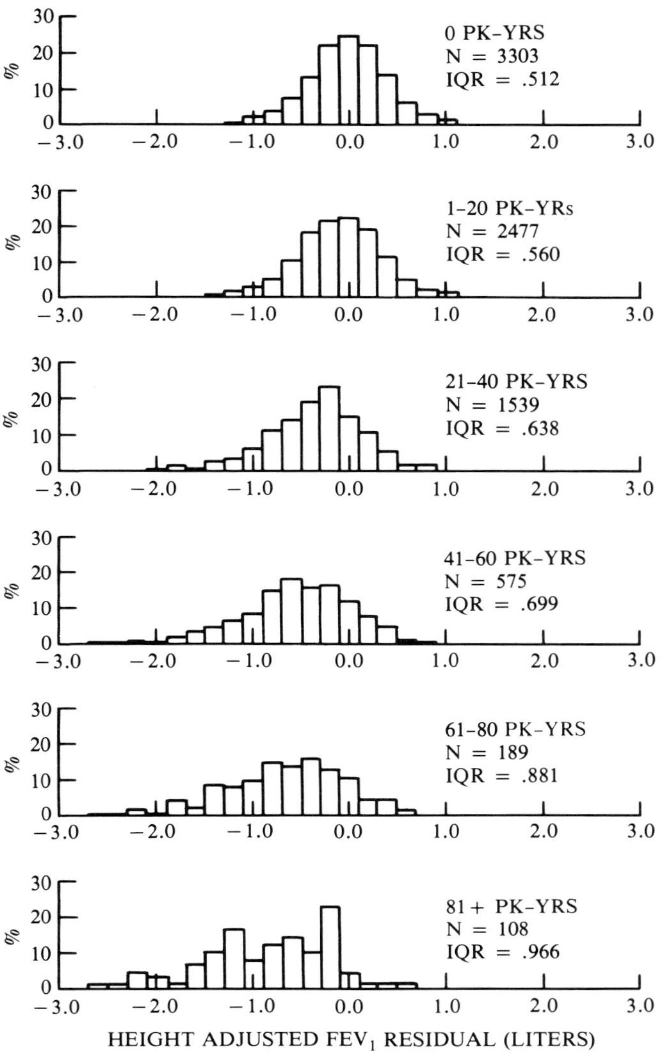

Figure 28–4. Distributions of height-adjusted deviations of FEV_1 from that predicted by cumulative pack-years of smoking in adults from six U.S. cities. (Reproduced with permission from Dockery DW, et al. Am Rev Respir Dis 1988; 137:286–292.)

the patients. Male patients were more often diagnosed with "emphysema," whereas females were more often diagnosed as "asthmatic" or "bronchitic."

Nationwide data collected in the National Health Interview Survey provide estimates of the proportion of U.S. adults affected by chronic bronchitis and emphysema. For example, in 1986, the prevalence of chronic bronchitis was estimated as 5.5% and that of emphysema as 6.5%.[37] These estimates are based on the clinical usage of the terms "chronic bronchitis" and "emphysema," and not on the more stringent definitions used for epidemiologic purposes. Furthermore, some persons might report both chronic bronchitis and emphysema. Nevertheless, these data illustrate the substantial burden of morbidity in the United States related to these cigarette smoking-caused diseases.

Only a few epidemiologic studies have addressed the relationship between cigarette smoking and physician diagnosis of COPD.[65] In a community survey in New Mexico, after considering age and sex, cigarette smoking was the only significant predictor of a physician diagnosis of chronic bronchitis and/or emphysema.[48] In the longitudinal epidemiologic study in Tucson, 82.5% of adults given a new diagnosis of emphysema during an 8-year follow-up period were cigarette smokers.[15]

COPD AND CIGARETTE SMOKING

Lung Function Level

Numerous surveys conducted throughout the world have shown that cigarette smoking is the predominant determinant of the prevalence of airflow obstruction.[65] The typical methodology for these studies included spirometry and a questionnaire on respiratory symptoms and illnesses and on cigarette smoking. Chronic airflow obstruction was considered to be present if the FEV_1 and/or the FEV_1 to FVC (forced vital capacity) ratio were lower than specified values.

The results of these epidemiologic studies show that COPD, regardless of the index used to assess its presence, is a common condition in the U.S. and other countries (Table 28–3). The studies also indicate that, in every U.S. population for which prevalence data are available, chronic airflow obstruction is more common among smokers than among nonsmokers.[13, 31, 35, 46]

Cigarette smoking is an equally strong determinant of the level of FEV_1 (Table 28–4). In cross-sectional studies, the level of FEV_1 was found to decline as the amount of smoking increased.[65] Multiple regression techniques have been applied to data from different populations to describe the quantitative relationship between amount smoked and loss of ventilatory function. These analyses indicate that ventilatory function declines linearly with the cumulative consumption of cigarettes, usually expressed as pack-years.[4, 8, 14] Analyzing data on 8191 men and women from six U.S. cities, Dockery and associates[14] found that male smokers of average height lose an average of 7.4 ml of their FEV_1 for each pack-year and that women smokers of average height lose 4.4 ml of FEV_1 per pack-year. Current smokers, compared with former smokers, tend to have a somewhat lower level of function, even after considering cumulative consumption.[4, 14] Although the decline in the mean level of FEV_1 appears small, the distributions of lung function level in smokers and in nonsmokers are different (Fig. 28–4); the distribution for smokers is skewed toward lower levels so that a much greater proportion of smokers than of nonsmokers have levels below the usual limit of normal.[4, 8, 14, 65]

Longitudinal Decline in Lung Function

In the commonly accepted conceptual model for the development of COPD (Fig. 28–3), clinically evident disease develops after sustained cigarette smoking has resulted in sufficient loss of ventilatory function to produce impairment. In nonsmokers without respiratory disease ventilatory function begins to decline, beginning at about 25 to 35 years of age. The FEV_1 drops by about 25 ml annually in nonsmokers.[65] In cigarette smokers, the average rate of loss of ventilatory function is much greater; some smokers can lose 100 ml or more annually (Fig. 28–5).[19, 65] The distribution of FEV_1 decline in smokers is broad (Fig. 28–5), however, and not all cigarette smokers develop COPD; it is the susceptible minority, with higher rates of decline, who are at greatest risk for the disease.

The factors influencing the rate of lung function decline in cigarette smokers have not yet been adequately characterized.[65] The rate of decline tends to increase with the amount smoked, and ex-smokers generally revert to the rate of loss of nonsmokers. In fact, the excessive decline observed in some smokers might represent a common physiologic consequence of different pathophysiologic mechanisms. Habib and colleagues[21] carefully characterized 13 subjects from the Tucson epidemiologic study with a mean annual decline in FEV_1 of more than 60 ml annually. Clinically, these subjects were

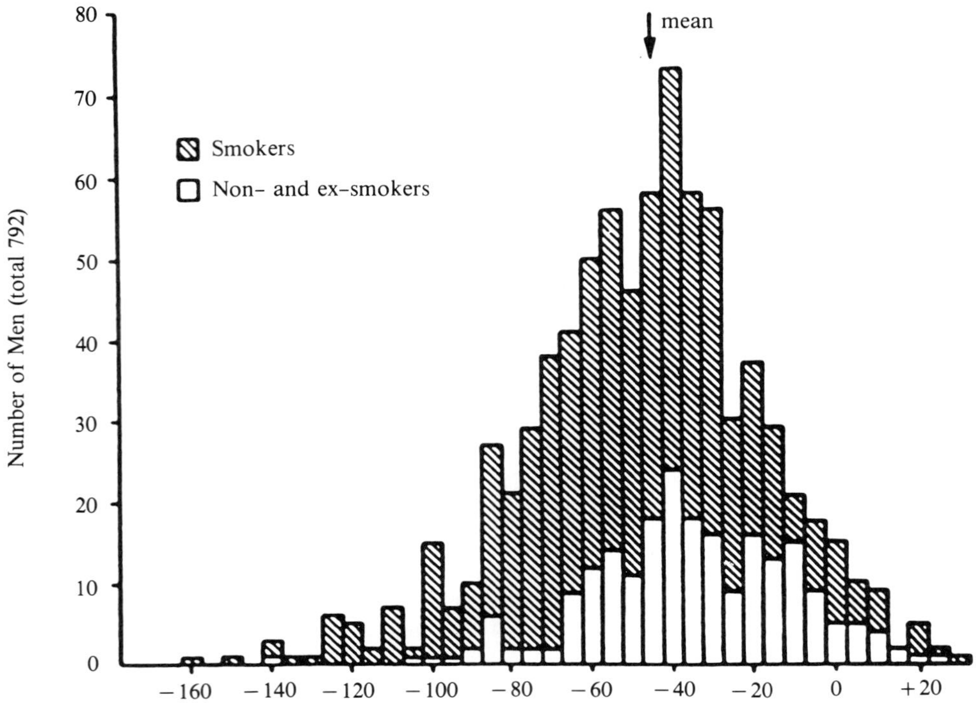

Figure 28–5. Distribution of 8-year slope of FEV_1 in a longitudinal study of 792 London men. (Reproduced with permission from Fletcher CM, et al. The Natural History of Chronic Bronchitis and Emphysema. An Eight-Year Study of Early Chronic Obstructive Lung Disease in Working Men in London. New York, Oxford University Press, 1976.)

not unique and none had alpha$_1$-antitrypsin deficiency. Physiologic assessment suggested that some were developing emphysema, whereas others appeared to have disease of the large or small airways or of both.

The studies of longitudinal change in lung function have only spanned segments of the full natural history of COPD, and many questions remain unanswered. It is unclear, for example, whether the excessive decline takes place at a constant rate in continuous smokers, as suggested by most epidemiologic evidence, or whether this decline occurs intermittently after some triggering event. In this regard, cases of COPD resulting from relatively steep and brief declines of lung function have been described.[3, 19, 29] The rate of functional decline might also accelerate with age.

If excessive loss of function occurs in smokers at a relatively constant rate, it should be possible to correlate the level of function measured at a particular time with the rate of loss of lung function. This relationship, named the "horse-racing effect" by Fletcher and colleagues,[19] has been demonstrated in several longitudinal studies.[9, 19, 65] Although the magnitude of the correlation between the level of function and rate of loss is small, and correlation has not been found in all studies, the horse-racing effect has important clinical implications. It implies that the level of function in smokers predicts future

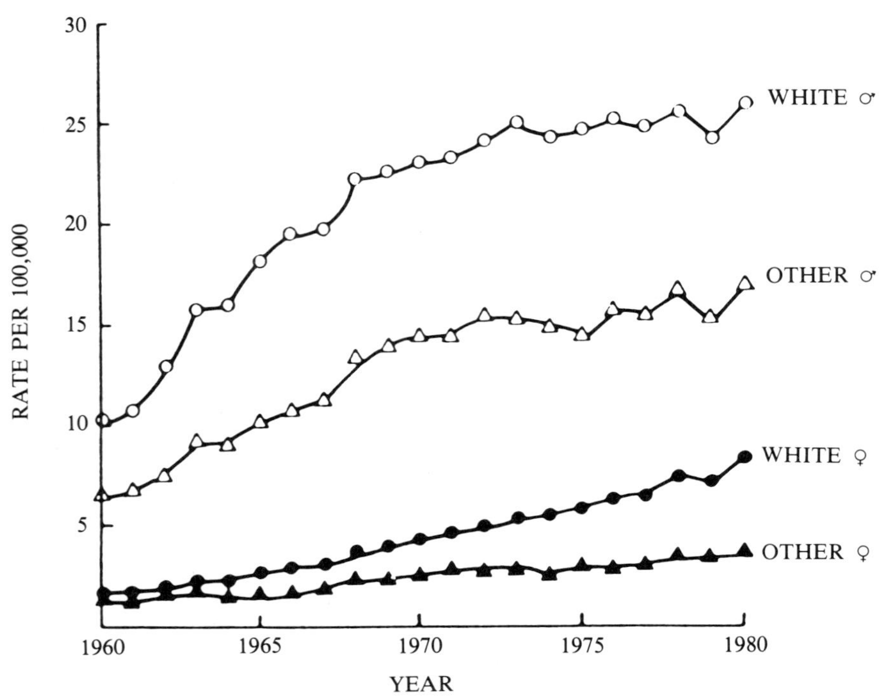

Figure 28–6. Age-adjusted COPD mortality rates for U.S. whites and nonwhites, 1960–1980.

decline; thus, more susceptible smokers should be identifiable prior to the development of COPD, as the level of function slowly diverges from the predicted value. The horse-racing effect supports the use of spirometric testing to screen for smokers likely to develop COPD, particularly middle-aged smokers who might have reached an abnormally low level of function without sufficient impairment to have clinically significant COPD.

Longitudinal studies on the incidence of COPD confirm the importance of a low level of function in predicting the development of disease. Higgins and associates[28] examined predictors of developing "obstructive airways disease," defined as an FEV_1 lower than 65% of that predicted and with an FEV_1 to FVC ratio lower than 80%, in the longitudinal study in Tecumseh, Michigan. The mathematical formulas that best predicted risk included baseline lung function level and measures of cigarette smoking habits. Similarly, in a longitudinal study in Tucson, initial lung function level was an important predictor of meeting the Tecumseh definition of obstructive airways disease and of having a new diagnosis by a physician of chronic bronchitis or emphysema.[32]

Mortality from COPD

In the United States, since 1950, the underlying cause of death has been classified according to the International Classification of Diseases, an international system that is revised every 10 years. Before 1950, the underlying cause of death was assigned according to a more rigid system that deemphasized chronic bronchitis and emphysema.[47] The Sixth and Seventh Revisions of the International Classification of Diseases included codes for "bronchitis unqualified," "chronic bronchitis," and "emphysema." Until the Eighth Revision of the International Classification of Diseases (1968), however, a code for COPD and similar conditions was not explicitly included. In the late 1960s, the National Center for Health Statistics introduced a unique code for COPD, as physicians increasingly began to use this term on death certificates. In the Ninth Revision of the International Classification of Diseases (1978), a death clinically caused by COPD might be assigned to one of the following: code 490, "bronchitis, not specified as acute or chronic"; code 491, "chronic bronchitis"; code 492, "emphysema"; or code 496, "chronic airways obstruction, not elsewhere classified."

Mortality rates for COPD must be considered in relation to the changing coding system for deaths assigned to chronic bronchitis, emphysema, and COPD or a similar condition.[38] Furthermore, deaths resulting from COPD can be misclassified on the death certificate because of lack of correlation between clinical status and the underlying disease. Studies have found that COPD has been underdiagnosed on death certificates.[34]

In spite of the limited accuracy of death certificates in investigating COPD, data on mortality from COPD strongly support the causal association of cigarette smoking with this disease. Since 1950, mortality rates for COPD have steadily risen (Fig. 28–6). In 1950, 3157 U.S. deaths were attributed to "bronchitis unqualified," "chronic bronchitis," or "emphysema"; by 1980, 52,348 deaths were assigned to "bronchitis unqualified," "chronic bronchitis," "emphysema," or "chronic airways obstruction, not elsewhere classified." The temporal patterns of the increasing rates (Fig. 28–6) are consistent with the patterns of cigarette smoking throughout the 20th century (Figs. 28–1 and 28–2). The patterns of increased cigarette smoking by men and women were both followed approximately 30 years later by an upsurge of COPD mortality as the smokers reached the age at which COPD becomes clinically manifest.

Longitudinal epidemiologic studies have confirmed the association of death from COPD with cigarette smoking.[65] For example, in a study of mortality in British physicians in relation to smoking habits, mortality rates for chronic bronchitis and emphysema over a 20-year follow-up period were dramatically increased for smokers as compared with nonsmokers (Table 28–5). Similarly, in the American Cancer Society's nationwide study of over 1,000,000 volunteer subjects, mortality in male cigarette smokers, as compared with nonsmokers, increased more than six-fold in the age group 45 through 64 years and more than eleven-fold in the age group 65 through 79 years.[23] Other prospective studies conducted worldwide, as well as retrospective studies, have shown similarly strong relationships between cigarette smoking and increased mortality from COPD.

Structural Changes in the Lungs of Smokers

Both the airways and lung parenchyma are extensively damaged by cigarette smoking (Table 28–2). The structural changes found in COPD are described in detail elsewhere in this volume. This section discusses the relationship between these changes and cigarette smoking. In patients with COPD, chronic airflow obstruction represents the functional manifestations of increased airflow resistance in the lung's smaller airways and of emphysema. The extent to which these two distinct pathophysiologic mechanisms contribute to airflow obstruction in a given patient is highly variable, but cigarette smoking has been demonstrated to cause extensive abnormalities in the small airways and to cause emphysema.

The conceptual model for the development of COPD proposed in Figure 28–3 suggests that changes should be evident in the lungs of smokers long before COPD develops. Abnormalities of the small airways, which are associated with reduced ventilatory function,[12] are present in the lungs of young smokers. Niewoehner and associates[39] examined the lungs of 20 smokers and 19 nonsmokers who had died suddenly at a mean age of 25 years. A pattern of small airways injury, termed "respiratory bronchiolitis," was readily identified in the lungs of the smokers, even at this early age. Clusters of brown pigmented macrophages were found in the respiratory bronchioles, which also displayed increased numbers of inflammatory cells and denuded epithelium. These observations have been confirmed by other investigators.[65]

With prolonged smoking the small airways are further damaged. Changes include fibrosis of the airways with narrowing, squamous metaplasia, increased muscle mass, plugging of the lumen by mucus and inflammatory cells, and a reduced number of airways.[65] The extent of abnormality in the small airways correlates with tests of small airways function and with standard spirometric measures of function.[12, 65]

TABLE 28–5. Age-Standardized Mortality Rate for Chronic Bronchitis and Emphysema in the Study of British Male Physicians

GROUP	MORTALITY RATE (per 100,000)
Smoking group	
Nonsmokers	10
Cigarettes only	140
Pipe and/or cigars only	58
Mixed*	82
Sustained cigarette smokers	
1–14 cigarettes/day	51
15–24 cigarettes/day	78
≥25 cigarettes/day	114

*Cigarettes with pipe, cigar, or both.

From Doll, R, Peto R. Br Med J 1976; 2:1525–1536.

Cigarette smoking is closely associated with the development of centrilobular emphysema.[65] Emphysema is uncommon in nonsmokers; in smokers, the frequency of occurrence of emphysema increases with age and with the amount smoked.[65] The extent of emphysema, like indexes of small airways damage, is associated with the degree of physiologic impairment.[22, 36]

These observations on structural changes in the lungs of smokers and on structure-function correlations complement the epidemiologic evidence on the association between cigarette smoking and COPD. The evolution of structural changes in the lung is consistent with the natural history of COPD, as described in epidemiologic investigations. The rarity of severe emphysema and airways abnormalities in nonsmokers confirms the predominant role of cigarette smoking as the cause of COPD.

Determinants of Susceptibility to Cigarette Smoke

Whereas a causal association of cigarette smoking with COPD has been firmly established,[65] determinants of susceptibility to cigarette smoke have not yet been identified, with the exception of alpha$_1$-antitrypsin deficiency. Current concepts of pathogenesis emphasize lung inflammation and an imbalance between protease activity and antiproteases.[40] These mechanisms of lung injury have primarily been investigated in animal models and in small numbers of volunteer subjects using bronchoalveolar lavage, a technique not readily applicable to large numbers of subjects in an epidemiologic study. Thus, the determinants of susceptibility to cigarette smoke, in regard to the protease-antiprotease hypothesis, have not yet been adequately examined epidemiologically.

Three hypotheses have been evaluated in epidemiologic investigations of the etiology of COPD. A hypothesis advanced by British investigators emphasized the potential role of recurrent respiratory infection in persons with mucous hypersecretion as the cause of lung destruction.[56, 57] This hypothesis was suggested by the cross-sectional association of chronic mucus hypersecretion with recurrent episodes of chest infection and lower level of lung function. Longitudinal investigations, however, have shown that lung function decline, after controlling for cigarette smoking, is not affected by respiratory infections.[19] Mucus hypersecretion and chronic airflow obstruction are separate entities that are associated because they have a common cause—cigarette smoking.[19, 45]

Orie and colleagues[41] advanced an alternative hypothesis, often referred to as the "Dutch hypothesis," that emphasized endogenous susceptibility. They suggested that bronchial hyper-reactivity increases susceptibility to environmental agents such as tobacco smoke. The results of several small longitudinal investigations[2, 7, 30] are consistent with this hypothesis, as are some cross-sectional observations.[53] Currently this hypothesis is being tested further in longitudinal investigations.

The third hypothesis has emphasized the role of childhood factors in determining susceptibility during adulthood.[8, 49] A reduced level of function at maturity because of events during childhood is thought to lead to the more rapid development of impairment during adulthood (Fig. 28–3). Changes in the lung related to childhood factors might also predispose to a steeper decline in lung function in cigarette smokers. Cross-sectional observations in adults generally support this hypothesis; adults reporting that they had respiratory trouble during childhood tend to have a lower level of lung function than those without childhood respiratory problems.[8, 49] Persistent abnormalities of ventilatory function and increased airways hyper-reactivity have been demonstrated in children who had various forms of lung injury during childhood.[49] This hypothesis has not yet been tested fully in longitudinal studies, but the available evidence is sufficiently compelling to warrant further investigation.

Less Hazardous Cigarettes

Since the 1950s, cigarette tar content and nicotine yield have declined markedly.[65] In 1955, the average American cigarette delivered 43 mg tar and 2.8 mg nicotine to the lung.[64] By 1980, the U.S. sales-weighted average tar yield was lower than 15 mg and the average nicotine yield was about 1 mg. These lower tar and nicotine yields, as measured by a smoking machine, have been achieved by changes in tobacco growing and processing methods, filtration, dilution of the tobacco smoke, and other changes in cigarette design.

It would seem that a lower yield of tar and nicotine implies a less hazardous cigarette. A reduced yield of tar, however, as measured by a machine, might not produce an equivalent reduction in the amount of toxic tobacco smoke components delivered to the lung.[6, 65] Compensatory changes in smoking behavior can increase the amount of smoke components inhaled above those predicted by machine yields of tar and nicotine. Smokers of lower yield cigarettes might compensate by smoking more cigarettes and by inhaling more deeply.[65] In experimental studies, levels of biologic markers of tobacco smoke components were not found to correlate strongly with tar and nicotine ratings.[5, 6, 65]

The lack of correlation between the machine yield of tar and nicotine and the amount of inhaled toxic materials might explain the weakness of the evidence for reduced disease risks for smokers of the lower yield cigarettes.[51, 65] For COPD, the 1984 Report of the Surgeon General[65] concluded that a reduction in cigarette tar content might not reduce the risk of dyspnea and chronic airflow obstruction. Furthermore, the extent of the data on newer cigarettes with extremely low yields is limited. In the longitudinal study conducted by the American Cancer Society from 1960 through 1972, smokers of cigarettes containing more than 2 mg of nicotine and 25.8 mg of tar had a higher mortality rate from emphysema.[33] A British case-control study showed a lower risk of bronchitis in men who switched from plain to filter cigarettes, but a similar protective effect was not found in women.[1] An American Cancer Society study of 1.2 million American men and women provides relevant evidence on mortality from COPD and other diseases in relation to the type of cigarette smoked.[54] The initial cross-sectional data from this study indicate the importance of determining the risks of lower yield products; one-third of male and one-half of female smokers reported using brands with tar yields lower than 12 mg.

Measures of cumulative tar consumption and tar yield are not strongly associated with lung function level.[25, 43, 44] In one study of U.S. males, the tar content of cigarettes smoked did not predict the rate of decline in pulmonary function over a 5-year period.[52] Although methodologic problems limit the use of the epidemiologic approach for evaluating the potential benefits of lower yield cigarettes,[50] most evidence to date weighs against a strong protective effect of the lower yield products in regard to the development of COPD.

CONCLUSIONS

Cigarette smoking is causally associated with the development of COPD and most cases in the U.S. can be attributed to this addictive behavior. The strong association of cigarette smoking with COPD has clinical and public health implications. Clinicians should be cautious in making the diagnosis of COPD in nonsmokers, particularly if the alpha$_1$-antitrypsin level is within normal limits. Conversely, a history of cigarette smoking, particularly if the daily level of consumption has been high, increases the likelihood of developing COPD. Only a minority of smokers develop COPD, however, so the disease should not be diagnosed on the basis of smoking history alone.

The clear association of cigarette smoking with COPD and other diseases provides a strong imperative for the prevention and cessation of smoking. Voluntary health agencies, state agencies, and the federal government have implemented prevention programs. Health care providers should instruct smoking patients about the risks of COPD and other diseases and should relentlessly counsel cessation. With continued progress toward a tobacco-free society, COPD could become an uncommon disease.

REFERENCES

1. Alderson MR, Lee PN, Wang R. Risks of lung cancer, chronic bronchitis, ischaemic heart disease, and stroke in relation to type of cigarette smoked. J Epidemiol Community Health 1985; 39:286–293.
2. Barter CE, Campbell AH. Relationship of constitutional factors and cigarette smoking to decrease in 1-second forced expiratory volume. Am Rev Respir Dis 1976; 113:305–314.
3. Bates DV. The fate of the chronic bronchitic: A report of the ten-year follow-up in the Canadian Department of Veteran's Affairs Coordinated Study of Chronic Bronchitis. Am Rev Respir Dis 1973; 108:1043–1065.
4. Beck GJ, Doyle CA, Schachter EN. Smoking and lung function. Am Rev Respir Dis 1981; 123:149–155.
5. Benowitz NL, Hall SM, Herning RI, et al. Smokers of low-yield cigarettes do not consume less nicotine. N Engl J Med 1983; 309:139–142.
6. Benowitz NL, Payton J, Kozlowski LT, Yu L. Influence of smoking fewer cigarettes on exposure to tar, nicotine, and carbon monoxide. N Engl J Med 1986: 315:1310–1313.
7. Britt EJ, Cohen B, Menkes H, et al. Airways reactivity and functional deterioration in relatives of COPD patients. Chest 1980; 77(Suppl):260–261.
8. Burrows B, Knudson RJ, Cline MG, Lebowitz MD. Quantitative relationships between cigarette smoking and ventilatory function. Am Rev Respir Dis 1977; 115:195–205.
9. Burrows B, Knudson RJ, Camilli AE, et al. The "horse-racing effect" and predicting decline in forced expiratory volume in one second from screening spirometry. Am Rev Respir Dis 1987; 135:788–793.
10. Camilli AE, Burrows B, Knudson RJ, et al. Longitudinal changes in forced expiratory volume in one second in adults. Am Rev Respir Dis 1987; 135:794–799.
11. Christie RV. Emphysema of the lungs. Br Med J 1944; 1:105–108, 143–146.
12. Cosio M, Ghezzo H, Hogg JC, et al. The relations between structural changes in small airways and pulmonary-function tests. N Engl J Med 1978; 298:1277–1281.
13. Detels R, Rokow SN, Coulson AH, et al. The UCLA population studies of chronic obstructive respiratory disease. I. Methodology and comparison of lung function in areas of high and low pollution. Am J Epidemiol 1979; 109:33–58.
14. Dockery DW, Speizer FE, Ferris BG Jr, et al. Cumulative and reversible effects of lifetime smoking on simple tests of lung function in adults. Am Rev Respir Dis 1988; 137:286–292.
15. Dodge R, Cline CG, Burrows B. Comparison of asthma, emphysema, and chronic bronchitis diagnoses in a general population sample. Am Rev Respir Dis 1986; 133:981–986.
16. Doll R, Peto R. Mortality in relation to smoking: 20 years' observations on male British doctors. Br Med J 1976; 2:1525–1536.
17. Ferris BG, Higgins ITT, Higgins MW, Peters JM. Chronic nonspecific respiratory disease in Berlin, New Hampshire, 1961 to 1967. A follow-up study. Am Rev Respir Dis 1973; 107:110–122.
18. Ferris BG Jr, Speizer FE, Spengler JD, et al. Effects of sulfur oxides and respirable particles on human health. Methodology and demography of populations in study. Am Rev Respir Dis 1979; 120:767–779.
19. Fletcher CM, Peto R, Tinker C, Speizer FE. The Natural History of Chronic Bronchitis and Emphysema. An Eight-Year Study of Early Chronic Obstructive Lung Disease in Working Men in London. New York, Oxford University Press, 1976.
20. Goodman N, Lane RE, Rampling SB. Chronic bronchitis: An introductory examination of existing data. Br Med J 1953; 2:237–269.
21. Habib MP, Klink ME, Knudson DE, et al. Physiologic characteristics of subjects exhibiting accelerated deterioration of ventilatory function. Am Rev Respir Dis 1987; 136:638–645.
22. Hale KA, Ewing SL, Gosnell BA, Niewoehner DE. Lung disease in long-term cigarette smokers with and without chronic airflow obstruction. Am Rev Respir Dis 1984; 130:716–721.
23. Hammond EC. Smoking in relation to the death rates in one million men and women. In: Haenszel W, ed. Epidemiological Approaches to the Study of Cancer and Other Chronic Diseases. U.S. Department of Health, Education, and Welfare, 1966, 127–204. National Cancer Institute Monograph No. 19. Washington, D.C.: U.S. Government Printing Office, 1966.
24. Harris JE. Cigarette smoking among successive birth cohorts of men and women in the United States during 1900–1980. J Natl Cancer Inst 1983; 71:473–479.
25. Higenbottam T, Shipley MJ, Clark TJH, Rose G. Lung function and symptoms of cigarette smokers related to tar yield and number of cigarettes smoked. Lancet 1980; 1:409–412.
26. Higgins MW, Kjelsberg M. Characteristics of smokers and nonsmokers in Tecumseh, Michigan. II. The distribution of selected physical measurements and physiologic variables and the prevalence of certain diseases in smokers and non-smokers. Am J Epidemiol 1967; 86:60–77.
27. Higgins MW, Keller JB, Metzner HL. Smoking, socioeconomic status and chronic respiratory disease. Am Rev Respir Dis 1977; 116:403–410.
28. Higgins MW, Keller JB, Becker M, et al. An index of risk for obstructive airways disease. Am Rev Respir Dis 1982; 125:144–151.
29. Howard P, Astin TW. Precipitous fall of the forced expiratory volume. Thorax 1969; 24:492–495.
30. Kanner RE, Renzetti AD Jr, Klauber MR, et al. Variables associated with changes in spirometry in patients with obstructive lung diseases. Am J Med 1979; 67:44–50.
31. Knudson RJ, Burrows B, Lebowitz MD. The maximal expiratory flow-volume curve: Its use in detection of ventilatory abnormalities in a population study. Am Rev Respir Dis 1976; 114:871–879.
32. Lebowitz MD, Knudson RJ, Burrows B. Risk factors for airways obstructive diseases: A multiple logistics approach. Chest 1984; 85:11S–12S.
33. Lee PN, Garfinkel L. Mortality and type of cigarette smoked. J Epidemiol Community Health 1981; 35:16–22.
34. Mitchell RS, Maisel JC, Dart GA, Silvers GW. The accuracy of the death certificate in reporting cause of death in adults. With special reference to chronic bronchitis and emphysema. Am Rev Respir Dis 1971; 104:844–850.
35. Mueller RE, Keble DL, Plummer J, Walker SH. The prevalence of chronic bronchitis, chronic airway obstruction, and respiratory symptoms in a Colorado city. Am Rev Respir Dis 1971; 103:209–228.
36. Nagai A, West WW, Thurlbeck WM. The National Institutes of Health Intermittent Positive Pressure Breathing Trial: Pathology Studies II. Correlation between morphologic findings, clinical findings, and evidence of expiratory air-flow obstruction. Am Rev Respir Dis 1985; 132:946–953.
37. National Center for Health Statistics. Current estimates from the National Health Interview Survey, United States, 1986. In: Dawson DA, Adams DF, eds. Vital and Health Statistics, Series 10, No. 164. Washington, DC: U.S. Government Printing Office, 1987. DHHS Publ. (PHS) 87-1592.
38. National Heart, Lung, and Blood Institute. Epidemiology of respiratory diseases. Task Force report. Bethesda, MD: U.S. Government Printing Office, 1980. NIH Publ. 81-2019.
39. Niewoehner DE, Kleinerman J, Rice B. Pathologic changes in the peripheral airways of young cigarette smokers. N Engl J Med 1974; 291:755–758.
40. Niewoehner DE. Cigarette smoking, lung inflammation, and the development of emphysema. J Lab Clin Med 1988; 111:15–27.

41. Orie NG, Sluiter HJ, deVries K, et al. The host factor in bronchitis. In: Orie NGM, Sluiter HJ, eds. Bronchitis, An International Symposium, April 27–29, 1960. Assen, The Netherlands: Royal Vangorcum Association, 1961, 43–59.
42. Oswald NC, Harold JT, Martin WJ. Clinical pattern of chronic bronchitis. Lancet 1953; 2:639–643.
43. Paoletti P, Camilli AE, Holberg C, Lebowitz MD. Respiratory effects in relation to estimated tar exposure from current and cumulative cigarette consumption. Chest 1985; 88:849–855.
44. Peach H, Hayward DM, Ellard DR, et al. Phlegm production and lung function among cigarette smokers changing tar groups during the 1970s. J Epidemiol Community Health 1986; 40:110–116.
45. Peto R, Speizer, FE, Cochrane AL, et al. The relevance in adults of air-flow obstruction, but not of mucus hypersecretion, to mortality from chronic lung disease. Am Rev Respir Dis 1983; 128:491–500.
46. Rokaw SN, Detels R, Coulson AH, et al. The UCLA population studies of chronic obstructive respiratory disease. 3. Comparison of pulmonary function in three communities exposed to photochemical oxidants, multiple primary pollutants, or minimal pollutants. Chest 1980; 78:252–262.
47. Rosenblatt MB. Emphysema. J Am Geriatr Soc 1970; 18:517–528.
48. Samet JM, Schrag SD, Howard CA, et al. Respiratory disease in a New Mexico population sample of Hispanic and non-Hispanic whites. Am Rev Respir Dis 1982; 125:152–157.
49. Samet JM, Tager IB, Speizer FE. The relationship between respiratory illness in childhood and chronic airflow obstruction in adulthood. Am Rev Respir Dis 1983; 127:508–523.
50. Samet JM. Less hazardous cigarettes and diseases of the lung. Chest 1985; 88:802–803.
51. Scarborough Conference on Preventive Medicine, Fourth Conference. Is there a future for lower-tar-yield cigarettes? Lancet 1985; 2:1111–1114.
52. Sparrow D, Stefos T, Bosse R, Weiss ST. The relationship of tar content to decline in pulmonary function in cigarette smokers. Am Rev Respir Dis 1983; 127:56–58.
53. Sparrow D, O'Connor G, Colton T, et al. The relationship of nonspecific bronchial responsiveness to the occurrence of respiratory symptoms and decreased levels of pulmonary function. Am Rev Respir Dis 1987; 135;1255–1260.
54. Stellman SD, Garfinkel L. Smoking habits and tar levels in a new American Cancer Society prospective study of 1.2 million men and women. J Natl Cancer Inst 1986; 76:1057–1063.
55. Stuart-Harris CH. The epidemiology and evolution of chronic bronchitis. Br J Tuberculosis Dis Chest 1954; 48:169–178.
56. Stuart-Harris CH. Chronic bronchitis, Part I. Abstr World Med 1968; 42:649–669.
57. Stuart-Harris CH. Chronic bronchitis, Part II. Abstr World Med 1968; 42:737–751.
58. Tager I, Speizer FE. Risk estimates for chronic bronchitis in smokers. A study of male-female differences. Am Rev Respir Dis 1976; 113:619–625.
59. Tager I, Tishler PV, Rosner B, et al. Studies of the familial aggregation of chronic bronchitis and obstructive airways disease. Int J Epidemiol 1978; 7:55–62.
60. United States Centers for Disease Control. Cigarette Smoking in the United States, 1986. MMWR 1987; 36:581–85.
61. United States Centers for Disease Control. Regional variation in smoking prevalence and cessation: Behavioral risk factor surveillance, 1986. MMWR 1987; 36:751–754.
62. United States Public Health Service. Smoking and health. Report of the Advisory Committee to the Surgeon General. Washington, DC: U.S. Government Printing Office, 1964, 44, 277. PHS Publ. 1103.
63. United States Public Health Service. The health consequences of smoking. A report of the Surgeon General. Washington, DC: U.S. Government Printing Office, 1972. DHEW Publ. HSM 72-7516.
64. United States Public Health Service. Smoking and health. A report of the Surgeon General. Washington, DC: U.S. Government Printing Office, 1979, 4:1–7; 5:1–74; 6:1–52; 8:1–93. DHEW Publ. PHS 79-50066.
65. United States Public Health Service. The health consequences of smoking. Chronic obstructive lung disease: A report of the Surgeon General. Rockville, MD: U.S. Government Printing Office, 1984, 9, 75–118, 185–260, 348–352, 361–412. DHHS Publ. (PHS) 84-50205.
66. United States Public Health Service. The health consequences of smoking. Cancer and chronic lung disease in the workplace. Rockville, MD: U.S. Government Printing Office, 1985. DHHS Publ. (PHS) 1986 0-157-964.
67. United States Public Health Service. The health consequences of involuntary smoking: A report of the Surgeon General. Rockville, MD: U.S. Government Printing Office, 1986, 19–118, 196–198. DHHS Publ. (CDC) 87-8398.

Chapter 29

EFFECTS OF AIR POLLUTION ON COPD

Michael A. Bauer   Mark J. Utell   Richard W. Hyde

Since the turn of the century, heavily industrialized areas have occasionally experienced dramatic epidemics with fatalities clearly related to high levels of air pollution. In December 1952, cold temperatures and a 5-day thermal inversion over industrial areas of London, England, resulted in increased numbers of physician house calls and emergency room visits, with more than 3500 to 4000 deaths.[59, 66] People older than 45 years with chronic respiratory or cardiac disease suffered the highest mortality, especially those with chronic bronchitis, for whom the death rate exceeded eight to ten times that expected. In the United States similar climatic conditions caused extremely high levels of atmospheric pollutants in Donora, Pennsylvania, in October 1948.[84] Twenty deaths in a population of 13,000 were attributed to inhalation of sulfur oxides and particulate matter. An estimated 6000 suffered less serious health effects. Analyses of these and similar health disasters indicate that the elderly and persons with underlying cardiac or respiratory diseases are most vulnerable. In addition, air pollution disasters usually result from abnormal concentrations of one or more materials commonly emitted into the atmosphere, and meteorologic conditions often contribute to the magnitude of the disaster.

Fortunately, the degree of exposure to high levels of atmospheric pollutants has decreased in many developed western countries. In the United States the Environmental Protection Agency (EPA), under the authority of the Clean Air Act, oversees the protection and enhancement of outdoor air quality. Statutory regulations specify ambient air quality standards and complex regulations control both mobile and stationary sources of air pollution. According to the EPA, from 1975 to 1983 the concentrations of many pollutants, including sulfur dioxide (SO_2), total suspended particulates (TSP), carbon monoxide (CO), and lead (Pb) substantially decreased, with the possible exception of nitrogen dioxide (NO_2).[71] Even so, there remains the need to study and recognize the potentially adverse health effects of air pollution. First, even though smoking might have a greater impact on health than inhalation of ambient air pollutants, a considerable number of cases of respiratory disease probably result from air pollution. For example, the National Center for Health Statistics has estimated that in 1979 to 1981 approximately 10,000,000 persons suffered from chronic obstructive pulmonary disease (COPD) in the United States.[37a] Thus, even if air pollution causes a small proportion of COPD cases, the absolute number of subjects with disease will be large. Epidemiologic experience clearly indicates that persons with underlying disease, especially COPD, are more sensitive to the adverse health effects of air pollution than normal subjects.[26, 59, 66, 84] Second, air pollution and cigarette smoking might have synergistic adverse health effects. The results of both animal and epidemiologic studies suggest that air pollution multiplies the risk of developing respiratory disease in smokers.[75, 100]

Supported in part by National Institute of Health Grants ES00143, ES01247, ES02679, HL-07216 and RR00044; Health Effects Institute Contracts 84-3 and 88-8; and Electric Power Research Institute Contract RP-3009.

Sources and Categories of Air Pollutants

In the normal atmosphere, dry air has a constant composition of 78% nitrogen (N_2), 21% oxygen (O_2), and 1% argon (Ar) by weight, up to altitudes of approximately 50 miles. Other components in the atmosphere are minor, with concentrations expressed in parts per million (ppm). For example, carbon dioxide (CO_2) typically has a concentration of 320 ppm. Other gases such as helium, neon, methane, krypton, oxides of nitrogen, hydrogen, xenon, and ozone constitute only 0.004% of the atmosphere. The concentration of atmospheric water vapor varies widely and depends on such factors as latitude, geography, nearness to large bodies of water, and ambient temperature. Water vapor composition can vary from 0.02% (200 ppm) in desert areas to 6% (60,000 ppm) in warm, humid climates.

Air pollution is the accumulation of substances, usually manmade, to levels that can be detrimental to the health of humans, animals, or plant life. Most of these pollutants are associated with fossil fuel consumption, either by stationary sources, such as power plants and factories, or by mobile sources, such as motor vehicles. Two main categories of outdoor air pollutants are recognized:

1. *Industrial smog* generally predominates in large industrial areas, such as New York and Tokyo. Smog is a combination of smoke and fog and is more of a problem in cold, humid climates. Industrial smog results from combustion of solid or liquid fossil fuels and consists primarily of sulfur oxides and particulate complexes.
2. *Photochemical smog* occurs in areas with a high density of motor vehicles and resultant auto emissions. This type of pollutant is more of a problem in warm, sunny climates, which facilitate photochemical reactions with nitrogen oxides, ozone, and carbon monoxide. The increasing use of the automobile catalytic converter has added sulfuric acid to the pollutants included in this category.

Table 29–1 lists common air pollutants and summarizes their major sources and adverse effects.

In industrial areas, high pollution levels occur most often in association with specific climatic factors. For example, low wind velocities can inhibit the dispersion of pollutants. Thermal inversions occur when warm layers of atmospheric air hold cold layers of polluted air beneath them at ground level.

TABLE 29–1. Principal Sources and Adverse Effects of Common Air Pollutants

POLLUTANT	SOURCE	EFFECTS
Sulfur oxides-particulate complexes	Fossil fuels; power plants, oil refineries, tobacco smoke, kerosene heaters, wood and coal stoves	Bronchoconstriction
Photochemical oxidants, oxides of nitrogen, ozone	Automobile exhaust, power plants, plus solar radiation	Airway irritation, impaired ventilatory function and lung defenses, airway injury
Carbon monoxide	Automobile exhaust, cigarette smoking	Tissue hypoxia, especially of cardiovascular and neurologic systems

Common Air Pollutants

Gases

Incomplete combustion of coal, natural gas, and other carbon-containing compounds emits carbon monoxide (CO) at concentrations as high as 6%. This production of CO from fossil fuels accounts for greater quantities of pollutants than from all other sources combined.

Hydrocarbons are compounds such as paraffins, olefins, acetylenes, and aromatics. There are more than 60 different hydrocarbons in smog; most are secondary to the combustion of oil and gasoline. These compounds, by themselves, are thought to have low toxicity. They are of concern, however, because photochemical activity in the presence of sunlight and oxides of nitrogen produces photochemical oxidants, especially ozone, which are responsible for many of the adverse health effects from smog.

Ozone is the main component of photochemical oxidants, contributing up to 90% of the total oxidants present in photochemical smog. It is the product of atmospheric reactions involving volatile organic compounds and oxides of nitrogen (NO_x), hydroxyl (OH^-) or other radicals, oxygen, and sunlight.

Nitrogen oxides include nitrous oxide (N_2O), nitric oxide (NO), and nitrogen dioxide (NO_2). They are produced mainly by fossil fuel combustion. In Los Angeles, NO levels are maximum during the early morning rush hour. Soon thereafter the sun initiates photochemical reactions, which convert NO to NO_2. After a few hours, NO_2 reaches maximum levels and can react photochemically to produce ozone (O_3). From outdoor monitoring stations, the mean NO_2 concentration for 24 hours has been found to be as high as 0.21 ppm and for 30 minutes as high as 0.45 ppm. Annual mean NO_2 concentrations in urban areas in the U.S. are generally about 0.01 to 0.04 ppm (Table 29–2). One-hour indoor NO_2 concentrations in kitchens with unvented gas stoves can exceed 1.0 ppm.

Sulfur dioxide (SO_2) is a major atmospheric pollutant in the U.S. It is colorless, with a pungent, irritating odor, and is normally oxidized to sulfur trioxide (SO_3) in the air. This reaction is facilitated by the presence of other oxidant pollutants or by aqueous aerosols that contain SO_2. Combustion of fossil fuels is the main source of SO_2. When sulfur-containing fuels are burned, the sulfur combines with O_2 in the air to form aqueous oxides of sulfur. Once SO_3 forms, it reacts instantaneously with water vapor in the atmosphere to become sulfuric acid (H_2SO_4). In addition, SO_2 can also combine with water vapor to form sulfurous acid (H_2SO_3), which is later oxidized to sulfuric acid. The highest levels of SO_2 in the U.S. are found in the northeastern and midwestern states, where there are concentrations of heavy industry that use large amounts of fossil fuels. The atmospheric concentration can range from 0.01 to 0.10 ppm, with occasional peaks from 1.0 to 1.5 ppm. For example, the lethal London smog of 1952 was associated with an estimated average SO_2 concentration of 1.34 ppm over a 48-hour period, probably derived from the widespread burning of coal and its by-products by heavy industry and households.[59, 66] Because SO_2 is highly soluble in water, only a small portion of this inhaled pollutant reaches the distal portions of the lung.[32]

Particulates

Suspended particulate pollutants generally occur in association with SO_2, and the ambient concentrations of the two often parallel each other. The exact composition of particulate pollutants varies, as does the actual size of the particles, but most suspended particles are respirable. They consist of mixtures of carbon, soot and tars, oxides of iron, aluminum, sulfates, and phosphates, as well as various organic compounds. The concentrations of these pollutants are commonly reported as a total concentration of respirable particles. Sulfur oxides and the suspended particulates are usually combined into one category, because they are commonly found together and because SO_2 itself is often a constituent of particulate aerosols. Various metallic and ammonium sulfate salts represent a large fraction of total suspended particulates. The atmospheric sulfates include ammonium bisulfate and ammonium sulfate; H_2SO_4 occurs as an aerosol mist. Nitrate aerosols are also part of suspended particulate matter. They are produced by the conversion of NO_2 and nitric acid through photochemical reactions. These particulates and mixtures of sulfur oxides can also be transported great distances by prevailing atmospheric wind conditions. Eventually they return to the earth's surface, "raining out" as an acidic mixture and having profound, harmful effects on some ecosystems.

In addition to considering the deleterious health effects of pollutants in outdoor air, it is now recognized that the ill effects of exposure to indoor air pollutants should be of equal concern, because urban residents, for example, spend up to 80% of their time indoors.[91] The major indoor pollutants can reach concentration levels that are significantly higher than those permitted by current National Ambient Air Quality Standards for outdoor levels (Table 29–2). For example, an average NO_2 level of 0.025 to 0.075 ppm is typical in homes with gas stoves, and can reach a peak value of 0.1 to 0.5 ppm with gas stoves or kerosene heaters (0.053 ppm = annual average EPA ambient standard). Carbon monoxide produced by gas ranges and pilot lights, tobacco smoke, and backdrafting of furnace or wood stoves can reach a level higher than 50 ppm. Indoor sources of total respiratory particulates include tobacco smoke, unvented kerosene heaters, wood and coal stoves, and fireplaces. Bars, meeting rooms, and waiting rooms with smoking can have levels of particulates higher than 500 $\mu g/m^3$. Homes with fireplaces can reach a level as high as 1000 $\mu g/m^3$, which is more than three times above the EPA 24-hour standard ambient air level of 265 $\mu g/m^3$ and 12-fold above the EPA annual standard ambient air level of 75 $\mu g/m^3$. Other indoor pollutants include carbon dioxide; formaldehyde fumes from foam insulation, plywood, particle board, carpet backing and fabrics; radon and radon daughters; volatile and semivolatile organic compounds; and asbestos fibers released from insulated pipes, furnaces, and structural beams. As buildings become more fuel-efficient to conserve heat, the turnover rate of the indoor air decreases, raising the levels of many of these indoor pollutants.

TABLE 29–2. National Ambient Air Quality Standards, 1987 Outdoor Concentration Ranges, and Principal Health Effects Attributable to Increased Pollutant Levels

POLLUTANT	PRIMARY STANDARDS*	AVERAGING TIME	CONCENTRATION RANGE†	HEALTH EFFECTS
Ozone	0.12 ppm (235 μg/m³)	1 hour	0.20–0.80 ppm	Decrements in lung function; chronic (?) lung disease
Particulate matter (PM_{10})‡	50 μg/m³ 150 μg/m³	Annual (arithmetic mean) 24 hour	30–80 μg/m³§	Chronic respiratory disease; altered lung function in children
Sulfur oxides (SO_2)	0.03 ppm (80 μg/m³) 0.14 ppm (365 μg/m³)	Annual (arithmetic mean) 24 hour	0.002–0.018 ppm	Exacerbation of asthma
Nitrogen dioxide	0.053 ppm (100 μg/m³)	Annual (arithmetic mean)	0.01–0.04 ppm	Increased respiratory infections; risk of acute lung disease
Carbon monoxide	9 ppm (10 mg/m³) 35 ppm (40 mg/m³)	8 hour 1 hour	3–13 ppm	Aggravation of coronary artery disease

*Primary standard: standard to protect against adverse health effects.

†Fifth to 95th percentiles, values from National Air Quality and Emissions Trend Report, 1987. Research Triangle Park, NC, U.S. EPA, 1989. EPA 450/4-89-001. Data represent range of second-highest concentration.

‡PM_{10}: particulate matter equal to or smaller than 10 μ in diameter.

§Reported as total suspended particulate matter; data not availble for PM_{10}.

Sites of Action and Defense Mechanisms

Atmospheric pollutants exist either in gaseous or particulate form. The penetration and retention of pollutant gases within the lung vary widely and depend on several factors, including the solubility of the gas, its concentration in inspired air, the duration of exposure, and the pattern of flow during breathing. For example, SO_2 is a highly soluble gas and is absorbed quickly and almost entirely in the nose and upper airway of a healthy subject during quiet breathing.[32] The mucosal surfaces of the nasal turbinates act as an efficient "scrubber" of SO_2 and thereby reduce levels at the glottis to less than 2% of the concentration measured at the nose. During exercise, with a more rapid inspiratory flow rate and greater tidal volume, SO_2 reaches the lower airways.

Another factor causing enhanced alveolar deposition of SO_2 is the conversion of nasal breathing to an oral-nasal pattern of breathing during exercise. The smaller surface area of mucosal membranes in the mouth, compared to that of the nasal passages, results in diminished efficiency as a defense mechanism under conditions of increased ventilatory rates during exercise. Exercising asthmatics using oral-nasal breathing instead of nasal breathing have an attenuated bronchoconstrictor response to inhaled SO_2.[12] These findings imply that subjects with diseases causing chronic nasal obstruction might have a greater susceptibility to the adverse effects of soluble pollutant gases. In contrast less-soluble gases, such as ozone and nitrogen dioxide, penetrate deeply into the respiratory tract, even with nasal breathing.

Pollutants in particulate form are usually found in nature as aerosols. These small liquid droplets or solid particles are dispersed in the atmosphere with sufficient stability to remain in an aerial suspension. Common aerosols include sulfuric acid mists, sulfate salts, and nitrate salts. The magnitude of their effect is influenced by the numbers of particles deposited in the lung, their sites of deposition, and their ultimate fate. These factors are in turn largely related to breathing patterns and levels of ventilation, as well as to the significant factor of particle size.

Based on the model of the Task Group on Lung Dynamics, the relationships between particle size and deposition in different lung regions can be calculated.[8] For example, all but a small fraction of particles larger than 10 μ in diameter are trapped in the nasal passages and do not penetrate into the more distal airways. The deposition onto nasal cilia is an efficient mechanism for removing these large particles. Those that are not removed in this way are effectively prevented from reaching the lower airways by retention on the mucosal surfaces of the upper respiratory tract and large airways at their points of bifurcation. Large particles have a high inertia and impact on such surfaces because they cannot change their direction as the airflow abruptly alters its direction in the nose, pharynx, and upper tracheobronchial tree. Particles deposited in this region of the lung are cleared by the mucociliary escalator, assisted by sneezing and coughing. Smaller particles are deposited primarily in the tracheobronchial region of the lung and in the pulmonary parenchyma. Intermediate-sized particles, ranging from 0.5 to 3.0 μ in diameter, are deposited by the force of gravitational sedimentation in more distal airways, where the airflow is slower. In the tracheobronchial tree, the most important defense mechanisms promoting the clearance of inhaled particles are mucociliary clearance and coughing. Mucociliary clearance operates down to the level of the terminal bronchioles. Cough reflexes are particularly effective in clearing particles deposited in the central airways. Particulate pollutants smaller than 2 μ in diameter undergo a constant random motion caused by the impact of the gas molecules surrounding the particles. This results in deposition by diffusion in the small airways and the alveoli. Particles deposited in the alveolar region of the lung are too distal for clearance by mucociliary transport and coughing. In these distal airways, solubilization and phagocytosis by cell scavengers represent the primary clearance mechanisms. The alveolar macrophage is the most active defender, and either digests particles or migrates with them to central areas of the lung, where mucociliary clearance takes place. Other particles ingested by the alveolar macrophage can migrate to the pulmonary interstitium where the clearance half-life is variable; it can be measured in many hours to weeks or even years, depending on the physical and chemical characteristics of the particulate matter.

Health Effects of Air Pollution

A scientific basis for predicting potential adverse side effects from a given level of air pollution rests on evidence obtained from three different types of studies: epidemiologic evaluation of exposed populations, short-term controlled human exposures, and experimental animal studies. Each has its advantages and disadvantages in helping to understand the impact of pollutants on human health.[53]

Epidemiologic Studies

Epidemiologic studies involve assessing relationships between exposure and health effects in large populations. Health effects are usually determined by analyzing questionnaire data and by measuring physiologic parameters, such as forced vital capacity (FVC) or 1-second forced expiratory volume (FEV_1). If adverse effects are unquestionably demonstrated, these types of studies offer strong evidence that a given pollutant causes a known adverse health effect. Unfortunately, inherent methodologic difficulties complicate the interpretation of these studies. A major problem is the lack of reliable studies on exposure levels in large populations. Also, many types of pollutants are found in association with other pollutants in outdoor environments. For example, the levels of atmospheric oxidants such as ozone can be increased concurrently with high levels of SO_2, thus confounding the interpretation of data, which might suggest adverse health effects. In addition, outdoor pollutant levels can change as a result of other factors, such as allergens, dusts, pollens, temperature, and relative humidity. These can all affect pulmonary performance, especially in susceptible populations. Other confounding variables such as age, cigarette use, housing environment, concurrent medical problems, occupation, and individual activity patterns contribute to the difficulty in interpreting questionnaires and physiologic data. Despite these problems, epidemiologic evidence has identified air pollution as a contributor to the aggravation of disease in certain populations. It has limited predictive power, however, in determining which pollutants produce the earliest risk of disease and at what concentrations.

Clinical Studies

Clinical studies involving short-term exposure to pollutants by small groups of subjects enable strict control over the experimental subject and the environment. The limitation of using environmental exposure chambers rests on ethical and practical considerations. The safety of volunteer subjects is of primary concern, so that chronic exposure tests cannot be carried out, and the investigator is limited to studying mild, acute, and reversible health effects. Exposures to pollutants are usually for a short duration, such as a few hours, and at a low concentration level. Only small groups of subjects can be studied, with limited end points, such as acute changes in pulmonary function, clinical blood tests, and other relatively noninvasive measurements. It is difficult to extrapolate findings from short-term to long-term effects. For example, whereas normal subjects might demonstrate no acute physiologic changes after exposure to low levels of NO_2 or ozone, the prediction that similar effects might be seen with chronic exposures cannot be made using this methodology.

Clinical studies are valuable, however, in helping to determine the threshold concentration of an individual pollutant that might cause specific health effects. These studies often look at groups thought to be at high risk from pollutants, such as asthmatics, individuals with COPD, and normal subjects who undergo periods of heavy exercise. Controlled alterations in the study protocol afford valuable insights into the relative sensitivities of different human populations to low levels of air pollution.

Animal Studies

Animal studies also offer methods for determining pathogenic mechanisms of injury following exposure to pollutants. Animal experiments can be performed under a wide range of concentrations and exposure regimens. Many biologic parameters and a wide variety of species can be used. The difficulty in interpreting data from animal exposures lies in extrapolating from animal to human health effects. Differences in respiratory tract morphology, regional deposition of pollution within the lung, and interspecies differences in biologic and physiologic sensitivities to given levels of pollutants contribute to the difficulties of extrapolating to the human model.

SPECIFIC POLLUTANTS

Almost 102 million people in the United States reside in counties that exceeded at least one air quality standard during 1987 (Table 29–3).[71] This summarizes our current understanding of the relationship between exposure to air pollution and respiratory disease. The ranges of responses for both healthy populations and populations with obstructive lung disease are included. Although the pollutants are discussed individually, it should be emphasized that exposure can be difficult to characterize and often involves a mixture of pollutants.

Carbon Monoxide

The results of many studies have provided considerable information about sources of carbon monoxide (CO) [20, 22, 42, 51, 60, 79, 86] and its pathologic effects on normal and diseased humans (Tables 29–4 and 29–5). Approximately 70% of CO detected in ambient air at the many monitoring stations in the United States comes from vehicular exhaust with a bimodal peak corresponding to the morning and evening rush hours. Catalytic converters on motor vehicles decrease CO in the exhaust from 3% to 8% to 0.1% or less,[51] and their increasing use provides a logical explanation for the 30% decrease in ambient CO levels in the past 15 years in many cities.[71] Standards promulgated by the Environmental Protection Agency are designed to keep blood carboxyhemoglobin levels (COHb) in nonsmokers at levels below 2% of the total hemoglobin capacity for O_2 or CO. To attain this goal, no more than a 1-hour level of 35 ppm of CO and an 8-hour level of 9 ppm should be reached once a year. Chronic exposure to 9 ppm

TABLE 29–3. Number of Persons Living in Counties with Air Quality Levels Above the Primary National Ambient Air Quality Standards (NAAQS) in 1987*

POLLUTANT	PERSONS (millions)	TOTAL OF U.S. POPULATION (%)†
Ozone	88.6	36.3
Carbon monoxide	29.4	12.0
Particulate matter (PM_{10})‡	21.5	8.8
Nitrogen dioxide	7.5	3.1
Sulfur dioxide	1.6	0.7
Any NAAQS	101.8	41.7

*Based on 1980 population data from the National Air Quality and Emissions Trend Report, 1987. Research Triangle Park, NC, U.S. EPA, 1989, p. 5. EPA 450/4-89-001.

†Total estimated population in the United States in 1987 was 244 million.

‡PM_{10}: particulate matter with aerodynamic diameter of 10 μ or less.

TABLE 29–4. Representative CO Concentrations in the Environment

SOURCE	CO CONCENTRATION (ppm by volume)
Fresh sea air	0.06–0.5
Hospital air (Sweden)	0.7
Hospital air (Philadelphia)	2±1
Los Angeles weekly averages, 1958	5–15
Smoky English pub	13
Street corner	5–50
Major interchange	50–100
Smoker in enclosed car	90
Alveolar concentration in smokers	
While smoking	300–500
Between cigarettes	15–70*
Automobile exhaust	
No catalytic converter	10,000–80,000
Catalytic converter	1000
Cigarette smoke	20,000–60,000

*Calculated using equations from Coburn and colleagues,[20] assuming alveolar air PCO is in equilibrium with pulmonary capillary blood.

CO in sedentary, healthy subjects would be expected to result in a COHb level of 1.8%.[20]

Because combustion from fires, stoves, and motor vehicles generates CO at concentrations of 1% to 6% (10,000 to 60,000 ppm), acute CO poisoning, in which the COHb level exceeds 15% to 20%, most commonly results from exposure to the products of combustion in an enclosed space, such as a garage, a poorly ventilated vehicular tunnel, the interior of a vehicle with a faulty exhaust system (which leaks into the vehicle), an enclosed space in a building contaminated by CO from fires, or an area with an improperly vented stove or furnace. Cigarettes, cigars and, to a lesser extent, pipe smoking, commonly result in blood COHb levels of 2% to 14%. We believe, and other studies support this, that patients with obstructive lung disease who continue to smoke tend to have higher COHb levels than smokers free of cardiopulmonary disease. Calverley and colleagues[16] reported that 24% of smokers with emphysema or bronchitis attending an afternoon clinic in Edinburgh had COHb levels of 10% or higher, compared to a 3% level in 11,249 men completing a comprehensive health screening examination in London.[102] The physiologic factors that control blood COHb levels can explain this finding. The equations published by Coburn and associates[20] permit calculation of blood COHb levels under steady state conditions. They indicate that the alveolar hypoxia commonly present in patients with severe obstructive lung disease results in increased COHb levels, both from CO inhaled from environmental sources and from that produced in the body as a product of the metabolism of hemoglobin, myoglobin, and other heme proteins.* In addition, the lower diffusing capacity and alveolar ventilation frequently seen in these patients impair the excretion of CO produced by the body and thereby elevate the blood COHb level. Alternatively, different patterns of smoking in patients with chronic obstructive lung disease, such as deeper inhalation and more frequent cigarette consumption, might explain the high levels of blood COHb seen in these patients.

When patients with COPD are suddenly exposed to elevated levels of CO, however, the blood CO level will probably increase less rapidly than in normal subjects, because their diminished diffusing capacity and alveolar ventilation slow the uptake of CO from the lungs into the blood. For example, according to the equations of Coburn and coworkers,[20] a normal resting subject exposed to 400 ppm of CO for 1 hour increases the COHb level from 2% to 13%, whereas a COPD patient, with a 50% reduction in pulmonary diffusing capacity and a 10% reduction in alveolar ventilation, increases the blood COHb to only 9%. Experimental studies have confirmed this effect. Patients with pulmonary emphysema of unspecified severity had a COHb level increase following experimental exposure to 300 ppm of CO for 45 minutes that was 19% lower than that observed in healthy controls.[76]

Adverse Effects

Acute CO poisoning, with blood COHb levels over 30% to 50%, results in secondary hypoxic damage, mainly to the heart

*At equilibrium, the relationship between the partial pressures of O_2 (PO_2) and of CO (PCO) in blood compared to O_2 carried on hemoglobin (O_2Hb) and CO on hemoglobin (COHb) is defined by Haldane's first law:[34]

$$\frac{COHb}{O_2Hb} = M\frac{P_{CO}}{P_{O_2}}$$

where M, the equilibrium constant, has a value of approximately 240. Note that if PO_2 in the capillary blood is reduced, but the environment supplies the same value for PCO, the ratio of PCO to PO_2 rises and COHb in relation to O_2Hb must also increase.

TABLE 29–5. Blood Carboxyhemoglobin (COHb) in Normal and Pathologic States

CONDITION	BLOOD COHb (%)	SOURCE OF DATA (Ref. No.)
Contribution to blood COHb by endogenous catabolism of heme proteins		
Normals	0.4	21
Hemolytic anemia	0.7–3*	20, 21
Nonsmokers	0.9	21
Nonsmokers: 1¼ hours in a smoke-filled room	2.6	42, 79
Cigarette smokers		
Median value	5	102
Upper tenth percentile	8	102
Exercising patients acutely exposed to CO		
Ischemic heart disease—shortening of time of onset of angina	2–5	1, 2, 3
COPD—decreased exercise time	4–12	4, 16
Atherosclerotic peripheral arterial disease—shortening of time of onset of intermittent claudication	3	5
Acute CO poisoning in humans		
Headache	10–30	44
Nausea, vomiting, dimmed vision	20–40	44
Tachypnea, tachycardia, syncope, convulsions, collapse	40–60	44
Depressed heart action, ventilation, respiratory failure, and death	50–80	44

*Calculated using equations from Coburn and associates,[20, 21] assuming normal lung function.

and brain.[44] This is partly because less oxygen is carried on hemoglobin secondary to the formation of COHb. More importantly, tissue hypoxia develops as a result of the shift of the oxygen dissociation curve to the left. This increased avidity for O_2 by hemoglobin means that the capillary Po_2 falls to lower levels before being released to the surrounding tissues. Some authors have also claimed that acute poisoning has a direct toxic effect on the lungs, attributed to the poisoning of mitochondrial respiratory enzymes such as cytochrome oxidase. Rhodes[77] has studied mouse lung slices exposed to 0.25% to 1% CO in air and showed reversible inhibition of O_2 consumption by these tissues. Electron micrographs have shown reduced or absent staining of cytochrome oxidase in the mitochondria, bizarre shapes in mitrochondrial configuration, and cytoplasmic blebs, as well as tissue edema. Chance and colleagues[17] have studied isolated pigeon heart mitochondria rendered anaerobic and found that CO levels as low as 100 ppm slowed in vitro oxidative responses of cytochrome C to a pulse of O_2. They cautioned, however, that a compensatory mechanism called branching and cushioning can diminish this inherently high vulnerability of the cytochrome system to CO poisoning.

Niden and Schulz[72] carried out electron microscopic studies of the lungs of rats who were killed or spontaneously died following exposure to 0.5% to 1% CO. Their blood COHb levels varied from 55% to 70%. Swelling of the mitochondria and endoplasmic reticulum of alveolar epithelial cells, swelling of capillary and alveolar endothelium, and platelet thromboses in the pulmonary capillaries were observed. Although it was acknowledged that all these effects can result from the hypoxia induced by CO poisoning, the severity of the changes was considered to be "out of proportion to an equivalent degree of hypoxemia alone,"[72] so they attributed their findings to a direct effect of carbon monoxide on pulmonary tissues. Fein and coworkers[24] demonstrated essentially identical electron microscopic findings in rabbits exposed to 0.8% CO for 45 minutes, but they also did not carry out control experiments with hypoxia.

To determine whether CO has a direct histotoxic effect on lungs independent of systemic hypoxia, Fisher and associates[27] ventilated the left lung of anesthetized dogs with 8% to 14% CO, 5% CO_2, and 17% O_2 for 15 minutes while temporarily occluding the left pulmonary artery to prevent systemic CO poisoning. They found no change in lung mechanics, diffusing ability, or light or electron microscopic findings when the lung was exposed to 8% to 14% CO. They concluded that the lung damage seen with CO poisoning is a result of impaired oxygen transport by the blood and is not the result of direct histotoxicity of the alveolar CO. Other evidence for possible histotoxic effects of CO comes from visual studies in humans acutely exposed to CO. Abnormalities of visual perception were found to persist long after blood COHb levels returned to normal.[35] These persistent abnormalities, however, are attributable to the continued binding of cytochromes, which have extremely slow dissociation constants for CO,[17] and are eventually reversible. To our knowledge, there are no data indicating damage or impaired function of the lungs from levels of COHb below 15%, a value that is rarely exceeded by heavy smokers.

Effects on Exercise Performance in COPD Patients

Exercising healthy subjects with blood COHb levels of 20% have a reduced oxygen uptake seen only with a heavy workload.[101] Two studies have shown that patients with COPD have decreased exercise tolerance at COHb levels of 4% to 9%. Aronow and colleagues[4] reported that patients with FEV_1 of 48% predicted or 1.5 L reduced their exercise time with increasing workloads on a bicycle ergometer by 33% when blood COHb levels were increased from 1.5% to 4%. Calverley and associates[16] studied 15 patients with FEV_1 of only 0.6 L with a Pao_2 of 51 mm Hg and a Pco_2 of 47 mm Hg. An increase in the blood COHb level from 3% to 12% reduced the distance they could walk in 12 minutes from 694 to 646 m ($p < 0.01$). Both groups attributed their findings to the effects of diminished O_2 delivery to exercising muscles.

Effects On Diseases Commonly Seen in COPD Patients

Cigarette smoking is a risk factor for atherosclerosis as well as COPD; this could explain why many COPD patients have coexisting atherosclerotic coronary artery disease and peripheral vascular disease. Several studies of 10 to 15 patients have claimed that an increase of the blood COHb level from only 1% to 2% or 3% shortens the duration of exercise before the onset of anginal chest pain.[2, 3] Another study of 30 patients with a blood COHb level of 3.8% could not confirm these findings.[83] More recently, a multicenter study of 63 patients essentially confirmed the original findings.[1] An acute increase of the COHb level from 0.6% to 2% or 4% was found, which significantly shortened both the time of onset of angina and ischemic ST changes on the electrocardiogram. In patients with intermittent claudication from atherosclerotic peripheral vascular disease, experimental elevations of the blood COHb level from 1% to 3% decreased the time for onset of leg pain while bicycling from 174 to 144 seconds ($p < 0.001$).[5]

Clarkson[19] has reviewed epidemiologic studies suggesting that environmental exposure to CO increases prevalence as well as death from atherosclerotic coronary artery disease. Cohen and coworkers[22] reported an increase in fatal myocardial infarctions among individuals living in districts with heavy air pollution in Los Angeles during periods of increased ambient CO levels compared to those in less polluted areas. Finnish foundry workers stratified by levels of CO exposure showed a clear dose-response curve between CO exposure and angina pectoris.[37] Clarkson concluded, on the basis of these studies and others, that COHb levels greater than 6% can exacerbate coronary artery atherosclerosis.[19] This interpretation should be regarded with caution, however, because epidemiologic studies are subject to errors from many confounding factors, such as cigarette smoking and choice of control subjects.

Controversy exists about the ability of CO exposure to induce atherosclerosis in humans and experimental animals. Early positive findings in rabbits and monkeys[92, 103] were not confirmed by subsequent studies,[13, 40] but many authorities believe that studies of high-cholesterol diet plus CO exposure in experimental animals, which reported induction of vascular atherosclerosis, are convincing.[6, 19, 94]

In conclusion, patients with COPD tend to have higher blood levels of COHb than healthy subjects with the same endogenous CO production and levels of CO exposure. A blood COHb level of 5% or higher probably reduces exercise tolerance and aggravates angina pectoris. Controversy still exists about the contribution of CO to the development of vascular atherosclerosis. No evidence indicates that CO by itself at the usual levels seen in COPD patients contributes to the development of pulmonary emphysema or other forms of lung injury.

Particulate Matter and Sulfur Oxides

The sulfur dioxide-particulate matter complex is formed mainly as a result of the combustion of sulfur-containing fossil fuels. Because of the complexity of particulate matter and the importance of particle size in determining dose, many terms are used to describe particulate matter. Terms such as suspended particulate matter (PM), total suspended particulates (TSP), and black smoke can be defined by sampling methods whereas others, such as PM_{10}, defined as particulate matter with an aerodynamic diameter of 10 μm or smaller, have both physiologic and sampling components. More sophisticated methods of monitoring further divide TSP into fine particulate matter (particulates <2.5 μm in aerodynamic diameter), sulfates, which are a major component of fine particulates, and hydrogen ion (H^+) concentration, which is presumably the active component of sulfates.

Despite this variable terminology, from a historical perspective a closer relationship exists between industrial pollution caused by elevated TSP levels and excess mortality and morbidity than that caused by other ambient pollutants. The large-scale pollution disasters in the middle of the 20th century in the Meuse Valley in 1930,[26] in London in 1952,[59, 66] and in Donora, Pennsylvania, in 1948[84] probably involved acid aerosols as well as primary pollutants, such as SO_2 and smoke. During the London fog episode of 1952, it was estimated that 4000 extra deaths occurred, primarily among elderly persons and those with pre-existing respiratory disease.[61, 62] More recently, existing data for daily mortality during nine winters in London, from 1963 to 1972, were re-examined.[93] The strongest correlations were observed between daily mortality and sulfuric acid (H_2SO_4) levels of the prior day. The offending agent in the large-scale pollution episodes was probably the acidity of particles in the stagnating air mass. Kitagawa[43] identified H_2SO_4 as the probable causative agent of approximately 600 cases of respiratory disease, including chronic bronchitis and asthma, in the Yokkaichi area of central Japan between 1960 and 1969. The average concentration of sulfur trioxide in a village near a titanium dioxide plant was 130 μg/m³, equivalent to a sulfuric acid concentration of 159 μg/m³. With the installation of control measures in 1967, the number of new cases of respiratory disease gradually declined. More recently, a consistent association was found among hospital admissions for respiratory disease in Southern Ontario and daily levels of sulfates, ozone, and temperature.[9] The respiratory effects, however, might not be attributable to ozone or sulfates, but rather some unmeasured species (H_2SO_4 being the prime candidate) or some pattern of sequential or cumulative exposures. These mortality and morbidity studies re-emphasize the difficulty in attributing adverse health effects to specific pollutants when populations are usually exposed to mixtures of pollutants.

An alternative epidemiologic approach involves examining differences in the prevalence of chronic respiratory symptoms or respiratory illnesses among communities with differing pollution levels. The ongoing Harvard Study of Air Pollution and Health in six eastern and midwestern U.S. cities (the Six Cities Study) has demonstrated important links between particulate exposure and respiratory diseases in children.[87] Sulfate levels were related to frequency of chronic cough, bronchitis, and other respiratory illnesses in young children, but not to decrements in pulmonary function.[104] Findings from four cities of the Harvard Six Cities Study, in which the H^+ concentrations (i.e., acidity rather than sulfate particles) were determined, indicated a better correlation of bronchitis prevalence with H^+ than with particulate matter (smaller than 15 μm).[87] In a four-city study of young adults in Utah, persistent cough and sputum production were related to SO_2 and sulfate levels.[18]

The bulk of the toxicologic data base on acid aerosols examines sulfate particles, primarily submicrometer H_2SO_4. Repeated daily exposures to acid aerosols depositing in the central and peripheral airways can lead to the development and progression of chronic bronchitis.[58] Similar to cigarette smoke, inhalation of acidic aerosols affects the airway primarily by direct irritation. Subacute exposure to acid aerosols in animals results in decreased bronchial mucociliary clearance rates, hypertrophy and hyperplasia of mucous secretory cells in airways, and airway hyper-reactivity. These are findings characteristic of chronic bronchitis and associated with cigarette smoke. For example, histologic examination of rabbits exposed to 250 μg/m³ of a sulfuric acid mist for 1 hour daily for only 4 weeks revealed increased numbers of secretory cells in distal airways and an increase in epithelial thickness, extending from medium-sized airways to terminal bronchioles.[82] Thus, the earliest stages of the effect of acidic aerosol exposure can be a change in secretory cell proportions in the airways, followed by thickening of the epithelium, which might initiate events in a pathogenic sequence leading to the development of chronic bronchitis.

In controlled clinical studies of normal humans, minimal changes in lung function were observed after acute exposure to an H_2SO_4 aerosol[97] up to 1000 μg/m³ or to SO_2 up to 2.0 ppm,[31] concentrations that far exceed high ambient levels. It appears, however, that asthmatics represent a "susceptible" subgroup responsive to the effects of SO_2 and H_2SO_4, at concentrations that have no effect on normal subjects. With both pollutants, exercise during exposure greatly enhances airway constriction, as assessed by measurements of pulmonary function. Exercise not only increases the volume of pollutant inhaled, but also shifts breathing from the nasal to oronasal route. This reduces the uptake of SO_2 and the deposition of sulfate particles in the nose, but increases pollutant delivery to the central airways. Using a moderate level of exercise, with minute ventilation in the range of 40 liters/minute, significantly increases airway resistance in asthmatics breathing SO_2 for 5 to 10 minutes at a concentration of 0.4 to 0.5 ppm.[12, 48] Other factors that have been implicated in potentiating the bronchoconstrictor effects of SO_2 include temperature and relative humidity of the inspired gas, in which dry air potentiates airway reactivity attributed at least in part to its cooling effect; mode of ventilation, in which mouthpiece exposures bypass nasal scrubbing; and total ventilation.[39]

In 1983, Koenig and colleagues[47] identified allergic, adolescent asthmatics as a subgroup responsive to inhalation of 100 μg/m³ H_2SO_4 aerosols delivered for 30 minutes at rest followed by 10 minutes of exercise. Other studies have indicated that exercising, allergic asthmatics develop mild bronchoconstriction by inhaling aerosols of H_2SO_4 at levels below 100 μg/m³.[11, 46] In addition to exercise, factors that modulate the intensity of the bronchoconstrictor response to acid aerosols include aerosol acidity or titratable acidity,[25, 99] particle size, and level of respiratory ammonia.[98] The protective effect of ammonia is attributed to its ability to cause partial neutralization of acid aerosols. Alterations in lung function in asthmatics in response to exposure to 1000 μg/m³ H_2SO_4 aerosols have correlated with the degree of airway constriction induced by inhalation of the parasympathomimetic agent carbachol.[99] If this airway hyper-reactivity is a significant risk factor for obstructive lung disease, then the relationship between changes induced by pharmacologic bronchoconstrictors and inhaled air pollutants might be significant. Although current data are insufficient to allow conclusive relationships, they do raise serious concern that acidic aerosols could account for past associations among particulate air pollution and the exacerbation and development of chronic bronchitis.

Ozone

Ozone, the major component of photochemical smog, represents the most pervasive ambient air pollutant. In 1987, nearly 90,000,000 people in the U.S. resided in counties in which the national ambient air quality standard for ozone was exceeded (Table 29–3).[71] Although considerable information is available about acute effects following a single exposure, current information about chronic health effects of ozone is sparse.

Ozone is a powerful oxidant. It is formed as a result of complex chemical interactions of reactive hydrocarbons with nitrogen oxides in the presence of sunlight. Because of its high reactivity, inhalation of ozone can result in damage to almost all parts of the respiratory tract, depending on concentration. At a relatively low concentration, damage is primarily confined to the junction between the alveoli and conducting airways. Using morphometric techniques, significant changes were observed in alveoli just distal to terminal bronchioles in rats exposed for 12 hours daily for 6 or 12 weeks to 0.12 or 0.25 ppm ozone.[7] Inflammation is another characteristic of exposure to ozone and has been observed in a number of species. Ozone-induced airway hyper-responsiveness in dogs is associated with an influx of neutrophils in airway epithelium[38] and hyper-responsiveness is diminished by prior neutrophil depletion.[73] Continuous exposure to ozone (0.50 ppm) unfavorably alters the course of influenza viral infection in mice.[41] Furthermore, repeated, intermittent exposure of monkeys to ozone concentrations as low as 0.25 ppm for 8 hours daily, 5 days weekly, on alternate months for 18 months resulted in increased lung collagen content.[95] The major limitation of the extensive information on the influence of inhaled ozone on infectivity, damage to lung cells, or development of chronic lung disease is that it involves inherent uncertainties in extrapolating from animal effects to possible effects in humans.

Although animals chronically exposed to ozone show evidence of pulmonary fibrosis and accelerated loss of lung function, epidemiologic studies examining these problems have so far been inconclusive. The results of one epidemiologic study of populations living in southern California in communities with high levels of oxidants suggested an accelerated rate of loss of lung function over a 5-year period.[23] These long-term population studies, however, often suffer from inadequate characterization of exposure, as well as from other potential confounding factors (detailed subsequently, in the discussion of oxides of nitrogen). In contrast, the so-called "field studies," evaluating natural populations acutely exposed to air pollutants, have provided more definitive information on characterizing ozone effects. Studies of children attending summer camps[89] and of adults exercising outdoors[90] showed decrements in lung function at or even below the level of the ozone standard. In these studies ozone levels were well characterized and correlated with changes of lung function on repeated measurements.

Findings from field studies of children's camps have been largely confirmed in human clinical studies. Inhalation of 0.12 ppm ozone for 6.6 hours with high levels of exercise resulted in progressive decrements in lung function in ten healthy adults.[29] At the end of the study, the decrease in FVC averaged 400 ml and the decrease in FEV_1 averaged 540 ml. In addition, acute exposure to ozone at or slightly above the standard was found to induce respiratory symptoms, including cough and chest discomfort, enhanced airway reactivity, changed airway permeability measured by clearance of inhaled technetium-99m–labelled diethylenetriaminepentoacetate (^{99m}Tc-DTPA), and altered performance by athletes.[57] Inflammatory and biochemical changes in the airways have also occurred following ozone exposure, similar to findings from animal studies. Koren and associates[49] found almost a ten-fold increase in neutrophils in bronchoalveolar lavage fluid 18 hours after a 2-hour exposure to 0.4 ppm ozone. In addition, the fluid had a two-fold increase in protein, albumin, and IgG levels. These findings indicate increased epithelial permeability. Markers of increased fibrogenic activity were also detected. Evidence of an inflammatory response has been observed in lavage fluid from subjects exposed to 0.1 ppm ozone for 6.6 hours.[50]

The progressive decrements in pulmonary mechanics during exposure, accompanied by persistent biochemical changes many hours after cessation of exposure, indicate the potential for the development of chronic effects from repeated inhalation. Other aspects of ozone exposure include the proposed mechanisms underlying the progressive decrements in forced vital capacity, the mechanism of reduced responses after repeated ozone exposures called "tolerances," and effects of ozone on the clearance of particles and fibers. These topics are beyond the scope of this chapter, but have been comprehensively reviewed by Lippmann.[57]

Given that ozone can cause airway inflammation, alter airway permeability, and produce heightened airway responsiveness, exacerbations of asthma and COPD with exposures to ozone might be predicted. Despite some epidemiologic evidence suggesting worsening of asthmatic symptoms with high ozone levels,[14] however, functional responses to ozone are typically no higher among asthmatics[45] and patients with COPD.[54] The lack of more definitive information on the chronic effects of exposure to ambient levels of ozone on humans is a serious problem. Carefully performed epidemiologic studies on the relationship of ozone exposure to accelerated aging of the lung and to the exacerbation of obstructive airway disease need to be carried out. If a further reduction of ambient ozone levels is advocated based on adverse health effects, it will be extraordinarily expensive and must be well justified.

Nitrogen Dioxide

Nitrogen dioxide (NO_2) is an oxidant gas that contaminates ambient air in many urban and industrial locations and indoor air in homes with appliances, such as gas stoves, that burn fossil fuels. Oxidant injury has been postulated to be the principal mechanism through which NO_2 damages the lung.[70] At high concentrations NO_2 causes fatal pulmonary edema and bronchopneumonia in humans and animals. Lower concentrations are associated with bronchitis, bronchiolitis, and pneumonia.[68] Sustained lower level exposure of animals is associated with emphysematous enlargements of the terminal air spaces.[74] In experimental animals, NO_2 reduces the efficacy of several lung defense mechanisms. It reduces lung clearance of inhaled bacteria and viruses and increases the mortality of experimental animals.[68] Gardner and coworkers[33] have demonstrated similar effects from the inhalation of NO_2 at levels near the ambient range of 0.50 ppm for several days, and suggested that concentration has a greater effect on susceptibility to respiratory infection than duration of exposure. The deposition of NO_2 throughout the lung, with the potential for injuring large and small airways and the effects on lung defense mechanisms, suggests diverse human health effects.[81]

Early epidemiologic studies focused on adverse respiratory effects from exposure to ambient NO_2.[85] Few of the studies directed at NO_2 exposure from ambient sources involved populations exposed primarily to NO_2.[81] Studies conducted during the 1970s revealed that indoor sources of combustion add NO_2 to indoor air, so that the NO_2 level in these homes often exceeds the outdoor concentration.[28, 64] In more recent investigations, exposure to NO_2 has been classified on the basis of the presence of a gas stove or other gas appliance in the home. For example, a major U.S. study involved children ranging in age from 6 to 10 years in six cities.[87] Children living in homes that used gas for cooking had significantly more serious respiratory illnesses before 2 years of age. In the initial analysis of this data, investigators observed average reductions of 16 and 18 ml in the FEV_1 and FVC, respectively, in children from homes with gas stoves compared to children from homes with electric stoves.[52] On expansion of the cohorts and with further adjustments for confounders, however, the relationships for respiratory illnesses and pulmonary function were found to be weaker and not statistically significant.[80] A series of studies of school children in the United Kingdom has shown a weak relationship between respiratory illness reported by the mother and the use of gas for cooking at home. There was some evidence of a relationship among the incidence of respiratory symptoms and NO_2 levels in bedrooms and living rooms but, after correcting for confounders, the association was no longer statistically significant.[28] Other studies examining the frequency of respiratory illness during the first year of life have shown variable effects of the use of appliances that burn gas.[63, 65]

Few epidemiologic studies have examined exposure to NO_2 and exacerbations of asthma or COPD. Lebowitz and colleagues[52] studied acute effects from the use of gas stoves in subjects with and without asthma, allergies, and airway obstruction. Their analysis indicated adverse effects of NO_2 on symptoms and peak flow in asthmatics, but not in normal subjects. Ussetti and associates[96] have linked asthma episodes in Barcelona with environmental and climatic factors. Although significant associations were not established with the analyzed pollution factors, the investigators reasoned that several findings from the episodic outbreaks suggested that environmental pollutants affected the incidence of asthmatic attacks, especially the high levels of NO_x. Oxides of nitrogen reached a peak of 0.5 ppm between 9 and 10 am, and asthma visits to the emergency room peaked at 10 am. However, more recent studies have linked outbreaks of asthma in Barcelona with inhalation of soybean dust released during the unloading of soybeans at the city harbor.[2a]

The overall impression provided by the epidemiologic studies is that the use of gas for cooking might have a small effect on the respiratory tracts of children and asthmatics. An increased incidence of respiratory illnesses during childhood predisposes to the development of chronic respiratory disease in adults.[36] Estimates of risk for acute or chronic respiratory disease from indoor or outdoor NO_2 exposure remain controversial. Samet and coworkers[80] have reviewed the methodologic limitations of the epidemiologic investigations of exposure to NO_2 and concluded that misclassification of exposure, inadequate sample size, and misclassification of disease outcome accounted in part for the lack of definitive findings.

Controlled clinical studies examining the effects of NO_2 on lung function have largely focused on populations with underlying obstructive lung disease because of their presumed increased risk from pollutant exposure. At levels below 1.5 to 2.0 ppm NO_2, no effects on lung function or enhanced responsiveness to bronchoconstrictors have been detected.[69] Other controlled clinical studies of NO_2 in the range of 0.1 to 4.0 ppm have obtained mixed and occasionally conflicting results concerning effects in asthmatics. Exposure to 0.30 ppm NO_2 with intermittent exercise demonstrated significant decrements in forced expiratory flow rates after exercise, but not after a sedentary exposure.[10, 78] Furthermore, after a 1-hour recovery period, airway function returned to baseline and rechallenge with isocapneic cold air hyperventilation elicited increased airway reactivity in the asthmatics exposed to NO_2.[10] Enhanced reactivity to aerosolized histamine and methacholine has been found in nonexercising asthmatics breathing 0.50 ppm NO_2 for 60 minutes or less.[15, 67] Despite evidence for the effects of low-level NO_2 on the lung function of asthmatics, there remains considerable controversy because of some inconsistencies in the data. Even using intermittent periods of exercise, no alterations in lung functions or symptoms were detected in mild asthmatics inhaling NO_2 at concentrations as high as 4.0 ppm.[56] The reason for inconsistent findings is most readily explained by differences in selecting the asthmatic subjects, including obstructed versus nonobstructed asthmatics, varying requirements for medication, differences in experimental protocols, such as exposure through a mouthpiece versus a chamber, and sedentary activity versus exercise. These problems have been reviewed in detail.[81]

Few studies have examined responses to NO_2 by subjects with COPD. No pulmonary effects of NO_2 were detected in patients with COPD after exposure to 0.5, 1.0, and 2.0 ppm for 1-hour periods.[55] However, 4-hour exposure to 0.3 ppm NO_2 with intermittent exercise resulted in progressive decrements in lung function during the exposure and significant decreases in FVC at the end of the 4-hour exposure.[69] It is noteworthy that changes in lung volume were typical of the "restrictive pattern" seen with ozone, and not the obstructive pattern found with inhalation of NO_2 by asthmatics.

Keeping in mind that dosimetric models indicate that exercise increases the uptake of NO_2, primarily in the distal lung, standard pulmonary function tests, most sensitive to large airway function, might be a relatively insensitive means of detecting the earliest responses. The adaptation of new clinical investigative tools, such as bronchoalveolar lavage following pollutant exposure, should permit the application of new approaches using advances in cell biology for understanding the mechanisms of low-level, pollutant-induced effects. For example, alveolar macrophages obtained by bronchoalveolar lavage 3½ hours after a 3-hour continuous exposure to 0.60 ppm NO_2 tend to inactivate influenza virus in vitro less effectively than cells collected after air exposure.[30] These techniques should offer new methods for assessing responses to toxic agents, identifying markers of exposure and injury, and discovering correlations between recurrent exposures to pollutants and the development of chronic lung disease.

Although the relationship between exposure to air pollutants and the development of chronic respiratory disease is complicated, considerable progress has been made, especially in understanding acute effects. In spite of decades of laboratory, clinical, and epidemiologic research, however, the health effects of exposure of humans to pollutants remain incompletely characterized. In 1987, almost 102,000,000 people in the United States were exposed to "dirty air," as defined by the National Ambient Air Quality Standards of the EPA (Table 29–3). The EPA is currently re-evaluating these standards. There might be a further reduction in the ozone standard, a new short-term SO_2 standard, and a listing of acid aerosols as specific pollutants. Such changes would serve to increase the population living in communities classified as not meeting the federal standards.

Finally, it should be recognized that these standards address only single pollutants, and unfortunately most environmental exposures involve multiple pollutants. In considering the issue of responses to mixtures of pollutants, it is important to remember the role of cigarette smoke in producing respiratory disease. Certainly it is the predominant risk factor. To date, the interactive role of cigarette smoke and exposure to pollutants in hastening the development of chronic lung disease has largely been ignored. Such studies seem necessary because, if research dictates more stringent standards to protect the health of millions of people, the cost to society could be billions of dollars annually to achieve compliance with the new standards.

REFERENCES

1. Allred EN, Bleecker ER, Chaitman BR, et al. Short-term effects of carbon monoxide exposure on exercise performance of sub-

jects with coronary artery disease. N Engl J Med 1989; 321:1426–1432.
2. Anderson EW, Andelman RJ, Strauch JM, et al. Effect of low-level carbon monoxide exposure on onset and duration of angina pectoris. Ann Intern Med 1973; 79:46–50.
2a. Anto JM, Sunyer J, Rodriguez-Roisin R, et al. Community outbreaks of asthma associated with inhalation of soybean dust. N Engl J Med 1989; 320:1097–1102.
3. Aronow WS. Aggravation of angina pectoris by two percent carboxyhemoglobin. Am Heart J 1981; 101:154–157.
4. Aronow WS, Ferlinz J, Glauser F. Effect of carbon monoxide on exercise performance in chronic obstructive pulmonary disease. Am J Med 1977; 63:904–908.
5. Aronow WS, Stemmer EA, Isbell MW. Effect of carbon monoxide exposure on intermittent claudication. Circulation 1974; 49:415–417.
6. Astrup P, Kjeldsen K, Wanstrup J. Enhancing influence of carbon monoxide on the development of atheromatosis in cholesterol-fed rabbits. J Atherosclerosis Res 1967; 7:343–354.
7. Barry BE, Miller FJ, Crapo JD. Effects of inhalation of 0.12 and 0.25 ppm ozone on the proximal alveolar region of juvenile and adult rats. Lab Invest 1985; 53:692–704.
8. Bates DV, Fish R, Hatch TE, et al. Task Group on Lung Dynamics: Deposition and retention models for internal dosimetry on the human respiratory tract. Health Phys 1966; 12:173–208.
9. Bates DV, Sizto R. The Ontario Air Pollution Study: Identification of the causative agent. Environ Health Perspect 1989; 79:69–72.
10. Bauer MA, Utell MJ, Morrow PE, et al. Inhalation of 0.30 ppm nitrogen dioxide potentiates exercise-induced bronchospasm in asthmatics. Am Rev Respir Dis 1986; 134:1203–1208.
11. Bauer MA, Utell MJ, Speers DM, et al. Effects of near ambient levels of sulfuric acid aerosol on lung function in exercising subjects with asthma and COPD [abstract]. Am Rev Respir Dis 1988; 137 (Part 2):167.
12. Bethel RA, Erle DJ, Epstein J, et al. Effect of exercise rate and route of inhalation on sulfur dioxide-induced bronchoconstriction in asthmatic subjects. Am Rev Respir Dis 1983; 128:592–596.
13. Bing RJ, Sarma JSM, Weishaar R, et al. Biochemical and histological effects of intermittent carbon monoxide exposure in cynomolgus monkeys (Macaca fascicularis) in relation to atherosclerosis. J Clin Pharmacol 1980; 20:487–499.
14. Boushey HA. Ozone and asthma: In: Utell MJ, Frank R, eds. Susceptibility to Inhaled Pollutants. Philadelphia: American Society for Testing and Materials, 1989, 214–217. ASTM STP 1024.
15. Bylin G, Lindvall T, Rehn T, Sundin B. Effects of short-term exposure to ambient nitrogen dioxide concentrations on human bronchial reactivity and lung function. Eur J Respir Dis 1985; 62:205–217.
16. Calverley PMA, Leggett RJE, Flenley D. Carbon monoxide and exercise tolerance in chronic bronchitis and emphysema. Br Med J 1981; 283:878–880.
17. Chance BC, Erecinska M, Wagner M. Mitochondrial responses to carbon monoxide. Ann NY Acad Sci 1970; 174:193–203.
18. Chapman RS, Calafiore DC, Hasselblad V. Prevalence of persistent cough and phlegm in young adults in relation to long-term ambient sulfur oxide exposure. Am Rev Respir Dis 1985; 132:261–267.
19. Clarkson TB. Evaluation of automotive emissions as risk factors for the development of atherosclerosis and coronary heart disease. In: Watson A, Bates RR, Kennedy D, eds. Air Pollution, The Automobile, and Public Health. Washington, DC: National Academy Press, 1988, 605–629.
20. Coburn RF, Forster RE, Kane PB. Considerations of the physiological variables that determine the blood carboxyhemoglobin concentrations in man. J Clin Invest 1968; 44:1899–1910.
21. Coburn RF, Williams WJ, Kahn SB. Endogenous carbon monoxide production in patients with hemolytic anemia. J Clin Invest 1966; 45:460–468.
22. Cohen SI, Deane M, Goldsmith JR. Carbon monoxide and survival from myocardial infarction. Arch Environ Health 1969; 19:510–517.
23. Detels R, Tashkin DP, Sayre JW, et al. The UCLA population studies of chronic obstructive respiratory disease. Nine lung function changes associated with chronic exposure to photochemical oxidants; a cohort study among neversmokers. Chest 1987; 92:594–603.
24. Fein A, Grossman RF, Jones JG, et al. Carbon monoxide effect on alveolar epithelial permeability. Chest 1980; 78:726–731.
25. Fine JM, Gosdon T, Thomson JE, Sheppard D. The role of titratable acidity in acid aerosol-induced bronchoconstriction. Am Rev Respir Dis 1987; 135:826–830.
26. Firket J. Fog along the Meuse Valley. Trans Faraday Soc 1936; 32:1192–1197.
27. Fisher AB, Hyde RW, Baue AE, et al. Effect of carbon monoxide on function and structure of the lung. J Appl Physiol 1969; 26:4–12.
28. Florey CV, Melia RJ, Chinn S, et al. The relation between respiratory illness in primary school children and the use of gas for cooking. III. Nitrogen dioxide, respiratory illness, and lung function. Int J Epidemiol 1979; 8:347–353.
29. Folinsbee LJ, McDonnell WF, Horstman DH. Pulmonary function and symptom responses after 6.6 hours exposure to 0.12 ppm ozone with moderate exercise. J Air Pollut Control Assoc 1988; 38:28–35.
30. Frampton MW, Ettensohn DB, Smeglin AM, et al. Inactivation of virus and interleukin-1 production by human alveolar macrophages and blood-derived macrophages after *in vitro* exposure to influenza virus [abstract]. Am Rev Respir Dis 1987; 135(Part 2):A208.
31. Frank NR, Ambur MO, Worcester J, Whittenberger JH. Effects of acute controlled exposure to SO_2 on respiratory mechanics in healthy male adults. J Appl Physiol 1962; 17:252–258.
32. Frank NR, Yoder RE, Brain JD, Yokoyama EL. SO_2 [^{35}S-labeled] absorption by the nose and mouth under conditions of varying concentration and flow. Arch Environ Health 1969; 18:315–322.
33. Gardner DE, Miller FJ, Illing JW, Graham JA. Non-respiratory function of the lungs: Host defenses against infection. In: Schneider T, Grant L, eds. Air Pollution by Nitrogen Oxides. New York: Elsevier Scientific Publishing Company, 1982; 401–415.
34. Haldane JBS. The dissociation of oxyhemoglobin in human blood during partial CO poisoning [abstract]. J Physiol 1912; 45:22–24.
35. Halperin MH, McFarland RA, Niven JI, Roughton FJW. The time course of the effects of carbon monoxide on visual thresholds. J Physiol 1959; 146:583–593.
36. Henderson FW, Collier AM. Childhood factors related potentially to respiratory health in adulthood. In: Utell MJ, Frank R, eds. Susceptibility to Inhaled Pollutants. Philadelphia: American Society for Testing and Materials, 1989, 141–147. ASTM STP 1024.
37. Hernberg S, Karava R, Kokela RS, Luoma K. Angina pectoris, ECG findings and blood pressure of foundry workers. Scand J Work Environ Health 1976; 2(Suppl 1):54–63.
37a. Higgins M. Epidemiology of COPD: State of the art. Chest 1986; 85(Suppl):3S–8S.
38. Holtzman MJ, Fabbri LM, O'Byrne PM, et al. Importance of airway inflammation for hyperresponsiveness induced by ozone. Am Rev Respir Dis 1983; 127:686–690.
39. Horstman DH, Folinsbee LJ. Sulfur dioxide-induced bronchoconstriction in asthmatics exposed for short durations under controlled conditions: A selected review. In: Utell MJ, Frank R, eds. Susceptibility to Inhaled Pollutants. Philadelphia: American Society for Testing and Materials, 1989; 195–206. ASTM STP 1024.
40. Hugod C, Hawkins LH, Kjeldsen K, et al. Effect of carbon monoxide exposure on aortic and coronary intimal morphology in the rabbit (a reevaluation). Atherosclerosis 1978; 30:333–342.
41. Jakab GJ. Influenza virus, ozone, and fibrogenesis [abstract]. Am Rev Respir Dis 1988; 137(Part 2):166.
42. Jarvis MJ, Russel RAH, Feyerabend C. Absorption of nicotine and carbon monoxide from passive smoking under natural conditions of exposure. Thorax 1983; 38:829–833.
43. Kitagawa T. Cause analysis of the Yokkaichi asthma episode in Japan. J Air Pollut Control Assoc 1984; 34:743–746.
44. Klaassen CD. Nonmetallic environmental toxicants: Air pollutants, solvents and vapors, and pesticides. In: Gilman AG, Goodman LSA, Rall TW, Murad F, eds. Goodman and Gilman's The Pharmacological Basis of Therapeutics. 7th ed. New York: Macmillan, 1985; 1631–1633.
45. Koenig JQ, Covert DS, Morgan MS. Acute effects of 0.12 ppm ozone or 0.12 ppm nitrogen dioxide on pulmonary function in healthy and asthmatic adolescents. Am Rev Respir Dis 1985; 132:648–651.

46. Koenig JQ, Covert DS, Pierson WE. Effects of inhalation of acidic compounds on pulmonary function in allergic adolescent subjects. Environ Health Perspect 1989; 79:173–178.
47. Koenig JQ, Pierson WE, Horike M. The effects of inhaled sulfuric acid on pulmonary function in adolescent asthmatics. Am Rev Respir Dis 1983; 128:221–225.
48. Koenig JQ, Pierson WE, Horike M, Frank R. Effects of SO_2 plus NaCl aerosol combined with moderate exercise on pulmonary function in asthmatic adolescents. Environ Res 1981; 25:340–348.
49. Koren HS, Devlin RB, Graham DE, et al. Ozone-induced inflammation in the lower airways of human subjects. Am Rev Respir Dis 1989; 139:407–415.
50. Koren HS, Devlin RB, Graham DE, et al. The inflammatory response in human lung exposed to ambient levels of ozone. In: Schneider T, Lee SD, Wolters GJR, Grant LD, eds. Atmospheric Ozone Research and its Policy Implications. Amsterdam: Elsevier, 1989; 745–753.
51. Landers D. Unsuccessful suicide by carbon monoxide: A secondary benefit of emissions control. West J Med 1981; 135:360–363.
52. Lebowitz MD, Holberg CJ, Boyer B, Hayes C. Respiratory symptoms and peak flow associated with indoor and outdoor pollutants in the Southwest. J Air Pollut Control Assoc 1985; 35:1154–1158.
53. Linn WS. Health Effects of Ambient Air Pollution. New York: American Lung Association, 1989, 1–85.
54. Linn WS, Fischer DA, Medway DA, et al. Short-term respiratory effects of 0.12 ppm ozone exposure in volunteers with chronic obstructive pulmonary disease. Am Rev Respir Dis 1982; 125:658–663.
55. Linn WS, Shamoo DA, Spier CE, et al. Controlled exposure of volunteers with chronic obstructive pulmonary disease to nitrogen dioxide. Arch Environ Health 1985; 40:313–317.
56. Linn WS, Solomon JL, Trim SC, et al. Effects of exposure to 4 ppm nitrogen dioxide in healthy and asthmatic volunteers. Arch Environ Health 1985; 40:234–238.
57. Lippmann M. Health effects of ozone: A critical review. J Air Pollut Control Assoc 1989; 39:672–695.
58. Lippmann M, Gearhart JM, Schlesinger RB. Basis for a particle size-selective TLV for sulfuric acid aerosols. Appl Ind Hyg 1987; 2:188–197.
59. Logan WPD. Mortality in London fog incident. Lancet 1953; 1:336–338.
60. Longo LD. The biological effects of carbon monoxide on the pregnant woman, fetus, and newborn infant. Am J Obstet Gynecol 1977; 129:69–103.
61. Martin AE. Mortality and morbidity statistics and air pollution. Proc Soc Med 1964; 57:969–975.
62. Mazumdar S, Schimmel H, Higgins ITT. Relation of daily mortality to air pollution: An analysis of 14 London winters, 1958/1959–1971/1972. Arch Environ Health 1982; 37:213–220.
63. Melia RJW, Florey CV, Altman DS, Swan AV. Association between gas cooking and respiratory disease in children. Br Med J 1977; 2:149–152.
64. Melia RJW, Florey CV, Darby SC, et al. Differences in NO_2 levels in kitchens with gas or electric cookers. Atmos Environ 1978; 12:1379–1381.
65. Melia RJW, Florey CV, Sittampalam Y, Watkins C. The relation between respiratory illness in infants and gas cooking in the UK: A preliminary report. In: Proceedings of the Sixth World Congress on Air Quality 16:209, August 1983. Paris: International Union of Air Pollution Prevention Associations, 1983, 263–269.
66. Ministry of Health. Mortality and morbidity during the London fog of December 1952. London: Her Majesty's Stationery Office, 1954. Reports on Public Health and Medical Subjects No. 95.
67. Mohsenin V. Airway responses to nitrogen dioxide in asthmatic subjects. J Toxicol Environ Health 1987; 22:371–380.
68. Morrow PE. Toxicological data on NO: An overview. J Toxicol Environ Health 1984; 13:205–227.
69. Morrow PE, Utell MJ. Responses of susceptible subpopulations to nitrogen dioxide. Montpelier, VT: Capital City Press, 1989, 1–52. Health Effects Institute, Research Report No. 23.
70. Mustafa MG, Tierney DF. Biochemical and metabolic changes in the lung with oxygen, ozone, and nitrogen dioxide toxicity. Am Rev Respir Dis 1978; 118:1061–1090.
71. National Air Quality and Emissions Trend Report, 1987. Research Triangle Park, NC: United States Environmental Protection Agency, 1989, 51–58. EPA 450/4-89-001.
72. Niden AH, Schulz H. The ultrastructural effects of carbon monoxide inhalation on the rat lung. Virchows Arch Pathol Anat 1965; 339:283–292.
73. O'Byrne PM, Waters EH, Gold BD, et al. Neutrophil depletion inhibits airway hyperresponsiveness induced by ozone exposure. Am Rev Respir Dis 1984; 130:214–219.
74. Pickrell JA, Hahn FF, Rebar AH, et al. Pulmonary effect of exposure to 20 ppm NO_2. Chest 1981; 80:50S–52S.
75. Rall DP. Review of the health effects of sulfur dioxides. Environ Health Perspect 1974; 8:97–121.
76. Ramsey JM. Carbon monoxide, tissue hypoxia, and sensory psychomotor response in hypoxaemic subject. Clin Sci 1972; 42:619–625.
77. Rhodes ML. The effect of carbon monoxide on mitochondrial respiratory enzymes in pulmonary tissue [abstract]. Am Rev Respir Dis 1976; 103:906.
78. Roger LJ, Horstman DH, McDonnell WF, et al. Pulmonary effects in asthmatics exposed to 0.3 ppm NO_2 during repeated exercise [abstract]. Toxicologist 1985; 5:70.
79. Russell MAH, Cole PV, Brown E. Absorption by non-smokers of carbon monoxide from room air polluted by tobacco smoke. Lancet 1973; 1:576–579.
80. Samet JM, Marbury MC, Spengler JD. Health effects and sources of air pollution. Part I. Am Rev Respir Dis 1987; 136:1486–1508.
81. Samet JM, Utell MJ. The risk of nitrogen dioxide: What have we learned from epidemiological and clinical studies? Toxicol Indust Health 1990; 6:247–262.
82. Schlesinger RB, Naumann BD, Chen LC. Physiological and histological alterations in the bronchial mucociliary clearance systems of rabbits following intermittent oral or nasal inhalation of sulfuric acid mist. J Toxicol Environ Health 1983; 12:441–465.
83. Sheps DS, Adams KF Jr, Bromberg PA, et al. Lack of effect of low levels of carboxyhemoglobin on cardiovascular function in patients with ischemic heart disease. Arch Environ Health 1987; 42:108–116.
84. Shrenk HH, Heimann H, Clayton GD, et al. Air pollution in Donora, PA: Epidemiology of the unusual smog episode of October 1948. Preliminary report. Washington, DC: Public Health Service, 1949. Publ. Health Bull. 306.
85. Shy CM, Goldsmith JR, Hackney JD, et al. Health effects of air pollution. ATS News 1978; 6:1–63.
86. Sjostrand T. Endogenous formation of carbon monoxide: The CO concentration in the inspired and expired air of hospital patients. Acta Physiol Scand 1951; 22:137–141.
87. Speizer FE. Studies of aerosols in six cities and in a new multi-city investigation. Design issues. Environ Health Perspect 1989; 79:61–67.
88. Speizer FE, Ferris B Jr, Bishop YM, Spengler J. Respiratory disease rates and pulmonary function in children associated with NO_2 exposure. Am Rev Respir Dis 1980; 121:3–10.
89. Spektor DM, Lippmann M, Lioy PJ, et al. Effects of ambient ozone on respiratory function in active normal children. Am Rev Respir Dis 1988; 137:313–320.
90. Sektor DM, Lippmann M, Thurston GD, et al. Effects of ambient ozone on respiratory function in healthy adults exercising outdoors. Am Rev Respir Dis 1988; 138:821–828.
91. Spengler JD, Sexton K. Indoor air pollution: A public health perspective. Science 1983; 221:9–17.
92. Thomsen HK. Carbon monoxide-induced atherosclerosis in primates. An electron-microscopic study on the coronary arteries of Macaca irus monkeys. Atherosclerosis 1974; 20:233–240.
93. Thurston GD, Ito K, Lippmann M, Hayes C. Reexamination of London, England, mortality in relation to exposure to acidic aerosols during 1963–1972 winters. Environ Health Perspect 1989; 79:69–72.
94. Turner DM, Lee PN, Roe FJC, Gough KJ. Atherogenesis in the white carneau pigeon: Further studies of the role of carbon monoxide and dietary cholesterol. Atherosclerosis 1979; 34:407–417.
95. Tyler WS, Tyler NK, Last JA, et al. Comparison of daily and seasonal exposures of young monkeys to ozone. Toxicology 1988; 50:131–144.
96. Ussetti P, Roca J, Agusti AGN, et al. Another asthma outbreak in Barcelona: Role of oxides of nitrogen [letter]. Lancet 1984; 1:156.
97. Utell MJ. Effects of inhaled acid aerosols on lung mechanics:

An analysis of human exposure studies. Environ Health Perspect 1985; 63:39–44.
98. Utell MJ, Mariglio JA, Morrow PE, et al. Effects of inhaled acid aerosols on respiratory function: The role of endogenous ammonia. J Aerosol Med 1989; 2:141–147.
99. Utell MJ, Morrow PE, Speers DM, et al. Airway responses to sulfate and sulfuric acid aerosols in asthmatics: An exposure-response relationship. Am Rev Respir Dis 1983; 128:440–450.
100. Vena JE. Air pollution as a risk factor in lung cancer. Am J Epidemiol 1982; 116:42–56.
101. Vogel JA, Glaser MA. Effect of carbon monoxide on oxygen transport during exercise. J Appl Physiol 1972; 32:234–239.
102. Wald NJ, Idle M, Boreham J, Bailey A. Carbon monoxide in breath in relation to smoking and carboxyhemoglobin levels. Thorax 1981; 36:366–369.
103. Wanstrup J, Kjeldsen K, Astrup P. Acceleration of spontaneous intimal-subintimal changes in rabbit aorta by a prolonged moderate carbon monoxide exposure. Acta Pathol Microbiol Scand 1969; 75:353–362.
104. Ware JH, Ferris BG, Dockery DW, et al. Effects of ambient sulfur oxides and suspended particles on respiratory health of preadolescent children. Am Rev Respir Dis 1986; 133:834–842.

Chapter 30

CHRONIC AIRFLOW LIMITATION AND OCCUPATION

W. K. C. Morgan R. B. Reger

Although the harmful effects of dust on the lungs have been known since the 15th century and even before, it was the observations of Ramazzini in the late 17th and early 18th centuries and of Thackrah[1] and Greenhow[2] in Victorian Britain that called attention to the magnitude of the problem. The increased frequency of lung disease in grinders, textile workers, weavers, tailors, and potters was noted by Thackrah. In a series of monographs and pamphlets, he effectively called the attention of Parliament to the sorry state of health that existed in workers at the time of the Industrial Revolution. Unfortunately, Thackrah died at the early age of 38 and it was left to Greenhow and others to carry on his mission.

The recognition of dust as a hazard in the mid 19th century led to the introduction in Britain and Europe of attempts to control its effects through the application of industrial hygiene measures. In the U.S., a comparable program did not come into existence until the pioneering efforts of Alice Hamilton in the first two decades of this century. In her autobiography, *Exploring the Dangerous Trades,* she describes the Fourth International Congress on Occupational Accidents and Diseases that took place in Brussels in 1910.[3] Her chagrin and disappointment at the absence of a U.S. program for the control of occupational disease, especially when compared with those of the various European nations, brought the deficiencies to the attention of legislators and the public and to some extent helped eliminate the complacency of U.S. industry. To use her words, "It (the Congress) was not an occasion for national pride." In 1914, as a result of her proselytizing, the U.S. Public Health Service set up the Office of Industrial Hygiene and Sanitation. The efforts of this office were to prove the stimulus for the development of a program for the prevention of occupationally related diseases in the U.S.

It is now clear that the so-called dust-induced diseases that were referred to as grinders' rot, miners' phthisis, and bronchitis, among other names, included a number of distinct diseases that it is now possible to diagnose with certainty. Not all were a consequence of the inhalation of dust. Included among them were tuberculosis, emphysema, bronchitis, silicosis, coalworkers' and other pneumoconioses, and lung cancer. It was not until the turn of the 20th century that the discovery of x-rays and their application to the diagnosis of disease along with advances in bacteriology, pathology, and epidemiology made it possible to separate with any precision the various diseases and conditions mentioned. Much of what is now known about the relationship of airways obstruction to occupation has come about through detailed studies of specific diseases affecting certain workers, viz., coalworkers' pneumoconiosis (CWP), silicosis, asbestosis, and byssinosis.

DUST, RESPIRATORY DISEASE, AND OCCUPATION

Occupational exposure may lead to a number of conditions or diseases, including cancer of the lung, other respiratory malignancies such as mesothelioma and nasal cancer, various parenchymal lung diseases, i.e., the pneumoconioses, and a group of conditions affecting the airways and characterized by chronic airflow limitation. The last includes occupational asthma, chronic bronchitis, and emphysema. Occupational asthma is not discussed in this chapter because it is a separate and distinct condition with a different pathogenesis from those conditions causing occupational nonallergic airways obstruction.

The Pneumoconioses

The early investigations of CWP and silicosis showed that workers with these conditions often had cough and sputum, with a lesser number affected by shortness of breath.[1, 2] Formerly the presence of cough and sputum and shortness of breath in a coal miner or slate worker was usually diagnosed as miner's phthisis or silicosis. Subsequent epidemiologic studies have shown that cough and sputum occur in the absence of pneumoconiosis, and their presence indicates bronchitis. Those occupations associated with prolonged exposure to either coal mine dust or silica were observed to be associated with a decreased life expectancy and an increased standardized mortality ratio (SMR) for respiratory diseases, and in particular, in the case of silicosis, an increased frequency of tuberculosis.[4–7] The precise contributions of pneumoconiosis, tuberculosis, emphysema, and bronchitis to the decreased longevity have been delineated in the last four decades.

It became clear as a result of the investigations carried out in South Wales by the Pneumoconiosis Research Unit of the Medical Research Council and by Gough and Heppleston at the National University of Wales Medical School that CWP existed in two forms, simple and complicated.[8–10] The former was recognized by the extent and profusion of small opacities in the chest radiograph and came to be grouped or graded into categories 1, 2, and 3 according to the profusion of such opacities. The presence of a large opacity or opacities on a background of simple pneumoconiosis is known as complicated pneumoconiosis or progressive massive fibrosis.

Later studies of the pathology of the lungs of coal miners showed that radiographic category was related to the weight of coal mine dust that had been deposited and retained in the lungs.[11–13] A similar relationship was found in subjects exposed to silica dust.[13, 14] Because the lungs of subjects with the higher radiographic categories had been shown to contain more dust, it was assumed that the higher categories of CWP and silicosis would be associated with a decrease in lung function and that magnitude of the decrement would also be related to increasing radiographic category. This did not prove to be the case, and miners with simple CWP showed no decrease in ventilatory capacity with the increasing category of pneumoconiosis.[8, 15–17] In contrast, complicated disease was associated with both restrictive and obstructive impairment and the size of the large opacities proved to be a rough indicator of the degree of impairment present.[18]

Epidemiologic studies using standard tests of ventilatory capacity, such as the forced vital capacity (FVC) and the forced expiratory volume in 1 second (FEV_1), have shown that the ventilatory capacity of coal and gold miners is unaffected by simple CWP and silicosis, but complicated CWP and complicated silicosis both produce a significant reduction of the FVC and FEV_1.[17–19] Thus the lung function of coal miners with clear chest radiographs does not differ from that of miners with simple CWP. This, however, is not the whole story, and studies comparing coal miners with similar groups of non-dust–exposed workers of the same socioeconomic status revealed that coal miners had a greater prevalence of cough and sputum than did the reference groups.[22, 23] Moreover, the ventilatory capacity of the coal miners tended to be somewhat less than that of the nonminers, and this was equally true of those miners with a normal chest radiograph.[23] Two possible explanations for the decreased ventilatory capacity in coal miners come to mind: (1) coal miners have a form of dust-induced airways obstruction that is independent of radiographic category; and (2) differential migration explains the lower ventilatory capacity observed in the dusty trades, and in particular in coal miners. Thus, were the fittest and youngest men to leave coal mining in the first 2 or 3 years of employment or before, those who remain would be less fit and would be more likely to have a lower ventilatory capacity. Such a situation would be likely to be extant when the industry was undergoing difficult times.

The second hypothesis will be considered first. Cochrane and coworkers[24] and others have suggested that when employment is high, the fittest and youngest tend to migrate and seek employment in another industry. For the past 30 years, however, there has been little evidence in either Britain or the U.S. to indicate that this situation was operative. Moreover, a study by McClintock[25] of new entrants into the British coal mines indicated that those who were less muscular, and by implication less fit, tended to leave coal mining first. In addition, he showed that the early leavers had more symptoms of all kinds. By the same token, it has been noted that miners with radiographic evidence of category 3, simple pneumoconiosis, often have a higher ventilatory capacity than do those in the lower categories, a phenomenon that is probably related to the healthy worker effect.[17, 18]

Turning to the first hypothesis, namely, that there is a form of occupationally related industrial lung disease that causes obstruction, then such obstruction could be accounted for by bronchitis, emphysema, or both conditions. This hypothesis will be considered in detail subsequently.

Bronchitis and Emphysema

It is now evident that, although bronchitis and emphysema are both related to cigarette smoking, they are distinct entities. Thus, the studies of Fletcher and Peto[26] and those of Bates[27] have shown that, while bronchitis and airways obstruction may result from cigarette smoking, they are separate responses to the same insult and have entirely different physiologic and pathologic effects. Moreover, bronchitis does not portend the development of disabling airways obstruction.

Subjects who have smoked more than half a pack of cigarettes a day for 5 years or more usually will admit to a smoker's cough, and bronchial biopsy will often show mucous gland hypertrophy and an increased Reid index.[28] Similar changes may be observed in nonsmoking subjects exposed to long-term high levels of gaseous pollutants and to dust.[29–31] The other response seen in cigarette smokers affects the smaller airways, namely those distal to the eleventh generation. This response is characterized by inflammatory changes in the form of bronchiolitis and by the development of irreversible airways obstruction and emphysema. Although bronchitis affects the majority of subjects who have smoked for any length of time, irreversible obstruction and associated significant emphysema occur in only 13% to 15% of cigarette smokers.[26] The more cigarettes the subject smokes, the more likely he or she is to develop emphysema with an increased rate of decline of respiratory function. Nonetheless, some long-term smokers of more than a pack a day never develop significant or disabling, irreversible obstruction or emphysema. Moreover, whereas chronic bronchitis, whether induced by cigarette smoke or by any other agent, tends to improve when the insult has been removed, the same cannot be said of emphysema, because the latter by definition indicates destruction of the alveolocapillary surface. It is also apparent that minor degrees of emphysema may be present in the lungs in the absence of detectable airways obstruction and that chronic airflow limitation can only be detected when at least 15% to 20% of the lungs is involved by emphysema. The severity of the emphysematous changes present and their relationship to cigarette smoking are far from predictable, as is evident from the work of Ryder and colleagues.[32] This study shows that although there is a general relationship between the severity of emphysema and cigarette smoking, the relationship is markedly skewed and is in the main unpredictable. Thus, some subjects smoke heavily for many years and yet develop either limited or no emphysema.

Emphysema, Airways Obstruction, and Dust Exposure

For the last 30 to 40 years, it has been apparent that the long-term inhalation of a variety of nonspecific dusts can induce focal emphysema. Such observations have been made in urban dwellers exposed to soot and in those exposed to nonfibrogenic dusts, such as stannic oxide.[33, 34] The anthracotic pigment from air pollution and other dusts is deposited in the alveoli but is taken up by macrophages and subsequently transported and deposited around the wall of the second division of the respiratory bronchiole at a centrilobular site. This condition, termed "focal dust emphysema," is seen par excellence in the lungs of coal miners.[9, 10, 33] A more detailed description of its pathogenesis follows.

After coal dust is deposited in the alveoli, it is phagocytized by macrophages and carried away from the alveoli and toward the respiratory bronchioles.[9, 34] Should exposure be intense and prolonged, small aggregations of dust start to accumulate around the lobular pulmonary arterioles and veins. Whereas some dust is deposited in pulmonary lymphoid tissue, most is conveyed to the regional lymph nodes. After some time, aggregations of dust begin to accumulate around the first and second divisions of the respiratory bronchiole and when they reach a certain size appear in macrosections as small black dots that are referred to as macules. The macule initially has little in the way of fibrosis, but has a large amount of dust. Over time, however, a little reticulin and later some collagenous fibrosis may develop. The macule enlarges, and as this occurs, the smooth muscle in the bronchial wall atrophies. The bronchiole, being subject to the normal stresses and strains acting on the lung, starts to dilate. As time goes by, the dilatation of the bronchiole becomes apparent and can be located in the center of the macule. This condition is usually referred to as focal emphysema. Unlike with the centrilobular emphysema that is seen in cigarette smokers, there is no associated bronchiolitis.[33]

The characteristic sequence of events leading to focal emphysema in coal miners was described many years previously. In 1968, Gough[33] wrote,

> In the young coal miner with short exposure to dust, dying of accident or of nonpulmonary disease, there is an accumulation of coal dust specifically related to the terminal and respiratory bronchioles. The lungs can evidently withstand this deposition without harm for some years. Emphysema then develops and in miners who have been exposed for 20 years, some degree of dilatation of the proximal orders of the respiratory bronchioles is usual and may be marked. After 40 years of exposure, the majority of miners show focal dust emphysema, although there is a surprising range in the quantity of dust deposited and the degree of emphysema in miners working under similar conditions.[33]

Ruckley and colleagues[35] related cumulative lifetime exposure to respirable mine dust to the presence of emphysema as determined at post-mortem. These investigators claimed that their study was the first demonstration of the relationship among centriacinar emphysema, exposure to coal dust in life, and the post-mortem quantification of emphysema. Nonetheless, such an assertion should be accepted with a modicum of skepticism in view of Gough's observations and the fact that a clear-cut relationship had been demonstrated many years previously among the coal content of the lungs, the extent of focal emphysema present at post-mortem, and radiographic evidence of pneumoconiosis during life.

Over the past 20 years, a series of papers from South Wales has put forward the thesis that coal miners have a greater prevalence of emphysema than do nonminers, and they go on to maintain that its presence is associated with airways obstruction.[36–39] The basis for their contention, that is, that the decreased ventilatory capacity of coal miners is a result of occupation, depended on relating the severity and extent of emphysema found at post-mortem with antemortem measurements of lung function that had been made in the last few years of the miner's life. Ryder and colleagues[36] claimed to have shown a correlation between the antemortem FEV_1 measurements and the presence of simple and complicated pneumoconiosis. The subjects they examined had all been referred to a pneumoconiosis panel and as a result had undergone a physical examination, chest radiography, and a series of lung function tests. These investigators went so far as to maintain that "there is no reason why these deaths should not provide a true sample of men with this disease," namely CWP. The last statement would imply that this specifically selected sample of subjects was representative of coal miners as a whole, not only from South Wales, but from elsewhere in the world, an assumption that can only be regarded as epidemiologic heresy. The contention that the disability claimants were representative of all miners was challenged by Gilson and Oldham.[40] In their first paper, Ryder and colleagues[36] attempted to relate the presence and extent of the emphysema found at post-mortem to the last radiograph prior to death.[36] In doing so, they made no distinction between simple and complicated CWP. In view of the fact that complicated CWP leads to both restrictive and obstructive impairment in the absence of cigarette smoking, clearly the reduction of the FEV_1 was more likely to be a consequence of complicated CWP than any concomitant emphysema. In the second paper, the investigators still did not exclude subjects with complicated CWP, and they were again criticized by Oldham and Berry.[41] Their paper shows that there was no relationship between the category of simple CWP and the FEV_1, and whereas men with categories 2 and 3 had an FEV_1 of 0.8 L below the predicted value, those with a clear chest radiograph had an FEV_1 that was 1.25 L below the predicted value.[37] Thus, there was no relationship between the coal dust content of the lung and the extent of the ventilatory impairment.

Additional studies relating the prevalence of emphysema in coal miners and nonminers dying of ischemic heart disease have been carried out.[42] Although the lungs were examined without knowledge of the subject's occupation, the appearance of a coal miner's lung invariably provides, even to the neophyte, an instant means of identification. Similarly, although the authors made an attempt to take into account the differences in cigarette smoking in their two groups, the smoking histories were obtained retrospectively, and it is well accepted that smoking histories obtained by panels or agencies that are charged with making decisions concerning compensation tend to be inaccurate and unreliable.[43]

A number of compelling arguments exist that indicate that the presence of focal dust emphysema does not explain the reduced ventilatory capacity noted in coal miners. Thus, it has been clearly established that increasing category of simple CWP is associated with increasing dust deposition in the lungs.[11–13] Moreover, it is equally apparent that with increased dust deposition a concomitant increase in the amount of focal emphysema is present in the lungs.[33, 35] Numerous studies have shown that increasing category of simple CWP is not associated with a fall in ventilatory capacity.[18, 34] Simple CWP, however, has been shown to cause abnormalities of the distribution of inspired gas, some overdistention, and a slight loss of retractive forces.[34] Similarly, in simple CWP the dimensions of the air spaces have been shown to be increased, but the increase was not associated with a decrease in the FEV_1.[44] By the same token, numerous other dust-exposed populations show a decreased ventilatory capacity in the absence of overt pneumoconiosis, and this includes both asbestos miners[45] and hard rock and metal miners exposed to silica particles.[19, 46] It is well recognized that both silica and asbestos exposure lead to the development of stiff lungs rather than to emphysema. Moreover, a well-designed epidemiologic study of U.S. coal miners showed that, although cigarette smoking leads to a loss of lung recoil, no such findings were present in nonsmoking coal miners. However, many bronchitic nonsmokers had significantly decreased flow rates at high lung volumes and symptoms of cough and sputum.[47]

Finally, it must be remembered that the post-mortem demonstration of emphysema bears a poor relationship to antemortem evidence of airways obstruction.[48]

Definition and Pathology of Bronchitis

The term bronchitis was used for many years to imply a condition characterized by cough and sputum, usually associated with a reduction in ventilatory capacity or likely to lead to one. When chronic airflow obstruction was present in a subject and he or she was noted to have cough and sputum plus an overdistended chest with decreased markings, then a diagnosis of chronic bronchitis and emphysema was attached to the patient. This by inference implied that the two diseases were invariably associated and were part and parcel of the same process. Thus, the MRC Committee that was set up by the Ministry of Pensions in Britain in the early 1960s, whose charge it was to examine the role of occupation in the etiology of bronchitis, although accepting the fact that not all subjects with chronic bronchitis demonstrated a decrease in their ventilatory capacity, nevertheless avoided defining bronchitis.[49] The text of their statement suggested that, *faut de mieux,* a relationship between symptoms of cough and sputum and a decreased ventilatory capacity existed, and that although cough and sputum could exist in the absence of any decrement, sooner or later most if not all subjects with chronic bronchitis would go on to develop irreversible chronic airflow limitation.

Subsequently, Fletcher and colleagues[50] suggested classifying bronchitis into simple and obstructive forms with the former characterized by cough and phlegm in the absence of airways obstruction and the latter accompanied by obstruction and emphysema. Nonetheless, it was the acceptance and general use of the MRC definition of chronic bronchitis in terms of symptoms without reference to lung function that made possible an appreciation of the pathophysiology of this condition.[51] Later, the American Thoracic Society accepted the MRC definition.[52] To persist in separating bronchitis into simple and obstructive as some still do serves to obfuscate rather than to clarify.

In humans, the mucous glands of the large airways are mostly responsible for mucus secretion, and in chronic bronchitis they are increased in number and in size. The goblet cells, which are located mainly in the smaller airways, are also increased in number, but the increase is less impressive. The seminal studies of Lynne Reid[28] provided a means of quantifying the extent and severity of any chronic bronchitis present.[28] She noted that the depth of the mucous glands (gland thickness), expressed as a fraction of the depth of the bronchial wall thickness as measured from the surface of the respiratory epithelium to the cartilage in the wall, provided a diagnostic yardstick. In a healthy subject, the ratio of this depth, i.e., glands to bronchial wall, is 25% or less. In subjects with severe chronic bronchitis, the ratio may be 50% or greater.

Mucous gland hypertrophy occurs as a result of exposure to any chronic irritant, be the irritant a particulate, a gas, or a mixture of the two.[53] The heavier and more prolonged the exposure, the greater the likelihood of the subject developing bronchitis, and the more obvious and gross the changes in the bronchial glands. By far the commonest cause of chronic bronchitis is cigarette smoke but, in addition, excellent evidence indicates that dust and other air pollutants, not to mention particulate matter, can all act as inciting factors.[53, 54]

In studies of working populations in which an attempt is being made to study the effects and frequency of bronchitis, two important confounding factors are always present, namely cigarette smoke and age. In smokers, the effects of cigarette smoking far outweigh those of dust and air pollutants. In women, the prevalence of bronchitis tends to be related to educational and social status inversely, and less well related to cigarette smoking and occupational exposure. This results from a reluctance on the part of middle and upper socioeconomic groups of women to admit to the production of sputum.

Bronchitis, Dust Exposure, and Airways Obstruction

Many of the studies that have related dust exposure to the prevalence of chronic bronchitis have been carried out in coal miners. This has come about as a consequence of the fact that coal miners are a well-defined and relatively large group of subjects who tend to stay in the same occupation. Ashford and colleagues[55] showed the prevalence of bronchitis in British coal miners, as determined by cough and sputum, increased with age and it may be assumed, because age and dust exposure are related, with cumulative dust exposure. This observation was subsequently confirmed by Rae and colleagues.[56] Similarly, Kibelstis and colleagues[57] were able to show in U.S. coal miners that cough and sputum were related to dust exposure and also to cigarette smoking. In nonsmoking coal miners there was increasing prevalence of bronchitis from the surface to the coal face, that is to say, from the least dusty to the most dusty jobs. This gradient was demonstrable in virtually all age groups.[57, 58] In smoking miners the effects of dust versus smoking could not be separated, since the effects of cigarette smoking completely overshadowed those of dust. Similar observations have also been reported in Belgian coal miners.[59]

Studies have shown that both cigarette smoke and dust increase bronchial mucous gland dimensions in coal miners.[53] Thus, good pathologic evidence indicates that both dust and cigarette smoke lead to mucus hypersecretion and to an increased prevalence of cough and sputum.

In 1973, Rogan and colleagues[60] demonstrated in British coal miners that ventilatory capacity was inversely related to lifetime cumulative exposure to coal dust. The presence of pneumoconiosis did not lead to an additional decrement of ventilatory capacity above and beyond those decrements due to cumulative dust exposure, smoking habits, and stature. Although smokers showed a more rapid decline in the FEV_1 than did nonsmokers, a cumulative effect of dust exposure was apparent in both smoking and nonsmoking miners. Among nonsmokers, the FEV_1 was generally lower in those subjects who were most dust exposed than it was in the less dust exposed miners, but the rate of decline per year for nonsmokers remained the same from age 30 to 60 in both high- and low-exposure groups. In smoking miners, the rate of decline with age was greater than that for nonsmokers in each exposure category, but in the smoking miners at any given age, the absolute FEV_1 was uniformly lower for the group with the most dust exposure.

Kibelstis and colleagues[57] were able, using surrogate measures of dust exposure, to demonstrate an effect on the ventilatory capacity of nonsmoking miners. These investigators subdivided their cohort according to whether the men worked at the face, on transportation, in miscellaneous other jobs, or on the surface. Prior dust measurements had shown a gradient from the face to the surface, with the lowest exposures occurring on the surface. It was apparent that the FEV_1 of nonsmoking surface workers was higher than that of the nonsmoking face workers. The difference, however, was only 4.3%, but because large numbers were involved it was statistically significant. In contrast, the difference in the FEV_1 between the smoking and nonsmoking face workers was 6% and the difference between the smoking surface workers and the nonsmoking surface workers was 10.6%. The effects of cigarette smoking were, therefore, substantially greater than those of dust exposure. Airways obstruction was three times more common in smokers than in nonsmokers.

An extensive West German study of nearly 7000 workers employed in a variety of dusty trades related symptoms and lung function to dust exposure, smoking habits, and other factors. This study showed that the most important factors related to the prevalence of bronchitis and airways obstruction were age and smoking habits.[61] In younger workers, there was an additive effect of smoking, age, and dust with the combined effect of all three equalling the sum of their separate effects. Thus, it is clear from these studies that increasing dust exposure is associated with a small decrement in ventilatory capacity.

At a later date, Hankinson and coworkers[47] characterized the physiologic impairments that are associated with the inhalation of dust and cigarette smoke. They studied the same 9000 working coal miners who had been studied by Kibelstis and colleagues.[57] The ventilatory capacity had been assessed with flow volume curves, but in addition lung volumes were calculated by a radiologic method using posteroanterior and lateral chest films. From a knowledge of the total lung capacity (TLC) it was possible to express flow rates, not only as a percentage of vital capacity, but also at absolute lung volumes. Four age- and height-matched groups were selected on the basis of the presence of bronchitis and on the basis of whether they were smokers or not. In each group, 428 subjects were included, and all were matched within 1 year of age and 1 centimeter in height. The mean flow volume curves are shown in Figures 30–1 to 30–3. It is apparent that cigarette smoking affects flows at all lung volumes. In nonsmoking bronchitic patients, the dominant effect was on flows at high lung volumes, although there was some reduction in flow rates at lower lung volumes, indicating that the small airways were not entirely spared. When the same flows were expressed at absolute lung volumes, smokers were noted to have an increased residual volume (RV) and an increased TLC. The nonsmoking subjects in contrast had a normal TLC and RV. The increased TLC suggests loss of elastic recoil in the lungs and the presence of subclinical emphysema. Industrial bronchitis was not associated with an increase in TLC.

A study by Kreiss and colleagues[61a] showed that hard rock mining exposures affected smokers and nonsmokers differently. In smokers, flow rates were decreased at all lung volumes and TLC and RV were increased. In nonsmokers, dust exposure was associated with decreased lung volumes and increased flow rates. The investigators further went on to state that their results differed from those of Hankinson and colleagues,[47] who had expressed the opinion that "industrial bronchitis is limited to the large airways." In practice, Hankinson and colleagues showed that, although flows in the large airways were predominantly affected, there was also a reduction in flows in the small airways. The apparent disparities in the findings of the two groups of investigators can be easily reconciled. Kreiss and colleagues[61a] were studying rock miners exposed to silica. Exposure to the latter leads to nodular fibrosis and increased lung stiffness, with a decrease in compliance and lung volumes. The opposite situation prevails in coal miners, and the focal dust emphysema that affects them, especially those with CWP, leads to an increased TLC and an increased RV.[17, 61b]

It is well recognized that maximal expiratory flow rates depend on (1) the elastic recoil of the lung, (2) the frictional resistance of the small airways, and (3) the cross-sectional area of the large airways. Thus, in a dust-exposed population, flow rates are influenced by the effects of both parenchymal and tracheobronchial deposition. Moreover, the lung parenchyma may become either more or less compliant viz. coalworkers' pneumoconiosis versus asbestosis or silicosis. The effects of industrial bronchitis on expiratory flow rates at various lung volumes are therefore going to be influenced significantly by the elastic properties of the lung parenchyma. Nevertheless, the predominant effect of industrial bronchitis is on the large airways, just as it is in cigarette smoke–induced bronchitis.[26] When the dust to which the subject is exposed is likely to have an effect on the mechanical properties of the lungs, the physiologic effects of industrial bronchitis may be dissimulated, and it therefore becomes essential to express the flows at absolute lung volumes.[47, 58]

The series of investigations described here is compelling evidence for the existence of industrial bronchitis. Thus, in summary, it is evident that industrial bronchitis is distinct from pneumoconiosis. In nonsmokers, bronchitis may occur as a response to a variety of agents, including inert dusts, various gases, and vapors, and is characterized by the presence of cough and sputum. The size of the particles responsible for the development of industrial bronchitis is almost certainly somewhat greater than the size of those that are responsible for pneumoconiosis and is predominantly between 3 and 10 microns.[54] Moreover, because such particles are removed by the mucociliary escalator, the subject does not develop an abnormal chest radiograph.

Physiologically, industrial bronchitis leads to decreased flows in the large airways with lesser effects on the small airways. The RV is usually slightly increased.[54] Changes in the mechanical properties of the lung will, however, modify the physiologic effects of industrial bronchitis. Although the decrease in ventilatory capacity that is seen in industrial bronchitis is related to cumulative dust exposure, the fact that the particles responsible for the condition differ in size from those that cause pneumoconiosis explains the poor correlation between respirable dust measurements and the prevalence of bronchitis.[62] There is no evidence that industrial bronchitis leads to emphysema. In addition, the prevalence and incidence of bronchitis are likely to be more closely associated with measurements of total dust and the number of particles, irrespective of size, than with measurements of respirable dust. Whether industrial bronchitis clears up with the cessation of exposure is uncertain, although there is some limited evidence to this effect.

Relative Contributions of Dust and Cigarette Smoke to Decline in Ventilatory Capacity

A number of studies involving serial measurements of lung function have been carried out in coal miners. A few longitudinal studies have also been carried out in subjects exposed to silica. Most studies suggest that the effects of dust are equal to about one quarter those of cigarette smoke.

Love and Miller[63] studied 1677 men from five British collieries (coal mines) for a period of 11 years. The loss of FEV_1 was found to increase with cumulative dust exposure after corrections had been made for age, smoking, and colliery

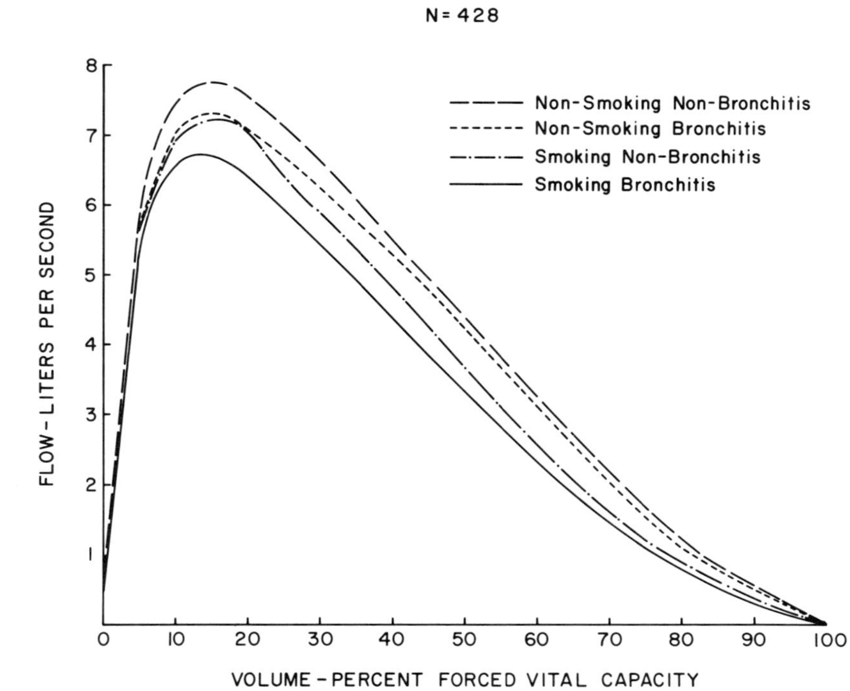

Figure 30–1. Mean flow-volume curves expressed as percentages of forced vital capacity. (Reproduced with permission from Hankinson JL, Reger RB, Morgan WKC. Maximal expiratory flows in coal miners. Am Rev Respir Dis 1977; 116:175.)

effect. Smoking was classified according to whether the subjects were nonsmokers, ex-smokers, or current smokers. Some adjustment was made for the duration and intensity of smoking. The investigators expressed the opinion that if men left the industry because of ill health and respiratory impairment, the average loss of FEV_1 would have been underestimated. There are a number of problems with this study, in particular that there were only 1667 survivors tested out of an original cohort of 6191. The FEV_1 was regressed against age, regular smoking habit, and dust. Smoking was treated as a static, unchanging variable, such as height. Clearly this is not the case. The effects of cigarette smoking increase with the number of pack-years.

A further study by Attfield[64] described his findings in a 9-year follow-up of U.S. coal miners. Again, only 1161 of the original 4139 were included in the analysis. Attfield noted that those who left coal mining tended to be older, showed more evidence of bronchitis and ill health, and were more likely to

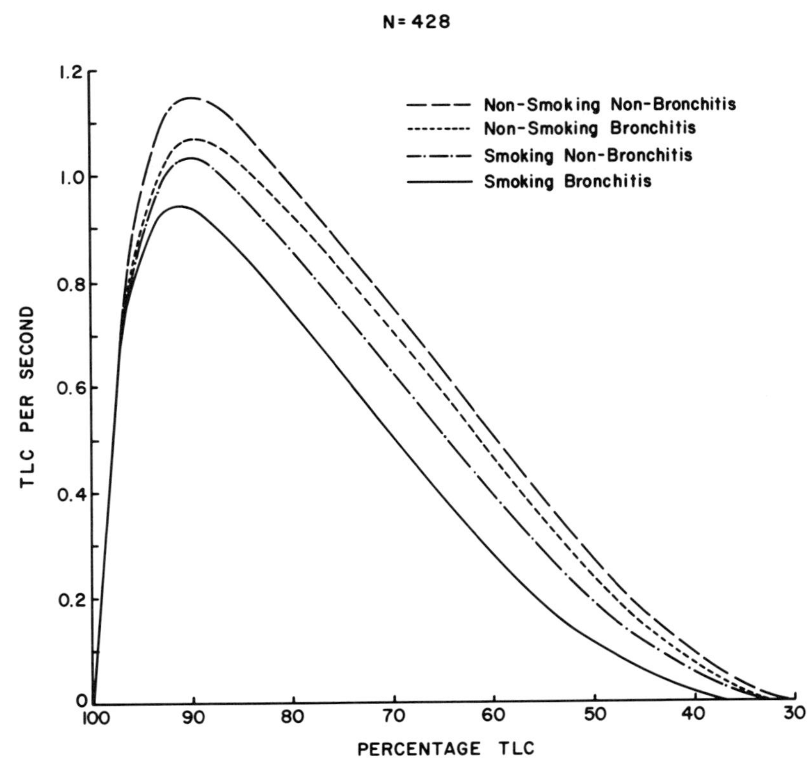

Figure 30–2. Mean flow-volume curves expressed as percentages of total lung capacity. (Reproduced with permission from Hankinson JL, Reger RB, Morgan WKC. Maximal expiratory flows in coal miners. Am Rev Respir Dis 1977; 116:175.)

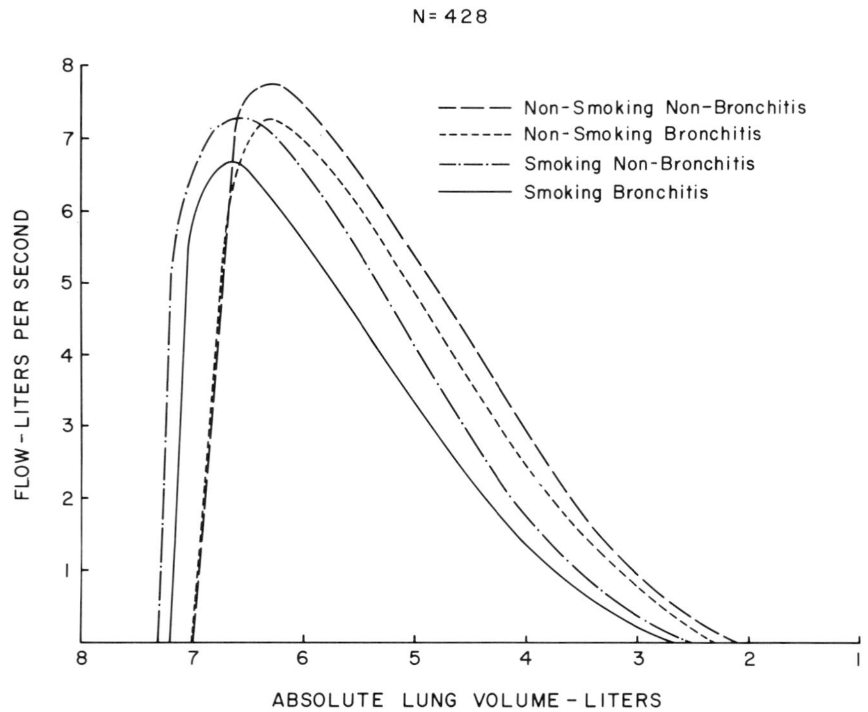

Figure 30–3. Mean flow-volume curves expressed at absolute lung volume. (Reproduced with permission from Hankinson JL, Reger RB, Morgan WKC. Maximal expiratory flows in coal miners. Am Rev Respir Dis 1977; 116:175.)

be smokers. Hence, because much of the difference between those who remained working and those who left could be accounted for by age, Attfield decided to include only those miners between 20 and 49 years of age. This is not acceptable in that the older age groups where the maximal effects of cigarette smoking are apparent were thereby excluded. He found that cigarette smoking had three to four times the effect of coal dust exposure. It is interesting to note, however, that dust exposures in the U.S. were far fewer than they were in Britain despite the relatively similar effects. A further study using the same subjects who had originally been studied by Rae and coworkers[56] and subsequently by Rogan and colleagues[60] has been published.[65] This again purports to show that both the FEV_1 and the forced vital capacity (FVC) are affected by dust and goes on to claim that chronic bronchitis is a potent cause of loss of lung function.

Comparisons made between the mean decrease in FEV_1 induced by cigarette smoking and that induced by dust are likely to lead to fallacious conclusions.[66] Whereas airways obstruction is present in only 12% to 13% of cigarette smokers, bronchitis, as diagnosed by cough and sputum, is present in almost 50% of nonsmoking miners who have worked underground for 20 years or more.[57] It therefore seems probable that Love and Miller and Attfield were comparing a significant and often disabling decrement in ventilatory capacity that affects a minority of smoking miners with a much smaller dust-induced decrement that affects a far greater percentage of nonsmoking miners and that in any individual produces a far lesser effect on the ventilatory capacity. Because only 12% to 15% of cigarette smokers develop airways obstruction,[26] the 11 ml decrease noted by Love and Miller is occurring solely in the susceptible minority, whereas the remaining smokers are unaffected.

Thus, the decrement due to cigarette smoking is much more likely to lead to a severe reduction in ventilatory capacity in some of those affected. This was made evident by Fletcher and colleagues[26] when they pointed out that were the whole population to smoke 20 cigarettes a day, the resultant mean reduction in FEV_1 would be relatively small, because the effects would be skewed, with most subjects showing a normal age-related decline. A minority of these subjects would show substantial but not disabling decrement in excess of that due to age and other factors, whereas a few would show severe loss of ventilatory capacity. This is evident from a study by Ryder and coworkers,[32] which relates emphysema found at post-mortem to age and cigarette smoking. Because more than 20% of the lung needs to be affected by emphysema before abnormal shortness of breath is present, the fact that only 19 of the 106 smokers' lungs that were examined by Ryder and coworkers showed more than 20% involvement renders it abundantly clear that the majority of smokers do not develop significant airways obstruction.

A further problem relates to the healthy worker effect. In general, it is assumed that workers leave their occupation because of exposure to dust or other occupationally related hazards. In reality, when one studies the percentage of nonsmokers, ex-smokers, and smokers in the various age groups who were included in the National Coal Study, it becomes apparent that the older the subjects are, the greater the percentage of nonsmokers and ex-smokers who continue to work. Thus, in the 30 to 39 years of age group, the percentages of nonsmokers, ex-smokers, and current smokers were 20.7%, 18%, and 61%, respectively. Comparable figures for the 50 to 59 years of age group were 31%, 38%, and 39%, respectively.[57] Moreover, Attfield[64] showed a greater attrition of smokers than nonsmokers in his follow-up study. This would imply that the smokers who leave the work force because of premature disability and the smokers who continue to work are likely to be relatively resistant to the effects of cigarette smoking. As such, they show lesser effects from smoking than those who have already dropped out because of pulmonary impairment, lung cancer, or heart disease.

Although there is little doubt that bronchitis is associated with an increased mortality from nonmalignant respiratory disease, providing an attempt is made to control for the effect of the reduced FEV_1 found concomitantly with bronchitis, it becomes evident that cough and sputum alone do not lead to premature death from respiratory disease other than cancer.[68–70] The increased death rate associated with bronchitis is a reflection of cigarette smoking and not an effect of bronchitis per se. Thus, while cigarette smoking causes bronchitis, it is also responsible for the development of cancer of the lung, larynx, and bladder, not to mention emphysema and coronary artery disease. Moreover, the studies of Thurlbeck and colleagues[71, 72] have made it quite clear that although bronchitis produces some symptoms, no correlation seems to exist between pathologic evidence of bronchitis and a decreased FEV_1. This matter is discussed in some detail elsewhere.[32, 67]

Were dust-induced airways obstruction to lead to disabling airways obstruction, one would expect the proportion of miners so affected to develop right ventricular hypertrophy and cor pulmonale. In reality, numerous studies have been made of the right ventricle during life and at post-mortem, and these make it evident that neither cor pulmonale nor right ventricular hypertrophy occurs except in cigarette-smoking coal miners with long-standing airways obstruction and in those with progressive massive fibrosis (PMF).[73–78] Moreover, a later study of a fairly large number of British coal miners showed that right ventricular hypertrophy did not occur in the absence of a history of cigarette smoking or PMF.[79] Finally, the relative importance of cigarette smoking versus dust and other factors in occupational lung disease has been reviewed by Elmes.[80] He concluded that although the control of occupational exposure to coal dust remains important, substantial future improvements in the respiratory health of coal miners can only be achieved by reducing the prevalence of smoking among miners.

Radiographic Opacities, Dust Exposure, and Airways Obstruction

The pneumoconioses are characterized by the presence of certain relatively specific radiographic abnormalities. These have been referred to earlier. In simple pneumoconiosis such opacities are small, being less than 1 cm in diameter, and either regular (rounded) or irregular.[81] Small opacities are subdivided according to their size. Those that are rounded are designated as p, q, or r, and those that are irregular are designated as s, t, or u. Small rounded opacities up to 1.5 mm in diameter are classified as p, opacities between 1.5 mm and 3 mm are classified as q, and r opacities are between 3 mm and 10 mm. Irregular opacities are classified in the same way with s opacities having a width of up to 1.5 mm, t opacities having a width between 1.5 mm and 3 mm, and u opacities having a width between 3 mm and 10 mm. Whereas silicosis, welders' siderosis, and coalworkers' pneumoconiosis are characterized by rounded opacities, asbestosis is recognized by the presence of irregular opacities.

The profusion of rounded opacities is closely related to the dust content of the lungs, be the dust silicon dioxide, coal mine dust, iron dust, or other mineral dusts.[10, 11] In asbestosis, a reasonable relationship also exists between the number of asbestos fibers present in the lungs and the category of asbestosis. With the exception of asbestosis, the significance of irregular opacities in the pneumoconioses is far less certain, and a number of investigations have been carried out over the past 15 or so years to try and identify those factors that lead to the development of irregular opacities in the chest radiographs of dust-exposed workers.

In 1974, Lyons and colleagues[82] carried out a post-mortem study in coal miners and pointed out that there was a positive association among the presence of irregular opacities, emphysema, and impairment of the FEV_1. Unfortunately, this was a post-mortem study and no smoking histories were available. It was, therefore, impossible to decide whether smoking contributed to the presence of emphysema. A further study purported to show that irregular opacities were related to age, smoking, and underground exposure.[83] The subjects studied in this instance were coal miners who were receiving disability benefits and as such could not be regarded as representative of the coal mining population as a whole. Subsequently, Cockroft and colleagues[84] carried out a study in which they related lung function abnormalities in 46 men who had subsequently died but who had been referred to a pneumoconiosis panel while still living for consideration for compensation for work-related disease.[84] Lung function abnormalities and appearance of the chest radiograph in living subjects were related to the presence and severity of emphysema found at death. It was shown that irregular opacities were associated with a reduced diffusing capacity of the lungs for carbon monoxide (DL_{CO}) and TLC, increased emphysema, and to a limited extent an increasing score for the presence of fibrosis quantified post mortem. Although there was a correlation between the TLC and emphysema, it was found that TLC decreased with increasing irregular opacities. The investigators suggested this decline in TLC was related to increasing fibrosis; however, no comparable fall in the FVC and FEV_1 occurred. Clearly a decrease in all three lung volumes should have been present were fibrosis responsible. The study suffered from the major drawback that only two subjects in the series were nonsmokers. Moreover, smoking was not associated with any particular defect in lung function or any specific pathologic finding, observations that indicated that the group was not representative and resulted from biased selection.

A further case control study has been published.[85] The investigators showed a relationship between the presence of irregular opacities and age but no such relationship was evident with smoking. Because they only had one nonsmoker in the coalworkers' cases, this is not surprising. Irregular opacities were also noted in noncoal miners, but the relative risk of such opacities being present was increased in coal miners (relative risk 2.45). The selection of subjects even here, however, was suspect in that there were a greater number of older coal miners than older noncoal miners.

A study relating irregular opacities to dust exposure based on the chest radiographs of 895 British coal miners has been published. Irregular opacities were associated with impairment in respiratory function. The investigators maintain that the deficits in lung function could not be explained by body size and smoking habits. Even so, the prevalence of irregular opacities was nearly twice as great among the smoking miners, with only 39 subjects out of 758 having predominant irregular opacities. Of these, 4 were nonsmokers while the remaining 35 were current or ex-smokers.

The best-designed study aimed at detecting the significance of irregular opacities in coal miners was carried out by Amandus and colleagues.[87] The prevalence of small irregular opacities in the chest radiographs of coal miners was related not only to lung function but to a surrogate measure of dust exposure, i.e., years spent working underground. Their study included 4479 smokers and 1687 nonsmokers, all of whom were then currently employed in coal mining. Subjects with predominantly rounded opacities were excluded from the analysis, even though scanty irregular opacities may have been present in their radiographs. Smoking was associated with the presence of irregular opacities, as were bronchitis, age, and years worked underground. These investigators also demonstrated that the mean FEV_1 and FVC were lower and that the mean RV and TLC were higher among smoking miners with irregular as opposed to rounded opacities. In nonsmoking miners, no matter the type of opacity, whether regular or irregular, no such decrease in ventilatory capacity could be demonstrated.

The vast weight of available evidence indicates that scanty irregular opacities are a not uncommon feature in the radiographs of cigarette smokers no matter their job. The frequency of such opacities increases with age, duration of cigarette smoking, and to a limited extent with dust exposure. Separation of these three confounding variables, although often assumed as relatively easily achieved, proves difficult because of the problem of collinearity. Although certain British investigators have suggested that the presence of irregular opacities in the radiographs of coal miners should be regarded as part and parcel of CWP, this hypothesis is based on a tenuous association that does not take into account the many confounding factors. Thus, virtually all of the British studies have been on cohorts or groups of coal miners, and in most instances, those selected for inclusion were either claiming or had already been awarded compensation.[82–86] Few attempts have been made in Britain to look at the frequency of irregular opacities in other dust-exposed workers, with the notable exception of slate miners[88] and a limited number of kaolin workers.[89] In both slate miners and kaolin workers, irregular opacities were noted to be present and in the former were clearly related to smoking.

In the U.S. it has been suggested that irregular opacities are relatively uncommon in nondust–exposed blue-collar workers.[90] The study on which this opinion was based involved an extraordinarily young working population with a mean age of 33.9 years. As such, the mode of selection would to a large extent exclude the effects of age and cigarette smoking because the frequency of irregular opacities is related both to age and to the duration of smoking. Clearly the inferences and conclusions drawn are questionable in view of the inadequate subject selection. Elsewhere, the presence of irregular opacities has been reported in those exposed to silica;[91] to synthetic mineral fibers;[92] to bauxite;[93] and indeed, it would seem, in the prolonged exposure to most inert dusts, not to mention cigarette smoke alone in the absence of dust exposure.[94]

When such opacities are associated with cigarette smoking, the FEV_1 and FVC are both reduced, although not concordantly, and the RV and TLC are both increased, although not to the same extent.[87, 95] When present in dust-exposed nonsmokers, irregular opacities are seldom associated with detectable impairments of ventilatory capacity, although there are probably some exceptions to this rule.[93] Even in asbestos-exposed populations it is clear that the presence of scanty irregular opacities, i.e., categories 0/1 and 1/0, is more likely these days to be a result of cigarette smoking than the development of early asbestosis.[96,97] With better control of asbestos levels and adoption of the most stringent standards, new cases of asbestosis are not being seen.

The precise pathologic changes that are responsible for the presence of irregular opacities in the chest radiograph remain a mystery. The problem is well reviewed by Weiss,[97] who points out that both animal studies and cross-sectional human studies have shown a relationship between the presence of irregular opacities and smoking.[97] Although it is tempting, as Weiss has done, to relate the presence of irregular opacities in the chest film to fibrosis, it is obviously incorrect to assume that the pathologic changes that are found in smokers are the same as those that are found in early asbestosis or other dust diseases. Clearly, the patchy alveolar fibrosis and emphysema that Auerbach and colleagues[98] described in their classic studies differ from the alveolitis and bronchiolitis observed in asbestosis and in other forms of interstitial fibrosis or alveolar injury. Nor is there any reason to believe that irregular opacities should be attributed to the presence of centrilobular emphysema. Thus, although irregular opacities are situated almost entirely at the bases, emphysema, whether induced by cigarette smoking or by dust exposure, has a characteristic apical localization. The relationship between the radiographic presence of "increased markings emphysema" and the pathologic changes present in such subjects is reviewed at some length by Fraser and Paré,[99] who were unable to explain the radiographic changes in terms of morbid anatomy. Little doubt exists, however, that irregular markings in the chest radiograph are associated with cigarette smoking and the presence of airways obstruction, and the possibility exists that peribronchial fibrosis, increased vascularity, or both, may in some instances account for their presence.

Chronic Airflow Limitation and the Role of Bronchial Hyperreactivity in the Development of Airways Obstruction

Although the physiologic mechanisms and pathologic features of established airflow obstruction have been exhaustively studied, those factors, be they related to habits or to occupational exposure, that initiate or predispose to the development of chronic airflow limitation are poorly understood and are the subject of fierce debate. When it comes to the pathogenesis of chronic airways obstruction two schools of thought exist, often referred to as the Dutch School and the British-Canadian-U.S. School.

The Dutch School and its adherents believe that chronic airflow limitation develops in the main in those who are inherently susceptible.[100, 101] They postulate that environmental exposures are at least as important as is cigarette smoking, and were the individual not predisposed or susceptible, cigarette smoking would not lead to airways obstruction. In favor of this hypothesis is the fact that only 13% to 15% of smokers develop chronic airflow obstruction.[26] The main epidemiologic support for the Dutch hypothesis comes from a study of two areas in the Netherlands, one of which was urban and heavily polluted, whereas the other was rural and pollution free.[100, 101]

The British-Canadian-U.S. hypothesis puts forward the notion that there are two separate responses to cigarette smoking, namely chronic bronchitis (mucus hypersecretion) and small airways disease, and by inference (see earlier discussion), emphysema.[26, 50] As such, the separate responses affect different anatomic regions of the lung, namely the dead space in the case of chronic bronchitis, and the bronchioles and lung parenchyma in the case of emphysema. Other irritants, including dusts and gases, may also produce bronchitis.[102] Becklake,[103] in her review of chronic airflow limitation and its relationship to working in the dusty occupations, states "The key factor which makes an individual susceptible may well be the capacity of his or her airways to become reactive to inhaled materials." She goes on to suggest that this capacity to react is related to individual susceptibility, and further endorses the concept of simple and obstructive bronchitis, an outmoded concept that serves only to obfuscate.

Bronchial hyperreactivity exists in about 3% of the general population, 30% of atopic patients in the absence of asthma, 70% of patients with asymptomatic asthma, and probably over 90% of patients with active asthma.[104–108] It is also known that exposure to irritants, such as sulfur dioxide, aluminum fluoride, and citric acid, may induce bronchial hyperreactivity.[109] In the case of acute irritant exposures, in healthy subjects such bronchial hyperreactivity is relatively ephemeral. The currently available evidence would suggest that prolonged exposures to irritants may lead to bronchial hyperreactivity persisting for months or years. Similar observations have been noted in nonasthmatic grain workers.[110] The various possible mechanisms of the induction of bronchial hyperreactivity have been well discussed by Simonsson[111] and include the following:

1. Increased sensitivity of afferent nerve endings
2. Changes in nerve transmission or modulation of transmission in the central nervous system
3. Changes in release and breakdown of acetylcholine
4. Changes in smooth muscle cell and its membrane receptors or internal metabolism

5. An altered wall-to-lumen ratio causing more deposition of histamine or methacholine and leading to an excess dose-effect curve in those subjects whose airways are narrow.

There seems little doubt that subjects with chronic bronchitis show increased airways reactivity and that those with airways obstruction can be shown to have more bronchial hyperreactivity than those without.[112–114] It has also been suggested that the nature of the bronchial hyperresponsiveness seen in subjects with chronic airflow limitation differs from that seen in asthmatic subjects.[106] The positions of the dose-response curves of the asthmatics and of subjects with nonspecific chronic airflow limitation overlap; however, the geometric mean values for the PC_{20} for the two groups differ significantly. There is a good correlation between the FEV_1/FVC and the PC_{20} FEV_1 values in the patients with chronic obstructive lung disease but not in the patients with asthma. Other studies have shown that, despite a wide range of PC_{20} values in chronic obstruction, *in vivo* airways responsiveness does not correlate with any of the *in vitro* responses examined, indicating that airways reactivity is not due solely to smooth muscle responsiveness to contractile agonists nor to a localized deficiency in the nonadrenergic inhibitory system, beta-adrenergic inhibition, or abnormal cyclic AMP–mediated pathways of relaxation.[115] Thus, the evidence would suggest that there is indeed a distinction between the mechanisms of bronchial hyperreactivity in cigarette smoke–induced chronic airflow limitation and those in asthma.

The relationship of bronchial activity and the annual rate of decline in ventilatory capacity in male smokers and ex-smokers has been studied by Taylor and colleagues.[114] They showed that bronchial reactivity to histamine was greater in smokers than in nonsmokers. Furthermore, an accelerated rate of decline in the FEV_1 was present in the smokers. This observation is compatible with the Dutch hypothesis in that bronchial reactivity is increased in smokers who also happen to have airways obstruction. Such a hypothesis postulates that the increased susceptibility in the hyperresponsive group is a consequence of hereditary factors. An alternative explanation would be that the enhanced bronchial reactivity might result from the reduced cross-sectional lumina that are present in smokers who happen to have a decreased FEV_1, i.e., the bronchial hyperreactivity is acquired and develops with the passage of time. Certainly it is now apparent that this is likely to be the case in occupational asthma, that is, the increased bronchial reactivity develops as a result of prolonged exposure to the antigen.[116, 117]

The Dutch hypothesis suggests that a minority of smokers are affected by a form of allergy akin to atopy and this predisposes them to a progressive reduction in FEV_1. Support for this thesis comes from the raised IgE levels and the increased eosinophil count found in some smokers; however, the correlation between skin test positivity and raised total IgE levels is poor.[118, 119] Moreover, measurement of bronchial reactivity in young symptomless smokers has, for the most part, failed to reveal any increased excitability of the airways. The bronchial hyperreactivity of smokers, therefore, seems to develop gradually and to be related to the duration of smoking. The exact cause remains uncertain, but perhaps the most feasible explanation is that it is related to changes in airways geometry. The finding of an increased PC_{20} in almost all subjects with an FEV_1 below 80% of the predicted is in favor of this hypothesis. When one compares bronchial hyperreactivity in smokers and nonsmokers who have an FEV_1 of greater than 80%, the airways of smokers demonstrate increased reactivity, but by the same token, smokers also have a mean FEV_1 that is lower than that of a nonsmoker.[120] For a given decrease in the FEV_1 in subjects otherwise matched for age and height, patients with asthma show much more bronchial hyperresponsiveness than do patients with chronic bronchitis. Similarly, whereas asthmatic patients show a good correlation between histamine-induced bronchoconstriction and that induced by hyperventilation or cold air, smokers with increased histamine responses do not develop bronchoconstriction with hyperventilation or cold air despite heat loss equivalent to that which produces a response in patients with asthma.[121, 122]

The hypothesis that bronchial hyperreactivity may be induced or increased by cigarette smoking also needs to be considered; however, no relationship appears to exist among total IgE, eosinophil count, and the level of FEV_1 or its rate of decline.[118] This would argue against the somewhat tenuous demonstration of allergic predisposition playing any role in the development of chronic airflow limitation or the rate of decline of FEV_1.

The weight of evidence thus suggests that bronchial hyperreactivity is acquired rather than inherited, and as such argues cogently against the Dutch hypothesis. Moreover, the studies that have been carried out so far have not revealed any allergic predisposition in those who show an increased rate of decline in the FEV_1, and more plausible explanations for the development of emphysema in smokers exist. These include the distribution of inhaled smoke and differences in the regional disposition of particles during cigarette smoking.[123]

CHRONIC AIRFLOW OBSTRUCTION: EXPOSURE TO SPECIFIC AGENTS

Cotton, Hemp, and Flax Fibers

Exposure to cotton, hemp, and flax may lead to the development of one or more of the following responses:[124]

1. Chest tightness and shortness of breath on first returning to work
2. A decline in ventilatory capacity over the first work shift of the week
3. An increased prevalence of bronchitis as manifested by cough and sputum
4. A clinical syndrome known as mill fever

With the exception of mill fever, the other three conditions are often loosely referred to as byssinosis. This term, however, should preferably be reserved for the acute response, that is, chest tightness. There is also some justification for using the term to apply to the associated decrease in ventilatory capacity that occurs on first returning to work, because frequently some concordance exists between the presence of chest tightness and a decrease in FEV_1.

For many years it was believed that those workers who showed an acute response on exposure to cotton fibers would, with repeated exposure, go on to develop chronic irreversible airways obstruction.[125, 126] It was further assumed that the abrupt onset on Monday morning of the acute response slowly became less obvious, and that the chest tightness that initially was present on Monday would persist through Tuesday and Wednesday, and throughout the week. Thus, the affected subject lost his awareness of the onset and presence of chest tightness. Irreversible obstruction in a cotton mill worker was often referred to as chronic byssinosis and was recognized by the presence of cough, sputum, and breathlessness. As such, it was indistinguishable clinically from chronic airflow obstruction induced by cigarette smoking.

A number of studies have indicated that the lungs of some cotton, hemp, and flax workers frequently showed the loss of recoil and the type of classic pulmonary impairment found in emphysema.[127, 128] Lung static recoil and airways obstruction have been studied in hemp workers by Guyatt and coworkers.[127] However, their study makes it quite clear that the majority of those who were severely affected were cigarette smokers or ex-smokers. Other studies have shown that cotton workers have significantly lower spirometric values than non-cotton workers,[129, 130] but it was not established whether the reduction in FEV_1 was permanent or simply a prolonged manifestation of acute exposure to cotton dust. It was also observed that those mill workers with reduced FEV_1 also usually have an increased prevalence of cough and sputum. However, it has become abundantly clear over the last 15 or so years that cough and sputum do not necessarily presage the onset of irreversible obstruction.[26, 54]

A number of studies have been done that suggest that cotton textile workers show a greater annual decrease in ventilatory capacity than would be expected in a similar control population.[131, 132] One such study reported a decrease of 54 ml/year (expected 25 to 30 ml).[131] Mill workers processing synthetic fibers were used as controls and showed a decrease of 32 ml/year; however, the two synthetic mills studied had vastly different rates of decline, and one mill seemed to be responsible for the overall relatively normal rate of decline of ventilatory capacity in the synthetic fiber workers. Similarly, in another study, a survivor population of active and retired workers in South Carolina were shown to have a lower mean FEV_1 and FVC than did the reference population from Connecticut.[130, 133] Although a series of papers have been published purporting to indicate that the South Carolina cotton workers showed a vastly increased rate of decline in FEV_1,[130–133] the method by which the original population was selected is open to question and indeed was invalid. The reference population was obtained from a precisely defined community by soliciting participation from the total group. The textile workers were drawn from a group out of whom 78% were recruited by uncontrolled referral or by self-selection from an undefined motley group, in short, those who felt that they had symptoms and indeed suspected or knew that they were unwell.[134] The original study design had been based on the assumption that sufficient cotton workers who had been randomly designated from the whole population would participate, but when it became apparent that this was not the case, additional workers were "recruited by word of mouth."[130] The percentage of smokers in those who were recruited by random selection and those who were recruited by word of mouth differed greatly. There were 30 nonsmokers, 52 ex-smokers, and 18 current smokers among the cardroom workers who were in the original selected cohort, whereas, in contrast, the cardroom workers who were recruited by word of mouth or self-selected comprised 22 nonsmokers, 34 ex-smokers, and 38 current smokers. Thus, there is an almost complete reversal of the proportions of nonsmokers versus smokers in the two groups. Much the same imbalance was apparent in the male weave room workers.

Over the last 10 to 15 years it has become evident that nonsmoking cotton workers do not develop emphysema and loss of elastic recoil. This is based on a number of post-mortem studies.[135–138] Moreover, a well-controlled study showed that the diffusing capacity in "byssinotic" female nonsmoking cotton workers was normal and only in smokers was there a significant reduction.[139] Thus, it would seem evident that cotton, flax, and hemp workers, when exposed to the high concentrations of dusts that are generated in the cardroom and elsewhere in the mill, are likely to develop chronic bronchitis but not emphysema. It is probably true that chronic bronchitis is associated with a minor decrement in the FEV_1, probably very similar to that seen in industrial bronchitis from other exposures in which emphysema is absent.[124, 140, 141] Long-term studies are presently under way to determine the magnitude of the decrement in FEV_1 that occurs in cotton workers but it is clear that it is not comparable to that resulting from cigarette smoking.[140, 141]

In addition, a series of mortality studies in which the standardized mortality ratio (SMR) of cotton workers has been compared with that of the general population has shown that there is no increased death rate from chronic nonmalignant respiratory disease in cotton and flax workers.[142–145] Were long-continued exposure to cotton, flax, and hemp to lead to significant and disabling chronic airflow obstruction, this would be reflected in the SMR for respiratory diseases.

Welding and Airways Obstruction

Over the past several years a number of studies have shed some light on the chronic effects of welding, especially in regard to the prevalence and effects of bronchitis. Hunnicutt and colleagues,[146] in a group of welders from the Newport News shipyard, found that the prevalence of symptoms, such as cough and sputum, was significantly higher in welders than in nonwelders. There was also an increased prevalence of airways obstruction, but only smoking welders were affected. Comparable findings resulted from a study of Boston shipyard welders.[147] In this study it was recognized that many welders had significant exposure to asbestos. Peters and colleagues[147] concluded that no detectable ventilatory defect was present in welders who did not smoke. Fogh[148] and colleagues observed similar findings in 156 Danish welders. They concluded that there was no significant difference between welders and control subjects in the occurrence of chronic bronchitis and ventilatory function after controlling for smoking. Similarly, Sjogren and Ulfvarson,[149] although able to show an increased prevalence of bronchitis, could detect no effect on lung function in a group of 269 welders of whom 64 were aluminium welders, 56 stainless steel welders, and 149 road track welders. Antti-Poika and coworkers[150] found similar findings in a group of Finnish arc welders.

In a series of well-executed and detailed studies, McMillan[151] investigated the health of welders employed in the Royal Navy dockyards in Britain. In a carefully controlled retrospective study, McMillan analyzed the morbidity and incidence of respiratory disease over a 5-year period. Five relatively comparable groups who also worked in the shipyard were included as a reference population. These included boiler makers, shipwrights, electrical fitters, painters, and joiners. He concluded that there was no evidence of a significant excess of chronic respiratory disease in the welders. Moreover, in 16 subjects who were discharged from the dockyards on account of respiratory disease, only two were welders, and in these there was nothing to suggest that the disease responsible for their stopping work was related to their job. He did, however, notice that welders had somewhat more upper respiratory illnesses than other groups, but that the absence on account of these illnesses was of the same duration.

McMillan[152] has also published a general review of the health of welders in Royal Navy dockyards and has concluded that there was no evidence of a causal relationship between welding and respiratory diseases or other ill health, with the exception of injuries. He believed there may be a small minority of welders who are unusually susceptible to the effects of fumes and gases, and that such persons have obstructive airways disease, such as asthma or emphysema. Neither the asthma nor the emphysema was, however, related to welding exposure.

Owing to the fact that most studies have been carried out in welders with relatively short exposures to welding fumes, that is to say, less than 15 years, McMillan and Pethybridge[153] decided to examine 135 welders aged 45 and over who had prolonged exposure. The average duration of welding in their group was 33.1 years. Those exposed had detailed clinical, radiologic, and pulmonary function examinations carried out and were compared with a comparable control group aged 45 and over. They concluded that prolonged exposure to welding fumes did not cause significant clinical abnormality nor any serious impairment of lung function. McMillan and Pethybridge expressed the opinion that minimal airways obstruction may result from exposure to welding fumes. Rather similar findings have been reported by Hayden and colleagues[154] in welders employed in three engineering factories in the British Midlands. These investigators concluded, however, that welders had no increased risk of chronic obstructive lung disease. Similar conclusions have been reached by others.[147, 148, 150]

Silica Exposure and Airways Obstruction

Simple silicosis is seldom associated with significant pulmonary impairment, and both the ventilatory capacity and diffusing capacities remain within the normal range.[155] However, there is some suggestion that the higher categories of simple silicosis may occasionally lead to a slight stiffening of the lungs.[156] In contrast, there is no doubt that categories B and C complicated silicosis lead to both restrictive and obstructive impairment.[157]

Theriault and coworkers[158] studied the effects of estimated lifetime dust exposure in 784 granite workers. They claimed, as a result of a cross-sectional study, to have shown a 2 ml annual excess decrement in the FVC. Many problems existed with their methodology, not least of which was a 30% radiographic prevalence of silicosis in those with no exposure. Moreover, the silica content of the dust samples was 9% lower than that found in prior analyses. Subsequent dust measurements have shown that Theriault and coworkers significantly underestimated exposure to silica. A follow-up paper described a longitudinal study in the same group of workers and purported to show a 70 to 80 ml mean annual decrement in the FVC and a 50 to 70 ml mean annual decrement in the FEV_1.[159] At the time these results were published the validity of these studies was questioned.[160] Were the average loss as high as had been suggested, a significant number of the work force would have been severely impaired by the time the subjects were 50 years old or would have left the workforce, and this was not the case. Similarly, the susceptible would have been respiratory cripples long before they were 50. Furthermore, the annual decline in the FVC is invariably less than that of the FEV_1, whether the subject is normal or not, or whether he or she has restrictive or obstructive impairment; this alone should have alerted the investigators. Even so, the investigators' analysis of variance still showed smoking as having the overriding effect on ventilatory capacity. Subsequently, Graham and coworkers[161] restudied the same group of Vermont granite shed workers and showed that from 1974 to 1979 the FVC had increased by 0.50 L and the FEV_1 by 0.030 L. In this paper, Graham and coworkers commented on the fact that the spirometer used by Theriault and colleagues[158] had a leak and that, as might be expected, the leak influenced the measured volume of the FVC more than that of the FEV_1. A well-designed study of the ventilatory capacity of South African gold miners showed that simple silicosis produced no ventilatory impairment in itself.[162] Although the miners with simple silicosis tended to have a lower FEV_1 and forced expiratory flow (FEF_{25-75}) than did those miners without silicosis, when corrections were made for cumulative dust exposure it became apparent that no significant difference existed in ventilatory capacity between those with and without silicosis. This suggested that another mechanism must explain the presence of the excess airways obstruction, and in this regard industrial bronchitis provides a plausible explanation.

Becklake and others[163] subsequently studied the predictors of the development of emphysema in South African gold miners. They showed that those subjects who were exposed to silica and who developed emphysema differed from exposed subjects who did not develop emphysema in that they smoked more cigarettes, were older at the time of death, and had a higher total dust exposure. Although it was suggested by Becklake and colleagues[163] that the extent of silicosis was about the same in those with and without emphysema, their data do not bear out this assertion, and the silicotic patients with emphysema in general had higher dust exposure and smoked more heavily. Their study indicates clearly that smoking is of paramount importance in the development of emphysema. Other problems exist in this study, in particular the collinearity of certain of the variables may well have invalidated the logistic regression analysis they used. Thus, as the subject ages, so his or her cigarette consumption goes up, and so also does his or her cumulative dust exposure. Multiple logistic regression analysis does not necessarily apportion the contribution of each of these factors.[164] Moreover, age alone in the absence of smoking and dust exposure is associated with increasing prevalence of emphysema, especially of the panlobular variety.[165] Finally, the characteristic lesion of silicosis is the silicotic nodule, a small, whorled fibrotic nodule that is located near the arteriole of the respiratory bronchiole, an entity that is likely to lead to stiff lungs, not the excessively compliant lungs of emphysema. In well-established silicosis occurring in middle-aged adults, a marked paucity of emphysema exists despite the presence of multiple small nodules throughout the lung parenchyma.

A 10-year follow-up of a group of silica-exposed workers in Hong Kong has also been published.[166] The study compared pulmonary function data in those who progressed radiographically, with those who did not. The data in this study suggested that the increased rate of decline in function in these workers was more strongly related to prior dust exposure than to smoking. These subjects were drawn from a Silicosis Register and over 90% were smokers. Closer study suggests, however, that those subjects whose radiographs showed the most rapid progression of the disease also showed the greatest decrement in lung function and are the same subjects who go on to develop complicated silicosis. Continued smoking and the development of the latter seem to predict an increased decrement in ventilatory capacity rather than any other factors.

In summary, the weight of evidence suggests that simple silicosis per se is associated with little in the way of pulmonary impairment. Subjects with prolonged exposure to silica, however, frequently develop cough and sputum even when they are nonsmokers. These symptoms are accompanied by minor decrements in the FEV_1 and FEV_1/FVC percentage, which should be attributed to bronchitis rather than emphysema or parenchymal fibrosis. When complicated silicosis develops, both restrictive and obstructive defects may be present and the magnitude of the impairment is related to the size of the conglomerate lesions.

Exposure to Isocyanates and Airways Obstruction

Repeated exposure to isocyanates is a recognized cause of occupational asthma. This has been known for considerable time and the features of this condition have been well described.[167, 168] Aside from reversible airways obstruction, some investigators have claimed that workers exposed to isocyanates show an increased rate of decline of ventilatory capacity, with the FEV_1 being particularly affected.[169–171] They maintain that the decrease in FEV_1 that occurs in such workers is not related to the presence of asthma but is a consequence of the development of irreversible obstruction, and the latter is dose related and occurs more frequently in those with long-continued cumulative exposure to isocyanates.

A series of papers has been published, the authors of which claim to have shown an increased rate of decline in the ventilatory capacity of workers exposed to relatively low levels of isocyanates that conformed to the former recommended time-weighted average for toluene diisocyanate (TDI).[169–171] Other studies failed to show any long-term effects of exposure to isocyanates other than those of asthma.[172, 173] In the past 3 to 4 years, it has become evident that little reliance can be placed on many of the investigations in which an excess decrement was reported. When spirometry was subsequently repeated 10 years later the mean FVC and FEV_1 of those exposed showed a significant improvement over the 10-year observation period.[174] Subsequent inspection of the tracings carried out at the first survey revealed that they were unsatisfactory and that the duration of the forced expiratory volume maneuvers in the main was less than 3 seconds.[174] By the same token, well-controlled studies conducted elsewhere have failed to show an increased rate of decline in the isocyanate workers when the effects of occupational asthma had been excluded.[172, 173]

The problem was later compounded in a carefully controlled study carried out by Diem and colleagues,[175] who claimed to have shown a 24-ml excess annual decrement in the FEV_1 in workers exposed to above 24 ppb toluene diisocyanate. Somewhat peculiarly, the comparable excess decline for smokers who were exposed to the same level was only 18 ml, suggesting that smoking had a protective effect. Whereas this was a carefully carried out study, the several anomalous findings, which included an across-the-board, unexplained improvement in FEV_1 during the study, make the results obtained somewhat questionable. Thus, at one survey the workers exposed to high and low levels of TDI, and also the controls, showed a sudden improvement in the FEV_1 for which no explanation was available. Moreover, the presence of symptoms in the high and low exposed groups showed certain rather bizarre features, in particular a higher prevalence of severer grades of shortness of breath in those with less exposure. In addition, in both the high and low exposure groups, the prevalence of bronchitis was unusually low—well below 5%—and much below what is to be expected with the proportion of smokers included in the study.

In summary, the evidence that long-continued exposure to isocyanates induces disabling irreversible obstruction is unconvincing, mainly because the various longitudinal studies have shown conflicting results and, moreover, those studies purporting to show a decrement have been shown to be flawed. The investigators who performed these studies concluded that long-continued exposure to TDI induces irreversible airways obstruction. Were this so, such obstruction would have to be a consequence of either a parenchymal destruction, such as emphysema, or an irreversible pathologic process involving the small airways, such as bronchiolitis obliterans. No evidence is available suggesting that exposure to isocyanates causes either of the two pathophysiologic responses, and morbid anatomic confirmation of the presence of either of these conditions is lacking. The possibility that isocyanates are sufficiently irritative to induce bronchitis must be borne in mind, but the low prevalence of cough and sputum in both of the exposed groups of workers described by Diem and colleagues[175] makes this hypothesis most unlikely. In the absence of unequivocal evidence that long-continued isocyanate exposure induces not only an increased rate of decline of ventilatory capacity but also persistent pathologic changes that can explain such a reduction in ventilatory capacity, it would seem prudent to reserve judgment rather than to assume that exposure to isocyanates causes irreversible obstruction.

REFERENCES

1. Thackrah CT. The effects of Arts, Trades and Professions and of the Civic States and Habits of Living on Health and Longevity (2nd ed). London: Longman, 1832.
2. Greenhow EH. (a) Report of the Medical Officer of the Privy Council. Third Report. London: H. M. Stationery Office, 1961. (b) Trans Path Soc London 12, 36, 186. (c) Report of the Medical Officer Local Government Board, 1865.
3. Hamilton A. Exploring the Dangerous Trades. Boston: Little, Brown & Co, 1943.
4. Hart P d'A, Aslett A. Medical Research Council, Special Report Series No. 243. London: H. M. Stationery Office, 1942.
5. Sutherland CL, Bryson S. Report on the Incidence of Silicosis in the Pottery Industry. London: H. M. Stationery Office, 1926.
6. Sutherland CL, Bryson S, Keating N: Report on the Occurrence of Silicosis among Granite Workers. London: H. M. Stationery Office, 1930.
7. McDonald JC, Gibbs GW, Liddell FDK, et al. Mortality following exposure to cummingtonite-grunerite. Am Rev Respir Dis 1978; 118:271.
8. Gilson JC, Hugh-Jones P. Lung Function in Coal Workers Pneumoconiosis. Medical Research Council, Special Report Series No. 290. London: H. M. Stationery Office, 1955.
9. Gough J. Pneumoconiosis in coal workers in Wales. Occup Med 1947; 4:86.
10. Heppleston AG. The essential lesion of pneumoconiosis in Welsh coal workers. J Pathol Bacteriol 1947; 59:453.
11. Rivers D, Wise ME, King EJ, Nagelschmidt G. Dust content, radiology, and pathology in simple pneumoconiosis of coal workers. Br J Ind Med 1960; 17:87.
12. Bergman I, Casswell C. Lung dust and lung iron contents of coal workers in different coalfields in Great Britain. Br J Ind Med 1972; 29:160.
13. Nagelschmidt G. The study of lung dust in pneumoconiosis. Am Ind Hyg Assoc J 1965; 26:1.
14. Strachan AS. Proceedings of Conference on Silicosis Pneumoconiosis and Dust Suppression in Mines. London: Institute of Mining Engineers and Institute of Mining and Metallurgy, 1947.
15. Cochrane AL, Higgins ITT. Pulmonary ventilatory function of coal miners in various areas in relation to the x-ray category of pneumoconiosis. Br J Prev Soc Med 1961; 15:1.
16. Ashford JR, Brown S, Morgan DC, Rae S. The pulmonary ventilatory function of coal miners in the United Kingdom. Am Rev Respir Dis 1968; 97:810.
17. Morgan WKC, Handelsman L, Kibelstis J, et al. Ventilatory capacity and lung volumes of U.S. coal miners. Arch Environ Health 1974; 28:182.
18. Morgan WKC, Lapp NL. Respiratory disease in coal miners. State of the art. Am Rev Respir Dis 1976; 113:531.
19. Irwig LM, Rocks P. Lung function and respiratory symptoms in silicotic and non-silicotic gold miners. Am Rev Respir Dis 1978; 117:429.
20. Cochrane AL, Haley TJL, Moore F, Hole D. The mortality of men in the Rhondda Fach, 1950–1970. Br J Ind Med 1979; 36:15.
21. Cochrane AL, Moore F. A 20-year follow-up of a population sample (aged 25–34) including coal miners and foundry workers in Staveley, Derbyshire. Br J Ind Med 1980; 37:230.
22. Enterline PE. The effects of occupation on chronic respiratory disease. Arch Environ Health 1967; 14:189.
23. Higgins ITT. Chronic respiratory disease in mining communities. Ann NY Acad Sci 1972; 200:197.
24. Cochrane AL, Higgins ITT, Thomas J. Pulmonary ventilation functions of coal miners in various areas in relation to x-ray category of pneumoconiosis. Br J Prev Soc Med 1961; 15:1.
25. McClintock JS. The selection of juvenile entrants to mining. Br J Ind Med 1971; 28:45.
26. Fletcher CM, Peto R, Tinker E, Speizer FE. The Natural History of Chronic Bronchitis and Emphysema. New York: Oxford University Press, 1976.
27. Bates DV. The fate of the chronic bronchitic: a report of the ten-year follow-up in the Canadian Department of Veteran's Affairs coordinated study of chronic bronchitics. Am Rev Respir Dis 1973; 108:1043.

28. Reid L. Measurement of the bronchial mucous gland layer: a diagnostic yardstick in chronic bronchitis. Thorax 1960; 132:141.
29. Fogh A, Frost J, Georg J. Respiratory symptoms and pulmonary function in welders. Ann Occup Hyg 1969; 12:213.
30. Ferris BG, Puleo S, Chen HY. Mortality and morbidity in a pulp and paper mill in the United States: a ten-year follow-up. Br J Ind Med 1979; 36:127.
31. Fernie JM, Douglas NA, Lamb D, Ruckley VA. Right ventricular hypertrophy in a group of coal miners. Thorax 1983; 38:436.
32. Ryder RC, Dunnill MS, Anderson JA. A quantitative study of bronchial mucous gland volume, emphysema and smoking in a necropsy population. J Pathol 1971; 104:59.
33. Gough J. The pathogenesis of emphysema in the lung. In: Liebow A, Smith DT, eds. Baltimore: Williams and Wilkins, 1968, 109.
34. Morgan WKC. Coalworkers' pneumoconiosis: In: Morgan WKC and Seaton A, eds. Occupational Lung Diseases. 2nd Ed. Philadelphia: W B Saunders Company, 1984, 377.
35. Ruckley VA, Gault SJ, Chapman JS, et al. Emphysema and dust exposure in a group of coal workers. Am Rev Respir Dis 1984; 129:528.
36. Ryder RC, Lyons JP, Campbell H, Gough J. Emphysema in coal workers' pneumoconiosis. Br Med J 1970; 3:481.
37. Lyons JP, Ryder R, Campbell H, Gough J. Pulmonary disability in coal worker's pneumoconiosis. Br Med J 1972; 1:713.
38. Lyons JP, Campbell H. Evaluation of disability in coal workers' pneumoconiosis. Thorax 1976; 31:527.
39. Cockroft A, Seal RME, Wagner JC, et al. Post-mortem study of emphysema in coal workers and noncoal workers. Lancet 1982; ii:600.
40. Gilson JC, Oldham PD. Coal workers' pneumoconiosis. Br Med J 1970; 4:305.
41. Oldham PD, Berry G. Coal miners' pneumoconiosis. Br Med J 1970; 2:292.
42. Cockroft A, Seal RME, Wagner JC, et al. Post-mortem study of emphysema in coal workers and non-coalworkers. Lancet ii:600. 1982;
43. Berry J, Newhouse ML, Antonis D. Combined effect of asbestos and smoking on mortality from lung cancer and mesothelioma in factory workers. Br J Ind Med 1985; 42:12.
44. Hankinson JL, Palmes ED, Lapp NL. Pulmonary air space size in coal miners. Am Rev Respir Dis 1979; 119:391.
45. Fournier-Massey G, Rossiter E. Respiratory symptoms in chrysotile asbestos mine and mill workers of Quebec. Arch Environ Health 1972; 24:358.
46. Manfreda J, Sidwall G, Maini K, et al. Respiratory abnormalities in employees of the hard rock mining industry. Am Rev Respir Dis 1982; 126:629.
47. Hankinson JL, Reger RB, Morgan WKC. Maximal expiratory flows in coal miners. Am Rev Respir Dis 1977; 116:175.
48. Fletcher C. Some observations of the bronchial and emphysematous types of patient with severe generalized airways obstruction. In: Cumming G, Hunt LB, eds. Form and Function in the Human Lung. Baltimore: Williams & Wilkins, 1968, 231.
49. Medical Research Council. Chronic bronchitis and occupation. Br Med J 1966; 1:101.
50. Fletcher CM, Elmes PC, Fairbairn AS, Wood CH. The significance of respiratory symptoms and the diagnosis of chronic bronchitis in a working population. Br Med J 1959; 2:257.
51. Medical Research Council, Committee on the Etiology of Chronic Bronchitis. Definition and classification of chronic bronchitis for clinical and epidemiological purposes. Lancet 1965; i:775.
52. American Thoracic Society. Chronic bronchitis, asthma, and pulmonary emphysema. Am Rev Respir Dis 1962; 85:762.
53. Douglas AN, Lamb D, Ruckley VA. Bronchial gland dimensions in coal miners: influence of smoking and dust exposure. Thorax 1982; 37:760.
54. Morgan WKC. Industrial bronchitis. Br J Ind Med 1978; 35:285.
55. Ashford JR, Morgan DC, Rae S, Sowden RR. Respiratory symptoms in British coal miners. Am Rev Respir Dis 1970; 102:370.
56. Rae S, Walker DD, Attfield ND. Chronic bronchitis in dust exposure in British coal miners. In: Walton WH, ed. Inhaled Particles III. Old Woking, Surrey: Unwin Bros, 1971, 883.
57. Kibelstis JA, Morgan EJ, Reger R, et al. Prevalence of bronchitis and airway obstruction in American bituminous coal miners. Am Rev Respir Dis 1973; 108:886.
58. Hankinson JL, Reger RB, Fairman RP, et al. Factors influencing expiratory flow rates in coal miners. In: Walton WH, ed. Inhaled Particles IV. Oxford: Pergamon Press, 1977, 737.
59. Vuylsteek K, Depoorter AM. Smoking, occupational dust exposure and chronic non-specific lung disease. Broncho-pneumologie 1978; 28:31.
60. Rogan JM, Attfield MD, Jacobsen M, et al. Role of dust in the working environment in development of chronic bronchitis in British coal miners. Br J Ind Med 1973; 30:217.
61. Deutsche Forschungsgemeinschaft. Research Report on Chronic Bronchitis and Occupational Dust Exposure. Boppard, West Germany: Harald Boldt Verlag KC, 1978.
61a. Kreiss K, Greenberg LM, Kogut SJH, et al. Hard-rock mining exposures affect smokers and nonsmokers differently. Am Rev Respir Dis 1989; 139:1487.
61b. Morgan WKC, Burgess DB, Lapp NL, Seaton A. Hyperinflation of the lungs in coal miners. Thorax 1971; 26:585.
62. Cochrane AL. Chronic bronchitis and occupation. Br Med J 1966; 1:85.
63. Love RG, Miller BG. Longitudinal study of lung function in coal miners. Thorax 1982; 37:193.
64. Attfield MD. Longitudinal decline in FEV_1 in United States coalminers. Thorax 1985; 40:132.
65. Marine WM, Gurr D, Jacobsen M. Clinically important respiratory effects of dust exposure and smoking in British coal miners. Am Rev Respir Dis 1988; 137:106.
66. Morgan WKC. On dust, disability, and death. Am Rev Respir Dis 1986; 134:639.
67. Matsuba K, Thurlbeck WM. Disease of the small airways in chronic bronchitis. Am Rev Respir Dis 1973; 107:552.
68. Foxman B, Higgins ITT, Oh MS. The effects of occupation and smoking on respiratory disease mortality. Am Rev Respir Dis 1986; 134:649.
69a. Liddell FDK. Morbidity of British coal miners in 1961–62. Br J Ind Med 1973; 30:1.
69b. Liddell FDK. Mortality of British coal miners in 1961. Br J Ind Med 1973; 30:15.
70. Peto R, Speizer FE, Cochrane AL, et al. The relevance in adults of airflow obstruction, but not of mucus hypersecretion, to mortality from chronic lung disease. Am Rev Respir Dis 1983; 128:491.
71. Jamal K, Cooney TP, Fleetham JA, Thurlbeck WM. Chronic bronchitis: correlation of morphologic findings to sputum production and flow rates. Am Rev Respir Dis 1984; 129:719.
72. Thurlbeck WM, Henderson JA, Fraser RG, Bates DV. Chronic obstructive lung disease. Medicine 1970; 49:81.
73. Kremer R, Timmerman G, Baudrez J, Lambrecht P. Hémodynamique pulmonaire dans les pneumoconioses des houilleurs. Rev Inst Hyg Mines 1967; 22:3.
74. Thomas AJ. The heart in the pneumoconiosis of coalminers. Br Heart J 1948; 10:282.
75. Thomas AJ. Right ventricular hypertrophy in the pneumoconiosis of coal miners. Br Heart J 1951; 13:1.
76. Wells AL. Pulmonary vascular changes in coal-workers' pneumoconiosis. J Pathol Bacteriol 1954; 68:573.
77. James WRL. Thomas AJ. Cardiac hypertrophy in coalworkers' pneumoconiosis. Br J Ind Med 1956; 13:24.
78. Lapp NL, Seaton A, Kaplan KC, et al. Pulmonary hemodynamics in symptomatic coal miners. Am Rev Respir Dis 1971; 104:418.
79. Fernie JM, Douglas NA, Lamb D, Ruckley VA. Right ventricular hypertrophy in a group of coal miners. Thorax 1983; 38:436.
80. Elmes PC. Relative importance of cigarette smoking in occupational lung disease. Br J Ind Med 1981; 38:1.
81. Guidlelines for the use of the ILO International Classification of radiographs of pneumoconiosis. No. 22 (Rev.), Occupational Safety and Health series. Geneva: International Labour Office, 1980.
82. Lyons JP, Ryder RC, Campbell H, et al. Significance of irregular opacities in the radiology of coal workers' pneumoconiosis. Br J Ind Med 1974; 31:36.
83. Cockcroft AE, Berry G, Cotes JE, Lyons JP. Shape of small opacities and lung function in coal workers. Thorax 1982; 37:765.
84. Cockcroft AE, Wagner JC, Seal RMF, et al. Irregular opacities in coalworkers' pneumoconiosis: Correlation with pulmonary function and pathology. Ann Occup Hyg 1982; 26:767.

85. Cockcroft AE, Andersson N. Radiological irregular opacities and coalwork exposure: a case-referent study. Br J Ind Med 1987; 44:484.
86. Collins HPR, Dick JA, Bennett JG, et al. Irregularly shaped small shadows in chest radiographs, dust exposure and lung function in coalworkers' pneumoconiosis. Br J Ind Med 1988; 45:43.
87. Amandus HE, Lapp NL, Jacobson G, Reger RB. Significance of irregular small opacities in radiographs of coalminers in the U.S.A. Br J Ind Med 1976; 33:13.
88. Glover JR, Bevan C, Cotes JE, et al. Effects of exposure to slate dust in North Wales. Br J Ind Med 1980; 37:152.
89. Wagner JC, Pooley FD, Gibb A, et al. Inhalation of China stone and China clay dusts. Relationship between minerology of dust retained in the lungs and pathological changes. Thorax 1986; 41:190.
90. Castellan RM, Sanderson WT, Petersen MR. Prevalence of the appearance of pneumoconiosis in an unexposed blue collar population. Am Rev Respir Dis 1985; 131:684.
91. Theriault GP, Peters JM, Johnson WM. Pulmonary function and roentgenographic changes in granite dust exposure. Arch Environ Health 1974; 28:23.
92. Weill H, Hughes JM, Hammad YY, et al. Respiratory health in workers exposed to man-made vitreous fibers. Am Rev Respir Dis 1983; 128:104.
93. Townsend MC, Sussman NB, Enterline PE, et al. Radiographic abnormalities in relation to total dust exposure at a bauxite refinery and alumina-based chemical products plant. Am Rev Respir Dis 1988; 138:90.
94. Carilli AD, Kotzen LM, Fischer MJ. The chest roentgenogram in smoking females. Am Rev Respir Dis 1973; 107:133.
95. Legg SJ, Cotes JE, Bevan C. Lung mechanics in relation to radiographic category of coalworkers' simple pneumoconiosis. Br J Ind Med 1983; 40:28.
96. Weiss W. Cigarette smoking and diffuse pulmonary fibrosis. Am Rev Respir Dis 1969; 99:67.
97. Weiss W. Smoking and pulmonary fibrosis. J Occup Med 1988; 30:33.
98. Auerbach O, Garfinkel L, Hammond EC. Relation of smoking and age to findings in lung parenchyma. Chest 1974; 65:29.
99. Fraser RG, Paré JAP. Airways disease. In: Fraser RG, Pare JAP, eds. Diagnosis of Diseases of the Lung. Philadelphia: WB Saunders Company 1979, 1364.
100. Orie NGM, Sluiter HJ, de Vries K, et al. The host factor in bronchitis. In: Bronchitis: an International Symposium, 27–29 April 1960. University of Groningen, The Netherlands. Assen Royal Van Gorcum, 1961, 43.
101. Van de Lende R, de Kroon JPM, van der Muelen GG, et al. Possible indicators of endogenous factors in the development of CNSLD. In: Orie NGM, van de Lende R, eds. Bronchitis III. Proceedings of the Third International Symposium on Bronchitis, 23–26 September 1969. University of Groningen, The Netherlands. Assen. Royal Van Gorcum, 1970, 52.
102. U.S. Public Health Service. The health consequences of smoking: cancer and chronic obstructive lung disease in the work place. A report of the Surgeon General. Chapter 5. Rockville, Md: Office of Smoking and Health, 1985, 183.
103. Becklake MR. Chronic airflow limitation: its relationship to work. Chest 1985; 88:608.
104. Cockcroft DW, Killian DN, Mellon JJA, Hargreave FE. Bronchial reactivity to inhaled histamine: a method and clinical survey. Clin Allerg 1977; 7:235.
105. De Vries K, Tammeling GJ. Discussion in the pathophysiology of chronic bronchitis. In: Orie NGM, Sluiter HJ, Eds. Bronchitis I. University of Groningen, The Netherlands. Assen Royal Van Gorcum, 1961, 221–226.
106. Yan K, Salome CM, Woolcock AJ. Prevalence and nature of bronchial hyperresponsiveness in subjects with chronic obstructive pulmonary disease. Am Rev Respir Dis 1985; 132:25.
107. Woolcock AJ, Coleman MH, Jones MW. Atopy and bronchial hyperreactivity in Australian and Melanesian populations. Clin Allerg 1978; 8:155.
108. Rijcken B, Schouten JP, Weiss ST, et al. The relationship between airway responsiveness to histamine and pulmonary function level in a random population sample. Am Rev Respir Dis 1988; 137:826.
109. Empey DW. Induced hyperreactivity in humans. Proceedings of International Conference on Bronchial Hyperreactivity. Chapter 3. Oxford: The Medicine Publishing Foundation, 1982, 9.
110. Mink JT, Gerrard JW, Cockcroft DW, et al. Increased bronchial reactivity to inhaled histamine in non-smoking grain workers with normal lung function. Chest 1980; 77:28.
111. Simonsson BG. Bronchial reactivity in relation to occupational bronchitis and asthma. Eur J Respir Dis 1982; 123(suppl):27.
112. Bahous J, Cartier A, Ouimet G, et al. Non-allergic bronchial hyperexcitability in chronic bronchitis. Am Rev Respir Dis 1984; 129:216.
113. Ramsdell JW, Nachtwey FJ, Moser KM. Bronchial hyperreactivity in chronic bronchitis. Am Rev Respir Dis 1982; 126:829.
114. Taylor RG, Joyce H, Gross E, et al. Bronchial reactivity to inhaled histamine and annual rate of decline in FEV_1 in male smokers and ex-smokers. Thorax 1985; 40:9.
115. Taylor SM, Pare PD, Armoor CL, et al. Airway reactivity in chronic obstructive pulmonary disease. Am Rev Respir Dis 1985; 132:30.
116. Thiel H, Ulmer WT. Baker's asthma: development and possibility for treatment. Chest 1980; 78(suppl):400.
117. Burge PS. Non-specific bronchial hyper-reactivity in workers exposed to toluene di-isocyanate, diphenylmethane di-isocyanate and colophony. Eur J Respir Dis 1982; 123(suppl):91.
118. Burrows B, Hasan FM, Barbee RA, et al. Epidemiologic observations on eosinophilia and its relation to respiratory disorders. Am Rev Respir Dis 1980; 122:708.
119. Taylor RG, Gross E, Joyce H, et al. Smoking, allergy, and the differential white blood cell count. Thorax 1985; 40:23.
120. Benson MK. Bronchial hyperreactivity. Br J Dis Chest 1975; 69:227.
121. Arnup ME, Mendella LA, Anthonisen NR. Effects of cold air hyperpnea in patients with chronic obstructive lung disease. Am Rev Respir Dis 1983; 128:236.
122. Ramsdale EH, Roberts RS, Morris M, Hargreave FE. Differences in responsiveness to hyperventilation and methacholine in asthma and chronic bronchitis. Thorax 1985; 40:422.
123. Pearson MG, Chamberlain MJ, Morgan WKC, Vinitski S. Regional deposition of particles in the lung during cigarette smoking in humans. J Appl Physiol 1985; 59:1828.
124. Morgan WKC, Vesterlund J, Burrell R, et al. Byssinosis: some unanswered questions. Am Rev Respir Dis 1982; 126:354.
125. Schilling RSF. Byssinosis in cotton and other textile workers. Lancet 1956; ii:319.
126. Bouhuys A, Heaphy LJ Jr, Schilling RSF, Welborn JW. Byssinosis in the United States. N Engl J Med 1967; 277:170.
127. Guyatt AR, Douglas JS, Zuskin E, Bouhuys A. Lung static recoil and airway obstruction in hemp workers with byssinosis. Am Rev Respir Dis 1973; 108:1111.
128. Bouhuys A, Van de Woestijne KP. Respiratory mechanics in dust exposure in byssinosis. J Clin Invest 1970; 49:106.
129. Berry G, Molyneux MKB, Tombleson JBL. Relationship between dust level and byssinosis and bronchitis in Lancashire cotton mills. Br J Ind Med 1974; 31:18.
130. Bouhuys A, Schoenberg JB, Beck GJ, Schilling RSF. Epidemiology of chronic lung disease in a cotton mill community. Lung 1977; 154:167.
131. Berry G, McKerrow CW, Molyneux MKB, et al. A study of the acute and chronic changes in ventilatory capacity in Lancashire cotton mills. Br J Ind Med 1973; 30:25.
132. Beck GJ, Schacter EN, Maunder LR, Schilling RSF. A prospective study of chronic lung disease in cotton textile workers. Ann Intern Med 1982; 97:645.
133. Beck GJ, Schacter EN, Maunder LR. The relationship of respiratory symptoms and lung function loss in cotton textile workers. Am Rev Respir Dis 1984; 130:6.
134. Jones RN. Cotton and chronic lung disease. Chest 1984; 85:587.
135. Moran TJ. Emphysema and other chronic lung disease in textile workers: An 8 year autopsy study. Arch Environ Health 1983; 38:267.
136. Edwards C, Macartney J, Rooke G, Ward F. The pathology of the lung in byssinosis. Thorax 1975; 30:612.
137. Rooke GB. The pathology of byssinosis. Chest 1981; 79(suppl):67.
138. Pratt PC. Comparative prevalence and severity of emphysema and bronchitis at autopsy in cotton mill workers versus controls. Chest 1981; 79(suppl):49.
139. Honeybourne D, Pickering CAC. Physiological evidence that emphysema is not a feature of byssinosis. Thorax 1986; 44:6.

140. Tockman MS, Baser M. Is cotton dust associated with chronic effects. Am Rev Respir Dis 1984; 130:1.
141. Elwood PC, McAulay IR, Elwood JH. The flax industry in Northern Ireland: Twenty years on. Lancet 1982; ii:1112.
142. Henderson VL, Enterline PE. An unusual mortality experience in cotton textile workers. J Occup Med 1973; 15:717.
143. Merchant JA, Ortmeyer CE. Mortality of employees of two cotton mills in North Carolina. Chest 1981; 79(suppl):6.
144. Berry G, Molyneux MKB. A mortality study of workers in Lancashire cotton mills. Chest 1981; 79(suppl):11.
145. Elwood PC, Thomas HF, Sweetman PM, Elwood JH. Mortality of flax workers. Br J Ind Med 1982; 39:18.
146. Hunnicutt TN, Cracovaner DJ, Myles JT. Spirometric measurements in welders. Arch Environ Health 1964; 8:661.
147. Peters JM, Murphy RLH, Ferris BG Jr. Pulmonary function in shipyard welders. Arch Environ Health 1973; 26:28.
148. Fogh A, Frost J, George J. Respiratory symptoms and pulmonary function in welders. Ann Occup Hyg 1969; 12:213.
149. Sjogren B, Ulfvarson U. Respiratory symptoms and pulmonary function among welders working with aluminium, stainless steel, and railroad tracks. Scand J Work Environ Health 1985; 11:27.
150. Antti-Poika M, Hassi J, Pyy L. Respiratory diseases in arc welders. Intern Arch Occup Environ Health 1977; 40:225.
151. McMillan GHG. Studies of the health of welders in naval dockyards. Ann Occup Hyg 1979; 21:377.
152. McMillan GHG. The health of welders in naval dockyards. Final Summary Report. J Royal Nav Med Serv 1983; 69:125.
153. McMillan GHG, Pethybridge RJ. A clinical, radiological and pulmonary function case-control study of 135 dockyard welders aged 45 years and over. J Soc Occup Med 1984; 34:3.
154. Hayden SP, Pincock AC, Hayden J, et al. Respiratory symptoms and pulmonary function of welders in the engineering industry. Thorax 1984; 39:442.
155. Morgan WKC. Airborne free silica: How much? (Chapter 5) In: Gee JBL, ed. Occupational Lung Disease. New York: Churchill Livingstone, 1984, 99–109.
156. Teculescu DB, Stanescu DC, Pilat L. Pulmonary mechanics in silicosis. Arch Environ Health 1967; 14:461.
157. Ziskind M, Jones RN, Weill H. State of the art–silicosis. Am Rev Respir Dis 1976; 113:643.
158. Theriault GP, Peters JM, Johnson WM. Pulmonary function and roentgenographic changes in granite dust exposure. Arch Environ Health 1974; 28:23.
159. Musk AW, Peters JN, Wegman DH, Fine LJ. Pulmonary function in granite dust exposure: a four-year follow-up. Am Rev Respir Dis 1977; 115:769.
160. Morgan WKC. The walrus and the carpenter or the silica criteria standard. J Occup Med 1975; 17:782.
161. Graham WGB, O'Grady RV, Dubuc B. Pulmonary function loss in Vermont granite workers. Am Rev Respir Dis 1981; 123:25.
162. Irwig LM, Rocks P. Lung function and respiratory symptoms in silicotic and nonsilicotic gold miners. Am Rev Respir Dis 1978; 117:429.
163. Becklake MR, Irwig L, Kielkowski D, et al. The predictors of emphysema in South African gold miners. Am Rev Respir Dis 1987; 135:1234.
164. McGee D, Reed D, Yano K. The results of logistic analyses when the variables are highly correlated: an empirical example using diet and CAD incidence. J Chronic Dis 1984; 37:713.
165. Heard BE, Izukawa T. Pulmonary emphysema in fifty consecutive male necropsies in London. J Pathol Bacteriol 1964; 88:423.
166. Ng T-P, Chan S-L, Lam K-P. Radiological progression and lung function in silicosis: A ten year follow-up. Br Med J 1987; 295:164.
167. Zapp JA, Jr. Hazards of isocyanates in polyurethane foam plastic production. AMA Arch Ind Health 1957; 15:324.
168. Gandevia B. Studies of ventilatory capacity and histamine response during exposure to isocyanate vapor in polyurethane foam manufacture. Br J Ind Med 1963; 20:204.
169. Peters JM, Murphy RHL, Pagnotto LD, VanGanse WF. Respiratory impairment in workers exposed to safe levels of toluene diisocyanate (TDI). Arch Environ Health 1970; 20:364.
170. Wegman DH, Peters JM, Pagnotto LD, et al. Chronic pulmonary function loss from exposure to toluene diisocyanate. Br J Ind Med 1975; 34:72.
171. Wegman DH, Musk AW, Main DM, Pagnotto LD. Accelerated loss of FEV_1 in polyurethane production workers; a four year prospective study. Am J Ind Med 1982; 3:209.
172. Adams WGF. Long term effects on the health of men engaged in the manufacture of toluene diisocyanate. Br J Ind Med 1975; 32:72.
173. Butcher BT, Jones RN, O'Neil CE, et al. Longitudinal study of workers employed in the manufacture of toluene-diisocyanate. Am Rev Respir Dis 1977; 116:411.
174. Gee JB, Morgan WKC. A ten year follow up study of a group of workers exposed to isocyanates. J Occup Med 1985; 27:15.
175. Diem JE, Jones RN, Hendrick DJ, et al. Five year longitudinal study of workers employed in a new toluene diisocyanate manufacturing plant. Am Rev Respir Dis 1982; 126:420.

Chapter 31

RELATIONSHIP OF NEONATAL AND CHILDHOOD LUNG DISEASE TO ADULT COPD

Richard J. Martin **Pamela B. Davis**

Although many of the factors that predispose to chronic obstructive pulmonary disease (COPD) are well known, the development of COPD is highly variable even among individuals with similar levels of alpha$_1$-antitrypsin deficiency or similar cumulative cigarette smoke exposure. Other explanations for this variability have been sought. One possibility is that damage to the lung in childhood renders the adult more vulnerable to such factors as the proteolytic damage of uninhibited elastases or to the toxic effects of cigarette smoke. This chapter presents evidence for the possibility that neonatal and childhood lung injury is associated with adult COPD. A number of different childhood lung diseases are possible risk factors for COPD, including chronic neonatal lung disease or bronchopulmonary dysplasia (BPD), viral bronchiolitis, and asthma. The predisposing factors for bronchiectasis, another type of COPD, are not discussed here; however, one of the most frequent causes of severe obstructive lung disease in childhood, cystic fibrosis, is discussed in Chapter 32.

The normal lifelong pattern of change in pulmonary function is one of growth during childhood and adolescence, steady function during young adulthood, and then gradual decline with age, possibly with acceleration of decline in very old age. It follows that development of COPD could be affected by childhood conditions that influence the attainment of maximal pulmonary function with growth, conditions that influence the rate of age-related decline in pulmonary function, or conditions that influence both. If lung damage in childhood prevents pulmonary function levels from ever reaching their expected values, the subject starts from a lower level, and even a normal rate of age-related decline in lung function may produce functional impairment. Thus, conditions that result in lower pulmonary function during childhood and that prevent catch-up growth might be predisposing factors for COPD. Also, conditions that set the stage for accelerated age-related decline in pulmonary function, possibly in combination with another disease promoter, such as tobacco smoke, would also increase risk for COPD. This chapter considers some of these possibilities.

NEONATAL LUNG DISEASE

It is only over the last 2 decades that assisted ventilation has become an integral part of neonatal intensive care. This has been associated with a remarkable decrease in mortality for very low birth weight infants, although longer term morbidity has remained relatively unchanged. Comprehensive follow-up data are emerging for the infant, preschool, and early school-age survivors of modern neonatal intensive care, focusing on both neurodevelopmental and respiratory outcome. Even though the earliest graduates of this era have reached adolescence, scant data exist that pertain to respiratory well-being or pulmonary function at that age. It follows that the impact of acute or chronic neonatal lung disease on adult COPD will remain speculative for many years to come. Nonetheless, the real potential for chronic pediatric lung disease to contribute to chronic disease in adults requires an increasing awareness of these disorders by pulmonologists who care for adult patients.

The Spectrum of Chronic Neonatal Lung Disease

The emergence of chronic neonatal lung disease as a common problem in infants presents a major challenge to pediatricians, including both neonatologists and pediatric pulmonologists. Fortunately most preterm infants with acute pulmonary disease, most commonly manifesting as respiratory distress syndrome (RDS), make a rapid and apparently complete recovery and subsequently appear to have entirely normal lungs. The term bronchopulmonary dysplasia (BPD) was introduced in 1967 by Northway and colleagues[1] to describe a sequence of clinical and radiographic pulmonary changes that developed over weeks in a group of infants with RDS following prolonged assisted ventilation and exposure to high inspired oxygen concentration. Subsequent reports have described a similar chronic course after prolonged assisted ventilation in infants for meconium aspiration syndrome, persistent fetal circulation, diaphragmatic hernia, or pneumonia due to a variety of pathogens.

Bronchopulmonary dysplasia is now recognized as a disease with a much broader spectrum of clinical severity than that of the acute cystic emphysema originally documented by Northway and colleagues. The typical case is characterized by a preterm infant recovering from RDS in whom weaning of inspired oxygen and assisted ventilation comes to a halt in as early as 7 days. A characteristic clinical picture of chronic lung disease then emerges at 20 to 30 days, when recovery from RDS should be long complete. Bancalari and Gerhardt and others have defined BPD as existing in infants who require mechanical ventilation during the first week, are oxygen dependent after at least 28 days, and exhibit persistent increased densities with or without hyperinflation on chest radiographs.[2]

The incidence of BPD in surviving infants who develop RDS and require assisted ventilation is estimated at between 10% and 20%. Thus, BPD represents a great medical and social challenge that could impact considerably on the incidence of chronic lung disease in childhood and adult life.

The exact mechanisms responsible for the morphologic and functional disruption of the lung in infants with BPD have not been clearly established, although many pathophysiologic events are contributory (Fig. 31–1). The macroscopic appearance (in the more severe examined cases at autopsy) constitutes a coarse pattern of scarring mixed with regional emphysema. Reid[3] has proposed that the emphysema arises from a combination of compensatory overinflation, hypoplasia secondary to failure of alveolar multiplication, and both alveolar and capillary destruction. Parts of the vascular bed become condensed in scar tissue, which, together with medial muscular hypertrophy, leads to pulmonary hypertension and an altered hemodynamic state. The real paucity in pathologic data is caused by limited autopsies represented by the most severe end of the BPD spectrum. Development of a primate model of BPD by Coalson and coworkers[4] has confirmed extensive atelectasis with regional overinflation and unique hyperplastic and obliterative changes in the respiratory bronchioles, which may be shown with further studies to contribute to the widespread atelectasis.

Factors Influencing the Progression of Disease

MECHANICAL VENTILATION. It has become widely accepted that barotrauma resulting from apparently excessive pressures used in assisted ventilation is the major culprit in the development of chronic lung injury. The key role played by mechanical ventilation is supported by the fact that BPD is an infrequent complication of the use of nasal continuous positive airway pressure despite prolonged requirements for increased inspired oxygen. The detrimental role of the endotracheal tube itself is difficult to ascertain, as mucosal and ciliary damage may ensue and the drainage of tracheal secretions may be hindered.

Combined morphometric and biochemical evidence for the injurious role of mechanical ventilation on lung growth comes from the work of Hislop and coworkers.[5] Based on 104 perinatal and infant autopsies they were able to characterize lung changes in the presence and absence of prior mechanical ventilation. Infant lungs subjected to mechanical ventilation revealed impaired alveolar number and surface area when related to body weight (Fig. 31–2). The fact that decreased alveolar number was seen in some ventilated infants who had not been exposed to high pressures is consistent with the clinical observation that BPD may develop in immature lungs not apparently exposed to excessive barotrauma. No such abnormality could be determined in the small number of lungs from preterm infants not subjected to assisted ventilation. Biochemical features of ventilated versus normal infant lungs included a high concentration of hydroxyproline, present in collagen and consistent with the structural appearance of thick interalveolar septa. The apparent increase in desmosine in the ventilated infant lungs was restricted to those lungs exhibiting severe damage and can be related to the thick bands of elastic tissue seen in the alveolar and bronchial walls.

Considerable variability exists in the techniques of assisted ventilation administered between various centers, but there is no consensus as to which measure of pressure (peak inspiratory, mean inspiratory, or positive end-expiratory) is most detrimental to the immature lung. A large multicenter trial of high frequency oscillation using a frequency of 900 cycles per minute has failed to demonstrate a decrease in the incidence of airleaks or BPD when compared with conventional ventilation. High frequency jet ventilation from 150 to 600 cycles per minute still holds some promise for decreasing lung injury, as it is possible to ventilate infants at lower peak and mean airway pressures with this technique, although gas exchange remains comparable to that during conventional ventilation.

INCREASED INSPIRED OXYGEN CONCENTRATION. Although pulmonary oxygen toxicity is a major factor in the etiology of BPD, the precise concentration that is toxic probably depends on many variables, such as maturation, nutritional and endocrine status, and duration of exposure to oxygen and other oxidants. The effects of oxygen toxicity appear to include impaired mucociliary transport, altered alveolar and capillary permeability, and influx of leukocytes containing proteolytic enzymes together with inhibition of the antiprotease defense system. To resist the detrimental effects of oxygen toxicity, the body has evolved various antioxidant enzymes, such as superoxide dismutase, while other compounds, such as vitamin E and selenium, also may offer endogenous antioxidant protection. Administration of superoxide dismutase or vitamin E to neonates has, however, failed to demonstrate any sustained benefit in preventing lung injury. Frank and Sosenko[6] have demonstrated in animal models that pulmonary antioxidant enzyme systems increase activity in late gestation in parallel with the enzymes involved in surfactant production. Furthermore, dexamethasone administration augments the pathways in both enzyme systems, suggesting a dual beneficial role in enhancing lung maturation and resisting lung injury in premature lungs. It remains to be determined whether this is a

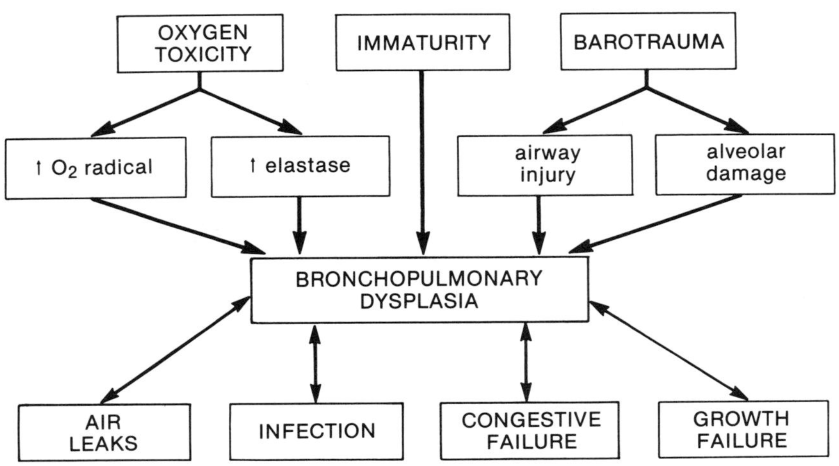

Figure 31–1. Multiple interrelated pathophysiologic events that are thought to contribute to bronchopulmonary dysplasia (BPD).

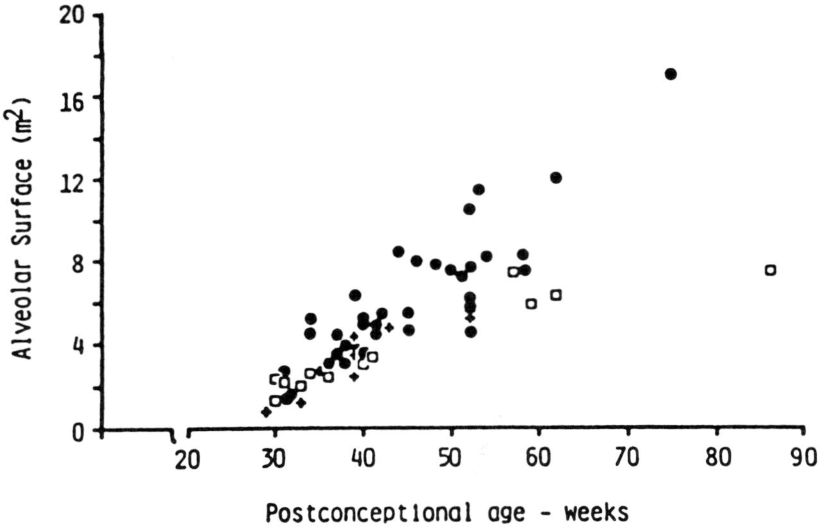

Figure 31–2. Alveolar surface area derived from autopsy data in ventilated versus nonventilated infants at various postconceptional ages. The + represents data from preterm infants with asphyxia or apnea who were ventilated at low pressures; □ represents data from preterm infants with respiratory distress syndrome (RDS) whose ventilator pressure requirements were generally greater than in the above group; and ● represents data from nonventilated control autopsies. The findings suggested that assisted ventilation caused decreased alveolar surface area at autopsy, regardless of the need for high ventilator pressures. (Reproduced with permission from Hislop AA, Wigglesworth JS, Desai R, Aber V. Early Hum Dev 1987; 15:147–164.)

mechanism contributing to the documented beneficial effect of steroids on BPD.

Exogenous surfactant therapy offers real promise as a technique to decrease both ventilatory and oxygen requirements and resultant lung injury. The issue of natural versus synthetic products is not entirely resolved, although purely synthetic surfactant has received less attention in human studies. Jobe and Ikegami[7] have summarized the results of seven clinical trials that enrolled 307 infants from various centers, excluding studies that used exclusively artificial surfactants. Overall there was a 2- to 4-fold decrease in the incidence of airleaks and mortality, although there was no difference in incidence of BPD between surfactant-treated and control groups (Fig. 31–3). Presumably more of the control infants who died would have developed BPD had they survived. Therefore, no evidence exists that the incidence of neonatal chronic lung disease is waning.

NUTRITIONAL DEFICITS. There is increasing recognition that altered nutritional status can impact directly on lung function in infants with chronic respiratory disease and that growth failure is an integral part of BPD. Expenditure of energy is elevated by about 25% over normal in infants with BPD, related in part to the increased work of breathing these infants exhibit. This problem is compounded by the limited possibilities for enteral feeding; poor tolerance for excessive glucose loads, which may result in hypercapnia; and need for strict fluid management. Thus, tissue growth in response to ongoing lung injury remains limited, whereas metal groups and vitamins that provide antioxidant potential become deficient.

Vitamin A has been shown in animal models to promote epithelial cell differentiation, and its deficiency causes squamous metaplasia and injury to the conducting airways. With this background Shenai and colleagues[8] conducted a controlled trial with vitamin A supplementation and demonstrated decreased morbidity associated with BPD in predisposed very low birth weight infants who received vitamin A. This initial report suggests that identification and correction of specific nutrient deficiencies may play a real role in decreasing vulnerability to continuing lung injury in BPD.

INFECTIOUS COMPLICATIONS. Viral, bacterial, and fungal sepsis can all result in profound setbacks for the infant with BPD. Of greater interest is the unknown role played by infection in the etiology of chronic lung injury. The radiographic picture of BPD is certainly indistinguishable from that caused by cytomegalovirus, *Candida*, staphylococci, or gram-negative organisms in infants. As indicated earlier, influx of protease-containing polymorphonuclear leukocytes or macrophages, or both, into the lung may be an important component of the emphysematous changes in these infants.

PULMONARY VASCULAR CHANGES. Infants with BPD frequently have evidence of cor pulmonale, which appears to resolve as lung function improves. Greater pulmonary blood flow secondary to a patent ductus arteriosus may increase interstitial fluid and further impair pulmonary mechanics. Susceptibility to pulmonary edema may relate to abnormal lymphatic drainage or the deleterious effects of right-sided heart failure on left ventricular function, necessitating fluid restriction and diuretic therapy. Capillary permeability may be increased in the lung secondary to endothelial cell injury. Thus, a vicious cycle is established whereby excessive lung fluid compromises lung function, prolonging the need for aggressive respiratory assistance and further aggravating lung injury. It has been proposed that leukotrienes and other vasoactive mediators, myocardial ischemia, and thromboem-

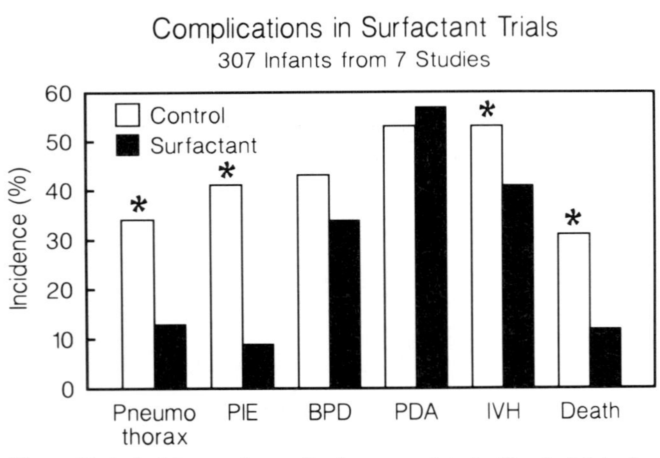

Figure 31–3. Incidence of complications associated with administration of surfactant to human infants with respiratory distress syndrome (RDS). The data are based on seven clinical trials from various centers, excluding studies that employed exclusively artificial surfactants. Surfactant caused significant reduction in airleaks, intraventricular hemorrhage, and mortality (*$P<0.05$). PIE = pulmonary interstitial emphysema; BPD = bronchopulmonary dysplasia; PDA = patent ductus arteriosus; IVH = intraventricular hemorrhage. (Modified from Jobe A, Ikegami M. Am Rev Respir Dis 1987; 136:1256–1275).

bolic phenomena all may contribute to this sequence of events. The extent to which increased pulmonary vascular resistance in infants with BPD is alleviated by increasing levels of partial pressure of oxygen (Po_2) appears variable and may be of prognostic significance.

Physiologic Parameters as Prognostic Indicators

Although BPD has emerged as a major clinical problem, methods for early diagnosis and grading of severity have been imprecise. This problem has hampered clinical trials that seek to perform early therapeutic interventions. Truog and coworkers[9] were unable to predict mortality during the first 2 years of life from need for supplemental oxygen of greater than or less than 40% at 1 month of age. Nonetheless, duration of supplemental inspired oxygen probably is a useful indicator of longer-term outcome, as discussed later.

Goldman and colleagues[10] performed pulmonary function studies during the first week of life to predict development of chronic lung disease in high-risk infants. All enrolled infants required mechanical ventilation for RDS for at least 3 days. There were no differences in lung compliance and distribution of ventilation between infants who did and did not develop BPD. However, mean pulmonary resistance in the infants who developed BPD was approximately 90% higher than that of those who did not. Unfortunately these data do not only allow us to speculate whether high resistance is contributing to lung damage or whether it is an early manifestation of the chronic lung disease itself. High resistance could result from mechanical airway damage or peribronchial edema secondary to heart failure. Use of early elevation of pulmonary resistance as a marker for BPD requires considerably more evidence and a clearer understanding of underlying mechanisms. Bronchodilators play an important role in acute management of BPD, indicating that airway obstruction is at least partially reversible; however, the impact of such therapy on longer-term outcome is unknown. Furthermore, theophylline has potential effects other than bronchodilatation, such as decreased respiratory pauses and enhanced diaphragmatic contractility.

Healthy preterm infants have been thought to have insufficient bronchial smooth muscle to produce significant bronchoconstriction, although objective data are lacking. Nonetheless, infants with BPD do have pathologic evidence of bronchiolar smooth muscle hypertrophy. Motoyama and colleagues[11] evaluated deflation flow volume curves, a possibly sensitive index of lower airway function, in sedated, ventilated preterm infants developing BPD. Airway reactivity was defined by an increase in respiratory flow at a fixed volume in response to a bronchodilator aerosol. Infants with developing chronic lung injury demonstrated relief of lower airway obstruction by 2 to 4 weeks postnatal age. Severity of airway reactivity at initial testing during the first postnatal weeks seemed to predict the severity and duration of respiratory failure. Thus, increased airway reactivity may lead to bronchospasm early in postnatal life; its role in the longer-term outcome of BPD needs further study.

Longer-Term Prognosis

The long-term outcome for infants with chronic lung disease clearly depends on the extent of their initial disease, which covers a broad spectrum of severity, as indicated. A small but significant proportion of infants with severe BPD die prior to, or shortly after, discharge from the hospital. Although often labeled as episodes of sudden infant death, this outcome may be associated with acute respiratory infections or cardiac failure triggered by myocardial ischemia or hypoxemia-induced pulmonary hypertension. The prolonged stay of severely affected infants may be reduced considerably if oxygen administration can occur at home, and this should be encouraged if the parents' abilities and home environment are optimal. Resultant benefits include improved parent-infant bonding and sensory stimulation, significant monetary savings, and decreased risk of nosocomially acquired respiratory pathogens.

Although the oldest survivors of BPD are barely 20 years old, increasing numbers of studies are being reported regarding the neurodevelopmental and pulmonary outcomes of these infants.

NEURODEVELOPMENTAL HANDICAP. The incidence of neurologic and developmental deficits in survivors with BPD varies widely, related in large part to differences in patient selection criteria. Shankaran and colleagues[12] related developmental indices to duration of time the infants received supplemental oxygen. In their small series they noted that infants with subnormal developmental scores had a mean time in oxygen of 84 days versus a mean of 46 days oxygen for those with subsequently normal scores. Thus, outcome could be related to severity of pulmonary disease as reflected in the need for prolonged oxygen therapy. Several studies have demonstrated a higher incidence of growth and developmental delays in infants with BPD, using the Northway[1] criteria for diagnosis of BPD. Later data have demonstrated less evidence for developmental impairment in BPD infants when diagnostic criteria for chronic lung disease have been liberalized and based primarily only on oxygen requirement at 28 days.

PULMONARY FUNCTION AND MORBIDITY. Sauve and Singhal[13] documented the outcome of a large number of infants diagnosed as having BPD between 1975 and 1982 in comparison to a control group who also received assisted ventilation during the first week of life. *Lower* respiratory tract infections and rehospitalization for respiratory illnesses were significantly more common in the BPD group but only during the first year of life. The incidence of multiple *upper* respiratory infections appeared comparable between groups of all ages. These data are encouraging for longer term morbidity and in keeping with the tendency for BPD to improve over time. Myers and coworkers[14] prospectively compared the frequency and severity of subsequent respiratory illness over the first 12 months in preterm infants with or without a history of RDS with similar events in term infants. Overall, preterm infants did not demonstrate an inherent risk for subsequent infection when compared with term infants. Infants who survived RDS and developed residual lung disease, however, had both more frequent and more severe subsequent lower respiratory illnesses over the first year. Thus, these data also suggest that later respiratory morbidity is a consequence of residual pulmonary abnormalities apparent on chest radiograph at discharge from the nursery and consistent with most diagnostic criteria for BPD.

Concurrent with these evaluations of persistent respiratory symptoms in infants, lung function has been systematically determined in infants with chronic lung disease. Tepper and colleagues[15] evaluated lung function during the first year of life in infants with BPD (as diagnosed by Northway's criteria[1]) and age-matched controls. In addition to a low functional residual capacity (FRC), BPD infants had flattened expiratory flow-volume curves and very limited expiratory flow reserve during rapid chest compression performed at about 1 year of age (Fig. 31–4). These data suggest abnormal functional development in the infants' small airways. Unlike the alveoli, the absolute number of conducting airways is fixed prior to the neonatal period. It is unclear whether the changes in resistance documented previously are the result of neonatal lung injury or whether the early injury has interfered with subsequent normal growth and development.

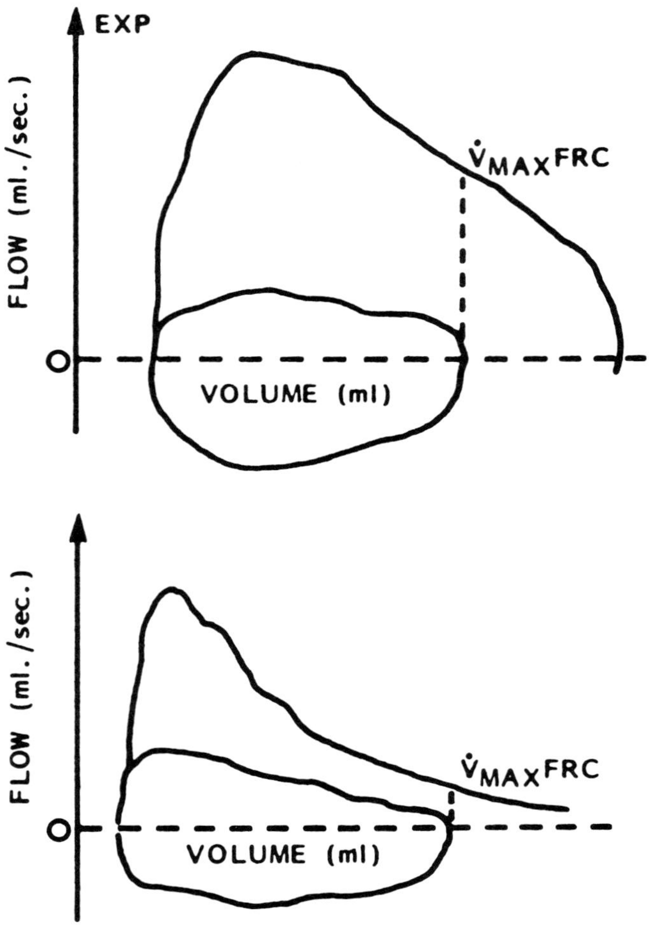

Figure 31–4. Partial expiratory flow-volume curve determinations in infants. The smaller inner curve represents tidal breathing, and the larger curve represents maximal expiratory flow generated by rapid chest compression. The data demonstrate both maximal expiratory flow at functional residual capacity, and the difference between flow during tidal breathing and maximal expiratory flow, also referred to as expiratory flow reserve. The healthy control infant (above) has a convex maximal expiratory flow-volume curve with a large expiratory flow reserve, whereas the infant with BPD (below) has a concave flow-volume curve, with decreased expiratory flow reserve. (Reproduced with permission from Tepper RS, Morgan WJ, Cota K, Taussig LM. J Pediatr 1986; 109:1040–1046.)

Gerhardt and coworkers[16] measured pulmonary function over the first 36 months in 39 infants with BPD and 40 normal growing infants who served as controls. Many of the infants with BPD did have milder disease defined as 28 days of supplemental oxygen and persistent but nonspecific radiographic changes. Functional residual capacity corrected for body weight was decreased over the first 6 months but then normalized with no evidence of gas trapping (Fig. 31–5). Lung compliance also began at subnormal levels but increased to near normal levels by 3 years. The close correlation between compliance and weight suggested that the observed increase in compliance with age related to lung growth and formation of new alveoli. Finally, pulmonary conductance began at low levels, increased little during the first 6 months, but then reached 85% of normal levels by 3 years of age. Thus, increased pulmonary resistance did not appear to be a major residual problem in these infants whose pulmonary function was steadily improving with growth.

Several years earlier Smyth and colleagues[17] studied nine infants with BPD at a mean age of 8 years. In this group persistent respiratory symptoms were common with both air trapping and abnormal chest radiographs. Spirometry demonstrated evidence of airway obstruction; salbutamol aerosol inhalation improved forced expiratory flow in many of the group. Thus, at least for some children, abnormal pulmonary function does not resolve in early childhood. Persistence of airway damage is the likely cause of their airway hyperreactivity and frequent wheezing episodes. Although a high incidence of asthma has been reported in the families of infants with BPD, suggesting a genetic predisposition to airway hyperreactivity in BPD, this remains controversial. Bertrand and colleagues[18] have studied 7- to 12-year-old survivors of RDS, comparable preterm infants without history of lung disease, and their siblings. Airway reactivity was positive in both preterm groups when compared with that in term infants. The investigators concluded that (1) infants with RDS have evidence of airway reactivity as a consequence of RDS severity and its treatment, and (2) preterm infants without RDS have airflow limitation related to familial airway hyperreactivity. This led the investigators to speculate that unexplained premature labor may share a common pathway with airway lability. In severely affected children pulmonary vascular resistance may remain elevated, and there may be a fall in response to oxygen administration, resembling the findings in adults with COPD.

Summary

Because the oldest survivors of chronic neonatal lung injury are only 20 years old, long-term outlook well into adult life must remain speculative. It may actually take a lifetime before its full impact on the incidence of adult COPD is established. As we await the results of long-term prospective studies of large numbers of BPD survivors, other factors, such as infection, atopic disposition, smoking, air pollution, and socioeconomic factors, inevitably complicate the issue. The prevention of further respiratory insult during childhood has become mandatory in these patients. The use of both standard and new pediatric immunizations should be important in minimizing further airway injury. Both parental smoking and smoking by the patients themselves as they grow into adolescence should be vigorously discouraged. Overall, the short- and medium-term outlook for pulmonary function in the majority of survivors of prematurity with chronic neonatal lung disease remains very encouraging.

CHILDHOOD LUNG DISEASE

Lower Respiratory Infections

As already indicated, survivors of neonatal lung devastation are only now reaching adulthood, so data directly linking the development of COPD (generally a phenomenon of middle to old age) and BPD are lacking. However, considerable circumstantial evidence is available that suggests that other lower respiratory diseases in childhood are associated with the development and progression of COPD in adults. Initial evidence came from epidemiologic investigations in adults, in whom childhood respiratory illnesses were documented by the taking of patients' histories.

Adults who report having had lung disease in childhood were found to have lower airflow in cross-sectional studies, more rapid age- and smoking-related decline in pulmonary function, or more current respiratory symptoms associated with COPD.[19–21] However, self-reports are subject to recall

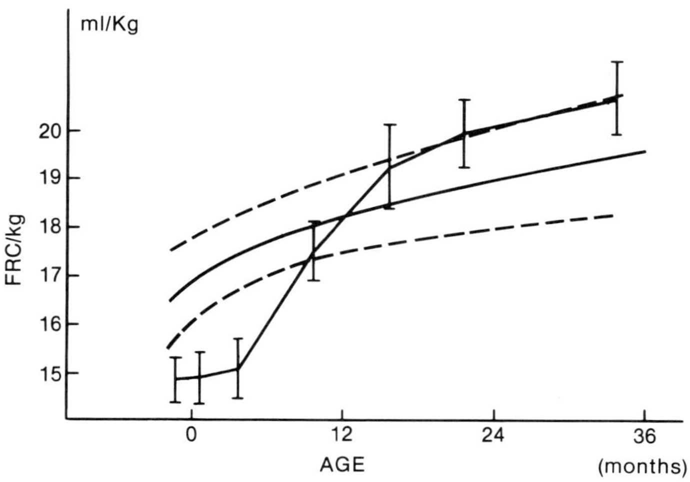

Figure 31–5. Sequential measurements of functional residual capacity (FRC) per kg bodyweight (with standard error of the mean for each point indicated by vertical bars) in infants with chronic lung disease. For comparison a curve is shown for healthy infants with its 95% confidence limits. The data indicate that FRC, corrected for weight, increases to the normal range by approximately 18 months in this group of infants. (Reproduced with permission from Gerhardt T, Hehre D, Feller R, et al. J Pediatr 1987; 110:448–456.)

bias, that is, the likelihood that current symptoms affect the recall of past events. Those with current symptoms are more likely to recall a similar illness in the past, and those who are currently well are less likely to report past illness, making these studies flawed. Recall bias may be reduced, although not eliminated, by using the parents as a source of information about childhood illness and making inquiries closer to the time of the illness. The published studies of this type are strikingly concordant. Several investigators in Great Britain and Australia have shown that children who had lower respiratory illness early in life by parental report have lower airflow later in childhood.[22–24] However, in these studies, the definitions of pneumonia and bronchitis were often imprecise. Still less recall bias is introduced in studies in which the questionnaire data on respiratory illness early in life are obtained from the parents early in the child's life, and pulmonary function or respiratory symptoms are measured longitudinally thereafter. In these studies as well, an excess of respiratory symptoms is present in children who had lower respiratory infections in infancy, and their airflow also appears to be slightly but significantly impaired.[25–32] Because of shifting symptom histories with time, imprecise definition of the childhood events, residual recall bias, lack of pulmonary function measurements in some cases, lack of follow-up into adulthood in most cases, and difficulties in extrapolating from pulmonary function in childhood to pulmonary function later in life, these studies are not definitive. Nevertheless, the data, taken together, are strongly suggestive that childhood lower respiratory illness is associated with COPD later in life.

A different strategy for approaching this question is to select as subjects a group of children hospitalized for bronchiolitis and a control group who were not hospitalized, track the patients, and follow pulmonary function tests and airway reactivity. Although this approach eliminates recall bias, it is subject to incomplete tracking of the subject pool. Also, interpretation of the results is limited by the study design, for only the most severely affected children with bronchiolitis are hospitalized, and thus the implications of milder illness for later functional impairment cannot be ascertained. Nevertheless the results are in accord with the questionnaire studies. Pulmonary function has been found to be impaired, airway reactivity more prevalent, and symptoms of airway reactivity increased in the bronchiolitis group.[33–38] Another viral infection that has been associated with later pulmonary sequelae is croup. Increased airway reactivity is found in children who had croup.[39, 40]

The association between childhood lower respiratory illness and later development of COPD may not be causal, although the childhood illness clearly predates the development of COPD. There might, for example, be some genetic predisposition to airways disease that makes both symptomatic childhood lower respiratory infection and development and progression of COPD in adulthood more likely in a particular individual. Airway reactivity is frequently observed at follow-up of children with BPD,[17] bronchiolitis,[35–38] and croup,[39, 40] and airway reactivity has been proposed as a risk factor for development and progression of obstructive pulmonary disease.[41] One can imagine that a child with increased airway reactivity would be more likely to become symptomatic from bronchiolitis, more likely to be hospitalized, or that his or her parents would be more likely to recall childhood bronchiolitis if it were severe or were accompanied by noisy, "wheezy" breathing. Thus, airway reactivity might link childhood respiratory illness and adult COPD. These relationships are at present just associations, however, and causality cannot be inferred.

Asthma

Certainly if airway reactivity is a risk factor for development and progression of COPD, then patients with the prototypic disease of airway reactivity, asthma, might be at increased risk. Because a substantial portion of childhood asthmatics remain asthmatic in adulthood, thus displaying persistently increased airway reactivity, at least these childhood asthmatics are probably at increased risk for COPD.

Airway reactivity in childhood, however, appears to be associated with poorer pulmonary function in children. In one study, children who were consistently hyperresponsive to cold air challenge had worse pulmonary function than those who never responded, and children who were intermittently responsive fell in between the two groups.[42] The close associations among lower respiratory infection, atopy, asthma, airway reactivity, personal and maternal cigarette smoking, and familial factors, however, make it hard to separate any one effect.

Mechanisms

A mechanism by which airway reactivity, or the tendency to develop reversible reduced airflow in response to an exogenous irritant, might develop into permanent functional impairment has not been established. Because airway reactivity implies a rapid response, the usual mechanism invoked is bronchial smooth muscle constriction, although edema formation, mucus secretion, and vascular engorgement are possibilities. Perhaps with repeated cycles smooth muscle hypertrophy occurs. One may also speculate that, because of the close association between inflammation and airway reactivity, airway reactivity represents an exaggerated tendency toward inflammation. Perhaps in reactive individuals the epithelium produces chemotaxins for neutrophils on irritation, and an inflammatory cycle is set up that is never entirely reversed but becomes cumulative day by day and year by year. The biochemical mechanisms, however, await further investigation.

A direct causal relationship is also possible between childhood respiratory infection and adult COPD, although the biochemical mechanisms are obscure. A precedent exists for a single devastating viral infection leaving permanent lung devastation in its wake; witness the development of bronchiectasis following infection with adenovirus or influenza.[43] Viral infections of sufficient severity might cause structural damage to the lower airways sufficient to predispose to later lung damage. In support of this hypothesis are studies in rats that show that animals infected in the first 5 days of life with Sendai virus have narrower airways at maturity than uninfected animals or animals infected later in life, although the histology of the airways appears to be normal to light microscopy.[44] It is also possible that physiologic changes are introduced into the airway by such infections. Viral infections might induce functional alterations, such as hypertrophy and hyperplasia of the smooth muscle, thereby increasing contractility and bronchial responsiveness, hypertrophy, and hyperplasia of the mucus-secreting apparatus, damage to the respiratory epithelium, alteration of neural innervation, and connective tissue alterations that could affect the quantity or geometry of lung growth.

It has also been speculated that viral infection leads to increased airway reactivity, or to atopy, which the Tucson epidemiologic study has associated with COPD.[45] Viral infections may lead to reduced beta-adrenergic responsiveness,[46] and if autonomic imbalance predisposes the patient to airway reactivity or to atopy,[47] this disturbance might provide a mechanism whereby viral infections could have far-reaching effects. Viral infection may have a greater impact on the airways of infants than those of older persons. Why infants are more vulnerable is unclear. If, however, airway reactivity increases vulnerability to long-term sequelae, findings that infants have greater decrement in airflow in response to irritants than adults[48] suggest one possible mechanism. Could this confer additional vulnerability to airway injury on infants? Again, the mechanisms are unclear.

Knowledge of the mechanism by which COPD develops following childhood infection or asthma is important for developing strategies for prevention of COPD. If severe lower respiratory infection in childhood is merely a marker for some underlying predisposition to COPD, then prevention or amelioration of the childhood infections, as with vaccines or aggressive immunotherapy or antiviral chemotherapy, will have little impact on the subsequent risk, and attention must be directed at the true predisposing factor. However, in this case severe lower respiratory infection may identify a child requiring special preventive efforts. If, on the other hand, the viral infection contributes directly to the subsequent lung damage, then prevention of infection may be critical in reducing lifetime morbidity. If childhood airway reactivity is strongly associated with later vulnerability to COPD, could treatment of airway reactivity (not merely optimizing pulmonary function in asthmatic patients but minimizing airways responsiveness pharmacologically) be of benefit? It would seem, in any case, that children with lower respiratory disease of any sort represent a special target population for antismoking campaigns.

REFERENCES

1. Northway WH Jr, Rosan RC, Porter DY. Pulmonary disease following respiratory therapy of hyaline-membrane disease. N Engl J Med 1967; 276:357–368.
2. Bancalari E, Gerhardt T. Bronchopulmonary dysplasia. Pediatr Clin North Am 1986; 33:1–23.
3. Reid L. Bronchopulmonary dysplasia-pathology. J Pediatr 1979; 95:836–841.
4. Coalson JJ, Kuehl TJ, Escobedo MB, et al. A baboon model of bronchopulmonary dysplasia. II. Pathologic features. Exp Mol Pathol 1982; 37:335–350.
5. Hislop AA, Wigglesworth JS, Desai R, Aber V. The effects of preterm delivery and mechanical ventilation on human lung growth. Early Hum Dev 1987; 15:147–164.
6. Frank L, Sosenko RS. Development of lung antioxidant enzyme system in late gestation: Possible implications for the prematurely born infant. J Pediatr 1987; 110:9–14.
7. Jobe A, Ikegami M. Surfactant for the treatment of respiratory distress syndrome. Am Rev Respir Dis 1987; 136:1256–1275.
8. Shenai JP, Kennedy KA, Chytil F, Stahlman MT. Clinical trial of vitamin A supplementation in infants susceptible to bronchopulmonary dysplasia. J Pediatr 1987; 111:269–277.
9. Truog WE, Jackson JC, Badura RJ, et al. Bronchopulmonary dysplasia and pulmonary insufficiency of prematurity. Am J Dis Child 1985; 139:351–354.
10. Goldman SL, Gerhardt T, Sonni R, et al. Early prediction of chronic lung disease by pulmonary function testing. J Pediatr 1983; 102:613–617.
11. Motoyama EK, Fort MD, Klesh KW, et al. Early onset of airway reactivity in premature infants with bronchopulmonary dysplasia. Am Rev Respir Dis 1987; 136:50–57.
12. Shankaran S, Szego E, Eizert D, Siegel P. Severe bronchopulmonary dysplasia: predictors of survival and outcome. Chest 1984; 86:607–610.
13. Sauve RS, Singhal N. Long-term morbidity of infants with bronchopulmonary dysplasia. Pediatrics 1985; 76:725–733.
14. Myers MG, McGuinness GA, Lachenbruch PA, et al. Respiratory illnesses in survivors of infant respiratory distress syndrome. Am Rev Respir Dis 1986; 133:1011–1018.
15. Tepper RS, Morgan WJ, Cota K, Taussig LM. Expiratory flow limitation in infants with bronchopulmonary dysplasia. J Pediatr 1986; 109:1040–1046.
16. Gerhardt T, Hehre D, Feller R, et al. Serial determination of pulmonary function in infants with chronic lung disease. J Pediatr 1987; 110:448–456.
17. Smyth JA, Tabachnik E, Duncan WJ, et al. Pulmonary function and bronchial hyperreactivity in long-term survivors of bronchopulmonary dysplasia. Pediatrics 1981; 68:336–340.
18. Bertrand JM, Riley SP, Popkin J, Coates AL. The long-term pulmonary sequelae of prematurity: The role of familial airway hyperreactivity and the respiratory distress syndrome. N Engl J Med 1985; 312:742–745.
19. Oswald NC, Harold JT, Martin WJ. Clinical pattern of chronic bronchitis. Lancet 1953; ii:639–643.
20. Fletcher C, Peto R, Tinker C, Speizer FE. The Natural History of Chronic Bronchitis and Emphysema. Oxford: Oxford University Press, 1976.
21. Burrows B, Knudson RJ, Lebowitz MD. The relationship of childhood respiratory illness to adult obstructive airway disease. Am Rev Respir Dis 1977; 115:751–760.
22. Colley JRT, Reid DD. Urban and social origins of childhood bronchitis in England and Wales. Br Med J 1970; 2:213–217.
23. Yarnell JWG, St Leger AS. Respiratory illness, maternal smoking habit and lung function in children. Br J Dis Chest 1979; 73:230–236.
24. Yarnell JWG, St Leger AS. Respiratory infections and their influence on lung function in children: a multiple regression analysis. Thorax 1981; 36:847–851.
25. Colley JRT, Douglas JWB, Reid DD. Respiratory disease in young adults: influence of early childhood lower respiratory tract

illness, social class, air pollution, and smoking. Br Med J 1973; 3:195–198.
26. Kiernan KE, Colley JRT, Douglas JWB, Reid DD. Chronic cough in young adults in relation to smoking habits, childhood environment and chest illness. Respiration 1976; 33:236–244.
27. Miller FJW, Court SDM, Know EG, Brandon S. The school years in Newcastle-upon-Tyne. London: Oxford University Press, 1974.
28. Lunn JE, Knowelden J, Roe JW. Patterns of respiratory illness in Sheffield junior school-children. A follow-up study. Br J Prev Soc Med 1970; 24:223–228.
29. Holland WW, Bailey P, Bland JM. Long-term consequences of respiratory disease in infancy. J Epidemiol Community Health 1978; 32:256–259.
30. Leeder SR, Corkhill RT, Irwig LM, et al. Influence of family factors on asthma and wheezing during the first five years of life. Br J Prev Soc Med 1976; 30:213–218.
31. Martin AJ, Landau LI, Phelan PD. Lung function in young adults who had asthma in childhood. Am Rev Respir Dis 1980; 122:609–615.
32. Woolcock AJ, Leeder SR, Peat JK, Blackburn CRB. The influence of lower respiratory illness in infancy and childhood and subsequent cigarette smoking on lung function in Sydney schoolchildren. Am Rev Respir Dis 1979; 120:5–14.
33. Stokes GM, Milner AD, Hodges IGC, Groggins RC. Lung function abnormalities after acute bronchiolitis. J Pediatr 1981; 98:871–884.
34. Kattan M, Keens TG, Lapierre JG, et al. Pulmonary function abnormalities in symptom-free children after bronchiolitis. Pediatrics 1977; 59:683–688.
35. Sims DG, Downham MPAS, Gardner PS, et al. Study of 8-year-old children with a history of respiratory syncytial virus bronchiolitis in infancy. Br Med J 1987; 1:11–14.
36. Gurwitz D, Mindorff C, Levison H. Increased incidence of bronchial reactivity in children with a history of bronchiolitis. J Pediatr 1981; 98:551–555.
37. Pullan CR, Hey EN. Wheezing, asthma, and pulmonary dysfunction 10 years after infection with respiratory syncytial virus in infancy. Br Med J 1982; 284:1665–1669.
38. Rooney JC, Williams HE. The relationship between proved viral bronchiolitis and subsequent wheezing. J Pediatr 1971; 79:744–777.
39. Zach M, Eiben A, Olinsky A. Croup, recurrent croup, allergy and airways hyperreactivity. Arch Dis Child 1981; 56:336–341.
40. Gurwitz D, Corey M, Levison H. Pulmonary function and bronchial reactivity in children after croup. Am Rev Respir Dis 1980; 122:95–99.
41. Weiss ST. Increased levels of airways responsiveness as a risk factor for development of chronic obstructive lung disease. Chest 1984; 86:3–4.
42. Redline S, Weiss ST, Tager IB, et al. Longitudinal assessment of the relationship between bronchial responsiveness and lung growth. Am Rev Respir Dis 1987; 135:A380.
43. Davis PB, Hubbard VS, Taussig LM, McCoy K. Medical progress: familial bronchiectasis. J Pediatr 1983; 102:177–185.
44. Castleman WL. Alteration in pulmonary ultrastructure and morphometric parameters induced by parainfluenza (Sendai) virus in rats during postnatal growth. Am J Pathol 1984; 114:322–335.
45. Burrows B, Bloom JW, Traverse GA, Cline MG. The course and prognosis of different forms of chronic airways obstruction in a sample from the general population. N Engl J Med 1987; 317:1309–1314.
46. Busse WW. Decreased granulocyte response to isoproterenol in asthma during upper respiratory infections. Am Rev Respir Dis 1977; 115:783–791.
47. Kaliner M, Shelhamer J, Smith L, et al. NIH Conference. Autonomic nervous system abnormalities and allergy. Ann Intern Med 1982; 96:349–357.
48. Geller DE, Morgan WJ, Cota KA, et al. Airway responsiveness to cold, dry air in normal infants. Pediatr Pulmonol 1988; 4:90–97.

Section VI

THE RELATIONSHIP OF CHRONIC OBSTRUCTIVE PULMONARY DISEASE TO OTHER RESPIRATORY DISEASES

Chapter 32

CYSTIC FIBROSIS: A MAJOR CAUSE OF OBSTRUCTIVE AIRWAYS DISEASE IN THE YOUNG

Pamela B. Davis

The most common cause of pulmonary insufficiency in the first 3 decades of life (and one of the top 15 causes of death in children) is cystic fibrosis (CF), an autosomal recessive genetic disorder. The main cause of death is respiratory insufficiency due to chronic obstructive pulmonary disease (COPD). About 30,000 people in America have CF: it affects about 1 in 2500 live births among whites, about 1 in 17,000 blacks, and about 1 in 90,000 orientals. These data imply that 4% to 5% of white Americans carry this lethal gene, though in heterozygotes it appears to have no serious consequences. At present, CF in its homozygous form is inevitably fatal, though the median survival age has increased from less than 1 year when it was first described in the 1930s to about 25 years in recent times. Because of its prevalence and severity, CF deserves consideration as a major cause of fatal airway obstruction in young people.

DIAGNOSIS
(Table 32–1)

Cystic fibrosis is recognized by the diagnostic triad of a high concentration of salt in the sweat in combination with chronic obstructive pulmonary disease of appropriate character, or exocrine pancreatic insufficiency, or both (Table 32–1).[1] The sweat chloride concentration is a laboratory test of remarkable discriminant power in clinical medicine (Fig. 32–1). Among children with CF 98% have a sweat chloride concentration of over 60 mEq/L, 1% to 2% have concentrations of 50 to 60 mEq/L, and only 0.1% have less than 50 mEq/L, whereas nearly all children who do not have CF have a sweat chloride concentration of less than 60 mEq/L.[2] The few disease states in which the sweat chloride concentration is high are easily distinguishable from CF on clinical grounds (untreated adrenal insufficiency, ectodermal dysplasia, untreated hypothyroidism, renal diabetes insipidus, some types of glycogen storage disease, and a few others). Though more adults have higher sweat chloride concentrations (in 4% the sweat chloride is over 60 mEq/L and in 1%, over 80 mEq/L), an elevated sweat chloride concentration in the appropriate clinical setting is still diagnostic for CF.[3]

TABLE 32–1. Diagnostic Criteria for Cystic Fibrosis

Sweat Cl concentration >60 mEq/L
and either
Pancreatic insufficiency
or
Chronic suppurative progressive pulmonary disease
or
Both
Alternative: Diagnosis by RFLP analysis (requires siblings' and parents' DNA)

An elevated sweat chloride concentration by itself is not sufficient to make the diagnosis of CF: it must be accompanied by either exocrine pancreatic insufficiency or chronic pulmonary disease. Exocrine pancreatic insufficiency occurs in 80% to 90% of patients with CF. The definitive test for exocrine pancreatic insufficiency—analysis of duodenal fluid for trypsin and chymotrypsin—is rarely performed because it is difficult, tedious, and invasive. However, in diagnostic dilemmas, this test can reveal a reduced bicarbonate output in response to secretin, even in patients who produce adequate quantities of enzymes,[4] and this may confirm an otherwise questionable diagnosis. A less invasive test, the determination of 72-hour stool fat, requires a high-fat diet and collection of stool for 3 days, a procedure that many patients find unacceptable. Alternative tests, such as the benzyltyrosyl para-aminobenzoic acid test, measurement of stool trypsin and chymotrypsin content (in infants), and measurement of immunoreactive trypsin or the pancreatic isozyme of amylase in the serum or the level of carotene in the serum, have been used to distinguish patients with pancreatic insufficiency, but each of these tests has some possibility of error and misclassification.[5–7]

The third diagnostic criterion for CF is chronic obstructive pulmonary disease of appropriate character—suppurative and progressive. The typical respiratory flora is often an important clue. The presence of mucoid *Pseudomonas aeruginosa* in the sputum of CF patients (though occasionally seen in other patients with bronchiectasis) is so characteristic of CF that it has been proposed as a diagnostic criterion itself.[8] Other features of the CF lung disease are chronic cough and sputum production, roentgenographic abnormalities consistent with bronchiectasis, often with upper lobe and right-sided predominance, and pulmonary function tests indicating an obstructive ventilatory defect.[9]

Although the presence of a sibling or first cousin with CF is of great diagnostic assistance, it is prudent to require some clinical manifestation of CF in addition to elevated sweat chloride concentration before making a definitive diagnosis. However, the quality and accuracy of restriction fragment length polymorphism (RFLP) analysis of DNA are such that if DNA is available from a known CF patient and both parents, and the family is informative (as over 98% now are), RFLP diagnosis of a sibling of a known CF patient may be accepted

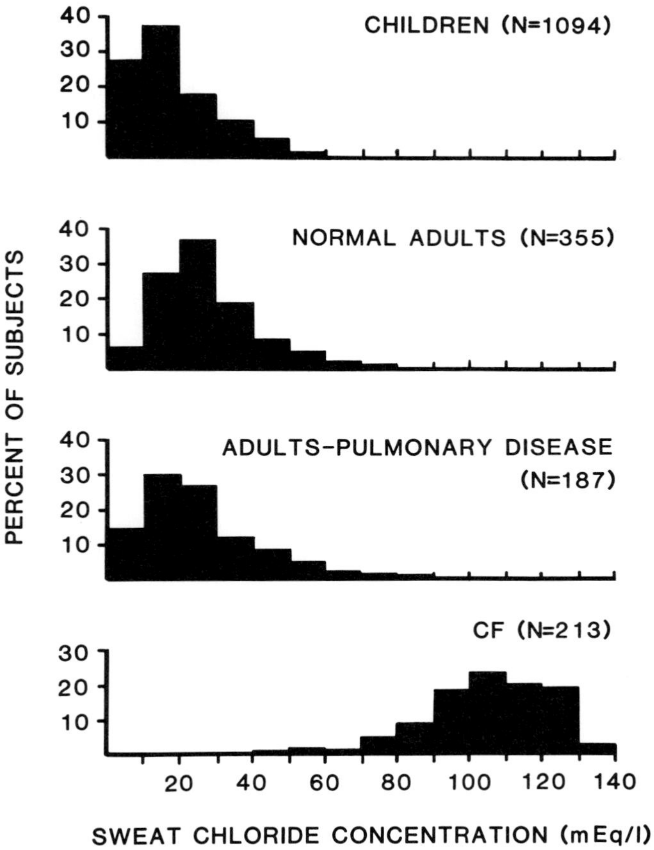

Figure 32–1. Distribution of sweat chloride concentrations in children who do not have CF, normal adults, adults with pulmonary disease who do not have CF, and patients with CF. There is almost no overlap between CF and non-CF children and only 4% of adults have a sweat chloride concentration greater than 60 mEq/L. (Reproduced with permission from Davis PB, di Sant'Agnese PA. Chest 1984; 85:802–809.)

as definitive. When the gene itself becomes available, it is likely that genetic (DNA) diagnosis of CF will be definitive for almost anyone.

Ancillary features of CF that are helpful in making the diagnosis (but are not diagnostic) include the presence of sinusitis (nearly universal in adults with CF in the United States), azoospermia in men, a history of intestinal obstruction or high fecal impaction, meconium ileus (very few babies with meconium ileus have diseases other than CF), unexplained cirrhosis, and gallstones outside of the usual epidemiologic setting.[1, 2, 8]

Several studies have been conducted on early diagnosis of CF patients by elevated serum immunoreactive trypsin (IRT) concentrations.[10–12] These analyses can be done on the blood spots collected from newborn infants for testing for phenylketonuria, are inexpensive (less than $1.00 per test), and identify a large portion (probably over 80%) of infants with CF. Unfortunately, the IRT test is not very specific (about four to five non-CF infants are identified for every child with CF), so an elevated sweat chloride concentration and a compatible clinical syndrome are still required for definitive diagnosis.

THE BASIC DEFECT

Cystic fibrosis is finally yielding to persistent efforts to understand the basic defect. At the gene level, the site of the error has been localized to within a million base pairs and will almost surely be known when this comes to print. All families studied so far have the CF lesion on the long arm of chromosome 7, between the *met* oncogene and an anonymous probe called J3.11 (D7S8), which lie 1 to 3 million base pairs apart.[13] Restriction fragment length polymorphism (RFLP) analysis can now identify the genotype of family members of a CF proband with great certainty, and when the gene itself is in hand, unambiguous identification of the CF genetic status of anyone will be possible. Identification of the gene also holds out the tantalizing prospect of being able to work from the abnormal gene to the abnormal protein and thus to obtain clues to the physiologic defect.

The genetic data also indicate that all CF patients studied so far have the lesion at the same site on the chromosome, suggesting a lesion in the same gene. In addition, other haplotypes on chromosome 7 are in linkage disequilibrium with CF,[14] possibly due to founder effect. This opens the interesting possibility that other genetic variations are preferentially transferred with the CF gene and may provide a biologic explanation for some of the phenomena associated with CF, which are apparently genetically based but inconsistent from family to family.

At the functional level, a block in passive chloride permeability at the epithelial surface appears to be the common denominator for tissues affected by CF. It now appears that this striking and regular elevation of the sweat chloride concentration is caused by a block of a chloride channel on the luminal surface of the duct, preventing reabsorption of salt as the sweat passes along the duct[15] (Fig. 32–2). This block in passive chloride permeability is sufficient to explain all the electrochemical observations that have been made in the CF sweat duct. A similar block in passive chloride conductance is present in the airway epithelium[16]—the first time a physiologic abnormality has been found to link the lung and the sweat duct. In the airway, however, all the electrochemical observations are not explained by passive chloride permeability alone, and other lesions must be postulated. In addition, how the abnormality in ion transport in the airway translates into the CF lung disease is unclear. The presence of a comparable ion transport abnormality in the pancreas has not been established, owing to the inaccessibility of the organ, but in the intestine, passive chloride permeability also appears to be blocked in CF.[17] A common functional characteristic of several affected tissues suggests that this physiologic lesion may be very close to the basic defect itself.

The failure of chloride to pass across epithelial surfaces may be due to the absence of a functional channel in these tissues, or to a failure of the channel to open. Patch-clamp studies

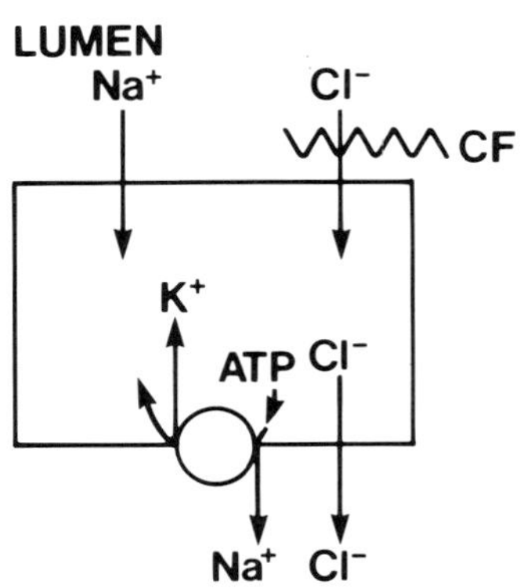

Figure 32–2. Diagram of sweat duct cell illustrating a CF lesion. Ordinarily sodium and chloride are resorbed across the apical membrane. In CF, apical chloride permeability is absent. Since chloride cannot be resorbed on the apical surface, the salt content of the sweat in the lumen is greatly elevated.

have demonstrated that chloride channels with electrical properties identical to normal are present in patches of CF airway epithelial cells that have been removed from the cell, but not in cell-attached patches, indicating that channels are present in CF tissues but are seldom open in the intact cell.[18, 19] These channels fail to respond to the major intracellular regulator for normal channels, cAMP, but the CF cells appear to be capable of responding to calcium, suggesting a lesion in signal transduction in the cAMP system in CF. However, CF epithelial cells have normal ability to generate cAMP and normal cAMP-dependent protein kinase. The addition of protein kinase and its substrate to CF membrane patches fails to increase their open time, as it does in a normal cell.[20] Therefore, the protein kinase mechanism is capable of regulating the chloride channel in normal cells but fails to do so in CF. Thus, the lesion in CF cells is most likely distal to the protein kinase. It will be important to distinguish a lesion in the chloride channel itself (inability to be modified and regulated) from a more general lesion in signal transduction, which could have broader implications for other regulated systems besides ion transport.

PULMONARY DISEASE

Babies born with CF who die of meconium ileus without developing lung infection have normal pulmonary histology.[21] Thus, unlike the pancreas, intestine, or vas deferens, the lung appears to suffer no structural damage *in utero*. However, infection occurs shortly after birth, and once bacterial infection becomes established it is difficult to eradicate, despite prolonged and intensive antibiotic treatment. It is uncertain how infection first occurs in children with CF, or whether viral infection precedes bacterial infection, or which bacteria are the initial invaders. It is clear, however, that many young patients have *Staphylococcus aureus* in their sputum. Rarely, staphylococcal emphysema or sepsis may complicate the course early in life. Since the *Staphylococcus* is such a tissue-destructive organism, the hypothesis has been advanced that antistaphylococcal prophylaxis early in life will delay the establishment of structural damage in the CF lung. This hypothesis is now being tested in a multicenter study of suppressive antibiotic therapy (cephalexin) in the first 2 years of life. No definitive data are yet available.

At some point in their course, most patients with CF become colonized with *Pseudomonas aeruginosa*. Mucoid transformation is frequent in the *Pseudomonas* that colonizes the CF lung, and in other gram-negative invaders as well.[8, 22] Another organism that has emerged as a major pathogen in CF is *Pseudomonas cepacia*.[23, 24] The mechanisms by which these "replacement" pathogens become established in the CF lung are uncertain. The intensive antibiotic therapy applied to CF patients has been blamed for the emergence of these invaders, but host factors cannot be excluded.

Viral infections occur in CF patients with a frequency comparable to that of their normal siblings. However, the CF child is more likely to become symptomatic than the unaffected sibling.[25] Also, viral infections frequently can be documented in association with pulmonary exacerbations,[26] and one study indicates that CF children with frequent viral infections have a more rapid decline in pulmonary function than do CF children with fewer infections.[27] Certain viral infections have been associated in the past with significant morbidity in CF, including influenza and rubeola, but these difficulties have been obviated by the widespread application of vaccination in the CF population.

Tuberculous organisms are recovered occasionally in CF—often atypical organisms, such as *Mycobacterium fortuitum*.[28] However, in most cases this is colonization and not infection.

The CF lung disease apparently begins in the small airways with inflammation and destruction of the airway wall. The alveolus is relatively spared, and alveolar simplification and remodeling (true emphysema) is unusual in CF.[29] Gradually, the damage spreads centripetally to the larger airways, and eventually all the conducting airways are involved. Persistent neutrophilic infiltrate is the hallmark of the CF inflammatory process, though some lymphocytic and monocytic infiltration occurs. There is hypertrophy and hyperplasia of the mucus-secreting apparatus, and thick secretions clog the airways. There is some sloughing of the epithelium, but in general the ultrastructure of the CF epithelium is remarkably intact.[30] There is some hypertrophy of bronchial smooth muscle as well, but this is not as prominent as it is in asthma. The pulmonary vasculature is also abnormal. With hypoxia, there is increase in the vascular musculature and intimal hypertrophy. The bronchial circulation becomes more prominent, and engorged, tortuous bronchial blood vessels develop. The airway wall is destroyed, and the airways become enlarged and floppy; bronchiectasis sets in. The enlarged airways are inflamed and have thickened walls; they become filled with purulent secretions and plugged. Air exchange is severely compromised (Fig. 32–3).

These abnormalities produce small airways dysfunction early in the course of the disease. Reduced midexpiratory flows and increased air trapping (increased residual volume) are early signs of pulmonary dysfunction. Later in the course, frank obstruction to airflow occurs, and the FEV_1 falls. The ratio of residual volume to total lung capacity increases dramatically. Gas exchange, however, is well preserved, even late in the course of the disease. Hypoxemia occurs relatively late in the course, and the diffusing capacity for carbon monoxide is well preserved. Hypercapnia occurs even later.[1]

The chest roentgenogram findings in CF are characteristic, though not pathognomonic. Hyperinflation is frequent in children and may be the only abnormality, but in adults hyperinflation is always accompanied by parenchymal abnormalities. The early parenchymal changes are increased pulmonary markings, but, as the disease progresses, peribronchial thickening with "tram tracks" and ring shadows becomes evident. Later, cystic changes occur (Fig. 32–4). Often these changes occur first in the right upper lobe, and it is common for the upper lobes to be more heavily involved than the lower lobes and the right side to be more heavily involved than the left.[1]

PATHOPHYSIOLOGY

In the sweat duct, the functional consequences of the CF defect follow directly from the lesion itself. The sweat duct is a very tight epithelium, and the failure of salt to pass across it (failure to resorb salt) results in elevated concentrations of salt in the sweat. How the CF lesion leads to the chronic lung disease is unclear. Since the airway is a more leaky epithelium than the sweat duct, blocking ion transport through one pathway may not absolutely prohibit the movement of salt or water across the epithelium. The chronic inflammation and infection in the CF lung introduce the additional variables of tissue damage, abnormal blood flow, and other effects whose consequences are difficult to predict. Besides, it is difficult to predict the consequences of a block in chloride permeability in the small airways where the CF disease begins, because what we know about the CF lesion is derived from study of the upper airway. Ion transport pathways and/or direction may be different in the lower airways. Thus the relation of the basic defect to the lung disease in CF remains speculative and awaits further work.

Several hypotheses are possible. First, if the CF lesion results

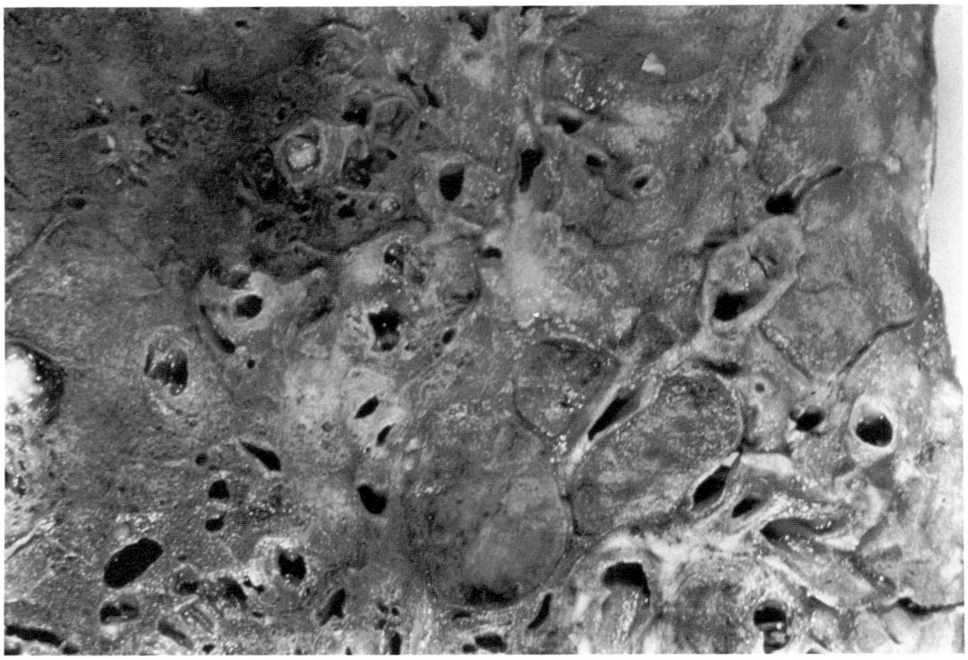

Figure 32–3. Specimen of CF lung post mortem, illustrating occupation of air-spaces by inflammatory infiltrate, lack of aeration, and tremendous dilation of airways, even close to the pleura.

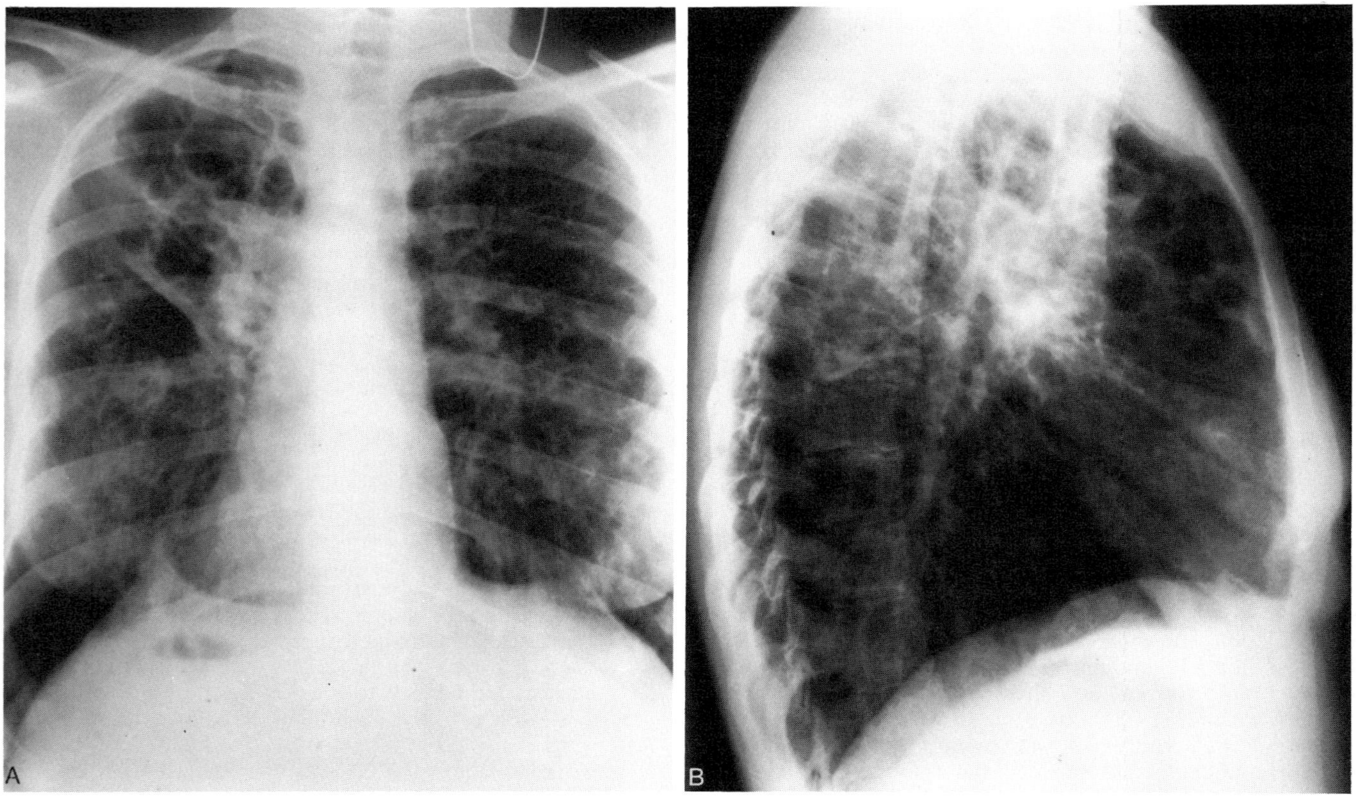

Figure 32–4. Chest roentgenogram of an adult CF patient, illustrating hyperinflation and formation of subpleural blebs and cysts. (Reproduced with permission from Davis PB, di Sant'Agnese PA. Chest 1984; 85:802–809.)

in too little salt and therefore water passing the airway epithelium, then either the hydration of mucus or the depth of periciliary fluid, or both, may be insufficient. The results, impaired mucociliary clearance and failure to clear the lower airways, could lead to recurrent or persistent infection, and infection leads to bronchiectasis. In support of this hypothesis is the fact that the lung disease of CF appears to be largely secondary to infection and inflammation. However, some data are not consistent with this hypothesis. Because patients with primary disorders of mucociliary clearance, such as the ciliary dyskinesia syndrome, do not develop lung disease as relentless and severe as that of CF, something other than (or in addition to) disordered mucociliary clearance is necessary to account for the severity of CF. Also, were mucociliary clearance the primary problem in CF, then all studies of mucociliary clearance should be able to demonstrate deficient clearance. In fact, in many CF patients, mucociliary clearance is normal or even increased.[31, 32]

Another possibility is that the failure of salt transport across the mucosa results in elevated osmolarity either in the basal state or under conditions of hydrothermal stress (increased minute ventilation), or both. Mast cells can degranulate under hyperosmolar conditions, with release of mediators of inflammation.[33] If this occurs regularly in CF patients, persistent inflammation could result, initiating and turning a vicious cycle in the airways.

A third possibility is that disordered ion transport results in abnormal salt composition or abnormal pH of the airways, which is especially hospitable to the typical CF flora, allowing establishment of bacterial infection and initiation of an inflammatory response, which subsequently becomes permanently established owing to the special properties of the pathogen and the host.

In any event, the weight of the evidence is that infection plays a role in the lung deterioration in CF. The association of more rapid lung deterioration with frequent viral infections[27] and the historical perspective of the disastrous consequences of influenza and measles pneumonia in CF attest to the contribution of viruses. The role of bacteria is not as easy to determine. Several studies indicate that either continuous or intermittent suppressive antibiotic treatment preserves pulmonary function.[34–37] It is more difficult to prove the role of the chronically colonizing bacteria in pulmonary exacerbations in CF, for there is usually no bacteriologic cure, and several studies suggest that antibiotics are not crucial in treatment of pulmonary exacerbations.[38, 39] Nevertheless, serum precipitins against the infecting organisms rise during pulmonary exacerbations,[40] several studies attest to the value of antibiotic treatment in exacerbations,[35, 37] and the weight of the evidence appears to be that in at least some exacerbations, the bacteria in the lung are responsible for the increased symptoms. The nature of the bacterial flora appears to make a difference in the course of the CF patient. Patients colonized with *Pseudomonas aeruginosa* do worse than those with no gram-negative organisms,[41] and those with *Pseudomonas cepacia* do worse than those with *Pseudomonas aeruginosa*.[23, 24]

The infecting organisms may have an impact on the course of the disease in other ways, however. They may initiate the inflammatory response, which has tremendous destructive potential, or they may serve as a continuous source of antigen in the airways for Type I or Type III allergic reactions. In support of the latter hypothesis is the demonstration of *Pseudomonas*-specific IgE in the serum of patients with CF, which might initiate a destructive bronchial response comparable to that of allergic bronchopulmonary aspergillosis.[42]

The host's response to infection may contribute in a major way to the CF lung disease. The observation that about 20% of CF patients under age 10 years have hypogammaglobulinemia—and it is these patients who are the least ill and have the best prognosis—[43, 44] stimulated consideration of the role of inflammation and immune complexes in CF lung disease. Neutrophils are an excellent source of destructive agents, including proteases and active oxygen species, and produce mediators, such as prostaglandins and leukotrienes, capable of sustaining and augmenting the inflammatory response. Examples of lung destruction due to neutrophils are numerous: both functional derangement (as in adult respiratory distress syndrome) and permanent damage (as in emphysema) have been observed. The persistent neutrophilic infiltrate in the lungs in CF, a hallmark of the pathology of the disease, may be the prime source of airways damage. The etiology of the persistence of neutrophilic response without clearance of *Pseudomonas* is a subject of intense investigation. Though *Pseudomonas* produces destructive exoproducts, such as elastases, and pigments that may inhibit some immune responses, persistence of the infection is still unexplained. Induction of nonopsonic antibodies may contribute to the problem, as may cleavage of antibodies by uninhibited elastases. The complement pathway may be crippled by elastolytic destruction of neutrophil receptors or bacterial ligands. The combination of a persistent stimulus and unmodulated response may be deadly in CF.

COMPLICATIONS

The lung disease of CF may be complicated by many of the problems that beset patients with bronchiectasis.

Clubbing and Hypertrophic Pulmonary Osteoarthropathy

Digital clubbing occurs early in the course of CF. At the time of diagnosis, most patients have some degree of clubbing, if only softening of the nailbeds. Occasionally the clubbing is striking and may prove embarrassing to young women. Hypertrophic pulmonary osteoarthropathy occurs in only about 3% of older patients.[9] This complication affects the distal portions of the long bones and the joints adjacent to them, such as the distal femur with the knee, the tibia and fibula with the ankle, and the radius and ulna with the wrist. Occasionally, other bones may be involved. Hypertrophic pulmonary osteoarthropathy is characterized by tenderness, warmth, redness, and swelling over the distal portions of the long bones, often with a noninflammatory effusion and pain in the adjacent joint. On x-ray examination there is periosteal elevation, but this may be absent in the acute phase and take several months to develop. Though nonsteroidal anti-inflammatory agents are of benefit, treatment of the underlying lung disease is essential.

It may be difficult, especially in the early phases before roentgenographic manifestations are evident, to distinguish hypertrophic pulmonary osteoarthropathy from other arthritides that may occur in CF patients, such as immune complex arthritis or erythema nodosum.[45] Perhaps because of longer survival and more protracted exposure to foreign antigens, immune-mediated arthritis is becoming more common in CF.

Hemoptysis

Blood streaking of the sputum is very common in patients over the age of 10 years, but massive hemoptysis is unusual, occurring in fewer than 10% of adults.[9] It may be a substantial clinical problem, however. The source of bleeding is tremendously dilated bronchial arteries, which, stressed by tissue damage from inflammation and pressure changes from coughing, rupture and bleed. Because bleeding comes from systemic arteries, blood loss may be considerable (and even fatal) and require supportive measures. Actual treatment of the problem is difficult, for it is often difficult to localize the site of bleeding, but resection of the bleeding area, and embolization of the largest and most prominent tortuous vessels have been successful.[46] However, hemoptysis may continue even after these measures because of the diffuse lung involvement in CF.

It is surprising that there is little negative prognostic import of even massive hemoptysis—the prognosis is determined by the underlying state of the lung as much as by the presence of the complication.

Pneumothorax

In contrast, pneumothorax appears to be a negative prognostic indicator. Of the patients reported in the literature, about one fifth did not survive the hospitalization during which pneumothorax was treated.[1] This may mean that pneumothorax occurs late in the course of the disease, or that the stress it represents exceeds the tolerance of patients. The pathology of pneumothorax has recently been elucidated.

Bronchiectatic cysts, interstitial cysts, and emphysematous bullae have all been identified in CF lungs at necropsy, in 15 of 21 patients aged 14 to 36 years at death. Bronchiectatic cysts are larger and more numerous than the other types of cysts. Blebs are more numerous in the upper lobes. However, there is no difference in number, type, or size of cysts between patients with and without a pneumothorax.[47] The presence of blebs or cysts is not related to the bacterial flora or the severity of bronchiectasis. It thus appears that subpleural blebs are a part of the pathology of long-standing CF lung disease, and rupture of these blebs may result in pneumothorax. Because there is a 50% chance of recurrence following the first pneumothorax, and because the consequences of collapse of a lobe or a lung may be disastrous in a CF patient, many experts recommend definitive treatment at the first episode. The use of chemical sclerosing agents is fraught with pain for the patient and may not prevent the recurrence of pneumothorax. Surgical treatment (pleurectomy, pleural abrasion, and oversewing of the rent) is definitive in most cases. Failure of the airleak to seal following surgery occasionally occurs, especially in patients on high-dose steroids. Chemical pleurodesis with talc may be useful for these patients.

Cor Pulmonale and Pulmonary Hypertension

Patients with CF, like others with lung disease, are vulnerable to the effects of intermittent or continuous hypoxemia on the pulmonary circulation. When the arterial oxygen tension is below 50 torr, pulmonary hypertension is universal,[48] and right heart strain soon follows. However, lesser degrees of hypoxemia or the desaturation that occurs during sleep in CF patients may produce lesser abnormalities in the pulmonary circulation; even mildly affected patients with CF display some echocardiographic abnormalities consistent with right heart strain.[49] Cor pulmonale is a poor prognostic indicator—when frank heart failure supervenes, more than half the patients are dead within 6 months.[50]

These complications are best treated by improvement of pulmonary function. Once oxygen desaturation is evident, however, there is no clear consensus on the best course of treatment. Even the provision of supplemental oxygen is controversial, for extension of the studies in adult COPD patients (which clearly demonstrate benefit from maintenance of near-normal blood oxygen tensions) to children with CF may not be valid. Digitalis preparations are indicated if there is left heart failure as well as right heart failure. Diuresis is often helpful and is a mainstay of conventional treatment, although, on theoretical grounds, loop diuretics may worsen the primary CF lesion. Whether pulmonary vasodilation is of benefit has not been proved, but anecdotal evidence suggests that a trial of nifedipine may be warranted in patients whose cardiac status is difficult to control with diuresis and maintenance of normoxia alone.[51]

TREATMENT

Although conventional treatment of the CF pulmonary disease has evolved with very little understanding of the basic pathophysiology of the disease, it has been remarkably successful, prolonging median survival age from less than 1 year in the 1940s to more than 20 years today. For the lung disease, the principles of conventional therapy are (1) the removal of secretions from the airways, and (2) combating infection, with (3) bronchodilation in selected patients. These principles translate into a comprehensive program of care that has become the standard at American Cystic Fibrosis Centers.

Removal of secretions is usually accomplished by percussion and postural drainage, that is, positioning the patients so that each lobe in turn can drain by gravity and then pounding on the chest above that lobe to accelerate drainage of mucus (also termed "the ketchup-bottle method").[52] Often postural drainage and percussion are preceded by aerosol treatment, either a bland aerosol to hydrate secretions (the efficacy of which has not been proved) or bronchodilator aerosol to enlarge the route by which the secretions drain. Mucolytics are popular with a few patients, but many find their irritant properties intolerable. Alternatives to postural drainage and clapping, such as deep breathing exercises and directed coughing or a regular exercise program, have been explored and may be effective. Though it is difficult experimentally to prove the efficacy of a single postural drainage and clapping treatment, several studies indicate that postural drainage and other pulmonary toilet strategies are of benefit when performed consistently over a period of weeks.[53, 54]

Prevention of respiratory infection is most desirable, and immunization against all the usual childhood illnesses as well as influenza each year is a critical part of a CF management program. Because of the potential for devastation from influenza in CF patients, amantadine prophylaxis and treatment during influenza A epidemics may be reasonable.

The role of suppression of bacterial infection is more controversial. Because even in successful treatment of pulmonary exacerbations the bacteria are seldom eradicated (and sometimes persist in the same numbers as before treatment), the argument has been made that antibiotic treatment may be superfluous in managing pulmonary exacerbations in CF.[55] This argument has been reinforced by a few studies that indicate that placebo or nonspecific antibiotic treatment is as efficacious as culture-specific antibiotics in controlling a pulmonary exacerbation. However, other studies find culture-specific antibiotics superior to placebo in exacerbations, and studies of long-term antibiotic suppression of bacterial growth, either by the oral or the aerosol route, generally suggest benefit from such treatment.[34, 36] So far, studies have not been directed at prospective identification of patients most likely to benefit from antibiotic therapy, nor have they addressed the means by which antibiotics benefit patients. However, because of the tremendous purulent response to bacterial infection and because of the clear benefit obtained by some patients from intensive antibiotic treatment, antibiotic therapy is a mainstay of therapeutic programs for the CF lung disease.

Most authorities administer antibiotics according to the sensitivities of the organisms recovered in culture. In patients who harbor only *Staphylococcus aureus* and *Haemophilus* species, oral antibiotics are quite efficacious. When *Pseudomonas* is present, often few oral antibiotics are appropriate: sometimes tetracycline, trimethoprim/sulfisoxazole, or cephalosporins show activity, but this is rare. The recent introduction of ciprofloxacin has provided a useful antipseudomonal drug that is effective orally, but the rapid development of resistance and the unproved safety in children are significant drawbacks. For this reason chronic suppression of *Pseudomonas* is often attempted by aerosolized antibiotics such as tobramycin, colistin, or cephalosporins. Otherwise, intensive antipseudomonas therapy is best delivered by the intravenous route. Aminoglycosides, semisynthetic penicillins, and cephalosporins are all useful. However, CF patients have unusual pharmacokinetics for most of these drugs, with both higher volumes of distribution and rates of excretion than normal subjects. In many instances this necessitates very high doses of antibiotics to achieve therapeutic serum levels. Whenever possible, serum levels should be monitored to assure optimal dosing. Therapy should be continued at high enough dosage for long enough to achieve adequate suppression of bacterial growth, usually a minimum of 10 to 14 days, and sometimes much longer.

Another therapeutic approach to the CF lung disease is the use of bronchodilators. Since at any given time about half of CF patients have increased airway reactivity, treatment of bronchospasm may be appropriate. Most patients either improve airflow or have no change upon administration of bronchodilators, but a few actually deteriorate,[56] and thus it is prudent to verify that benefits are obtained from bronchodilators by a therapeutic trial in the pulmonary function laboratory. Because CF patients seem to have a high prevalence of gastroesophageal reflux under the best of circumstances, theophyllines may be poorly tolerated. Aerosolized or systemic beta-adrenergic agents are often better tolerated. Aerosolized anticholinergic agents are of comparable efficacy in short-term trials.[57, 58] For patients with stubborn airway reactivity, a short course of steroids may be useful; a few patients receive steroids chronically. Treatment of respiratory allergy is controversial: though CF patients have a higher prevalence of increased IgE, higher mean IgE levels, and an increased prevalence of positive allergic skin tests,[59] the contribution of allergic asthma to the CF lung disease is difficult to assess, for the symptoms and signs of CF and asthma overlap. No systematic studies have been conducted on desensitization against inhalant antigens in CF.

In summary, clearance of secretions, antibiotic therapy, and bronchodilation are the main conservative therapies for the CF lung disease. Inspection of the median survival age curves for CF shows a remarkable increase over the 1960s and 1970s but a much slower rate of increase in recent years despite the introduction of newer, more potent antipseudomonas antibiotics and the increasingly aggressive attitude at CF centers (Fig. 32–5). The limits of aggressive conventional therapy may be reached. New strategies must be sought if the survival curve is to be pushed upward yet again. Several such strategies are now under investigation.

Because so much of the lung damage appears to result from the tissue destruction of inflammation, and because children with less immunoglobulin G response appear to do better than those with greater response,[43, 44] anti-inflammatory therapy might be of benefit in CF if given early in the course of the disease, before extensive structural damage has occurred. A preliminary 4-year clinical trial of alternate-day steroid therapy was sufficiently promising[60] to warrant launching a much more extensive trial, which is now in progress. In the preliminary

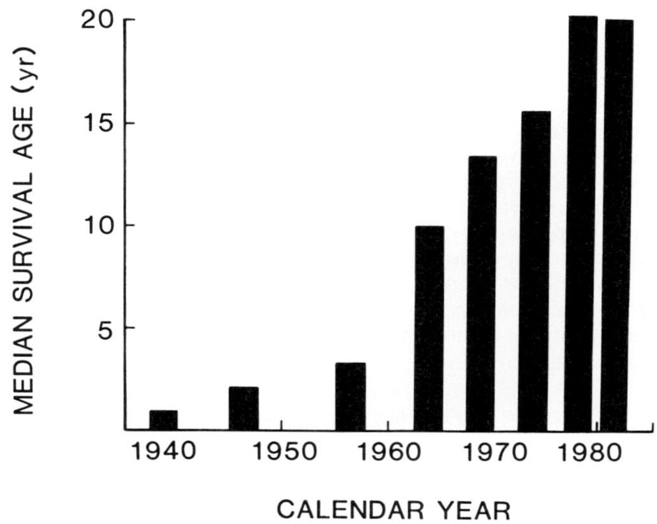

Figure 32–5. Median survival age of patients with CF in the United States since description of the disease in 1938. (Reproduced with permission from Davis PB, di Sant'Agnese PA. Chest 1984; 85:802–809.)

trial, children 2 to 12 years of age were treated with placebo or prednisone (2 mg/kg) on alternate days, and at the end of 4 years, the children on prednisone had greater height and weight for age and better pulmonary function.[60] However, small numbers of subjects and incomplete pulmonary function data complicate interpretation of the results. A much larger trial is in progress now. A potentially less toxic alternative to steroids is also being tested in a clinical trial. Ibuprofen was effective in limiting the area of lung inflammation in a rat model of chronic *Pseudomonas* bronchitis.[61] Preliminary clinical studies indicate lack of toxicity, but no information on its clinical efficacy in CF is yet available.

Another strategy being applied to CF is the modification of ion transport pathways in the airway. If the high amiloride-sensitive potential difference across the airway interferes with water secretion in CF, reducing that potential may be of benefit. Knowles and coworkers[16] have launced a placebo-controlled trial of aerosolized amiloride in patients with CF. This or other strategies directed at bypassing the deleterious effects of the primary defect have considerable intellectual appeal, but since the pathogenetic mechanisms linking the ion transport defect to the lung destruction in CF are poorly understood, more basic investigations will be necessary before the definitive treatment can be proposed.

COMPARISON OF CYSTIC FIBROSIS AND CHRONIC BRONCHITIS/EMPHYSEMA

Though both the lung disease of CF and chronic bronchitis/emphysema are characterized by obstructive physiology, chronicity, and disease progression, there are striking differences between the disease processes. The etiology of the obstructive physiology in emphysema is largely the loss of elastic recoil due to alveolar damage, but this is a minor mechanism of airways obstruction in CF, in which true emphysema is unusual. The pathophysiology of airways obstruction in CF is largely bronchiectasis and narrowing of the airstream from mucus, edema, and bronchospasm. Infection probably plays a major role in the progression of the CF lung disease but only a minor role in the progression of emphysema/chronic bronchitis. Patients with CF die *of* their lung disease, but patients with emphysema often die *with* their disease: since the patients with emphysema are usually older they have more degenerative diseases, and since the etiology of the emphysema is often cigarette related, lung cancer and arteriosclerotic cardiovascular disease are frequent concomitants of emphysema. The complications are different, too: the incidence of pneumothorax, massive hemoptysis, and hypertrophic osteoarthropathy is much higher in CF than in emphysema. Cystic fibrosis is a multisystem disease and affects many organs outside the lung: emphysema is often confined to the lung. CF is genetically caused but may be profoundly affected by environmental or adventitious factors (such as influenza or allergy). Although there is almost surely genetic vulnerability to emphysema, a major cause is environmental—inhalation of cigarette smoke.

INVOLVEMENT OF OTHER ORGANS

Although the lung disease contributes much of the morbidity and nearly all the mortality in CF patients, many other organs are involved by the disease process.

Upper Airway

Rhinosinusitis is common in patients with CF. Most patients have some abnormalities on roentgenogram of the paranasal sinuses, but acute sinusitis is rare. Sometimes the organisms recovered from the sinuses correspond to those recovered from the lower airways, and sometimes they do not. Nevertheless, it is unusual to have to treat the sinusitis in CF patients separately from the lung infection.[1, 9]

Nasal polyposis is also very common, occurring in 10% to 15% of the children and half the adults with CF at some point in the course.[9] The polyps may be quite large and may obstruct the nasal passages and demand resection. However, spontaneous regression occurs, conservative therapy (with nasal steroids) is sometimes effective, and recurrence after resection is common. Therefore a conservative approach to these polyps is often rewarded. Unfortunately, repeated resections are necessary in some patients.

Pancreas

One of the major organ involvements in CF is that of the pancreas, which may begin before birth and progresses throughout life, so that most adults (95%) have exocrine pancreatic insufficiency. The pathogenesis of this organ involvement is unclear, but plugging of the ducts with eosinophilic material is frequently observed. Acinar degeneration occurs, and eventually the acini are completely replaced by fat and fibrosis,[62] which come to strangle the islets as well. Sometimes the progressive loss of pancreatic function is marked by episodes of pancreatitis. Indeed, unexplained pancreatitis may be a presenting symptom of CF.[9]

Early in the course of the pancreatic involvement there are derangements of electrolyte transport. Even in patients with normal pancreatic enzyme release, the production of bicarbonate and water by the pancreas is reduced compared with that of controls.[3] This is a very consistent feature of the CF pancreatic disease.

The clinical consequences of these abnormalities are substantial. First, due to the reduced bicarbonate content of the pancreatic secretions, neutralization of gastric acid fails to occur normally, and the enzymes supplied to the patient for digestion (either endogenously or exogenously) must work at suboptimal pH. Second, in the majority of patients adequate quantities of enzymes are not released, resulting in maldigestion and malabsorption of food, steatorrhea and azotorrhea, malabsorption of fat-soluble vitamins (A, D, E, and K), and malabsorption of bile salts leading to imbalance of cholesterol and bile salts in bile and predisposition to gallstones, and to abnormal fatty acid composition of lipid in blood and cells. The deficiency of vitamin E is particularly striking and of potential clinical import because of its neurologic sequelae. The consequences of modest essential fatty acid deficiency have not yet been elucidated. In animal models, essential fatty acid deficiency can lead to impairment of host defenses against pulmonary infection with *Pseudomonas*.[63] On the other hand, deficiency of arachidonate may inhibit generation of inflammatory mediators in the lung.

The need to assure adequate nutrition in CF patients is clear, for they have the disadvantage of malabsorption coupled with the increased caloric demands of chronic infection and respiratory insufficiency. This is often accomplished by the provision of pancreatic enzyme supplements and additional vitamins. To increase the effectiveness of the pancreatic enzyme supplements, the addition of inhibitors of gastric acid production has been tested. Though they are efficacious, their long-term safety in children has not been established.[64] Specific provision of vitamin E in water-miscible form is recommended in CF patients, and double doses of ordinary multivitamins are usually enough to prevent other vitamin deficiencies. Particularly in patients with liver disease, specific supplemental vitamin K should be provided.

The progressive anatomic damage to the pancreas in CF eventually disrupts the islets of Langerhans. The consequences of this, insulinopenia and glucagonopenia, give rise to glucose intolerance and hyperglycemia that are usually *not* complicated by ketoacidosis. The osmotic effects of hyperglycemia are present, but renal, retinal, and microvascular damage, as occurs in diabetes, appears to be unusual. It is possible, however, that the duration of hyperglycemia in CF has not been sufficient for development of microangiopathy, and that as survival lengthens, this complication will arise. Hyperglycemia is worse during stress and may be exacerbated by steroid therapy. Insulin treatment is sometimes required, but often diet is sufficient.

Gastrointestinal Tract

Histologic abnormalities are regularly observed along the gastrointestinal tract and consist of hypertrophy and hyperplasia of the mucous glands in the gut. Physiologic abnormalities are only now being elucidated. It is likely that the ion transport defects observed elsewhere in CF are also present in the gut[17] and that this results in reduced water content of the intestinal contents. The clinical result of this defect appears at birth in 10% to 15% of patients in the form of meconium ileus, or neonatal intestinal obstruction. Although this obstruction may be relieved by hypertonic enemas, often surgical intervention is required. If ileal resection is necessary, the malabsorptive difficulties of the patient are compounded by reduced absorptive surface.

Later in life, CF patients may also develop intestinal obstruction.[9] The intestinal contents are solid or semisolid when they should be liquid, and feces may accumulate at the ileocecal junction, resulting in high fecal impaction. Alternatively, feces may become densely adherent to the bowel wall and serve as a lead point for intussusception. Some 20% of adults with CF suffer some form of intestinal obstruction. This complication presents as abdominal pain, obstipation, and usually a right lower quadrant mass. Early intervention with meglumine diatrizoate (Hypaque, Gastrografin) enemas may obviate the problem. Such conservative treatment is much to be preferred, for resection of the gut only complicates the malabsorptive problems, and manipulation of the inflamed gut predisposes to adhesions in a patient already susceptible to obstructive complications. Adhesions may create additional physical barriers to passage of gut contents. Preventive measures for intestinal obstruction consist of assiduous use of pancreatic enzyme supplements, sometimes use of stool softeners like dioctyl sodium sulfosuccinate, and, in some clinics, oral *N*-acetylcysteine.

Male Reproductive System

The male reproductive tract is affected in nearly all men with CF. Early in life, the vas deferens disappears, either because of primary maldevelopment or secondary to plugging of the passage with abnormal secretions.[65] The functional result of this is that sperm cannot pass into the ejaculate. Thus, more than 98% of men with CF are sterile. However, sexual development, desire, and hormone production are quite normal. Because a few men with CF are fertile, the reproductive status should be determined by semen analysis before sexual activity begins.

Female Reproductive System

Menarche occurs later in women with CF, but despite their thinness, women with CF do begin menses.[66] However, CF patients appear to be less fertile than other women. The cervical mucus has reduced water content compared with normal and fails to undergo the usual midcycle thinning that favors sperm penetration. However, pregnancy is possible and has been carried to term in hundreds of instances. In general, the outcome of pregnancy for the mother is better the better the initial lung status. In women who have right heart strain or even moderate pulmonary disease with hypoxemia, pregnancy (especially the blood volume increase in the second trimester) is poorly tolerated. During pregnancy in a patient with mild lung disease, extra attention to nutrition and weight gain and meticulous pulmonary care are crucial. Though antibiotics and other therapeutic measures should be selected with the presence of the fetus in mind, adequate care of the mother's pulmonary disease must not be compromised. Congenital malformation of children of women with CF attributable to drug treatment during pregnancy must be unusual, for there are no reports, but fetal wastage of 10% to 15% is reported.[67] Children of mothers with CF have a 2% chance of having the disease.

Contraception is appropriate for many women with CF. Barrier methods carry little health risk but have a higher failure rate than oral contraceptives. Oral contraceptives are well tolerated by most women with CF but as in other cases should be prescribed at the lowest effective dose with careful pulmonary function monitoring after initiating treatment.

Heat Prostration

One of the consequences of the CF sweat defect is heat prostration, which is frequent in babies (with a high surface area-to-volume ratio) and in young men who exercise in hot weather with little attention to salt and fluid replacement. Indeed, it was the high incidence of heat prostration among babies with CF in the 1949 New York heat wave that caused Paul di Sant'Agnese to recognize the sweat abnormality in CF patients.[68] Pursuit of this observation ultimately led to the diagnostic test for the disease, and finally to the unraveling of its physiologic basis.

Prevention of heat prostration is achieved by careful attention to salt and fluid intake when the level of sweating is increased. Once it develops, treatment of heat prostration must be prompt and vigorous and usually permits no time for transfer to a center. Administration of saline, 15 ml/kg in the first 30 minutes, is essential to prevent cardiovascular collapse. This complication is potentially fatal and requires urgent attention.

Liver Disease

About one third of CF patients display abnormal liver function tests at any one time, and the presence of focal eosinophilic concretions in the bile ducts is very frequent post mortem or at liver biopsy.[9, 69] However, only a small portion of CF patients develop clinical manifestations of liver disease—biliary cirrhosis, which can be severe enough to cause disability and death. The complications are those of portal hypertension, including hypersplenism, esophageal verices and gastrointestinal hemorrhage, and ascites. Hepatocellular complications, such as encephalopathy, are relatively unusual. For this reason, many centers perform portal-systemic shunting early in the course of the liver disease, because the risk of encephalopathy is considered to be low and the risk of death from variceal hemorrhage, high.[70] However, a contolled study has not been reported, and may not be because of the rarity of the complication.

Liver disease may occur secondary to other problems in CF patients. Acute fatty metamorphosis, often secondary to malnutrition, is observed in some CF patients and usually responds to institution of pancreatic enzyme therapy and nutritional repletion. Cardiac cirrhosis due to chronic or acute right heart failure is also obseved in patients with severe pulmonary disease. In pure right heart failure, diuresis is the approach of choice, if improvement of pulmonary status and correction of hypoxemia are impossible and fail to yield improvement in the heart failure.

Gallbladder Disease

The gallbladder is frequently involved in CF. Microgallbladder is observed in about 20% of patients, and the gallbladder may be filled with thick mucus.[71] In addition, because of the malabsorption of bile salts, bile may be lithogenic, and gallstones are frequent (13% of adults).[72] It is unclear what should be done about asymptomatic gallstones in CF patients: a case can be made that as lung disease worsens, the risk of acute cholecystectomy (should the stones becomes symptomatic) increases, and thus elective cholecystectomy is preferable. However, the risk of subsequent symptoms from silent gallstones in CF has not been established. In the presence of symptoms referable to cholelithiasis, cholecystectomy is reasonable.

SUMMARY

Cystic fibrosis, the most frequent lethal genetic disease in America, kills its victims by progressive respiratory insufficiency due to chronic obstructive pulmonary disease. Though survival has increased to over 20 years, the disease is still fatal. Increased understanding of the basic error in recent years gives reason for hope for specific therapeutic strategies to circumvent it, and better knowledge of the pulmonary inflammatory response affords new approaches to nonspecific treatment. For the present, though, clearance of secretions, antibacterial therapy, and bronchodilators remain the fundamental therapeutic strategies.

Since this chapter was prepared, the CF gene has been located and sequenced, and the major mutation (which accounts for 75% of the abnormal CF genes in whites) identified. The major mutation is a deletion of three base pairs causing one amino acid to be eliminated from the protein, without a shift in reading frame. More than 50 other mutations have been identified. This plethora of "private" mutations has made the prospects for mass screening more remote. The protein encoded by the CF gene, called the "cystic fibrosis transmembrane conductance regulator," or CFTR, is predicted from its amino acid sequence to have two membrane spanning regions, two intracellular nucleotide-binding folds, and another intracellular region, termed the "R" domain of unique sequence and unknown function. The specific function of CFTR is not yet known.

REFERENCES

1. Davis PB, di Sant'Agnese PA. Diagnosis and treatment of cystic fibrosis: An update. Chest 1984; 85:802-809.
2. Davis PB, Hubbard VS, di Sant'Agnese PA. Low sweat electrolytes in a patient with cystic fibrosis. Am J Med 1980; 69:643-646.
3. Davis PB, Del Rio S, Muntz J, Dieckman L. Sweat chloride concentrations in adults with pulmonary diseases. Am Rev Respir Dis 1983; 128:34-37.
4. Gaskin KJ, Durie PR, Corey M, et al. Evidence for a primary defect of pancreatic HCO_3-secretion in cystic fibrosis. Pediatr Res 1982; 16:554-557.
5. Nousia-Arvanitakis S, Arvanitakis C, Greenberger NJ. Diagnosis of exocrine pancreatic insufficiency in cystic fibrosis by the synthetic peptide *N*-benzoyl-L-tyrosyl-*p*-aminobenzoic acid. J Pediatr 1978; 92:734-737.
6. Jacobson DG, Curington C, Connery K, Toskes PP. Trypsin-like immunoreactivity as a test for pancreatic insufficiency. N Engl J Med 1984; 310:1307-1309.
7. Wong LTK, Turtle S, Davidson AGF. Secretin pancreozymin stimulation test and confirmation of the diagnosis of cystic fibrosis. Gut 1982; 23:744-750.
8. Stern RC, Boat TF, Doershuk CF. Obstructive azoospermia as a diagnostic criterion for the cystic fibrosis syndrome. Lancet 1982; i:1401-1404.
9. di Sant'Agnese PA, Davis PB. Adults with cystic fibrosis: 75 cases and a review of 232 cases in the literature. Am J Med 1979; 66:121-132.
10. Wilcken B, Brown ARD, Urwin R, Brown DA. Cystic fibrosis screening by dried blood spot trypsin assay: Results in 75,000 newborn infants. J Pediatr 1983; 102:383-387.
11. King DN, Walsh MP, Heeley AF, Kuzemxo JA. Sensitive trypsin assay for dried-blood specimens as a screening procedure for early detection of cystic fibrosis. Lancet 1979; ii:1217-1218.
12. Davidson AGF, Wong LTK, Kirby LT, Applegarth DA. Immunoreactive trypsin in cystic fibrosis. J Pediatr Gastroenterol Nutr 1984; 3(1):S79-S88.
13. White R. The search for the cystic fibrosis gene. Science 1986; 234:1054-1055.
14. Tsui LC. Genetic analysis of cystic fibrosis with linked DNA markers. Pediatr Pulmonol 1987; 1(Suppl):31-33.
15. Quinton PM. Missing Cl conductance in cystic fibrosis. Am J Physiol 1986; 251:C649-C652.
16. Knowles M, Gatzy J, Boucher R. Relative ion permeability of normal and cystic fibrosis nasal epithelium. J Clin Invest 1983; 71:1410-1417.
17. deJonge HR, Bijman J, Sinaasappel M. Relation of regulatory enzyme levels to chloride transport in intestinal epithelial cells. Pediatr Pulmonol 1987; 1(Suppl):54-56.
18. Frizzell RA, Techkemmer G, Shoemaker RL. Altered regulation of airway epithelial cell chloride channels in cystic fibrosis. Science 1986; 233:558-560.
19. Welsh MJ, Liedtke CM. Chloride and potassium channels in cystic fibrosis airway epithelia. Nature 1986; 322:467-470.
20. Li M, McCann JD, Liedtke CM, et al. Cyclic AMP-dependent protein kinase opens chloride channels in normal but not cystic fibrosis airway epithelium. Nature 1986; 331:358-360.
21. Sturgess J, Imrie J. Quantitative evaluation of the development of tracheal submucosal glands in infants with cystic fibrosis and control infants. Am J Pathol 1982; 106:303-311.
22. Macone AB, Pier GB, Pennington JE, et al. Mucoid *Escherichia coli* in cystic fibrosis. N Engl J Med 1981; 304:1445-1449.
23. Isles A, Machesky I, Corey M, et al. *Pseudomonas cepacia* infection in cystic fibrosis; an emerging problem. J Pediatr 1984; 104:206-208.
24. Thomassen ML, Demko CA, Klinger L, Stern RC. *Pseudomonas cepacia* colonization among cystic fibrosis patients: A new opportunist. Am Rev Respir Dis 1985; 131:791-796.
25. Wong EEL, Probs CG, Manson B, et al. Association of respiratory viral infections with pulmonary deterioration in patients with cystic fibrosis. N Engl J Med 1984; 311:1653-1658.
26. Petersen NT, Hoiby N, Mordhorst CH, et al. Respiratory infections in cystic fibrosis patients caused by virus, chlamydia, and mycoplasma—possible synergism with *Pseudomonas aeruginosa.* Acta Paediatr 1981; 70:623-628.
27. Efthimiou J, Hodson ME, Taylor P, et al. Importance of viruses and *Legionella pneumophilia* in respiratory exacerbations of young adults with cystic fibrosis. Thorax 1984; 39:150-154.
28. Boxerbaum B. Isolation of rapidly growing mycobacteria in patients with cystic fibrosis. J Pediatr 1980; 96:689-691.
29. Bedrossian CWM, Greenberg SD, Singer DB, et al. The lung in cystic fibrosis. Hum Pathol 1976; 7:195-204.
30. Jeffery PK, Brain APR. Surface morphology of human mucosa: normal, carcinoma or cystic fibrosis. Scan Microsc 1988; 2(1):553-560.
31. Wood RE, Wanner A, Hirsch J, Farrell PM. Tracheal mucociliary transport in patients with cystic fibrosis and its stimulation by terbutaline. Am Rev Respir Dis 1975; iii:733-738.
32. Yeates DB, Sturgess JB, Kahn SR, et al. Mucociliary transport in treachea of patients with cystic fibrosis. Arch Dis Child 1976; 51:28-33.
33. Eggleston PA, Kagey Sobotka A, Lichtenstein LM. A comparison of the osmotic activation of basophils and human lung mast cells. Am Rev Respir Dis 1987; 135:1043-1048.
34. Loenig-Baucke VA, Mischler E, Myers MG. A placebo-controlled trial of cephalexin therapy in the ambulatory management of patients with cystic fibrosis. Chest 1979; 95:630-637.
35. Wientzen R, Prestidge CB, Kramer RI, et al. Acute pulmonary exacerbations in cystic fibrosis. A double-blind trial of tobramycin and placebo therapy. Am J Dis Child 1980; 134:1134-1138.
36. Hodson ME, Penketh AR, Batten JC. Aerosol carbenicillin and gentamicin treatment of *Pseudomonas aeruginosa* infection in patients with cystic fibrosis. Lancet 1981; ii:1137-1139.
37. Hyatt AC, Chipps BE, Kumor KM, et al. A double-blind controlled trial of antipseudomonas chemotherapy of acute respiratory exacerbations in patients with cystic fibrosis. J Pediatr 1981; 99:307-311.
38. Beaudry PH, Markes MI, McDougall D, et al. Is antipseudomonas therapy warranted in acute respiratory exacerbations in children with cystic fibrosis? J Pediatr 1980; 97:144-147.
39. Gold R, Carpenter S, Heurter H, et al. Randomized trial of ceftazidime versus placebo in the management of acute respiratory exacerbations in patients with cystic fibrosis. J Pediatr 1987; 111:907-913.
40. Brut MM, Ghonheim ATM, Littlewood JM. Serum antibodies to *Pseudomonas* in cystic fibrosis. Arch Dis Child 1986; 61:1114-1120.
41. Wilmott RW, Tyson SL, Matthew DJ. Cystic fibrosis survival rates: The influence of allergy and *Pseudomonas aeruginosa.* Am J Dis Child 1985; 139:669-671.
42. Moss RB, Lewiston NJ. Immune complexes and humoral response to *Pseudomonas aeruginosa* in cystic fibrosis. Am Rev Respir Dis 1980; 121:23-29.
43. Matthews WJ, Williams M, Oliphint B, et al. Hypogammaglobulinemia in patients with cystic fibrosis. N Engl J Med 1980; 302:245-249.
44. Wheeler WB, Williams M, Matthews WJ, Colten HR. Progression

of cystic fibrosis lung disease as a function of serum immunoglobulin G levels: A 5 year longitudinal study. J Pediatr 1984; 104:695-699.
45. Dixey J, Redington AN, Butler RC, et al. The arthropathy of cystic fibrosis. Ann Rheum Dis 1988; 47:218-223.
46. Fellows KE, Khaw KT, Schuster S, Shwachman H. Bronchial artery embolization in cystic fibrosis: Technique and long-term results. J Pediatr 1979; 95:959-963.
47. Tomashefski JF, Bruce M, Stern RC, et al. Pulmonary air cysts in cystic fibrosis. Hum Pathol 1985; 16:253-261.
48. Moss AJ. The cardiovascular system in cystic fibrosis. Pediatrics 1982; 70:728-741.
49. Lester LA, Egge AC, Hubbard VS, et al. Echocardiography in cystic fibrosis: A proposed scoring system. J Pediatr 1980; 97:742-748.
50. Stern RC, Borkat G, Hirschfeld SS, et al. Heart failure in cystic fibrosis: Treatment and prognosis of cor pulmonale with failure of the right side of the heart. Am J Dis Child 1980; 134:267-272.
51. Michael JR, Kennedy TP, Fitzpatrick S, Rosenstein BJ. Nifedipine inhibits hypoxic pulmonary vasoconstriction during rest and exercise in patients with cystic fibrosis and cor pulmonale. Am Rev Respir Dis 1984; 130:516-519.
52. Murray JF. The ketchup-bottle method. N Engl J Med 1979; 300:1155-1157.
53. Desmond KJ, Schwenk WF, Thomas E, et al. Immediate and long-term effects of chest physiotherapy in patients with cystic fibrosis. J Pediatr 1983; 103:538-542.
54. DeBoeck C, Zinman R. Cough versus chest physiotherapy. A comparison of the acute effect on pulmonary function in patients with cystic fibrosis. Am Rev Respir Dis 1984; 129:182-184.
55. R.E.M. Commentary. J Pediatr 1980; 97:148.
56. Shapiro GG, Bamman J, Kanarek P, et al. The paradoxical effect of adrenergic and methylxanthine drugs in cystic fibrosis. Pediatrics 1976; 58:740-743.
57. Kattan M, Mansell A, Levison H, et al. Response to aerosol salbutamol, SCH 1,000 and placebo in cystic fibrosis. Thorax 1980; 35:531-535.
58. Larsen GL, Barron RJ, Cotton EK, Brooks JG. A comparative study of inhaled atropine sulfate and isoproterenol hydrochloride in cystic fibrosis. Am Rev Respir Dis 1979; 119:399-407.
59. Moss RB. Immunology of cystic fibrosis: Immunity, immunodeficiency and hypersensitivity. In: Lloyd-Still JD, ed. Textbook of Cystic Fibrosis. Boston: John Wright/PSG, 1983.
60. Auerbach HS, Williams M, Kirkpatrick JA, Colten HR. Alternate-day prednisone reduces morbidity and improves pulmonary function in cystic fibrosis. Lancet 1985; ii:686-688.
61. Konstan MW, Davis PB, Vargo KM, et al. Ibuprofen attenuates inflammation in an animal model of chronic pulmonary *Pseudomonas* infection/inflammation. Am Rev Respir Dis 1987; 135:A284.
62. Oppenheimer EH, Esterly JR. Pathology of cystic fibrosis—review of the literature and comparison with 146 autopsied cases. Perspect Pediatr Pathol 1975; 2:241-278.
63. Harper TB, Chase HP, Henson J, Henson DM. Essential fatty acid deficiency in the rabbit as a model of nutritional impairment in cystic fibrosis. In vitro and in vivo effects on lung defense mechanisms. Am Rev Respir Dis 1982; 126:540-547.
64. Hubbard VS, Dunn GD, Lester LA. Effectiveness of cimetidine as an adjunct to supplemental pancreatic enzymes in patients with cystic fibrosis. Am J Clin Nutr 1980; 33:2281-2286.
65. Taussig LM, Lobeck CC, di Sant'Agnese PA, et al. Fertility in males with cystic fibrosis. N Engl J Med 1972; 287:586-589.
66. Davis PB. Reproductive complications of CF. Semin Resp Med 1985; 6:314-318.
67. Cohen LF, di Sant'Agnese PA, Friedlander J. Cystic fibrosis and pregnancy. A national survey. Lancet 1980; ii:842-844.
68. di Sant'Agnese PA, Darling RC, Perera GA, et al. Abnormal electrolyte composition of sweat in cystic fibrosis of the pancreas. Pediatrics 1953; 12:549-563.
69. Hubbard VS. Gastrointestinal complications in cystic fibrosis. Semin Resp Med 1985; 6:299-307.
70. Stern RC, Stevens DP, Boat T, et al. Liver physiology and disease: Symptomatic hepatic disease in cystic fibrosis: Incidence, course and outcome of portal systemic shunting. Gastroenterology 1976; 70:645-649.
71. L'Heureux PR, Isenberg JN, Sharp HL, Warwick W. Gallbladder disease in cystic fibrosis. AJR 1977; 128:953-956.
72. Roy CC, Weber AM, Morin CL, et al. Abnormal biliary lipid composition in cystic fibrosis. Effect of pancreatic enzymes. N Engl J Med 1977; 297:1301-1305.

Chapter 33

THE RELATIONSHIP OF COPD TO ASTHMA

Steven R. White **Alan R. Leff**

The relationship of chronic obstructive pulmonary disease (COPD) to asthma is both complex and controversial. In the past, these two disorders have been thought to be two distinct but related processes, having airflow obstruction in common.[1] Conventionally, the obstruction of asthma is defined as reversible and acute, whereas the obstruction of COPD is defined as irreversible and chronic; however, some patients with COPD are capable of a response to bronchodilators.[2] It has been suggested that COPD is the result of a genetic predisposition to airway hyperreactivity combined with the deleterious effects of smoking.[3] This chapter will explore the differences between COPD and asthma and summarize efforts

Supported by National Heart, Lung and Blood Institutes Grants HL–32495 and HL–35718 and grants from the American Lung Association and the Schweppe Foundation.

currently being made to determine whether these diseases are, in fact, differing manifestations of the same pathophysiologic process.

Historical Perspective

Both asthma and emphysema have been recognized for centuries. The word asthma is derived from the Greek ασθμα, meaning panting or a short-drawn breath.[4] Asthma was recognized by Greek, Egyptian, and Hebrew physicians and was described by Hippocrates.[5] Thomas Willis in 1678 believed asthma to be due "to cramps of the moving fibres of the bronchi."[4,6] The classic description of the symptoms of asthma is given by Sir John Floyer in his *A Treatise of the Asthma.* Floyer also recognized that the mechanism was due to bronchospasm;[7,8] he provided the first detailed description of the morphology of emphysema in a broken-winded mare, which was later confirmed by Laennec.[8,9]

Emphysema was recognized as a pathologic entity in the 17th century, and the first detailed descriptions were made in the late 18th century by Watson[10] and Morgagni.[11] Laennec's classic description of emphysema[9] provides the modern basis for understanding the disease, and numerous pathologic studies developed the notion that emphysema was caused by a destruction of alveolar spaces.[12] The hereditary nature of emphysema first was recognized by James Jackson, Jr., and published by Louis in 1837.[13,14] However, until the late 19th century, many practicing physicians confused both asthma and emphysema. Osler separated the two diseases in his text and ascribed asthma to a "nervous condition."[15] This view persisted well into the 20th century. Emphysema, chronic bronchitis, and asthma came to be regarded as distinct clinical entities; however, these terms often were interchanged and confused. Patients with persistent dyspnea on exertion and chronic expectoration have been diagnosed as having emphysema, even without a smoking history or the pathologic manifestations of emphysema at autopsy.[16]

The 1959 report of the Ciba International Symposium,[17] and a subsequent report by the American Thoracic Society[18] defined the terms used today. Emphysema was defined in anatomic terms as an "increase beyond the normal in the size of the airspaces distal to the terminal bronchiole either from dilatation or from destruction of their walls." Chronic bronchitis was defined in clinical terms as "chronic or recurrent excessive mucous secretion in the bronchial tree." A new functional definition, *airflow obstruction,* was introduced.[17] Asthma was defined as reversible airflow obstruction with a compatible clinical history. However, there has been considerable controversy in distinguishing patients with asthma from those with a component of reversible obstruction superimposed upon irreversible obstruction.[16–18] Especially problematic was the elderly, nonsmoking patient with a long history of asthma and no demonstrable reversible airflow obstruction. The Ciba Symposium proposed that asthma and emphysema were two manifestations of a generalized, obstructive disorder of airways. However, the term *chronic obstructive pulmonary disease* was introduced in the United States shortly thereafter to refer to patients with minimal reversibility of airflow obstruction and without the atopy and acute episodes of bronchospasm characteristic of asthma. This term presumed that emphysema and asthma were indeed two different diseases with some shared clinical symptoms and that, in most cases, a proper distinction could be made.

There have been numerous investigations of the etiology of emphysema. Clinicopathologic correlations of patients with similar degrees of airflow obstruction have demonstrated remarkable differences in pathology. At one end of the spectrum are those patients with advanced emphysema; at the other end are those with little emphysema but significant degrees of bronchial pathology, including mucous plugging, narrowed airways, and mucous gland hypertrophy.[19,20] This has led to the concept of distinct emphysematous and bronchial types of chronic airflow obstruction, and the conclusion that chronic peripheral bronchial infection may cause airflow obstruction.[21,22] Chronic infection could damage either the bronchi or the alveoli, causing either chronic bronchitis or emphysema. This became regarded as "irritative" chronic airflow obstruction, in contrast to the "allergic" pathogenesis of airflow obstruction of asthma.

During 1960 to 1965, physicians in the Netherlands developed an alternative hypothesis for the pathogenesis of airflow obstruction.[23,24] Asthma and emphysema were regarded as two manifestations of the same pathologic process. This hypothesis was based upon two important observations: (1) only a small minority of people who smoke actually develop symptomatic chronic airflow obstruction; and (2) some individuals with airflow obstruction demonstrate increased sensitivity to inhaled bronchoconstricting agents, i.e., airway hyperreactivity typical of asthmatic patients. It was hypothesized that cigarette smokers with chronic, irreversible airflow obstruction shared with asthmatics a similar genetic predisposition to increased airway hyperreactivity. This theory is labeled commonly as the "Dutch" hypothesis.[25,26] It diverges from the "British" hypothesis, which holds that COPD is the direct result of the deleterious effects of smoking upon the airways and does not require pre-existing airway hyperreactivity.[25] The Dutch hypothesis states that airway hyperreactivity and atopy precede the onset of smoking but are not of sufficient magnitude to produce the usual symptoms and signs of asthma. However, a longitudinal study to resolve this hypothesis might require generations to conduct. A weakness of the British hypothesis is the fairly frequent demonstration of reversible airflow obstruction in some patients thought on clinical grounds to have emphysema.[27,28] In such cases, patients have been described as having both asthma and COPD to explain partially reversible airflow obstruction. However, significant airway hyperreactivity to methacholine has been demonstrated in patients with COPD,[29–31] and significant bronchodilatation has been demonstrated in patients previously thought to have "irreversible" obstruction.[32]

The central question in the relation of COPD to asthma, then, is whether the airway hyperreactivity that characterizes both syndromes stems from the same or different defects. If the former, identification of asymptomatic individuals with airway hyperreactivity would identify a subset of patients with an increased risk of irreversible, chronic airflow obstruction. This could lead to useful interventions, if these patients could be convinced to quit smoking. Aggressive treatment with bronchodilating agents and corticosteroids might be warranted, because of the possibility that control of hyperreactivity might slow or arrest the progression of subsequent, irreversible disease.

CONTROVERSIES IN THE STUDY OF AIRWAY HYPERREACTIVITY

Given that reversible airflow obstruction can be demonstrated both in asthma and COPD, is it possible to separate the two diseases based on the patient's bronchodilator response? This question poses both methodologic and physiologic problems.

Epidemiologic bias in population descriptors, such as sex, race, and age, have confounded the evaluation of the prevalence of airway hyperreactivity in patients with COPD. Dodge and colleagues have demonstrated that male subjects developing new dyspnea, wheezing, and shortness of breath were more likely to be labeled by physicians as having emphysema, particularly if they smoked.[33] In contrast, women were more likely to be diagnosed as having asthma or chronic bronchitis when presenting with the same symptoms. Other epidemiologic factors are important in studying airway hyperreactivity. For example, the predicted normal spirometric values, which are of critical importance in determining obstruction to airflow, vary with race. Black and Asian patients have normal predicted values for lung volumes and flow that differ from those for white subjects.[34–36]

Older patients are more likely to be labeled as having COPD, whereas younger patients, regardless of sex, are more likely to be called asthmatic. Age is also an important factor affecting lung function. Populations with COPD may be considerably older than populations from which "normal" data are derived. Inappropriate use of nomograms derived from younger subjects may introduce bias into the data. Most nomograms incorporate age in a multiple linear regression model; however, the use of either curvilinear regression[34] or a second regression equation for differing ages[37] has been explored. In addition, there is considerable evidence showing that poor lung function is highly predictive of mortality, so that subjects with a low FVC or FEV_1 tend not to survive to old age.[38] Those subjects surviving presumably have better lung function, and thus studies focusing on such subjects discriminate against those with poor lung function. Age also creates bias in clinical definitions of asthma and COPD. Older patients are more likely to be labeled as having COPD, whereas younger patients, regardless of sex, are more likely to be called asthmatic.

Proper categorizing of the older patient with evidence of both irreversible obstruction and hyperreactivity can be difficult. Previously the term asthmatic bronchitis was applied to such conditions.[39] Nonsmokers are more likely to be called asthmatic, although the rates of smoking among asthmatic subjects do not differ significantly from those of subjects with COPD.[33]

The definition of airflow obstruction as determined by spirometry has varied. Obstruction has been defined by some as an FEV_1 of less than 60% of predicted.[40] Some investigators have defined obstruction as an FEV_1 of less than 60% of the FVC[41] or have combined these criteria.[32, 41] Others have defined obstruction as an FEV_1 of 500 to 1500 ml.[42] Accepting an absolute FEV_1 of less than 60% might include patients with restrictive, as well as obstructive, lung disease, since FEV_1 is reduced in both. Limiting a study to patients with an FEV_1 of less than 1500 ml excludes taller patients, who necessarily have a higher FEV_1 than shorter subjects but nevertheless may have true airflow obstruction. Such a limitation also may introduce a bias toward older patients, owing to the natural decrease in FEV_1 with age.[43]

There also is no consensus on the definition of reversibility of airflow obstruction. Most investigators use a 15% improvement in FEV_1 following administration of a bronchodilating agent.[40, 42, 44] However, this degree of improvement does not have equal significance in patients with severe airflow obstruction compared with subjects with relatively mild obstruction.[43] This is because of the occurrence of regression to the mean: the lower the initial parameter of interest is, e.g., FEV_1, the greater the likelihood that a subsequent measurement will be higher than the initial value; and conversely, the higher the initial value, the more likely a subsequent measurement will be lower. The significance of a change is exaggerated by expressing it as a per cent change of the initial value. If a subject with an initial FEV_1 of 0.50 L improves to 0.60 L after administration of a bronchodilating drug, a 20% increase in FEV_1 is obtained. If a second subject with an initial FEV_1 of 2.00 L has the same absolute response (0.1 L) following a bronchodilator, the increase is only 5%. Since a common laboratory criterion for reproducibility of spirometry is ± 3% to 5%, the response in our second subject could be dismissed as "no apparent change." The result of these effects is that subjects with the greatest degree of airflow obstruction initially will tend to show the most improvement after bronchodilator, and this effect is exaggerated by expressing the improvement as a per cent change from the initial value.

Definition of airway hyperreactivity by responses to bronchial provocation instead of responses to bronchodilators has been attempted, but, as in bronchodilator trials, the decision of whether the response to a bronchoconstricting agent is abnormal may be difficult, particularly in patients who have increased airway resistance under baseline conditions. Airway resistance is inversely proportional to the fourth power of the radius of the airway. Therefore, a relatively small change in airway diameter elicits a large change in airway resistance in subjects with initially narrowed airways. The subject thereby reaches the predefined cutoff (usually a 20% decrease in FEV_1 or a 35% decrease in specific conductance) after receiving much less provocation agent, compared with a normal subject, even though the intrinsic activity of the agent in airway smooth muscle may not differ between the two subjects. Further, the distribution, deposition, and retention of the inhaled provocative agent differs between normal subjects and patients with chronic airflow obstruction,[45] confounding comparisons between these two groups.

There is also a significant day-to-day variation in both the determination of spirometric values and the response to bronchodilating drugs.[37, 46] All these variations taken together make interstudy comparisons of data difficult, and perhaps impossible. Eliasson and colleagues demonstrated that after calculating the response to bronchodilator therapy in obstructed patients by four different criteria, the likelihood of properly assigning a subject to the appropriate diagnostic category (response versus no response) was little better than random.[43] An attempt has been made to define norms for research purposes.[47]

In conclusion, serious methodologic and epidemiologic problems have hampered the evaluation of reversibility of airflow obstruction in patients with chronic airflow obstruction. Careful attention to the definitions of airflow obstruction and reversibility, and to the expression of data, is essential in deriving conclusions about the role of airway hyperreactivity in COPD.

COMPARISONS IN NATURAL HISTORY AND EPIDEMIOLOGY

DEMOGRAPHICS. Both asthma and COPD are common in most populations in the world. Asthma is a disease of both the young and of older adults,[48] whereas COPD is principally a disease of older persons, which reaches a peak incidence in the sixth decade of life.[49] The actual prevalence of both diseases may be obscured partially by the difficulty of separating asthma and emphysema in older adults. There is a male predominance in COPD, principally because of the high prevalence of smoking in men. The prevalence of both diseases is increased in lower socioeconomic groups.[50] There also may be racial predilections to asthma. When controlled for socioeconomic status and sex, the prevalence of asthma in black children has been found to be almost twice that of whites.[51]

GENETIC DISTRIBUTION. Both asthma and COPD may have genetic predispositions. Asthma has a strong correlation with other immunologic states such as allergy and eczema, which are hereditary. Asthma also has a strong family concordance. COPD also has familial concordance, although less substantial.[52, 53] Prevalence is greater in offspring of affected parents and in siblings of affected subjects. Both airway hyperreactivity and decrements in pulmonary function have been noted in young male relatives of patients with COPD[54] but could be related to similarities in body habitus[55] as well as other genetic and environmental factors.

The best-known genetic defect causing emphysema is deficiency of alpha$_1$-antitrypsin (AAT). Deficiency in AAT is responsible for approximately 2% of all cases of emphysema in the United States.[56] There is evidence that this protein is essential; loss of AAT leads to uncontrolled elastase enzymatic activity and eventual destruction of alveoli. In contrast, AAT determinations in children with asthma have been normal,[57] and elastase-mediated destruction of peripheral lung units does not occur in asthma. Since only a small percentage of patients with COPD have demonstrable AAT deficiency, and since patients with a heterozygote phenotype (only one allele for deficiency) are not thought to be at increased risk for COPD,[58] other factors are responsible for the pathogenesis of COPD. Other genetic abnormalities associated with COPD are controversial, most notably the presence of the A allele in the ABO blood group.[49] No such abnormality has been reported in association with asthma.

ATOPY. The importance of atopy, the hereditary predisposition to a clinical hypersensitivity state, or clinical allergy, in both asthma and COPD has been debated. Earlier in this century asthma largely was attributed to allergy, whereas atopy was not considered to be important in the pathogenesis of COPD. In recent years, the significance of atopy in the pathogenesis of asthma and immunologic factors in the pathogenesis of COPD have been reappraised (see later). Extrinsic asthma has been defined as asthma caused by IgE immune hyperreactivity to an allergen. Although as many as half of all asthmatics may have evidence for extrinsic disease,[59] immune mechanisms do not cause bronchospasm in the remainder. Extrinsic asthma and skin reactivity are less prevalent in older adults compared with children.[60, 61] As patients age, the pattern of their asthma often changes from an extrinsic to a perennial pattern.

A number of immunologic abnormalities are found in smoking subjects. Smokers have diminished skin test reactivity but higher serum IgE concentrations and higher numbers of eosinophils, compared with nonsmokers.[62–64] Both serum IgE and eosinophils increase with the number of cigarettes smoked.[65] Smokers are more likely than nonsmokers to develop skin test reactivity when exposed to new allergens in an industrial setting.[66] Further, qualitative differences may exist between serum IgE concentrations of smokers and those of atopic, nonsmoking subjects.[67] However, it is not certain that the increased serum IgE concentrations observed in cigarette smokers are related to the pathogenesis of COPD. Serum IgE that is specific for tobacco antigen can be found only in a small percentage of smokers.[68] Further, such specific IgE would have to be present in high quantities to affect materially total IgE concentrations (in comparison, the elevations in specific IgE titers in allergic bronchopulmonary aspergillosis are 100 to 1000 times those seen in COPD). It has been suggested that the elevated IgE concentrations and eosinophilia seen in smokers may play a causal role in some patients with persistent airways obstruction and symptoms of asthma, thus linking both reversible and irreversible airways obstruction.[67] However, there is no prospective evidence to support this contention.

Asthma has a strong atopic component in some patients, although this may diminish in time. Patients with COPD can have immunologic abnormalities resembling those seen in atopic patients. It has not been established whether these changes are the result of the deleterious effects of smoking, or whether they cause airflow obstruction. In either case, the interaction of smoking with these pathologic processes conceivably could establish a true syndrome of "chronic asthmatic bronchitis."

VIRAL ILLNESS IN CHILDHOOD. Lower respiratory tract illness in childhood has been proposed as a potential risk factor for the development of COPD. This hypothesis is supported by epidemiologic, physiologic, and microbiologic observations of the subtle, long-term effects of childhood respiratory illness.[69–72] These studies have demonstrated that infection with respiratory syncytial virus (RSV) or other pathogens during infancy was associated with a higher incidence of bronchial hyperreactivity later in childhood and respiratory symptoms, including airflow obstruction, in adult life. However, there may be methodologic problems in these studies, i.e., recall bias and incomplete follow-up.[73] Adults with chronic airflow obstruction have a higher recollection of childhood respiratory tract infection,[71] but this must be balanced against the fact that almost all children contract such infections in their early years. Viral illness also could interact with atopic or other host factors[74] and could predispose to airway hyperreactivity.[73, 75]

Viral infections also are associated with asthma in children; again, the difficulty is determining whether such infections predispose to the development of asthma later in life. There is a strong association between children hospitalized with bronchiolitis and wheezing or asthma on follow-up evaluation,[76–78] as well as between respiratory infection and atopy.[74] These studies support the notion that infant bronchiolitis might subsequently lead to asthma, but they could also support the alternative hypothesis that asthma and susceptibility to infant respiratory infection result from the same pathophysiologic defect.[73]

AIRWAY HYPERREACTIVITY. Having defined the major problems involved in the investigation of airway hyperreactivity, it is not surprising that disparate results have emerged from studies of airway hyperreactivity in chronic airflow obstruction. Are patients with COPD simply occult asthmatics with superimposed cigarette-induced lung disease? Or, alternatively, is the airway hyperreactivity seen in COPD a result of the chronic inflammation induced by the products of cigarette smoke?

Even with the current controversies in methodology, certain conclusions can be drawn. Airway reactivity differs among patients with chronic airflow limitation. Many studies demonstrate a strong correlation between the presence of airway hyperreactivity and the rate of decline in pulmonary function over time.[29, 31, 79] When subjects are grouped according to baseline function, those with hyperreactivity have the greatest loss of function over time.[80, 81] Recent literature suggests that appropriate bronchodilator therapy in patients manifesting hyperreactivity in COPD may lead to a markedly improved prognosis, compared with patients without a significant airway response.[82, 83]

The response to bronchodilating drugs may be different in patients with COPD than in those with asthma. Ramsdale and colleagues have shown that subjects with chronic airflow obstruction do not respond to cold air hyperventilation, as opposed to asthmatics who do.[84] Subjects with COPD may respond less to certain provocative agonists, such as methacholine or methoxamine, when compared with asthmatics,[85] though their response clearly is greater than that of normal subjects.[86] Airway responsiveness *in vivo* does not correlate with a number of pharmacologic *in vitro* responses, suggesting that airway reactivity *in vivo* in these patients may be due more to factors that modulate bronchial smooth muscle rather than intrinsic defects in the muscle itself.[87, 88] Immunoglobulins, the products of eosinophils and other cells infiltrating the airways, and other mediators could alter the response of smooth muscle in subjects with COPD, as is postulated in asthma,[89] or could result from smoking. When stratified for current and ex-smokers, patients with airway hyperreactivity actually have a lower percentage of positive skin test reactions.[90] Although serum IgE concentrations are greater in smokers than in nonsmokers,[64, 67] there are no long-term, longitudinal studies demonstrating either a pre-existing elevation or the development of an elevated IgE concentration in the serum of subjects who smoke cigarettes. While it would be intriguing to do so, it is not possible to define the relationship between these immunologic markers and airway hyperreactivity in the pathogenesis of COPD. It seems certain that a certain percentage of patients with COPD have significant airway hyperreactivity and certain immunologic anomalies. However, these may be different than those associated with asthma and may be the result of smoking, rather than the cause of COPD.

COMPARISONS IN PATHOLOGY

Asthma and COPD share some epidemiologic and physiologic similarities, but their pathologic presentations differ considerably and offer the firmest evidence that the two syndromes are, in fact, different diseases.

The greatest source of information concerning the pathology of asthma comes either from patients dying of status asthmaticus or from subjects with chronic asthma who died of other causes. A significant concern is whether these pathologic changes in patients dying of asthma reflect the usual asthmatic state in life. The pathologic data for emphysema and chronic bronchitis are abundant. Like asthma, however, relatively few studies are available concerning the early stages of COPD, the so-called "small airways disease" state.

CENTRAL AIRWAYS. Pathologically, asthma is a disease of chronic inflammation of the major airways. Upon gross examination, the most striking change in patients dying in status asthmaticus is the hyperinflation, which results from air trapping. This is caused by extensive mucous plugging of the airways,[91] which is present but less extensive in mild-to-moderate chronic asthma. Vascular dilatation, increased vascular permeability, mucosal edema, migration of inflammatory cells, shedding of epithelial cells, and excess secretion of mucus are the hallmarks of the chronic inflammatory state. This is accompanied by secretion and the release of mediators from the various cells involved in the inflammatory process, producing smooth muscle hyperreactivity.

Chronic bronchitis is defined as the hypersecretion of mucus caused by hypertrophy and hyperplasia of the tracheobronchial submucosal glands. In severe cases, the epithelium may consist almost entirely of goblet cells from the largest airways to the terminal bronchioles, accompanied by loss of ciliated epithelium.[92] The peripheral destructive changes of emphysema, which are almost never seen in asthma, commonly accompany chronic bronchitis. In addition, subsegmental bronchi may undergo extensive loss of bronchial cartilage, muscle, and peribronchial connective tissue.[93] This loss of peribronchiolar alveolar tissue, which normally holds these bronchi open, increases the likelihood of narrowing and collapse during expiration. The cause of airflow obstruction in emphysema thus differs substantially from that of asthma.

PERIPHERAL AIRWAYS. Emphysema, by definition, is the result of destruction of the terminal airways. These changes generally are not seen in asthma, even in patients dying of status asthmaticus.[94] In early disease associated with inflammation in the terminal airways, careful partitioning of resistance to airflow demonstrates that much of the increased airflow resistance is in the peripheral, as opposed to central, airways.[20, 95, 96] This correlates with the lesions seen in small airways disease[97] and is distinctly different from the obstruction to airflow in asthma. These lesions, in smokers, correlate positively with airflow obstruction[98] and provide further evidence for the differing etiologies of airflow obstruction in COPD compared with asthma.

INFLAMMATION. The inflammatory response differs between asthma and COPD. Besides the differences noted in the actual site (asthma in predominantly central airways versus emphysema in small airways), there may be substantial differences in the mediators and cells involved in each process.

In both asthma and chronic bronchitis, inflammatory changes can be observed in the central airways. Epithelial cells are sloughed, and large areas of denuded bronchial mucosa can be demonstrated. It has been suggested that airway hyperreactivity in both asthma and chronic bronchitis is caused by an increase in epithelial permeability produced by disruption of epithelial tight junctions.[99] These breaks would permit allergens and mediators to gain contact with the afferent neural receptors, mast cells, and smooth muscle within the mucosa and submucosa of the airway. However, it has been demonstrated that smokers, some of whom have increased epithelial permeability, have normal airways reactivity;[100] conversely, asthmatics with documented hyperreactivity may have normal epithelial permeability.[101]

Inflammatory cell infiltrates in the submucosa may be similar in the two disease processes. In both asthma and COPD, neutrophils and macrophages are found in abundance in areas of inflammation. However, in asthma, there is an excess of eosinophils not seen in either the central airways inflammation of chronic bronchitis or the small airways inflammation of emphysema. Bronchoalveolar lavage following allergen challenge in asthmatics yields an excess of eosinophils as well as neutrophils,[102] whereas lavage in smoking subjects with COPD yields excess neutrophils.[103] Numerous mediators secreted by both cells have been identified; the role of these mediators in the pathogenesis of both asthma and COPD is an area of intense investigation at this time.

Unlike asthma, emphysema results from destructive inflammatory changes that may be related to neutrophil or macrophage elastase activity. These enzymes solubilize native lung elastin. Endogenous protease inhibitors prevent this process, and deficiency of these inhibitors causes classic emphysema. Toxic constituents of cigarette smoke recruit neutrophils and macrophages into the peripheral airways and stimulate secretion of elastases, while simultaneously interfering with protease inhibitors.[104] Similar defects have not been demonstrated in asthma.

In conclusion, important differences exist in the pathologic presentations of asthma and COPD. These differences are the clearest evidence that these two diseases are in fact two distinct processes.

COMPARISONS IN THERAPEUTICS

Therapeutic agents such as theophylline, beta-adrenergic agonists, and corticosteroids are used commonly in both syndromes. However, some important differences in therapeutic approaches and responses to treatment have been defined recently.

THEOPHYLLINE. Theophylline has been a mainstay in the treatment of both asthma and COPD. Despite imprecise definition of its mechanism of action, it has become one of the most widely prescribed therapeutic agents in the management of airflow obstruction.

Despite its wide use, questions have been raised about the efficacy of theophylline in the treatment of "irreversible" airflow obstruction. Eaton and coworkers demonstrated that while theophylline increased FEV_1, it did not provide clinically significant relief of dyspnea, nor did it improve exercise capacity.[42, 105] Some investigators have demonstrated improvement in air flow rates but no improvement in symptoms following theophylline administration[106, 107] whereas others[108] have demonstrated the opposite. Guyatt and coworkers demonstrated significant improvements in exercise capacity and spirometric flows as well as dyspnea after theophylline therapy.[109] Theophylline increased FEV_1 significantly even in patients pretreated with inhaled beta-adrenergic agonists.[110] A problem with such studies is that patients with significant airway hyperreactivity are often excluded from further testing; therefore, there would be less response to any bronchodilating agent in the remaining subjects with minimal hyperreactivity. Studies in patients who have acute exacerbations of COPD in emergency rooms also have raised questions concerning the efficacy of theophylline.[111] In contrast to COPD, the efficacy of theophylline in asthma is uncontested; numerous studies have established efficacy in a variety of clinical settings.[112–116]

BETA-ADRENERGIC AGONISTS. Beta-adrenergic agonists are effective in treating both COPD and asthma. There is some evidence that beta-adrenergic agonists are somewhat less effective than anticholinergic agents (see later) in COPD, whereas sympathomimetic agents are more efficacious in asthma. Sympathetic neural innervation modulates cholinergic postganglionic activity, but there is no direct sympathetic innervation to airways.[117] Beta-adrenergic modulation of the airways depends on sympathetic modulation of cholinergic tone and the effect of circulating catecholamines.[118] Thus, beta-adrenergic stimulation may modulate several important pathways in the genesis of bronchoconstriction in asthma.

As the principal cause of airflow obstruction in emphysema is destruction of alveoli, sympathetic modulation of airway tone might be expected to play a lesser role in the management of COPD. Beta-adrenergic agonists have a considerable bronchodilating effect in many patients with COPD, however, indicating their importance in modulating cholinergic airway tone (see later).[119] In addition, beta-adrenergic agonists may affect the secretion of mucous glands.[120]

PARASYMPATHOLYTIC AGENTS. Endogenous parasympathetic activity is the source of resting bronchomotor tone in normal individuals. The use of anticholinergic agents in the treatment of asthma is centuries old. British physicians introduced the smoking of "asthma cigarettes" from the *Datura* plant in the early 19th century; the principal alkaloid extract from this plant is atropine.[121] This practice suffered from the considerable side effects of atropine (as well as the cigarette smoke itself!) and fell into disfavor in the early 1900s upon the introduction of adrenergic agents. Interest in anticholinergic agents was revived in the past 20 years with the introduction of synthetic analogues of atropine, which avoid many of the undesirable side effects.

There is considerable controversy over the importance of parasympathetic regulation of airway smooth muscle in the pathogenesis of asthma. In clinical asthma, synthetic parasympathomimetics, such as ipratropium bromide, dilate airways, but their effect is less than that of beta-adrenergic agonists.[121] The additive administration of ipratropium to maximal beta-adrenergic therapy may add additional bronchodilatation.[122] Ipratropium has provided better results in older asthmatics;[123] however, in this group, it is more difficult to distinguish asthma from COPD (see earlier). The overall results of clinical studies with ipratropium in asthma indicate some efficacy.

There is some evidence that parasympatholytic agents are more potent bronchodilators than beta-adrenergic agents in the treatment of COPD.[121, 124] Other investigators have found ipratropium to be equipotent to albuterol.[125] Ipratropium and similar drugs have less use in asthma, in which beta-adrenergic therapy clearly is superior. These differences in therapy illustrate fundamental differences between COPD and asthma.

CORTICOSTEROIDS. In recent years there has been considerable new information about the mechanisms by which corticosteroids affect both asthma and COPD. Much of this information comes from research in asthma and has led to the identification of biochemical mediators responsible for the pathophysiologic manifestations of this disease. Some of these mediators may also contribute to the manifestations of COPD. The addition of corticosteroids to the treatment of asthma has proved invaluable. Patients with COPD benefiting from therapy frequently have historical or physiologic findings similar to those of asthmatic patients, including a component of reversible airflow obstruction. Yet the use of corticosteroid therapy in COPD remains controversial.

In the setting of acute airflow obstruction, corticosteroids suppress the inflammatory response by inhibiting each of the essential components of the inflammatory reaction.[126] Corticosteroids block the margination of neutrophils into the lung and suppress leukocyte function.[127] Synthesis of a number of lipid and protein mediators that work to enhance chemotaxis, increase permeability of vessels, and dilate vessels, most notably the synthesized products of arachidonic acid, are inhibited by corticosteroids.[126] Corticosteroids also inhibit release of several lipid mediators, e.g., platelet-activating factor. By inhibiting the intermediate steps of inflammation, corticosteroids contribute to reversal of chronic inflammation in airways.

Corticosteroids modulate the response to a number of inflammatory mediators by influencing the availability and binding affinity of the various receptors and the coupling of the receptors to the intracellular enzymes. These agents potentiate the response to beta-adrenergic agonists commonly employed in the treatment of asthma[128] and prevent tachyphylaxis to these agonists.[129] Corticosteroids also attenuate the airway responses to constrictor agonists such as histamine[130] and suppress the binding of IgE to mast cells, neutrophils, and other inflammatory cells.[126] Corticosteroids thus inhibit bronchoconstriction and facilitate bronchodilatation at a number of intermediate points in the early phase of asthma. There is considerable evidence that corticosteroids also inhibit the late phase of nonspecific bronchoconstriction following exposure to a specific allergen.[131]

Besides their usefulness in acute asthma, corticosteroids suppress airway hyperreactivity in the long-term setting of chronic asthma.[132, 133] Such effects require continued therapy and are dose-dependent. Corticosteroids also suppress bronchorrhea associated with asthma[134] and reduce the frequency and severity of acute episodes of asthma.

Although corticosteroids are very efficacious in the management of both chronic, severe asthma and acute exacerbations of asthma, the utility of corticosteroids in the management of COPD is somewhat more controversial. Reports on the efficacy of corticosteroids in emphysema date back to 1951.[135] Since then, a number of studies have demonstrated the usefulness of corticosteroids, both oral and aerosol.[136] However, many of the earlier studies were not properly controlled. More recent studies have demonstrated a substantial benefit from corticosteroids in a variety of doses and schedules.[40, 137–139] Treatment with corticosteroids may even slow the progression of airflow obstruction.[140] However, these data are disputed because of the substantial risk of bias due to the random variation in spirometric values and in the referencing of study patients to populations that may lack the similar severity of airflow obstruction.[141] Further, one could claim that patients who respond to corticosteroids, generally about 20% to 30% of those studied, have undiagnosed asthma rather than (or in addition to) COPD.

It is evident that the response of some patients with COPD to corticosteroids is comparable to the response seen in asthmatic subjects. Whether these changes indicate a potential relationship between COPD and asthma is controversial.

ANTIBIOTICS. Antibiotics long have been part of the standard treatment of acute exacerbations of COPD. Their use has grown out of a conviction that infection participated in the pathogenesis of airflow obstruction (see earlier). The routine use of antibiotics has been questioned since the 1970s;[142] a recent, carefully controlled study demonstrated the usefulness of prophylactic antibiotics in the acute setting.[143] This differs from asthma, in which most acute exacerbations are caused by viral infections, noncompliance with medication, or exposure to a stimulating agent—none of which are amenable to antibiotic therapy.

OTHER PHARMACOLOGIC AGENTS. Disodium cromoglycate, an agent thought to stabilize mast cell membranes, is effective in the treatment of exercise-induced asthma, some cases of occupational asthma, and some younger asthmatics.[144] It has no demonstrated efficacy in patients with COPD.

Calcium channel antagonists, e.g., nifedipine and verapamil, have been studied in asthma, with contradictory results.[145–148] Nifedipine has been shown to protect against exercise-induced asthma.[149, 150] These agents have not been studied extensively in patients with COPD.

OXYGEN THERAPY. Patients with COPD constitute the largest group of patients with chronic hypoxemia. Continuous oxygen therapy clearly is of benefit in reducing the sequelae of chronic hypoxemia.[151, 152] Patients with asthma do not develop cor pulmonale and do not require oxygen therapy unless in the midst of status asthmaticus, or unless their asthma is compounded by severe hypoxemia.

CONCLUSIONS

Both asthma and COPD are complex diseases that share a number of similarities but have important differences in presentation, natural history, pathology, and management. For the present, asthma and COPD may best be considered and managed as distinct syndromes.

REFERENCES

1. American Thoracic Society. Chronic bronchitis, asthma and pulmonary emphysema. A statement by the committee on diagnostic standards for nontuberculous respiratory diseases. Am Rev Respir Dis 1962; 85:762–768.
2. Curtis JK, Liska AP, Rasmussen HK, Cree EM. The bronchospastic component in patients with chronic bronchitis and emphysema. JAMA 1966; 197:693–696.
3. Gross NJ. COPD: a disease of reversible air-flow obstruction. Am Rev Respir Dis 1986; 133:725–726.
4. Ellul-Micalluf R. Asthma: a look at the past. Br J Dis Chest 1976; 70:112–116.
5. Chadwick J, Mann WN. The Medical Works of Hippocrates. Oxford: Blackwell Scientific, 1950.
6. Willis T. Practice of Physick, Pharmaceutice Rationalis or the Operations of Medicine in Humane Bodies. London, 1678.
7. Floyer T. A Treatise of the Asthma. London: R Wilkin, 1698.
8. Sakula A. Sir John Floyer's A Treatise of the Asthma (1698). Thorax 1984; 39:248–254.
9. Laennec RTH. De l'auscultation mediate. Vol 1. Paris: JA Brosson and JS Chaude, 1819, 225.
10. Watson W. An account of what appeared on opening the body of an asthmatic person. Philos Trans 1746; 54:239–245.
11. Morgagni J. The Seats and Causes of Disease Investigated by Anatomy. (Alexander B, translator.) London: Millar, 1769, Vol 1, Book II, Letter XII, Articles 12, 13.
12. Rosenblatt MB. Emphysema: historical perspective. Bull NY Acad Med 1972; 48:823–841.
13. Louis M. Researches sur l'emphyseme des poumons. Soc Med Observ Paris Mem 1837; 1:160–261.
14. Louis M. Researches on emphysema of the lungs. Dunglison's American Medical Lib 1838; 8:491–552.
15. Osler W. The Principles and Practice of Medicine. Edinburgh and London: Young J. Pentland, 1892.
16. Fletcher CM, Pride NB. Definitions of emphysema, chronic bronchitis, asthma and airflow obstruction: 25 years on from the Ciba Symposium. Thorax 1984; 39:81–85.
17. Ciba Guest Symposium. Terminology, definitions and classifications of chronic pulmonary emphysema and related conditions. Thorax 1959; 14:286–289.
18. American Thoracic Society. Chronic bronchitis, asthma, and pulmonary emphysema: a statement by the committee on diagnostic standards for nontuberculous respiratory diseases. Am Rev Respir Dis 1962; 85:762–768.
19. Burrows B, Fletcher CM, Heard BE, et al. The emphysematous and bronchial types of chronic airways obstruction. Lancet 1966; i:830–835.
20. Hogg JC, Macklem PT, Thurlbeck WM. Site and nature of airway obstruction in chronic obstructive lung disease. N Engl J Med 1968; 278:1355–1360.
21. Lees AW, McNaught W. Bacteriology of lower respiratory tract secretions, sputum and upper respiratory tract secretions in "normals" and chronic bronchitics. Lancet 1959; ii:1112–1115.
22. Brumfitt W, Willoughby MLN, Bromley LL. An evaluation of sputum examination in chronic bronchitis. Lancet 1957; ii:1306–1309.
23. Orie NGM, Sluiter HJ, de Vries K, et al. The host factor in bronchitis. In: Bronchitis: An International Symposium, April 1960, University of Groningen. Assen: Royal Van Gorcum, 1961, 43–59.
24. Van der Lende R, de Kroon JPM, van der Muelen GG. Possible indicators of endogenous factors in the development of CNSLD. In: Orie NGM, van der Lende R, eds. Bronchitis III. Proceedings of the Third International Symposium on Bronchitis, September 1969, University of Groningen. Assen: Royal Van Gorcum, 1970, 52–70.
25. Fletcher C, Peto R, Tinker C, Speizer FE. The Natural History of Chronic Bronchitis and Emphysema. Oxford: Oxford University Press, 1976.
26. Pride N. Smoking, allergy and airways obstruction: revival of the 'Dutch hypothesis.' Clin Allergy 1986; 16:3–6.
27. Curtis JK, Liska AP, Rasmussen HK, Cree EM. The bronchospastic component in patients with chronic bronchitis and emphysema. JAMA 1966; 197:693–696.
28. Moron JW, Turnbull KW. The reversibility of chronic bronchitis, asthma and emphysema. Dis Chest 1968; 53:126–132.
29. Barter CE, Campbell AH. Relationship of constitutional factors and cigarette smoking to decrease in 1-second forced expiratory volume. Am Rev Respir Dis 1976; 115:305–314.
30. Gerrard JW, Cockcroft DW, Mink JT, et al. Increased nonspecific bronchial reactivity in cigarette smokers with normal lung function. Am Rev Respir Dis 1980; 122:577–581.
31. Ramsdell JW, Nachtwey FJ, Moser KM. Bronchial hyperreactivity in chronic obstructive bronchitis. Am Rev Respir Dis 1982; 126:829–832.
32. Anthonisen NR, Wright EC, IPPB Trial Group. Bronchodilator response in chronic obstructive pulmonary disease. Am Rev Respir Dis 1986; 133:814–819.
33. Dodge R, Cline MG, Burrows B. Comparisons of asthma, emphysema and chronic bronchitis diagnoses in a general population sample. Am Rev Respir Dis 1986; 133:981–986.
34. Schoenberg JB, Beck GJ, Bouhuys A. Growth and decay of pulmonary function in healthy blacks and whites. Respir Physiol 1978; 33:367–393.
35. Seltzer C, Seigelaub AB, Freidman GD, Collen MF. Differences in pulmonary function related to smoking habits and race. Am Rev Respir Dis 1974; 110:598–608.
36. Clausen JL. Prediction of normal values. In: Pulmonary Function Testing: Guidelines and Controversies. Orlando: Grune and Stratton, 1984, 51–62.
37. Knudson RJ, Slatin RC, Lebowitz MD, Burrows B. The maximal expiratory flow-volume curve. Normal standards, variability, and effects of age. Am Rev Respir Dis 1976; 113:587–600.
38. Burr M, Phillips KM, Hurst DN. Lung function in the elderly. Thorax 1985; 40:54–59.
39. Dodge RR, Burrows B. The prevalence and incidence of asthma and asthma-like symptoms in a general population sample. Am Rev Respir Dis 1980; 122:567–575.
40. Mendella LA, Manfreda J, Warren CPW, Anthonisen NR.

Steroid response in stable chronic obstructive pulmonary disease. Ann Intern Med 1982; 96:17–21.
41. Detels R, Tashkin DP, Simmons MS, et al. The UCLA population studies of chronic obstructive pulmonary disease. 5. Agreement and disagreement of tests in identifying abnormal lung function. Chest 1982; 82:630–638.
42. Eaton ML, Green BA, Church TR, et al. Efficacy of theophylline in "irreversible" airflow obstruction. Ann Intern Med 1980; 92:758–761.
43. Eliasson O, DeGraff AC. The use of criteria for reversibility and obstruction to define patient groups for bronchodilator trials. Influence of clinical diagnosis, spirometric and anthropometric variables. Am Rev Respir Dis 1985; 132:858–864.
44. Eaton ML, MacDonald FM, Church TR, Niewoehner DE. Effects of theophylline on breathlessness and exercise tolerance in patients with chronic airflow obstruction. Chest 1982; 82:538–542.
45. Dolovich MB, Sanchis J, Rossman C, Newhouse MT. Aerosol penetrance: a sensitive index of peripheral airways obstruction. J Appl Physiol 1976; 40:468–471.
46. Turner-Warwick M. Observing patterns of airflow obstruction in chronic asthma. Br J Dis Chest 1977; 71:73–86.
47. American College of Chest Physicians. Criteria for the assessment of reversibility in airways obstruction. Chest 1974; 65:552–553.
48. Wilder CS. Prevalence of selected chronic respiratory conditions. Vital Health Stat 1973; 10:1–49.
49. Epidemiology of Respiratory Diseases. Task Force Report. U.S. Department of Health and Human Services, NIH publication no. 81–2019, 1980.
50. Cohen BH, Ball WC, Brashears S, et al. Risk factors in chronic obstructive pulmonary disease (COPD). Am J Epidemiol 1977; 105:223–231.
51. Mak H, Johnson P, Abbey H. Prevalence of asthma and health service utilization of asthmatic children in an inner city. J Allergy Clin Immunol 1982; 70:367–372.
52. Sibbald B, Turner-Warwick M. Factors influencing the prevalence of asthma among first degree relatives of extrinsic and intrinsic asthmatics. Thorax 1979; 34:332–337.
53. Sibbald B, Horn ME, Brain EA, Gregg I. Genetic factors in childhood asthma. Thorax 1980; 35:671–674.
54. Britt EJ, Cohen B, Menkes H, et al. Airways reactivity and functional deterioration in relatives of COPD patients. Chest 1980; 77(Suppl):260–261.
55. Lebowitz MD, Knudson RJ, Burrows B. Family aggregation of pulmonary function measurements. Am Rev Respir Dis 1984; 129:8–11.
56. Gadek JE, Crystal RG. α_1-Antitrypsin deficiency. In: Stanbury JB, Wyngaarden JB, Fredrickson DS, et al., eds. The Metabolic Basis of Inherited Disease. 5th ed. New York: McGraw-Hill, 1983, 1450–1467.
57. Schwartz RH, Van Ess JD, Johnstone DE, et al. Alpha-1-antitrypsin in childhood asthma. J Allergy Clin Immunol 1977; 59:31–34.
58. Bruce RM, Cohen BH, Diamond EL, et al. Collaborative study to assess risk of lung disease in Pi MZ phenotype subjects. Am Rev Respir Dis 1984; 130:386–390.
59. Kiviloog J, Irnell L. The prevalence of bronchial asthma and chronic bronchitis in Uppsala, Sweden. Scand J Respir Dis 1974; 89[Suppl]:35–40.
60. Ford RM. Aetiology of asthma: a review of 11,551 cases (1958 to 1968). Med J Aust 1969; 1:628–631.
61. Hendrick DJ, Davies RJ, D'Souza MF, Pepys J. An analysis of skin prick test reactions in 656 asthmatic patients. Thorax 1975; 30:2–8.
62. Burrows B, Lebowitz MD, Barbee RA. Respiratory disorders and allergy skin test reactions. Ann Intern Med 1976; 84:134–139.
63. Burrows B, Halonen M, Barbee RA, Lebowitz MD. The relationship of serum immunoglobulin E to smoking. Am Rev Respir Dis 1981; 124:523–525.
64. Warren CPW, Holford Streven V, Wong C, Manfreda J. The relationship between smoking and total immunoglobulin E levels. J Allergy Clin Immunol 1982; 69:370–375.
65. Halonen M, Barbee RA, Lebowitz MD, Burrows B. An epidemiologic study of the interrelationships of total serum immunoglobulin E, allergy skin-test reactivity, and eosinophilia. J Allergy Clin Immunol 1982; 69:221–228.
66. Zetterstrom O, Osterman K, Machado L, Johansson SGO. Another smoking hazard: raised serum IgE concentration and increased risk of occupational allergy. Br Med J 1981; 283:1215–1217.
67. Burrows B, Halonen M, Lebowitz MD, et al. The relationship of serum immunoglobulin E, allergy skin tests, and smoking to respiratory disorders. J Allergy Clin Immunol 1982; 70:199–204.
68. Lehrer SB, Wilson MR, Karr RM, Salvaggio JE. IgE antibody response of smokers, nonsmokers and "smoke-sensitive" persons to tobacco leaf and smoke antigen. Am Rev Respir Dis 1980; 121:168–170.
69. Reid DD. The beginning of bronchitis. Proc R Soc Med 1969; 62:311–316.
70. Leeder SR. Role of infection in the cause and course of chronic bronchitis and emphysema. J Infect Dis 1975; 131:731–742.
71. Burrows B, Knudson RJ, Lebowitz MD. The relationship of childhood respiratory illness to adult obstructive airway disease. Am Rev Respir Dis 1977; 115:751–760.
72. Sims DG, Downham MAPS, Gardner PS, et al. Study of 8-year-old children with a history of respiratory syncytial virus bronchiolitis in infancy. Br Med J 1978; 276:11–14.
73. Samet JM, Tager IB, Speizer FE. The relationship between respiratory illness in childhood and chronic air-flow obstruction in adulthood: state-of-the-art. Am Rev Respir Dis 1983; 127:508–523.
74. Laing I, Riedel F, Yap PL, Simpson H. Atopy predisposing to acute bronchiolitis during an epidemic of respiratory syncytial virus. Br Med J 1982; 284:1070–1072.
75. Stempel DA, Boucher RC. Respiratory infection and airway reactivity. Med Clin North Am 1981; 65:1045–1053.
76. Wittig HJ, Cranford NJ, Glaser J. The relationship between bronchiolitis and childhood asthma. J Allergy 1959; 30:19–23.
77. Rooney JC, Williams HE. The relationship between proved viral bronchiolitis and subsequent wheezing. J Pediatr 1971; 79:744–747.
78. Zweiman B, Schoenwetter WF, Pappano JE, et al. Patterns of allergic respiratory disease in children with a past history of bronchiolitis. J Allergy Clin Immunol 1971; 48:283–289.
79. Barter CE, Campbell AH, Tandon MK. Factors affecting the decline of FEV_1 in chronic bronchitis. Aust NZ J Med 1974; 4:339–345.
80. Kanner RE. The relationship between airways responsiveness and chronic airflow limitation. Chest 1984; 86:54–57.
81. Vollmer WM, Johnson LR, Buist AS. Relationship of response to a bronchodilator and decline in forced expiratory volume in one second in population studies. Am Rev Respir Dis 1985; 132:1186–1193.
82. Postma DS, De Vries K, Koeter GH, Sluiter HJ. Independent influence of reversibility of air-flow obstruction and nonspecific hyperreactivity on the long-term course of lung function in chronic air-flow obstruction. Am Rev Respir Dis 1986; 134:276–280.
83. Burrows B, Bloom JW, Traver GA, Cline MG. The course and prognosis of different forms of chronic airways obstruction in a sample from the general population. N Engl J Med 1987; 317:1309–1314.
84. Ramsdale EH, Morris MM, Roberts RS, Hargreave FE. Bronchial responsiveness to methacholine in chronic bronchitis: relationship to airflow obstruction and cold air responsiveness. Thorax 1984; 39:912–918.
85. Du Toit JI, Woolcock AJ, Salome CM, et al. Characteristics of bronchial hyperresponsiveness in smokers with chronic air-flow limitation. Am Rev Respir Dis 1986; 134:498–501.
86. Bahous J, Cantier A, Quimet G, et al. Nonallergic bronchial hyperreactivity in chronic bronchitis. Am Rev Respir Dis 1984; 129:216–220.
87. Taylor SM, Pare PD, Armour CL, et al. Airway reactivity in chronic obstructive pulmonary disease. Am Rev Respir Dis 1985; 132:30–35.
88. Armour CL, Lazar NM, Schellenberg RR, et al. A comparison of in vivo and in vitro human airway reactivity to histamine. Am Rev Respir Dis 1984; 129:907–910.
89. Leff AR. State of the art: endogenous regulation of bronchomotor tone. Am Rev Respir Dis 1988; 137:1198–1216.
90. Welty C, Weiss ST, Tager IB, et al. The relationship of airways responsiveness to cold air, cigarette smoking, and atopy to respiratory symptoms and pulmonary function in adults. Am Rev Respir Dis 1984; 130:198–203.

91. Hogg JC. The pathology of asthma. Clin Chest Med 1984; 5:567–571.
92. Spencer H. Diseases of the bronchial tree. In: Pathology of the Lung, 3rd ed. Oxford: Pergamon Press, 1985, 131–166.
93. Spencer H. Emphysema. In: Pathology of the Lung, 3rd ed. Oxford: Pergamon Press, 1985, 557–594.
94. Spencer H. Bronchial asthma. In: Pathology of the Lung, 3rd ed. Oxford: Pergamon Press, 1985, 758–764.
95. Niewoehner DE, Kleinerman J. Morphologic basis of pulmonary resistance in the human lung and effects of aging. J Appl Physiol 1974; 36:412–418.
96. van Brabrandt H, Cauberghs M, Verbeken E, et al. Partitioning of pulmonary impedance in excised human and canine lungs. J Appl Physiol 1983; 55:1733–1742.
97. Cosio M, Ghezzo H, Hogg JC, et al. The relations between structural changes in small airways and pulmonary-function tests. N Engl J Med 1978; 298:1277–1281.
98. Hale KA, Ewing SL, Gosnell BA, Niewoehner DE. Lung disease in long-term cigarette smokers with and without chronic air-flow obstruction. Am Rev Respir Dis 1984; 130:716–721.
99. Hogg JC. Bronchial mucosal permeability and its relationship to airways hyperreactivity. J Allergy Clin Immunol 1981; 67:421–425.
100. Kennedy SM, Elwood RK, Wiggs BJR, et al. Increased airway mucosal permeability of smokers: relationship to airway reactivity. Am Rev Respir Dis 1984; 129:143–148.
101. Elwood RK, Kennedy S, Belzberg A, et al. Respiratory mucosal permeability in asthma. Am Rev Respir Dis 1983; 128:523–527.
102. Metzger WJ, Richerson HB, Worden K, et al. Bronchoalveolar lavage of allergic asthmatic patients following allergen bronchoprovocation. Chest 1986; 89:477–483.
103. Martin TR, Raghu G, Maunder RJ, Springmeyer SC. The effects of chronic bronchitis and chronic air-flow obstruction on lung cell populations recovered by bronchoalveolar lavage. Am Rev Respir Dis 1985; 132:254–260.
104. Snider GL. Pathogenesis of emphysema and chronic bronchitis. Med Clin North Am 1981; 65:647–665.
105. Eaton ML, MacDonald FM, Church TR, Niewoehner DE. Effects of theophylline on breathlessness and exercise tolerance in patients with chronic airflow obstruction. Chest 1982; 82:538–542.
106. Anderson G, Peel ET, Pardoe T, Jones R. Sustained-release theophylline in chronic bronchitis. Br J Dis Chest 1982; 76:261–265.
107. Alexander MR, Dull WL, Kasik JE. Treatment of chronic obstructive pulmonary disease with orally administered theophylline. JAMA 1980; 244:2286–2290.
108. Mahler DA, Matthay RA, Snyder PE, et al. Sustained-release theophylline reduces dyspnea in nonreversible obstructive airway disease. Am Rev Respir Dis 1985; 131:22–25.
109. Guyatt GH, Townsend M, Pugsley SO, et al. Bronchodilators in chronic air-flow limitation. Effects on airway function, exercise capacity, and quality of life. Am Rev Respir Dis 1987; 135:1069–1074.
110. Filuk RB, Easton PA, Anthonisen NR. Responses to large doses of salbutamol and theophylline in patients with chronic obstructive pulmonary disease. Am Rev Respir Dis 1985; 132:871–874.
111. Rice KL, Leatherman JW, Duane PG, et al. Aminophylline for acute exacerbations of chronic obstructive pulmonary disease. A controlled trial. Ann Intern Med 1987; 107:305–309.
112. Jackson RH, McHenry JI, Moreland FB, et al. Clinical evaluation of elixophyllin with correlation of pulmonary function studies and theophylline serum levels in acute and chronic asthmatic patients. Dis Chest 1964; 45:75–85.
113. Weinberger MM, Bronsky EA. Evaluation of oral bronchodilator therapy in asthmatic children. J Pediatr 1974; 84:421–427.
114. Wolfe JD, Tashkin DP, Calvarese B, Simmons M. Bronchodilator effects of terbutaline and aminophylline alone and in combination in asthmatic patients. N Engl J Med 1978; 298:363–367.
115. Rossing TH, Fanta CH, McFadden ER, Medical House Staff of Peter Bent Brigham Hospital. A controlled trial of the use of single versus combined-drug therapy in the treatment of acute episodes of asthma. Am Rev Respir Dis 1981; 123:190–194.
116. Nassif EG, Weinberger M, Thompson R, Huntley W. The value of maintenance theophylline in steroid-dependent asthma. N Engl J Med 1981; 304:71–75.
117. Richardson JB. Nerve supply to the lungs. Am Rev Respir Dis 1979; 119:758–802.
118. Garrity ER, Stimler NP, Munoz NM, et al. Sympathetic modulation of biochemical and physiological response to immune degranulation in canine bronchial airways in vivo. J Clin Invest 1985; 75:2038–2046.
119. Gross NJ, Skorodin MS. Role of the parasympathetic system in airway obstruction due to emphysema. N Engl J Med 1984; 311:421–425.
120. Santa Cruz R, Landa J, Hirsch J, Sackner MA. Tracheal mucous velocity in normal man and patients with obstructive lung disease; effects of terbutaline. Am Rev Respir Dis 1974; 109:458–463.
121. Hertz CW. Historical aspects of anticholinergic treatment of obstructive airways disease. Scand J Respir Dis 1979; 103:105–109.
122. Bryant DH. Nebulized ipratropium bromide in the treatment of acute asthma. Chest 1985; 88:24–29.
123. Ullah MI, Newman GB, Saunders KB. Influence of age on response to ipratropium and salbutamol in asthma. Thorax 1981; 36:523–529.
124. Gross NJ, Skorodin MS. Anticholinergic, antimuscarinic bronchodilators. Am Rev Respir Dis 1984; 129:856–870.
125. Easton PA, Jadue C, Dhingra S, Anthonisen NR. A comparison of the bronchodilating effects of a beta-2 adrenergic agent (albuterol) and an anticholinergic agent (ipratropium bromide) given by aerosol alone or in sequence. N Engl J Med 1986; 315:735–739.
126. Morris HG. Mechanisms of glucocorticoid action in pulmonary disease. Chest 1985; 88:133S–141S.
127. Fauci AS. Immunosuppressive and anti-inflammatory effects of glucocorticoids. In: Baxter JD, Rousseau G, eds. Glucocorticoid Hormone Action. New York: Springer Verlag, 1979, 449–465.
128. Ellul-Micallef R, Lefkowitz RJ. Agonist-promoted high affinity state of the β-adrenergic receptor in human neutrophils: modulation by corticosteroids. Lancet 1975; ii:1269–1271.
129. Davies AO, Lefkowitz RJ. In vitro desensitization of beta-adrenergic receptors in human neutrophils: attenuation by corticosteroids. J Clin Invest 1983; 71:565–571.
130. Ahmed T, King MM, Kramson JP. Modification of airway histamine receptor function with methylprednisolone succinate. J Allergy Clin Immunol 1983; 71:224–229.
131. Abraham WM, Lanes S, Stevenson JS, Yerger LD. Effect of an inhaled glucocorticosteroid (budesonide) on post-antigen induced increases in airway responsiveness. Bull Eur Physiopathol Respir 1986; 22:387–392.
132. Hartley JPR, Charles TJ, Seaton A. Betamethasone valerate inhalation and exercise-induced asthma in adults. Br J Dis Chest 1977; 71:253–258.
133. Clarke PS. The effect of beclomethasone dipropionate on bronchial hyperreactivity. J Asthma 1982; 19:91–93.
134. Agnew JE, Bateman JR, Sheaham NF, et al. Effect of oral corticosteroids on mucus clearance by cough and mucociliary transport in stable asthma. Bull Eur Physiopathol Respir 1983; 19:37–41.
135. Lucas DS. Some effects of adrenocorticotrophic hormone and cortisone on pulmonary function of patients with obstructive emphysema. Am Rev Tuberc 1951; 64:279–294.
136. Sahn SA. Corticosteroids in chronic bronchitis and pulmonary emphysema. Chest 1978; 73:389–396.
137. Albert RK, Martin TR, Lewis SW. Controlled clinical trial of methylprednisolone in patients with chronic bronchitis and acute respiratory insufficiency. Ann Intern Med 1980; 92:753–758.
138. Shim CS, Williams MH. Aerosol beclomethasone in patients with steroid-responsive chronic obstructive pulmonary disease. Am J Med 1985; 78:655–658.
139. Blair GP, Light RW. Treatment of chronic obstructive pulmonary disease with corticosteroids: comparison of daily vs alternate-day therapy. Chest 1984; 84:524–528.
140. Postma DS, Steenhuis EJ, Van der Weele LT, Sluiter HJ. Severe chronic airflow obstruction: can corticosteroids slow down progression? Eur J Respir Dis 1985; 67:56–64.
141. Eliasson O, Hoffman J, Trueb D, et al. Corticosteroids in COPD. A clinical trial and reassessment of the literature. Chest 1986; 89:484–490.
142. Tager I, Speizer FE. Role of infection in chronic bronchitis. N Engl J Med 1975; 292:563–570.
143. Anthonisen NR, Manfreda J, Warren CPW, et al. Antibiotic

therapy in exacerbations of chronic obstructive pulmonary disease. Ann Intern Med 1987; 106:196–204.
144. George RB, Payne DK. Anticholinergics, cromolyn, and other occasionally useful drugs. Clin Chest Med 1984; 5:685–693.
145. Williams DO, Barnes PJ, Vickers HP, Rudolf M. Effect of nifedipine on bronchomotor tone and histamine reactivity in asthma. Br J Med 1981; 283:348.
146. McIntyre E, Fitzgibbon B, Otto H, et al. Inhaled verapamil in histamine-induced bronchoconstriction. J Allergy Clin Immunol 1983; 71:375–381.
147. Popa VT, Somani P, Simon V. The effect of inhaled verapamil on resting bronchial tone and airway contractions induced by histamine and acetylcholine in normal and asthmatic subjects. Am Rev Respir Dis 1984; 130:1006–1013.
148. Ahmed T, Abraham WM. Role of calcium-channel blockers in obstructive airway disease. Chest 1985; 88:142s–151s.
149. Barnes PJ, Wilson NM, Brown MJ. A calcium antagonist, nifedipine, modifies exercise-induced asthma. Thorax 1981; 36:726–730.
150. Cerrina J, Denjean A, Alexandre G, et al. Inhibition of exercise-induced asthma by a calcium antagonist, nifedipine. Am Rev Respir Dis 1981; 123:156–160.
151. Nocturnal Oxygen Therapy Trial Group. Continuous or nocturnal oxygen therapy in hypoxemic chronic obstructive lung disease: a clinical trial. Ann Intern Med 1980; 93:391–398.
152. Medical Research Council Working Party. Long-term domiciliary oxygen therapy in chronic hypoxic cor pulmonale complicating chronic bronchitis and emphysema. Lancet 1981; i:681–686.

Chapter 34

BRONCHIECTASIS

Anne Logan Davis **Steve H. Salzman**

Although bronchiectasis is an old disease, first described by Laennec in 1819,[1] and considered by many a dying or "orphan" disease,[2] it still presents a diagnostic and therapeutic challenge. It remains a major problem in less-developed populations[3, 4] but still occurs in the United States and other developed countries and may be overlooked as a possible diagnosis when the presentation is unusual. It may be a clue to the presence of other congenital, genetic, or acquired abnormalities that affect host defenses and lead to bronchial wall damage.

The precise prevalence or annual incidence of bronchiectasis is unknown. Better prevention and prompt effective treatment of childhood infections have helped reduce the clinical prevalence in the United States to a number too small (less than 120,000) to be included any longer in the National Health Interview Survey estimates of disease prevalence.[5] Nevertheless, bronchiectasis can still cause considerable morbidity, disability, and even death despite the best currently available medical and surgical therapy. In the past 20 to 25 years the mean age of those dying from bronchiectasis in the United States has remained around 53.[2] On the other hand, bronchiectasis can be asymptomatic, an incidental finding at postmortem examination.

DEFINITION

Bronchiectasis is an abnormal permanent dilatation of the medium-sized cartilaginous bronchi, accompanied by variable destruction of muscular and elastic components of the walls. It is not to be confused with the temporary, reversible dilatation that often accompanies pneumonia or transient atelectasis.[6]

Bronchiectasis may be focal or diffuse. It is not a single disease, but it is a pathologic entity resulting from a variety of pathogenetic mechanisms and now recognized to be associated with many different conditions.

It can occur with chronic bronchitis and emphysema. Patients with bronchiectasis often show mucous gland hyperplasia and other pathologic and physiologic characteristics of chronic bronchitis, whereas patients with chronic bronchitis may exhibit some degree of bronchial dilatation.

CLASSIFICATION

Most classifications of bronchiectasis are based on pathologic or radiographic characteristics. The most widely used system is the Reid Classification based on pathologic and bronchographic findings in 45 bronchiectatic lobes.[7] Reid divided bronchiectasis into cylindrical, varicose, and saccular (or cystic types) (Figs. 34–1 to 34–3). Although this classification helps describe the radiologic features, it is not particularly useful in improving our understanding of the epidemiology or of the clinical and physiologic features of bronchiectasis.

PATHOLOGY

Pathologically, the cartilage-containing segmental and subsegmental bronchi are most commonly involved. The bronchi are dilated and may be filled with purulent secretions or mucous plugs. Bronchi and bronchioles distal to the dilated bronchi are often obliterated and appear as fibrotic strands.[7–10] There is thus a reduction in the number of bronchial

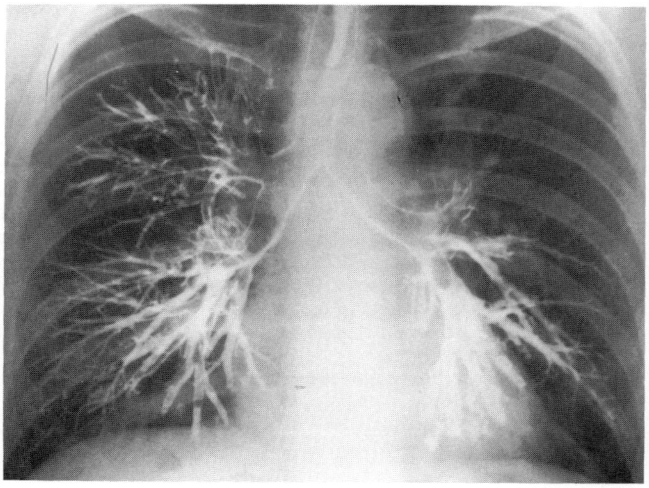

Figure 34–1. Cylindrical Bronchiectasis. Bronchogram demonstrates cylindrical bronchiectasis of both lower lobes, especially the left. The bronchi are regular in outline, but instead of tapering gradually as in the normal right middle and right upper lobe anterior segment, they end squarely and abruptly. Mucous plugs or fibrotic obliteration prevent normal filling with contrast material. The normal fine, side-branching pattern is lost, giving a "stripped-twig" appearance. (Reproduced with permission from Davis AL, Bronchiectasis. In: Fishman AP, ed. Pulmonary Diseases and Disorders. New York: McGraw-Hill Inc., 1980.)

subdivisions. This obliteration contributes to the airflow obstruction and gas exchange abnormalities often observed in cases of bronchiectasis. Gross mucosal inflammatory changes may extend to the adjacent undilated proximal bronchi. Mucous gland hyperplasia in the central airways is common. Transverse ridging of bronchial smooth muscle is prominent,

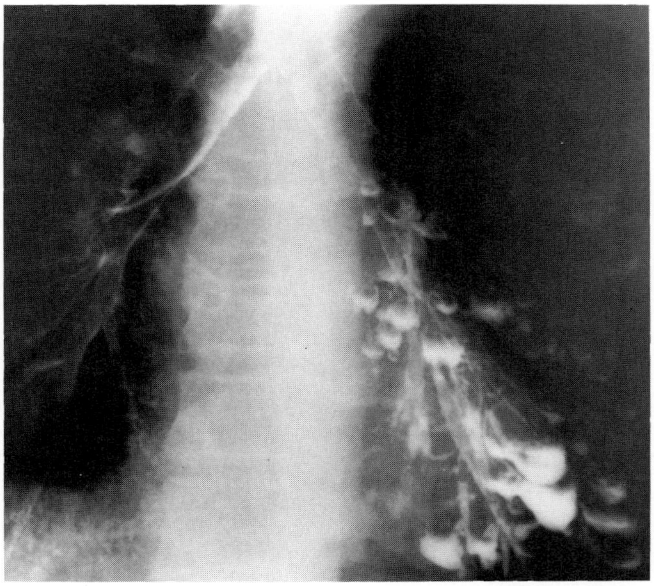

Figure 34–2. Varicose Bronchiectasis. Oblique bronchogram of right lung. Dilated bronchi present an irregular outline resembling varicose veins. In varicose bronchiectasis the bronchi are more dilated than in cylindrical bronchiectasis, and as in cystic bronchiectasis, terminate in bulbous ends. The characteristic irregularity is due to areas of local bronchial constriction alternating with dilation. (Reproduced with permission from Davis AL, Bronchiectasis. In: Fishman AP, ed. Pulmonary Diseases and Disorders. New York: McGraw-Hill Inc., 1980.)

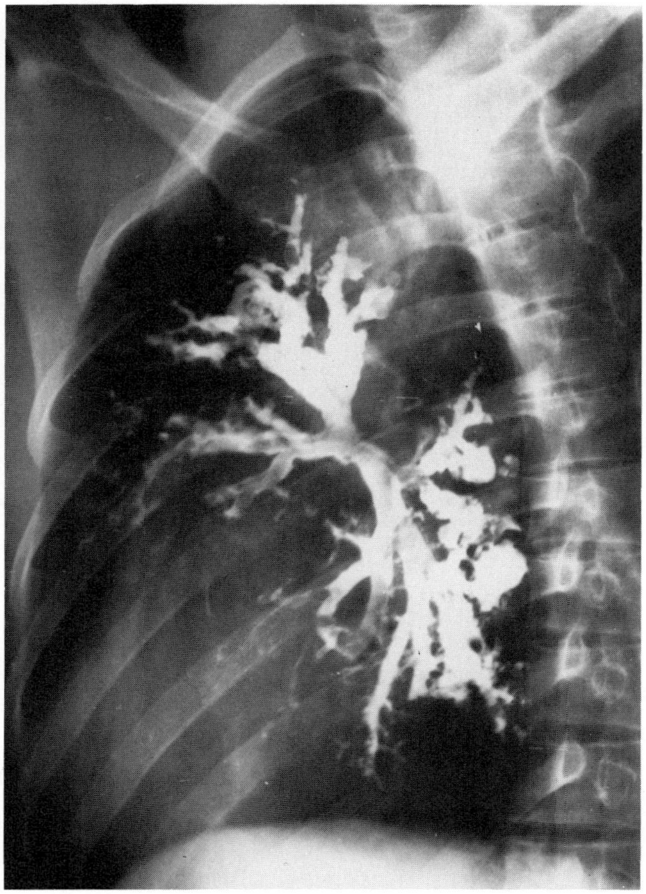

Figure 34–3. Cystic (Saccular) Bronchiectasis. Bronchogram reveals disease predominantly in the basilar segments of the left lower lobe. The bronchial dilatations, increasing progressively from the segmental bronchus, end in blind sacs as a result of obliteration of the bronchi and bronchioles beyond the dilated bronchi. The dilatations are responsible for the characteristic ballooned appearance on bronchograms. (Reproduced with permission from Davis AL, Bronchiectasis. In: Fishman AP, ed. Pulmonary Diseases and Disorders. New York: McGraw-Hill Inc., 1980.)

and pits representing dilated ducts of bronchial mucous glands are evident in the walls (Fig. 34–4).

Microscopically, there are varying degrees of bronchial wall destruction and inflammation (Fig. 34–5). In saccular bronchiectasis particularly, all components of the wall—cartilage, muscle, and elastic tissue—may be lost and replaced by fibrous tissue.[11] Chronic inflammatory cells and lymphoid follicles are often but not invariably prominent. Ulceration can occur. Squamous metaplasia may be seen, but bronchiectasis does not by itself appear to be a risk factor for bronchogenic carcinoma. Clusters of Kultchitsky or argentaffin cells are often found in the distal airways, thought to be stimulated by inflammation and fibrosis.[12]

Although the principal pathologic abnormalities are in the airways, parenchymal and peribronchial inflammation and fibrosis accompany the bronchial changes and help explain some of the radiographic features and functional impairment.[9] Parenchymal lesions in bronchiectasis include combinations of emphysema, fibrosis, and loss of alveoli. Collateral ventilation from adjacent normal bronchi probably explains the aeration of some alveoli present in the area normally fed by the obstructed bronchus.[8, 10]

Enlargement of bronchial arteries in bronchiectasis is striking.[13] The bronchial inflammation and new growth of granu-

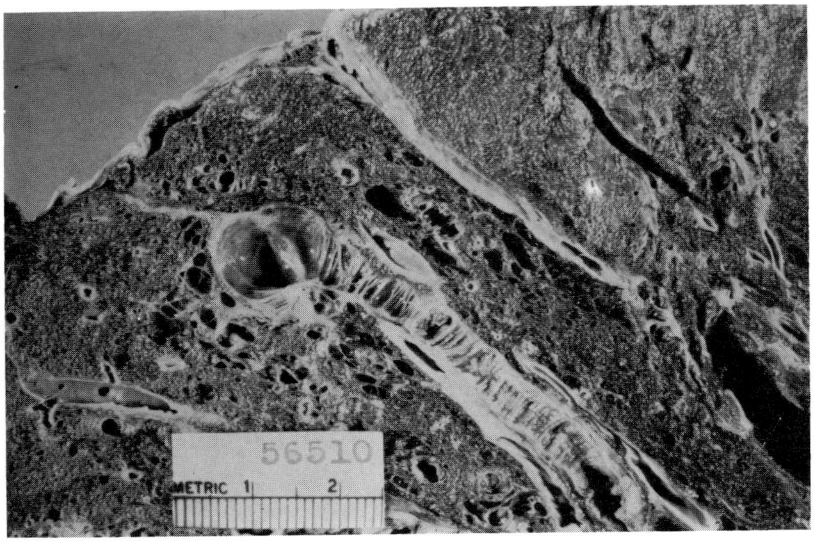

Figure 34–4. Postmortem Slice of Lung. This shows marked transverse ridging in a bronchiectatic bronchus, which extends almost to the pleural surface. Saccular dilation is seen at the end of the patent bronchus with obliteration of the bronchus distal to this appearing as a fibrotic strand. Dilated smaller bronchioles are present above, and dilated respiratory bronchioles (localized emphysema) may be seen below the abnormal bronchus. The extent of disease is often much greater than is suspected from bronchography. Inflammatory changes typical of diffuse chronic bronchitis are often found proximal to the dilated bronchi, and lung parenchyma may be totally replaced by ectatic bronchi or may show varying degrees of collapse, fibrosis, organizing bronchopneumonia, or patchy to extensive emphysema. (Reproduced with permission from Davis AL, Bronchiectasis. In: Fishman AP, ed. Pulmonary Diseases and Disorders. New York: McGraw-Hill Inc., 1980.)

lation and fibrotic tissue probably account for the increased vascularity. Bronchial veins are also enlarged. Anastomoses between the bronchial and pulmonary arterial systems have been demonstrated by Liebow, Hales, and Lindskog[13] and are believed to represent expansion of pre-existing channels as well as development of new capillary links between the two circulations. The large precapillary bronchopulmonary anastomoses are occasionally thought to be an important causative factor in pulmonary hypertension and right ventricular hypertrophy in bronchiectasis. Pathologically, bronchiectasis is usually more extensive than one suspects clinically. It may be an incidental finding at autopsy in those dying of other diseases not suspected during life. Even when bronchiectasis was diagnosed during life, a study of resected lung tissue from affected children showed pathologic findings to be more extensive than bronchograms had suggested.[14]

The lower lobes are the commonest sites of bronchiectasis, especially the left lower lobe, presumably because of poor gravitational drainage.[5a, 9, 15, 16, 25] In one series, the posterior basal segment of the left lower lobe was almost always affected.[9] The lingula of the left upper lobe and the right middle lobe are frequently involved, but the distribution probably depends on the specific pathogenetic factors. Upper lobe bronchiectasis is often secondary to prior tuberculosis or lung

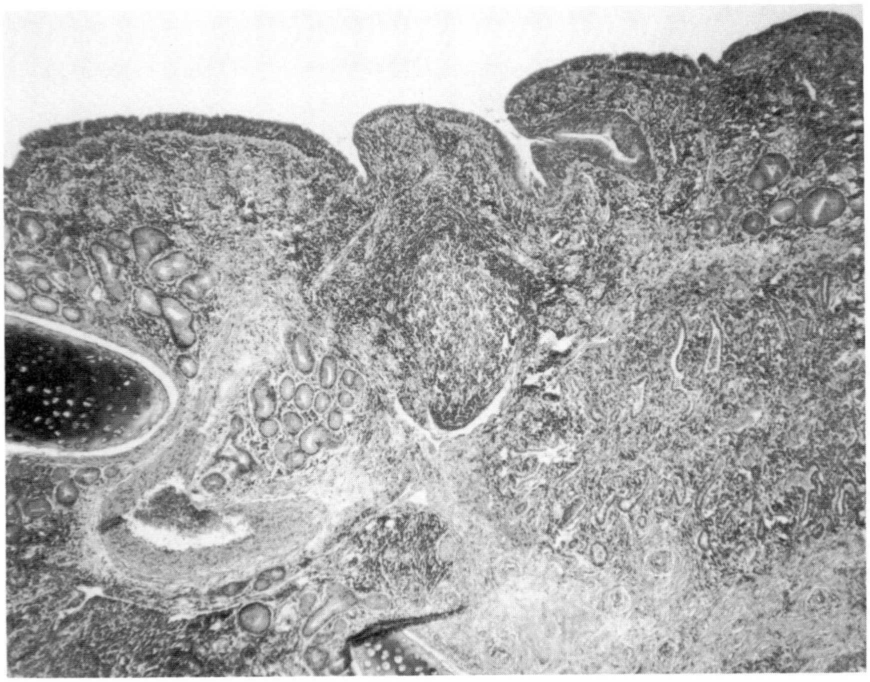

Figure 34–5. Microscopic Section of Bronchial Wall. This shows irregular contour of the luminal surface, dilated mucous ducts and glands, with some suggestion of hyperplasia, marked inflammatory infiltration of the wall, and lymphoid follicle formation, 120×. (Reproduced with permission from Davis AL, Bronchiectasis. In: Fishman AP, ed. Pulmonary Diseases and Disorders. New York: McGraw-Hill Inc., 1980.)

abscess but can be seen in cystic fibrosis as well. Bronchiectasis and chronic bacterial pneumonia in the right middle lobe were recognized as a syndrome by Graham and colleagues in 1948.[18] The middle lobe bronchus tends to be vulnerable because of its angular takeoff, poor collateral ventilation, and peribronchial nodes at its origin, which can be involved in various pathologic processes. Eighteen to 41% of cases have been reported to have bilateral bronchiectasis.[5a, 15, 19] Approximately one third have bilateral lower lobe involvement.[17]

In allergic bronchopulmonary aspergillosis, a characteristic "proximal" form of bronchiectasis may occur.

PATHOGENESIS

Initiating Factors

Bronchiectasis is generally considered to be acquired. Although congenital abnormalities and genetic alterations may predispose to its development, no data show that bronchiectasis is present at birth. Acquired infection appears to be an important factor. Lesions previously reported as "congenital bronchiectasis" are now considered a separate entity, congenital cystic adenomatoid malformation.[20–22]

Several hypotheses have attempted to explain the development of the bronchial wall inflammation, destruction, and dilatation. Possible initiating factors are summarized in Table 34–1. Primary or secondary infection, either recurrent or persistent, has almost always been implicated. Experimental induction of bronchiectasis in animals has required bronchial infection with concomitant bronchial obstruction.[23, 24]

Clinical observations have also supported the pathogenetic role of infection. Bacteria, viruses, mycoplasmas, and mycobacteria have all been implicated. Among more than 1000 cases of bronchiectasis in children reported in the 1940s and 1950s,[5a, 9, 25–29] the majority had a recognizable event such as measles, pertussis, severe pneumonia, or aspiration at the onset of symptoms. Seventy-seven percent of newly diagnosed cases of bronchiectasis at Boston Children's Hospital between 1940 and 1960 began with an infectious episode, but the number of new cases dropped dramatically with the increased use of antimicrobial agents in the 1950s.[30]

In some cases, antibody titers and autopsy studies have implicated viruses[31–39, 41–43] and mycoplasma[44, 45] in the development of necrotizing airway lesions and bronchiectasis. Some adenovirus types seem to be particularly destructive, not only in children, but in adults as well,[38] specifically types 3,[35] 7,[37] and 21.[33, 34, 36, 39] However, recent *in situ* hybridization studies of adenoviral infection by Hogg and colleagues[40] failed to show adenovirus in resected lung with follicular bronchiectasis.[40]

Tuberculosis used to be a much more important cause of bronchiectasis than it is today, but the bronchial implications still persist in some portions of the population and remain a therapeutic challenge in many other parts of the world. In the absence of early and effective antituberculosis therapy and prophylaxis, factors contributing to bronchiectasis are endobronchial necrosis, focal stenosis from endobronchial inflammation, lymph node involvement producing extensive compression or endobronchial obstruction, and parenchymal scarring producing distortion of airways.[46–48]

TABLE 34–1. Initiating Factors in Bronchiectasis

Infection: primary or secondary
Inhaled chemical toxins or immunoactive substances
Abnormal immune responses: genetic or acquired
Mechanical factors
Bronchial obstruction: focal or diffuse
Parenchymal traction on bronchi
Miscellaneous inherited or congenital abnormalities

A connection between infections of the upper respiratory tract with those of the lower has been recognized for a long time, but an etiologic role for nasal sinusitis in bronchiectasis has not been established. It is probable that infection occurs in both directions and that infected sinuses can lead to lower airway exacerbations and persistence of infection there.[15]

About a third of cases of bronchiectasis, however, develop insidiously or without definite initial infection. Some other damaging insult appears to be implicated. Inhalation of a toxic chemical or immunoactive substance, or an autoimmune reaction, may induce bronchiectatic changes. Inhalation of noxious fumes, gases, or particles has resulted in diffuse bronchiectasis. Anhydrous ammonia fumes,[49–51] sulfur oxides,[52, 53] talc,[55] cork,[56] bakelite,[57] and smoke[58] are a few examples.

Aspiration of gastric contents results in intense inflammation[59] and has been followed by development of bronchiectasis.[60] In 400 consecutive hospitalized patients with proved benign esophageal disease, including hiatal hernia, motility disorders, and diverticuli, 35% of the patients had pulmonary complications.[61] There was a 2% incidence of bronchiectasis. Aspiration of saliva, gastric contents, or food can produce chronic contamination of the airways and at times recurrent or even massive pneumonia. Chronic tracheoesophageal fistulas are also associated with bronchiectasis.[62, 63]

Heroin pulmonary edema or intoxication has been followed by development of bronchiectasis.[60, 64–66] Heroin appears to induce damage even without aspiration of gastric contents. The mechanism is unknown but may be related to altered immunologic defenses, impaired lymphatic clearance because of injected particulates, or microbial contamination of the heroin.

A few reports of airways disease, including bronchiectasis, occurring in ulcerative colitis,[67–71] rheumatoid arthritis,[72, 73] Sjögren's syndrome,[74] cutaneous vasculitis,[75] Hashimoto's thyroiditis,[76, 77] pernicious anemia,[76] primary biliary cirrhosis,[76] celiac disease,[76] and sarcoid,[78–80] have suggested that bronchiectasis may be part of a systemic disorder in which these are abnormal immunologic manifestations, often reflecting hyper- or autoimmune responses.

The role of abnormal mechanical forces, as in atelectasis or parenchymal fibrosis, has aroused considerable controversy.[9, 15, 16, 81, 82] Dilatation and distortion of bronchi *per se* do not constitute bronchiectasis, but they can impair mucociliary clearance, promote retained secretions, and allow infection with eventual destruction of bronchial wall elements characteristic of true bronchiectasis. Lander and Davidson demonstrated experimentally that pulmonary collapse can produce dilation of bronchi that reverses when the lung re-expands.[81] That parenchymal scarring might cause dilatation by putting traction on the bronchi was suggested by Corrigan in 1838[83] and others[82] since then, but pathologic evidence does not support this theory, as fibrosis can be seen without bronchiectasis and bronchiectasis can be found without significant parenchymal scarring.[15, 81] The cases of "traction bronchiectasis" reported by Westcott and Cole[82] were similar to postinfectious bronchiectasis, but the pattern of involvement was less segmental and marked dilation of bronchi was rarely present.

Congenital and genetic abnormalities provide a favorable stage for the other pathogenetic factors to play out their roles. (See section on Conditions Associated with Bronchiectasis.)

Although the exact sequence of events leading to the bronchial wall changes and clinical manifestations of bronchiectasis is still unclear, electron microscopy and newer immunologic and molecular and cellular biologic techniques have helped extend our knowledge of the pathologic changes in bronchiectasis and improve understanding of how some of the associated conditions may contribute to the development of the characteristic bronchial wall defects.

Role of Host Responses and Products of Infecting Agents

Bacterial products such as endotoxins, cilioinhibitory substances, and proteases seem to be involved, along with host products of inflammation and immunity such as chemotactic factors, neutrophil elastase, other serine proteases, superoxide radicals, immune complexes, and possibly in some cases eosinophil products. Whatever the initiating event or defect is, tissue damage occurs, mucociliary clearance usually is impaired,[84, 85] mucus is retained, bacterial colonization is present, and neutrophils appear in the bronchial secretions, probably by recruitment from the blood with the help of increased chemotactic activity. With ^{111}indium-labeling techniques, polymorphonuclear leukocytes have been observed to migrate from the blood to the lungs in bronchiectasis,[86] and increased chemotactic activity, demonstrated in the sol phase of purulent sputum, has been shown to decline after successful antimicrobial therapy.[87, 88]

The presence of neutrophils in the sputum of patients with chronic bronchial suppuration is thought by some to have pathogenetic implications.[89] Elastolytic activity, present in secretions of patients with chronic bronchial sepsis,[90] may not reflect only an inflammatory *response* to injury; neutrophil elastase itself can *injure* respiratory epithelium, leading to bronchial secretory cell metaplasia and emphysema in hamsters[91] and tracheal mucosal damage and impaired mucociliary activity *in vitro*.[92]

Furthermore, purulent secretions from bronchiectatic patients can impair ciliary beating *in vitro,* and the effect can be reduced when elastolytic activity is removed with alpha$_1$-antiproteinase.[93] Elastase activity in secretions may possibly enhance bacterial colonization by interfering with IgA function, allowing greater bacterial adherence to respiratory epithelium.[94] In the study of Niederman and colleagues,[94] the majority of sputum elastase degrading IgA was a serine proteinase derived from neutrophils.

Oxygen-derived free radicals released by activated neutrophils and phagocytes can cause tissue injury. Their effect may be direct or mediated by inactivation of proteinase inhibitors.[95] Their role in bronchial damage is unknown.

Whether eosinophils play a role in some cases of bronchiectasis, e. g., allergic bronchopulmonary aspergillosis, is unknown. Several eosinophil granule proteins have been demonstrated to produce respiratory epithelial damage and ciliostasis *in vitro*.[96] Histologically, eosinophils are often abundant at the site of bronchial involvement in allergic bronchopulmonary aspergillosis, mucoid impaction,[97] and some cases of bronchocentric granulomatosis.[98, 99]

Defective immunologic responses may predispose to bronchiectasis.[100–109] Abnormalities in number, maturation, or function of B or T cells or both, whether due to regulatory factors (often genetic) or to autoantibodies or other acquired influences, have been described in patients with chronic sinopulmonary disease, including bronchiectasis.[101] Opsonization, phagocytic function, and other defense mechanisms may be altered. A cell-mediated immune response has also been suggested by the abnormal mononuclear cell infiltration in human bronchiectasis and by immunopathologic studies in a rat model of experimental bronchiectasis.[110]

The role of circulating immune complexes in the pathogenesis of bronchiectasis is unclear. Circulating immune complexes have been reported in severe bronchiectasis,[75] but they could result from persistent chronic antigenic stimulation, either from bacterial products that are inadequately cleared or from products of tissue destruction. However, the association of bronchiectasis with several "autoimmune" diseases and the finding of antibodies to bronchial mucosa[67] and smooth muscle,[67, 68] and clinical improvement with corticosteroid therapy,[67] raise the tantalizing possibility of a pathogenetic role in some cases. Nevertheless, deposition of immune complexes in bronchiectatic areas and correlation with disease activity have not been demonstrated to our knowledge. There is some evidence that circulating immune complexes can deposit in alveolar capillary walls and interstitium of lung as they do in kidney and cause tissue injury, the severity of which depends on such factors as increased vascular permeability[111] and the degree and duration of antibody responses.[112] Furthermore, by activating complement, immune complexes have been demonstrated to lead to epithelial damage.[113]

Microbial organisms, apart from the host immune responses they can induce, can directly injure airway epithelium and alter ciliary function *in vitro*.[114, 115] *Pseudomonas,*[116–120] *Haemophilus influenzae,*[121–123] *Staphyloccus aureus,*[124] *Streptococcus pneumoniae,*[125] and *Bordetella pertussis*[126] are some of the bacteria reported to produce factors that damage ciliary function and airway epithelium. A glycolipid hemolysin derived from the cell wall of *Pseudomonas aeruginosa* affects ion transport and can increase mannitol permeability.[116] Several hydrophobic low-molecular-weight products of *Pseudomonas* inhibit ciliary beating.[115, 117–119] Whereas 1-hydroxyphenazine rapidly caused dyskinesia and ciliostasis with little epithelial disruption, pyocyanin pigment had a slower effect with eventual epithelial disruption as well as ciliostasis. *Pseudomonas* also produces a metalloelastase and an alkaline protease that experimentally can cause epithelial necrosis, but their role in human airway damage is unclear.[115] *Pseudomonas* bacterial elastase can digest IgG and affect opsonic function.[127] *H. influenzae* (both encapsulated and nonencapsulated) produces a toxin that damages tracheal epithelial cells and causes sloughing,[121, 122] and a purified lipopolysaccharide that has been shown to disrupt epithelium.[123]

Mycoplasma and certain respiratory virus infections have been followed by development of bronchiectasis. The mechanisms of injury to respiratory epithelium and ciliary function by these agents are still being investigated.[128, 129] *Mycoplasma* organisms can attach to both ciliated and nonciliated cells, alter cell metabolism, and produce ciliary dyskinesia and ultimate cellular necrosis. Influenza virus also interacts with receptors on airway epithelium with resultant injury.[130] The immunologic responses evoked, as well as viral-bacterial interactions[131] and genetic factors, probably help determine the type and severity of tissue damage.

The proximal bronchiectasis observed in allergic bronchopulmonary aspergillosis is thought to result from an immune response to inhaled fungus (usually *Aspergillus* spores). Usually some factor favoring colonization, such as airflow obstruction, or excessive mucus is present. The fungus growing in the airways releases antigen. It is postulated that IgE-sensitized mast cells in the bronchi react with the fungal antigen and release mediators that permit penetration of antigen. The absorbed antigen may then react with IgG to form immune complexes and activate complement. Chronic inflammation and destruction could result.[132] Histologic findings of mononuclear cells and granulomas suggest a cell-mediated component may also be implicated.[133]

Other Factors

Noninfectious agents, such as inhaled exogenous particles or gases, can exert their toxicity on the airway epithelium either through immunologic pathways or through direct interaction with the epithelium. Ion transport, permeability of the paracellular areas (tight junctions), or in some cases metabolic pathways may be affected.[134]

To summarize current concepts of pathogenesis, it appears that some insult, infectious or noninfectious, damages the bronchial mucosa, disturbs mucociliary, immunologic, or other host defenses, and permits microorganisms to thrive. Both host and external infectious and noninfectious agents or their products probably contribute to the damage. Endotoxins, mediators of inflammation, antigen-antibody complexes, and other factors still to be elucidated may contribute to bronchial mucosal injury and eventually to deeper destruction of bronchial wall components. Present hypotheses will undoubtedly be revised when new data become available.

CONDITIONS ASSOCIATED WITH BRONCHIECTASIS

Recognition of increasing numbers of conditions and defects associated with bronchiectasis has gradually been improving our understanding of how and why it may develop. Table 34–2 summarizes the most commonly associated conditions and possible mechanisms for the relationship.

A history of **severe infection,** either poorly treated or untreated or caused by a particularly necrotizing agent such as *Klebsiella, Staphylococcus aureus, Bordetella pertussis, Mycobacterium tuberculosis,* influenza or adenovirus, *Mycoplasma,* or fungus has often been reported in cases of bronchiectasis.[9, 15, 17, 25, 46, 135] On the other hand, bronchiectasis itself may be associated with recurrent pneumonia. It was associated in 23 of 158 reported patients with recurrent pneumonia.[136] With necrotizing pneumonias, bronchial distortion, and dilatation are common, but whether bronchial dilatation results in chronic bronchial sepsis with destructive changes in the wall depends on adequacy of drainage of the affected bronchi and the degree of obstruction. Recognizable signs of the cause of the original necrotizing process are often gone by the time the bronchiectasis is diagnosed.[46]

Bronchial obstruction may be associated with focal bronchiectasis. Endobronchial obstruction from a foreign body, neoplasm, granuloma, or mucoid impaction; stenosis following endobronchial inflammation from tuberculosis or other necrotizing infections or injury; or external compression or kinking from enlarged lymph nodes or parenchymal scarring can lead to postobstructive pneumonitis, slow resolution, and bronchiectasis. Bronchiectasis as a sequela of foreign body aspiration is particularly common in children, with a reported incidence of 3.5% to 16%.[2, 137] Bronchiectasis is rare with an obstructing bronchogenic carcinoma because the tumor is either resected or the patient has expired before bronchiectasis becomes evident. With partially obstructing benign tumors, however, bronchiectasis is more common.[138]

The precise relationship of **chronic bronchitis, emphysema,** and **asthma** to bronchiectasis needs further clarification, but the three conditions are often associated.[12, 139, 140] Mucous gland hyperplasia and dilated bronchial gland ducts characteristic of chronic bronchitis are often found in central, nonbronchiectatic airways of patients with bronchiectasis. Varying degrees of emphysema are commonly found in bronchiectatic lobes,[140]

TABLE 34–2. Some Conditions Associated with Bronchiectasis

CONDITION	POSSIBLE MECHANISMS FOR BRONCHIECTASIS
Infection Bacteria: *K. pneumoniae, S. aureus, B. pertussis* Mycobacteria Mycoplasma Viruses: Influenza, adenoviruses, measles Fungi	Impaired mucociliary clearance, disruption of respiratory epithelium. Effects of microbial products such as endotoxins, cilioinhibitory substances, and proteases. Effects of host immune responses and inflammatory products
Focal bronchial obstruction Foreign body Endobronchial tumor or granuloma, mucoid impaction External compression from lymph node, aneurysm, tumor Bronchial stenosis	Poor drainage of secretions, recurrent or slowly resolving infections with potential for prolonged exposure to damaging bacterial and host inflammatory products
Chronic bronchitis	Increased mucous secretion, impaired mucociliary clearance, airflow obstruction in some, impaired macrophage function. Bacterial colonization and recurrent infections. Increased number of neutrophils. Increased proteolytic enzymes and other products of bacteria and viruses, and inflammation that can impair defenses and cause tissue injury
Emphysema	Probable proteinase-antiproteinase imbalance. Genetic deficiency in $alpha_1$-antiproteinase in a few
Asthma	Abnormal inflammatory response of airways to variety of stimuli. (See also Allergic bronchopulmonary aspergillosis, Mucous impaction, and Bronchocentric granulomatosis)
Allergic bronchopulmonary aspergillosis (ABPA)	Immunologic response (mainly Type I and Type III and perhaps Type IV) to fungus in the bronchial lumen (most often *A. fumigatus*)
Mucoid impaction	Overlaps with ABPA, bronchocentric granulomatosis. Immunologic response suspected, but antigen not yet identified. *Aspergillus* or other fungi present in some but not all
Bronchocentric granulomatosis	Overlaps with ABPA. Immunologic response suspected, but antigen not yet identified. *Aspergillus* or other fungi present in some, but not all. Possible role of eosinophils in destruction of airways
Cystic fibrosis	Genetic defect resulting in an altered transport protein (cystic fibrosis transport regulator) and abnormal airway epithelial Cl^- transport, and mucus secretion. Recurrent infection, perpetuated by damaging microorganisms such as *Staphylococcus* and *Pseudomonas*

Table continued on following page

TABLE 34–2. Some Conditions Associated with Bronchiectasis *Continued*

CONDITION	POSSIBLE MECHANISMS FOR BRONCHIECTASIS
Ciliary dyskinesia (includes Kartagener's syndrome)	Genetic defect in ciliary ultrastructure with absent or dyskinetic ciliary beating, impaired mucociliary clearance, and potential for recurrent or persistent infections
Young's syndrome (obstructive azoospermia)	Unknown. Normal mucociliary function and ultrastructure. Normal sweat chloride
Immunodeficiency states IgG deficiency, IgG subclass deficiencies, IgA deficiency, leukocyte dysfunction, lymphocyte dysfunction, complement deficiencies	Genetic or acquired predisposition to recurrent or persistent infections and in some cases to allergic and autoimmune diseases
Autoimmune or hyperimmune disorders Rheumatoid arthritis, ulcerative colitis, cutaneous vasculitis, Hashimoto's thyroiditis, pernicious anemia, primary biliary cirrhosis, celiac disease	Unknown. Bronchiectasis may be part of systemic autoimmune disorder or reaction to persistent foreign antigen
Pulmonary sequestration	Congenital abnormal development of portion of lung tissue and its blood supply, predisposes to infection
Yellow nail syndrome	Unknown. Congenital lymphatic hypoplasia associated with poor lymphatic drainage and sometimes immunologic deficiency, may promote infection
Diseases of tracheal or bronchial cartilage Williams-Campbell syndrome	Congenital deficiency of cartilage in 4th to 8th bronchial divisions, interference with airway mechanics leading to airflow obstruction, impaired clearance and recurrent infections
Tracheobronchomegaly (Mounier-Kuhn syndrome)	Unknown, but probably congenital enlargement of tracheal rings and membranous portion of trachea, with recurrent infections as above. Possible disease of abnormal elastic tissue, cartilage and muscle
Unilateral hyperlucent lung (Swyer-James syndrome)	Severe infection in infancy leading to hypoplasia of lung, smaller pulmonary artery on involved side, and cystic changes in proximal bronchi
Inhalation of noxious fumes or dusts Anhydrous ammonia, sulfur dioxide, talc, cork, bakelite, silica	Direct damage to epithelium possibly affecting tight junctions, metabolic function, and ion transport. Also immunologic effect in some
Chronic fibrosing diseases	Bronchial distortion can occur, but destructive inflammation necessary for true bronchiectasis
Aspiration of gastric contents	Products of inflammation evoked
Heroin use, especially with pulmonary edema	Unknown. Possible impaired lymphatic clearance, and/or microbial contamination of the heroin. Gastric aspiration in some
Marfan's syndrome	Unknown. Genetic connective tissue disease. Structural bronchial defect or chest deformity might explain tendency to recurrent infections
Heart-lung transplant	Bronchiolitis obliterans. Inflammatory process may be factor in development of bronchiectasis.

and localized bronchiectasis has been found in 18% to 27% of patients dying of chronic airflow obstruction, most of whom had extensive emphysema.[139] Whether bronchiectasis is primary and some bronchitis and emphysema secondary, or whether the bronchiectasis is secondarily associated with bronchitis and emphysema, is sometimes difficult to distinguish. The distribution and extent of dilatation may help.[12] In bronchiectasis, emphysema is localized to the area of bronchiectasis. In chronic bronchitis and emphysema, the dilatation is milder and widespread rather than focal. In patients dying of status asthmaticus, the distribution of cystic bronchiectasis was found to be similar to the distribution of focal areas of collapse, suggesting that asthmatic bronchial inflammatory occlusion was the mechanism for the bronchiectasis in asthma.[141]

Alpha$_1$-antiproteinase deficiency, associated with certain genetic phenotypes[142] and most commonly related to panacinar emphysema, also has been reported in severe diffuse bronchiectasis.[142–146] In some of the reported cases, other factors have contributed to the bronchiectasis, such as pertussis or recurrent pneumonia. In 60 cases of bronchiectasis, Varpela and colleagues[146] found six patients with low levels of alpha$_1$-antitrypsin and the Pi MZ phenotype, but all had other potential causes for the bronchiectasis. In the necropsy case of panacinar emphysema with diffuse dilation of small bronchi and bronchioles and alpha$_1$-antitrypsin deficiency reported by Glascow and colleagues,[143] the elastic lamina was not intact in any of the bronchi examined, suggesting the role of elastase and inadequate proteinase inhibition as a factor in the airways dilatation. Proteinases are helpful in host defense, but it is also postulated that proteinase inhibition protects the lung from injury, especially during inflammation or infection, when high local concentrations of proteinases may be present. If the inhibition is deficient, there is greater potential for tissue destruction.

Allergic bronchopulmonary aspergillosis has been reported in as many as 20% of patients with chronic asthma.[147] The characteristic "central" or "proximal" bronchiectasis, a characteristic complicating feature,[98] is thought to be responsible for much of the morbidity: the repetitive pneumonic episodes, some episodes of hemoptysis, enhancement of colonization with fungi (especially *Aspergillus* species), chronicity of infection, and ultimate mortality in the "BEAP" syndrome, characterized by bronchiectasis, eosinophilia, asthma, and pneumonitis.[148] Although sensitization to *Aspergillus* seems to lead to bronchiectasis, Bahous and colleagues[149] postulated that at least occasionally pre-existing bronchiectasis leads to colonization and sensitization to the fungus. Occasionally an invasive necrotizing form of aspergillosis occurs, with purulent sputum, infiltrates seen radiographically, and cavitary lesions.[150] Some of these may represent bronchiectatic cysts with fungal invasion of the wall.

Bronchiectasis is also associated with other airway diseases, such as **mucoid impaction**[151] and **bronchocentric granulomatosis,**[152] which show clinical symptoms similar to those of allergic bronchopulmonary aspergillosis and have other overlapping features. Hypersensitivity to *Aspergillus* and probably other fungal agents can probably be manifested in several different ways: as mucoid impaction,[151] bronchocentric granulomatosis,[152] or other pathologic reactions[153] that are associated with bronchiectasis. With mucoid impaction, a history of asthma is common (80% of cases). Proximal bronchiectasis may be seen after resolution of the proximal mucous plug, and eosinophilic infiltration of the bronchial walls is common.[97, 151] *Aspergillus* or other noninvasive fungi may be found in the plugs, but *Aspergillus* skin tests and precipitins may be negative. In bronchocentric granulomatosis there may or may not be a history of asthma and blood and tissue eosinophilia. Sometimes neutrophils predominate in the lung. Noninvasive fungi may or may not be found. Bronchiolar epithelium may be replaced by granulomatous inflammation, and destruction of distal airways is characteristic.[152]

Bronchiectasis is a prominent feature of **cystic fibrosis** in both children and adults (see Chapter 32). This genetic disease occurs in about 1:2000 white and 1:17,000 black live births.[154] The abnormal CF gene that affects chloride transport and leads to inspissated mucus has been identified.[155–157] Adolescents and adults with the disease are now seen with increasing frequency.[158–161] Bronchial changes are more common than parenchymal changes.[154, 160, 161] Inspissated secretions, bronchial obstruction, atelectasis, and occasionally allergic bronchopulmonary aspergillosis may contribute to the bronchiectatic changes. Studies of pulmonary specimens suggest that the pulmonary involvement begins as a bronchiolitis and progesses to a mucopurulent bronchitis, invasion of airways by inflammatory cells, and progressive destruction leading to bronchiectasis. Hypertrophy and hyperplasia of the mucous glands, plugging of peripheral airways, and infection occur early in the course. Large bronchiectatic abscess cavities separated by bands of tissue are seen later on autopsy sections.[162]

The association of bronchiectasis with sinusitis and *situs inversus,* first described by Kartagener in 1933, is well known. **Kartagener's syndrome** is inherited as an autosomal recessive condition with incomplete penetrance and is present in about 1 in 30,000 to 1 in 60,000 births.[163] The earliest and most striking feature is situs inversus, occurring in about 1 in 10,000 births,[164] and 16% to 25% of patients with this manifestation have been reported to have bronchiectasis, as opposed to 0.05% to 0.3% of the general or hospital population without situs inversus.[165] The explanation for the association of the triad of sinusitis, situs inversus, and bronchiectasis was obscure until the discovery in 1975 that these patients have a congenital abnormality of their cilia that may account for the situs inversus, respiratory manifestations, and infertility frequently observed.[166, 167, 176] Since then, Kartagener's syndrome has been recognized as a subset of a larger group of heterogeneous conditions with variable clinical manifestations but having in common **primary ciliary dyskinesia.** A variety of ultrastructural and functional abnormalities in cilia have been reported, including absence of and reduction of dynein arms.[166, 168] Dynein is an ATPase protein arranged along the length of the outer microtubules and believed to relate to ciliary motility. The dynein arm abnormalities, defective radial spokes[169] and abnormalities of microtubules,[170] have correlated with abnormalities in ciliary beat frequency and wave form[171] and are associated with poor or no mucociliary transport. The range of clinical manifestations includes chronic cough, expectoration, chronic rhinitis, often with nasal polyposis, chronic or recurrent sinusitis, chronic or recurrent otitis media (usually most severe in childhood and adolescence), and recurrent pneumonia. Infertility, especially in men but seen also in some women, and various degrees of *situs inversus* from none to total[171] are present. Bronchiectasis is common, occurring in 19 of 24 patients studied by Mossberg and colleagues.[172] Some patients have mild symptoms; others develop bronchiectasis early in childhood and become incapacitated. However, some patients with Kartagener's syndrome have survived into their 80s.[173] In general, patients with ciliary dyskinesia syndrome have a better prognosis than patients with cystic fibrosis.[174] Pulmonary function is variable, from normal to restrictive, but most often shows airflow obstruction, suggesting that impaired mucociliary transport may be a contributing factor in development of chronic obstructive lung disease (COPD).[167, 172, 174]

Although the dyskinetic cilia syndrome is usually inherited as an autosomal recessive gene,[175] with a frequency in Caucasians of about 1:16,000 to 1:20,000,[174] *acquired* abnormalities in bronchial cilia, similar to the changes seen in primary immotile cilia syndrome, have been observed in patients with respiratory neoplastic disease or chronic sinusitis, in smokers, and during respiratory infections.[177–179] Such changes might account for recurrent respiratory infections and bronchiectasis in some individuals.[177]

Other syndromes with some clinical features similar to those of cystic fibrosis and primary ciliary dyskinesia syndrome, but also with some differing features, have been reported and may be associated with bronchiectasis.

Young's syndrome, obstructive azoospermia, was first described in 1970 in 28 men attending an infertility clinic, who had azoospermia and lung defects. Ten had bronchiectasis.[180] In subsequent reports, bronchiectasis has been a frequent finding.[181, 182] It is estimated that Young's syndrome is more prevalent than either cystic fibrosis or the ciliary dyskinesia syndrome.[182] Like the other two conditions, it is characterized by chronic sinopulmonary infections and fertility problems, but the mechanisms are different. Young's syndrome does not have the abnormal sweat or pancreatic function patterns of cystic fibrosis nor the cilial ultrastructual disorders of the dyskinesia syndrome. Spermatogenesis is normal, and the azoospermia is due to obstruction of the epididymis by inspissated secretions. The maldevelopment of Wolffian duct structures characteristic of cystic fibrosis is not present. The nature of the defect is not known. Whether an immunologic defect contributes to the tendency to respiratory infections is unknown. The respiratory involvement is often mild and does not necessarily progress with age, but the epididymal obstruction, which may not develop until after puberty, seems to be progressive.

Additional variant syndromes are reported, in which chronic infections or bronchiectasis or both are a feature.[183, 184] The nature of the fundamental genetic defects still needs to be worked out.

Bronchiectasis is also associated with a variety of **immunologic abnormalities,** both genetic and acquired. In one series of 53 patients with chronic purulent sputum and bronchiectasis of unknown cause, 42 (79%) had immunogloblin abnormalities, usually elevation of IgA, IgG, or IgM. Elevations tended to be significantly greater than those observed in patients with chronic bronchitis, emphysema, or asthma. Autoantibodies were also more prevalent (rheumatoid factor in 52%, antinuclear antibodies in 10%), and one or more autoimmune disorders were commonly associated (19%). IgA deficiency was noted in two of the ten cases with autoimmune disease.[76] None of the abnormalities correlated with disease activity.

The most common immunodeficency associated with bronchiectasis is panhypogammaglobulinemia.[100–103] Persistent cough, recurrent pneumonia, and bronchiectasis are characteristic. Symptomatic IgA deficiency is said to account for 10% to 15% of clinically serious immunodeficiency.[101] The deficiency can be primary or related to other factors, such as phenytoin administration or some immunologic abnormality, and occurs in 1 in 700 people in the general population.

In a Japanese survey of primary immunodeficiency, more than half the patients with IgA deficiency had frequent infections, and a quarter had autoimmune or collagen vascular diseases.[185] Gastrointestinal malabsorption, malignant neoplasms, and allergies also have been reported.[105] Abnormalities in IgA subclasses or in the secretory component may determine the range of clinical expression. IgA deficiency has been reported to be associated with other deficiencies, such as IgG_2 and IgG_4, and these immunoglobulin subclass deficiencies seem to be related to increased susceptibility to infection.[108, 109, 186–188] Isolated IgA deficiency is more likely to be associated with chronic respiratory disease when IgE is normal or increased. IgE deficiency alone or IgE plus IgA deficiency do not seem to predispose to chronic respiratory disease.[189] About half of selected IgA-deficient patients are also IgE deficient.[189]

In addition to an association with hypo- or agammaglobulinemia and other immunoglobulin aberrations, bronchiectasis has been reported in the "bare lymphocyte syndrome," in which lymphocytic expression of HLA-A, HLA-B, and HLA-C antigens, important to recognition of immunogenic antigen, was lacking.[190] Bronchiectasis also occurs with acquired immunoglobulin abnormalities in lymphosarcoma,[191] leukemia, or thymomas.[191–193]

The association of bronchiectasis with various **autoimmune or collagen vascular diseases** is intriguing and not yet clearly understood. Reports of rheumatoid arthritis with bronchiectasis are uncommon.[2] In 516 patients with rheumatoid arthritis reported by Walker and Wright, 16 had bronchiectasis.[73] The respiratory symptoms generally preceded the onset of arthritis by years. Mathieu and associates reported that 5 of 11 patients with bronchiectasis and/or cystic fibrosis developed a polyarthritis with positive rheumatoid factor.[72] Bronchiectasis also has been associated with Sjögren's syndrome.[74]

When cutaneous vasculitis and bronchiectasis have been associated, circulating immune complexes were present and deposition of C3, IgG, and IgA was demonstrated in dermal blood vessels.[75] The skin lesions occurred only during exacerbations of respiratory symptoms, suggesting to the investigators that possibly *H. influenzae* (isolated from sputa in all four cases) could be the antigenic component of the immune complexes. If immune complex deposition occurred in the lung as it did in the skin, it might perpetuate and increase tissue damage in the lung.

The association of sarcoidosis and bullous and bronchiectatic air cysts has been reported by several observers,[78–80] as a complication of sarcoidosis occurring in 5.8% to 24.5% of cases, and contributes to morbidity and mortality. How immunologic characteristics of sarcoidosis relate to the roentgenologic and pathologic changes is speculative. Sarcoidosis occurring in two patients with cystic fibrosis has been reported.[194]

The association of inflammatory bowel disease and chronic bronchopulmonary disease, including bronchiectasis, has been recognized since the report by Kraft and associates[69] in 1976 of six patients who developed chronic respiratory disease from 3 to 13 years after the onset of the colon disease. Among 1400 patients in a registry for inflammatory bowel disease who were seen between 1930 and 1970, 94 (approximately 6%) had pulmonary diagnoses, but unexplained bronchopulmonary disease was rare (6 of 94 cases). At least 31 cases of unexplained pulmonary disease associated with ulcerative colitis have now been reported.[68] Bronchiectasis has been most frequent, with extensive changes noted on bronchograms and vasculitis on lung biopsy. Mild airways obstruction and reduction in carbon monoxide diffusion capacity have been demonstrated respectively in 50% and 25% of 36 patients with inflammatory bowel disease, suggesting that pulmonary involvement may be more common than is reported. Generally, the cases with pulmonary involvement tended to have severe colitis. The higher frequency of a positive family history for inflammatory bowel disease in the cases with pulmonary involvement than in those without pulmonary disease, the frequency of other extraintestinal complications,[67, 69–71] and the temporal relationship to the inflammatory bowel disease raise the question of a common pathogenesis. Chronic bronchial suppuration has been reported soon after colectomy, coincident with the colitis, and in some cases before the onset of colitis. Antinuclear antibodies, smooth muscle antibodies, and circulating immune complexes have been reported.[67]

In all these conditions with immunologic abnormalities, whether the immunologic changes play a pathogenetic role in the bronchiectasis or whether some of the immunologic findings may be secondary to bacterial products,[195] chronic infection, and tissue damage associated with bronchiectasis still needs evaluation.

Bronchiectasis has been associated with a variety of congenital abnormalities. **Pulmonary sequestration,**[196–198] one of the most common developmental malformations of the foregut, is an area of lung that has no or incomplete communication with the tracheobronchial tree and that has an aberrant systemic arterial blood supply. The sequestrated area usually contains dilated bronchial elements and other bronchoalveolar tissue. Intralobar sequestrations that occur within the pleural covering of a pulmonary lobe, usually the lower lobe, frequently become infected. Recurrent pneumonia or abscesses and bronchiectasis are characteristic. Infection and obstructive changes are uncommon in extrapulmonary sequestrations that are outside the pleural covering and isolated from the normal lung, often resting between the diaphragm and lower lobe. They are usually asymptomatic but may be associated with other malformations, such as diaphragmatic hernia or pectus excavatum.

The **yellow nail syndrome,** first described by Samman and White in 1964,[199] is thought to result from underdeveloped hypoplastic lymphatics. In addition to the characteristic primary lymphedemas, yellow dystrophic nails, and pleural effusions, which may be present in various combinations, bronchiectasis[200, 201] and sinusitis[201] have been associated in some cases. Bronchiectasis is thought to be related to defective lymphatic clearance and perhaps to an increased susceptibility to infection because of associated immunologic deficiency,[200, 201] although the latter has rarely been demonstrated. The time between the development of the various manifestations is variable from months to many years.[200] Yellow nails are not always present, and pleural effusions tend to occur after the other manifestations. There may be a propensity to malignant disease, especially lymphomas or sarcomas.[200] The lymphedema is often precipitated initially by an infection or injury.

Several disorders affecting airway cartilage are associated with bronchiectasis. The **Williams-Campbell syndrome,**[201a, 202] described in 1960, is characterized by deficiency in bronchial cartilage from the 4th to 8th generation bronchi (0 generation = trachea; first generation = mainstem bronchi), leading to persistent cough and wheezing first noticed in infancy. Chest deformity, clubbed fingers, and small stature are common. Ballooning and collapse of segmental bronchi are apparent. It is thought to be congenital and it may be familial.[203]

The early onset of symptoms, the extension of the bronchiectasis proximally to the first and second order bronchi (rare in acquired bronchiectasis), the uniformity of the defect, the lack of destruction of the bronchial wall elements, and the disproportionate amount of structural change in relation to the duration of infection have supported a congenital origin. It is uncertain whether bronchiectasis is present at birth or develops because of predisposing conditions. Diffuse congenital bronchomalacia without bronchiectasis has been reported.[204]

Tracheobronchomegaly, a rare condition characterized by dilation of the trachea and bronchial tree, is usually associated with bronchiectasis, which accounts for the clinical symptoms. Although the first bronchial abnormality was recorded in 1897 by Czylarz, the first clinical description was made by Mounier-

Kuhn in 1932. The trachea may be 30 to 45 mm wide instead of the normal 15 to 22 mm seen in normal adult men.[205] The longitudinal muscles are thinned, and atrophy of the elastic fibers of the pars membranacea has been observed histologically.[205] About one third of cases have tracheal diverticuli as well.

Although the abnormality has been postulated to be a congenital defect in cartilage, elastic tissue, and muscle, the respiratory symptoms, typical of bronchiectasis, tend to occur in the third and fourth decades of life, suggesting an acquired abnormality.[206] However, cases have been reported in children.[205] Other connective tissue diseases, such as Ehlers-Danlos syndrome and cutis laxa, as well as other anatomic variations of the tracheobronchial tree, are reported to be associated.

Bronchiectatic changes have been observed in cases of **unilateral hyperlucent lung,** first described by Swyer-James and MacLeod in the 1950s.[207, 208] Radiographically, the condition is recognized by the small, hyperlucent, relatively devascularized lung with little volume change during respiration. It has been thought to result from some childhood injurious event that causes bronchitis, obliterative bronchiolitis, lung parenchymal destruction, and impaired pulmonary perfusion. Cases have been reported after viral, especially adenoviral, pneumonitis in infancy.[209] Bronchography usually shows a pattern of bronchitic and bronchiectatic abnormality, particularly peripherally. The normal caliber of the main stem bronchi and branches tends to distinguish this syndrome from congenital hypoplastic lung.[210] However, damage has been demonstrated in bronchi more proximal than the typical location for bronchitis obliterans.[209]

Bronchiectasis has been reported in patients with **Marfan syndrome,**[211–213] a disorder of connective tissue inherited as an autosomal dominant of variable expression. Skeletal, cardiovascular, and ocular abnormalities are most common, but pulmonary abnormalities, including especially spontaneous pneumothorax and emphysema, occur in about 10% of patients.[211] Bronchiectasis in Marfan syndrome was first described by Katz in 1952.[214] Since then other cases have been reported, but in one series of 100 hospital cases, only two patients had bronchiectasis.[212] Bronchiectasis may result from a basic bronchial defect, or from the high incidence of recurrent respiratory infections or pneumonia that often accompanies associated thoracic cage deformity. The reason for bronchiectasis is not fully understood. Defects in biosynthesis of two polypeptide chains necessary for collagen type I have been reported in Marfan syndrome,[215, 216] as well as abnormal elastic tissue.[217]

FUNCTIONAL CHANGES

Airway Dynamics

Normally the intrathoracic portion of the trachea and the bronchi widen on inspiration and elongate as a result of the arrangement of the myoelastic tissue in the bronchial wall. On expiration, active contraction of the muscles and natural recoil of the elastic tissue cause the bronchi to narrow and shorten.[15] Cinebronchography, manometric studies of intrabronchial and pleural pressures, and measurements of airflow at the mouth have shown that on forced expiration, instead of uniform reduction in caliber of bronchial divisions seen in normal people and in patients with cylindrical bronchiectasis, patients with cystic and varicose bronchiectasis tend to collapse their lobar or segmental origins without changing the caliber of bronchiectatic spaces or segments.[218] Intrabronchial pressures in the bronchiectatic segments are generally high in these cases. The altered dynamics in varicose and cystic bronchiectasis are similar to those seen in chronic bronchitis and emphysema, in which morphologic reduction in cartilage, smooth muscle, and fibrous tissue has been described by Wright in the walls of segmental bronchi.[219] These mechanical aberrations in bronchiectasis have important clinical implications. Inadequate airflow velocity and widened bronchiectatic spaces in relation to particle size can limit cough effectiveness and promote retention of secretions and perpetuation of chronic infection.[218]

Tracheobronchial Deposition and Clearance

Deposition and clearance patterns also tend to resemble those seen in chronic bronchitis. Studies using tagged particles or radiocontrast material have shown a more central pattern of deposition than expected from the size of the inhaled particles or pattern of breathing, and clearance has tended to be slow.[84, 85] With tantalum, Gamsu and colleagues demonstrated delayed clearance specifically from bronchiectatic areas.[220] In one study, clinical features relating to greater impairment of clearance were generalized airway symptoms, earlier onset, and continuity of symptoms.[221]

Several factors probably contribute to these abnormalities. In addition to less effective cough (for the aforementioned reasons), abnormalities of ciliary function and viscoelastic properties of bronchial secretions play a role. Ciliated epithelium is replaced by squamous cells (metaplasia) or granulation tissue in some cases. Also, *in vitro* studies have shown slower ciliary beat frequency in some patients with bronchiectasis, compared with controls or patients with cystic fibrosis,[222] and structurally and functionally defective cilia have been described in some cases, such as in those with Kartagener's triad or other variants of the ciliary dyskinesia syndrome.[223, 224] Host responses and microbial agents themselves may contribute to the ciliary slowing or stasis. Cilia from sites of purulent secretions beat more slowly *in vitro* than cilia from normal people or patients with bronchiectasis without purulent infection.[225] A serine protease, possibly elastase, released from neutrophils during the inflammation may be a possible factor, as the slowing effect has been inhibited by alpha$_1$-antitrypsin.[93] Bacterial products from microorganisms such as *P. aeruginosa* and *H. influenzae* are capable of producing slowing and disorganization of normal human mucociliary beat function, and as they are prevalent in patients with bronchiectasis, these microorganisms might accentuate the clearance problems.[114, 115, 117–121, 226, 227] (See Section on Pathogenesis.)

Pulmonary Physiology and Hemodynamics

Most patients with bronchiectasis have abnormalities of pulmonary function.[12] The pattern and severity of derangement reflect the variable extent, topography, and type of bronchiectasis, as well as any additional airway and parenchymal disease present. Some degree of airflow obstruction is common; it occurred in more than two thirds of 42 patients studied by Cherniack and Carton [228] and of 31 patients studied by Pande and associates.[4] Thurlbeck believes that it is not the dilated airways but the obliterated distal bronchi and bronchioles and mucous plugging that produce the airflow limitation.[12] Bronchospasm, mucosal edema, and increased dynamic compression are also possible factors. Limitation of airflow at low lung volumes[229] and reduced dynamic compliance and frequency dependence have been demonstrated[4, 228, 229] in some cases. These abnormalities probably result from small airways disease[229] and nonuniformity of airway resistance, although some degree of lung stiffening from fibrosis also has been postulated.[4, 228] Vital capacity and total lung capacity often are reduced but may be normal. The pattern of dysfunction can be similar to that in emphysema or chronic bronchitis with airflow limitation, but in bronchiectasis the residual volume and functional residual capacity tend to be smaller.[4, 12, 228] The carbon monoxide diffusion capacity may be reduced,[4, 12, 228–230] but the alveolar-arterial Po_2 gradient is increased even in those with a normal diffusion capacity.[228]

Inhomogeneity of ventilation and increased venous admixture are common,[4, 228] but carbon dioxide retention is infrequent. True right-to-left shunts have been demonstrated in patients with extensive bronchiectasis.[4] Pulmonary hypertension and cor pulmonale are late findings and contribute significantly to mortality. Hypoxemia, primarily from ventilation perfusion maldistribution but also from arterial-venous shunting, is a major factor. Occasionally bronchial arterial flow through anastomoses with the pulmonary arterial system may be large enough to produce retrograde flow in the pulmonary artery,[231] but these left-to-right shunts usually do not contribute to the pulmonary hypertension.

The pulmonary function derangements correlate significantly with the extent of bronchiectasis; the highest correlations in Pande's series were with steady state diffusion capacity ($r = 0.559$, $P < 0.001$), maximal midexpiratory flow rate (MMFR), maximal breathing capacity (MBC), and dynamic compliance,[4] but in the patients of Cherniack and Carton, MBC, residual volume/total lung capacity ratio, pulmonary resistance, and 7-minute N_2 index correlated best with the number of segments involved.[228] However, both series disclosed that pulmonary function was not always inversely related to the extent of disease. Even with extensive disease, functional impairment was sometimes minimal, and yet with localized disease abnormalities in pulmonary function could be considerable. Saccular bronchiectasis was no different from cylindrical bronchiectasis in respect to the average results or the regression coefficients for each lung function test.[228]

The obstructed airways in bronchiectasis sometimes respond to bronchodilators. In a group of 16 patients studied by Nogrady and colleagues, peak expiratory flow rate (PEFR) and FEV_1 increased after salbutamol aerosol inhalation 25.8% and 16.4%, respectively.[232] Reversibility was related to baseline severity of the flow limitation and was greatest in those with moderate obstruction. To what extent chronic bronchitis and emphysema play a role in the functional impairment in bronchiectasis is unclear.

BRONCHIAL SECRETIONS

Understanding of how bronchial secretions are formed and their specific characteristics in different diseases is incomplete and still evolving. Bronchial secretions are usually studied as sputum, which is a mixture of bronchial secretions and saliva, but even when bronchial secretions are aspirated they represent a mixture of transudate or inflammatory exudate, immunoglobulins, secretion of mucus from serous and mucous submucosal glands and the goblet cells of the surface epithelium, and some alveolar fluid.[233]

Patients with bronchiectasis are generally thought to have increased secretions. The gland/wall ratio (Reid index),[234] believed to reflect the degree of hypersecretion, is increased in bronchiectasis as it is in simple chronic bronchitis, but an increase in the size of mucous gland acini is not necessarily a feature, as it is in chronic bronchitis.[235] The proportion of serous cells to mucous cells in the bronchial submucosal glands seems to be increased in bronchiectasis.[235] In addition, histochemical studies also have shown alterations in the pattern of glycoproteins secreted by mucous cells, with more sulfated mucin and a marked reduction in sialomucin production.[236, 237]

Studies using chemical markers of mucous and serum glycoproteins have suggested that differences in concentrations of these glycoproteins related more to the macroscopic type of sputum than to the specific disease. Purulent sputum from patients with chronic bronchitis, cystic fibrosis, or bronchiectasis had similar concentrations of mucous and serum glycoproteins. The range in absolute concentrations of *mucous* glycoprotein markers seemed to reflect the degree of gland hypertrophy and change in intracellular glycoprotein, i.e., whether sialylated or sulfated, whereas *serum* glycoprotein markers reflected the degree of inflammation, especially in asthma.[238] In their study of COPD patients, including cases of bronchiectasis, Lopata and colleagues concluded that patients with COPD produce sputum that is similar to induced sputum from "normal" subjects, suggesting merely hypersecretion.[239] However, when sputum becomes purulent, the alterations in DNA, water content, and type of cross-linking reflect the accompanying inflammatory process.

Lipids are present in bronchial mucus, and there is evidence for airway synthesis. The profile in hypersecretory states is different from that in normals.[240] In hypersecretory states such as chronic bronchitis and cystic fibrosis, there is a shift from neutral lipids, which predominate in normal mucus, to glycolipids.

The biochemical characteristics of bronchial secretions affect the physical properties, which in turn influence mucociliary transport. The mucoid properties of bronchial secretions are thought to be due to the presence of glycoprotein mucins. Their length and carbohydrate groups permit secondary bonding between molecules, which contributes to formation of a coherent viscoelastic gel. Disulfide bonds are involved in the cross-linking, and hydrogen bonding with water and other elements also occurs.[241]

With infection and inflammation, the bronchial secretions are augmented by leukocytes, macrophages, shed epithelial cells, abnormal effusion of blood proteins, and products from infecting bacteria. Deoxyribose nucleoprotein fibrils are liberated from disintegrating cells and are believed to become incorporated in the gel structure and contribute to the tenacious consistency. However, viscosity does not always correlate with purulence.[242] Increased pulmonary epithelial permeability has been demonstrated in bronchiectatic patients with purulent sputum and significant colonization of the respiratory tract by bacterial pathogens.[243] Under such circumstances, dilution of the bronchial components by serum components might decrease viscosity. In mucoid sputum, the mucous glycoprotein seems to be most important in determining viscosity, whereas in infected sputum both mucus and serum components contribute.[238] Furthermore, the increased enzymic activity in purulent sputum can result in breakdown of mucopolysaccharides and may contribute to lowering viscosity. Dulfano and Adler,[244] in a study of patients with COPD, found that for maximal transport velocity, low viscosity and high elastic recoil represent the best rheologic combination. Undoubtedly the rheologic properties of respiratory secretions in bronchiectasis affect mucous transport. In fact, the rheologic properties rather than the biochemical characteristics, *per se,* seem to determine the interaction between ciliary activity and mucus.[245]

Studies of protein fractions present in bronchial secretions have provided variable results even for the same disease. The concentrations seem to be related largely to the presence and intensity of the inflammatory response, but differences in patient populations and techniques might account for some of the discrepant findings. In the study by Gawel and colleagues,[246] secretory immunoglobulin A was decreased in children with chronic lung diseases, including cystic fibrosis and bronchiectasis, and lysozyme levels were increased. Considerable variation was observed in IgG and lactoferrin. Immunoglobulin G, lactoferrin, and lysozyme increased during infection, but not secretory IgA. On the other hand, a necropsy study by Burnett and colleagues,[247] using the immunoperoxidase technique, showed that the total number of IgA-positive cells was increased in bronchiectatic and bronchitic lungs compared with lungs from those with no history of lung disease. IgA1 cells predominated in the major bronchi and were more increased in the bronchitic lungs. IgA2 cells were also increased in both disease groups and were proportionately greater in the bronchi than in nonmucosal lymphoid tissues. More needs to be known about immunoglobulin and enzyme patterns in normals and disease states, both in the respiratory secretions as well as in serum, to be able to interpret the significance of these different proteins in secretions of people with bronchiectasis.

In addition to lysozyme, lactoferrin, and neutrophil elastase, cathepsin B–like cysteine proteinase activity has also been described in sputum and bronchoalveolar lavage (BAL) samples from patients with bronchiectasis and patients with chronic bronchitis.[248] It has correlated with neutrophil counts in BAL fluid, and the activity has decreased with antibiotic or corticosteroid therapy that resulted in a change of sputum from purulent to mucoid. Beta-lactamase activity also has been identified in sputum from patients with bronchographically proved bronchiectasis during a period of clinical stability.[249] Since the activity was significantly higher in sputum than in saliva, and highest in purulent specimens, the β-lactamase activity was believed to be derived mainly from bronchial bacterial flora, even perhaps from bacteria commonly considered nonpathogenic.

These and perhaps other enzymes yet to be observed may be important in perpetuating the inflammatory process. Fibronectin-cleaving activity has been found in bronchial secretions from patients with cystic fibrosis and from patients with chronic bronchitis with acute exacerbations. Bronchial secretions from individuals with cystic fibrosis were found to have proteolytic activity against surface airway mucosal cells.[250] Neutrophil elastase and cathepsin G accounted for most of this activity. However, in contrast to patients with chronic bronchitis, in whom the activity was present only during exacerbations, the fibronectin-cleaving activity persisted over a follow-up period of several years. Since *Pseudomonas* adheres better to cell surfaces devoid of fibronectin, this fibronectin activity in cystic fibrosis and during exacerbations of chronic bronchitis may help explain the frequency of this microorganism in cystic fibrosis and bronchiectasis without cystic fibrosis.

CLINICAL FEATURES

Initial Presentation

Bronchiectasis can present in a variety of ways and can mimic other diseases. Frequently, patients describe a severe pneumonia with subsequent chronic cough and phlegm. Bronchiectasis also commonly presents insidiously with chronic, productive cough[15, 27] and is symptomatically indistinguishable from other chronic inflammatory pulmonary diseases such as chronic bronchitis or pulmonary tuberculosis. Recurrent lower respiratory infections, especially pneumonia in the same anatomic location, is another important mode of presentation. Hemoptysis may be the first and only complaint,[251] and in some asymptomatic individuals with "dry bronchiectasis" and usually upper lobe disease, the chest radiograph may provide the first clue. When bronchiectasis presents as pleuritic chest pain and hemoptysis, it can be mistaken for pulmonary embolism.[252] A fluid-filled bronchus can mimic a coin lesion.[253] Accompanying inflammatory infiltrates can sometimes be confused with mycobacterial infection or even bronchoalveolar cell carcinoma.

When childhood infections were the major cause of bronchiectasis, symptoms typically began in childhood.[5a, 9, 27] Now, however, with childhood immunizations and better antimicrobial control of infection, bronchiectasis may not be recognized until adolescence and even much later adulthood, even though inherited or congenital predisposing factors are predominant and the process may begin early.

Symptoms

The symptoms are variable, depending on the severity of disease, the presence of infection and degree of inflammation, and the presence of other associated or predisposing conditions. Chronic productive cough is the most common symptom. It may be persistent or intermittent but is typically productive. Hemoptysis has been reported in up to 50% to 70% of cases, but in some series the incidence is considerably lower. Sputum is usually blood streaked from erosion of capillaries in inflamed mucosa, but bleeding can be massive when bronchial arteries are the source of bleeding. Acute exacerbations of cough and sputum associated with fever occur in approximately one third of patients. Shortness of breath and wheezing are variable complaints that reflect the clinical state (more common during exacerbations) and the presence of associated obstructive airways disease. Sinusitis with nasal complaints may be present, particularly when the underlying etiology of bronchiectasis is cystic fibrosis, ciliary dyskinesia, or immunoglobulin deficiencies.

Signs

Findings on physical examination are nonspecific. Localized persistent rales are the most characteristic. The rales are typically loudest in early and mid-inspiration but are also present in expiration.[254] Rhonchi, wheezes, and signs of consolidation also may be present. Other signs, such as cachexia, cyanosis, and clubbing, are present in advanced cases and are no longer commonly seen in the United States. In sequential studies by Field, clubbing decreased in frequency from 44% in 1949 to 13% in 1961, and then to 7% in 1969.[283] She attributed this to the use of antibiotics. Signs of cor pulmonale may be present in severe cases with respiratory failure.

Sputum

Sputum is similar to that in chronic bronchitis. It may be mucoid, mucopurulent, or purulent, depending on the clinical state. In advanced cases the sputum, on standing, separates into a frothy top layer, a mucoid middle layer, and a yellow-to-green layer of pus and debris at the bottom.

Gram stain usually shows numerous polymorphonuclear leukocytes and mixed bacterial flora. *H. influenzae, S. pneumoniae, Staphylococcus aureus,* and a variety of gram-negative bacteria are frequently reported.[255–263] Nontuberculous mycobacteria and anaerobes also have been identified in bronchiectatic cavities. With increasing severity of disease, the mucoid strain of *Pseudomonas* tends to appear in some cases.

RADIOLOGIC CHARACTERISTICS

Chest Radiograph

The routine chest radiograph usually is abnormal, but mild bronchiectasis may be present despite a normal radiograph.

In Gudbjerg's study in 1955, only 7% of patients with bronchiectasis had a normal chest radiograph,[264] and others have found similar results. A later study suggests that the sensitivity of the plain chest radiograph may be only 47%.[265] Another group found a sensitivity of 73% and a specificity of 76%.[266]

Mixtures of increased and decreased radiographic density are seen, depending on underlying pathology. Early changes include increased size and loss of definition of the bronchial markings in specific segmental areas of the lung.[264, 267] Gudbjerg attributed this to peribronchial fibrosis and to a lesser extent to retained secretions.[264] When present as a linear lucency associated with thin radiodense lines ("tram tracks"), these changes have greater diagnostic significance. These same shadows seen in cross-section may appear as ring shadows. When these dilated bronchi are filled with secretions, they may present as a thick linear density ("mucous plug") or a branching Y or V-shaped density ("gloved-finger sign"). When atelectasis or parenchymal fibrosis becomes prominent, there is crowding together of the thickened bronchial markings (Fig. 34–6). When disease is more advanced, there may be complete atelectasis of a lobe with compensatory hyperinflation of remaining lung tissue.

When cystic bronchiectasis is present (Fig. 34–7), cystic spaces up to 3 cm in diameter may be seen. These may have air-fluid levels or, if completely filled, may present as pulmonary nodules. A coarse honeycomb pattern may result from emphysematous spaces surrounded by fibrosis, rather than from dilated airways (Fig. 34–8). These will not be visualized on bronchography, since they are in the parenchyma rather than in the bronchi. Recurrent pneumonia in the same segmental or lobar distribution is another radiographic feature suggestive of the diagnosis.

Bronchography

Bronchography with instillation of radiocontrast material via a catheter or bronchoscope, despite its diagnostic value, is no longer routinely performed in the evaluation of patients with possible bronchiectasis. Unless surgery is being considered, it will not usually contribute to patient management. It is contraindicated in patients with severely compromised pulmonary function or acute bronchospasm. Potential complications include allergic reactions to the local anesthetic or contrast material, acute worsening of pulmonary function, or both.[267]

The radiographic pathologic classification of Reid[7] is generally used to classify the abnormalities as cylindrical, varicose, or cystic (or saccular) (see Figs. 34–1 to 34–3).

True bronchiectasis should be distinguished from the reversible dilation that can be seen after an acute pneumonia. This "pseudobronchiectasis" presumably results from reversible bronchial inflammation or associated atelectasis.[267–270] Retained secretions also may result in false-positive or false-negative results. These problems can be minimized by proper timing of the procedure, preferably 4 to 6 months after a pneumonia and by the use of antimicrobials, bronchodilators, and postural drainage beforehand.

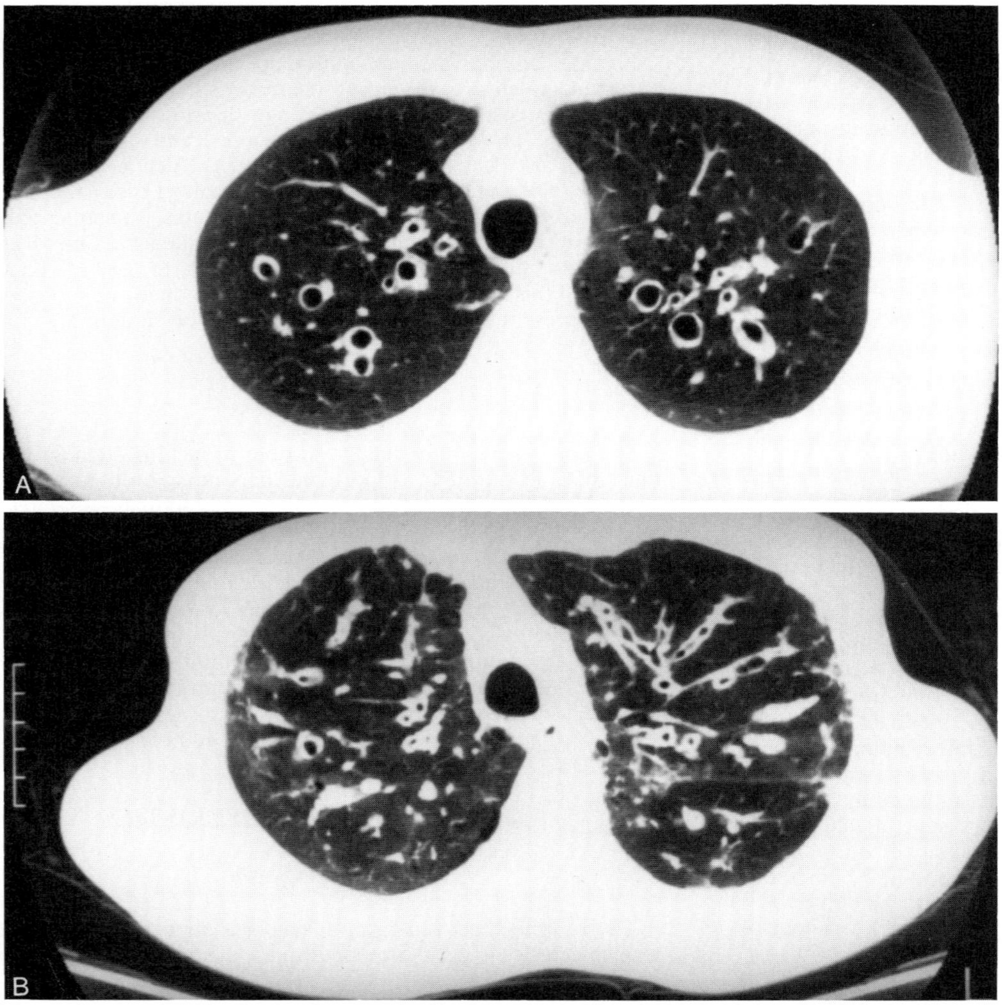

Figure 34–6. Posteroanterior Radiograph of Bronchiectasis. Thickening and crowding of bronchovascular markings in both lower lobes, especially the right.

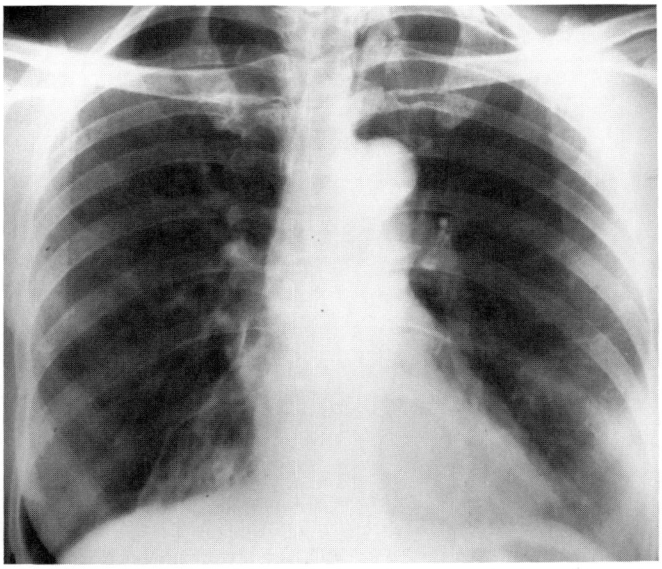

Figure 34–7. Posteroanterior Radiograph of Cystic Bronchiectasis. Multiple cysts, ranging from 1.5 to 2.5 cm, are seen in the left lower lobe. Bronchogram is seen in Figure 34–3.

COMPUTED TOMOGRAPHY

Computed tomographic criteria for the diagnosis of bronchiectasis have been described by Naidich and Phillips and their coworkers.[271, 272] Cylindrical and varicose bronchiectases are recognized by dilated and thick-walled bronchi extending toward the lung periphery, an area where they are not normally visualized on CT. Cylindrical bronchiectasis causes smooth dilation, which is recognized as "tram lines" when oriented horizontally in the CT section. When the bronchus is oriented longitudinally or obliquely to the CT section, the transverse section gives the appearance of a "signet ring," a large, round, thick-walled, air-containing structure (bronchus) accompanied by a smaller round density (accompanying pulmonary artery) (Fig. 34–9). Varicose bronchiectasis results in a similar appearance, except that the dilated bronchi have an irregular, beaded contour. Cystic bronchiectasis results in more grossly enlarged cystic spaces. These may present as a string of cysts when a single bronchus is seen longitudinally or as a cluster of cysts, similar to a cluster of grapes, when bronchi crowded together are seen in cross-section.

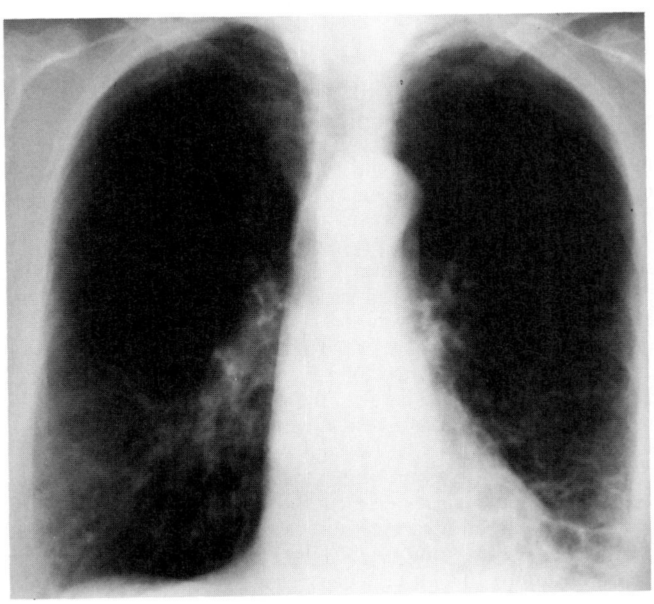

Figure 34–8. Posteroanterior Radiograph of Bronchiectasis. Thickened interstitial markings in a honeycomb pattern are demonstrated, particularly in the left lung. In the right lower lobe, areas of thickened markings and lucencies suggesting emphysema are seen.

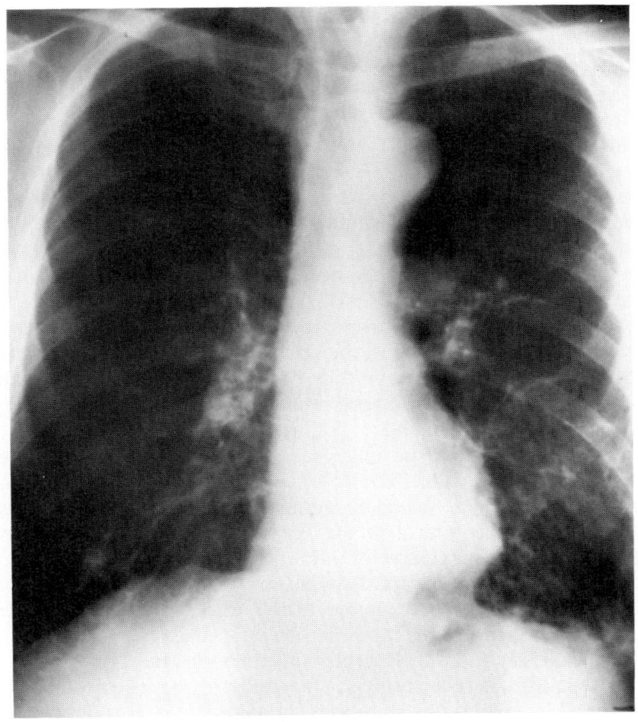

Figure 34–9. Computed Tomography (CT) of Bronchiectasis. *A*, CT of upper lobes shows cross section of dilated bronchi with thickened walls. Accompanying vessel causing "signet-ring" appearance identifies the structures as bronchi. *B*, CT of upper lobes shows dilated, thick-walled bronchi seen both in cross section and longitudinally. Bronchi containing air appear black. White "blob" or "flame-shaped" densities are secretion-filled bronchiectatic airways. They are distinguished from vessels by their shape or by lack of enhancement with contrast (courtesy of Dr. D.P. Naidich).

Studies comparing computed tomography with bronchography, using the latter as the standard,[272–278] have shown a sensitivity ranging from 63% to 97% and a specificity ranging from 92% to 100%, except for one study that had a sensitivity and specificity of 50% each.[273]

Bronchiectasis may be overlooked on CT when there are areas of collapse, consolidation, interstitial disease, or emphysema; when mild disease is studied with thick or noncontiguous CT sections; or when secretion-filled dilated bronchi are not recognized as such.[271, 279] Mucoid impaction may be mistaken for an abnormal blood vessel, but it will not enhance with intravenous contrast material. Varicose and cylindrical bronchiectases are more easily missed than cystic bronchiectasis.

False-positive diagnosis can result from failure to distinguish bronchiectasis from peribronchial thickening owing to interstitial fibrosis with peripheral visualization of bronchi. Emphysematous blebs, also mistaken for bronchiectasis, are distinguished by their extremely thin walls, usually subpleural location, lack of linear arrangement, and absence of an accompanying vessel (i.e., no signet ring appearance).

DIAGNOSIS

A presumptive diagnosis based on the characteristic clinical and radiograph findings is sometimes sufficient for management, but when diagnostic certainty is required, as in a patient with unexplained hemoptysis or when surgical resection is contemplated and the distribution and extent of bronchiectasis must be known, computed tomography is often a helpful and noninvasive alternative to bronchography. When thin contiguous sections are used CT may be the equal of bronchography in diagnostic accuracy,[277, 279] but even advocates for CT recommend the use of bronchography if surgery is being considered[277, 279] (see Radiologic Characteristics).

After bronchiectasis has been diagnosed, evaluation is directed at identifying a predisposing condition. Male infertility is suggestive of cystic fibrosis, Young's syndrome, or ciliary dyskinesia. Upper lobe bronchiectasis, gastrointestinal symptoms, and *Pseudomonas* in the sputum are suggestive of cystic fibrosis, although *Pseudomonas* occurs in other patients with bronchiectasis.[258] Central (proximal) bronchiectasis, wheezing, eosinophilia, and transient infiltrates are typical of allergic bronchopulmonary aspergillosis.[280] Although sinusitis can be seen in cystic fibrosis, Young's syndrome, ciliary dyskinesia, immunoglobulin deficiencies, and neutrophil disorders, otitis media is more common in the last three diseases. Recurrent skin infection is suggestive of immunoglobulin and complement deficiencies and neutrophil disorders. The underlying conditions associated with bronchiectasis and tests helpful in their diagnosis are found in Table 34–3.

When disease radiologically appears to be localized or unilateral, or of recent onset, fiberoptic bronchoscopy to rule out focal bronchial obstruction is indicated. It is also important for localizing the bleeding site in cases of hemoptysis.

Macroscopic and microscopic characteristics of sputum and the sputum flora are not specific for bronchiectasis but are helpful in identifying other diseases, such as lung carcinoma, tuberculosis, or allergic bronchopulmonary aspergillosis, and in monitoring the course and results of therapy.

The routine laboratory tests are not diagnostic but provide information about the severity and development of complications. The CBC may suggest increased infection, lymphoproliferative disease, or certain immunodeficiency diseases. Eosinophilia points to allergic bronchopulmonary aspergillosis. Anemia of chronic disease may be identified in long-standing cases. Serum protein electrophoresis may point to possible immunologic abnormalities and to homozygous alpha$_1$-antiproteinase deficiency. Urinary protein may be a clue to development of secondary amyloidosis, which is an uncommon complication today. Electrocardiogram, and particularly echocardiogram, may reveal evidence of right ventricular strain, hypertrophy or dilation.

Spirometry before and after bronchodilator is useful for assessing pulmonary function impairment, especially any obstructive component, and for monitoring the course and effects of treatment. Additional assessment of lung volumes, diffusion capacity, arterial blood gases, and pH is helpful in characterizing the pattern of impairment and evaluating the severity of the bronchiectasis and any accompanying chronic bronchitis, emphysema, and fibrosis.

Sinus radiographs are useful, especially if nasal symptoms are present. Thickening of the mucous membrane but especially opacification or the presence of air fluid levels require further attention.

The search for an underlying cause of bronchiectasis may require extensive and costly studies. The intensity of the evaluation should be guided by the likelihood that a *specific* diagnosis will result in an alteration in therapy. The diagnosis of cystic fibrosis, allergic bronchopulmonary aspergillosis, immunoglobulin deficiencies, or alpha$_1$-antitrypsin deficiency fits this description.

Patients without any of the clinical features suggestive of a specific underlying diagnosis probably should have a sweat test by the quantitative pilocarpine iontophoresis method and quantitative measurement of serum immunoglobulins, including subclasses, and alpha$_1$-antiproteinase. The other studies in Table 34–3 are relevant in selected cases.

TABLE 34–3. Diagnostic Studies for Specific Conditions Causing Bronchiectasis

CONDITION	DIAGNOSTIC CRITERIA
Cystic fibrosis	Sweat test (child > 60 mEq/L; adult > 80 mEq/L), DNA probe
Allergic bronchopulmonary aspergillosis	Elevated serum IgE, eosinophilia, immediate skin hypersensitivity to aspergillin, (+) serum precipitin to *Aspergillus,* refractory asthma, central bronchiectasis, transient infiltrates, mucous plugs
Ciliary dyskinesia	Bronchial biopsy or sperm for ultrastructure examination, ciliary motility and transport studies
Young's syndrome	Normal sweat chloride, spermatozoa, and testicular function; no sperm antibodies; intraluminal epididymal obstruction
Immunoglobulin deficiencies	Quantitative immunoglobulin measurements
Alpha$_1$-antiproteinase deficiency	Serum alpha$_1$-antiproteinase measurement, phenotyping
Neutrophil disorders	Neutropenia (possibly intermittent), neutrophil function studies
Complement deficiencies	Total hemolytic complement (CH_{50}) and serum C_3 level reduced
Pulmonary sequestration	Mass or polycystic opacity—typically left lower lobe posterior basal segment; CT scan, angiogram
Unilateral hyperlucent lung (Swyer-James, MacLeod syndrome)	Small-to-normal hyperlucent lung or lobe, decreased vascular markings, small pulmonary artery; fluoroscopy (delayed emptying), angiography (small vessels), bronchography (poor peripheral filling, areas of beading and dilation)
Williams-Campbell syndrome	Bronchography with expiratory collapse of proximal bronchi
Tracheobronchomegaly (Mounier-Kuhn syndrome)	Tracheal width twice normal, large main stem bronchi, normal distal bronchi

The sweat test must be performed with an adequate amount of sweat (100 mg minimum). One must be certain that the sweat test is performed by experienced personnel. The concentration of sweat sodium and chloride is high in people with cystic fibrosis and increases slightly with age.[281] Values of sweat chloride of between 45 and 60 mEq/L in children and between 50 and 80 mEq/L in adults are borderline and should be repeated.[281] A false-positive test can occur in malnutrition and some rare conditions.

Ultrastructural examination of cilia is not always reliable. As ciliary abnormalities also can be acquired and transient, it is important to do ultrastructural examinations of a number of sections over time and to be aware that nonspecific ciliary defects in up to 10% of cilia can occur even in normal people.

Alpha$_1$-antiproteinase is an acute phase reactant that can rise with infection, smoking, pregnancy, or malignancy. Many commercial assays overestimate the true level. Recent assay improvements have allowed definition of a threshold level,

11 μM, above which there is no increased risk of emphysema, and presumably bronchiectasis. When the level is low or borderline, phenotyping can be performed by electrophoresis to confirm the presence of abnormal alleles for alpha$_1$-antiproteinase. The technique requires skill and experience.[282]

Measurement of serum immunoglobulin does not necessarily identify all deficiencies. IgG subclass deficiencies may be present despite a normal total serum IgG, and specific secretory IgA deficiency can occur with a normal serum IgA. The clinical usefulness of measuring subclasses and of measuring immunoglobulins in respiratory secretions obtained by BAL is currently being debated.

COURSE AND PROGNOSIS

In the era before antibiotics and widespread childhood immunization, bronchiectasis was a highly lethal disease. Childhood bronchiectasis had a high mortality rate in the first 5 years of life. In one series, two thirds of the subjects were dead by 30 years of age.[16] In another series, only 9.4% of those with onset in the first decade lived past age 40 years.[5a] Others confirmed the dismal prognosis.[6a] Patients with onset at an older age had a somewhat better prognosis.[5a, 16] The majority died of infectious complications of bronchiectasis: lung abscess, empyema, brain abscess, sepsis, and amyloidosis due to chronic bronchial infection. About 5% died of massive hemoptysis.[5a, 6a] Cor pulmonale was frequently present in advanced cases.

By 1969, Field was able to report that most children with bronchiectasis improved in their teenage years and stabilized thereafter.[283] One third of surgically treated and medically treated children were symptom-free after long-term follow-up. In the same year Konietzko and colleagues reported that the average age at death was 55 years. Only two patients died before age 40 years.[284] Only half the deaths were related to bronchiectasis. Cor pulmonale and infection contributed equally.

Factors reported to affect severity and prognosis have included "wheezing or asthma," associated chronic bronchitis, repeated and protracted lower respiratory infections, the number of segments involved, and the degree of ventilatory impairment when first tested.[285, 286] Worsening of bronchiectasis has been reported with increasing age in some studies[287] but not in others.[283, 285] In fact, most patients tend to improve symptomatically or to show only a mild decline in FEV_1.[285] Presumed causes of bronchiectasis and the type of bronchiectasis generally were not related to severity,[285] although post-tuberculous bronchiectasis has been considered more benign.[283] Bronchiectasis from cystic fibrosis tends to be more severe. In ciliary dyskinesia, it tends to be mild and compatible with normal survival.[288]

It seems likely that associated chronic bronchitis significantly influences the prognosis, although it has been difficult to identify and separate bronchitis in cases of bronchiectasis clinically or bronchographically.[218] The rate of decline of pulmonary function in a significant subgroup of bronchiectasis patients has been no greater than that predicted by aging.[285] Patients with localized disease may have significant pulmonary function abnormalities; on the other hand, some patients with considerable bronchographic bronchiectasis have normal function. These observations suggest that respiratory insufficiency in bronchiectasis is caused by associated chronic bronchitis with airways obstruction rather than the bronchiectasis *per se*.

PREVENTION

Childhood immunization against pertussis and measles and improvement in living conditions and nutrition, when such measures are needed, can reduce prevalence and morbidity from the disease. Influenza vaccine should be given yearly; and pneumococcal vaccine, in those high-risk groups likely to respond, should be given at least once. Other preventive measures include early detection and removal or alleviation of bronchial obstruction and corticosteroids in difficult-to-control asthma. Prompt and effective management of treatable lower respiratory infections, especially severe bacterial, mycoplasmal, and mycobacterial infections, is indicated. Immunoglobulin replacement is sometimes beneficial when specific deficiencies have been demonstrated.[289, 290] Alpha$_1$-antiproteinase replacement may be considered when homozygous deficiency is identified, but long-term effects are unknown.[282] (See Chapter 54 on alpha$_1$-antiproteinase.) Recurrent sinusitis should be treated appropriately with antimicrobials or sinus drainage and surgery or both. When gastroesophageal reflux is believed to be a factor in respiratory symptoms, it should be treated. Inhalation of noxious gases and particulates and cigarette smoke should be avoided totally or minimized.

TREATMENT

The goals of treatment are to control acute and chronic infection, secretions, airway obstruction, and complications, such as hemoptysis, respiratory failure, and cor pulmonale in order to prolong life, improve the quality of life, and prevent further progression of disease. Antimicrobial agents for associated infection, pharmacologic tools, and physical therapy techniques to promote bronchial clearance of secretions are the major components that apply to all cases.

The effects of antibiotics have been studied in acute exacerbations and during periods of stability over a period of time, but the long-term effects on pulmonary function and mortality have not been satisfactorily demonstrated. Nevertheless, it seems likely that antibiotics have helped reduce the incidence and severity of the disease and mortality from it.[283, 284] Between 1925 and 1969, infection decreased as a cause of death in bronchiectasis from approximately 90% to 20%.[284] Median survival in cystic fibrosis has increased from age 2 years in the late 1940s to age 27 years in 1988.[291] A multidisciplinary aggressive aproach beginning early in the course is believed to be responsible. Treatment of infection has been the major component.

Although Gram stain and culture of sputum are often done, they are not helpful in many cases. Occasionally patients fail to respond when the cultured organism is sensitive to the administered drug. Conversely, good clinical response can occur despite the presence of resistant organisms.[260, 262]

Antimicrobials for acute febrile exacerbations or pneumonia are generally given empirically. Ampicillin, amoxicillin, tetracycline, trimethoprim-sulfamethoxazole or cefaclor are often efficacious in terms of reducing cough, sputum volume, and purulence, but with the usual short course of 5 to 14 days[260, 261] recurrences are frequent.

The role of antimicrobials in the stable patient with bronchiectasis who has chronic purulent sputum production is less widely accepted. In a British Medical Research Council trial of long-term tetracycline administered twice weekly for a year, mild improvement in symptoms and missed work days occurred, but this was not believed to warrant a recommendation for this regimen in all patients with bronchiectasis.[292]

More recently, Cole's "vicious cycle" hypothesis of pathogenesis of bronchiectasis has provided a rationale for treatment of stable patients who produce purulent sputum.[89, 260, 261] In this model, once chronic bacterial colonization or infection is established, bacterial products and the host inflammatory response are postulated to produce further bronchial damage, favoring impaired clearance and more colonization and infection. Antimicrobial agents that reduce the bacterial load might interrupt the pathogenetic cycle.

Although Cherniack and colleagues[286] suggested that recurrent infection may contribute to deterioration of pulmonary function over time, improvement in pulmonary function with long-term antimicrobial therapy has not been demonstrated. In a number of studies antibiotics have been shown to reduce sputum purulence and elastase activity,[262] bacterial load,[259] and symptoms,[263] but an alteration in long-term morbidity and mortality has not yet been demonstrated.

Most promising regimens have been of longer duration, because conventional 2-week courses have been associated with recurrence of purulent sputum.[257, 260, 261, 263] Higher doses and alternate routes of administration have met with success in some cases.[257, 260, 261, 263] Thick secretions in the airways, harboring of microorganisms within phagocytes, and substances in secretions that may inactivate antimicrobial agents need to be overcome. Aerosol carbenicillin or gentamicin in the treatment of *Pseudomonas aeruginosa* infection in patients with COPD caused some clinical improvement in a group reported by Hodson and colleagues.[293] Work by Cole and others suggests that colonizing *Haemophilus influenzae* in the bronchial tree can be reduced with sufficient doses of antibiotic over a prolonged period with either oral amoxicillin, 3 g twice weekly for 6 months, or with aerosol amoxicillin, 1 g twice daily for 6 months.[259] It is interesting that when *H. influenzae* was reduced, even antibiotic-resistant *Pseudomonas* was also reduced. It was thought that reduction of the numbers of colonizing organisms that were antibiotic sensitive might have turned off or down the inflammatory response and permitted some recovery of host clearance mechanisms.[89, 259]

Chest physical therapy has been shown to be effective in patients with copious secretions in excess of 30 ml/day but of no benefit in those with scant secretions. The primary benefit appears to be mobilization of sputum and improved mucociliary clearance.[294–296] Only one study showed an improvement in pulmonary function.[297] No study to date has demonstrated a beneficial effect on the natural history of the disease.

Postural drainage combined with a forced expiratory technique is most important and superior to directed coughing alone. The forced expiratory technique begins at mid to low lung volumes and proceeds with one to two forced expirations without glottic closure. Vibration and percussion do not improve the results of postural drainage with the forced expiration technique.[298, 299] The use of nebulized saline and a beta-agonist prior to chest physical therapy improves sputum yield.[300]

Bronchodilators are frequently used in bronchiectasis to improve airflow, facilitate mucociliary clearance, and enhance the effects of chest physiotherapy. (See chapters in Section VIII on treatment of COPD.)

Mucolytic-expectorant therapy has fallen out of favor because of difficulties documenting its efficacy and side effects, such as bronchospasm from acetylcysteine and other complications from iodinated compounds. A recent controlled trial of iodinated glycerol in chronic obstructive bronchitis suggested a benefical effect.[301] Corticosteroids are used for severe bronchospasm as in COPD or asthma. They are particularly important in allergic bronchopulmonary aspergillosis,[280] but their role in preventing progressive bronchial damage by reducing airway inflammation remains speculative.[260] A few studies in patients with bronchiectasis and other systemic and/or autoimmune disease have suggested that the pulmonary symptoms and sputum abnormalities improved with corticosteroids.[67]

The major indications for resectional surgery are (1) localized disease with significant morbidity despite conservative management, and (2) massive hemoptysis. Surgery for localized disease is rarely performed today. Most patients have mild symptoms that respond well to medical therapy. Those with more severe symptoms typically have a contraindication to surgery because extensive disease leaves inadequate pulmonary reserve. When a systemic or familial disease has caused bronchiectasis, surgery is generally contraindicated because bronchiectasis cannot be considered truly localized. Some thoracic surgeons recommend a more aggressive, surgical approach to localized, symptomatic bronchiectasis.[287, 302, 303] Occasionally, bilateral disease is sufficiently localized for successful resection of segments or lobes from both lungs.[304–306]

Intermittent mild hemoptysis, primarily blood-streaked sputum, often occurs in bronchiectasis. Fortunately, life-threatening massive hemoptysis, commonly defined as greater than 600 ml in 24 hours, occurs far less frequently. Hemoptysis is the cause of death in about 5% of patients.[5a, 6a, 284] It is nonetheless one of the more common causes of massive hemoptysis.[307]

Prompt surgical resection for massive hemoptysis has generally been considered important because conservative management is associated with a mortality exceeding 50%.[307] Initial management includes bed rest with the bleeding side dependent, antibiotics, and cough suppressants. Even massive hemoptysis will sometimes subside with these measures. Prior to surgical intervention the bleeding site must be localized, generally by bronchoscopy. Most prefer the rigid to the fiberoptic bronchoscope because active bleeding usually obscures vision with the latter instrument. Though not commonly undertaken, endobronchial tamponade with a Fogarty balloon can be used as temporizing or definitive therapy.[308]

Bronchial artery embolization is an alternative to surgery in the patient with massive hemoptysis, particularly if there is a contraindication to resection.[309] The technique controls bleeding in 75% to 90% of cases. Approximately 20% recur in the first 6 months. The major complications—bronchial necrosis and spinal cord infarction—are rare with current techniques. There have been no randomized trials comparing the results of surgery with embolization. Local expertise and features of the particular patient likely will influence the choice between these two approaches.

Respiratory failure and cor pulmonale are common accompaniments of extensive disease, especially when chronic bronchitis and emphysema are present. Oxygen, diuretics, and mechanical ventilation are used as in COPD (see relevant chapters). When patients are intubated, careful attention to suctioning is vital because of copious bronchial secretions.

REFERENCES

1. Laennec RTH. De l'auscultation mediate ou traite du diagnostic des maladies des poumons et du coeur, fonde, principalement sur ce nouveau moyen d'exploration. Vol 1. Paris, Brosson et Chaude, 1819, 124–138.
2. Barker AF, Bardana EJ. Bronchiectasis: update of an orphan disease. State of the art. Am Rev Respir Dis 1988; 137:969–978.
3. Adebonojo SA, Grillo IA, Osinowo O, Adebo OA. Suppurative diseases of the lung and pleura: a continuing challenge in developing countries. Ann Thorac Surg 1982; 33:40–47.
4. Pande JN, Jain BP, Gupta RG, Guleria JS. Pulmonary ventilation and gas exchange in bronchiectasis. Thorax 1971; 26:727–733.
5. National Center for Health Statistics. Unpublished data, 1989.
5a. Perry K, King D. Bronchiectasis: a study of prognosis based on a follow-up of 400 patients. Am Rev Tuberc 1940; 41:531–548.
6. Blades B, Dugan DJ. Pseudobronchiectasis. J Thorac Surg 1944; 13:40–48.
6a. Bradshaw HH, Putney FJ, Clerf LH. The fate of patients with untreated bronchiectasis. JAMA 1941; 116:2561–2563.
7. Reid LM. Reduction in bronchial subdivision in bronchiectasis. Thorax 1950; 5:233–247.

8. Churchill ED. The segmental and lobular physiology and pathology of the lung. J Thorac Surg 1949; 18:279–293.
9. Whitwell F. A study of the pathology and pathogenesis of bronchiectasis. Thorax 1952; 7:213–239.
10. Culiner MM. Obliterative bronchitis and bronchiolitis in bronchiectasis. Dis Chest 1963; 44:351–361.
11. Hayward J, Reid LMcA. The cartilage of the intrapulmonary bronchi in normal lungs, in bronchiectasis, and in massive collapse. Thorax 1952; 7:98–110.
12. Thurlbeck WM. Chronic airflow obstruction. In: Bennington JL, ed. Lung Disease. Philadelphia: WB Saunders, 1976, 60–95.
13. Liebow AA, Hales MR, Lindskog GE. Enlargement of the bronchial arteries and their anastomoses with the pulmonary arteries in bronchiectasis. Am J Pathol 1949; 25:211–231.
14. Moore JR, Kobernick SD, Wiglesworth FW. Bronchiectasis. A study of the segmental distribution of the pathologic lesions. Surg Gynecol Obstet 1949; 89:145–153.
15. Ogilvie AG. The natural history of bronchiectasis. A clinical, roentgenogologic and pathologic study. Arch Intern Med 1941; 68:395–465.
16. Moll HH. A clinical and pathological study of bronchiectasis. Q J Med 1932; 25:457–469.
17. Jaffe HJ, Katz S. Current ideas about bronchiectasis. Am Fam Phys 1973; 7:69–76.
18. Graham EA, Burford TH, Mayer JH. Middle lobe syndrome. Postgrad Med 1948; 4:29–34.
19. Diamond S, Van Loon EL. Bronchiectasis in childhood. JAMA 1942; 118:771–778.
20. Taber P, Schwartz DW. Cystic lung lesion in a newborn: congenital cystic adenomatoid malformation of the lung. J Pediatr Surg 1972; 7:366–368.
21. Wexler HA, Dapena MV. Congenital cystic adenomatoid malformation. Radiology 1978; 126:737–741.
22. Landing BH, Dixon LG. Congenital malformations and genetic disorders of the respiratory tract. Am Rev Respir Dis 1979; 120:151–185.
23. Croxatto OC, Lanari A. Pathogenesis of bronchiectasis. Experimental study and anatomic findings. J Thorac Surg 1954; 27:514–528.
24. Cheng K-K. The experimental production of bronchiectasis in rats. J Pathol Bacteriol 1954; 67:89–98.
25. Field CE. Bronchiectasis in childhood. Part I. Clinical survey of 160 cases. Pediatrics 1949; 4:21–46.
26. Field CE. Bronchiectasis in childhood. Part II. Aetiology and pathogenesis, including a survey of 272 cases of doubtful irreversible bronchiectasis. Pediatrics 1949; 4:231–254.
27. Avery ME, Riley MC, Weiss A. The course of bronchiectasis in childhood. Bull Johns Hopkins Hosp 1961; 109:20–34.
28. Lindskog GE, Hubbell DS. An analysis of 215 cases of bronchiectasis. Surg Gynecol Obstet 1955; 100:643–650.
29. Strang C. The fate of children with bronchiectasis. Ann Intern Med 1956; 44:630–655.
30. Glauser EM, Cooke CD, Harris GBC, Shaw JH. Bronchiectasis: a review of 187 cases in children with follow-up pulmonary function studies in 58. Acta Paediatr Scand 1966; 165(Suppl):3–16.
31. MacFarlane PS, Sommerville RG. Non-tuberculous juvenile bronchiectasis; a virus disease? Lancet 1957; i:770–771.
32. Gold R, Wilt JC, Adhikari PK, MacPherson RI. Adenoviral pneumonia and its complications in infancy and childhood. J Can Assoc Radiol 1969; 20:218–224.
33. Lang WR, Howden CW, Laws J, Burton JF. Bronchopneumonia with serious sequelae in children with evidence of adenovirus type 21 infection. Br Med J 1969; 1:73–79.
34. Becroft DMO. Pulmonary sequelae of epidemic type 21 adenovirus infection. A 13 year follow-up. Arch Dis Child 1979; 54:155–156.
35. Herbert FA, Wilkinson D, Burchak E, Morgante O. Adenovirus type 3 pneumonia causing lung damage in childhood. Can Med Assoc J 1977; 116:274–276.
36. James AG, Lang WR, Liang AY, et al. Adenovirus type 21 bronchopneumonia in infants and young children. J Pediatr 1979; 95:530–533.
37. Simila S, Linna O, Lanning P, et al. Chronic lung damage caused by adenovirus type 7: a ten year follow-up study. Chest 1981; 80:127–131.
38. Rytel MW, Conner GH, Welch CC, et al. Infectious agents associated with cylindrical bronchiectasis. Dis Chest 1964; 46:23–28.
39. Becroft DMO. Bronchiolitis obliterans, bronchiectasis and other sequelae of adenovirus type 21 infection in young children. J Clin Pathol 1971; 24:72–82.
40. Hogg JC, Irving WL, Porter H, et al. In situ hybridization studies of adenoviral infections of the lung and their relationship to follicular bronchiectasis. Am Rev Respir Dis 1989; 139:1531–1535.
41. Schonland M, Strong ML, Wesley A. Fatal adenovirus pneumonia. Clinical and pathological features. S Afr Med J 1976; 50:1748–1751.
42. Kipps A, Kaschula ROC. Virus pneumonia following measles. A virological and histological study of autopsy material. S Afr Med J 1976; 50:1083–1088.
42a. Kaschula ROC, Druker J, Kipps A. Late morphologic consequences of measles; a lethal and debilitating lung disease among the poor. Rev Infect Dis 1983; 5:395–404.
43. Laraya-Cuasay LR, DeForest A, Huff D, et al. Chronic pulmonary complications of early influenza virus infection in children. Am Rev Respir Dis 1977; 116:617–625.
44. Halal F, Brochu P, Delage G, et al. Severe disseminated lung disease and bronchiectasis probably due to *Mycoplasma pneumonia*. Can Med Assoc J 1977; 117:1055–1056.
45. Whyte KF, Williams GR. Bronchiectasis after mycoplasma pneumonia. Thorax 1984; 39:390–391.
46. Rosenzweig DW, Stead WW. The role of tuberculosis and other forms of bronchopulmonary necrosis in the pathogenesis of bronchiectasis. Am Rev Respir Dis 1966; 93:769–785.
47. Shek JL, Cope JA. Bronchiectatic sequelae of pulmonary tuberculosis and its subsequent complications. Dis Chest 1956; 30:566–569.
48. Jones EM, Peck WM, Woodruff CE, Willis HS. Relationships between tuberculosis and bronchiectasis. Am Rev Tuberc 1950; 61:387–398.
49. Kass I, Zamel N, Dobry CA, Holzer M. Bronchiectasis following ammonia burns of the respiratory tract. A review of two cases. Chest 1972; 62:282–285.
50. Hoeffler HB, Schweppe I, Greenberg SD. Bronchiectasis following pulmonary ammonia burn. Arch Pathol Lab Med 1982; 106:686–687.
51. Flury KE, Dines DE, Rodarte JR, Rodgers R. Airway obstruction due to inhalation of ammonia. Mayo Clin Proc 1983; 58:389–393.
52. Bates DV, Macklem PT, Christie RV. Case 48. "Chemical" bronchiectasis; acute exposure to oxides of sulfur. In: Respiratory Function in Disease. 2nd ed. Philadelphia: WB Saunders, 1971, 395.
53. Fraser RG, Pare JAP. Pulmonary disease resulting from sulfur dioxide inhalation. In: Fraser RG, et al. Diagnosis of Diseases of the Chest. 2nd ed. Vol III. Philadelphia: WB Saunders, 1979, 1537.
54. Deleted in press.
55. Gould SR, Barnardo DE. Respiratory distress after talc inhalation. Br J Dis Chest 1972; 66:230–233.
56. Pimentel JC, Avila R. Respiratory disease in cork workers ('suberosis'). Thorax 1973; 28:409–423.
57. Pimentel JC. A granulomatous lung disease produced by bakelite. Am Rev Respir Dis 1973; 108:1303–1310.
58. DiVicenti FC, Pruitt BA, Reckler JM. Inhalation injuries. J Trauma 1971; 2:109–117.
59. Sladen A, Zanca P, Hadnott WH. Aspiration pneumonitis, the sequelae. Chest 1971; 59:448–450.
60. Warnock ML, Ghahremani GG, Rattenborg C, et al. Pulmonary complication of heroin intoxication. JAMA 1972; 219:1051–1053.
61. Iverson LIG, May IA, Samson PC. Pulmonary complications in benign esophageal disease. Am J Surg 1973; 126:223–228.
62. Dakaraju P, Mansfield RE, Shatapathy P. Undiagnosed congenital oesophago-bronchial fistulas in adults and older children. Anaesthesia 1974; 29:169–174.
63. Kiser JC, Peterson TA, Johnson FE. Chronic recurrent tracheo-oesophogeal fistula. Chest 1972; 62:222–224.
64. Schachter EN, Basta W. Bronchiectasis following heroin overdose. A report of two cases. Chest 1973; 63:363–366.
65. Banner AS, Muthuswamy P, Shah R, et al. Bronchiectasis following heroin-induced pulmonary edema. Chest 1976; 69:552–555.

66. Banner AS, Rodriguez J, Sunderrajan EV, et al. Bronchiectasis: a cause of pulmonary symptoms in heroin addicts. Respiration 1979; 37:232–237.
67. Butland RJA, Cole P, Citron KM, Turner-Warwick M. Chronic bronchial suppurative and inflammatory bowel disease. Q J Med 1981; 197:63–75.
68. Moles KW, Varghese G, Hayes JR. Pulmonary involvement in ulcerative colitis. Br J Dis Chest 1988; 82:79–83.
69. Kraft SC, Earl RH, Roesler M, Esterly JR. Unexplained bronchopulmonary disease with inflammatory bowel disease. Arch Intern Med 1976; 136:454–459.
70. Wilcox P, Miller R, Miller G, et al. Airway involvement in ulcerative colitis. Chest 1987; 92:18–22.
71. Gibb WRG, Dhillon DP, Zilkha KJ, Cole PJ. Bronchiectasis with ulcerative colitis and myelopathy. Thorax 1987; 42:155–156.
72. Mathieu JP, Stack BHR, Dick WC, et al. Pulmonary infection and rheumatoid arthritis. Br J Dis Chest 1978; 72:57–61.
73. Walker WC, Wright V. Pulmonary lesions and rheumatoid arthritis. Medicine 1968; 47:501–520.
74. Fairfax AJ, Haslam PL, Pavia D, et al. Pulmonary disorders associated with Sjögren's syndrome. Q J Med 1981; 199:279–295.
75. Hilton AM, Hasleton PS, Bradlow A, et al. Cutaneous vasculitis and immune complexes in severe bronchiectasis. Thorax 1984; 39:185–191.
76. Hilton AM, Doyle L. Immunological abnormalities in bronchiectasis with chronic bronchial suppuration. Br J Dis Chest 1978; 72:207–216.
77. Shneerson JM. Lung bullae, bronchiectasis, and Hashimoto's disease associated with ulcerative colitis treated by colectomy. Thorax 1981; 36:313–314.
78. Freundlich IM, Libshitz HI, Glassman LM, Israel HL. Sarcoidosis. Typical and atypical thoracic manifestations and complications. Clin Radiol 1970; 21:376–383.
79. Felson B. Uncommon roentgen patterns of pulmonary sarcoidosis. Dis Chest 1958; 34:357–367.
80. Mayock RL, Bertrand P, Morrison CE, Scott JH. Manifestations of sarcoidosis. Am J Med 1963; 35:67–89.
81. Lander FPL, Davidson M. The aetiology of bronchiectasis (with special reference to pulmonary atelectasis). Br J Radiol 1938; 11:65–89.
82. Westcott JL, Cole SR. Traction bronchiectasis in end-stage pulmonary fibrosis. Radiology 1986; 161:665–669.
83. Corrigan DJ. On cirrhosis of the lung. Dublin J Med Sci 1838; 13:266–286.
84. Lourenco RV, Loddenkemper R, Carton RW. Patterns of distribution and clearance of aerosols in patients with bronchiectasis. Am Rev Respir Dis 1972; 106:857–866.
85. Currie DC, Pavia D, Agnew JE, et al. Impaired tracheobronchial clearance in bronchiectasis. Thorax 1987; 42:126–130.
86. Currie DC, Saverymuttu W, Peters AM, et al. Indium-111-labeled granulocyte accumulation in respiratory tract of patients with bronchiectasis. Lancet 1987; i:1335–1339.
87. Falk F, Goodwin RH Jr, Leonard EJ. A 48-well micro chemotaxis assembly for rapid and accurate measurement of leukocyte migration. J Immunol Methods 1980; 33:239–247.
88. Stockley RA, Shaw J, Hill SL, Burnett D. Neutrophil chemotaxis in bronchiectasis: a study of peripheral cells and lung secretions. Clin Sci 1988; 74:645–650.
89. Cole PJ. Inflammation: a two-edged sword—the model of bronchiectasis. Eur J Resp Dis 1986; 69(Suppl 147):6–15.
90. Stockley RA, Hill SL, Morrison HM, Starkie CM. Elastolytic activity of sputum and its relation to purulence and to lung function in patients with bronchiectasis. Thorax 1984; 39:408–413.
91. Snider GL, Stone PJ, Lucey EC, et al. Eglin-c, a polypeptide derived from the medicinal leech, prevents human neutrophil elastase-induced emphysema and bronchial secretory cell metaplasia in the hamster. Am Rev Respir Dis 1985; 132:1155–1161.
92. Tegner H, Ohlsson K, Toremalm NG, Von Mecklenburg C. Effect of human leukocyte enzymes on tracheal mucosa and its mucociliary activity. Rhinology 1979; 17:199–206.
93. Smallman LA, Hill SL, Stockley RA. Reduction of ciliary beat frequency in vitro by sputum of patients with bronchiectasis: a serine proteinase effect. Thorax 1984;39:663–667.
94. Niederman MS, Merrill WW, Polomski LM, et al. Influence of sputum IgA and elastase on tracheal cell bacterial adherence. Am Rev Respir Dis 1986; 133:255–260.
95. Weiss SJ. Tissue destruction by neutrophils. N Engl J Med 1989; 320:365–376.
96. Motojima S, Frigas E, Loegering DA, Gleich GJ. Toxicity of eosinophil cationic proteins for guinea pig tracheal epithelium in vitro. Am Rev Respir Dis 1989; 139:801–805.
97. Braman SS, Whitcomb ME. Mucoid impaction of the bronchus. JAMA 1973; 223:641–644.
98. Scadding JG. The bronchi in allergic aspergillosis. Scand J Resp Dis 1967; 48:372–377.
99. Spencer H. Pulmonary diseases of uncertain etiology. In: Spencer H. Pathology of the Lung. 3rd ed. Vol. 2. Philadelphia: WB Saunders, 1977, 708–709.
100. Kirkpatrick CH, Ruth WE. Chronic pulmonary disease and immunologic deficiency. Am J Med 1966; 41:427–439.
101. Rosen FS, Cooper MD, Wedgwood RJP. The primary immunodeficiencies (Parts I and II). N Engl J Med 1984; 311:235–242, 300–310.
102. Phelan PD, Landau LI, Williams HE. Lung disease associated with infantile agammaglobulinaemia. Aust Paediatr J 1973; 9:147–151.
103. Suhs RH, Dowling HF, Jackson GG. Hypogammaglobulinaemia with chronic bronchitis or bronchiectasis. Arch Intern Med 1965; 116:29–39.
104. Dukes RJ, Rosenow EC, Herman PE. Pulmonary manifestations of hypogammaglobulinemia. Thorax 1978; 33:603–607.
105. Chipps BE, Talamo RC, Winkelstein JA. IgA deficiency, recurrent pneumonias, and bronchiectasis. Chest 1978; 73:519–526.
106. Stanley PJ, Cole PJ. The concentrations of IgA and free secretory piece in the nasal secretions of patients with recurrent respiratory infection. Clin Exp Immunol 1985; 59:197–202.
107. Heiner DC, Mayer AS, Beck AS. Deficiency of IgG4: a disorder associated with frequent infections and bronchiectasis that may be familial. Clin Rev Allergy 1983; 1:259–266.
108. Beck CS, Heiner DC. Selective immunoglobulin G4 deficiency and recurrent infections of the respiratory tract. Am Rev Respir Dis 1981; 124:94–96.
109. Heiner DC. Significance of immunoglobulin G subclasses. Am J Med 1984; 76:1–6.
110. Lapa e Silva JR, Gurreiro D, Noble B, et al. Immunopathology of experimental bronchiectasis. Am J Respir Cell Mol Biol 1989; 1:297–304.
111. Henson PM, Cochrane CG. Acute immune complex disease in rabbits. The role of complement and of a leukocyte-dependent release of vasoactive amines from platelets. J Exp Med 1971; 133:554–571.
112. Brentjens JR, O'Connell DW, Pawlowski IB, et al. Experimental immune complex disease of the lung: the pathogenesis of a laboratory model resembling certain human interstitial lung diseases. J Exp Med 1974; 140:105–125.
113. Etievant M, Chevance LG, Lesourd M, Ohayon H. Complement activation and cytoimmunological alterations of the respiratory mucosa. Ann Immunol (Paris) 1980; 131d:13–42.
114. Wilson R, Roberts D, Cole P. Effect of bacterial products on human ciliary function in vitro. Thorax 1985; 40:125–131.
115. Wilson R, Cole PJ. The effect of bacterial products on ciliary function. Am Rev Respir Dis 1988; 138:S49–S53.
116. Stutts MJ, Schwab JH, Chen MG, et al. Effects of *Pseudomonas aeruginosa* on bronchial epithelial ion transport. Am Rev Respir Dis 1986; 134;17–21.
117. Reimer A, Klementsson K, Ursing J, Wretlind B. The mucociliary activity of the respiratory tract. I. Inhibitory effects of products of *Pseudomonas aeruginosa* on rabbit trachea *in vitro*. Acta Otolaryngol (Stockh) 1980; 90:462–469.
118. Hingley ST, Hastie AT, Kueppers F, et al. Effect of ciliostatic factors from *Pseudomonas aeruginosa* on rabbit respiratory cilia. Infect Immun 1986; 51:254–262.
119. Wilson R, Pitt J, Taylor G, et al. Pyocyanin and 1-hydroxy phenazine produced by *Pseudomonas aeruginosa* inhibit the beating of human respiratory cilia in vitro. J Clin Invest 1987; 79:221–229.
120. Sykes DA, Wilson R, Watson D, et al. *Pseudomonas aeruginosa* phenazine pigments in the sputum in chronic bronchial sepsis (CBS) inhibit human ciliary beat frequency in vitro. Thorax 1986; 41:729.
121. Denny FW. Effect of a toxin produced by *Haemophilus influenzae* on ciliated respiratory epithelium. J Infect Dis 1974; 129:93–100.

122. Johnson AP, Clark JB, Osborn MF. Scanning electron microscopy of the interaction between *Haemophilus influenzae* and organ cultures of rat trachea. J Med Microbiol 1983; 16:477–482.
123. Wilson R, Sykes D, Rutman A, et al. The effect of *Haemophilus influenzae* lipopolysaccharide on human respiratory epithelium in vitro. Thorax 1986; 41:728–729.
124. Hoorn B, Lofkvist T. The effect of staphylococcal alpha toxin and preparations of staphylococcal antigens on ciliated respiratory epithelium. Acta Otolaryngol (Stockh) 1965; 60:452–460.
125. Steinfort C, Wilson R, Sykes D, Cole PJ. Effect of *Streptococcus pneumoniae* on human ciliary function in vitro. Thorax 1986; 41:253.
126. Rosenthal RS, Nogami W, Cookson BP, et al. Major fragment of soluble peptidoglycan released from growing *Bordetella pertussis* is tracheal cytotoxin. Infect Immun 1987; 55:2117–2120.
127. Fick RB, Baltimore RS, Squier SU, Reynolds HY. IgG proteolytic activity of *Pseudomonas aeruginosa* in cystic fibrosis. J Infect Dis 1985; 151:589–598.
128. Chandler DKF, Barile MF. Ciliostatic, hemagglutinating and proteolytic activities in a cell extract of *Mycoplasma pneumoniae.* Infect Immun 1980; 29:1111–1116.
129. Carson JL, Collier AM, Hu S-C. Ultrastructural observations on cellular and subcellular aspects of experimental *Mycoplasma pneumoniae* disease. Infect Immun 1980; 29:1117–1124.
130. Reeve P, Pibermann M, Gerendas B. Studies with some influenza B viruses in cell cultures, hamsters, and hamster tracheal organ culture. Med Microbiol Immunol 1981; 169:179–186.
131. Jakab GJ. Viral-bacterial interactions. In: Bienstock J, ed. Immunology of the Lung and Upper Respiratory Tract. New York: McGraw-Hill, 1984, 298–310.
132. Casale TB, Kaliner M. Allergic reactions in the respiratory tract. In: Bienstock J, ed. Immunology of the Lung and Upper Respiratory Tract. New York: McGraw-Hill, 1984, 326–344.
133. Chan-Yeung M, Chase WH, Trapp W, Grzybowski S. Allergic bronchopulmonary aspergillosis: clinical and pathological study of three cases. Chest 1971; 59:33–39.
134. Boucher RC, Van Scott MR, Willumsen N, Stutts MJ. Mechanisms and cell biology of airway epithelial injury. Am Rev Respir Dis 1988; 138:S41–S44.
135. Barnett TB, Herring CL. Lung abscess. Arch Intern Med 1971; 127:217–227.
136. Winterbauer RH, Bedon GA, Ball WC. Recurrent pneumonia. Ann Intern Med 1969; 70:689–700.
137. Kurklu EU, Williams MA, le Roux BT. Bronchiectasis consequent upon foreign body retention. Thorax 1973; 28:601–602.
138. Peleg H, Pauzner Y. Benign tumors of the lung. Dis Chest 1965; 47:179–186.
139. Dunnill MS. An assessment of the anatomical factor in cor pulmonale in emphysema. J Clin Pathol 1961; 14:246–258.
140. Thurlbeck WM, Henderson JA, Fraser RG, Bates DV. Chronic obstructive lung disease. Medicine 1970; 49:81–145.
141. Dunnill MS. The pathology of asthma, with special reference to changes in the bronchial mucosa. J Clin Pathol 1960; 13:27–33.
142. Talamo RC. Basic and clinical aspects of the alpha–1-antitrypsin. Pediatrics 1975; 56:91–99.
143. Glasgow JFT, Lynch MJ, Hercz A, et al. Alpha–1-antitrypsin deficiency in association with both cirrhosis and chronic obstructive lung disease in two sibs. Am J Med 1973; 54:181–194.
144. Longstreth GF, Weitzman SA, Browning RJ, Lieberman J. Bronchiectasis and homozygous alpha-1-antitrypsin deficiency. Chest 1975; 67:233–235.
145. Jones DK, Godden D, Cavanagh P. Alpha-1-antitrypsin deficiency presenting as bronchiectasis. Br J Dis Chest 1985; 79:301–304.
146. Varpela E, Koistinen J, Korhola O, Kiskinen H. Deficiency of alpha-1-antitrypsin and bronchiectasis. Ann Clin Res 1978; 10:79–82.
147. Hoehne JH, Reed CE, Dickie HA. Allergic bronchopulmonary aspergillosis is not rare. Chest 1973; 63:177–181.
148. Goodman DH. Bronchiectasis, eosinophilia, asthma, pneumonitis (BEAP syndrome). Ann Allergy 1974; 33:289–292.
149. Bahous J, Malo JL, Paquin R, et al. Allergic bronchopulmonary aspergillosis and sensitization to *Aspergillus fumigatus* in chronic bronchiectasis in adults. Clin Allergy 1985; 15:571–579.
150. Binder RE, Faling J, Pugatch RD, et al. Chronic necrotizing pulmonary aspergillosis: a discrete clinical entity. Medicine 1982; 61:109–124.
151. Case records of the Massachusetts General Hospital. N Engl J Med 1983; 309:1501–1511.
152. Case records of the Massachusetts General Hospital. N Engl J Med 1982; 306:1471–1479.
153. Katzenstein AL, Liebow AA, Friedman PJ. State of the art: Bronchocentric granulomatosis, mucoid impaction, and hypersensitivity reactions to fungi. Am Rev Respir Dis 1975; 111:497–537.
154. Wood RE, Boat TF, Doershuk CF. Cystic fibrosis. Am Rev Respir Dis 1976; 113:833–878.
155. Rommens JM, Iannuzzi MC, Kerem B, et al. Identification of the cystic fibrosis gene: chromosome walking and jumping. Science 1989; 245:1059–1065.
156. Riordan JR, Rommens JM, Kerem B, et al. Identification of the cystic fibrosis gene: cloning and characterization of complementary DNA. Science 1989; 245:1066–1073.
157. Kerem B, Rommens JM, Buchanan JA, et al. Identification of the cystic fibrosis gene: genetic analysis. Science 1989; 245:1073–1080.
158. Rosenstein BJ, Levine J, Langbaum TS, Kennedy T. Cystic fibrosis in adults: delayed diagnosis in three siblings. South Med J 1986; 79:319–322.
159. Evensen SA. A 69 year-old man with chronic obstructive pulmonary disease, pancreatic insufficiency and elevated sweat electrolytes. Acta Med Scand 1981; 209:141–143.
160. Schwachman H, Kowalski M, Khaw K-T. Cystic fibrosis: a new outlook. 70 patients above 25 years of age. Medicine 1977; 56:129–149.
161. di Sant'Agnese PA, Davis PB. Cystic fibrosis in adults. 75 cases and a review of 232 cases in the literature. Am J Med 1979; 66:121–132.
162. Andersen DH. Pathology of cystic fibrosis. Ann NY Acad Sci 1962; 93:500–517.
163. Rott HD. Kartagener's syndrome and the syndrome of immotile cilia. Hum Genet 1979; 46:249–261.
164. Torgersen J. Transposition of viscera—bronchiectasis and nasal polyps. Acta Radiol 1947; 28:17–24.
165. Katsuhara K, Kawamoto S, Wakbayashi T, Belsky JL. Situs inversus totalis and Kartagener's syndrome in a Japanese population. Chest 1972; 61:56–61.
166. Afzelius B, Eliasson R, Johnsen O, Lindholmer C. Lack of dynein arms in immotile human spermatozoa. J Cell Biol 1975; 66:225–232.
167. Eliasson R, Mossberg B, Camner P, Afzelius B. The immotile-cilia syndrome. N Engl J Med 1977; 297:1–6.
168. Waite D, Steele R, Ross I, et al. Cilia and sperm tail abnormalities in Polynesian bronchiectasis. Lancet 1978; ii:132–133.
169. Sturgess JM, Chao J, Wong J, et al. Cilia with defective radial spokes: a cause of human respiratory disease. N Engl J Med 1979; 300:53–56.
170. Sturgess JM, Chao J, Turner JAP. Transposition of ciliary microtubules: another case of impaired ciliary motility. N Engl J Med 1980; 303:318–322.
171. Rossman CM, Forrest JB, Lee RMKW, et al. The dyskinetic cilia syndrome. Abnormal ciliary motility in association with abnormal ciliary ultrastructure. Chest 1981; 80(Suppl):S860–S865.
172. Mossberg B, Camner P, Afzelius BA. The immotile-cilia syndrome compared to other obstructive lung diseases: a clue to their pathogenesis. Eur J Respir Dis 1983; 64(Suppl 127):129–136.
173. Amjad H, Richburg FD, Adler E. Kartagener syndrome. JAMA 1974; 227:1420–1422.
174. Mossberg B. Immotile-cilia syndrome: clinical features. Eur J Resp Dis 1982; (Suppl) 118:111–115.
175. Mossberg B, Hanngren A. Kartagener's syndrome—a ciliary immotilility syndrome. M Sinai J Med 1977; 44:837–843.
176. Afzelius BA. A human syndrome caused by immotile cilia. Science 1976; 193:317–319.
177. Corbeel L, Cornillie F, Lauweryns J, et al. Ultrastructural abnormalities of bronchial cilia in children with recurrent airway infections and bronchiectasis. Arch Dis Child 1981; 56:929–933.
178. Katz SM, Danjanov I, Carver J, et al. Kartagener's syndrome and abnormal cilia (letter). N Engl J Med 1977; 297:1011–1012.
179. Afzelius BA. Immotile-cilia syndrome and ciliary abnormalities induced by infection and injury (editorial). Am Rev Respir Dis 1981; 124:107–109.

180. Young D. Surgical treatment of male infertility. J Reprod Fertil 1970; 23:541–542.
181. Hendry WF, Knight RK, Whitfield HN, et al. Obstructive azoospermia: respiratory function tests, electron microscopy, and the results of surgery. Br J Urol 1978; 50:598–604.
182. Handelsman DJ, Conway AJ, Boylan LM, Turtle JR. Young's syndrome. Obstructive azoospermia and chronic sinopulmonary infections. N Engl J Med 1984; 310:3–9.
183. Davis PB, Hubbard VS, Garvin AJ. Bronchiectasis and oligospermia: two families. Thorax 1985; 40:376–379.
184. Greenstone MA, Dewar A, Cole PJ. Ciliary dyskinesia with normal ultrastructure. Thorax 1983; 38:875–876.
185. Hayakawa H, Iwata T, Yata J, Kobayashi N. Primary immunodeficiency syndrome in Japan. I. Overview of a nationwide survey on primary immunodeficiency syndrome. J Clin Immunol 1981; 1:31–39.
186. Umetsu DT, Ambrosino DM, Quinti I, et al. Recurrent sinopulmonary infection and impaired antibody response to bacterial capsular polysaccharide antigen in children with selective IgG-subclass deficiency. N Engl J Med 1985; 313:1247–1251.
187. Oxelius V. Chronic infections in a family with hereditary deficiency of IgG2 and IgG4. Clin Exp Immunol 1974; 17:19–27.
188. Reynolds HY. Host defense impairments that may lead to respiratory infections. Clin Chest Med 1987; 8:339–358.
189. Polmar SH, Waldmann TA, Balestra ST, et al. Immunoglobulin E in immunologic deficiency diseases. J Clin Invest 1972; 51:326–330.
190. Sugiyama Y, Maeda H, Okumura K, Takaku F. Progressive sinobronchiectasis associated with the "bare lymphocyte syndrome" in an adult. Chest 1986; 89:398–401.
191. Ultmann JE, Fish W, Osserman E, Gellhorn A. The clinical implications of hypogammaglobulinemia in patients with chronic lymphocytic leukemia and lymphosarcoma. Ann Intern Med 1959; 51:501–516.
192. Knowles GK, Stanhope R, Green M. Bronchietasis complicating chronic lymphatic leukeumia with hypogammaglobulinemia. Thorax 1980; 35:217–218.
193. Tan RS-H. Thymoma, acquired hypogammaglobulinaemia, lichen planus, alopecia areata. Proc R Soc Med 1974;67:196–198.
194. Cooper TJ, Day AJ, Weller PH, Geddes DM. Sarcoidosis in two patients with cystic fibrosis: a fortuitous association? Thorax 1987; 42:818–820.
195. Horan MA, Leahy BC, Fox RA, et al. Immunological abnormalities in patients with chronic bronchial suppuration: a possible relationship with endotoxaemia. Br J Dis Chest 1984; 78:66–74.
196. Thurlbeck W. Pathology of the Lung. New York: Thieme Medical Publishers, 1988, 118–120.
197. Luck SR, Reynolds M, Raffensperger JG. Congenital Bronchopulmonary Malformations. Chicago: Year Book Medical Publishers, 1986, 268–274.
198. Savic B, Birtel FJ, Tholen W, et al. Lung sequestration: report of seven cases and review of 540 published cases. Thorax 1979; 34:96–101.
199. Samman PD, White WF. The "yellow nail" syndrome. Br J Dermatol 1964; 76:153–157.
200. Dilley JJ, Kierland RR, Randall RV, Shick RM. Primary lymphedema associated with yellow nails and pleural effusions. JAMA 1968; 204:122–125.
201. Hiller E, Rosenow EC, Olsen AM. Pulmonary manifestations of the yellow nail syndrome. Chest 1972; 61:452–458.
201a. Williams H, Campbell P. Generalized bronchiectasis associated with deficiency of cartilage in the bronchial tree. Arch Dis Child 1960; 35:182–190.
202. Williams HE, Landau LI, Phelan PD. Generalized bronchiectasis due to extensive deficiency of bronchial cartilage. Arch Dis Child 1972; 47:423–428.
203. Wayne KS, Taussig LM. Probable familial comgenital bronchiectasis due to cartilage deficiency (Williams-Campbell syndrome). Am Rev Respir Dis 1976; 114:15–22.
204. Agosti E, DeFilippi G, Fior R, Chiussi F. Generalized familial bronchomalacia. Acta Paediatr Scand 1974; 63:616–618.
205. Rahbar M, Tabatabai D. Tracheobronchomegaly. Br J Dis Chest 1971; 65:65–67.
206. Bateson EM, Woo-Ming M. Tracheobronchomegaly. Clin Radiol 1973; 24:354–358.
207. Swyer PR, James GCW. A case of unilateral pulmonary emphysema. Thorax 1953; 8:133–136.
208. MacLeod WM. Abnormal transradiancy of one lung. Thorax 1954; 9:147–153.
209. MacPherson RI, Cumming GR, Chernick V. Unilateral hyperlucent lung: a complication of viral pneumonia. J Can Assoc Radiol 1969; 20:225–231.
210. Kogutt MS, Swischuk LE, Goldblum R. Swyer-James syndrome (unilateral hyperlucent lung) in children. Am J Dis Child 1973; 125:614–618.
211. Foster ME, Foster DR. Bronchiectasis and Marfan's syndrome. Postgrad Med J 1980; 56:718–719.
212. Wood JR, Bellamy D, Child AH, Citron KM. Pulmonary disease in patients with Marfan syndrome. Thorax 1984; 39:780–784.
213. Teoh PC. Bronchiectasis and spontaneous pneumothorax in Marfan's syndrome. Chest 1977; 72:672–673.
214. Katz HL. Thoracic manifestation in the Marfan's syndrome (arachnodactyly). Q Bull Sea View Hosp 1952; 13:95–106.
215. Boucek RJ, Nobel NL, Gunja-Smith Z, Butler WT. The Marfan syndrome: a deficiency in chemically stable collagen crosslinks. N Engl J Med 1981; 305:988–991.
216. Pyeritz RE, McKusick VA. Basic defects in the Marfan syndrome (editorial). N Engl J Med 1981; 305:1011–1012.
217. Sayers CP, Goltz RW, Mottaz J. Pulmonary elastic tissue in generalized elastolysis (cutis laxa) and Marfan's syndrome. A light and electron microscopic study. J Invest Dermatol 1975; 65:451–457.
218. Fraser RG, Macklem PT, Brown WG. Airway dynamics in bronchiectasis. A combined cinefluorographic manometric study. AJR 1965; 93:821–835.
219. Wright RR. Bronchial atrophy and collapse in chronic obstructive pulmonary emphysema. Am J Pathol 1960; 37:63–71.
220. Gamsu G, Weintraub RM, Nadel JA. Clearance of tantalum from airways of different caliber in man evaluated by a roentgenographic method. Am Rev Respir Dis 1973; 107:214–224.
221. Svartengren M, Mossberg B, Philipson K, Camner P. Mucociliary clearance in relation to clinical features in patients with bronchiectasis. Eur J Respir Dis 1986; 69(Suppl 146):303–310.
222. Rutland J, Cole PJ. Nasal mucociliary clearance and ciliary beat frequency in cystic fibrosis compared with sinusitis and bronchiectasis. Thorax 1981; 36:654–658.
223. Camner P, Mossberg B, Afzelius BA. Evidence for congenitally nonfunctioning cilia in the tracheobronchial tract in two subjects. Am Rev Respir Dis 1975; 112:807–809.
224. Rossman CM, Forrest JB, Ruffin RE, Newhouse MT. Immotile cilia syndrome in persons with and without Kartagener's syndrome. Am Rev Respir Dis 1980; 121:1011–1016.
225. Wilson R, Sykes DA, Currie D, Cole PJ. Beat frequency of cilia from sites of purulent infection. Thorax 1986; 41:453–458.
226. Sykes DA, Wilson R, Greenstone M, et al. Deleterious effects of purulent sputum sol on human ciliary function in vitro: at least two factors identified. Thorax 1987; 42:256–261.
227. Hingley ST, Hastie AT, Kueppers F, et al. Bacterial ciliostatic factors; effect on respiratory cilia. Eur J Respir Dis 1986; 69(Suppl 146):291–293.
228. Cherniack NS, Carton RW. Factors associated with respiratory insufficiency in bronchiectasis. Am J Med 1966; 41:562–571.
229. Landau LI, Phelan PD, Williams HE. Ventilatory mechanics in patients with bronchiectasis starting in childhood. Thorax 1974; 29:304–312.
230. Bass H, Henderson JAM, Heckscher T, et al. Regional structure and function in bronchiectasis. Am Rev Respir Dis 1968; 97:598–609.
231. Pump KK. The bronchial arteries and their anastomoses in the human lung. Dis Chest 1963; 43:245–255.
232. Nogrady SG, Evans WV, Davies BH. Reversibility of airways obstruction in bronchiectasis. Thorax 1978; 33:635–637.
233. Charman J, Lopez-Vidriero MT, Keal E, Reid L. The physical and chemical properties of bronchial secretion. Br J Dis Chest 1974; 68:215–227.
234. Reid L. Measurement of the bronchial mucous gland layer: a diagnostic yardstick in chronic bronchitis. Thorax 1960; 15:132–141.
235. Lamb D. Mucous secretion in hypersecretory states. Bronches 1968; 18:453–465.
236. Lamb D, Reid L. The tracheobronchial submucosal glands in cystic fibrosis: a qualitative and quantitative histochemical study. Br J Dis Chest 1972; 66:239–247.
237. Lamb D. Histochemical identification of acidic glycoproteins

with special reference to bronchial submucosal glands. Proc R Soc Med 1972; 65:825.
238. Lopez-Vidriero MT, Reid L. Chemical markers of mucous and serum glycoproteins and their relation to viscosity in mucoid and purulent sputum from various hypersecretory diseases. Am Rev Respir Dis 1978; 117:465–477.
239. Lopata M, Barton AD, Lourenco RV. Biochemical characteristics of bronchial secretions in chronic obstructive pulmonary disease. Am Rev Respir Dis 1974; 110:730–739.
240. Bhaskar KR, O'Sullivan DD, Opaskar-Hincman H, Reid L. Lipids in airway secretions. Eur J Respir Dis 1987; 71(Suppl 153):215–221.
241. Barton AD, Lourenco RV. Bronchial secretions and mucociliary clearance. Arch Intern Med 1973; 131:140–144.
242. Picot R, Das I, Reid L. Pus, deoxyribonucleic acid, and sputum viscosity. Thorax 1978; 33:235–242.
243. Chan TB, Arm JP, Anderson J, Eiser NM. Pulmonary epithelial permeability in bronchiectasis. Br J Dis Chest 1988; 82:56–63.
244. Dulfano MJ, Adler KB. Physical properties of sputum. VII. Rheologic properties and mucociliary transport. Am Rev Respir Dis 1975; 112:341–347.
245. Barnett B, Miller CE. Flow induced by biological mucociliary systems. Ann NY Acad Sci 1966; 130:891–901.
246. Gawel J, Rudnik J, Pryjma J, et al. Proteins in bronchial secretion of children with chronic pulmonary diseases. Scand J Resp Dis 1979; 60:63–68.
247. Burnett D, Crocker J, Stockley RA. Cells containing IgA subclasses in bronchi of subjects with and without chronic obstructive lung disease. J Clin Pathol 1987; 40:1217–1220.
248. Burnett D, Stockley RA. Cathepsin B-like cysteine proteinase activity in sputum and bronchoalveolar lavage samples: relationship to inflammatory cells and effects of corticosteroids and antibiotic treatment. Clin Sci 1985; 68:469–474.
249. Dragicevic P, Hill SL, Burnett D, et al. Activities and sources of beta-lactamase in sputum from patients with bronchiectasis. J Clin Microbiol 1989; 27:1055–1061.
250. Suter S, Schaad UB, Morgenthaler JJ, et al. Fibronectin- cleaving activity in bronchial secretions of patients with cystic fibrosis. J Infect Dis 1988; 158:89–100.
251. Jones DK, Cavanaugh P, Shneerson JM, Flower CDR. Does bronchography have a role in the assessment of patients with haemoptysis? Thorax 1985; 40:668–670.
252. Owens GR, Rogers RM. Bronchiectasis masquerading as pulmonary embolus. Am J Med 1985; 79:667–669.
253. Rogers PM, Ayres SM, Ribaudo CA. Extensive multisegmental bronchiectasis presenting as a transient parahilar coin lesion. Chest 1972; 62:499–501.
254. Nath AR, Capel LH. Lung crackles in bronchiectasis. Thorax 1980; 35:694–699.
255. Franklin AW, Garrod LP. Chloramphenicol treatment of bronchiectasis in children. Br Med J 1953; 2:1067–1069.
256. Helm WH, May JR, Livingstone JL. Long-term oxytetracycline (terramycin) therapy in advanced chronic respiratory infections. Lancet 1954; ii:630–633.
257. Allibone EC, Allison PR, Zinnemann K. Significance of *H. influenzae* in bronchiectasis of children. Br Med J 1956; 1:1457–1460.
258. Rivera M, Nicotra MB. *Pseudomonas aeruginosa* mucoid strain: I. Its significance in adult chest diseases. Am Rev Respir Dis 1982; 126:833–836.
259. Currie DC, Higgs E, Metcalfe S, et al. Simple method of monitoring colonising microbial load in chronic bronchial sepsis: pilot comparison of reduction in colonising microbial load with antibotics given intermittently and continuously. J Clin Pathol 1987; 40:830–836.
260. Stockley RA. Bronchiectasis—new therapeutic approaches based on pathogenesis. Clin Chest Med 1987; 8:481–494.
261. Stockley RA. Bronchiectasis—a management problem? Br J Dis Chest 1988; 82:209–219.
262. Stockley RA, Hill SL, Morrison HM. Effect of antibiotic treatment on sputum elastase in bronchiectatic outpatients in a stable clinical state. Thorax 1984; 39:414–419.
263. Hill SL, Morrison HM, Burnett D, Stockley RA. Short term response of patients with bronchiectasis to treatment with amoxicillin given in standard or high doses orally or by inhalation. Thorax 1986; 41:559–565.
264. Gudbjerg CE. Roentgenologic diagnosis of bronchiectasis: an analysis of 112 cases. Acta Radiol 1955; 43:209–226.
265. Currie DC, Cooke JC, Morgan AD, et al. Interpretation of bronchograms and chest radiographs in patients with chronic sputum production. Thorax 1987; 42:278–284.
266. Vandevivere J, Spehl M, Dab I, et al. Bronchiectasis in childhood: comparison of chest roentgenograms, bronchography and lung scintigraphy. Pediatr Radiol 1980; 9:193–198.
267. Fraser RG, Pare JAP, Pare PD, et al. Diagnosis of Diseases of the Chest. Vol III. 3rd ed. Philadelphia: WB Saunders, 1990, 2192–2201.
268. Bachman AL, Hewitt WR, Beekley HC. Bronchiectasis: a bronchographic study of 60 cases of pneumonia. Arch Intern Med 1953; 91:78–96.
269. Nelson SW, Christoforidis A. Reversible bronchiectasis. Radiology 1958; 71:375–382.
270. Pontius JR, Jacobs LG. The reversal of advanced bronchiectasis. Radiology 1957; 68:204–207.
271. Naidich DP, McCauley DI, Khouri NF, et al. Computed tomography of bronchiectasis. J Comput Assist Tomogr 1982; 6:437–444.
272. Phillips MS, Williams MP, Flower CDR. How useful is computed tomography in the diagnosis and assessment of bronchiectasis? Clin Radiol 1986; 37:321–325.
273. Muller NL, Bergin CJ, Ostrow DN, Nichols DM. Role of computed tomography in the recognition of bronchiectasis. Am J Roentgenol 1984; 143:971–976.
274. Silverman PM, Godwin JD. CT/bronchographic correlations in bronchiectasis. J Comput Assist Tomogr 1987; 11:52–56.
275. Cooke JC, Currie DC, Morgan AD, et al. Role of computed tomography in diagnosis of bronchiectasis. Thorax 1987; 42:272–277.
276. Mootoosamy IM, Reznek RH, Osman J, et al. Assessment of bronchiectasis by computed tomography. Thorax 1985; 40:920–924.
277. Grenier P, Maurice F, Musset D, et al. Bronchiectasis: assessment by thin-section CT. Radiology 1986; 161:95–99.
278. Joharjy IA, Bashi SA, Adbullah AK. Value of medium-thickness CT in the diagnosis of bronchiectasis. Am J Roentgenol 1987; 149:1133–1137.
279. Stanford W, Galvin JR. The diagnosis of bronchiectasis. Clin Chest Med 1988; 9:691–699.
280. Glimp RA, Bayer AS. Fungal pneumonias. Part 3. Allergic bronchopulmonary aspergillosis. Chest 1981; 80:85–94.
281. Jones JD, Steige H, Logan GB. Variations of sweat sodium values in children and adults with cystic fibrosis and other diseases. Mayo Clin Proc 1970; 45:768–773.
282. American Thoracic Society Statement. Guidelines for the approach to the patient with severe hereditary alpha–1-antitrypsin deficiency. Am Rev Respir Dis 1989; 140:1494–1497.
283. Field CE. Bronchiectasis. Third report on a follow-up study of medical and surgical cases from childhood. Arch Dis Child 1969; 44:551–561.
284. Konietzko NFJ, Carton RW, Leroy EP. Causes of death in patients with bronchiectasis. Am Rev Respir Dis 1969; 100:852–858.
285. Ellis DA, Thornley PE, Wightman AJ, et al. Present outlook in bronchiectasis: Clinical and social study and review of factors influencing prognosis. Thorax 1981; 36:659–664.
286. Cherniack NS, Dowling HF, Carton RW, McBryde VE. The role of acute lower respiratory infection in causing pulmonary insufficiency in bronchiectasis. Ann Intern Med 1967; 66:489–497.
287. Sanderson JM, Kennedy MCS, Johnson MF, Mabley DCE. Bronchiectasis: results of surgical and conservative management. A review of 393 cases. Thorax 1974; 29:407–416.
288. Davis PB, Hubbard VS, McCoy K, Taussig LM. Familial bronchiectasis. J Pediatr 1983; 102:177–185.
289. Cunningham-Rundles C, Siegal FP, Smithwick EM, et al. Efficacy of intravenous immunoglobulin in primary humoral immunodeficiency disease. Ann Intern Med 1984; 101:435–439.
290. Berger M. Immunoglobulin G subclass determination in diagnosis and management of antibody deficiency syndromes. J Pediatr 1987; 110:325–328.
291. National Cystic Fibrosis Registry Patients. Bethesda, MD, 1988.
292. Scadding JG, Crofton JW, Anderson T, et al. Prolonged antibiotic treatment of severe bronchiectasis. A report of the Antibiotics Clinical Trials Committee of the Medical Research Council. Br Med J 1957; 2:255–259.

293. Hodson ME, Penketh ARL, Batten JC. Aerosol carbenicillin and gentamicin treatment of *Pseudomonas aeruginosa* infection in patients with cystic fibrosis. Lancet 1981; ii:1137–1139.
294. Kirilloff LH, Owens GR, Rogers RM, Mazzocco MC. Does chest physical therapy work? Chest 1985; 88:436–444.
295. Sutton PP. Chest physiotherapy: time for reappraisal. Br J Dis Chest 1988; 82:127–137.
296. Mazzocco MC, Owens GR, Kirilloff LH, Rogers RM. Chest percussion and postural drainage in patients with bronchiectasis. Chest 1985; 88:360–363.
297. Cochrane GM, Webber BA, Clarke SW. Effects of sputum on pulmonary function. Br Med J 1977; 2:1181–1183.
298. Sutton PP, Parker RA, Webber BA, et al. Assessment of the forced expiration technique, postural drainage and directed coughing in chest physiotherapy. Eur J Respir Dis 1983; 64:62–68.
299. Sutton PP, Lopez-Vidriero MT, Pavia D, et al. Assessment of percussion, vibratory-shaking and breathing exercises in chest physiotherapy. Eur J Respir Dis 1985; 66:147–152.
300. Sutton PP, Gemmell HG, Innes N, et al. Use of nebulised saline and nebulised terbutaline as an adjunct to chest physiotherapy. Thorax 1988; 43:57–60.
301. Petty TL. The national mucolytic study: results of a randomized, double-blind, placebo-controlled study of iodinated glycerol in chronic obstructive bronchitis. Chest 1990; 97:75–83.
302. Wilson JF, Decker AM. The surgical management of childhood bronchiectasis. A review of 96 consecutive pulmonary resections in children with nontuberculosis bronchiectasis. Ann Surg 1982; 195:354–363.
303. Annest LS, Kratz JM, Crawford FA. Current results of treatment of bronchiectasis. J Thorac Cardiovasc Surg 1982; 83:546–550.
304. Sealy WC, Bradham RR, Young WG. The surgical treatment of multisegmental and localized bronchiectasis. Surg Gynecol Obstet 1966; 123:80–90.
305. George SA, Leonardi HK, Overholt RH. Bilateral pulmonary resection for bronchiectasis: a forty-year experience. Ann Thorac Surg 1979; 28:48–53.
306. Laros CD, Van den Bosch JMM, Westermann CJJ, et al. Resection of more than 10 lung segments. A 30-year survey of 30 bronchiectatic patients. J Thorac Cardiovasc Surg 1988; 95:119–123.
307. Winter SM, Ingbar DH. Massive hemoptysis: Pathogenesis and management. J Intens Care Med 1988; 3:171–188.
308. Saw EC, Gottlieb LS, Yokoyama T, Lee BC. Flexible fiberoptic bronchoscopy and endobronchial tamponade in the management of massive hemoptysis. Chest 1976; 70:589–591.
309. Stoll JF, Bettmann MA. Bronchial artery embolization to control hemoptysis: A review. Cardiovasc Intervent Radiol 1988; 11:263–269.

Chapter 35

BRONCHIOLITIS OBLITERANS

Paul M. Dorinsky **James E. Gadek**

Bronchiolitis obliterans is a rapidly progressive form of obstructive, and occasionally restrictive, lung disease that was initially described by Lange in 1901.[37] Although numerous terms (including adult bronchiolitis,[17, 33] bronchiolitis obliterans,[3, 14, 22, 32, 38] bronchiolitis fibrosa obliterans,[5, 7, 25, 35] cryptogenic obliterative bronchiolitis,[54] diffuse panbronchiolitis,[27] and bronchiolitis with organizing penumonia[18, 23, 43]) have been used to describe this entity, each of these terms emphasizes the profound bronchiolar inflammation that is responsible for the severe airflow obstruction.

Historically, bronchiolitis obliterans is a disease entity that was diagnosed by the pathologist. There was thought to be no radiographic, therapeutic, or physiologic means by which to distinguish this entity from more common obstructive lung diseases such as asthma, chronic bronchitis, emphysema, alpha$_1$-antitrypsin deficiency, bronchiectasis, and cystic fibrosis. However, in recent years, several studies have focused the attention of clinicians on the unique features of this disease and have emphasized that its rapid course, the absence of a major association with cigarettes, the degree of acute airway inflammation, and the response to anti-inflammatory therapy are different from other forms of obstructive lung disease.[17, 23, 25, 30, 31, 33, 39, 48, 52]

In this chapter, we review the etiology, pathology, pathogenesis, and clinical characteristics of patients with bronchiolitis. We emphasize the clinical features of this disorder as they relate to the diagnosis and management of patients with bronchiolitis. Finally, we suggest criteria for the diagnosis of bronchiolitis obliterans that do not require an open lung biopsy.

ETIOLOGY/CLINICAL ASSOCIATIONS

Bronchiolitis obliterans has been reported to occur in a wide range of clinical settings, summarized in Table 35–1. Despite the occasional identification of risk factors (e.g., adenovirus infection, toxic fume inhalation, heart-lung transplantation), no specific factor can be found in the majority of patients. Although it is estimated that bronchiolitis obliterans causes approximately 4% of obstructive lung disease,[33] the true incidence of idiopathic bronchiolitis obliterans may be even greater, since this disease may be confused with cigarette-induced obstructive lung disease.

TOXIC FUME INHALATION. The list of environmental agents capable of producing bronchiolitis obliterans includes agents such as nitrogen dioxide, sulfur dioxide, phosgene, cocaine,

TABLE 35–1. Known Causes or Clinical Associations for Bronchiolitis Obliterans

CLINICAL SETTING	EXAMPLE
Toxic fumes	Nitrogen dioxide, sulfur dioxide, cleaning agents, cocaine
Infection	Adenovirus, *Legionella, Mycoplasma, Nocardia*
Connective tissue disease	Rheumatoid arthritis, systemic lupus, scleroderma
Transplantation	Bone marrow transplantation, heart-lung transplantation
Idiopathic	—

cleaning agents, and combustion products. However, many of these substances can cause other forms of lung injury, including acute pulmonary edema (e.g., ARDS) and pulmonary fibrosis.[2, 36, 41, 42, 44, 47] Several of these substances (such as sulfur dioxide and nitrogen dioxide) have been used to induce bronchiolitis obliterans in experimental animals.[36, 42] Most of the studies looked at here confirm the fact that exposure to these toxic substances results in a self-limited disease. These experimental studies of bronchiolitis obliterans also allow specific treatment modalities to be assessed and have shown benefits of treatment with glucocorticoids but not antibiotic treatment.[41]

INFECTION. Bronchiolitis obliterans can be caused by adenovirus pneumonia, and several adenovirus serotypes (e.g., 3, 7, 21) seem to be of special importance.[6, 9, 59] Although infection with adenovirus is most common in children, it also occurs in adults and can be responsible for large outbreaks of disease. Bronchiolitis also has been reported to occur after nonadenoviral respiratory infections that are presumed to be viral in origin because of their "atypical" course. In addition, many patients with idiopathic bronchiolitis obliterans report the development of symptoms several weeks to months after viral respiratory infections. However, the link between these putative viral infections and the development of bronchiolitis obliterans is not clear.

Other infectious agents (e.g., *Nocardia, Mycoplasma, Legionella*) also can cause bronchiolitis obliterans.[4, 11, 51] However, bronchiolitis obliterans is an uncommon sequela of these infections.

CONNECTIVE TISSUE DISEASE. Lung involvement in association with the connective tissue diseases has been well described and usually takes the form of interstitial pulmonary fibrosis, pulmonary vascular disease with pulmonary hypertension, or pleural disease. However, recent studies have also documented the occurrence of bronchiolitis obliterans in association with the connective tissue diseases.[19, 21, 24, 26, 34] Although most of these cases of bronchiolitis obliterans have been reported in patients with rheumatoid arthritis, it has also been observed in patients with eosinophilic fasciitis, systemic lupus erythematosus, polymyositis, and scleroderma. It is likely of some significance that many of these patients with connective tissue disease and bronchiolitis obliterans had received penicillamine.[45, 55] The precise mechanism by which penicillamine may act as a cause or cofactor for the development of bronchiolitis obliterans is unknown. However, since penicillamine interferes with cross-linkage of collagen and elastin, it is postulated that penicillamine may impair the orderly repair process in the airways of these patients following bronchial infections.[19]

TRANSPLANTATION. Bronchiolitis obliterans has become an important cause of mortality and morbidity in patients who have undergone either bone marrow transplantation or heart-lung transplantation.[1, 8, 10, 46, 49, 50] Clark and associates[10] recently evaluated pulmonary function tests in 281 adult patients, 1 year after bone marrow transplantation. These investigators identified a strong association between chronic graft-versus-host disease, methotrexate use, or both and the subsequent development of airflow obstruction. In some patients, viral disease may be a cause. Although glucocorticoids and bronchodilators have been used with some success in the treatment of bronchiolitis obliterans in heart-lung transplantation patients,[1] these agents appear to have minimal benefit in bone marrow transplant patients. However, more aggressive protocols may be necessary before anti-inflammatory therapy is rejected as an approach to this syndrome in allograft recipients.

PATHOLOGY

In bronchiolitis obliterans, polypoid masses of granulation tissue are found within the bronchioles (Fig. 35–1). These lesions tend to involve all layers of the bronchiolar wall so that the lumen of the bronchiole is totally or partially occluded. When bronchioles are completely occluded, the alveoli subtended by the bronchiole become atelectatic or fibrotic or both. However, when the bronchioles are only partially occluded, distal alveoli become overdistended, with the result that alveolar emphysema is seen.

The distribution of the bronchiolar lesions is patchy and on gross inspection the lungs are usually distended, with nodules palpable throughout the parenchyma. Occasionally, focal lesions consistent with bronchiolitis obliterans are observed in open lung biopsy specimens. These lesions are thought to occur in areas of previous pneumonias and are not accompanied by the other clinical or physiologic features that characterize bronchiolitis obliterans. The early bronchiolar lesions are cellular and may contain neutrophils and/or lymphocytes. An organizing alveolar infiltrate also may be present. However, involvement of the alveolar spaces is generally limited to the peribronchiolar region of the involved bronchioles.[7, 22, 23, 41] This is an important feature and distinguishes the lesion of bronchiolitis obliterans from the lesions of organizing pneumonia and idiopathic pulmonary fibrosis, diseases that share many features with bronchiolitis obliterans.[23, 43] The peribronchial accumulation of dust or pigment, which may be seen in cigarette smokers or patients with pneumoconiosis, is usually absent in bronchiolitis obliterans.

An entity in which there is an airway lesion similar to that of bronchiolitis obliterans has been called "bronchiolitis obliterans with organizing pneumonia" (BOOP). In spite of compelling histologic similarities, several clinical and structural features appear to distinguish bronchiolitis obliterans from BOOP.[18, 43] Specifically, bronchiolitis obliterans rarely involves the interstitium or alveoli and most often manifests the clinical characteristics of severe airway obstruction and the chest film findings of air trapping. By contrast, patients with BOOP usually display physiologic evidence of restriction and chest film evidence of patchy alveolar consolidation. In addition, BOOP is characterized pathologically by bronchiolar inflammation and fibrosis, as well as significant alveolar disease and chronic inflammatory cell infiltration in the interstitium.[18]

A recent morphometric study by Guerry-Force and associates[23] has helped clarify the differences between bronchiolitis obliterans and BOOP and how these differences may explain the distinct clinical features of these two diseases. The data from their study indicate that BOOP, like bronchiolitis obliterans, has its focus within the small airways. However, true airway obliteration is very patchy in BOOP but not in bronchiolitis obliterans. The investigators logically hypothesized that the patchy distribution of the airway lesions in BOOP would have the effect of functionally subtracting lung units, thereby leading to the restriction. By contrast, the remaining lung units, which display few pathologic changes, are patent and offer minimal obstruction to expiratory airflow.

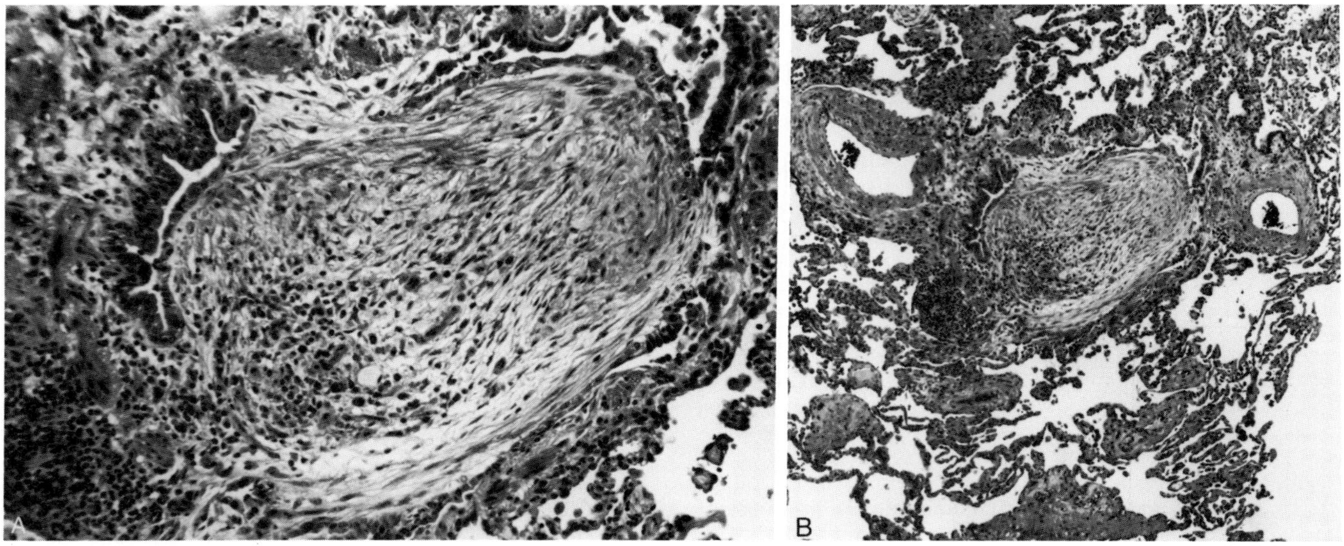

Figure 35–1. High (*A*) and low (*B*) power views of an open lung biopsy specimen from a patient with bronchiolitis obliterans. Note the bronchiole containing intraluminal granulation tissue that completely obliterates the lumen of the bronchiole. In addition, there is mild alveolar and interstitial inflammation which is limited to the peribronchiolar region. Hematoxylin-eosin, × 175 and 435.

Guerry-Force and colleagues also demonstrated significantly greater involvement of the bronchioles in patients with BOOP, compared with patients with idiopathic pulmonary fibrosis.[23] Although the small airways can be abnormal in idiopathic pulmonary fibrosis, the primary lesion is in the interstitium.

BRONCHOALVEOLAR LAVAGE

Bronchoalveolar lavage has proved to be useful in patients with a variety of acute (e.g., the adult respiratory distress syndrome) and chronic (e.g., sarcoidosis, idiopathic pulmonary fibrosis) lung diseases.[12, 13, 15, 29, 56] In each of these infiltrative lung diseases, cells recovered by bronchoalveolar lavage appear to be a valid reflection of the inflammation present in the parenchyma (i.e., alveolar and interstitial structures) of the lung. However, studies of bronchoalveolar lavage cells in airway diseases such as bronchiolitis obliterans are relatively few.

The normal cellular constituents of the lower respiratory tract, as determined by bronchoalveolar lavage, have been established for normal, nonsmoking subjects.[29] The majority of recovered cells are alveolar macrophages (90% to 95%) and lymphocytes (5% to 10%). By contrast, less than 1% of the cells recovered from the normal human lower respiratory tract are neutrophils or eosinophils. In patients with emphysema and chronic bronchitis associated with cigarette smoking, neutrophils may comprise as much as 10% to 15% of the recovered cells (mean neutrophil proportion is 4%).[28] This low-grade inflammatory process in the airways and alveoli of these patients is thought to contribute to the lung damage.

Inflammatory cell populations in the lower respiratory tract are even more strikingly altered in patients with bronchiolitis obliterans (Fig. 35–2). Dorinsky and associates[17] and Kindt and associates[33] have shown that neutrophils comprise an average of 55% of the cells recovered by bronchoalveolar lavage in patients with bronchiolitis obliterans. In almost every individual with bronchiolitis obliterans evaluated by bronchoalveolar lavage, neutrophil percentages exceeded 25%. In some individuals, neutrophils make up as many as 90% of the recovered cells.

The percentage of neutrophils in bronchoalveolar lavage fluid from bronchiolitis obliterans patients far exceeds that seen in other obstructive lung diseases, such as emphysema and cigarette-induced chronic bronchitis. The inflammatory cells recovered by bronchoalveolar lavage in these patients reflect the inflammatory process present at the level of the bronchioles. As discussed in the next section, these findings may also have important implications for the pathogenesis of the inflammatory and obliterative lesions of the small airways in bronchiolitis patients.

PATHOGENESIS

The precise sequence of events in which seemingly diverse risk factors lead to damage that is primarily confined to the bronchiolar compartment of the lung is unknown. However, based on morphologic and bronchoalveolar lavage studies, a

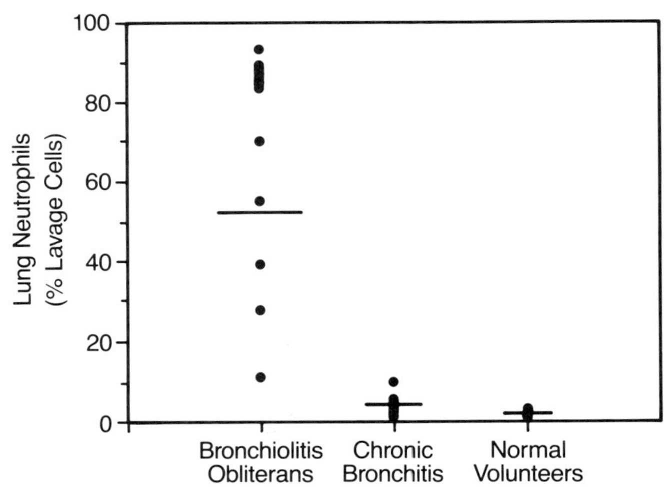

Figure 35–2. Bronchoalveolar lavage neutrophils in bronchiolitis obliterans patients, chronic bronchitis patients, and normal volunteers. Lung neutrophils are expressed on the ordinate as a per cent of total bronchoalveolar lavage cells. Neutrophils comprised 55 ± 10 per cent of the bronchoalveolar lavage cells in bronchiolitis patients. Lung neutrophils in the bronchiolitis patients far exceeded the neutrophil percentages observed in chronic bronchitis patients or normal volunteers.

plausible pathogenetic schema can be deduced (Fig. 35–3). Like idiopathic pulmonary fibrosis, bronchiolitis obliterans may begin with an inflammatory process. In idiopathic pulmonary fibrosis the inflammatory process begins in the alveoli (e.g., alveolitis),[12, 13, 15] whereas an inflammatory process in the bronchioles (e.g., bronchiolitis) is likely to be the initial event in the development of bronchiolitis obliterans. Once airway damage has occurred, the repair process can result in the characteristic pathologic lesions of bronchiolitis obliterans.

This pathogenetic scheme invests the neutrophil with a central role in the lesion of bronchiolitis obliterans. In support of this premise is the well-established evidence for the ability of neutrophil's oxidative and proteolytic mediators to damage the lung parenchyma.[16, 20, 53, 56–58] These neutrophil products have been shown capable of damaging epithelial cells and tracheal explants.[16] The case for the neutrophil as a central participant in the pathogenesis is strengthened by the observation that the specific neutrophil products, myeloperoxidase and collagenase, have been recovered from the lower respiratory tract of patients with bronchiolitis obliterans.[33] Greater amounts of these neutrophil oxidative and proteolytic products can be found in patients with bronchiolitis obliterans compared with patients with other forms of obstructive lung disease.[33]

In summary, the evidence available to date supports the postulate that once airway epithelial injury of sufficient degree develops, an inflammatory bronchiolitis, comprised largely of neutrophils, develops. As this inflammatory process becomes established, neutrophil oxidative and proteolytic products cause further damage to airway structures. Fibroblast proliferation and collagen deposition ensue, with the result that fibrotic, obliterative airway damage develops. It is likely that the relative degree of inflammation versus fibrosis will determine response to therapy.

CLINICAL PRESENTATION

The clinical signs and symptoms present in patients with bronchiolitis obliterans are listed in Table 35–2. The most common presenting symptoms are dyspnea on exertion and cough. Fever and chest pain, except in the acute stages following infection or toxic fume inhalation, are absent. In addition, although most patients with bronchiolitis obliterans experience cough, sputum production is minimal.

The most striking physical findings are tachypnea and prolonged expiration. Wheezing may be present, but rales are distinctly uncommon. Cyanosis is usually limited to patients with severe physiologic impairment, in whom both hypoxia and hypercapnia are present.

The most important clinical feature of bronchiolitis obliterans is its natural history. Unlike most chronic obstructive lung disorders in which significant lung obstruction develops over many years, the lung obstruction of bronchiolitis obliterans is telescoped into a comparatively short interval, ranging from several months to 5 years. This feature cannot be overemphasized, since often it is the only characteristic that distinguishes bronchiolitis obliterans from other chronic obstructive lung diseases. However, bronchiolitis should be suspected in any individual with significant lung obstruction that is out of keeping with the smoking history (e.g., less than 40 pack years). In the final analysis, only the clinician's high index of suspicion provides an opportunity for detecting this disease.

Bronchiolitis obliterans must be distinguished from several other chronic obstructive lung diseases, including asthma, chronic bronchitis, emphysema, alpha$_1$-antitrypsin deficiency, cystic fibrosis, and bronchiectasis. In general, only the exclusion of chronic bronchitis/emphysema provides a major challenge to the experienced physician (and then only in the patient who is a smoker). In this situation, bronchiolitis should be suspected in individuals with significant lung obstruction who have less than a 40-pack-year history of smoking. This distinction is of clinical significance, since patients with bronchiolitis obliterans can respond favorably to appropriate treatment.

As recently summarized by Epler and colleagues,[18] patients with BOOP, unlike patients with bronchiolitis obliterans, most often present with a flulike illness consisting of cough, fever, sore throat, and lethargy.[17, 18] In addition, the onset of symptoms is much more rapid in these individuals and rarely exceeds 3 months. Moreover, patients with BOOP demonstrate restriction on pulmonary function tests, patchy alveolar infiltrates on chest film, and rales rather than wheezing on physical examination. Taken together, these features should enable these two entities to be distinguished.

CHEST RADIOGRAPH

A number of chest x-ray patterns have been described in patients with bronchiolitis obliterans.[22, 43] Most common among these is hyperinflation. In addition, bronchiolitis patients also may have varying amounts of interstitial infiltrates. However, this pattern of hyperinflation and interstitial infiltrates also may be seen with bronchiectasis, cystic fibrosis, lymphangio-

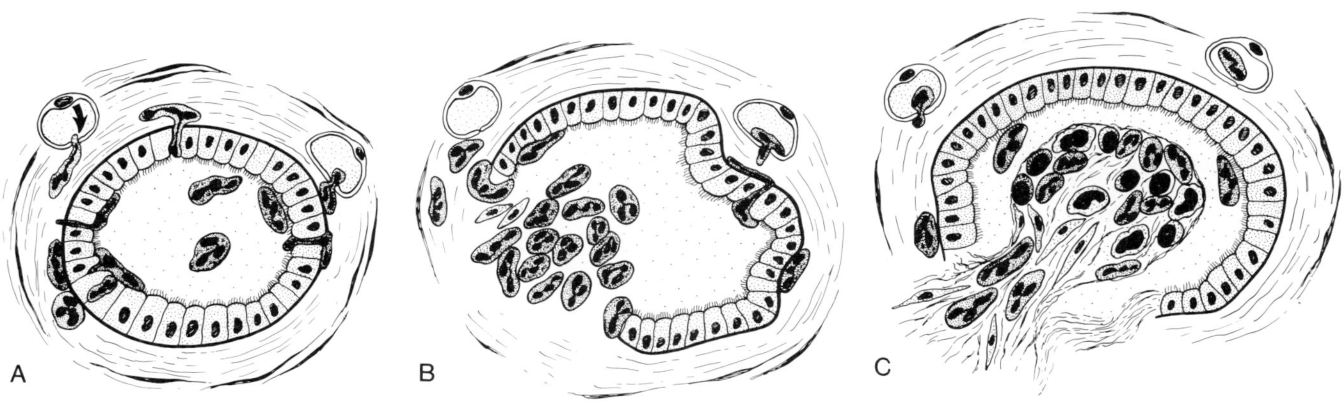

Figure 35–3. Proposed pathogenetic mechanisms of airway injury in bronchiolitis obliterans. *A, Neutrophil recruitment.* In response to a number of processes that mediate airway epithelial injury, neutrophils are recruited into the small airways of the lung. *B, Injury to airway.* Consequent to the recruitment of neutrophils, the release of inflammatory mediators (e.g., proteases and reactive oxygen species) contributes to damage of the airway epithelium and matrix. *C, Airway obliteration.* Persistence of the injury ultimately leads to less reversible architectural changes, which are manifest by intramural and intraluminal fibrosis, and result in obliteration of the bronchiole.

TABLE 35–2. Comparison of Clinical, Physiologic, and Roentgenographic Features of Bronchiolitis Obliterans and Bronchiolitis Obliterans Organizing Pneumonia (BOOP)

	BRONCHIOLITIS OBLITERANS	BOOP
Cough	Common	Common
Sputum	Minimal	Frequent
Dyspnea	Common	Common
Fever	Rare	Frequent
Onset of symptoms	Months, years	Weeks, months
Rales	Rare	Common
Rhonchi	Occasionally	Rare
Chest radiograph	Hyperinflation ± Interstitial infiltrates	Alveolar infiltrates
Pulmonary function	Usually obstruction	Restriction

leiomyomatosis, and eosinophilic granuloma. Nodular densities and alveolar infiltrates also have been described in bronchiolitis obliterans but are much less common. By contrast, patchy alveolar infiltrates are common in patients with BOOP.[18] Finally, pleural involvement is extremely rare in patients with bronchiolitis obliterans.

PULMONARY FUNCTION TESTS

Physiologic impairment in bronchiolitis obliterans is variable and may include severe obstruction, restriction, or a mixed obstructive-restrictive pattern.[17, 40] The diffusing capacity for carbon monoxide has been reported to be normal or decreased in patients with bronchiolitis obliterans, and variable degrees of hypoxemia and hypercapnia may also be present. Some of these differences in the pattern of physiologic impairment may be explained morphologically. Physiologic impairment in bronchiolitis obliterans reflects the net effect of the relative number of airways that are partially versus totally occluded. Lesions ranging from minimal to complete occlusion can be found in specimens obtained by open lung biopsy from bronchiolitis obliterans patients. This spectrum of occlusion may account for pure obstructive, pure restrictive, or mixed patterns.

DIAGNOSIS

Since bronchiolitis obliterans is a bronchiolar-based disease, bronchoscopy with transbronchial biopsy is inadequate for the diagnosis. Bronchiolitis obliterans requires an open lung biopsy for definitive diagnosis. However, Kindt and colleagues recently reported excellent diagnostic results for bronchiolitis obliterans using bronchoalveolar lavage.[33] In their series of 18 patients, the combination of (1) rapid progression, (2) severe airflow obstruction that is not explained by other entities associated with chronic airflow obstruction (namely, asthma, chronic bronchitis, emphysema, $alpha_1$-antitrypsin deficiency, cystic fibrosis, or bronchiectasis), (3) lack of physiologic improvement following bronchodilators, and (4) a large percentage of neutrophils (e.g., 25%) by bronchoalveolar lavage was sufficient to make the diagnosis of bronchiolitis obliterans in most patients (i.e., they predicted the diagnostic biopsy findings in 100% of these patients). These diagnostic criteria may be very useful in the patient with suspected bronchiolitis obliterans who has severe physiologic impairment, in whom a surgical biopsy would be perilous. Nonetheless, since treatment for this disorder requires prolonged, high-dose glucocorticoid therapy, open lung biopsy should be performed if the diagnosis is in question or if there are substantial risks in the use of glucocorticoids.

TREATMENT

A number of clinical studies have demonstrated successful treatment of bronchiolitis obliterans patients with oral prednisone in as much as 50% of the cases.[17, 25, 33] In addition, at least one clinical study reports successful treatment of bronchiolitis obliterans with cyclophosphamide.[55] The rationale of the use of these potent anti-inflammatory agents for suppression of the inflammatory process is similar to the rationale for their use in patients with idiopathic pulmonary fibrosis. Although adjuvant therapy with oral theophylline and inhaled bronchodilators also appears useful in some patients, glucocorticoids are the principal therapeutic modality and offer the only chance of preventing the progression to fibrosis of the airway inflammatory process.

Based on our clinical observations and greater than 24-month follow-up in 18 bronchiolitis patients seen at our institution,[33] we treat patients with oral prednisone at a dose of 1 mg/kg/day for 12 to 16 weeks or until maximal physiologic and clinical improvement occurs. The prednisone is then tapered to 20 mg/day over the next several months and the dose then maintained at this level or tapered to an alternate-day regimen for a period of 2 years. Although information concerning long-term follow-up without treatment is not available, we have observed some individuals to experience recurrent symptoms after prednisone is discontinued. Further studies are needed to address these long-term managment issues. However, patients should be followed closely with serial clinical examinations and pulmonary function tests once prednisone is discontinued.

The ultimate response to treatment is likely to reflect the amount of inflammation versus fibrosis that is present in the airways prior to treatment. Patients with predominantly airway inflammation (e.g., minimal fibrosis) are likely to respond better to anti-inflammatory agents than patients in whom airway fibrosis is far advanced. However, patients may also deteriorate if the anti-inflammatory agent fails to suppress the airway inflammation adequately. There is clear precedent for this in patients with idiopathic pulmonary fibrosis. Patients who do not respond to treatment should be re-evaluated. Presently, bronchoalveolar lavage is the only readily available technique for this purpose. Kindt and colleagues have shown that the percentage of bronchoalveolar lavage cell neutrophils decreases in bronchiolitis patients who demonstrate significant physiologic improvement with glucocorticoids.[33] In contrast, the percentage of lavage cell neutrophils does not change in patients with bronchiolitis who do not improve with glucocorticoids. Although additional studies are needed, bronchoalveolar lavage promises to be a useful technique for evaluating treatment response in these patients. Moreover, failure to respond to prednisone treatment, coupled with continued inflammation on bronchoalveolar lavage, may constitute criteria for the use of more potent anti-inflammatory agents, such as cyclophosphamide.

REFERENCES

1. Allen MD, Burke CM, McGregor CGA, et al. Steroid-responsive bronchiolitis after human heart-lung transplantation. J Thorac Cardiovasc Surg 1986; 92:449–451.
2. Arora NS, Aldrich TK. Bronchiolitis obliterans from a burning automobile. South Med J 1980; 73:507–510.
3. Azizirad H, Polgar G, Borns DF, Chatten J. Bronchiolitis obliterans. Clin Pediatr 1975; 14:572–584.
4. Barnett TB, Knowles MR. Diffuse bacterial broncholitis with bronchiolar pneumonia in adults. South Med J 1987; 80:10–15.
5. Barr HS, Galindo J. Bronchiolitis fibrosa obliterans. Thorax 1966; 21:209–214.

6. Becroft DMO. Bronchiolitis obliterans, bronchiectasis and other sequelae of adenovirus type 21 infection in young children. J Clin Pathol 1971; 24:72–82.
7. Blumgart HL, McMahon HE. Bronchiolitis fibrosa obliterans: A clinical and pathologic study. Med Clin North Am 1929; 13:197–208.
8. Burke CM, Theodore J, Dawkins KD, et al. Post-transplant obliterative bronchiolitis and other late lung sequelae in human heart-lung transplantation. Chest 1984; 86:824–829.
9. Castleman WL. Bronchiolitis obliterans and pneumonia induced in young dogs by experimental adenovirus infection. Am J Pathol 1985; 119:495–504.
10. Clark JG, Schwartz DA, Flournoy N, et al. Risk factors for airflow obstruction in recipients of bone marrow transplants. Ann Intern Med 1987; 107:648–656.
11. Coultas DB, Samet JM, Butler G. Bronchiolitis obliterans due to *Mycoplasma pneumoniae*. West J Med 1986; 144:471–474.
12. Crystal RG, Bitterman PB, Rennard SI, et al. Interstitial lung diseases of unknown cause (Parts 1 and 2). N Engl J Med 1984; 310:154–166.
13. Crystal RG, Gadek JE, Ferrans VJ, et al. Interstitial lung disease: current concepts of pathogenesis, staging and therapy. Am J Med 1981; 70:542–568.
14. Dale RC, Auchincloss JH, Gilbert R, Markarian B. Bronchiolitis obliterans. NY State J Med 1977; 77:1485–1488.
15. Davis WB, Crystal RG. Chronic interstitial lung disease. In Simmons DH, ed. Current Pulmonology. New York: John Wiley and Sons, 1984, 347–473.
16. Davis WB, Mohammed JR, Mohammed BS, Baker NR. Neutrophil myeloperoxidase: a mediator of airway epithelial damage. Clin Res 1986; 34:934A.
17. Dorinsky PM, Davis WB, Lucas JG, et al. Adult bronchiolitis: evaluation by bronchoalveolar lavage and response to prednisone therapy. Chest 1985; 88:58–63.
18. Epler GR, Colby TV, McCloud TC, et al. Bronchiolitis obliterans organizing pneumonia. N Engl J Med 1985; 312:152–158.
19. Epler GR, Snider GL, Gaensler EA, et al. Bronchiolitis and bronchitis in connective tissue disease. JAMA 1979; 242:528–532.
20. Gadek JE, Kelman JA, Fells G, et al. Collagenase in the lower respiratory tract of patients with idiopathic pulmonary fibrosis. N Engl J Med 1979; 301:737–742.
21. Geddes DM, Corrin B, Brewerton DA, et al. Progressive airway obliteration in adults and its association with rheumatoid disease. Q J Med 1977; 46:427–444.
22. Gosink BB, Friedman PJ, Liebow AA. Bronchiolitis obliterans. Am J Roentgenol 1973; 117:816–832.
23. Guerry-Force ML, Muller NL, Wright JL, et al. A comparison of bronchiolitis obliterans with organizing pneumonia, usual interstitial pneumonia, and small airways disease. Am Rev Respir Dis 1987; 135:705–712.
24. Hakala M, Paakko P, Sutinen S, et al. Association of bronchiolitis with connective tissue disorders. Ann Rheum Dis 1986; 45:656–662.
25. Hawley PC, Whitcomb ME. Bronchiolitis fibrosa obliterans in adults. Arch Intern Med 1981; 141:1324–1327.
26. Herzog CA, Miller RA, Hoidal JR. Bronchiolitis and rheumatoid arthritis. Am Rev Respir Dis 1981; 124:636–639.
27. Homma H, Yamanaka A, Tanimoto S, et al. Diffuse panbronchiolitis. Chest 1983; 83:63–69.
28. Hunninghake GW, Crystal RG. Cigarette smoking and lung destruction: accumulation of neutrophils in the lungs of cigarette smokers. Am Rev Respir Dis 1983; 128:833–838.
29. Hunninghake GW, Gadek JE, Kawanami O, et al. Inflammatory and immune processes in the human lung in health and disease: evaluation by bronchoalveolar lavage. Am J Pathol 1979; 91:149–206.
30. Iannuzzi MC, Farhi DC, Bostrom PD, et al. Fulminant respiratory failure and death in a patient with idiopathic bronchiolitis obliterans. Arch Intern Med 1985; 145:733–734.
31. Katzenstein AL, Myers JL, Prophet WD, et al. Bronchiolitis obliterans and usual interstitial pneumonia. Am J Surg Pathol 1986; 10:373–381.
32. Khan B, Cox GE, Taylor CB. Comparison of bronchiolitis obliterans with several other uncommon pulmonary diseases. Aerospace Med 1961; 32:695–700.
33. Kindt G, Gadek JE, Weiland JE, Dorinsky PM. Neutrophil mediators in adult bronchiolitis/bronchiolitis obliterans. Clin Res 1988; 36:506A.
34. Kinney WW, Angelillo VA. Bronchiolitis in systemic lupus erythematosus. Chest 1982; 82:646–649.
35. Ladue JS. Bronchiolitis fibrosa obliterans. Arch Intern Med 1941; 68:663–673.
36. Lam C, Kattan M, Collins A, Kleinerman J. Long-term sequelae of bronchiolitis induced by nitrogen dioxide in hamsters. Am Rev Respir Dis 1983; 128:1020–1023.
37. Lange W. Über eine eighenthumliche Erkrankung der kleinen Bronchien und Bronchiolen. Deutsches Arch Klin Med 1901; 70:342–364.
38. McAdams AJ. Bronchiolitis obliterans. Am J Med 1955; 19:314–322.
39. Meier-Sydow J, Schneider M, Rust M. Chronic bronchiolitis in adults. Eur J Respir Dis (Suppl) 1986; 146:337–344.
40. Mink SN, Coalson JJ, Whitley L, et al. Pulmonary function tests in the detection of small airway obstruction in a canine model of bronchiolitis obliterans. Am Rev Respir Dis 1984; 130:1125–1133.
41. Moran TJ, Hellstrom AR. Bronchiolitis obliterans. Arch Pathol 1958; 66:691–707.
42. Morgenroth K. Morphological alterations to the bronchial mucosa in high-dose long-term exposure to sulfur dioxide. Respiration 1980; 39:39–48.
43. Muller NL, Guerry-Force ML, Staples CA, et al. Differential diagnosis of bronchiolitis with organizing pneumonia and usual interstitial pneumonia: clinical, functional and radiologic findings. Radiology 1987; 162:151–156.
44. Murphy DMF, Fairman RP, Lapp NL, Morgan WKC. Severe airway disease due to inhalation of fumes from cleansing agents. Chest 1976; 69:372–376.
45. Murphy KC, Atkins CJ, Offer RC, et al. Obliterative bronchiolitis in two rheumatoid arthritis patients treated with penicillamine. Arthritis Rheum 1981; 24:557–560.
46. Ostrow D, Buskard N, Hill RS, et al. Bronchiolitis obliterans complicating bone marrow transplantation. Chest 1985; 87: 828–830.
47. Patel RC, Dutta D, Schonfeld SA. Free-base cocaine use associated with bronchiolitis obliterans organizing pneumonia. Ann Intern Med 1987; 107:186–187.
48. Perez-Guerra F, Walsh RE, Sagel SS. Bronchiolitis obliterans and tracheal stenosis. JAMA 1971; 218:1568–1570.
49. Ralph DD, Springmeyer SC, Sullivan KM, et al. Rapidly progressive air-flow obstruction in marrow transplant recipients. Am Rev Respir Dis 1984; 129:641–644.
50. Rosenberg ME, Vercellotti GM, Snover DC, et al. Bronchiolitis obliterans after bone marrow transplantation. Am J Hematol 1985; 18:325–328.
51. Sato P, Madtes DK, Thorning D, Albert RK. Bronchiolitis obliterans caused by *Legionella pneumophila*. Chest 1985; 87:840–842.
52. Seggev JS, Mason UG, Worthen S, et al. Bronchiolitis obliterans. Chest 1983; 83:169–174.
53. Slivka A, Lobuglio AF, Weiss SJ. A potential role for hypochlorous acid in granulocyte-mediated tumor cell cytotoxicity. Blood 1980; 55:347–350.
54. Turton CW, Williams G, Green M. Cryptogenic obliterative bronchiolitis in adults. Thorax 1981; 36:805–810.
55. Van De Laar MA, Westermann CJ, Wagenaar SS, Dinant HJ. Beneficial effect of intravenous cyclophosphamide and oral prednisone on D-penicillamine–associated bronchiolitis obliterans. Arthritis Rheum 1985; 28:93–97.
56. Weiland JE, Davis WB, Holter JF, et al. Lung neutrophils in the adult respiratory distress syndrome: clinical and pathophysiologic significance. Am Rev Respir Dis 1986; 133:218–225.
57. Weiland JE, Garcia JGN, Davis WB, Gadek JE. Neutrophil collagenase in rheumatoid interstitial lung disease. J Appl Physiol 1987; 62:628–633.
58. Weiss SJ, Slivka A. Monocyte and granulocyte-mediated tumor cell destruction. A role for the hydrogen peroxide–myeloperoxidase–chloride system. J Clin Invest 1982; 69:255–262.
59. Wohl MEB, Chernick V. Bronchiolitis. Am Rev Respir Dis 1978; 118:759–781.

Chapter 36

COPD AND LUNG CANCER

William Weiss

Every clinician with experience in the management of lung cancer recognizes that chronic obstructive pulmonary disease (COPD) is a common complication of this disease. This is to be expected since cigarette smoking is the major cause of both conditions. However, the association between COPD and lung cancer can be examined only epidemiologically. Papers describing the association began to appear in the 1950s, but studies that took into account the confounding factor of smoking habits as well as age and sex were not published until the 1960s.

This chapter reviews the epidemiologic investigations documenting the relationship between COPD and lung cancer, but these are limited to those studies adjusting for at least the confounders of age, sex, and smoking habits to some degree. The association is essentially in the temporal direction from COPD to cancer, since COPD has a much longer course than lung cancer. The issue as to whether COPD plays at least a partial role in the causation of lung cancer is considered during the review and in a discussion of possible mechanisms for a causal relationship. Finally, the clinical implication of COPD in the management of lung cancer is mentioned.

EPIDEMIOLOGIC INVESTIGATIONS

A list of the reports considered is given in Table 36–1. There were eight case-control studies, of which six were published before 1970, and in six the researchers concluded that there was an elevated risk of lung cancer in people with manifestations of COPD. Of seven cohort studies, only one was published before 1970, and all showed an elevated risk. The earlier appearance of case-control studies is probably due to the fact that they are easier to do, less time-consuming, and cheaper than the cohort studies. However, cohort studies are more reliable, less subject to bias, and provide exact measures of risk, i.e., incidence rather than estimates of relative risk. Therefore cohort studies will receive greater emphasis.

TABLE 36–1. Epidemiologic Studies of Lung Cancer Relative Risk Among People with Chronic Bronchitis or Chronic Obstructive Pulmonary Disease Adjusted for Age, Sex, and Smoking Habits

AUTHOR AND YEAR	ELEVATED RISK
Case-Control Studies	
Campbell 1963[5]	yes
Boucot 1964[2]	yes
Lombard 1965[12]	yes
Dean 1966[8]	yes
van der Wal 1966[20]	yes
Wynder 1966[23]	no
Stavraky 1971[17]	no
Samet 1986[15]	yes
Cohort Studies	
Boucot 1966[3] and 1977[4]	yes
Kubik 1970[9]	yes
Rimington 1971[14]	yes
Peto 1983[13]	yes
Skillrud 1986[16]	yes
Tockman 1987[19]	yes
Lange 1990[11]	yes

Case-Control Studies

The first report was made by Campbell and Lee in 1963.[5] They studied the prevalence of chronic bronchitis, defined as cough with sputum on most days of the year for at least 2 years, in 99 lung cancer cases and 166 controls over the age of 50 years. All were hospital admissions, with the controls being surgical or dermatologic patients. Age distributions were similar. Chronic bronchitis was found in 74% of the lung cancer cases and 46% of the controls ($\chi^2 = 20.08$, $P < 0.001$). The bronchitis had been present more than 6 years in 92% of 74 lung cancer cases and 82% of 77 controls. The excess of chronic bronchitis in the cases persisted across smoking categories (Table 36–2), but the difference was smaller among heavy cigarette smokers than among light cigarette smokers and nonsmokers of cigarettes.

The following year Boucot and colleagues reported the results of a case-control study nested in a cohort from the Philadelphia Pulmonary Neoplasm Research Project.[2] The cohort consisted of 6137 men aged 45 years and over who were screened every 6 months with a chest film and questionnaire about respiratory symptoms and smoking habits. At the time of this report the cohort had been followed 7 to 10 years, and 67 new lung cancer cases had developed among men who

TABLE 36–2. Case-Control Study of the Relationship Between Chronic Bronchitis and Lung Cancer by Daily Cigarette Consumption

NO. CIGARETTES	CASES			CONTROLS		
		Bronchitis			Bronchitis	
(Day)	N	*(No.)*	*(%)*	N	*(No.)*	*(%)*
0	12	7	58	44	11	25
1–19	36	28	78	67	32	48
20+	49	37	76	55	34	62
TOTAL	97	72	74	166	77	46

From Campbell AH, Lee EJ. The relationship between lung cancer and chronic bronchitis. Br J Dis Chest 1963; 57:113–119.

had no detectable lung cancer at the start of observation (entry). Two control groups were matched to the lung cancer cases by age, race, date of entry, and length of follow-up. One control group consisted of nonsmokers and the other was matched to the cancer cases by type, degree, and duration of smoking. The percentages of visits prior to cancer detection, with cough having a duration of months or years, were lung cancer cases, 38%; control smokers, 30%; and control nonsmokers, 4%. Thus, smokers without cancer had a prevalence of chronic cough that was a little lower than that of the cancer patients, all of whom were smokers. However, the analysis did not provide any information on the temporal relationship between chronic cough and cancer. This is of some importance because lung cancer may cause cough for months or years prior to its detection, so the relationship between chronic cough and the risk of cancer should be examined more than at least 2 years before cancer detection,[22] i.e., at a time before the chronic cough can be attributed to the cancer.

In 1965, Lombard reported a case-control study with partial regression analysis.[12] Chronic bronchitis and emphysema were found to be significant factors for lung cancer risk.

The following year Dean published a population-based case-control study of lung cancer deaths in Northern Ireland.[8] Controls were matched by age, sex, and area of residence. To control for smoking habit, a survey of the general population was done for smoking as well as for morning cough so that rates could be estimated. Table 36–3 shows the results. In all smoking categories regardless of sex, the lung cancer rates were considerably higher among the coughers than among the noncoughers. Unfortunately, those whose cough was due to the lung cancer were not distinguished from those whose cough was caused by COPD.

In 1966, van der Wal and colleagues reported a relatively small case-control study of 100 lung cancer cases compared with 100 controls matched by smoking habit as well as by age, sex, and neighborhood.[20] The investigators tabulated the percentages of chronic cough that began at least 10 years before cancer detection and found the frequencies by degree of daily cigarette consumption to be much higher among the lung cancer cases than among the controls: 0 to 9 cigarettes, 83.1% of cases and 10.5% of controls; 10 to 19 cigarettes, 87.3% and 33.3%, respectively; and 20+ cigarettes, 94.4% and 19.2%, respectively.

In the same year, Wynder and Fairchild[23] pointed out that other characteristics of smoking habit besides type and degree should be used to match cases and controls if one is to approach adequate control for inhaled dose of smoke: duration, degree of inhalation, butt length, number of puffs per cigarette, tar content of tobacco, and volume of draw. They defined a cougher as a person with cough on most days of the year beginning 3 or more years before cancer diagnosis. They found the prevalence of cough was higher among cancer cases than among controls only for those who smoked less than 30 cigarettes per day, but the lighter smokers showed a tendency to higher consumption within each category, longer duration of smoking, and shorter butt length among the cancer cases than among the controls. They felt that no conclusions could be drawn from their data and that it was not established that a history of long-term cough increases the risk of lung cancer independent of smoking intensity.

In 1971, Stavraky examined the frequency of a history of hospitalization for chronic bronchitis 2 to 12 years before cancer diagnosis in 526 cases and 525 controls among Canadian pensioned veterans who participated in a study of smoking and health.[17] The controls were matched by age, occupation, residence, and smoking habit. She concluded that her data did not support the hypothesis that differences in illness present long enough prior to death to be evident before symptoms of lung cancer emerged are useful predictors of lung cancer risk. Hospitalization for chronic bronchitis may have been too crude a measure of the risk factor.

Finally, Samet and colleagues recently published a population-based case-control study of white men in New Mexico.[15] The controls were a random sample of the state population matched by age, sex, ethnicity, and smoking habits. Using multiple logistic analysis, the relative risks measured by the odds ratios were 1.69 for chronic bronchitis, 1.63 for emphysema, and 1.97 for chronic bronchitis or emphysema. Although the data analysis was more elegant than that of previous investigators, stratification by smoking was limited to ever and never categories.

While the sophistication of these case-control studies has increased with time, the results leave some doubt as to whether COPD plays a substantial role in the risk of lung cancer independent of smoking.

TABLE 36–3. Age-Adjusted Lung Cancer Death Rates in Northern Ireland Among People Aged 35 Years and Over by Sex, Presence or Absence of Morning Cough, and Smoking Habit

SMOKING HABIT	LUNG CANCER RATE—NO./100,000/YEAR			
	Men		Women	
	Noncoughers	*Coughers*	*Noncoughers*	*Coughers*
Nonsmokers	17	33	8	31
Cigarettes only				
No. per day				
1–10	42	196	14	45
11–22	78	235	26	138
23+	174	471	96	378
Cigarettes and pipe/cigar	55	166		
Pipe/cigar only	30	85		

From Dean G. Lung cancer and bronchitis in Northern Ireland, 1960–1962. Br Med J 1966; 1:1506–1514.

Cohort Studies

Prospective examination of cohorts provides a more reliable source of information with regard to the issue than case-control studies. The first report to appear was from the aforementioned Philadelphia Pulmonary Neoplasm Research Project.[3] In this paper the 9- to 10-year cumulative incidence of lung cancer was tabulated among 6071 males aged 45 years and over, according to the presence or absence of chronic cough and smoking habit by both degree and duration on entry into the Project. No lung cancer occurred among nonsmokers or cigarette smokers of less than 20 years. Among men who smoked cigarettes for 20 to 39 years, the incidence was 1.7% among 583 coughers compared with 0.7% of 1258 noncoughers, but the higher risk was limited to those who smoked less than half a pack or more than 1 pack per day. Among smokers of 40 or more years, the differences were insignificant.

Eleven years later, after data coding for computer analysis permitted more careful evaluation, the results were easier to interpret.[4] The 10-year probability of lung cancer diagnosis was adjusted for age, race, and smoking habits by type, degree, and duration. Twenty-nine per cent of 6027 older men had cough for months or years on entry into the Project. The probability of developing lung cancer in the next 10 years was 2.98% among coughers and 2.05% among noncoughers ($P < 0.05$). A history of expectoration was not a factor. Figure 36–1 shows the curves for cumulative probability in the two groups, and it is apparent that the difference in absolute risk

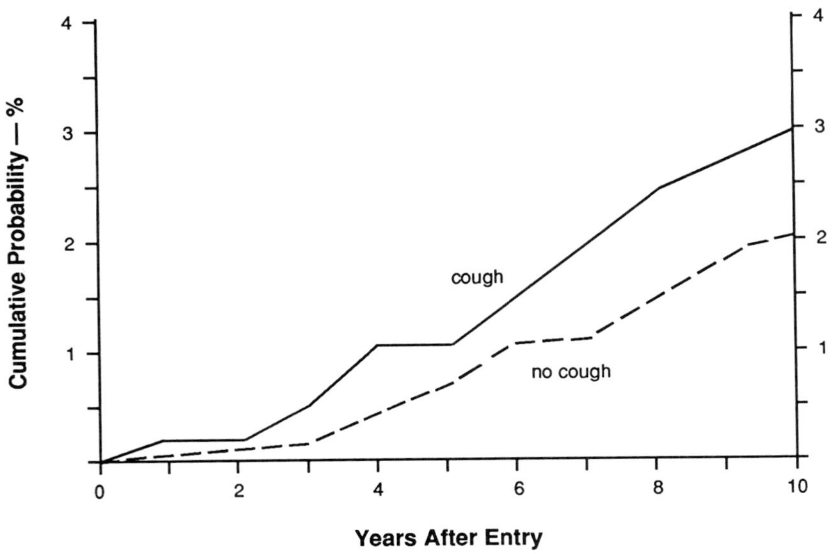

Figure 36–1. Cumulative probability of developing lung cancer through 10 years after entry into the project by presence or absence of chronic cough at entry, adjusted for age, race, and smoking habits at entry among 6027 older men. Data from the Philadelphia Pulmonary Neoplasm Research Project.[4]

tends to increase with time after the record of chronic cough. Thus, it may be assumed that cough due to the cancer itself played little role in the results.

When the data were stratified by duration of smoking, the adjusted probability for those smoking one or more packs per day was 6.23% among coughers and 2.51% among noncoughers ($P < 0.05$). The difference disappeared after smoking for 40 or more years. Among exsmokers of cigarettes there were large differences between coughers and noncoughers: 4.17% and 0.19% respectively for smokers of less than one pack per day ($P < 0.001$); 7.76% and 2.50% respectively for smokers of one pack or more per day ($P < 0.05$).

Kubik and colleagues presented positive results in a cohort of 12,322 men aged 40 to 64 years but measured only crude incidence in broad smoking categories by degree without considering duration of smoking, and the follow-up was limited to 3.5 years.[9]

Rimington reported positive results in terms of cumulative incidence among 21,579 male volunteers aged 40 years and over for those complaining of sputum on most days for at least 5 years.[14] Duration of smoking was not considered, and follow-up was limited to 36 to 56 months.

In the past 7 years, emphasis has shifted from symptoms of COPD to evidence of obstructive airway disease. Peto and associates reported a 20- to 25-year follow-up of random population samples in Britain.[13] A total of 2718 men was assessed in 1954 to 1961 by FEV_1 and questionnaires regarding mucus hypersecretion and smoking habits. The comparisons were internal. The FEV_1 was standardized for age and the cube of height (H^3) and categorized according to the number of standard deviations below the average in each group. The logrank method for cause-specific mortality was used. Expected numbers of deaths were calculated from death rates for all men, and the ratio of observed to expected deaths (O/E) was studied in relation to FEV_1 and to a history of phlegm production. The risk of lung cancer was twice as high among men with FEV_1/H^3 lower than average, compared with those with values above average. The O/E for those with phlegm adjusted for FEV_1/H^3 was 1.4 compared with 0.6 for those without phlegm ($P < 0.001$), and this association remained highly significant after adjustment for amount smoked.

Skillrud and associates at the Mayo Clinic followed 113 cases of COPD, chronic bronchitis, or emphysema with an FEV_1 of 70% or less of predicted normal for 10 to 12 years.[16] An equal number of controls—patients with uncomplicated fractures or dental extractions—were matched by age, sex, broad occupational category, and smoking habit in pack years; they were restricted to people with an FEV_1 of 85% or more. Cases and controls were all aged 45 to 59 years. The lung cancer endpoint required histologic or cytologic proof. Nine cases and two controls developed lung cancer. The actuarial cumulative probability at 10 years was 8.8% among the cases and 2.0% among the controls ($P = 0.024$). This increased risk occurred despite the shorter survival of the COPD cases.

More recently Tockman and colleagues reported a study of the relationship between COPD and lung cancer incidence in two cohorts: (1) 667 white men with COPD enrolled in a trial of intermittent positive pressure breathing (IPPB) followed for an average of 3 years, and (2) 3728 white men in the Johns Hopkins Lung Project (JHLP), a study of periodic screening for lung cancer, limited to those men who had a spirogram.[19] The follow-up in the latter group was only 1.2 years on average. All the JHLP group were heavy smokers of at least one pack per day. Airway obstruction was defined by an FEV_1 of 60% or less of predicted. This criterion was met by all the men in IPPB but only a minority of men in JHLP. The lung cancer incidence rate as the number per 1000 man-years was 11.0 in the IPPB and 11.4 in the obstructed men of JHLP, compared with 3.5 in the unobstructed men of JHLP. The odds ratio after adjustment for pack years of smoking was 6.07 for the obstructed men, and after adjustment for age it was 4.88 by the Mantel-Haenszel method.

Using the proportional hazards model, the risk factor seemed to be confined to obstruction with no independent effect of bronchitis. The relative risk of lung cancer increased with increasing degree of obstruction, and there was little additional effect from smoking. The log-linear method was used to develop a hierarchical model of lung cancer risk to circumvent the problem of a combination of both cross-sectional and prospective data. This showed that airway obstruction was more important than age or pack years, but it should be noted that the subjects were generally heavy smokers so the smoking effect was minimized by restriction of the participants.

Tockman and colleagues expressed several caveats about the association between obstruction and lung cancer in their data: (1) since they started with obstructed people, progression from normal function to obstruction could not be seen, (2) the precision of the relative risk estimates from odds ratios was dependent on the selection of categorical boundaries, and (3) there may have been confounding by misclassification of the smoke dose delivered to the tissues because of unmeasured aspects of smoking habits or airway geometry. Nevertheless, the consistency of the results suggests that among middle-aged smokers, ventilatory obstruction identifies those with the highest risk of lung cancer.

In 1990, Lange and colleagues[11] reported a cohort study of 13,946 people, a random sample of the general population of Copenhagen. During an average 10 years of follow-up, 225 died of lung cancer. Using multiple regression analysis and adjusting for age, sex, pack-years of smoking, and inhalation, FEV_1 as percent of predicted (FEV_1%) and chronic phlegm production at the start of observation were significant predictors of lung cancer mortality. In both sexes the relative risk of lung cancer death was 1.5 for those with chronic phlegm compared with those without this symptom. The degree of obstruction was a more important predictor; compared with people with FEV_1 of 80% or more, those with FEV_1 of 40% to 79% had a relative risk of 2.1, whereas those with FEV_1 of less than 40% had a relative risk of 3.9.

DISCUSSION

With all its shortcomings, the epidemiologic evidence described above meets to a considerable degree the criteria for judging an association to be causal, as outlined in the Surgeon General's 1982 Report on the Health Consequences of Smoking.[18] Although the association is not specific, it is consistent for the most part and strong in some studies. The temporal relationship is correct in that COPD precedes the cancer. And the association is coherent with what we already know about the natural history and biology of both COPD and lung cancer. The studies that have been reported are less than perfect, so there remains some doubt about causality. Yet the association has predictive properties and is therefore useful for this reason alone.

On the microscopic level, there is an association between nonspecific changes in bronchial epithelium and lung cancer in both humans[1] and animals.[10] Kuschner[10] raised the question as to whether nonspecific damage to the epithelium leads to carcinogenesis through cellular proliferation and regeneration, as well as interference with clearance of carcinogens by several pathophysiologic effects. Cohen has hypothesized that impaired pulmonary function may be self-accelerating and interferes with elimination of noxious agents so that cellular exposure is prolonged, thus serving as a modifying factor of cancer risk.[6] A vicious cycle results in people who are susceptible because of intrinsic and/or extrinsic influences. The molecular mechanism may involve the activity of oxygen radicals.[7] At this time much of this thinking is speculative.

From a clinical viewpoint, the association between COPD and lung cancer means that patients with the former disease should be watched for evidence of the latter disease. This association often poses a therapeutic problem. Patients with moderate-to-severe COPD who develop lung cancer are often difficult to treat definitively, since surgery and even radiation may reduce pulmonary function in impaired individuals to an intolerable level. Thus, COPD is one of a number of conditions that thwart successful management of patients with lung cancer.[21]

There remain unanswered questions that might have clinical significance, such as the relationship of age and cancer cell type to the presence or absence of COPD. The answers must await further investigation.

REFERENCES

1. Auerbach O, Stout AP, Hammond EC, Garfinkel L. Changes in bronchial epithelium in relation to cigarette smoking and in relation to lung cancer. N Engl J Med 1961; 256:253–267.
2. Boucot KR, Cooper DA, Weiss W, Carnahan WJ. The natural history of lung cancer. Am Rev Respir Dis 1964; 89:519–527.
3. Boucot KR, Cooper DA, Weiss W, Carnahan WJ. Cigarettes, cough, and cancer of the lung. JAMA 1966; 196:985–990.
4. Boucot KR, Seidman H, Weiss W. The Philadelphia Pulmonary Neoplasm Research Project: the risk of lung cancer in relation to symptoms and roentgenographic abnormalities. Environ Res 1977; 13:451–469.
5. Campbell AH, Lee EJ. The relationship between lung cancer and chronic bronchitis. Br J Dis Chest 1963; 57:113–119.
6. Cohen BH. Chronic obstructive pulmonary disease: a challenge in genetic epidemiology. Am J Epidemiol 1980; 112:274–288.
7. Cross CE, Halliwell B, Borish ET, et al. Oxygen radicals and human disease. Ann Intern Med 1987; 107:526–545.
8. Dean G. Lung cancer and bronchitis in Northern Ireland, 1960–1962. Br Med J 1966; 1:1506–1514.
9. Kubik A, Krivinka R, Sasek V, et al. Screening for lung cancer high-risk groups. Scand J Respir Dis 1970; 51:290–300.
10. Kuschner M. The J. Burns Amberson Lecture: The causes of lung cancer. Am Rev Respir Dis 1968; 98:573–590.
11. Lange P, Nyboe J, Appleyard M, et al. Ventilatory function and chronic mucus hypersecretion as predictors of death from lung cancer. Am Rev Respir Dis 1990; 141:613–617.
12. Lombard HL. An epidemiological study in lung cancer. Cancer 1965; 18:1301–1309.
13. Peto R, Speizer FE, Cochrane AL, et al. The relevance in adults of air-flow obstruction, but not of mucus secretion, to mortality from chronic lung disease. Am Rev Respir Dis 1983; 128:491–500.
14. Rimington J. Smoking, chronic bronchitis, and lung cancer. Br Med J 1971; 2:373–375.
15. Samet JM, Humble CG, Pathak DR. Personal and family history of respiratory disease and lung cancer risk. Am Rev Respir Dis 1986; 134:466–470.
16. Skillrud DM, Offord KP, Miller RD. Higher risk of lung cancer in chronic obstructive pulmonary disease. Ann Intern Med 1986; 105:503–507.
17. Stavraky KM. A study of precursor illness in lung cancer patients. J Chron Dis 1971; 23:691–705.
18. Surgeon General's Report on the Health Consequences of Smoking. Cancer. Rockville, Md: U.S. Department of Health and Human Services, Office on Smoking and Health, 1982, 16–20.
19. Tockman MS, Anthonisen NR, Wright EC, Donithan MG. Airways obstruction and the risk of lung cancer. Ann Intern Med 1987; 106:512–518.
20. van der Wal AM, Huizinga E, Orie NGM, et al. Cancer and chronic nonspecific lung disease. Scand J Resp Dis 1966; 47:161–172.
21. Weiss W, Seidman H, Boucot KR. The Philadelphia Pulmonary Neoplasm Research Project: thwarting factors in periodic screening for lung cancer. Am Rev Respir Dis 1975; 111:289–297.
22. Weiss W, Seidman H, Boucot KR. The Philadelphia Pulmonary Neoplasm Research Project: symptoms in occult lung cancer. Chest 1978; 73:57–61.
23. Wynder EL, Fairchild EP Jr. The role of a history of persistent cough in the epidemiology of lung cancer. Am Rev Respir Dis 1966; 94:709–720.

Section VII

DIAGNOSIS OF CHRONIC OBSTRUCTIVE PULMONARY DISEASE

Chapter 37

THE DIAGNOSIS OF EMPHYSEMA

David C. Flenley

Emphysema was redefined in 1985 as "a condition of the lung characterized by abnormal, permanent enlargement of air spaces distal to the terminal bronchioles, accompanied by destruction of their walls, without obvious fibrosis."[1] This diagnosis thus clearly depends on pathologic examination of the whole of both lungs, which have been fixed in inflation. The definition also requires that the range in size of normal distal air spaces be established, so as to determine when this is abnormal.

PATHOLOGIC DIAGNOSIS

Weibel[2] used the mean chord length, later renamed the mean linear intercept (Lm), to estimate the alveolar surface area in five normal lungs, and related this to the lung volume. They suggested that the alveolar surface area was some 40 square meters at a lung volume of 2.5 liters, rising to around 60 square meters at a lung volume of 5 to 6 liters, as in the normal adult. The mean linear intercept is the average distance between the intersections of alveolar walls on a line of known length thrown randomly on a random lung section. This method has been used to assess the size of distal air spaces in sections cut from paraffin-embedded blocks taken from inflation-fixed lungs, after correction for the shrinkage and distortion of such specimens from cutting.[3, 4] Alternatively, the degree of macroscopic emphysema (Fig. 37–1) has been assessed by comparing the naked eye appearance of a cut slice of a fixed inflated lung (possibly assisted by immersion under water and use of a hand lens) with that seen in a standard picture (picture grading).[5] Similar methods have been applied to lungs or lobes that have been resected at thoracotomy for lung cancer.[6] However, such surgical studies inevitably raise the problem of the uniformity of distribution of emphysema, particularly when such surgical measurements are related to physiologic studies, which inevitably depend on the function of the whole of both lungs, *in vivo,* prior to surgery.

CLINICAL DIAGNOSIS

Emphysema has traditionally been difficult to diagnose accurately in life and almost impossible to quantify. In the 48 autopsy lungs that were available from the 228 patients who died during the National Institutes of Health (NIH) Trial of Intermittent Positive Pressure Breathing, involving 935 non-hypoxemic patients with air flow limitation (FEV_1 varying from 11% to 57% of predicted normal), no significant relationships could be established between symptoms (breathlessness, wheeze, cough, sputum production) or hematocrit, arterial P_{CO_2}, and the picture grade of emphysema as assessed at autopsy.[4] There was also no correlation between these clinical or physiologic variables and either the alveolar wall thickness or the alveolar surface area, as calculated from measurements of the mean linear intercept.

Nonetheless, hyperinflation of the chest, as assessed by clinical examination, is often associated with emphysema, at least in patients with more severe disease. However, hyperinflation can also occur in an acute attack of bronchial asthma, and indeed the chronic asthmatic may also have chronically hyperinflated lungs. Hyperinflation can best be recognized at the bedside by a combination of three signs: indrawing of intercostal spaces (Fig. 37–2A), absence of the normal area of cardiac dullness behind the lower left border of the sternum, and shortening of the cricoid sternal distance to less than the usual three fingerbreadths (Fig. 37–2B).

RESPIRATORY FUNCTION IN EMPHYSEMA

Hyperinflation, however, can be more accurately measured by lung volumes, e.g., an increase in residual volume to total lung capacity ratio (RV/TLC), but this is commonly associated with airways obstruction arising from any cause, such as the classic "obstructive" pattern of respiratory function. These measurements do not necessarily relate to emphysema, as assessed pathologically, for as already noted an acute attack of asthma is associated with hyperinflation with the airway obstruction. Nonetheless, chronic airways obstruction, presumably diagnosed by the physical signs of hyperinflation, was one of the most repeatable diagnoses made in a recent study of the reliability of physical signs in the chest.[7]

If clinical diagnosis based on traditional history taking and physical examination is so unreliable, can respiratory function tests do any better in diagnosing emphysema? The low FEV_1/FVC ratio or a low peak expiratory flow rate (PEFR), both indicating airway obstruction, combined with a high RV/TLC ratio, which together form the classic obstructive pattern in respiratory function, relates to the airflow obstruction but not necessarily to the emphysema of chronic obstructive lung disease. However, in patients with persistent air flow obstruction, as shown by persistently low FEV_1 or PEF measurements when made several times per day over many days, if not months, some studies have shown that FEV_1 does correlate with the degree of emphysema.[8]

Diffusing Capacity in Emphysema

Traditionally the diffusing capacity for carbon monoxide (synonym: transfer factor) has been thought to relate to the

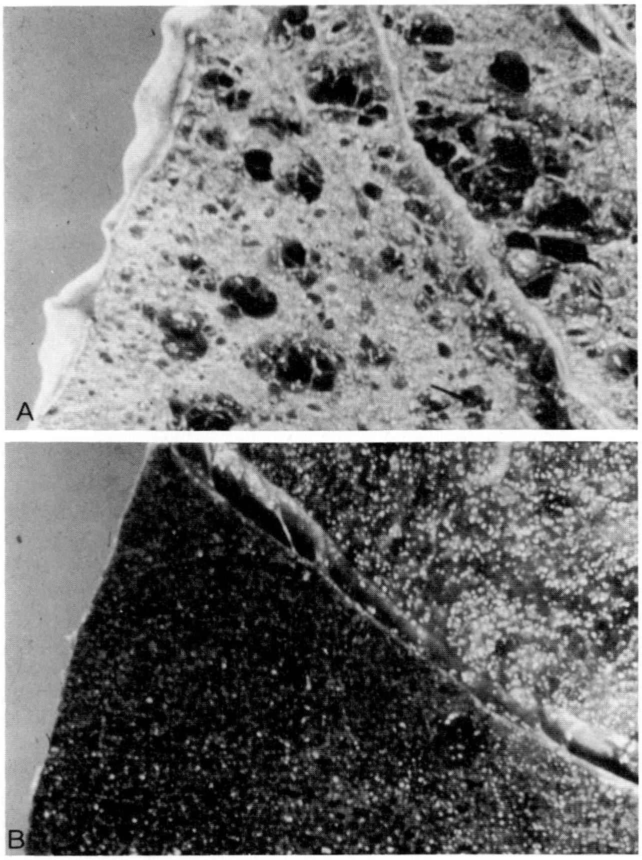

Figure 37–1. Macroscopic appearance of the fixed inflated specimen of two upper lobes. *A,* Obvious macroscopic emphysema of centrilobular type, with a small area of paraseptal emphysema. *B,* Essentially normal macroscopic appearance.

extent of emphysema. The results of two studies using diffusing capacity measurements [5,6] show that although diffusing capacity does indeed fall as the macroscopic emphysema score (assessed by the picture grading method) increases, there was clearly a wide variation in diffusing capacity measurements, even in patients with no macroscopic emphysema (Fig. 37–3). Indeed, a summary of previous studies using either steady-state[5,6,9,10] or single-breath[9–11] measurements of carbon monoxide diffusing capacity, expressed either as D_LCO in absolute terms or as a percentage of the predicted normal value, or as D_LCO/VA, or as the fractional uptake of carbon monoxide, shows that correlation coefficients between these measurements and the extent of macroscopic emphysema vary between studies from −0.36 to −0.73. Thus, as far as macroscopic emphysema is concerned, measurement of the diffusing capacity does not provide a particularly reliable means of assessing the extent of macroscopic emphysema in any individual case.

Lung Pressure-Volume Curves

The emphysematous lung is traditionally "floppy," resulting from loss of elastin, as this has been proteolytically digested by neutrophil elastase.[12] Thus lungs with emphysema would be expected to have a different pressure-volume relationship to that of normal lungs. The *in vivo* static pressure volume curve of the lungs, which conventionally uses the pressure recorded from a balloon in the lower esophagus as a measure of pleural pressure, is best described by the exponential equation

$$V = A - Be^{-kP}$$

where V is lung volume, P is static recoil pressure, and A, B, and k are constants.[13] In this equation, k is an index of lung distensibility, which describes the shape of the pressure volume curve in the upper half of the lung volume. This constant k mainly depends on the mean size of peripheral air spaces[14] and has thus been proposed to relate most closely to the severity of emphysema,[15] both in post-mortem studies and also in preoperative studies using *in vivo* measurements, when compared with the degree of emphysema as "scored" by macroscopic examination of the resected lobes or lungs.[6] However, neither of these studies, nor any of the earlier studies using less precise estimates of the shape of the pressure volume curve, has actually related pressure volume curves *in vivo* to the extent of emphysema, as assessed by either mean linear intercept measurements or macroscopic scoring, made from the whole of both lungs of patients as assessed post mortem.

RADIOLOGIC DIAGNOSIS

The notion that plain chest radiography is of clinical value in the diagnosis of emphysema has been challenged by Thurlbeck and Simon,[16] who studied the accuracy of this diagnosis in 696 patients who had had a chest radiograph within 6 months of death, and in whom paper-mounted whole lung sections were then available for study post mortem. The radiologic diagnosis of emphysema was made principally by recognition of the arterial deficiency pattern, but lung height, width, and size of the retrosternal space, heart size, and the position of the diaphragm were also recorded. In those patients in whom the pathologic specimen showed moderately severe or severe emphysema, only 41% were diagnosed correctly by radiology. Centriacinar emphysema was usually present when emphysema was diagnosed as being present in the upper lobes on the radiograph, whereas panacinar emphysema was more likely to be present when the disease was diagnosed as being only in the lower lobes. These investigators concluded that the chest radiograph was not a precise method of diagnosing emphysema, as occasional patients with no, trivial, or only mild emphysema would be diagnosed as having the disease, whereas a fairly high proportion of patients with severe emphysema were missed entirely on these radiologic criteria, which particularly emphasized the arterial deficiency pattern.

This problem has been reviewed.[17] Pratt questions the statement in a recent textbook on diagnostic radiology that "early diagnosis of emphysema by radiographic methods is most unsatisfactory."[18] Pratt reviews previous studies and concludes that opinion is varied, from those who found emphysema could be diagnosed accurately from the plain chest radiograph, to those who joined with Thurlbeck and Simon[16] in finding the radiograph of little value in this diagnosis. Pratt suggests that depression and flattening of the diaphragm, with blunting of the costophrenic angles, irregular translucency of the lung fields in the PA film, an abnormally large retrosternal space, and flattening or concavity of the diaphragm contour as seen in the lateral film, are of diagnostic value. He appears to base these conclusions on a study of 33 cases, carried out in 1965, using pathologic criteria for determining the extent of emphysema that were less precise than those currently employed, both for estimating macroscopic emphysema and for measuring alveolar or distal air space size, which is now the recognized defining characteristic of emphysema.[1] Sutinen and colleagues propose that hyperinflation, as recognized on the chest radiograph, is the most reliable sign of emphysema, but the figure

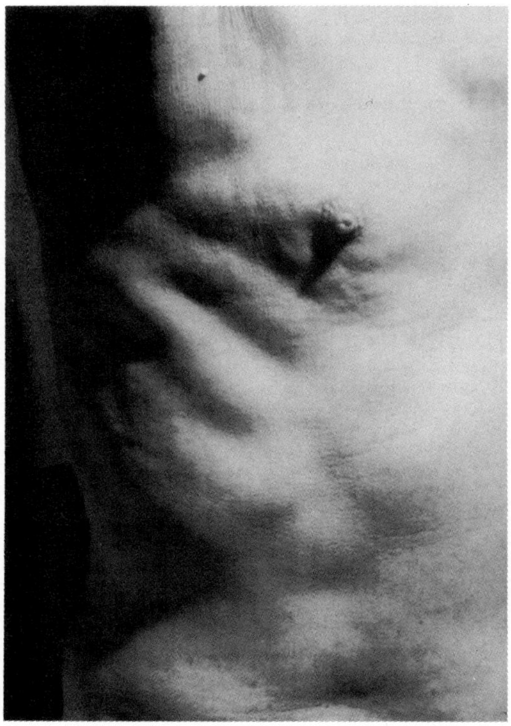

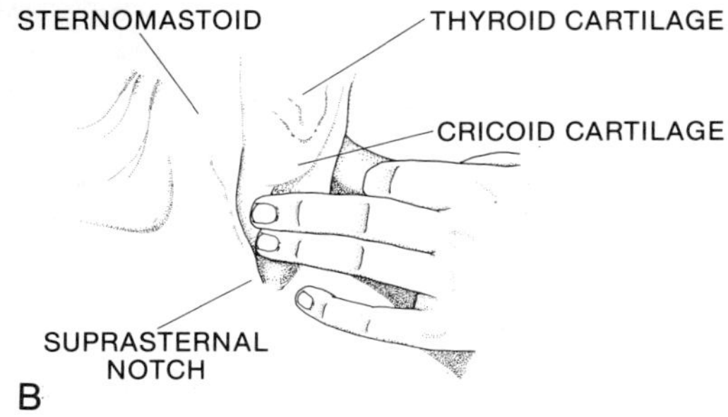

Figure 37–2. ***A,*** **Indrawing of intercostal spaces—a reliable sign of hyperinflation of the chest—but this also can occur in asthma as well as in COPD with emphysema.** ***B,*** **Shortening of the cricosternal distance to a value of less than the normal of three fingerbreadths— a reliable sign of hyperinflation when combined with indrawing of intercostal spaces (see** ***A*****)—but, again, not necessarily due to emphysema alone.**

illustrating this point in his 1965 paper[19] shows that, even in those patients with no emphysema (as shown pathologically by the point counting method he applied in 1965), there was a wide range of total lung capacities, encompassing the range of values found in 13 of his cases in which definite emphysema was shown by this pathologic estimation. Because Thurlbeck and Simon,[16] studying many more cases, found that radiologic hyperinflation (as measured by the retrosternal distance and diaphragmatic contour) was no better than their "arterial deficiency pattern," which identified only 41% of cases with severe emphysema, I conclude that the chest radiograph remains unreliable for the exclusion of emphysema; however, if emphysema is diagnosed from the radiograph, this will probably be found to be present at autopsy.

COMPUTER TOMOGRAPHY DIAGNOSIS

The CT scan presents a visual display, conventionally as a gray scale, which depends on the electron density of the tissue contained within the pixel (or unit) of the display. As air has a lower electron density than that of lung tissue, an emphysematous space that occupies several pixels will be shown as a black area in this gray scale display of the transthoracic CT scan, in contrast to the lighter areas representing tissues with a higher density—as in the extreme case for the bone in vertebrae and the rib cage. Using a window setting on the CT scan close to that of lung tissue, emphysematous spaces can indeed be distinguished from lung parenchyma visually.[20] However, the scan is derived from numerical information that represents the radioabsorbance of each pixel, which is expressed as either the Hounsfield unit or EMI number. Thus quantitative differences in lung density can be related to the presence of emphysema.[21] In a careful comparison of transthoracic CT scans with subsequent pathologic evidence of macroscopic emphysema (scored by a modified picture grading method)[5] in 32 patients aged 32 to 78 years who underwent thoracotomy for peripheral lung lesions following the scan, Bergin and colleagues[22] concluded that visual assessment from

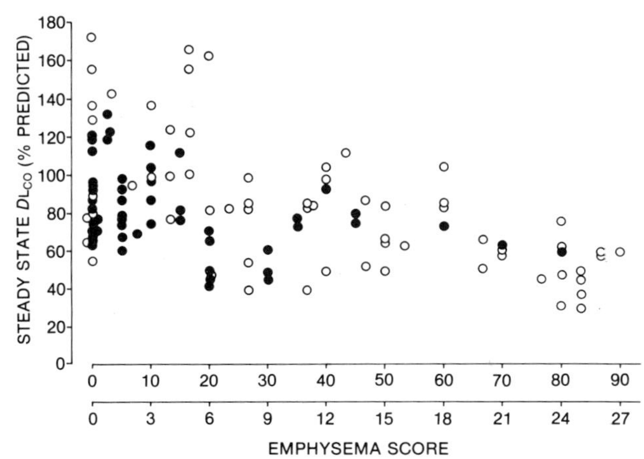

Figure 37–3. The relationship between the steady state diffusing capacity for carbon monoxide (expressed as per cent of predicted normal value) and the macroscopic emphysema score assessed by the picture grading method. Data plotted from ●, upper horizontal scale,[5] and ○, lower horizontal scale.[6]

A

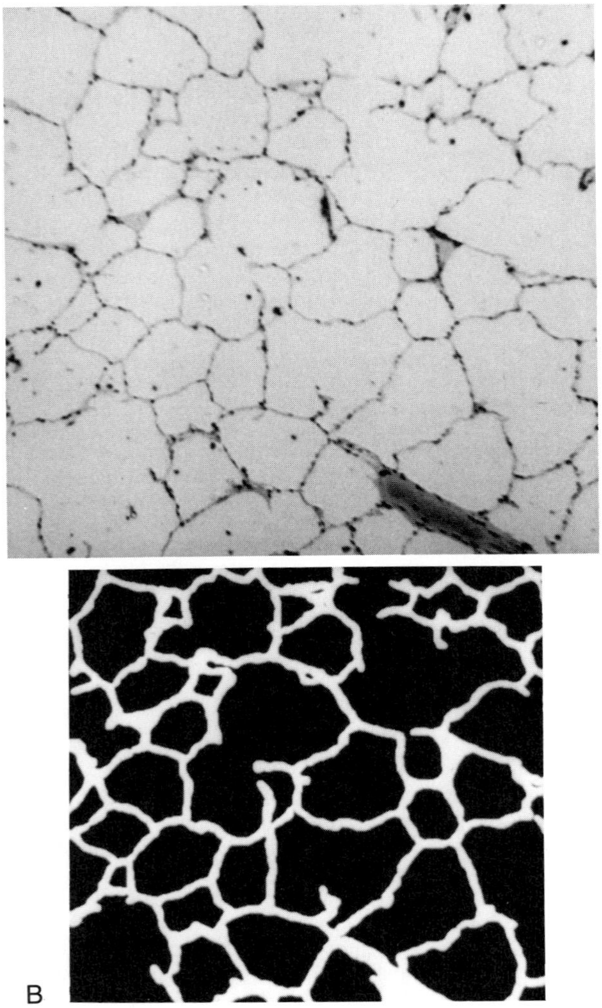

B

Figure 37–4. ***A***, **Histologic appearance of a random section taken from a methacrylate-embedded random block selected from a fixed inflated lobe resected from a patient with no clinical, radiologic, or functional evidence of emphysema, showing a relatively normal size of distal air spaces in the section.** ***B***, **A corresponding computer-enhanced image derived from this specimen; the air space wall per unit of lung volume (AWUV) was calculated from this computer image.**

the CT scan was "a useful method of assessing the presence and severity of emphysema." They made their visual assessment on the CT scan of the lobe or lung to be resected and then compared this with the pathologic appearance of the fixed inflated lung or lobe studied postoperatively.

We have recently used a computerized microscopic image analysis system to measure directly the surface area of distal air spaces in lungs or lobes resected for treatment of peripheral lung lesions.[23] We have made these measurements in sections taken from methacrylate-embedded blocks randomly selected from the inflation-fixed lungs or lobes resected from 45 patients (Figs. 37–4 and 37–5). In 28 of these, a preoperative CT scan was carried out, using two horizontal slices 6 and 10 cm below the sternal notch. This CT scan was then used to generate frequency histograms of CT numbers (measured as EMI units) using the EMI 5005 scanner. This scanner has been shown to provide a linear measurement of the electron density of air and water and a range of hydrocarbons whose physical density ranged from 0.001 (air) to 1.00 (water). Electron density within this range was also a linear function of the physical density, so that between EMI units of 0 (water) and −500 (air) the EMI 5005 scanner yields a linear measurement of physical density.

However, emphysema is defined as an increase beyond the normal in distal air space size, so that clearly regions of the lungs involved in emphysema will contain more air and less tissue and thus have a lower density. Since it was the low density regions we specially sought, we used the EMI number that defines the lowest fifth percentile of the frequency distribution histogram of EMI numbers within a lung field to characterize the extent of emphysema in that lung field (Figs. 37–6 and 37–7). We compared these numbers with direct measurements of the air space wall/unit lung volume (AWUV) derived by direct morphometric assessment of air space size in 26 to 32 fields randomly selected from the resected lobe or lung, following inflation after resection. The mean value of the surface area of the wall of the distal air spaces per unit of lung volume (AWUV) in the five fields yielding the lowest AWUV measurements was linearly correlated with the EMI unit defining the lowest fifth percentile of the frequency distribution, taken from the CT scan in the same area of the lobe or lung as that examined pathologically (Fig. 37–8). Since direct microscopy showed that the alveolar walls were not thickened in these regions, we conclude that this use of the CT scan can provide a quantitative estimate of the extent of emphysema within a given lung region.

A

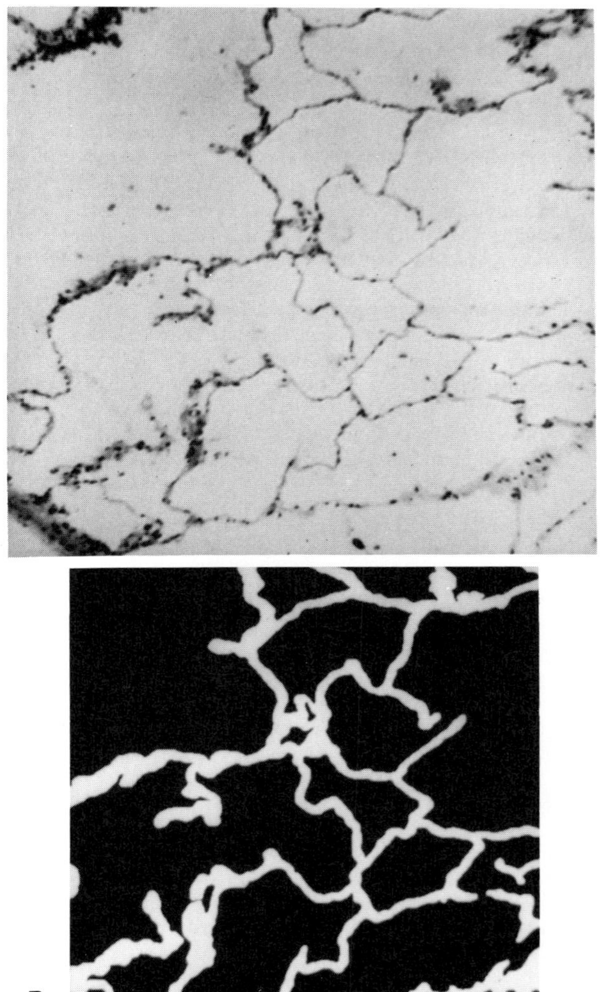

B

Figure 37–5. As in Figure 37–4 (at the same magnification), except that the specimens were taken from a patient with moderately severe emphysema, showing the greatly increased size of distal air spaces and the corresponding reduction in AWUV.

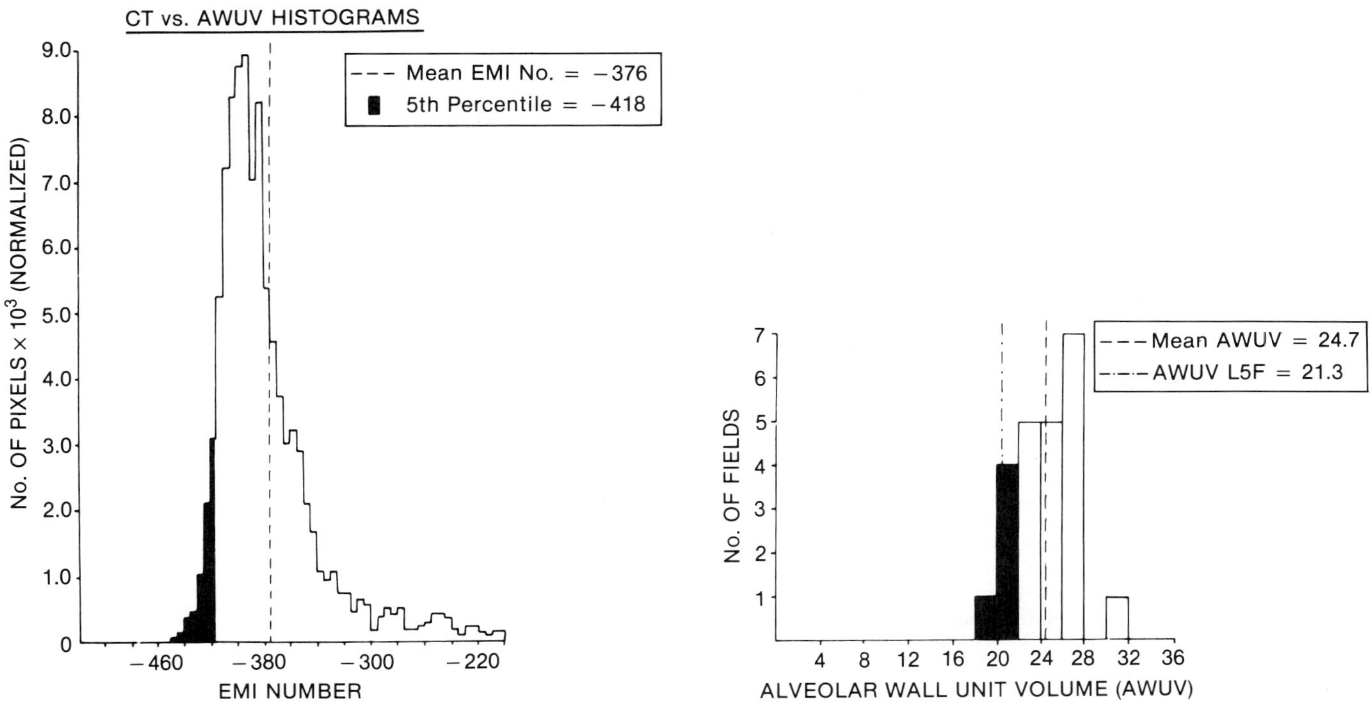

A B

Figure 37–6. ***A,*** **Frequency distribution of CT numbers (expressed as EMI units) in pixels derived from the lateral two fifths of the lung field in the horizontal CT scans taken 6 and 10 cm below the sternal notch. The distribution is obtained from those scans taken only from the lung field of the side from which a lung or lobe was later resected. Pixels forming the lowest fifth percentile of the distribution are shaded.** ***B,*** **Frequency distribution of the surface area of distal air spaces per unit of lung volume (AWUV: mm^2/mm^3) among fields randomly selected from the randomly selected blocks taken from the lateral two parasagittal slices of the resected lung or lobe. The five fields with the lowest AWUV values are shaded. (From Gould GA, MacNee W, McLean A, et al. Am Rev Respir Dis 1988; 137:380–392.)**

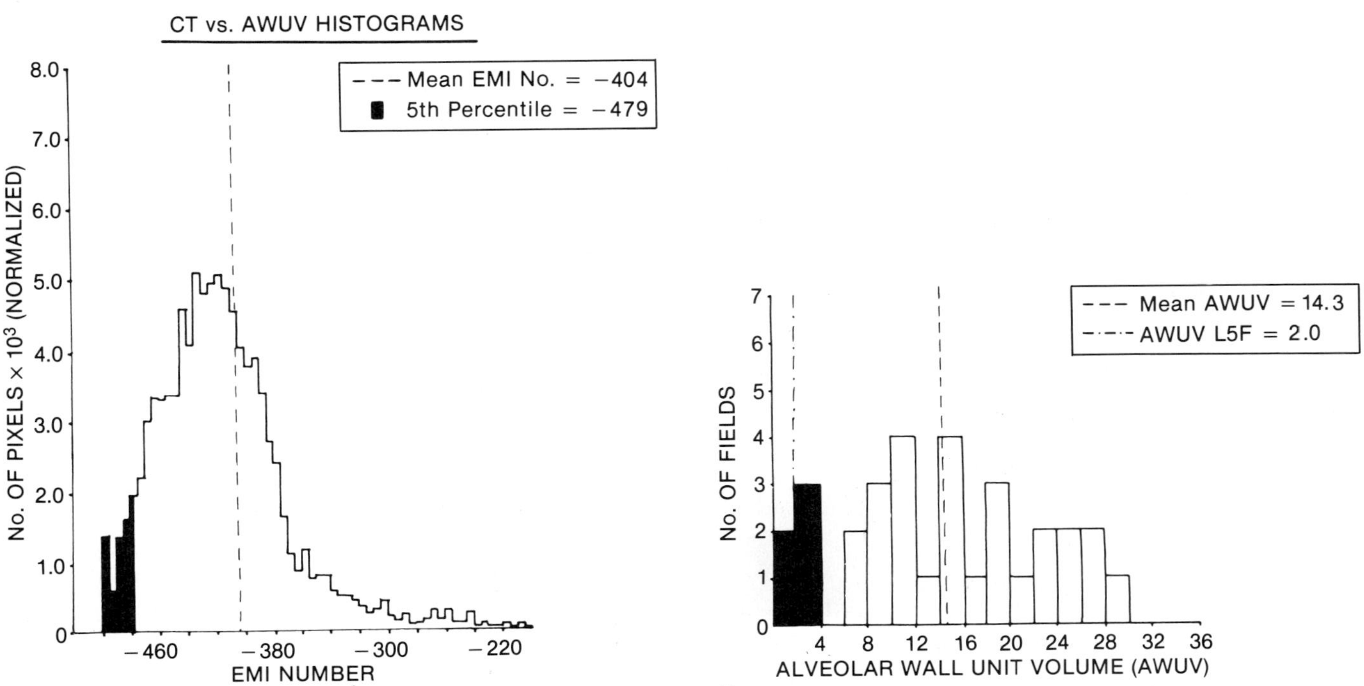

A B

Figure 37–7. As in Figure 37–6, but from a patient with emphysema, as shown by pixels in the CT histogram with values close to air (i.e., EMI unit values of −500) and the corresponding air space wall/unit lung volume (AWUV) values down to zero. (From Gould GA, MacNee W, McLean A, et al. Am Rev Respir Dis 1988; 137:380–392.)

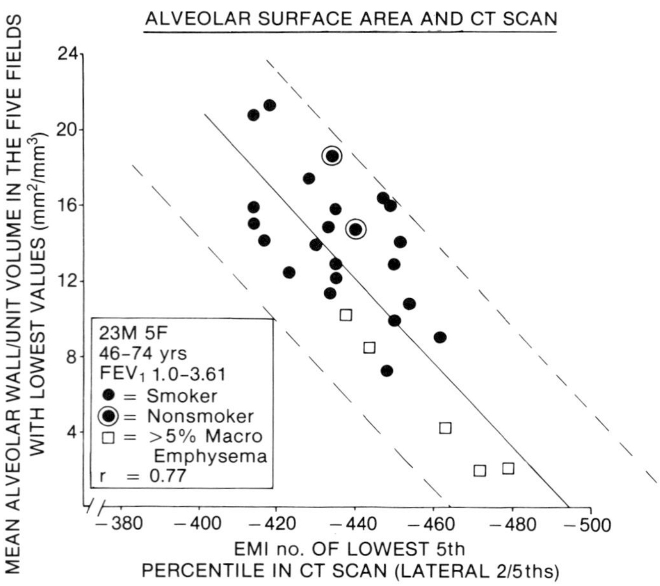

Figure 37–8. The relationship between the mean value of surface area of the walls of distal air spaces/unit of lung volume (AWUV) in the five fields with the lowest values in each case, and the value of the EMI unit that defined the lowest fifth percentile of the frequency distribution of EMI units. The relationship is significant (n = 28, r = −0.77, P <0.001).

Furthermore, by highlighting pixels of the CT display with low density numbers (arbitrarily selected as EMI units from −450 to −500, where 0 = water, and −500 = air), we can also use the CT scan to demonstrate zones in the lung field in which confluent emphysema occupies several pixels. This is confirmed by direct comparison between this highlighted CT scan and an emphysematous space, as shown in a transversely cut resected lobe or lung from the same patient (Fig. 37–9). Further studies, using fourth generation scanners with shorter scan time and improved resolution, are in progress. Nonetheless, it appears that the quantitative CT scan, by direct comparison with morphometric measurements in the same resected lobe or lung, can diagnose, quantify, and locate emphysema accurately in human lungs in life, noninvasively.

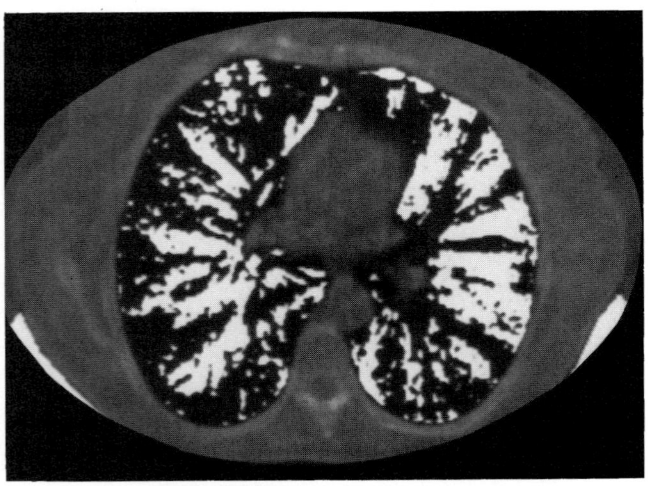

Figure 37–9. Computer-enhanced CT image from a patient with emphysema, in which pixels with EMI unit values lying in the range of −450 to −500 are shown in white, i.e., the lower density end of the range, extending down to pixels entirely occupied by air (EMI values −500). Comparison of such preoperative *in vivo* scans with subsequent resected specimens shows that this method can highlight areas of confluent emphysema.

In a further application of this *in vivo* CT method, we have found that the clinicopathologic pattern of the blue and bloated patient (airways obstruction, hypoxemia with CO_2 retention, pulmonary hypertension, and a history of cor pulmonale) can exist in patients with varying degrees of anatomic emphysema (Fig. 37–9), whereas other patients with the clinicopathologic pattern of the pink puffer (similar airway obstruction, but only modest hypoxemia and a low or normal arterial P_{CO_2}, little pulmonary hypertension, and no cor pulmonale) can also show some, much, or only a little emphysema. These results thus contradict the older notion that blue bloaters had mainly chronic bronchitis and pink puffers mainly emphysema.[24] However, they confirm the earlier physiopathologic studies that found that the degree of emphysema, as assessed by pathologic examination of both lungs post mortem, did not relate to the pattern of pink puffer or blue bloater.[25]

In summary, emphysema, which is clinically associated with air flow obstruction, cannot be precisely diagnosed in an individual patient from either physical signs, plain chest radiograph, or respiratory function studies. Although measurements of diffusing capacity corrected for alveolar volume do correlate well with the extent of anatomic emphysema as revealed by morphometry,[23] these do not relate closely to the extent of macroscopic emphysema in any individual patient. However, a new development, using the CT scan to measure regional lung density, can diagnose, quantify, and locate emphysematous regions in human lungs in life, noninvasively. The role of this new method remains to be fully assessed, but it appears that it will allow the relationship between the degree of emphysema and clinicopathologic patterns of chronic obstructive pulmonary disease to be re-evaluated. Furthermore, it provides the potential for quantitative assessment of the value of new potential agents for treating emphysema, e.g., antioxidants, genetically engineered $alpha_1$-proteinase inhibitor and/or synthetic antielastases.

REFERENCES

1. Snider GL, Klienerman J, Thurlbeck WM, Bengali ZH. The definition of emphysema. Report of a National Heart, Lung and Blood Institute. Division of Lung Diseases Workshop. Am Rev Respir Dis 1985; 132:182–185.
2. Weibel WR. Morphometry of the human lungs. Berlin: Springer-Verlag, 1963.
3. Thurlbeck WM. Measurement of pulmonary emphysema. Am Rev Respir Dis 1967; 95:752–764.
4. Nagai A, West WW, Paul JL, Thurlbeck WM. The National Institutes of Health Intermittent Positive-Pressure Breathing Trial: pathology studies. II. Correlation between morphologic findings, clinical findings and evidence of expiratory airflow obstruction. Am Rev Respir Dis 1985; 132:946–953.
5. Thurlbeck WM, Dunnill MS, Hartung W, et al. A comparison of three methods of measuring emphysema. Hum Pathol 1970; 1:215–226.
6. Pare PD, Brooks LA, Bates J, et al. Exponential analysis of the lung-pressure volume curve as a predictor of pulmonary emphysema. Am Rev Respir Dis 1982; 126:54–61.
7. Spiteri MA, Cook DG, Clarke SW. Reliability of eliciting physical signs on examination of the chest. Lancet 1988; i:873–875.
8. Thurlbeck WM, Henderson JA, Fraser RG, Bates DV. Chronic obstructive lung disease. A comparison between clinical, roentgenologic, functional and morphologic criteria in chronic bronchitis, emphysema, asthma and bronchiectasis. Medicine 1970; 49:81–145.
9. Berend A, Woolcock AJ, Marlin GE. Correlation between the function and structure of the lung in smokers. Am Rev Respir Dis 1979; 119:695–705.
10. Burrows B, Fletcher CM, Heard BE, et al. The emphysematous

and bronchial types of chronic airways obstruction: a clinico pathological study of patients in London and Chicago. Lancet 1966; i:830–835.
11. Symonds G, Renzetti AD, Mitchell MM. The diffusing capacity in pulmonary emphysema. Am Rev Respir Dis 1974; 109:391–394.
12. Janoff A. Elastases in emphysema: current assessment of the protease/antiprotease hypothesis. Am Rev Respir Dis 1985; 132:417–433.
13. Salazar E, Knowles JH. An analysis of pressure volume characteristics of the lungs. J Appl Physiol 1964; 19:97–104.
14. Greaves JA, Colebatch HJH. Observations on the pathogenesis of chronic airflow obstruction in smokers: implications for detection of "early" lung disease. Thorax 1986; 41:81–87.
15. Greaves JA, Colebatch HJH. Elastic behavior and structure of normal and emphysematous lungs post mortem. Am Rev Respir Dis 1981; 121:127–136.
16. Thurlbeck WM, Simon G. Radiographic appearance of the chest in emphysema. Am J Roentgenol 1978; 130:429–440.
17. Pratt CP. Role of conventional chest radiography in diagnosis and exclusion of emphysema. Am J Med 1987; 82:998–1116.
18. Heitzman AR. The Lung: Radiology. Pathologic Correlations. St Louis: CV Mosby, 1984.
19. Sutinen S, Christoforidis AJ, Clugh GA, Pratt PC. Roentgenologic criteria for the recognition of nonsymptomatic pulmonary emphysema: correlation between roentgenographic findings and pulmonary pathology. Am Rev Respir Dis 1965; 91:69–75.
20. Goddard PR, Nicolson EM, Laszlo G, et al. Computed tomography and pulmonary emphysema. Clin Radiol 1982; 33:379–387.
21. Hayhurst MD, MacNee W, Flenley DC, et al. Diagnosis of pulmonary emphysema by computerised tomography. Lancet 1984; ii:320–322.
22. Bergin C, Muller N, Nicholas DM, et al. The diagnosis of emphysema. A computer tomographic-pathologic correlation. Am Rev Respir Dis 1986; 133:541–546.
23. Gould GA, MacNee W, McLean A, et al. Measurements of lung density in life can quantitate distal air space enlargement—an essential defining feature of human emphysema. Am Rev Respir Dis 1988; 137:380–392.
24. McFadden ER, Braunwald E. Cor pulmonale and pulmonary thromboembolism. In: Braunwald E, ed. Heart Disease. A Textbook of Cardiovascular Medicine, 2nd ed. Philadelphia: WB Saunders, 1984, 1572–1604.
25. Mitchell RS, Stanford RE, Johnson JM, et al. The morphologic features of the bronchi, bronchioles, and alveoli in chronic airway obstruction: a clinico pathologic study. Am Rev Respir Dis 1976; 114:137–145.

Chapter 38

SYMPTOMS AND SIGNS OF COPD

D. Georgopoulos N. R. Anthonisen

The diagnosis of chronic obstructive pulmonary disease (COPD) is usually made on the basis of the history and physical examination with laboratory studies being used to validate the initial clinical impression. Though laboratory studies are essential, patients with COPD are often managed symptomatically—that is, therapies are applied to alleviate symptoms and also are evaluated in these terms. It therefore follows that eliciting and quantifying symptoms and physical signs are important in patients with COPD or suspected COPD.

The clinical and laboratory manifestations of COPD can be thought of as due to three independent processes, all related to cigarette smoking. Emphysema is characterized by dissolution of the lung parenchyma with loss of pulmonary surface area and recoil.[66] Small airways disease is characterized by inflammation and fibrosis of the smaller airways with obstruction.[35] Both these lesions may cause the expiratory slowing typical of the disease, and neither can be diagnosed with certainty without examination of tissue. Chronic mucous hypersecretion, or chronic bronchitis, is a term defining the symptom complex of chronic cough and sputum production; its anatomic basis is goblet cell hypertrophy and hyperplasia in the larger airways that do not *per se* cause airways obstruction or expiratory slowing.[65] Many efforts have been made to separate patients with COPD into groups based on the probabilities of emphysema or airways disease being the predominant lesion. Though these have been of interest, they are not helpful therapeutically, and 80% to 90% of patients with COPD have the clinical features of both airways disease and emphysema. "Pure" cases of airways disease or emphysema, therefore, are uncommon and represent the opposite ends of a spectrum. We shall not emphasize such differentiations in this chapter.

By far the most important cause of COPD is tobacco smoking.[74] Though emphysema and small airway disease may occur in nonsmokers, these conditions are extremely rare, and usually when chronic airways obstruction occurs in nonsmokers it can be ascribed to other diseases, such as asthma or bronchiectasis. Thus a history of smoking, usually in excess of 20 cigarettes a day for 20 years, is virtually essential to the diagnosis.

HISTORY—SYMPTOMS OF COPD

Classically the patient with COPD presents with dyspnea that has been gradually progressive over years. This is usually accompanied by a history of chronic cough and sputum and often by a history of wheezing. There is often a history of exacerbations of symptoms with respiratory infections. Patients almost always present when they are more than 50 years of age, and at present approximately 80% of them are male. This sex distribution will probably change, however, as more women accumulate the necessary exposure to tobacco smoke.

Though smoking is the most important risk factor for COPD, several other factors should be sought. A strong family history, especially one marked by disease before the age of 50 years, is suggestive of hereditary alpha$_1$-antitrypsin deficiency.[43] The disease also tends to be familial in people without this deficiency. An occupational history, with emphasis on exposure to respirable dusts and fumes, should be sought. Many such agents have been shown to be associated with loss of lung function or symptoms of chronic mucous hypersecretion[7, 16, 69] and probably augment the harmful effects of tobacco smoke.

COPD patients usually present because their dyspnea is severe enough to interfere with their usual daily activity. The symptom has almost always been slowly progressive for years and signifies major loss of lung function. Dyspnea at rest indicates severe respiratory impairment; the forced expiratory volume in one second (FEV_1) is usually less than 30% of predicted normal and the oxygen uptake (VO_2 max) less than 15 ml (kg min).[2] When dyspnea is the only symptom, pulmonary emphysema is likely to predominate, suggesting a large irreversible component.[14, 26, 31] In such patients cough and sputum production are often minimal unless respiratory infection occurs. The dyspnea of COPD should be differentiated from other causes of chronic dyspnea, particularly heart diseases. Orthopnea and paroxysmal nocturnal dyspnea, common in congestive heart failure, are not usually present in COPD.[64] Platypnea, defined as dyspnea on assuming the upright position, is rarely present in patients with COPD and might be due to postural changes in blood gases, although this has not been confirmed.[6]

The mechanism of dyspnea in patients with COPD has not been fully explained. Factors thought to contribute to the development of this subjective sensation include length-tension inappropriateness of the respiratory muscles,[15] quantitative disturbances in the sensing of respiratory loads,[40] fatigue of respiratory muscles,[27] abnormal control of breathing with excessive ventilatory drive,[12, 39, 40] and increased oxygen cost of breathing.[45] Hypoxia and hypercapnia may intensify the degree of breathlessness, through afferent inputs to the brain from peripheral chemoreceptors and mechanoreceptors.[1, 71]

The quantification of dyspnea is an important goal in the overall assessment of the patient with COPD. Quantitative measurements of dyspnea provide baseline data to assess the efficacy of various therapeutic regimens and the stability of the patient over time. The visual analog scale (VAS),[49] the oxygen cost diagram,[54] the baseline dyspnea index (BDI),[50] and the Borg category scale[11] are some of the techniques used for this purpose. The visual analog scale consists of a vertical 100-mm line connecting two points that represent "no breathlessness" and "greatest breathlessness." The patient marks a point in the line that corresponds to his or her breathlessness, and the distance above the "no breathlessness" point is an index of the severity of dyspnea. The oxygen-cost diagram is a type of VAS in which everyday activities are placed proportional to their oxygen cost along the 100-mm vertical line (Fig. 38–1). The baseline dyspnea index quantifies the intensity of dyspnea based on grades for components, including task magnitude, effort, magnitude, and functional impairment. The Borg category scale is used for rating breathlessness during exercise testing. The clinical measurement of dyspnea by these methods is reproducible and can be completed in a few minutes; results generally correlate with lung function and respiratory muscle strength.[50]

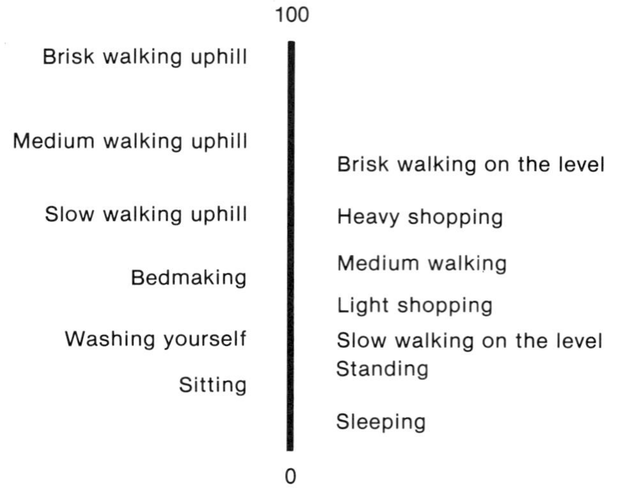

Figure 38–1. Oxygen-cost diagram. Everyday activities are placed along the 100-mm vertical line proportional to their oxygen cost. The patient is asked to mark the line at a point above which he or she will become breathless. The distance from the bottom of the scale (zero point) to the patient's mark is measured, and it represents an index of the subject's dyspnea. (Adapted from McGavin CR, et al. Dyspnoea, disability, and distance walked: comparison of estimates of exercise performance in respiratory disease. Br Med J 1978; 2:241–243.)

Acute increases in the severity of dyspnea in patients with COPD may indicate an exacerbation of the disease or another disease process, such as pulmonary embolism or pneumothorax.[25, 28, 44] The diagnosis of pulmonary embolism and pneumothorax should be made as soon as possible, because these complications are often fatal due to decreased lung function reserves.

Dyspnea is usually associated with a cough, which may be denied by patients who consider it a normal finding, attributed to cigarette smoking.[32] In over 75% of COPD patients either the cough antedates the onset of dyspnea or the two symptoms appear together.[14] The cough is chronic, usually productive, occasionally episodic, and worse in the morning upon rising. The patient is seldom awakened from sleep by coughing, a finding that differentiates patients with COPD from asthmatic patients. Asthmatic patients tend to be awakened by dry cough at 3 or 4 a.m. owing to increased bronchoconstriction at that time.[21] The cough of COPD may be required to clear abnormal amounts of mucus deposited in the airways by the hypertrophied bronchial glands. Cigarette smoking might contribute via direct stimulation of cough receptors.[47]

The amount, character, viscosity, and odor of the sputum can provide useful information. A normal person produces about 10 ml of sputum in 24 hours, an amount that is unnoticed and swallowed. Therefore, as a general rule any sputum production reported by the patient is abnormal. Patients are often able to estimate the amount of sputum production, although some may swallow large amounts of sputum unconsciously and thus give a negative history. Characterization of the sputum is important and always should be done. Patients with stable COPD usually produce white mucoid sputum, usually in the morning and often throughout the day. Increases in sputum volume and change in color to yellow or green are probably the most reliable symptoms of endobronchial infection treatable with antibiotics. It should be noted that changes in sputum color do not always denote purulence, since eosinophil accumulation may cause yellow sputum and a yellow-green color may be imparted by myeloperoxidase.[67] Foul-tasting or foul-smelling sputum is rare in COPD and strongly suggests superinfection with anaerobic organisms.

A history of wheezing is not unusual in patients with COPD and may indicate a reversible component of the disease. The Intermittent Positive-Pressure Breathing Trial Group examined 1000 patients with COPD and reported that symptomatic wheezing correlated negatively with the annual rate of decline of the FEV_1 and positively with the bronchodilator response to beta-agonists.[3, 4] However, bronchospasm is not the sole cause of wheezing. Many patients experience wheeze with exertion, presumably because of increased gas flow through airways narrowed by inflammation or scarring. Nocturnal dyspnea and wheeze are uncommon in COPD and suggest asthma or heart failure.[64]

Anorexia and weight loss are common complaints in patients with advanced disease. The etiology of the weight loss is not clear. An increase in body metabolism,[72] an adaptive mechanism to minimize metabolic demands and oxygen consumption, or inadequate caloric intake[75] are mechanisms that could contribute to weight loss. Whatever the mechanism, weight loss in a patient with COPD is probably a poor prognostic sign. Vandenbergh and colleagues[75] reported that patients with COPD who had lost about 20% of their initial body weight in 5 years had higher mortality than those without weight loss. Some studies have attempted to correlate the degree of weight loss with the severity of emphysema.[60, 61, 72, 75, 79] Openbrier and colleagues[60, 61] have observed that patients with emphysema are frequently undernourished, and there was an association between the weight loss and the decline in pulmonary function, as measured by the FEV_1 and the diffusion capacity for carbon monoxide.

Occasionally COPD patients complain of chest pain or hemoptysis. Chest pain usually is not due to the disease. A gradual onset of chest pain with or without cough, fever, or sputum production indicates the possibility of an infiltrative process involving the pleura or chest wall. A sudden onset of pain, pleuritic and sharp in character, associated with worsening of dyspnea and diaphoresis, strongly suggests pulmonary embolism or pneumothorax.[25, 28, 44] Pneumothorax, although not very common in patients with COPD, may have serious consequences because of the limited respiratory reserves.[20] Pulmonary embolism may complicate COPD, particularly when right heart failure and pulmonary hypertension are present. Chest pain also can be caused by reflux esophagitis or peptic ulcer, which occur frequently in patients with COPD,[25, 76, 78] perhaps because of gastric hypersecretion secondary to hypoxia, hypercapnia, and the use of xanthines.[24] David and colleagues[18] reported that approximately 40% of patients with chronic bronchitis have gastroesophageal reflux. This could be due to cigarette smoking and theophylline, both of which significantly reduce the lower esophageal sphincter pressure.[9, 19]

Hemoptysis is common in COPD, particularly during exacerbations involving increases in dyspnea, cough and sputum volume, and purulence.[38, 63] The blood presumably originates in inflamed airways, and the typical episode of hemoptysis is the production of blood-streaked purulent sputum. Other causes of hemoptysis, such as pneumonia, tumor, bronchiectasis, or heart failure, always should be considered, particularly when the patient produces "pure" blood.

Attention should be given to symptoms related to sleep. Nightmares, morning headaches, excessive daytime somnolence, and loud snoring in a patient with COPD suggest sleep disturbances with severe hypoxia and CO_2 retention during the night.[23] Obstructive sleep apnea may occur in COPD and should be sought in patients with hypersomnolence and snoring, particularly if they are obese.[30] On the other hand, episodic nocturnal hypoxemia and hypercapnia occur frequently in COPD without obstructive apnea and often are accompanied by arrhythmias and pulmonary hypertension.[23]

COPD is associated with psychiatric disturbances, which often are not recognized. Limitation of activity, as occurs in severe COPD, causes feelings of depression, hopelessness, and pessimism.[13] Hypoxia, breathlessness, or both may produce symptoms such as memory loss and reduced attention. Indeed, 43% of patients with an average PaO_2 of 68 mmHg showed moderate cognitive impairment, and the prevalence was 65% among patients with a PaO_2 of 45 mmHg.[29] In addition, psychogenic and organic sexual dysfunctions are associated with COPD and are related to the severity of the airways obstruction.[73]

A patient with COPD who presents with an exacerbation of symptoms needs special attention. These patients are at high risk of developing acute respiratory failure with severe hypoxia and hypercapnia during exacerbations. A history of increasing dyspnea, increasing use of bronchodilators, increasing sputum volume and purulence, and deterioration of mental status may signal the onset of acute respiratory failure. The possibility of sedative administration, which may seriously depress ventilation and lead to hypoxic hypercapnic respiratory failure, should always be considered as a cause of a patient's deterioration.

PHYSICAL EXAMINATION—SIGNS OF COPD

The physical examination is the second step in evaluation of COPD patients. Signs elicited by examination of these patients may be quite specific and sensitive, and they serve as a guide in following the progress of the disease and the efficacy of treatment.

Central to the examination of COPD patients is the assessment of dyspnea, hyperinflation, and respiratory muscle function by inspection. Patients with severe dyspnea may demonstrate tachypnea and respiratory distress with trivial exertion, such as undressing or entering the examining room. Such patients speak in an interrupted fashion, unable to sustain long sentences because of breathlessness. Patients with COPD almost always demonstrate resting breathing rates of over 16/min, which is abnormal, and the breathing rate is roughly proportional to the disease severity; hypercapnia frequently is associated with rates of 25 or more per minute.[48, 59] A minority of patients with COPD spontaneously develop pursed lip breathing—pursing the lips during expiration. This phenomenon has been studied on several occasions, but its physiologic function remains obscure. By increasing the luminal pressure in large intrathoracic airways, it may prevent sensations of discomfort due to collapse of these airways during expiration. Pursed lip breathing tends to slow respiratory frequency and by doing so increases the lung's gas exchange efficiency. Attempts are often made to teach COPD patients to use pursed lip breathing; these are seldom successful in patients who do not spontaneously employ this strategy.

The pattern of breathing should be noted. Use of accessory muscles is easily noted in the form of inspiratory contractions of the sternocleidomastoid muscle; this in general occurs in patients with an FEV_1 of less than 1.0.[53] Patients with very severe airways obstruction commonly increase the effectiveness of accessory muscles when sitting by leaning forward with their arms resting on a stationary object. By fixing the thoracic girdle, they allow muscles connecting the girdle and the rib cage, such as the latissimus dorsi, to perform an inspiratory function. Contraction of the abdominal rectus muscles during expiration is also abnormal and common in severe obstructive disease. By increasing abdominal pressure during expiration, these muscles displace the chief muscle of inspiration, the diaphragm cephalad, increasing its curvature and efficiency during the subsequent inspiration.[8, 52] Several breathing patterns have been associated with fatigue of the inspiratory muscles. Because such fatigue is extremely difficult to characterize accurately, this association has not been verified, but it is clear that both paradoxical breathing and respiratory alternans occur in patients with very severe ventilatory limitations, usually with respiratory failure.[5, 17, 68]

Paradoxical breathing consists of an inward motion of the upper abdominal wall with inspiration.[68] This can occur only if the diaphragm does not descend normally and thereby increase abdominal pressure, and it indicates inefficiency of diaphragmatic contraction relative to that of the muscles of the rib cage. Such inefficiency, while possibly due to fatigue, could also be due to hyperinflation with shortening of diaphragmatic fiber length, so that less tension is produced for a given stimulus, and to diaphragmatic flattening, so that increases in tension are less effective in generating pressure across the diaphragm (Fig. 38–2). Though more common in the erect position, paradoxical breathing is more easily detected when the patient is supine.

Respiratory alternans is a cyclic alteration in breathing movements so that a series of breaths are taken largely by the diaphragm with inspiratory outward movement of the abdomen, and then a series of breaths are taken using largely rib cage muscles with expansion of the rib cage and reduced or paradoxical abdominal motion.[5, 17] This sign is uncommon in COPD but has been observed in patients with respiratory failure. The Hoover sign[36] is an inward motion of the lower lateral rib cage with inspiration and is seen in severe COPD. It is probably similar in significance to paradoxical breathing, though other potential causes have been cited.[55, 68]

Hyperinflation can be assessed in qualitative fashion. With hyperinflation, the rib cage is in a more inspiratory position than normal, causing the well-known increase in thoracic anteroposterior diameter of COPD. Anteroposterior motion of the rib cage is reduced and, in severe cases, inspiration is associated with cephalad motion of the rib cage, presumably due to accessory muscle contraction. Diaphragmatic position may be assessed by percussion and is commonly low in COPD.[70, 77] Other signs of hyperinflation are tracheal tug and pulsus paradoxus. The former is a downward pull on the trachea with inspiration, possibly due to traction on mediastinal structures exerted by contraction of the low-lying diaphragm. Pulsus paradoxus is frequently observed in severe airways obstruction, with the systolic blood pressure at least 10 mmHg lower during inspiration than expiration.[34] It is due to abnormally low inspiratory pleural pressures that are transmitted to the cavity of the left ventricle, so ventricular pressure during inspiration is low in relation to that in extrathoracic arteries. Signs of hyperinflation, although useful, are not very sensitive. Many patients with substantially increased functional residual capacity and total lung compliance do not demonstrate unequivocal evidence of hyperinflation on physical examination.

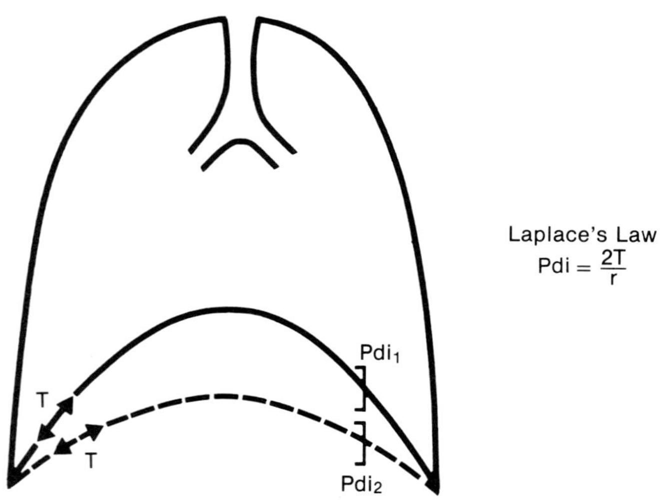

Figure 38–2. Schematic representation of the effect of diaphragmatic curvature on the generation of transdiaphragmatic pressure (Pdi). According to Laplace's law, a given tangential tension (T) developed by the diaphragm is translated into a smaller Pdi when the radius of the diaphragmatic curvature is large (dashed line) compared with a smaller radius (solid line).

Patients with severe COPD frequently develop pulmonary hypertension and right ventricular failure (cor pulmonale).[22, 33] Hypoxic pulmonary vasoconstriction plus obliteration of the pulmonary vascular bed is thought to be the cause of this syndrome, and it is commonly present in patients with hypoxemia and CO_2 retention.[22] On the other hand, it is unwise to ascribe signs of right ventricular failure to cor pulmonale in patients with COPD who are not hypoxemic (Pa_{O_2} greater than 60 mm Hg). Central cyanosis and peripheral edema are the most obvious signs of cor pulmonale, and other signs of pulmonary hypertension and right ventricular failure may be difficult to elicit in patients with severe COPD.[34] Right ventricular heaves are frequently obscured by hyperinflation, with the cardiac impulse being most evident in the subxiphoid area where it is difficult to relate to pulmonary artery pressure. Bedside assessment of jugular venous pressure is difficult in patients with vigorous accessory muscle contraction during inspiration. Nevertheless, an effort should be made to estimate the height of the jugular venous pulse. When this is more than 3 cm above the sternal notch in a patient whose head and thorax are 45 degrees from the horizontal, it is an excellent sign of right ventricular failure. Hepatomegaly is also difficult to assess in patients with COPD since the liver is often displaced downward due to pulmonary hyperinflation. Though in many patients with COPD the clinical diagnosis of cor pulmonale rests on the presence of arterial hypoxemia and ankle edema, in a minority signs of cor pulmonale—cardiomegaly, right ventricular heaves, jugular venous distention, and hepatomegaly—may dominate the physical examination. These patients usually have relatively little hyperinflation and severe blood gas disturbances and are thought to have predominantly airways disease as opposed to emphysema.

Inguinal hernias are a common finding in patients with COPD and may be found in up to 50% of them.[25] Inguinal hernias are probably related to the increased abdominal pressure associated with coughing.

Percussion of the chest is not very helpful in patients with COPD. Patients with severe hyperinflation may have a tympanic percussion note. However, in this case, pneumothorax must be ruled out as a cause of tympany. Some physicians use percussion to estimate diaphragmatic motion. Normally the diaphragm moves 5 to 6 cm during maximal inhalation and exhalation. In patients with a flat diaphragm, as in COPD, the excursion is 3 to 4 cm or even less.[70] However, there is considerable disagreement as to whether diaphragmatic motion can be determined accurately by percussion.[77]

Unlike percussion, auscultation of the chest can give valuable information regarding the severity of the disease and even the response to therapy. Patients with COPD generally have noisy chests because of the frequent occurrence of adventitious sounds. However, the intensity of vesicular breath sounds is decreased when not obscured by adventitious sounds.[10, 56, 70] Breath sound intensity has been related to the degree of emphysema and indices of airflow obstruction. Schneider and Anderson[70] demonstrated that decreased breath sounds were the most reliable physical sign of emphysema. Pardee and colleagues[62] and Bohadana and colleagues[10] showed that breath sound intensity related to FEV_1, specific conductance, and forced expiratory volume in one second/forced vital capacity

(FEV_1/FVC) (Fig. 38–3). The intensity of breath sounds was evaluated in these studies with the patient seated and performing fast deep inspirations from residual volume through the mouth. Sound intensity was assessed in the upper anterior and midaxial regions and the posterior bases bilaterally and classified on a simple 5-point scale. In 20 patients, the ratings of two independent observers showed a correlation coefficient of 0.97.[10] Nair and Turner-Warwick[56] also showed that decreased intensity of breath sounds was accompanied by poor regional ventilation, as measured by radioactive xenon. Accurate estimation of breath sound intensity required disregarding adventitious sounds that often are louder than normal sounds, which requires some practice and limits the method's utility.

Measurement of the forced expiratory time (FET), defined as the time of hearing airflow while listening with the stethoscope over the trachea as the patient performs a FVC maneuver, is a simple bedside technique to detect and assess airflow obstruction.[42] The duration of audible expiration is timed in seconds. An FET of less than 5 seconds suggests that severe airflow obstruction is absent and that FEV_1/FVC is greater than 60%. An FET of greater than 6 seconds indicates airways obstruction and an FEV_1/FVC of less than 50%.

Wheezing, a high-pitched continuous sound, is an important sign of airflow obstruction. Wheezing is best heard over the trachea or in the neck region, because high-frequency sounds are more clearly detected in these areas than through the chest wall.[46] The relationship among wheezing intensity, severity of

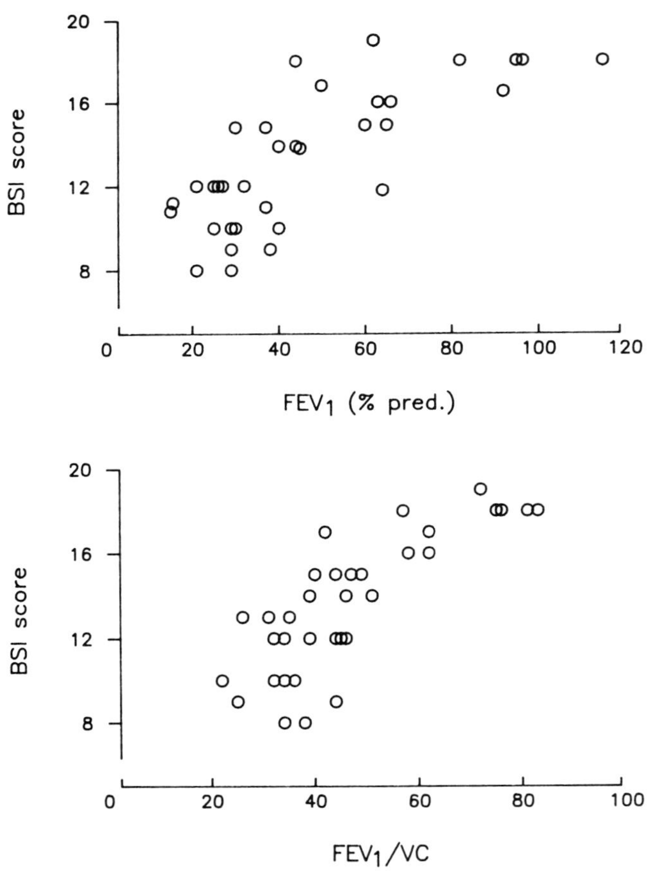

Figure 38–3. Relationship between breath sound intensity (BSI score) and forced expiratory volume in 1 second (FEV_1) and between BSI score and the ratio of FEV_1 to vital capacity (FEV_1/VC) in 34 subjects. Although the relationships were linear, there was a considerable scatter in the data. (Adapted from Bohadana AB, et al. Breath sounds in the clinical assessment of airflow obstruction. Thorax 1978; 33:345–351.)

obstruction, and response to bronchodilator was examined by Marini and colleagues[51] in 83 patients with COPD and 17 normal people. Wheezing heard during unforced breathing was specific for airflow obstruction, and the intensity correlated with severity of obstruction and bronchodilator response. However, wheezing was not sensitive for COPD, in that obstruction could be present in the absence of wheeze. Wheezing during forced breathing did not correlate with either the degree of obstruction or the bronchodilator response. In patients with confirmed COPD, the absence of wheezing during quiet breathing may indicate a degree of irreversible airway obstruction.

Discontinuous adventitious sounds are commonly found on auscultation of the chest of COPD patients. These sounds last for less than 20 msec and are heard as a series of brief explosive sounds (crackles or rales). They usually begin with the onset of inspiration, are few in number, and are generally heard at the lung bases.[46] Early inspiratory crackles are not changed by altering the patient's position and are thought to represent the bubbling of air through secretions. The sudden opening of small airways with rapid equilibration of pressures also may contribute to the generation of these sounds. However, sounds generated by the latter mechanism are heard late in the inspiratory cycle and may present in congestive heart failure or restrictive lung disease. Indeed, the most important aspect in describing crackles is the timing of their occurrence during inspiration, and this may help differentiate between COPD and congestive heart failure or restrictive lung disease.[57, 58] A combination of diseases, such as restrictive and obstructive lung disease, may produce crackles heard during early, middle, and late inspiration.

Cardiac auscultation is an essential part of the examination in patients with COPD, though the heart sounds may be difficult to hear because of hyperinflation and adventitious lung sounds. Frequently the heart sounds are best heard in the subxiphoid area.[34] Heart rate and rhythm constitute valuable information; severe COPD is associated with resting tachycardia, and arrhythmias are common and should be treated.[37, 41] Signs of cor pulmonale, such as right ventricular gallop or increases in the pulmonic second sound, may be heard, and murmurs of pulmonic or tricuspid insufficiency indicate very severe right ventricular failure.

CONCLUSION

The history and physical examination provide valuable information in patients with COPD. They do not supplant quantitative laboratory assessments, such as spirometry and blood gas analysis; these are, in general, the standards by which severity and progress of the disease are judged. Expensive or dangerous forms of therapy, such as systemic steroids or oxygen, require careful laboratory assessment. On the other hand, exacerbations of COPD are not always attended by distinct changes in spirometry and blood gases, and clinical decisions must be based on symptoms and signs. Decisions regarding low-risk therapies such as inhaled bronchodilators, diuretics, and broad-spectrum antibiotics are frequently and properly based on data gathered from the history and physical examination. It follows that these assessments should be carried out carefully and systematically.

REFERENCES

1. Adams L, Chronos N, Lane R, Guz A. The measurement of breathlessness induced in normal subjects: validity of two scaling techniques. Clin Sci 1985; 69:7–16.

2. American Medical Association. The respiratory system. In: Guides to the Evaluation of Permanent Impairment, 2nd ed. Chicago, 1984, 85–101.
3. Anthonisen NR, Wright EC, Hidgin JE, IPPB Trial Group. Prognosis in chronic obstructive pulmonary disease. Am Rev Respir Dis 1986; 133:14–20.
4. Anthonisen NR, Wright EC, IPPB Trial Group. Bronchodilator response in chronic obstructive pulmonary disease. Am Rev Respir Dis 1986; 133:814–820.
5. Ashutosh K, Gilbert R, Auchincloss JH, Peppi D. Asynchronous breathing movement in patients with chronic obstructive pulmonary disease. Chest 1975; 67:553–557.
6. Ault M, Robin EM. Platypnea (diffuse zone I phenomenon). N Engl J Med 1969; 281:1347–1348.
7. Becklake MR. State of the art. Asbestos-related diseases of the lung and other organs: their epidemiology and implications for clinical practice. Am Rev Respir Dis 1976; 114:187–227.
8. Bellemare F, Grassino A. Evaluation of human diaphragm fatigue. J Appl Physiol 1982; 53:1196–1206.
9. Berquist WE, Rachelefsky GS, Kadden M, et al. Effect of theophylline on gastroesophageal reflux in normal adults. J Allergy Clin Immunol 1981; 67:407–411.
10. Bohadana AB, Peslin R, Uffholtz H. Breath sounds in the clinical assessment of airflow obstruction. Thorax 1978; 33:345–351.
11. Borg G. Psychophysical bases of perceived exertion. Med Sci Sports Exerc 1982; 14:377–381.
12. Bradley CA, Fleetham JA, Anthonisen NR. Ventilatory control in patients with hypoxemia due to obstructive lung disease. Am Rev Respir Dis 1979; 120:21–30.
13. Burns BH, Howell JB. Disproportional severe breathlessness in chronic bronchitis. QJ Med 1969; 38:277–294.
14. Burrows B, Niden AH, Barclay WR, Kasik JE. Chronic obstructive lung disease. II. Relationship of clinical and physiologic findings to the severity of airways obstruction. Am Rev Respir Dis 1965; 91:665–678.
15. Campbell EJM, Freedman S, Smith PS, Taylor ME. The ability of man to detect added elastic loads to breathing. Clin Sci 1961; 20:223–231.
16. Churg A, Wright JL, Wiggs B, et al. Small airways disease and mineral dust exposure: prevalence, structure and function. Am Rev Respir Dis 1985; 131:139–143.
17. Cohen AC, Zagelbaum G, Gross D, et al. Clinical manifestations of inspiratory muscle fatigue. Am J Med 1982; 73:308–316.
18. David P, Denis P, Nouvet G, et al. Lung function and gastroesophageal reflux during chronic bronchitis. Bull Eur Physiopathol Respir 1982; 18:81–86.
19. Dennish GW, Castell DO. Inhibitory effect of smoking on the lower esophageal sphincter. N Engl J Med 1971; 284:1136–1137.
20. Dines DE, Clagett OT, Payne WS. Spontaneous pneumothorax in emphysema. Proc Mayo Clin 1970; 45:481–487.
21. Douglas NJ. Asthma at night. Clin Chest Med 1985; 6:663–674.
22. Fishman AP. State of the art. Chronic cor pulmonale. Am Rev Respir Dis 1976; 114:775–794.
23. Flenley DC. Sleep in chronic obstructive lung disease. Clin Chest Med 1985; 6:652–661.
24. Foster LJ, Trudeau WL, Goldman AL. Bronchodilator effects on gastric acid secretion. JAMA 1979; 241:2613–2615.
25. Fraser RG, Pare PJA. Diagnosis of Diseases of the Chest, 2nd ed. Vol III. Philadelphia: WB Saunders, 1979, 1770–1776.
26. Gaensler EA, Lindgren I. Symposium on emphysema and the "chronic bronchitis" syndrome. Chronic bronchitis as an etiologic factor in obstructive emphysema. Preliminary report. Am Rev Respir Dis 1959; 80:185–193.
27. Gandevia SC, Killian KJ, Campbell EJM. The effect of respiratory muscle fatigue on respiratory sensation. Clin Sci 1981; 60:463–466.
28. Goodwin JF. The clinical diagnosis of pulmonary thromboembolism. In: Sasahara AA, Stein M, eds. Pulmonary Embolic Disease. New York: Grune and Stratton, 1965, 239–255.
29. Grant I, Heaton RK, McSweeny JA, et al. Neuropsychologic findings in hypoxemic chronic obstructive pulmonary disease. Arch Intern Med 1982; 142:1470–1476.
30. Guilleminault C, Cummiskey J, Motta J. Chronic obstructive air flow disease and sleep studies. Am Rev Respir Dis 1980; 122:397–406.
31. Guliner MM. The hyperlucent lung; a problem in differential diagnosis. Dis Chest 1966; 49:578.
32. Haynes WF Jr, Krstulovic VJ, Bell ALL Jr. Smoking habit and incidence of respiratory infections in a group of adolescent males. Am Rev Respir Dis 1966; 93:730–735.
33. Heath D, Brewer D, Hicken P. Cor Pulmonale in Emphysema. Springfield, Ill: Charles C Thomas, 1968, 1.
34. Hill NS. The cardiac exam in lung disease. Clin Chest Med 1987; 8:273–285.
35. Hogg JC, Macklem PT, Thurlbeck WM. Site and nature of airway obstruction in chronic obstructive lung disease. N Engl J Med 1968; 278:1355–1360.
36. Hoover CF. Diagnostic significance of inspiratory movements of costal margins. Am J Med Sci 1920; 159:633.
37. Hudson LD, Kurt TL, Petty TL, Geuton E. Arrhythmias associated with acute respiratory failure in patients with chronic airway obstruction. Chest 1973; 63:661–665.
38. Johnston RN, Lockhart W, Ritchie RT, Smith DH. Haemoptysis. Br Med J 1960; 1:592–595.
39. Jones NL, Jones G, Edwards RHT. Exercise tolerance in chronic airway obstruction. Am Rev Respir Dis 1971; 103:477–491.
40. Killian KJ, Campbell EJM. Dyspnea and exercise. Annu Rev Physiol 1983; 45:465–479.
41. Kleiger RE, Senior RM. Long-term electrocardiographic monitoring of ambulatory patients with chronic airway obstruction. Chest 1974; 65:483–487.
42. Lal S, Ferguson AD, Campbell EJM. Forced expiratory time: a simple test for airways obstruction. Br Med J 1964; 1:814–817.
43. Larsson C. Natural history and life expectancy in severe alpha-1-antitrypsin deficiency PiZ. Acta Med Scand 1978; 204:345–351.
44. Leading article. Prevention of pulmonary embolism. Br Med J 1973; 2:1–2.
45. Levison H, Cherniack RM. Ventilatory cost of exercise in chronic obstructive pulmonary disease. J Appl Physiol 1968; 25:21–27.
46. Loudon R, Murphy RLH Jr. State of the art. Lung sounds. Am Rev Respir Dis 1984; 130:663–673.
47. Loudon RG. Smoking and cough frequency. Am Rev Respir Dis 1976; 114:1033–1036.
48. Loveridge B, West P, Kryger MH, Anthonisen NR. Alteration in breathing pattern with progression of chronic obstructive pulmonary disease. Am Rev Respir Dis 1986; 134:930–934.
49. Mahler DA. Dyspnea: Diagnosis and management. Clin Chest Med 1987; 8:215–230.
50. Mahler DA, Weinberg DH, Well CK, Freistein AR. The measurement of dyspnea: contents, interobserver agreement, and physiologic correlates of two new clinical indexes. Chest 1984; 85:751–758.
51. Marini JJ, Pierson DJ, Hudson LD, Lakshminaranyan S. The significance of wheezing in chronic airflow obstruction. Am Rev Respir Dis 1979; 120:1069–1072.
52. Marshall R. Relationship between stimulus and work of breathing at different lung volumes. J Appl Physiol 1962; 17:917–921.
53. McFadden ER, Kiser R, Degroot WJ. Acute bronchial asthma: Clinical and physiologic relations. N Engl J Med 1973; 288:221.
54. McGavin CR, Artvinli M, Naoe H, McHardy GJR. Dyspnoea, disability and distance walked: comparison of estimates of exercise performance in respiratory disease. Br Med J 1978; 2:241–243.
55. Mead J. Functional significance of the area of apposition of diaphragm to rib cage. Am Rev Respir Dis 1979; 119(No 2, Part 2, Suppl):31–39.
56. Nair JR, Turner-Warwick M. Breath sounds in emphysema. Br J Dis Chest 1969; 63:29–37.
57. Nath AR, Capel LH. Inspiratory crackles. Early and late. Thorax 1974; 29:223–227.
58. Nath AR, Capel LH. Inspiratory crackles and mechanical events of breathing. Thorax 1974; 29:695–698.
59. Oliven A, Cherniack NS, Deal EC, Kelsen SG. The effects of acute bronchoconstriction on respiratory activity in patients with chronic obstructive pulmonary disease. Am Rev Respir Dis 1985; 131:236–241.
60. Openbrier DR, Irwin MM, Rogers RM, et al. Nutritional status and lung function in patients with emphysema and chronic bronchitis. Chest 1983; 83:17–22.
61. Openbrier DR, Irwin MM, Dauber JH, et al. Factors affecting nutritional status and the impact of nutritional support in patients with emphysema. Chest 1984; 85(Suppl):67S–69S.
62. Pardee NE, Martin CJ, Morgan EH. A test of the practical value of estimating breath sound intensity. Chest 1976; 70:341–344.
63. Pode G, Stradling P. Routine radiography for haemoptysis. Br Med J 1964; 1:341–342.

64. Raffin TA, Theodore J. Separating cardiac from pulmonary dyspnea. JAMA 1977; 238:2066–2067.
65. Reid L. Measurement of the bronchial mucous gland layer: a diagnostic yardstick in chronic bronchitis. Thorax 1960; 15:132.
66. Reid L. The Pathology of Emphysema. Chicago: Year Book Medical Publishers, 1967.
67. Robertson AJ. Green sputum. Lancet 1952; i:12–15.
68. Roussos C. Function and fatigue of respiratory muscles. Chest 1985; 88(Suppl):124S–132S.
69. Schacter EN, Maunder LR, Beck GJ. The pattern of lung function abnormalities in cotton textile workers. Am Rev Respir Dis 1984; 129:523–527.
70. Schneider IC, Anderson AE. Correlation of clinical signs with ventilatory function in obstructive lung disease. Ann Intern Med 1965; 62:477–485.
71. Stark FD, Gambles SA, Lewis JA. Methods to assess breathlessness in healthy subjects: a critical evaluation and application to analyze the acute effects of diazepam and promethazine on breathlessness induced by exercise or by exposure to raised levels of carbon dioxide. Clin Sci 1981; 61:429–439.
72. Sukumalchantra Y, Williams MH Jr. Serial studies on pulmonary function in patients with chronic obstructive pulmonary disease. Am J Med 1965; 39:941–945.
73. Timms RM. Sexual dysfunction and chronic obstructive disease. Chest 1982; 81:398–399.
74. U.S. Public Health Service. The health consequences of smoking. Washington, DC: U.S. Department of HEW, DHEW Publication (CDC) 74-8704, 1974.
75. Vandenbergh E, Van de Woestijne KP, Gyselen A. Weight changes in the terminal stages of chronic obstructive pulmonary disease. Am Rev Respir Dis 1967; 95:556–566.
76. Watabe T, Ozaki K, Suzuki S. Peptic ulcer in pulmonary emphysema. Intern Med Pediatr 1961; 16:1149.
77. Williams TJ, Ahmad D, Morgan WKC. A clinical and roentgenographic correlation of diaphragmatic movement. Arch Intern Med 1981; 141:878–880.
78. Zasly L, Baum GL, Rumball JM. The incidence of peptic ulceration in chronic obstructive pulmonary emphysema. A statistical study. Dis Chest 1960; 37:400.
79. Ziegenspeck D, Sundermann A, Roth W. Das Korpergewicht beim Lungenemphysem (ein Klinishstatistishe Studie). Allerg Immunol 1963; 9:233–242.

Chapter 39

PULMONARY FUNCTION TESTS FOR DIAGNOSIS AND EVALUATION OF COPD

Frederic G. Hoppin, Jr.

Other chapters in this book and reviews[44] have dealt extensively with the nature of the abnormalities of ventilation and gas exchange characteristic of chronic obstructive pulmonary disease (COPD). This chapter addresses similar issues but from a different standpoint: how can such abnormalities be measured? What is worthwhile measuring?

For the purposes of this chapter, pulmonary function tests (PFTs) are those that evaluate the exchange of gas between atmosphere and blood. Figure 39–1 sets a framework for considering how PFTs can evaluate the multiple interactive pathophysiologic processes of COPD. The primary pathologic damage is to the airway wall in chronic bronchitis and to the alveolar structures in emphysema, although most commonly both pathologic processes are present. Various functional abnormalities ensue. Pathologic changes in the airways narrow them, and this limits and redistributes ventilation. Loss of alveolar structures disrupts the integrity of the tensile structure of the lung, and this leads to redistribution of ventilation, enlargement and distortion of the airspaces, and, again, narrowing of the airways. The narrowing of airways markedly reduces the maximal expiratory flow and, primarily because expiratory flow limitation is volume-dependent, breathing occurs at higher lung volumes at which the inspiratory muscles are less effective. The loss of alveolar structures also compromises the pulmonary vasculature, and this leads to an increase of pulmonary vascular resistance (PVR), impairment of diffusive transport of respiratory gases, and redistribution (maldistribution) of blood flow. These functional abnormalities combine to impair and limit ventilation, gas exchange, and cardiac output: ventilation because of the expiratory flow limitation and less effective inspiratory muscles; gas exchange because of the increased diffusion distances, the reduced vascular bed, and the nonuniformity of ventilation and perfusion; and cardiac output because of the increased afterload to the right side of the heart. The end results are respiratory acidosis, hypoxemia, and limitation of gas transport.

Pulmonary function tests can characterize many of these functional abnormalities, as indicated in Figure 39–1. The most widely used tests (Table 39–1) will be surveyed next with some attention to their functional significance, specificity, sensitivity, and practicality of performance. Detailed descriptions of the tests are available.[3]

TESTS OF LUNG AND CHEST WALL MECHANICS

VENTILATION. The rate of bulk transport of gas in the respiratory system can be measured by a timed collection of

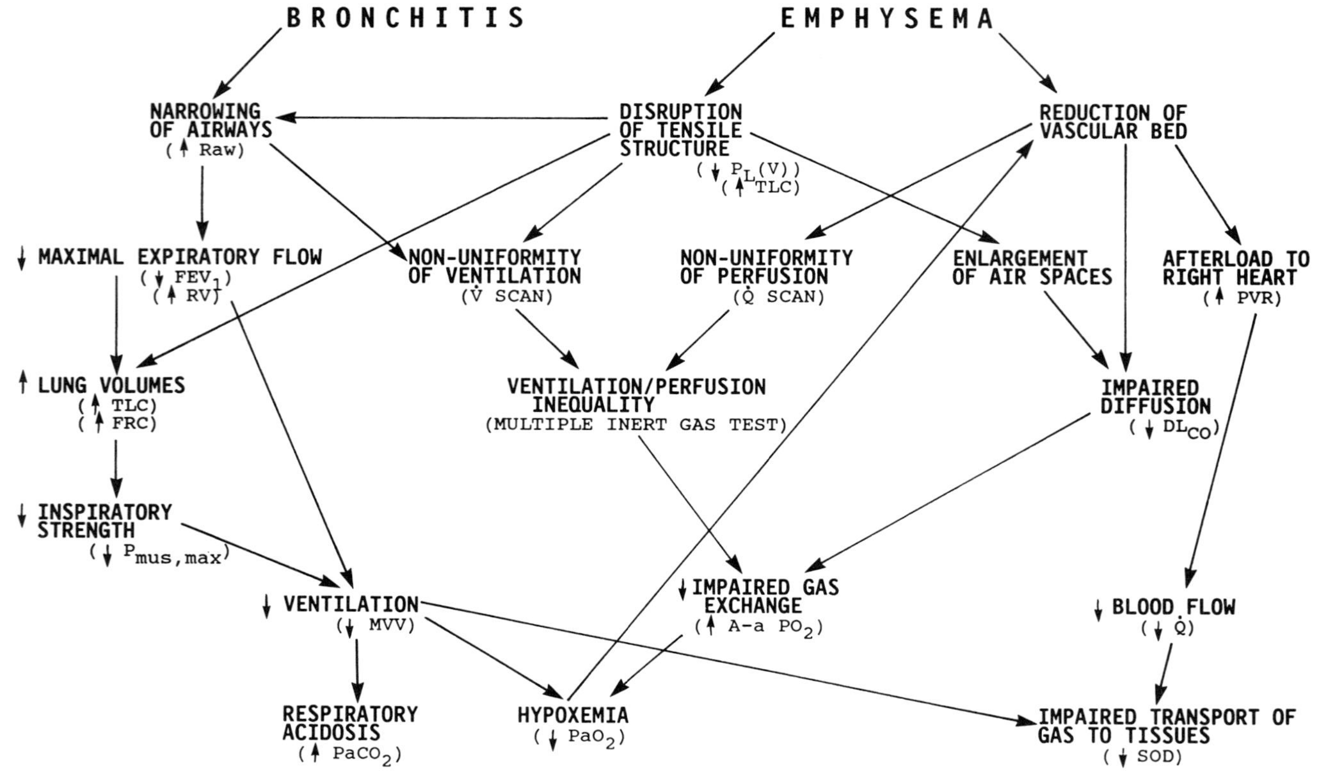

Figure 39–1. The pathophysiologic mechanisms in COPD in which primary damage to the alveolar septa and airways leads to impaired oxygen delivery and acidosis. Some common PFTs of use in evaluating these mechanisms are indicated in parentheses.

expired gas or summation of the excursions of a spirometric tracing. At rest, it is reported as the *minute ventilation* ($\dot{V}_E$). Its upper limit, the *maximal voluntary ventilation* (MVV), is evaluated while the subject breathes as hard and fast as possible, usually for 12 or 15 seconds. These measurements require a mouthpiece and are often done with a noseclip in place. They are usually well tolerated, although occasionally the MVV maneuver may itself induce bronchospasm.

TABLE 39–1. Pulmonary Function Tests

VENTILATION	**MUSCLE STRENGTH**
$\dot{V}_E$	$P_{mus,max}$
MVV	**SMALL AIRWAYS FUNCTION**
LUNG VOLUME	ΔSBNT
TLC	Frequency-dependence of compliance
RV	CV
FRC	$\Delta\dot{V}_{max50}$
VC	VisoV
LUNG TENSIONS	**GAS EXCHANGE AND TRANSPORT**
V/P curve	Pa_{O_2}
$P_{L,max}$	Pa_{CO_2}
$P_{L,\ max/TLC}$	$\dot{V}_A$
$C_{st,\ L}$	$V_{D,phys}/V_T$
K	Sa_{O_2}
AIRWAYS RESISTANCE	Ca_{O_2}
R_{aw}, G_{aw}	$\dot{Q}$
SR_{aw}, SG_{aw}	SOD
EXPIRATORY FLOW LIMITATION	A-aDO_2
FEV_1	DL_{CO}
FVC	$\dot{Q}_S/\dot{Q}_T$
FEF_{50}, FEF_{75}	$\dot{V}$ Scintigraphy
$FEF_{25\text{-}75}$	$\dot{Q}$ Scintigraphy
PEF	Multiple inert gas excretion and retention
$\dot{V}$/V curve	

Although resting $\dot{V}_E$ might be expected to be a useful parameter because it is a main determinant of baseline CO_2 retention and hypoxemia, interpretation of the test is limited by variabilities of behavior ("put this in your mouth and this on your nose and now (try to!) breathe naturally"), gas exchange efficiency, and metabolic load. By contrast, the MVV does not depend on those variables and gives relatively reproducible values. Its use differs from that of $\dot{V}_E$. MVV does not directly assess the baseline state, but rather probes the functional reserves of ventilation. The maneuver calls on multiple components of the ventilatory apparatus, i.e., the central nervous system, peripheral nerves, neuromuscular junction, inspiratory muscles, chest wall, lung distensibility, and airways. For this reason, MVV is a broad test; a good performance documents substantial reserves of each of these functions. Conversely, MVV is nonspecific; more discriminating tests are necessary to sort out the specific underlying abnormalities.

LUNG VOLUMES. There are three good techniques for determining the volume of gas in the lung (V_L). The most common is indicator dilution. The subject breathes through a mouthpiece on a closed spirometer circuit containing a known initial volume of a gas mixture containing helium. Initial and equilibration (about 7 minutes) helium concentrations are used to calculate the additional volume into which the helium has been diluted. As helium is inert and insoluble, this additional volume is that of the communicating airspaces. Alternatively, V_L can be measured by body plethysmography. The subject sits in a closed box (plethysmograph) for several minutes until the plethysmograph's gas temperature is equilibrated, and then the subject makes gentle inspiratory and expiratory efforts against a closed mouthpiece. The gas pressures within the box and at the mouth are measured. On the basis of Boyle's law, which relates the pressure and volume of a fixed quantity of gas under isothermal conditions, the volume of gas undergoing compression and decompression is calculated. The least-used alternative is analysis of chest posteroanterior (PA) and lateral radiographs taken at full inflation. Dimensions of the lung's profiles are measured, and V_L is then computed by one of several algorithms.[5, 25] Most patients carry out the helium dilution maneuvers with ease. Occasional patients find the body plethysmograph confining. For valid radiography, it is important to pay more attention to the full inspiratory effort than is routinely achieved.

These three methods in healthy subjects give very similar results, generally within about 5% of each other.[6] In disease, however, they may differ systematically. V_L by helium dilution, in particular, does not include poorly communicating volumes such as emphysematous bullae unless the test is substantially prolonged. V_L by body plethysmography, by contrast, includes all the gas undergoing compression. Body plethysmography actually may overestimate V_L in obstructive lung disease, probably because there are poorly communicating regions that undergo greater pressure cycles than the rest of the lung. This has been thought to account for overestimation of V_L by plethysmography in some patients with airway obstruction.[7] The test is then frequency-dependent, with marked increases in values for total lung capacity (TLC) when panting frequency is increased.[8] It is appropriate, therefore, to standardize panting frequency at about 1 cycle per second.

Very important information is gained from V_L at the limits of maximal inspiration (*total lung capacity,* TLC) and maximal expiration (*residual volume,* RV). V_L is first measured by one of the aforementioned techniques, usually at resting end-expiration (*functional residual capacity,* FRC), and then spirometry is performed so that TLC and RV can be calculated by reference to the measured V_L. A typical spirometric tracing is shown in Figure 39–2. Most patients can perform such maneuvers with adequate reproducibility. If the two steps (spirometry and measurement of absolute V_L) are not performed in direct juxtaposition, the reference volumes in the two steps could differ, introducing an error in the calculated TLC and RV[50]. Total lung capacity and RV are inherently stable; repeated careful measurements may vary by only 100 to 200 ml.[33] On the other hand, FRC is potentially performance-dependent, if the subject does not reliably relax the muscles of respiration.

Values of TLC and RV give relatively specific information about essential structural and functional changes of COPD.

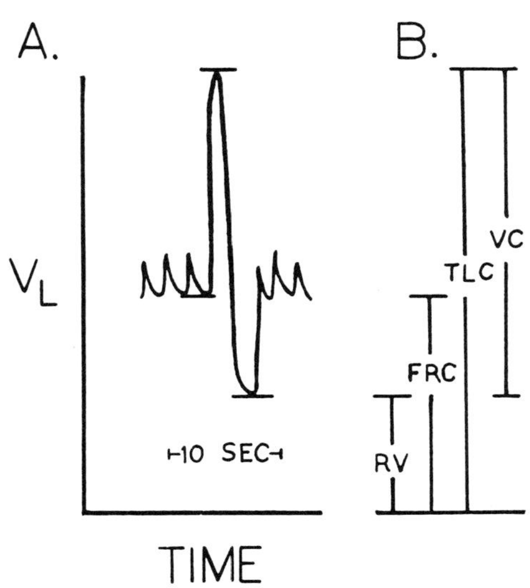

Figure 39–2. ***A,*** **Spirogram showing volume of gas displaced in and out of the mouth against time during quiet breathing, followed by inspiration to TLC, expiration to RV, and resumption of quiet breathing.** ***B,*** **Arrows indicate VC and the absolute V_L at TLC, RV, and FRC. Information in addition to that on the spirogram is needed for obtaining the absolute V_L, e.g., FRC by helium dilution.**

To understand their significance, it is important to know the mechanisms that determine them. Total lung capacity depends on two factors: the integrity of the tension-bearing structures of the lung parenchyma and the effectiveness of the inspiratory muscles. The first of these is directly compromised in emphysema, and, because the lung then can be readily stretched to a higher volume, TLC is increased. The only other recognized cause of a high TLC is asthma during the growing years (possibly a consequence of increased lung growth induced by the unusual persistent distending forces to which they were submitted[23]). The second factor, muscle strength, perhaps surprisingly, does not appear to be a primary cause of abnormally high TLCs; the muscles of inspiration, like other skeletal muscles, can be trained to substantially greater strength, but the TLC is very little increased,[33] perhaps because their operating range of lengths is not changed by strength training. This is not to say that there are not substantial secondary adaptations in the inspiratory muscles in COPD. Indeed, many patients with COPD breathe at V_L far greater than those where their inspiratory muscles would have been able to function prior to developing COPD; it appears that some length adaptation must have taken place.

The determinants of RV in healthy young individuals are analogous to those of TLC, namely strengths of the muscles of expiration and of the opposing forces passively developed in the chest wall. By middle age, however, maximal expiratory flows have fallen somewhat; the subject can no longer breathe down to a statically determined RV, but instead wheezes, with ever-diminishing expiratory flows, down to a slightly higher, dynamically determined RV.[34] In COPD, the fall of maximal expiratory flows is greatly exaggerated and RV is correspondingly increased; this may be a relatively early sign of the development of COPD.

Functional residual capacity is generally less directly informative than are TLC and RV. Functional residual capacity ordinarily represents the resting position of the respiratory system, in which the inspiratory pull of the relaxed chest wall equals the expiratory pull of the lung. Functional residual capacity is therefore predictably but modestly changed by changes in the volume/pressure characteristics of either lung or chest wall: e.g., FRC is somewhat increased by the loss of lung tensions in emphysema. A more important mechanism, however, takes over when expiratory flow limitation is severe. Functional residual capacity then is dynamically determined; expiration is so impeded that it is interrupted by the next inspiration before the static resting position is reached. Substantial increases in FRC may follow, and they are significant on two main grounds. First, they indicate severe reduction of maximal flow. Second, they indicate that the subject is breathing at lung volumes at which the inspiratory muscles may have diminished effectiveness and that any increase of ventilation will require further increase in V_L.

The *vital capacity* (VC) is defined as the maximal volume of gas expired from a point of maximal inspiration; it is the difference between TLC and RV and is easily obtained by spirometry (Fig. 39–2). Among the disadvantages of this parameter, any parallel changes of TLC and RV are missed, e.g., emphysema could substantially increase both TLC and RV, and, if the changes were equal, the VC would be unchanged. Furthermore, as VC does not contain direct information about absolute V_L, it cannot specify pathologic processes; decreased VC, for example, could result from either an increase of RV or a decrease in TLC, changes that reflect very different pathophysiologic processes. On the other hand, VC has the major advantage of great reproducibility (because of the inherent stability of TLC and RV) and simplicity of measurement. Vital capacity, then, may be sensitive in an individual to changes in airway obstruction (i.e., primarily in RV) due to bronchospasm or congestive heart failure.

LUNG TENSIONS. Lung tensions can be directly assessed from esophageal pressure. A thin-walled latex balloon on the end of a light polyethylene catheter is passed per nares with or without topical anesthesia. The difference between the pressure at the mouth and that in the esophagus is taken as the *transpulmonary pressure* (P_L), representing the sum of the volume-dependent *elastic recoil of the lung* ($P_{el,L}$) and the flow-dependent *resistive pressure drop* along the airways ($P_{res,aw}$). When measurements are taken statically, $P_{res,aw}$ is eliminated; thus $P_{el,L}$ is obtained by recording P_L, with the airway occluded at various (static) lung volumes or with the subject expiring against an airway with a leak controlled to allow slow (pseudo-static) expiration. The resulting static *volume/pressure relationship* (V/P curve) for the lung is illustrated in Figure 39–3 *A*. Ideally a full description of the V/P curve would include its position, slope, and curvature. Parameters currently in use, however, give only partial information; they include the *maximal transpulmonary pressure at TLC* ($P_{L,max}$), the *coefficient of retraction,* which is the $P_{L,max}$ divided by TLC, the *static compliance* ($C_{st,L}$), which is the slope of the linear portion of the V/P curve above FRC, and the *shape factor* (K), which is obtained by fitting the V/P curve to the function $V = A - Be^{-KP}$, where A and B are constants.[22]

The static V/P curve is a highly specific test. The elastic recoil of the lung reflects the tensions in the lung's elastic force-bearing structures, primarily the fibrous collagen, elastin, and the air-liquid alveolar interface. In emphysema there is loss of both tissue and interface, and the recoil, therefore, is reduced at any given V_L (compare dashed and continuous curves in Figure 39–3*A*). This displaces the V/P curve to the left, increases its slope (C_L), permits TLC to be somewhat higher, and raises the intersection with the V_L axis. Because the inspiratory muscles are less effective at the increased TLC, $P_{L,max}$ is decreased. The coefficient of retraction is decreased both because of the decrease in $P_{L,max}$ and the increase in TLC. The configuration of the curve, perhaps because of relative reduction of elastin, is relatively more convex to the volume axis, and the shape factor K is increased.[12, 22] Despite the specificity of the V/P curve and its various parameters, its utility is limited in clinical practice because the procedure entails mild discomfort, and the necessary maneuvers are difficult to perform reliably.

AIRWAYS RESISTANCE. The pressure cost of moving air through the airways can be readily measured with the body plethysmograph. The subject first pants gently against a mouthpiece with the shutter closed to establish the relationship of changes of alveolar gas pressure to changes of plethysmographic gas pressure. The shutter is then opened to permit airflow as the subject continues to pant gently. The changes of alveolar gas pressure during panting are now inferred from the changes of plethysmographic pressure, and flow is measured with a pneumotachograph. *Airways resistance* (R_{aw}) is the ratio of the alveolar pressure to flow. Its reciprocal is *airways conductance* (G_{aw}). To suppress the systematic effects of lung volume, R_{aw} is commonly multiplied by V_L and is reported as the *specific airways resistance* (SR_{aw}) and its reciprocal as *specific airways conductance* (SG_{aw}).

The major determinant of R_{aw} is airway diameter. R_{aw}, then,

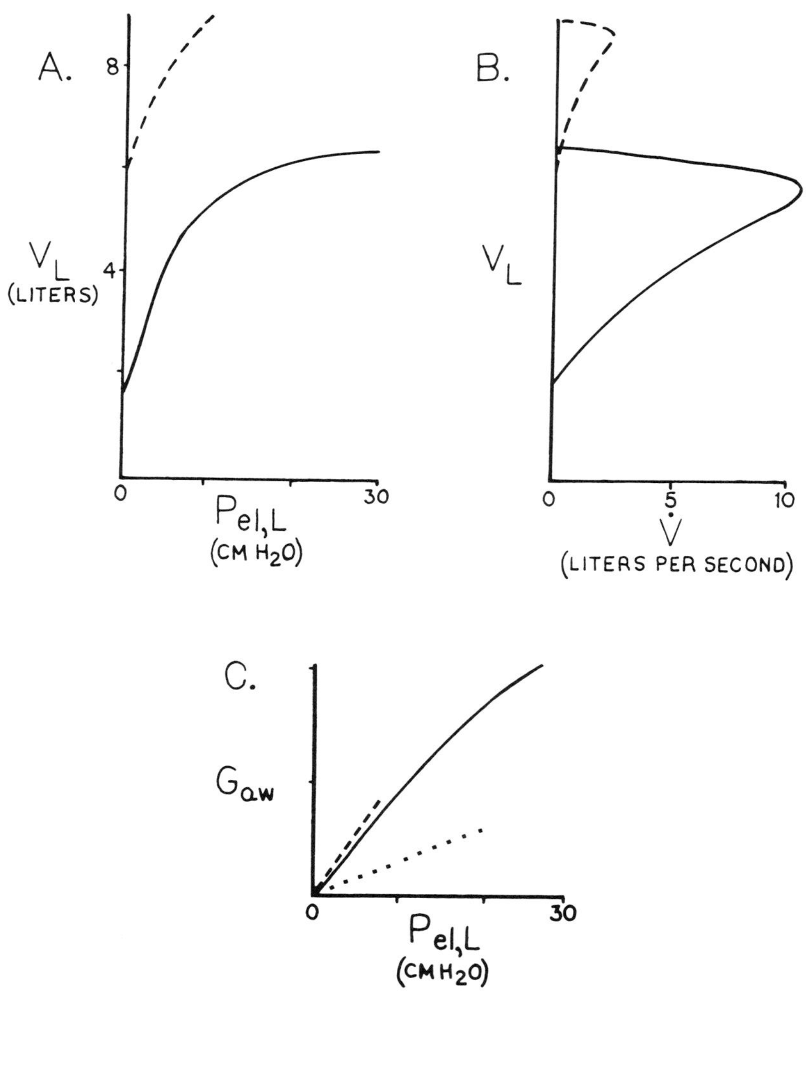

Figure 39–3. *A,* **Idealized static volume/pressure curves for the lung: normal (continuous line) and emphysema (dotted line). Note in emphysema the reduction of the elastic recoil at all lung volumes. The maximal pressure attainable (at TLC) is less because of the lesser pressures that can be developed by the inspiratory muscles.** *B,* **Corresponding maximal expiratory flow/volume curves. TLC and RV are higher because of the reduced elastic recoil of the lung.** *C,* **Corresponding plots of airway conductance versus static lung recoil. In the emphysematous patient (dashed line), conductance is reduced as a result of the reduction of elastic recoil, and the relationship is the same as in the normal (continuous line). By contrast, in chronic bronchitis (dotted line), intrinsic changes in the airways decrease the conductance at any given elastic recoil.**

may be increased in COPD due to retained secretions, mucosal hyperplasia, smooth muscle hypertrophy or constriction, or reduction of elastic recoil. To some degree, the two factors can be sorted out. In some patients with a predominance of emphysema, airway conductance can be shown to be reduced in proportion to elastic recoil (dashed curve in Figure 39–3*C*). With bronchitis, however, the narrowing is greater than can be explained by the reduction in elastic recoil alone, and G_{aw} is lowered at a given elastic recoil (dotted curve in Figure 39–3*C*).[32]

There are two main limitations to this test. First, R_{aw} is substantially variable (e.g., within individual coefficient of variation of 15% to 25%), probably largely because of involuntary changes in the configuration of the upper airway, particularly in the glottal aperture.[13] Second, R_{aw} may be relatively insensitive to changes in the peripheral airways in early chronic bronchitis; increases in the pressure drop along the peripheral airways may not be discernible, because they are only part of the total pressure drop being measured and therefore the change in total R_{aw} is small. Despite these limitations, R_{aw} retains two advantages over the standard tests of forced expiration. It is obtained at ordinary V_L, at which most breathing takes place, and it avoids the constricting or dilating effects on the airways that can result from inspiration to TLC.[35]

EXPIRATORY FLOW LIMITATION. "COPD is defined as a disorder characterized by abnormal tests of expiratory flow. . . ."[1] This is demonstrated by the forced vital capacity (FVC) maneuver, in which the subject inspires to TLC and then breathes out as hard, fast, and fully as possible into a spirometer. Typical tracings of volume against time and of volume against flow are given in Figures 39–4 and 39–3*B*. Most patients can perform these maneuvers with ease and reproducibility, although occasionally bronchospasm is induced.

Although FVC maneuvers have been jokingly called "unnatural acts" because they are probably never performed in daily living, they are invaluable in evaluating the abnormal flow limitation that is central to the dysfunction and disability of obstructive lung disease. Various parameters of the FVC can be obtained directly from the timed tracing, as indicated in Figure 39–4. The most common are the *volume expired in the first second* (FEV_1), the volume of the *forced vital capacity* itself (FVC), the *forced expiratory flows* at various fractions of FVC (e.g., FEF_{50}, FEF_{75}), the mean *flow over the middle of the FVC* (FEF_{25-75}), formerly called the *maximal midexpiratory flow rate* (MMEFR), and *peak expiratory flow* (PEF). The *flow-volume plot* ($\dot{V}$/V) (Fig. 39–3*B*), although it contains exactly the same information as the volume-time plot, has additional conceptual merit because it directly depicts flow, which is physiologically the dependent variable of volume. It is also more readily superimposed for purposes of comparison and may reveal configurations of significance.

The several parameters of the FVC have distinct merits. Peak expiratory flow has a degree of variability because peak flow occurs on the effort-dependent portion of the forced expiration. Nonetheless, this parameter is particularly useful for ambulatory use because it is so readily obtained with a hand-held device (the Wright peak flow meter). Important circadian patterns of flow-limitation and fluctuations over longer periods have been clearly and readily followed with this device used by the patient at home.

Forced expiratory volume in one second is the standard parameter for assessing flow limitation. Its merits include the ease of registering it reliably with a range (mechanical, graphic, electronic) of devices and its high reproducibility. Most important, it captures the portion of the curve that applies when breathing is severely stressed, namely near-maximal ventilatory efforts at 30 or more breaths per minute.

It is often useful to normalize the FEV_1 to the FVC by taking the ratio FEV_1/FVC; in the presence of processes other than obstructive (e.g., neuromuscular dysfunction or fibrotic lung disease), the FEV_1 and FVC are generally reduced proportionately, maintaining a normal FEV_1/FVC, whereas in obstructive lung disease, whether alone or in addition to restrictive disease, the FEV_1 is usually reduced proportionately more than is the FVC, and the FEV_1/FVC is therefore reduced.

Other frequently used parameters are FEF_{25-75} and FEF_{75}. They are of interest because they reflect changes in flow limitation at lower V_L, a region which is not well reflected by the FEV_1, particularly in the presence of modest obstruction.[24]

The functional significance of expiratory flow limitation in the COPD patient comes from two cardinal features. First, maximal flow is virtually *effort-independent* above a relatively modest expiratory effort; this has the effect of setting an absolute limit to ventilation. Second, maximal flow is strongly *volume-dependent,* as is emphasized on the $\dot{V}$/V plot (Fig. 39–3*B*); this is important because of its effect on operating lung volumes. Because of these two features, when the flow limit is sufficiently low there are only two recourses for maintaining or increasing ventilation: (1) increasing the time of expiration relative to that of inspiration, and (2) increasing V_L. Both are characteristic of COPD and can be readily noted in patients with moderate obstruction by watching them breathe. Most important, the failure of patients with COPD to maintain adequate ventilation results in large part from failure of these two adaptations to fully compensate for their flow limitation.

The detailed mechanism of expiratory flow limitation is

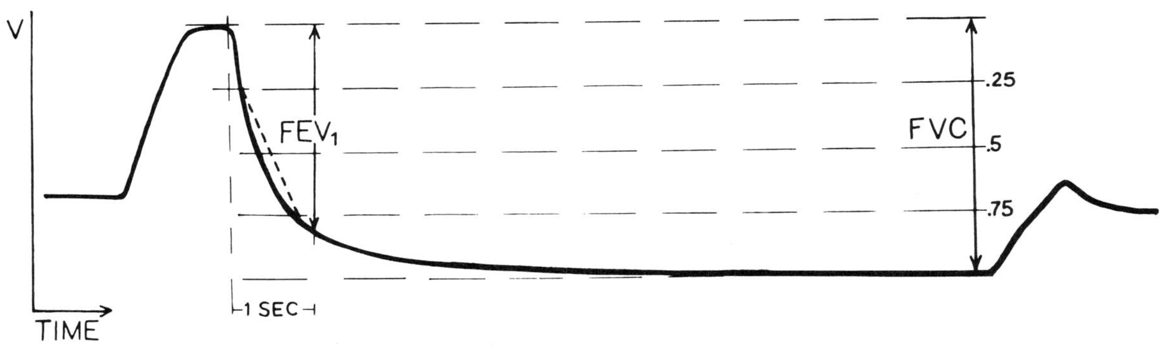

Figure 39–4. Spirogram showing inspiration to TLC, a forced expiratory vital capacity maneuver, and return to quiet breathing in a normal subject. The forced expired volume in the first second (FEV_1) is indicated, with the starting point determined by extrapolation.[3] The forced vital capacity (FVC) is indicated, and horizontal lines have been drawn to indicate the four quarters of the FVC. The flow at any point (e.g., FEF_{75}) is the slope of the tracing. Forced expiratory flow over the middle half of the FVC (FEF_{25-50}) is seen as the slope of the dashed line connecting the tracing at those two volumes.

beyond the scope of this chapter, but it is important to note the two primary functional changes that lower this limit in COPD—namely, lowered lung elastic recoil and narrowed airways. Under conditions of flow limitation, flow is absolutely dependent on elastic recoil; it is the elastic tension in the alveolar parenchyma that tethers the airways open and, to oversimplify somewhat, it is the elastic tension (not the expiratory effort) that drives airflow from the alveoli to the so-called choke points, the short airway segments where flow-limiting dynamic narrowing occurs. As a result, when elastic recoil at a given V_L is reduced in emphysema (Fig. 39–3*A*), maximal expiratory flow is also reduced at a given V_L (Fig. 39–3*B*). Indeed, maximal expiratory flow is volume-dependent *because* elastic recoil is volume-dependent.

Under conditions of flow limitation, flow depends not only on elastic recoil but also on the properties of the airways and is reduced in emphysema more than can be accounted for by the loss of elastic recoil alone.[32] With greater damage to the airways, maximal flows are reduced more than in patients without airway symptoms.[32]

Two additional mechanisms may reduce the flow limit and in particular change the configuration of the $\dot{V}/V$ curve. The first is the importance of the peripheral airways to the maximal flows at low V_L. With narrowing of these airways, there is a disproportionate effect on the flows at lower lung volumes, and this results in a characteristic convexity of the $\dot{V}/V$ curve toward the volume axis (dashed curve in Fig. 39–3*B*). The second is nonuniformity of expiration. Portions of the lung with less disease contribute substantial flow at the beginning of the forced expiration and, having deflated quickly, contribute relatively less flow during the remainder of expiration; the consequence, again, is convexity of the $\dot{V}/V$ curve.

Much effort has been expended to develop parameters of the FVC maneuver that discriminate dysfunction with better sensitivity. One approach is "size-correction," i.e., dividing flows by the FVC. Perhaps surprisingly, however, the variability of FEF_{50}/FVC is not much less than that of FEF_{50}.[24] Another approach is to choose parameters that are inherently keyed to the FVC, i.e., FEF_{25-75}, FEF_{75}, and FEV_1/FVC. Although this approach may increase discriminating ability,[28] the relationships are complex and warrant a thoroughly skeptical consideration. The definitions of these three FVC-keyed parameters are deceptively simple (the mean flow over the middle half of expired volume, the flow at three quarters expired volume, and the fraction expired in 1 second, respectively). Their interpretations, however, are complicated by changes of the FVC itself. An example of the problem that can arise is the subject who responds to a bronchodilator, increasing FEV_1, increasing flows at all absolute V_L, lowering RV, and increasing the FVC. These are all clearly favorable changes. Yet the increase of the FVC reduces the apparent improvement in all three FVC-keyed parameters and not infrequently actually decreases them, which then becomes a clearly misleading result.

Because the flow limit is volume dependent, it is tempting to compare flows at the same *absolute* V_L, as in Figures 39–3*B* and 39–4. However, even a small error in measuring absolute V_L would then introduce a substantial change in the flow that is not seen when flows are compared at the same fractions of the FVC. Furthermore, the variability of TLC and RV among normal subjects would introduce a large and unwanted variability in flow rates when evaluated at absolute, rather than FVC-keyed, volumes. The validity of FVC-keyed flows in discerning disease comes from the fact that the changes that occur in disease are generally not pure translations of the flow curve along the V_L axis but also involve distinct reductions of flow relative to the FVC itself. There are two main reasons for this. First, although TLC is increased in emphysema, as alluded to earlier, the lung recoil at TLC ($P_{L,max}$) is reduced. This is because the inspiratory muscles lose effectiveness with increasing V_L and only partially adapt to chronic operation at high V_L. As a result of the lower lung recoil, expiratory flow limits at all parts of the FVC are less. Second, small airways disease involvement and nonuniformity of expiration substantially change the configuration of the $\dot{V}/V$ curve.

There has been ongoing concern about what, at first glance, appears to be a technical problem in obtaining valid measurement of expiratory limits—namely, variable patient performance. To address this issue, the American Thoracic Society has set limits on reproducibility,[2] recommending that at least three maneuvers be performed and that the difference between the best and second best FEV_1 should be no greater than 5% or 100 ml. Ironically, failure of test reproducibility turns out to be almost as strong a predictor of mortality as is poor FEV_1 itself.[18] The possible explanations include induction of bronchospasm and inverse effort-dependence.[46] The latter deserves comment. Although the effort-independency of the FVC is very impressive when the volume is registered by body plethysmography, an inverse effort-dependence appears when volume is registered by that expired at the mouth (the most common procedure in PFT laboratories). This discrepancy occurs because the volume changes at the mouth do not account for the volume changes associated with thoracic gas compression. The stronger the expiratory effort, the more compression and the smaller the *actual* lung volume (and therefore elastic recoil) at a given *expired* volume; the effect is to lower the maximal flow at a given *expired* volume.[26] Making measurements by plethysmography would take care of the problem, but this is not nearly as practical as spirometry for routine use. In an effort to get around the problem of inverse effort-dependence, an alternative to the American Thoracic Society recommendations has been proposed. Based on the assumption (not well-established) that subjects will readily standardize their maximal expiratory efforts, it is suggested that subjects be instructed to expire with fullest effort and that, among several FVC efforts, the FEV_1 should be chosen from the FVC with the greatest PEF, because PEF is known to be positively effort-dependent.[31]

THE RESPIRATORY MUSCLES. The strength of the muscles of inspiration can be assessed as the difference of pressures recorded when the subject first relaxes and then makes a maximal inspiratory or expiratory effort ($P_{mus,max}$). The efforts are maintained for several seconds against a special mouthpiece designed to optimize the seal with the lips under high inspiratory or expiratory pressures. Such measurements are highly reproducible in trained subjects but require some coaching in the untrained. A more practical maneuver may be measurement of mouth pressure during a maximal inspiratory sniff.[30]

$P_{mus,max}$ is highly volume-dependent for two reasons: the classic length-dependency of force developed by the sarcomere, and the effect of configuration of the chest wall on the mechanical advantage of the inspiratory muscles. Thus at high V_L, inspiratory $P_{mus,max}$ is sharply reduced because the muscles are short and the configuration of the thorax is less favorable—the diaphragm becomes flatter. With the progressive increase of V_L in COPD, however, the inspiratory apparatus adapts. It is thought that, with persistent hyperinflation, the muscles of inspiration, as a result of operating chronically at short lengths, drop out some sarcomeres, allowing the remaining sarcomeres, being arranged in series, to operate again at more effective, longer lengths.[16, 19] This compensation, however, does not correct the loss of mechanical advantage at higher V_L, and the maximal transpulmonary pressure at TLC ($P_{L,max}$) is reduced (Fig. 39–3*A*). $P_{mus,max}$ is usually obtained at FRC. Marked reductions of $P_{mus,max}$ in COPD are usually associated with very high FRC and indicate decreased ventilatory reserve. They may also reflect loss of muscle mass and frank fatigue of the inspiratory muscles, which are often contributors to the disability and respiratory failure of COPD.

TESTS OF SMALL AIRWAYS

Small airways have been thought to be the sites of early changes in chronic bronchitis.[14] R_{aw} appears to be relatively insensitive to these changes, and more sensitive indices have been sought among the following:

- Abnormal indices of forced expiration. With small airway narrowing, *maximal expiratory flows* are reduced, particularly at low V_L where the properties of the small airways dominate the flow; the $\dot{V}/V$ curve, thus, shows a convexity to the flow axis, and FEF_{50}, FEF_{75}, and FEF_{25-75} are particularly reduced.
- Nonuniformity of ventilation. This can be expected with nonuniform changes in parallel peripheral airways. It can be qualitatively assessed by the pattern of nitrogen washout during a single expiration after a single inspiration of oxygen, i.e., the *single-breath nitrogen test* (SBNT). After the dead space gas is expired, the nitrogen concentration rises to an "alveolar plateau" (Phase III) on which the expired gas is thought to contain varying contributions from different regions and different depths in the lung. An increase in the slope of the nitrogen concentration (ΔSBNT) in Phase III is taken as indicating increased nonuniformity of ventilation.
- Effects of breathing frequency. The asynchrony of ventilation due to nonuniformity among small airways increases with increasing frequency of breathing, which in turn causes looping on a V/P plot and a decreased compliance between the no-flow points. *Frequency-dependence of compliance,* then, reflects nonuniformity and suggests small airways disease. This is a delicate measurement requiring an esophageal balloon and substantial cooperation of the subject.
- Airway closure. Some of the small airways close near the end of expiration, and this closure can be detected in the SBNT as a terminal rise in the nitrogen concentration (Phase IV). The volume above RV at which Phase IV starts is called the *closing volume* (CV); an elevated CV suggests premature closure of small airways.
- Density-dependence of forced expiratory flow. Sensitivity of maximal expiratory flow limits to changes of gas density suggests that the "choke points" (the sites of critical dynamic narrowing) are located in the central airways. In the early portions of the FVC, in which the choke points are known to be central, maximal expiratory flows are greater with a helium-oxygen mixture than with air. Later in expiration, however, the choke points migrate out to the peripheral small airways, the flows are no longer density-dependent, and the $\dot{V}/V$ curves with air and a helium-oxygen mixture can be superimposed. By this analysis it is thought that equalization of flows identifies the V_L at which the choke points migrate peripherally. This migration is thought to occur at higher V_L in small airways disease and is quantified by a reduced difference of the maximal flows at midvital capacity (ΔV_{max50}) and a higher volume below which maximal flows are equal for the two gases, the *volume of isoflow* (Viso$\dot{V}$). Reduced density-dependence, in the presence of a normal FEV_1, suggests small airway disease. In one epidemiologic study, density-dependence was more useful than FEF_{25-75}.[46]

TESTS OF GAS EXCHANGE AND TRANSPORT

Arterial blood gases (ABGs) refer to the *partial pressures of* O_2 (Pa_{O_2}) and CO_2 (Pa_{CO_2}) measured by electrodes on directly sampled arterial blood. Elevated Pa_{CO_2} and decreased Pa_{O_2} characterize respiratory failure and go far to assess the mechanisms that contribute to the failure.

CARBON DIOXIDE. The level of CO_2 depends on the *alveolar ventilation* ($\dot{V}_A$) (the effective rate at which the gas in the alveolar compartment is exchanged with fresh air) relative to metabolic CO_2 production. This relationship is formally expressed by the alveolar gas relationship for CO_2, which relates $\dot{V}_A$ to the rate of elimination of CO_2 ($\dot{V}_{CO_2}$) and the partial pressure of CO_2 in alveolar gas (PA_{CO_2}):

$$PA_{CO_2} \sim \dot{V}_{CO_2}/\dot{V}_A$$

$\dot{V}_A$ can be evaluated from this relationship by measuring the amount of CO_2 in expired gas collected over a measured interval ($\dot{V}_{CO_2}$) and the partial pressure of CO_2 in arterial blood (Pa_{CO_2}), which can be taken to be equivalent to the PA_{CO_2}. The absolute value of $\dot{V}_A$, however, is not as useful as is the Pa_{CO_2} itself; one usually foregoes collecting the expired gas and formally calculating $\dot{V}_A$ and instead simply uses the Pa_{CO_2} to answer the more tractable question of whether or not $\dot{V}_A$ is appropriate to the (unmeasured) $\dot{V}_{CO2}$, e.g., elevated Pa_{CO_2} is seen when $\dot{V}_A$ is inappropriately low for the subject's (metabolic) CO_2 production.

$\dot{V}_A$ may be impaired in COPD (and Pa_{CO_2} increased) for two reasons: reduced total ventilation ($\dot{V}_E$) and impairment of gas exchange. The reduced ventilation may be traceable to impaired lung and chest wall mechanics by the tests discussed earlier. The reduced efficiency of gas exchange also can be evaluated. A parameter of the effectiveness of ventilation is the *physiologic deadspace* ($V_{D,phys}$). This includes both the portion of total ventilation that is "wasted" in ventilating the anatomic deadspace volume and also the additional ventilation that goes to ventilate unperfused alveoli or, more generally, by nonuniformity of ventilation/perfusion ratios. $V_{D,phys}$ can be calculated from the tidal volume (V_T) and the partial pressures of CO_2 in the mixed expirate (PE_{CO_2}) and the arterial blood.

$$V_{D,\,phys} = V_T\,(1 - [PE_{CO_2}/Pa_{CO_2}])$$

This parameter is of conceptual value but is not much used for evaluation of the individual, perhaps because of the variability of the anatomic deadspace. The ratio of $V_{D,phys}$ to the V_T, however, is often calculated. Representing the fraction of ventilation that does not effectively ventilate gas-exchanging alveoli, it is increased not only with increased wasted ventilation (as with increased ventilation/perfusion inequality) but also with decreases of V_T, as seen in the shallow tachypnea of impending respiratory failure. $V_{D,phys}/V_T$, therefore, reflects the effectiveness of ventilation to gas exchange generally.

OXYGEN. Among the parameters of blood oxygenation and transport, the least invasively measured is arterial hemoglobin *saturation* (Sa_{O_2}), estimated by ear or finger pulse oximetry. Oximeters are now sufficiently comfortable and portable to be worn while walking or sleeping. The measurement is based on pulsatile changes in transmission of specific wavelengths of light in tissue that has been rendered hyperemic by warmth. Sa_{O_2} can also be directly measured on an arterial sample by oximeter or can be reasonably estimated, particularly with an Sa_{O_2} greater than 90%, from Pa_{O_2} and an oxyhemoglobin saturation curve. *Content* (Ca_{O_2}), in turn, can be calculated as the product of saturation and the hemoglobin concentration. For calculation of *systemic oxygen delivery* (SOD), a substantially more invasive test, catheterization of the pulmonary artery, is required for determining cardiac output ($\dot{Q}$); SOD then is the product of Ca_{O_2} and $\dot{Q}$.

These foregoing parameters of blood oxygenation are appealing because they address an ultimate function of the respiratory system—namely, quantitative oxygen transport. The most generally used parameter, however, is the partial pressure in arterial blood (Pa_{O_2}). It appeals, perhaps, because it points more directly to mechanism. It is important to understand the physiologic determinants of Pa_{O_2}. It is lower than inspired oxygen (PI_{O_2}) by two steps: first, dilution from inspired gas (PI_{O_2}) to alveolar gas (PA_{O_2}), and second, gas exchange from alveolar gas (PA_{O_2}) to the arterial blood (Pa_{O_2}). The steps can be distinguished. In the first step, PA_{O_2} depends on the inspired oxygen fraction (FI_{O_2}) and $\dot{V}_A$ relative to the (metabolic) oxygen utilization ($\dot{V}_{O_2}$). By the alveolar gas relationship for oxygen,

$$PA_{O_2} \sim FI_{O_2} - (\dot{V}_{O_2}/\dot{V}_A)$$

PA_{O_2} thus may be reduced in COPD, just as PA_{CO_2} is increased, by decreases in alveolar ventilation relative to metabolic needs. In the second step, arterial oxygen (Pa_{O_2}) is less than PA_{O_2} because of the costs of gas exchange, which depend on (1) a gradient for passive diffusion, (2) $\dot{V}/\dot{Q}$ nonuniformity, and (3) pulmonary vascular shunting. All three may be abnormal in COPD. To sort out the causes of a low arterial oxygen, then, one first assesses the role of inspired oxygen and ventilation by calculating PA_{O_2}; with an assumption for respiratory quotient (R) between O_2 consumption and CO_2 production, it is approximately true that

$$PA_{O_2} = PI_{O_2} - (Pa_{CO_2}/R)$$

Next, compare the calculated PA_{O_2} with the measured Pa_{O_2}. This *alveolar-arterial oxygen difference* (A-aDO_2) is an index of the effectiveness of gas exchange. (It is important to recognize that the values considered normal for this parameter are valid only for a Pa_{O_2} greater than approximately 60 torr, because for a Pa_{O_2} of less than about 60 torr, in which the oxyhemoglobin dissociation curve is steep, a large content difference (i.e., substantial gas exchange dysfunction) gives only a small difference of partial pressure.) If the A-aDO_2 is widened, its cause (diffusion impairment, shunting, or abnormal ventilation/perfusion ratios) can be more specifically assessed as follows.

Passive diffusion is the means of transport of gas from alveolar gas to pulmonary capillary blood. Carbon monoxide is generally used as a stand-in for oxygen. The *diffusing capacity of the lung for carbon monoxide* (DL_{CO}) is commonly measured in the single-breath study, in which the subject inspires a gas mixture, which includes carbon monoxide and an inert tracer gas, holds the breath for about 10 seconds, and then expires. Comparison of inspired and expired gases permits calculation of a conductance for passive diffusion—that is, the rate of carbon monoxide transfer per torr of partial pressure.

The major value of the measurement is in its strong dependence on the area of functioning pulmonary vascular bed that is available for gas exchange. For example, it is diminished in emphysema, in which the vascular bed is restricted by loss of alveolar septa, but not in asthma, which does not impair the vascular bed.

Pulmonary vascular shunting refers to blood entering the pulmonary vein without passing through ventilated alveoli. It can be quantified from three oxygen contents: (1) that of a mixed venous sample ($C\bar{v}_{O_2}$), obtained from the pulmonary artery by cardiac catheterization, (2) that of an arterial sample (Ca_{O_2}), and (3) that of the pulmonary capillary (Cpc_{O_2}), which can be assumed to have equilibrated with the calculated PA_{O_2}. The fraction of the cardiac output that passes through the shunt then is calculated as

$$\dot{Q}_S/\dot{Q}_T = (Cpc_{O_2} - Ca_{O_2})/(Cpc_{O_2} - C\bar{v}_{O_2})$$

To evaluate true shunts, the measurement should be made while the patient breathes pure O_2; otherwise, the result also includes effects of $\dot{V}/\dot{Q}$ nonuniformity and losses due to diffusion. For practical purposes, the requirements for invasive blood sampling and for breathing of 100% oxygen restrict this measurement to patients with indwelling cardiac catheter and endotracheal tube.

Nonuniformity of $\dot{V}/\dot{Q}$. Several means are available for evaluating the distributions of ventilation directly. (1) Ventilation can be directly visualized by scintigraphy, i.e., *ventilation scan* of an inhaled radioactive gas such as technetium. (2) Nonuniformity of ventilation can be supported by *nitrogen washout* as an increased ΔSBNT. (3) Sequential breaths can be analyzed for *nitrogen washout* or for *helium washin* and are examined for delay and departure from the ideal exponential behavior.

Nonuniformity of perfusion can also be depicted and quantified regionally by scintigraphy *(perfusion scan)* after venous injection either of radioactive aggregates of albumin or of a solution of a highly insoluble gas such as xenon.

The distributions of $\dot{V}$ and of $\dot{Q}$ themselves, however, are not as interesting as their *relative* distributions, because of the adverse effects of $\dot{V}/\dot{Q}$ nonuniformity *per se* on gas exchange. In the absence of a true shunt (generally the case in COPD), the A-aDO_2 can be taken to represent $\dot{V}/\dot{Q}$ nonuniformity. More detail can be gained with a mass spectrometer to record the retentions and excretions of multiple inert gases of widely differing solubilities. From such data, plots characterizing the general configurations of the *distributions of $\dot{V}/\dot{Q}$* can be generated.[48] This is a complex procedure, not likely to be applied in routine care of patients.

LIMITS AND PROBES

Whereas some of the aforementioned tests characterize function in the unstressed individual, others evaluate functional limits. Particular examples from tests of pulmonary mechanics include MVV, TLC, RV, $P_{mus,max}$, and FEV_1. Similarly, many tests can be repeated under conditions of stress (exercise, sleep, cold air) to reveal limits that were not apparent under baseline conditions—limits that may be particularly relevant to the patient. For example, gas exchange can be studied during exercise, such as walking or pedaling a stationary bicycle. Finger or ear pulse oximetry, a negligibly invasive procedure, can document desaturation with exercise and the degree of protection given by administering oxygen at various flow rates. Resting DL_{CO} is a less stressful alternative as it is tightly correlated with exercise desaturation,[39] but it is not clear that it adds to the direct demonstration of desaturation, which is the more pertinent parameter. Arterial blood can be directly sampled during exercise; although this is distinctly more invasive than oximetry, the electrode is more precise than the oximeter, and additional information (pH and Pa_{CO_2}) is gained, showing, for example, if the patient exceeded the anaerobic threshold or if ventilation was inadequate during the exercise. DL_{CO} also can be measured during exercise (with a steady-state method so that the breath need not be held). A large increase of DLCO with exercise, greater than doubling, documents appropriate recruitability of the pulmonary vascular bed.

Similarly, in COPD patients sleep can induce substantial changes of ventilation and desaturation that are not apparent in studies performed at rest.[21,51] The simplest approach is a continuous recording of oximetry during sleep, but more elaborate polysomnography may then be warranted.

Nonspecific bronchial provocation has enjoyed considerable attention over the past decade. Parameters of forced expiration and R_{aw} are studied at baseline and during administration of graded exposures to nonspecific agents, such as cold air, histamine, or methacholine. The dose-response curve can be characterized, or the result may be expressed more simply as the dose required to cause a given fractional change, such as a 20% decrease in FEV_1. Similarly, studies may be performed after inhalation of bronchodilators such as isoproterenol or metaproterenol.

Small changes are seen in the normal subject after bronchoconstrictors or bronchodilators; the responsiveness to both may be increased in COPD. Some of this may represent augmented hyperresponsiveness to the bronchoconstrictor or biologically significant reversibility by the bronchodilator. The latter is important to establish for several reasons: demonstration of reversibility may guide therapy, the best FEV_1 provides a standard against which to compare a patient's subsequent function, and changes in test performance over time can add the perspective of changes in reversibility rather than in lung structure. Beyond this, however, the demonstration of increased airway responsiveness is of uncertain meaning at present, as it has not as yet been established what the roles are of a low baseline FEV_1, or of smoking, or whether there is a causal or prognostic link between airway responsiveness and COPD.[45]

SIGNIFICANCE

What is normal? What identifies the presence of disease? What is predictive?

For most PFTs, the results in large numbers of normal patients have generated regression equations with age, sex, height, and race as the independent variables.[15,29,38] With the assumption of Gaussian distributions of the results, the 95% confidence limits can be derived as 1.65 times the coefficient of variation. Thus, for example, values of FEV_1, FVC, and FEF_{25-75} that fall below 80%, 80%, and 60% of predicted, respectively, have a less than 5% chance of being normal.[42]

Severe disease is accompanied by function on PFTs well below these limits. More problematic are patients with disease but with tests within the normal range.

Interest in the natural history of the disease and concern for identifying individuals who have early disease have prompted efforts to learn to what extent subjects with COPD are hiding within the normal range of PFTs and to find ways of identifying them. For example, a subject who starts with pulmonary function near the top of the normal range may have substantial progression of disease process before emerging below the normal threshold. The presence of the disease process, however, may be detected with greater sensitivity by looking for significant changes in test results performed serially in an individual or performed before and after inhalation of bronchodilator agents. Because the coefficients of variation for repeated tests in a single individual are smaller than those within a population, significance can be attributed to FEV_1, FVC, and FEF_{25-75} that *differ* by more than 23%, 21%, and 30%, respectively, over a longer term and 13%, 11%, and 23% after bronchodilation.[42] For example, values of FEV_1 of 114 and 90% of predicted in an individual would fall well in the normal range, but the change clearly would not.

Generally, the abnormal physiology that can be documented by PFTs is correlated with pathologic evidence of disease.[41] Even in a relatively uniform population, there was correlation of indices of flow limitation, DLCO, TLC, and the K of the P/V curve obtained within a few months of death with indices of emphysema on autopsied lungs.[49] Parenthetically, there may be better correlation when TLC is obtained with body plethysmography than with helium dilution, reflecting the underestimation of TLC by the dilution studies if not sufficiently prolonged.[49]

While most PFTs address physiologic function directly, tests of small airways function are distinctly indirect. Their meaning, then, must rest only on their ability to identify disease. Early, there were encouraging results.[14] Tests of density-dependence of expiratory flow were shown to differ in populations of smokers and nonsmokers[17,36] and were correlated with inflammatory changes in airways of subjects with generally normal PFTs.[14,40] Many subsequent studies, however, have been disappointing. The SBNT is of limited use in predicting the rate of decline of FEV_1 in smokers.[9] Small airways tests did not correlate with pathology scores[37] or respiratory problems.[27] In practice, furthermore, their usefulness is limited by variability due to technical and biologic factors.[11,46]

Indeed "abnormalities of lung mechanics usually will be present for many years before significant breathlessness on exertion becomes apparent,"[20] and to some extent, these functional tests can be predictive of the subsequent decline of function. In smokers, the initial FEV_1[10] and the SBNT[9,47] are correlated with the subsequent fall in FEV_1. More important, the FEV_1 is extraordinarily strongly correlated with death from COPD.[4,43] Incidentally, this association is better with the postbronchodilator FEV_1 than it is with the prebronchodilator FEV_1, perhaps because it represents the degree of fixed obstruction.

CHOICES OF TESTS

All PFTs surveyed have been widely applied in studying COPD. For research purposes, the choice among them may be dictated by specificity (e.g., CV for small airways dysfunction) and ease of administration in the field (e.g., PEF for circadian patterns of obstruction) and may permit some degree of complexity of measurement (e.g., frequency-dependence of compliance) or even of variability (e.g., R_{aw}), because variability, if random, can be overcome by studying a sufficiently large population.

In the individual, however, a relatively small selection will suffice for diagnosis and management.

- The simplest, most familiar, and probably the most informative of airways obstruction tests is recording of a forced expiration to obtain the FEV_1 and (less important) the FVC.
- The ultimate physiologic consequences of COPD are reduced or limited oxygen delivery and acidosis. Therefore it may be warranted to obtain ABGs; a recent American Thoracic Society task force recommends doing so for individuals with a FEV_1 of less than 1.5 liters.[1] Pa_{CO_2} above 45 torr may be considered hypercapnia. Pa_{O_2} less than 60 torr (below which the oxyhemoglobin dissociation curve begins to fall rapidly) can be considered hypoxemia. The A-aDO_2 "comes free" with the ABG and should be routinely calculated as it may be more sensitive to the presence or absence of a gas exchange abnormality than are the absolute levels of Pa_{O_2}.
- If there is significant reduction in the FEV_1 or abnormality

of the ABGs, or if there is motivation to look further (anticipated surgery, differential diagnosis, and so on), measurements should also be made of TLC, RV, and D_{LCO} (the TLC and DLco for documenting the presence and severity of emphysema and the FRC and RV for obstruction and hyperinflation). Tests of small airways function are not helpful in the individual, given the poor association with progression as documented by serial FEV_1s.

The choice of PFTs may be broadened for the differential diagnosis between COPD and other entities with similar clinical presentations. For example, dyspnea on exertion and cough are common presenting symptoms of cardiac dysfunction, pulmonary embolism, and interstitial lung disease, as well as of COPD. Normal or reduced TLC in the presence of good inspiratory $P_{mus,max}$ and normal or increased DLco point away from COPD. A distinction of COPD from asthma can be attempted by repeating tests after bronchodilator administration, although the absence of a response on one occasion does not rule out reversibility over a longer period or recovery of reversibility at a later date. DLco may be of particular assistance here, since a normal value in an obstructed patient is strongly against the loss of alveolar structure characteristic of emphysema.

Pulmonary function tests also may be of help in guiding therapy, particularly by documenting the utility of bronchodilators, of oxygen, or of other agents or by documenting the need for oxygen during exercise or during sleep.

REFERENCES

1. American Thoracic Society statement. Standards for the diagnosis and care of patients with chronic obstructive pulmonary disease (COPD) and asthma. Am Rev Respir Dis 1986; 136(1):225–244.
2. American Thoracic Society statement. Standardization of spirometry—1987 update. Am Rev Respir Dis 1987; 136:1285–1298.
3. Anthonisen NR. Tests of mechanical function. APS Handbook, Section 3, Volume III: Mechanics of Breathing, Part 2. Baltimore: Williams and Wilkins, 1986, 753–784.
4. Anthonisen NR, Wright EC, Hodgkin JE, IPPB Trial Group. Prognosis in chronic obstructive pulmonary disease. Am Rev Respir Dis 1986; 133(1):14–20.
5. Barnhard HJ, Pierce JA, Joyce JW, Bates JH. Roentgenographic determination of TLC. A new method evaluated in health, emphysema, and congestive heart failure. Am J Med 1960; 28:51–60.
6. Barrett WA, Clayton PW, Lambson CR, Morris AH. Computerized roentgenographic determination of total lung capacity. Am Rev Respir Dis 1976; 113:239–244.
7. Brown R, Ingram RH Jr, McFadden ER Jr. Problems in the plethysmographic assessment of changes in total lung capacity in asthma. Am Rev Respir Dis 1978; 118:685–692.
8. Brown R, Slutsky AS. Frequency dependence of plethysmographic measurement of thoracic gas volume. J Appl Physiol 1984; 57(6):1865–1871.
9. Buist AS, Vollmer WM, Johnson LR, McCamant LE. Does the single-breath N_2 test identify the smoker who will develop chronic airflow limitation? Am Rev Respir Dis 1988; 137(2):293–301.
10. Burrows B, Knudson RJ, Camilli AE, et al. The "horse-racing effect" and predicting decline in forced expiratory volume in one second from screening spirometry. Am Rev Respir Dis 1987; 135(4):788–793.
11. Camilli AE, Burrows B, Knudson RJ, et al. Longitudinal changes in forced expiratory volume in one second in adults: Effects of smoking and smoking cessation. Am Rev Respir Dis 1987; 135(4):794–799.
12. Colebatch HJ, Greaves IA, Ng CKY. Exponential analysis of elastic recoil and aging in healthy males and females. J Appl Physiol 1979; 47:683–691.
13. Collett PW, Brancatisano T, Engel LA. Changes in the glottic aperture during bronchial asthma. Am Rev Respir Dis 1983; 128:719–723.
14. Cosio M, Ghezzo MS, Hogg JC, et al. The relations between structural changes in small airways and pulmonary function tests. N Engl J Med 1978; 298(23):1277–1281.
15. Crapo RO, Morris AH, Gardner RM. Reference spirometric values using techniques and equipment that meet ATS recommendations. Am Rev Respir Dis 1981; 123:659–664.
16. Deal EC, Kelsen SG, Eberlin LB, et al. Respiratory effects of bronchoconstriction in anesthesized dogs. Am Rev Respir Dis 1983; 127(3):310–314.
17. Dosman J, Bode F, Urbanetti J, et al. The use of a helium-oxygen mixture during maximum expiratory flow to demonstrate obstruction in small airways in smokers. J Clin Invest 1975; 55:1090–1099.
18. Eisen EA, Dockery DW, Speizer FE, et al. The association between health status and the performance of excessively variable spirometry tests in a population-based study in six U.S. cities. Am Rev Respir Dis 1987; 136(6):1371–1376.
19. Farkas GA, Roussos C. Diaphragm in emphysematous hamsters: sarcomere adaptability. J Appl Physiol 1983; 54:1635–1640.
20. Fletcher C, Peto R. The natural history of chronic airflow obstruction. Br Med J 1977; 1:1645–1648.
21. Flick MR, Block AJ. Continuous *in vivo* monitoring of arterial oxygenation in chronic obstructive lung disease. Ann Intern Med 1977; 86(6):725–730.
22. Greaves IA, Colebatch HJH. Elastic behavior and structure of normal and emphysematous lungs post mortem. Am Rev Respir Dis 1980; 121:127–136.
23. Greaves IA, Colebatch HJH. Large lungs after childhood asthma: a consequence of enlarged airspaces. Aust NZ J Med 1985; 15:427–434.
24. Green M, Mead J, Hoppin FG Jr, Wohl ME. Analysis of the forced expiratory maneuver. Chest 1973; 63(4):335–365.
25. Harris TR, Pratt RC, Kilburn KH. Total lung capacity measured by roentgenograms. Am J Med 1971; 50:756–763.
26. Ingram RH Jr, Schilder DP. Effect of thoracic gas compression on the flow-volume curve of the forced vital capacity. Am Rev Respir Dis 1966; 94:56–63.
27. Knudson RJ, Bloom JW, Kaltenborn WT, et al. Assessment of air vs. helium-oxygen flow-volume curves as an epidemiologic screening test. Chest 1984; 86(3):419–423.
28. Knudson RJ, Burrows B, Lebowitz MD. The maximum expiratory flow-volume curve: its use in the detection of ventilatory abnormalities in a population study. Am Rev Respir Dis 1976; 114(19):871–878.
29. Knudson RJ, Slatin RC, Lebowitz MD, Burrows B. The maximal expiratory flow-volume curve. Normal standards, variability, and effects of age. Am Rev Respir Dis 1976; 113(5):587–600.
30. Koulouris N, Mulvey DA, Laroche CM, et al. The measurement of inspiratory muscle strength by sniff, esophageal, nasopharyngeal, and mouth pressure. Am Rev Respir Dis 1989; 139:641–646.
31. Krowka MJ, Enright PL, Rodarte JR, Hyatt RE. Effect of effort on measurement of forced expiratory volume in one second. Am Rev Respir Dis 1987; 136(4):829–833.
32. Leaver DG, Tattersfield AE, Pride NB. Contributions of lung recoil and of enhanced airways collapsibility to the airflow obstruction of chronic bronchitis and emphysema. J Clin Invest 1973; 52:2117–2128.
33. Leith DE, Bradley M. Ventilatory muscle strength and endurance training. J Appl Physiol 1976; 41(4):508–516.
34. Leith DE, Mead J. Mechanisms determining residual volume of the lungs in normal subjects. J Appl Physiol 1967; 23:221–227.
35. Lim TK, Pride NB, Ingram RH Jr. Effects of volume history during spontaneous and acutely induced air-flow obstruction in asthma. Am Rev Respir Dis 1987; 135:591–596.
36. Malo JL, Leblanc P. Functional abnormalities in young asymptomatic smokers with special reference to flow-volume curves breathing various gases. Am Rev Respir Dis 1975; 111:623–629.
37. Matsuba K, Shirakusa T, Kuwano K, et al. Small airways disease in patients without chronic air-flow limitation. Am Rev Respir Dis 1987; 136:1106–1111.
38. Morris JF, Koski A, Johnson LC. Spirometric standards for healthy nonsmoking adults. Am Rev Respir Dis 1971; 103:57–67.
39. Owens GR, Rogers RM, Pennock BM, Levin D. The diffusing capacity as predictor of arterial oxygen desaturation during exercise in patients with COPD. N Engl J Med 1984; 310(19):1218–1221.

40. Pare PD, Brooks LA, Coppin CA, et al. Density-dependence of maximal expiratory flow and its correlation with small airway disease in smokers. Am Rev Respir Dis 1985; 131(4):521.
41. Pare PD, Brooks LA, Bates J, et al. Exponential analysis of the lung pressure-volume curve as a predictor of pulmonary emphysema. Am Rev Respir Dis 1982; 126(1):54–61.
42. Pennock BE, Rogers RM, McCaffree DR. Changes in measured spirometric indices; what is significant? Chest 1981; 80:97–99.
43. Peto R, Speizer FE, Cochrane AL, et al. The relevance in adults of air-flow obstruction, but not of mucus hypersecretion to mortality from chronic lung disease. Am Rev Respir Dis 1983; 128:491–500.
44. Pride NB, Macklem PT. Lung mechanics in disease. APS Handbook, Section 3, Volume III: Mechanics of Breathing, Part 2. Baltimore: Williams and Wilkins, 1986, 659–692.
45. Redline S, Tager IB. The relationships of airway reactivity to the occurrence of chronic obstructive lung disease—an epidemiologic assessment. In: Lenfant C, Hensley M, eds. Lung Biology in Health and Disease; Clinical Epidemiology of COPD. New York: Marcel-Dekker, 1989, 169–199.
46. Redline S, Tager IB, Castile RG, et al. Assessment of the usefulness of helium-oxygen maximal expiratory flow curves in epidemiologic studies of lung disease in children. Am Rev Respir Dis 1987; 136(4):834–840.
47. Stanescu DC, Robenstein DO, Hoeven C, Robert A. "Sensitive tests" are poor predictors of the decline in forced expiratory volume in one second in middle-aged smokers. Am Rev Respir Dis 1987; 135:585–590.
48. Wagner PD, Smith CM, Davies NJ, et al. Estimation of ventilation-perfusion inequality by inert gas elimination without arterial sampling. J Appl Physiol 1985; 59:376–383.
49. West WW, Nagel A, Hodgkin JE, Thurlbeck WM. The National Institutes of Health intermittent positive pressure breathing trial—pathology studies. III. The diagnosis of emphysema. Am Rev Respir Dis 1987; 135:123–129.
50. Williams JH, Bencowitz HZ. Differences in plethysmographic lung volumes; effects of linked vs. unlinked spirometry. Chest 1989; 95(1):117–123.
51. Wynne JW, Block AJ, Hemenway J, et al. Disordered breathing and oxygen desaturation during sleep in patients with chronic obstructive lung disease (COLD). Am J Med 1979; 66:573–579.

Chapter 40

LABORATORY EVALUATION OF THE PATIENT WITH CHRONIC OBSTRUCTIVE PULMONARY DISEASE

Michael Donahoe Robert M. Rogers

In addition to abnormalities of lung function, patients with chronic obstructive pulmonary disease (COPD) develop other laboratory abnormalities. These abnormalities are important in the evaluation and treatment of COPD patients.

HEMATOLOGY

Red Blood Cells

Erythrocytosis is seen in certain patients with COPD, as well as in smokers without significant airflow obstruction. A hematocrit at sea level above 52% in men and 47% in women warrants evaluation, because higher hematocrits are seen in less than 5% of normal individuals. Upper normal limits for hemoglobin are 17.7 g/dl for men and 15.7 g/dl for women.[56] A normal red cell volume with a decreased plasma volume is characteristic of patients with relative erythrocytosis. An increased red cell volume with a normal or decreased plasma volume is found in those patients with absolute erythrocytosis (Table 40–1).[207] This division is somewhat arbitrary because of the wide range of reported normal values for the red cell volume.[207]

Absolute erythrocytosis is further subdivided into a primary form, known as polycythemia vera, and a secondary form, which is characteristic of patients with chronic lung disease and hypoxemia. In addition to lung disease, other causes of secondary absolute erythrocytosis include congenital heart disease and erythropoietin-producing tumors. The red cell volume is elevated in all forms of absolute erythrocytosis and the specific diagnosis is based on well-described clinical and laboratory findings.[11]

The importance of smoking in the development of erythrocytosis was ignored until the 1970s.[157, 171] Chronic cigarette smoking can produce significant elevations in blood carboxyhemoglobin levels, resulting in a functional anemia.[19] Hemoglobin bound to carbon monoxide cannot carry oxygen. This factor, combined with an associated shift to the left of the oxyhemoglobin dissociation curve, can significantly impair oxygen delivery to the tissues.

Smith and Landau,[171] in a study of 22 patients with erythrocytosis and elevated blood carboxyhemoglobin levels secondary to chronic smoking, showed that 12 of the patients had an elevated red cell mass and that 14 of the patients demonstrated a reduction in plasma volume. These results support the classification of smokers' polycythemia as both a relative

TABLE 40–1. Classification of Increased Hemoglobin or Packed Cell Volume in the COPD Patient

TYPE OF ERYTHROCYTOSIS	EXAMPLES
Relative erythrocytosis (decreased plasma volume, normal red cell volume)	Volume depletion—i.e., diuretic therapy, gastrointestinal disease, dehydration Smokers' polycythemia Chronic relative erythrocytosis
Absolute erythrocytosis Secondary erythrocytosis	Appropriate erythropoietin secretion—i.e., high-altitude, abnormal hemoglobin function, smokers' polycythemia, cardiopulmonary disease (COPD) Inappropriate erythropoietin secretion—i.e., renal disease (cysts, hypernephroma), cerebellar hemangioblastoma, hepatoma, etc.
Primary erythrocytosis (polycythemia vera)	

and an absolute polycythemia. A progressive shift to the left of the oxyhemoglobin dissociation curve was noted as the carboxyhemoglobin level increased. Five patients were able to reduce or stop smoking and all demonstrated normalization of their blood hematocrits. Smith and Landau suggested that, in addition to obtaining a reliable smoking history, smokers with erythrocytosis should be evaluated for venous carboxyhemoglobin levels at the end of the day to allow for the progressive rise in the serum value during the awake smoking hours ($t_{1/2}$ for carboxyhemoglobin, 3 to 5 hours).[171] The combination of erythrocytosis and elevation of the blood carboxyhemoglobin level, in the presence of a normal or elevated red blood cell (RBC) volume, should suggest the diagnosis of smokers' polycythemia. Because the changes in plasma volume associated with smoking are prompt, they believe that a 4% decrease in a patient's venous hematocrit after 2 to 3 days of smoking cessation strongly favors a low plasma volume, secondary to smoking, as a cause of the high hematocrit. Doll and Greenberg[37] have reported two cases of smokers' polycythemia and cerebrovascular occlusive disease, suggesting that these patients may be subject to the same risk of thrombotic episodes as patients with polycythemia vera or chronic relative erythrocytosis.

In addition to smokers' polycythemia, a relative erythrocytosis is seen under conditions of volume depletion and in chronic relative erythrocytosis (also referred to as Gaisböck's syndrome, stress polycythemia, spurious polycythemia, or pseudopolycythemia). As described by Lawrence and Berlin,[101] chronic relative erythrocytosis is thought to occur predominantly in middle-aged, slightly obese men, often with a history of hypertension. The existence of this abnormality, distinct from smoker's polycythemia, is unclear, because most reports of relative erythrocytosis do not include a smoking history or carboxyhemoglobin levels in the patient analysis. It is likely that a significant proportion of the patients described with chronic relative erythrocytosis actually had significant elevations of blood carboxyhemoglobin levels from smoking.

The clinical syndrome of chronic relative erythrocytosis has been seen in two groups of patients: those with a high-normal red blood cell volume and a low-normal plasma volume, and patients with a normal red blood cell volume and a low plasma volume. The importance of this distinction is that the latter group may have an increased predisposition to thrombotic disease, which has been reported in up to 30% of these patients.[200]

An absolute erythrocytosis in patients with COPD arises from inappropriate oxygen delivery to the tissues in association with arterial blood oxygen desaturation. The relationship between the level of arterial oxygen desaturation and the elevation of the blood hemoglobin level, hematocrit, and erythrocyte cell volume in patients with COPD has received much attention. Controversy exists as to whether patients with chronic airflow obstruction demonstrate an appropriate erythrocyte response to hypoxemia. The erythrocyte mass response of the hypoxemic COPD patient is most frequently compared to the erythocytic response seen in high-altitude dwellers.[197] In high-altitude residents, there is an inverse relationship between the erythrocyte cell volume and the arterial O_2 saturation. Various investigators have suggested that the erythrocyte response in hypoxemic COPD patients is normal,[77, 104, 162, 190] reduced,[55, 64, 130, 192, 206] or even excessive.[68] In most studies, the hypoxemic COPD patients have been reported to have an elevation in the mean red cell volume (MCV) and a reduction in the mean cell hemoglobin concentration (MCHC).[64, 190, 192, 206]

A number of factors contribute to the variability in the erythrocyte response noted in hypoxemic COPD patients. Comparison studies of matched hypoxemic COPD patients with and without erythrocytosis have revealed no differences in blood erythropoietin levels[61, 196] or in the sensitivity of bone marrow red cell precursors to erythropoietin.[61] A reduced erythrocyte response in some series has been attributed to chronic infection[206] or to decreased red cell survival time,[192] neither of which has been confirmed.

As suggested by Stradling and Lane,[180] the variability in erythrocyte response probably results from differences in the methods used in these investigations. First, the reported series used various parameters to assess the hematologic response, from isolated blood hematocrits to measures of the actual red cell volume. Clearly, the blood hemoglobin level and hematocrit alone are poor indicators of the hematologic response to hypoxemia because of the wide variations of plasma volume in the COPD patient population.

A second factor is the use of random sampling of oxygen saturation as the measure of tissue oxygen delivery. A single measurement of oxygen saturation is almost certainly an unreliable indicator of a patient's mean daily saturation. Intermittent desaturation, which could be missed by random sampling, has proven to be a potent stimulus for erythropoietin production.[159] Both sleep[15, 94, 144] and exercise[136] can produce episodes of desaturation in patients with normal arterial oxygen saturation (SaO_2) at rest. Wedzicha and colleagues[196] studied 20 hypoxemic COPD patients and found those patients that developed polycythemia spent a greater time with their arterial SaO_2 <80% during sleep than patients without polycythemia. Further investigation is necessary to define the importance of sleep and exercise desaturation in the development of erythrocytosis.

Arterial saturation and the erythrocyte cell mass are only two measures of the balance between oxygen supply and oxygen demand. Hemoglobin concentration, levels of erythrocyte 2,3-diphosphoglycerate, blood carboxyhemoglobin concentration, cardiac output, blood pH, and local tissue blood flow are all factors that influence oxygen delivery to the tissues.[69] Given the many factors that determine the adequacy of tissue oxygen supply and the variety of influences that can affect the compensatory mechanisms of the host, a variable relationship between arterial saturation and erythrocyte mass in COPD patients should be expected.[69, 180]

The treatment of erythrocytosis requires proper identification of the underlying disorder. A blood hematocrit above 60% reliably predicts an elevated RBC volume, but elevations below this level may be associated with a normal or low red cell volume in the presence of a reduced plasma volume.[11] Determination of erythrocyte volume, generally using ^{51}Cr, is required in these patients. Once an increased red cell volume has been established, the diagnosis of secondary polycythemia in patients with chronic lung disease is confirmed by clinical and laboratory criteria, including the presence of hypoxemia (or elevated carboxyhemoglobin levels in smokers) and the absence of the characteristic clinical findings of polycythemia vera.[11] The therapeutic options in patients with erythrocytosis secondary to chronic lung disease include smoking cessation, O_2 therapy (where indicated) and, less commonly, phlebotomy.

The role of phlebotomy remains controversial. In COPD patients, phlebotomy has generally not been associated with improvements in standard measures of resting pulmonary function. Although a reduction in pulmonary resistance,[67, 161, 201] improved exercise tolerance,[27, 67] increased cerebral blood flow,[212] improvement in right ventricular function,[27, 45, 201] and a decrease in respiratory drive[137] have all been observed following phlebotomy in COPD, no controlled studies have determined the true benefit of phlebotomy in these patients. In addition, the timing and method of bleeding are unresolved. A hematocrit level above 60% is frequently chosen as the point at which phlebotomy may be beneficial.[69] Systemic oxygen transport probably decreases significantly at this level, and this tends to correlate with the onset of hyperviscosity symptoms in these patients. Phlebotomy appears to have the most significant beneficial effects in patients with a hematocrit above 60% prior to treatment.[161, 201]

Controversy also exists as to the methods of phlebotomy. The most common method is simple, repeated venesection.[161] Concern regarding the hemodynamic shifts associated with bleeding the COPD patient has led some investigators to advocate simultaneous volume replacement with normal saline or exchange transfusion.[56, 69]

White Blood Cells

Leukocytosis in patients with COPD may result from either a complicating event (e.g., infection) or a therapeutic intervention (e.g., steroid therapy). Blood[42, 65, 111] and sputum[165] eosinophilia have been associated with a therapeutic response to steroid administration in some series. These patients frequently have, in addition, other markers of disease reversibility, such as variability in spirometry testing,[111] a response to inhaled bronchodilator,[124] or an elevated serum IgE level.[165] In contrast, Mendella and colleagues found that the therapeutic response to steroid administration did not correlate with the presence of blood or sputum eosinophilia, although a therapeutic benefit was most frequently seen in patients with a bronchodilator response during spirometry testing.[124]

Leukocytosis with a marked eosinophilia ($>3000\ mm^3$) suggests a complicating disorder, such as allergic bronchopulmonary aspergillosis, eosinophilic pneumonia, Churg-Strauss vasculitis, or the hypereosinophilic syndrome.

Platelets

Patients with COPD and hypoxemia may demonstrate subtle abnormalities of platelet function. Decreased platelet survival time,[176] shortened regeneration time,[188] and increased platelet aggregation[32] with elevations of the plasma beta-thromboglobulin level[32, 132] (an in vivo marker of platelet activation) have all been reported in hypoxemic COPD patients. The association of these platelet function abnormalities with the presence of hypoxemia is supported by the reversal of the decreased platelet survival time with supplemental oxygen.[85] Nenci and colleagues[132] studied 12 hypoxemic COPD patients and found that in vivo markers of increased platelet activation (increased plasma beta-thromboglobulin level and decreased platelet malondialdehyde production) were present. These findings disappeared with the administration of the platelet inhibitor dipyridamole. The investigators suggested that increased platelet activation, with release of platelet mediators, may play a role in the development of thromboembolic disease and pulmonary hypertension in hypoxemic COPD patients.

CHEMISTRY

Electrolytes

Hyponatremia in patients with COPD can arise in several different ways (mechanisms). Complicating disorders such as lung tumors and pulmonary infection may produce hyponatremia by inappropriate secretion of antidiuretic hormone. Most commonly, however, hyponatremia occurs as a result of salt and water retention.

Although frequently attributed to right heart failure, edema formation in these patients may occur in association with normal cardiac function.[23, 152] This is most frequently seen in the setting of hypercarbia. Recognition of these factors has prompted investigation into the mechanisms affecting salt and water balance in COPD patients.

Severe hypoxemia and hypercarbia are associated with reduced renal blood flow, as well as with salt and water retention.[10, 87] White and Woodings,[202] using a standard H_2O load in COPD patients, demonstrated decreased free H_2O clearance and decreased solute and creatinine clearance. The ability to excrete a water load was inversely correlated with the P_{CO_2}.

Farber and colleagues[49] have confirmed a decrease in free water and solute clearance during a water load in hypercapnic COPD patients compared to normocapnic, hypoxic patients. Hypercapnic COPD patients have an increased stimulus for Na^+ and water retention because of increased tubular secretion of H^+ and reabsorption of $NaHCO_3$ in the collecting system, which is required for buffering the respiratory acidosis. In addition, these hypercapnic patients often have elevated levels of plasma renin activity and plasma aldosterone.[49, 50] These patients may also have levels of plasma arginine vasopressin inappropriately elevated for the serum osmolality.[50] This combination of factors would promote salt and water retention. The role of the renin-angiotensin system has been supported by improvement in solute clearance in hypercapnic COPD patients following the administration of an angiotensin-converting enzyme inhibitor.[48] The interrelationships and mechanisms of reduced renal blood flow and the stimulated renin-angiotensin system require further investigation to determine their role in the edema formation and hyponatremia seen in COPD.

A second electrolyte abnormality often seen in chronic obstructive pulmonary disease is hypokalemia. Patients with hypokalemia are at increased risk for the occurrence of cardiac arrhythmias and respiratory muscle weakness.[91] Hypokalemia may be present in COPD patients as a result of poor oral intake, gastrointestinal loss from vomiting or diarrhea, or renal tubular defects with K^+ wasting. The possible iatrogenic precipitation of hypokalemia is also important in this patient population.

A hyper-renin state with secondary hyperaldosteronism, as previously suggested for hypercapnic COPD patients,[48] would promote renal tubular potassium excretion. This tendency would be augmented by concomitant steroid administration.

Diuretics, often used in the treatment of edema in COPD patients, produce hypokalemia. This complication occurs in 30% to 50% of patients taking thiazide diuretics.[92] A major complication of their use is a hypokalemic metabolic alkalosis.

In addition to the complications of hypokalemia, a significant alkalemia in COPD patients could decrease ventilatory drive and promote CO_2 retention.

Beta-agonist therapy, almost universally prescribed in these patients, can also promote hypokalemia. Epinephrine has been known to precipitate hypokalemia through beta$_2$-receptor stimulation.[31, 43] In similar fashion, intravenous beta$_2$-agonists (terbutaline and salbutamol) have also been shown to decrease serum K^+ levels acutely, primarily by causing a shift of potassium from extracellular to intracellular sites.[6, 103, 143] Beta$_2$-agonists, when given by aerosol, produce significantly decreased plasma levels compared to intravenous adminstration but theoretically could also aggravate tendencies to hypokalemia.

Hypophosphatemia is a frequent electrolyte abnormality in hospitalized patients with chronic obstructive pulmonary disease. Hypophosphatemia usually results from a combination of insults. Malnutrition with decreased oral intake of phosphate, phosphate-binding antacids, glucose administration (especially in the form of parenteral nutrition poorly supplemented with phosphate), an associated history of alcohol abuse, and respiratory acidosis, either acute or chronic, are common factors that can combine to precipitate hypophosphatemia in the hospitalized COPD patient.[90] In a retrospective review of 308 admissions to a chest ward, Fisher and colleagues found that 17% of patients had at least one episode of hypophosphatemia, compared to a 5% incidence in patients admitted to the general medical ward.[51] The incidence increased to 28% in patients with respiratory infections.

Hypophosphatemia is especially important in the population of patients with acute respiratory failure. The canine diaphragm shows increased susceptibility to fatigue under conditions of phosphate depletion.[146] In humans, hypophosphatemia has been reported to interfere with weaning from mechanical ventilation.[133] Aubier and colleagues[4] studied eight hypophosphatemic patients with acute respiratory failure requiring mechanical ventilation. Respiratory muscle strength was assessed by measurement of the transdiaphragmatic pressure (P_{di}) during supramaximal phrenic nerve stimulation. Correction of the serum phosphate concentration from a mean pretreatment level of 0.55 ± 18 mmol/L (normal value, 1.20 ± 0.10 mmol/L) to a level of 1.33 ± 0.21 mmol/L was associated with significant improvements in the P_{di} (preinfusion mean P_{di} = 9.75 ± 3.8 cm H_2O versus postinfusion mean P_{di} = 17.25 ± 3.8 cm H_2O).

Hypomagnesemia and hypocalcemia have also been associated with respiratory muscle weakness. Although most frequently a complication of alcohol abuse, hypomagnesemia may also result from the frequent administration of diuretics.[73] Dhingra and colleagues[35] demonstrated significant improvement in respiratory muscle force in 17 patients (11 alcoholics) following magnesium replacement therapy. Hypocalcemia in a canine model produced a progressive decline in diaphragm force output during low-frequency supramaximal stimulation.[5]

The complete clinical implications of these electrolyte abnormalities have not been firmly established in the COPD patient. The significant effect that electrolyte disturbances may have on respiratory muscle function, however, dictates close monitoring of these variables in the COPD patient. This concept is especially important in the hospitalized patient with respiratory failure.

Alpha$_1$-Antitrypsin

The link between the absence of antiprotease activity and the development of human pulmonary disease was first suggested by Laurell and Eriksson[100] from routine electrophoretic analysis of serum proteins. They noted an absent alpha$_1$-globulin peak in certain patients with severe emphysema. Since that time, a large body of literature has accumulated on the subject of alpha$_1$-antitrypsin (AAT).

Biochemical analysis has confirmed that AAT exists in multiple variants. These collectively have been termed the Pi (protease inhibitor) system. Genetic studies have suggested that inheritance of the specific Pi phenotypes follows the principles of simple mendelian genetics for codominant alleles at a single locus.[46, 97] This locus has been termed the Pi locus and the individual alleles given such names as Pi^M, Pi^Z, and Pi^S. The labels correlate with the phenotypic labeling of each biochemical variant by its electrophoretic mobility in acid-starch gel: F, fast; S, slow; Z, very slow; and M, intermediate. The frequency of individual alleles is highly dependent on the population investigated.[96]

Pi^M is the most common allele in the U.S. population (seen in approximately 90% of individuals).[129] Patients homozygous for the Pi^M allele have normal levels and function of AAT. Of the less common alleles, those most fequently recognized are Pi^S, Pi^Z, and, rarely, Pi^- (Pi^{null}). Individuals homozygous for Pi^- are completely deficient in AAT, whereas patients homozygous for Pi^S and Pi^Z have approximately 55% and 15% of the normal serum trypsin inhibitory capacity, respectively.[109, 129] The most common deficiency state encountered in the U.S. is homozygous Pi^Z, which occurs in approximately 0.05% to 0.1% of the population. The contribution of the heterozygote state (Pi^{MZ} or Pi^{MS}), characterized by a partial AAT deficiency, to the pathophysiology of emphysema has been a controversial area.[20, 109, 129] The preponderance of evidence suggests that the modest reductions in AAT characteristic of the heterozygote patient do not pose a risk for COPD.[20, 129]

Levels of AAT should be measured in patients who develop COPD at a relatively young age, have smoked sparingly or not at all, or have siblings or parents with emphysema. Serum protein electrophoresis may provide an important clinical clue to the presence of AAT deficiency. The absence of the alpha$_1$-globulin peak, as noted previously, suggests the possibility of this disorder. This finding, however, does not provide an accurate quantitative measure of serum AAT activity in the homozygote-deficient patient. Both quantitative and qualitative assays exist to assess AAT in the clinical laboratory.

Although rarely used clinically, the functional activity of a patient's serum AAT activity can be assessed by measurement of the serum trypsin inhibitory capacity (STIC). This method involves the hydrolysis of synthetic substrates of trypsin in the presence of various dilutions of the patient's serum.[47, 74] Because 90% of the STIC activity is caused by alpha$_1$-antitrypsin, a close correlation exists between the measurement of serum AAT levels by standard immunologic methods and the measured STIC.[107] The normal AAT serum level of 180 to 280 mg/100 ml correlates with a trypsin inhibitory activity of 0.9 to 1.5 mg trypsin inhibited/ml serum.[96]

Radioimmunodiffusion (RID) provides an accurate quantitative method of measuring AAT levels in serum.[112] In this technique, a fixed amount of a patient's serum is placed in the well of an agar gel that contains a specific antibody for AAT. The area of the resulting immune precipitate from the antigen diffusion into the agar is proportional to the antigen concentration.

Rate nephelometry is a more recently described technique for the quantitative assessment of AAT. Rate nephelometry uses the maximum rate of change of scattered light intensity in an antigen-antibody reaction as a measure of the antigen concentration (AAT).[177] Comparison of the three quantitative techniques (RID, STIC, and rate nephelometry) available for AAT deficiency screening provides comparable results if appropriate reference values are chosen.[54] Problems exist, however, when the quantitative measurement of AAT is used for identification of the heterozygote patient.

Alpha$_1$-antitrypsin is an acute phase reactant and, as a result, the serum value can be elevated in various conditions, including infection, inflammation, and pregnancy. In addition, exogenous estrogens have been shown to elevate the serum levels of AAT.[108] Although heterozygotes (Pi^{MZ}) may elevate their serum AAT levels into the normal range in the presence of factors associated with elevated acute phase reactants, Pi^{Z} homozygotes do not.[95] Also recognized is a significant overlap in AAT levels and STIC between patients with homozygote MM and heterozygote MS and MZ.[107, 182] Only the homozygote patient has clearly been associated with disease, and these patients can reliably be detected with the less expensive quantitative assays. If low levels of AAT are identified, this is confirmed with Pi typing. Qualitative techniques for Pi typing are required exclusively in situations that require identification of heterozygote populations, such as genetic counseling.

Starch-gel electrophoresis is the most frequently used qualitative technique for the determination of AAT variants. Each AAT variant shows a characteristic rate of migration with a pattern of bands that allows phenotype characterization.[79] Atypical patterns are further analyzed using the technique of crossed antigen-antibody electrophoresis. The initial starch-gel electrophoresis is transferred to an agarose gel containing specific AAT antisera. Application of the current at right angles to the initial electrophoresis allows further separation of the AAT bands.[99] A final technique, isoelectric focusing in polyacrylamide gel, has increased the ability to subtype certain alleles and eliminates the need for two-dimensional electrophoresis.[26]

Drug Levels

Theophylline

Theophylline (1,3-dimethylxanthine) has gained a prominent role in the therapy of patients with COPD. Its narrow therapeutic range and variable pharmacokinetics make monitoring of serum theophylline levels essential to avoid drug toxicity.[121] The various factors affecting theophylline metabolism that are present in most patients do not allow accurate prediction of serum levels by clinical parameters.[82, 123]

The older spectrophotometric assays for theophylline have been replaced in most clinical and research settings by the use of high-pressure liquid chromatography (HPLC), enzyme immunoassays, fluorescence polarization techniques, and enzyme immunochromatography. These techniques generally require specialized equipment and training. The introduction of simplified automated systems, which combine the principles of monoclonal enzyme immunochemistry and dry reagent chemistry, has allowed the monitoring of theophylline levels to be extended to physician's offices or emergency rooms, with reasonably accurate results.[39, 63, 149, 193]

The spectrophotometric assay may still be used in certain clinical situations. This assay system is subject to interference from other foods or drugs that the patient may be taking. Methylxanthine derivatives found in such foods as coffee, tea, or chocolate can produce small elevations in the theophylline measurement using this analytic method. A number of medications, including allopurinol, barbiturates, propylthiouracil, coumadin, folic acid, and chloramphenicol, have been proposed as possibly interfering with the spectrophotometric assay.[118, 209] Barbiturates, acetaminophen, and phenytoin may produce falsely low values by as much as 10 μg/ml. Salicylates can interfere with the spectrophotometric absorption spectrum.[7] In the presence of these additional medications, other assay systems for theophylline should be employed.

HPLC is also subject to measurement interference as a result of the presence of other drugs. Acetazolamide, methicillin, ampicillin, and cephalothin have all been shown to interfere with the HPLC assay of serum theophylline levels.[86, 153, 172] Once recognized, this problem can generally be overcome by altering the methods of drug extraction or column conditions.

The automated systems developed for rapid theophylline assay generally use whole blood for the sample specimen, rather than the more traditional use of plasma. Habib and colleagues[63] found that whole blood theophylline levels are significantly lower than plasma values and that the difference depends on the patient's hematocrit. The accurate use of these simplified automated systems may require adjustment for variations in individual hematocrit values.

Once the dosage has been established in clinically stable patients, the serum concentration of theophylline tends to remain constant over time.[83] Drug levels should be measured to confirm adequate dosing in patients who do not demonstrate a therapeutic benefit from theophylline administration. Stable patients need to have serum theophylline levels monitored only if symptoms or side effects occur. Introduction of any variable recognized as influencing theophylline pharmacokinetics into a patient's course would warrant more frequent monitoring of serum drug levels.

The type of oral drug formulation can affect the rate and amount of drug absorbed. Even sustained-release preparations show wide variability in drug absorption.[34] Theophylline elimination is dose-dependent but tends to deviate from first-order kinetics at higher plasma levels. Small changes in dosage may result in marked elevations in the theophylline serum concentration.[199]

Other medications may alter theophylline pharmacokinetics. These effects range from the decreased absorption of theophylline seen in the presence of certain commercially available antacids[3] to the alteration in hepatic metabolism associated with cimetidine administration.[81] A decreased rate of theophylline clearance has been reported to occur in the presence of erythromycin,[150] allopurinol,[113] cimetidine,[81] oral contraceptives,[187] troleandomycin,[194] ciprofloxacin,[148] and caffeine. An increased rate of theophylline clearance has been associated with the administration of phenytoin[117] and phenobarbital.[98] The significance and mechanisms of many of these interactions remain controversial.[121]

Smoking has consistently been recognized as increasing theophylline clearance.[147] Discontinuation of smoking might result in a gradual accumulation of theophylline with the risk of drug toxicity if serum drug levels are not monitored.

Finally, increased age,[134] congestive heart failure,[33] the presence of liver disease[114] and infection[25] may decrease theophylline clearance. All these factors must be considered when deciding on appropriate times for theophylline level monitoring.

The initial loading dose for intravenous theophylline administration can be determined from knowledge of the serum theophylline level using the following formula:[126]

$$\text{loading dose (mg/kg)} = \text{desired serum level (mg/L)} - \text{existing level (mg/L)} \times 0.5 \text{ L/kg body weight}$$

The serum concentration rises approximately 2 mg/L for each mg/kg of theophylline administered as a bolus.[70]

A serum level obtained 30 minutes following an intravenous loading dose provides a guide for determining the rate of constant infusion needed to maintain a target serum concentration. Because of individual variations in theophylline metabolism, serum theophylline levels should be monitored during the first 6 to 12 hours of an intravenous infusion to allow dosage adjustment.

Weinberger and colleagues have recommended that adjustment of outpatient oral theophylline doses be aided by measuring the serum theophylline level 4 hours after the preceding dose, in the absence of medication changes for the preceding 72 hours.[198]

Digitalis

The clinical impression of an increased risk of digitalis toxicity in COPD patients is supported by the available literature.[60] This effect may be secondary to an enhanced digitalis sensitivity rather than to alterations in drug metabolism.[36] The contribution to this enhanced sensitivity of hypoxia, hypokalemia, and a hyperadrenergic state, all of which are frequently present in these patients, is unclear. Although serum levels provide an index to dosing in those patients in whom digitalis is used, clinical features of digitalis toxicity may appear, even when the serum level is in the therapeutic range.

SPUTUM ANALYSIS

Cellular analysis of the sputum can be helpful in the evaluation of patients with COPD. Macroscopic examination of sputum is often misleading, because both neutrophils and eosinophils produce purulent sputum.[119, 127] Medici and colleagues have suggested that the sputum of patients with chronic bronchitis undergoes three phases: a stable phase, an infectious phase, and a resolution or postinfection phase.[122] During acute exacerbations, sputum neutrophils and bronchial epithelial cells increase. The bronchial epithelial cells remain elevated in the postinfectious phase, whereas the neutrophils decrease to stable phase levels. Alveolar macrophages, which do not increase during the infectious phase, increase significantly during the resolution period.[122]

A wet preparation of the sputum or an appropriately stained specimen allows detailed analysis of the cellular elements (alveolar macrophages, neutrophils, and eosinophils). The cellular analysis helps to determine the adequacy of the sputum specimen and to distinguish between an infectious exacerbation characterized by a neutrophilic predominance and an allergic exacerbation characterized by an eosinophilic predominance (occasionally associated with Curschmann's spirals and Charcot-Leyden crystals).[28, 44]

Many criteria have been proposed to determine the adequacy of a sputum specimen for bacteriologic analysis.[208] The goal is to distinguish tracheobronchial secretions from oropharyngeal flora. The presence of alveolar macrophages and few squamous epithelial cells suggests that the specimen originated from below the larynx. Murray and colleagues[131] have suggested that sputum specimens with fewer than ten squamous epithelial cells per high-powered field closely resemble transtracheal aspirates. This criterion is subject to inconsistencies because of variations in the thickness of the material in different areas of the same slide. To overcome these limitations, Barry[8] has proposed that a minimum ratio of white blood cells to epithelial cells of 5 to 1 be used to determine the adequacy of the sputum collection.

Diplococcus pneumoniae and *Hemophilus influenzae* are the most common bacterial organisms isolated from patients with increased production of purulent sputum.[52, 120, 145] They are also found as regular inhabitants of the upper respiratory tract of normal individuals. In addition, they are frequently present in the tracheobronchial secretions of asymptomatic COPD patients.[102, 128] Therefore, the significance of isolating these organisms in the COPD patient with chronic bronchitis and purulent sputum, even with "adequate" specimens, is unclear.[2, 155, 181]

Transtracheal aspiration represents an alternative technique for obtaining specimens of tracheobronchial secretions for bacteriologic evaluation in the COPD patient.[140] The technique involves the insertion of a needle catheter system through the cricothyroid membrane, with aspiration of tracheobronchial secretions. Transtracheal aspiration should only be carried out by trained personnel because of the increased risk of complications associated with this technique, such as bleeding, infection, and subcutaneous emphysema.[174]

Although generally recognized to be more reliable than expectorated sputum, interpretation of the results of cultures of transtracheal aspirates in patients with chronic lung disease is again limited as a result of a high incidence (85%) of positive cultures, even in clinically stable patients.[13] Schreiner and colleagues,[160] using transtracheal aspirates in 76 patients with chronic sputum production, found that 80% of the aspirates grew *Hemophilus influenzae* or *Diplococcus pneumoniae*. Haas and associates,[62] studying patients with chronic bronchitis, compared three methods for the evaluation of tracheobronchial secretions in patients with chronic sputum production: oropharyngeal sampling, transtracheal aspiration, and bronchoscopy. They found a high degree of correlation in the culture results using all three techniques. As expected, patients with chronic bronchitis most commonly grew *H. influenzae* and *D. pneumoniae*, regardless of the sampling method.

Finally, bronchoscopy and related techniques, including transbronchial lung biopsy, protected catheter brush specimens, and bronchoalveolar lavage, are available for the evaluation of infection in the COPD patient. Because of the increased risk of morbidity and mortality with these procedures, they are generally reserved for the COPD patient with undiagnosed pneumonia or for the immunocompromised host. The risks and benefits of these techniques have been reviewed elsewhere.[186]

Despite the many techniques available for sputum analysis of the COPD patient, the most appropriate indications and technique for microbiologic analysis have yet to be determined. The consistent isolation of identical organisms, regardless of the sampling technique or clinical status of the patient, has prompted some clinicians to conclude that sputum microbiologic evaluation in the absence of pneumonia is unrewarding.[139]

In addition to microbiologic criteria, biochemical characteristics of sputum have been proposed for the evaluation of COPD patients. Inflammatory bronchial secretions may contain elevated levels of deoxyribonucleic acid (DNA), lactate dehydrogenase (LDH), fibrinogen, and albumin.[9, 21] Stockley and colleagues have suggested that levels of 11S (locally produced) and 7S (serum-derived) IgA are increased in infectious sputum. In addition, the free secretory piece of IgA seen in noninfected sputum is apparently absent in infected specimens.[178] The value of these biochemical parameters in the evaluation and treatment of patients with COPD remains to be determined.

Other proteins such as albumin, the immunoglobulins, transferrin, AAT, alpha$_2$-macroglobulin, and alpha$_1$-antichymotrypsin may also be present. Under conditions of chronic bronchial irritation, these proteins may exist in a partially fragmented or denatured form. Albumin and AAT appear to enter lung secretions by passive diffusion, whereas alpha$_1$-antichymotrypsin and alpha$_2$-macroglobulin are secreted locally.[179, 203]

MUCOCILIARY CLEARANCE

Several methods are currently in use to assess mucociliary function. Two parameters proposed to evaluate lung mucous clearance are the measurement of the tracheal mucous velocity and of tracheobronchial clearance. The complexity of these techniques has restricted their use to the research environment.

Tracheal mucous velocity (TMV) can be measured by placing radiopaque Teflon discs at the tracheal bifurcation using a bronchoscope, and then recording the movement of these particles with a bronchoscope and cinematography[156] or by radiography.[53] An alternative approach involves the use of radioisotopes. Boluses of labeled albumin microspheres are aerosolized into the trachea and their movement is detected using a gamma camera.[211] TMV in those with chronic bronchitis appears to be reduced.[58, 158] Direct comparison to normals is limited because of the wide range of normal values observed for the TMV.

Tracheobronchial clearance provides a more global assessment of mucociliary clearance.[1] Following inhalation of a radioisotopically labeled aerosol, the clearance of the particles is recorded using a gamma camera located over the chest. This technique is limited by the marked influence of particle deposition on the rate of clearance. A more central initial deposition of inhaled particles results in a faster clearance rate. Inhaled tracers are more centrally deposited in patients with obstructive airway disease than they are in normal individuals, giving the false impression in some earlier investigations of an increased rate of tracheobronchial clearance.[38, 184] The variation in aerosol distribution has made comparative studies between COPD patients and normals difficult to interpret. When an index of particle deposition is used to control for this variable in patients with airflow obstruction, clearance in chronic bronchitic patients appears reduced.[22, 38, 167] Similar findings have been noted in patients with bronchiectasis.[110]

ELECTROCARDIOGRAPHY

The electrocardiogram (ECG) is abnormal in approximately 75% of patients with significant obstructive airway disease.[175, 195] The characteristic ECG findings in these patients are summarized in Table 40–2. Although none of the individual criteria is specific, the simultaneous finding of characteristic P-wave and QRS changes strongly supports the presence of underlying COPD.[24]

Hyperinflation with flattening of the diaphragm is associated with a more vertical position of the heart and a clockwise rotation along its longitudinal axis. The ECG frequently shows a rightward shift of the P and QRS axes in the frontal plane and a posterior displacement of the QRS axis in the horizontal plane. The mean QRS forces are directed posteriorly and perpendicular to the frontal plane, resulting in a decreased amplitude of the QRS complex in the limb and left precordial leads. Hyperinflation also reduces the electrical conductivity of the lung, further contributing to a decreased ECG amplitude.

TABLE 40–2. Electrocardiographic Changes in Chronic Obstructive Pulmonary Disease

ECG CHANGES	CHARACTERISTICS
P wave	Rightward deviation of the P-wave axis; P wave > 2.5 mm in leads II, III, aV_F; prominent negative P wave in lead I
QRS	Tendency for right axis deviation of the QRS vector and marked clockwise rotation of the electrical axis; QRS amplitude in all limb leads < 5mm; QRS amplitude < 5 mm in leads V_5 and/or V_6, or R wave < 7 mm in lead V_5, or R wave < 5 mm in lead V_6; R to S ratio < 1 in leads V_5 and/or V_6; R to S amplitude ratio in V_1 < 1; S_1Q_3 or $S_1S_2S_3$ pattern with R to S ratio < 1 in leads I, II, and III; incomplete (and, rarely) complete right bundle branch block
Other	Lead I sign with an isoelectric P wave, QRS amplitude less than 1.5, and T-wave amplitude less than 0.5 mm; pseudoinfarction pattern with large Q waves or QS in the inferior or precordial leads

(Adapted from material in Chou TC, ed. Electrocardiography in Clinical Practice. 2nd ed, New York: Grune & Stratton, 1979; and from Holford F, *In* Fishman AP, ed. Pulmonary Diseases and Disorders. New York: McGraw-Hill, 1988.)

The more vertical P-wave axis, characteristic of patients with significant airflow obstruction, results in a biphasic or isoelectric P wave in lead I and/or a V_L. This shift of the P-wave axis correlates with the severity of the airflow obstruction in some series.[24, 175] P pulmonale, characterized by peaked P waves (greater than 2.5 mm) in the inferior leads, occurs in patients with more severe airflow obstruction.[175]

The QRS axis is shifted to the right, usually by less than +90°.[88, 175] This shift of the QRS axis may be associated with an $S_1S_2S_3$ pattern.[175] The orientation of the mean QRS axis posteriorly, superiorly, and to the right can result in an "apparent" left axis deviation.[29, 71] An S_2 greater than S_3 helps to distinguish this finding from true left axis deviation.[29]

The posterior orientation of the mean QRS vector is reflected in the precordial leads, where the R to S ratio is usually less than 1 as far as V_5. The movement of the transitional zone is thus clockwise.

Wasserburg and colleagues have observed an electrocardiographic pattern, termed the "pentology of pulmonary emphysema," in patients with advanced emphysema. This pattern consists of the following: (1) exaggerated P waves in leads II, III, and aV_F; (2) prominent T-a waves in leads II, III, and aV_f; (3) vertical cardiac position, which at times may be extreme; (4) clockwise rotation on the longitudinal cardiac axis; and (5) tendency to low voltage, particularly in the left ventricular leads.[195]

Kok-Jensen[93] studied the ECG features of 228 patients with chronic bronchial obstruction.[93] A decreased survival was seen in patients with a QRS axis of +90° to +180° and a P-wave amplitude in lead II of 0.20 mV or greater; only 37% and 42%, respectively, of the patients with these features were alive at 4 years. Smit and colleagues[170] found that a higher P-wave amplitude in lead II and/or S amplitude in lead V_6 was associated with a decreased 5-year survival.

Cor Pulmonale

Chronic obstructive pulmonary disease is frequently complicated by chronic cor pulmonale, although the exact incidence of this complication is unknown. This diagnosis is generally based on electrocardiographic criteria. The classic determinants of right ventricular hypertrophy, developed from patients with congenital heart disease, include a right axis shift of the QRS (greater than +110°), an R to S ratio in V_1 greater than 1, and an R to S ratio in V_6 of less than 1.[59] However, these have proven to be relatively poor criteria for the diagnosis of cor pulmonale in patients with COPD.[88, 141] Some electrocardiographic features of cor pulmonale may be seen in patients with emphysema in the absence of right ventricular hypertrophy. These include the P-pulmonale pattern, the $S_1S_2S_3$ pattern, and the leftward shift of the transitional zone.[29] The presence of an RSR or QR pattern in V_1, marked clockwise rotation of the electrical axis, a frontal plane QRS axis of 110° or more, large Q waves or QS waves in the inferior or midprecordial leads, and ST- and T-wave changes in the right precordial or inferior leads are more suggestive of right ventricular hypertrophy in those with obstructive airway disease.[29, 71]

Kilcoyne and associates[88] have suggested that a progressive change in the ECG occurs in response to hypoxemia (arterial saturation below 85%) and pulmonary hypertension (mean

PA pressure 25 or greater). These changes consist of the following: (1) inverted, biphasic, or flattened T waves in the right precordium; (2) depressed ST segments in leads II, III, and aV_F; (3) a rightward shift of the mean QRS axis of 30° or more from its previous position; and (4) complete or incomplete right bundle branch block. These abnormalities frequently resolved with improvement of the arterial saturation. If the pulmonary hypertension persisted, the rightward rotation of the QRS axis and the T-wave changes in the right precordial leads remained. If pulmonary function was not reversed with therapy, then true right axis deviation (a frontal plane axis greater than +90°) and increased R-wave voltage in the right precordial leads developed. These abnormalities tended to be nonreversible.

Noninvasive techniques, such as echocardiography and radionuclide imaging, can also be used to confirm the diagnosis of pulmonary hypertension complicating COPD. M-mode echocardiography is of limited usefulness because the hyperinflation of the chest that occurs with COPD interferes with adequate visualization of the right ventricle. Two-dimensional echocardiography (2-D echo), however, permits visualization of both right venticular chamber and pulmonary artery dimensions.[115, 173, 213] Investigations in small numbers of patients have suggested that 2-D echo[213] or Doppler echocardiography[115] may accurately predict the severity of pulmonary hypertension in COPD patients.

The adequacy of radionuclide investigation of the heart with thallium-201 imaging depends on the amount of muscle mass and the blood flow to the organ to allow visualization. The nondominant right ventricle is usually not visualized in most patients studied with this technique. The right ventricle of patients with COPD and right ventricular enlargement and/or hypertrophy, however, may be visualized at rest.[168] Right ventricular visualization with thallium-201 imaging suggests the presence of pulmonary hypertension.[168, 210] Measurement of the right ventricular ejection fraction by radionuclide imaging may be another useful test for the noninvasive diagnosis of pulmonary hypertension in COPD.[18]

Arrhythmia

Patients with COPD are reported to have a variable incidence of arrhythmias complicating this disorder. As expected, the longer the monitoring period, the more arrhythmias are reported.[72]

Both supraventricular and ventricular arrhythmias complicate the course of patients with COPD. The type of arrhythmia may be influenced by the clinical state of the patient.[16] During exacerbations, supraventricular arrhythmias are more common.[76] In acute respiratory failure, up to 80% of arrhythmias may be supraventricular in origin.[169] In contrast, ventricular ectopic arrhythmias have been reported to be more frequent in stable COPD patients.[16, 89]

Severe COPD may be complicated by multifocal atrial tachycardia (MAT; Fig. 40–1).[142, 166] Significant obstructive lung disease is recognized in 30% to 80% of patients presenting with this rhythm abnormality. MAT is frequently confused with other supraventricular tachyarrhythmias, (i.e., atrial fibrillation). Unlike other supraventricular tachyarrhythmias, though, digitalis administration in MAT does not produce ventricular slowing and continued administration can lead to digitalis toxicity and further malignant arrhythmias.[166] The rhythm may respond favorably to treatment with verapamil.[105] Although MAT has been associated with a poor prognosis in the COPD patient, this may simply reflect the more frequent occurrence of this rhythm in patients with severe lung disease.

Two factors that exacerbate a tendency to arrhythmias in the COPD patient are hypoxemia and therapy with certain drugs. Nocturnal hypoxemia has been associated with increased ventricular ectopy in these patients.[163, 185] The prognostic implications of this finding, as well as the therapeutic benefit of oxygen supplementation, remain to be determined.

Theophylline is the drug most frequently implicated in producing a greater number of ventricular and atrial ectopic beats.[30, 40, 116, 138] Evidence from a canine model has suggested that theophylline does reduce the threshold for ventricular fibrillation.[75]

DETERMINATION OF NUTRITIONAL STATUS

The association between weight loss and severe chronic pulmonary disease has been recognized since the late 1960s.[151, 191] More recent recognition of the negative impact of weight loss on the course of these patients has led to a growing interest in the nutritional evaluation of emphysematous patients with COPD.[204] This section focuses on nutritional parameters in the evaluation of these patients (Table 40–3).

Anthropometric Measurements

Body weight provides a reasonable index of the patient's nutritional status in the absence of edema formation or dehydration. The measured body weight is compared to standard weight-for-height tables (e.g., as published by the Metropolitan Life Insurance Company)[125] to give percentage of ideal body weight (actual weight/ideal weight × 100). Additional indices include the percentage of usual weight (actual weight/usual weight × 100) and the percentage weight change (usual weight − (actual weight/usual weight) × 100).[14] Most investigations of malnourished COPD patients have defined malnourished as less than 90% ideal body weight.[41, 106, 205] Unfortunately, body weight often provides a poor index of body composition (i.e., muscle mass versus fat stores) and detailed studies on malnourished COPD patients in this area are lacking.

Additional anthropometric measurements used in the nutritional assessment include triceps skin fold thickness to estimate body fat stores, and arm muscle circumference to estimate skeletal muscle mass. The triceps skin fold (TSF) is usually measured in the nondominant upper arm at a point midway between the acromion process and the olecranon. The skin fold parallel to the long axis of the arm is firmly grasped and slightly lifted between the finger and thumb of the left hand. Standard calipers are applied at the midpoint of the arm, approximately 1 cm below the fingers. Three measurements are made and the results are averaged. The measurements obtained can be compared with standard values for age and sex.[14]

Mid-upper arm circumference is measured using a nonstretchable tape. The position for the measurement is similar to that described for the TSF. When this measurement is combined with the TSF thickness, an estimate of the arm muscle circumference can be made (AMC = arm circumference − 3.14 [TSF]). This parameter correlates well with estimates of the body cell mass.[189]

Biochemical Parameters

Visceral protein stores can be assessed by measurement of serum protein levels, such as albumin and transferrin. Many

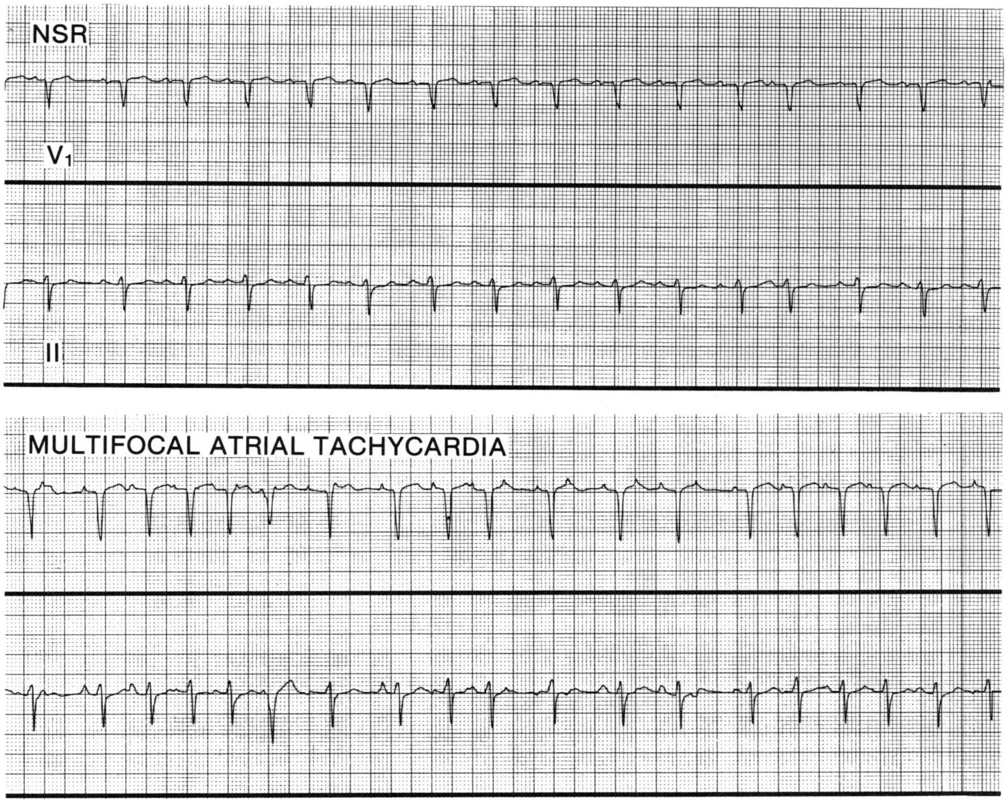

Figure 40–1. Continuous electrocardiographic rhythm strip demonstrating normal sinus rhythm and multifocal atrial tachycardia. In contrast to normal sinus rhythm (NSR), multifocal atrial tachycardia is characterized by multiple P-wave morphologies and a variable PP interval. (Courtesy of Edward Curtiss, MD.)

factors affect the level of serum albumin, such as liver disease and proteinuria, making it less reliable as a specific measure of nutritional status. In addition, albumin has a long half-life ($t_{1/2}$ = 12 to 14 days), so it is a poor parameter for evaluating the effects of short-term nutritional intervention. The transferrin level ($t_{1/2}$ = 8 days) appears to decrease under conditions of protein calorie malnutrition, but its value is affected by concomitant iron deficiency states, liver disease, and conditions associated with elevations of levels of acute phase reactants.[183]

Prealbumin and retinol-binding protein ($t_{1/2}$ = 12 hours) are serum proteins with shorter half-lives; their levels are also reduced in those with protein calorie malnutrition.[164] These proteins, unlike albumin and transferrin, appear to be sensitive to acute changes in dietary protein intake, suggesting that they may be more reliable indicators of effective short-term nutritional intervention.[80]

Twenty-four hour urine collections to help determine N_2 balance and the creatinine level are also used in the nutritional evaluation of the COPD patient. N_2 balance studies have been used to confirm an anabolic state during periods of nutritional repletion. The creatinine-height index is a parameter used to estimate total muscle mass. It is defined as the ratio of 24-hour creatinine excretion by the patient to the 24-hour creatinine excretion of a normal subject of the same height. Determination of both the creatinine-height index and N_2 balance require the careful collection and preservation of a 24-hour urine specimen. Because of this, and the knowledge that these parameters are heavily influenced by changes in dietary protein intake, they are probably best restricted to very controlled settings.

A decreased total lymphocyte count (< 1200) is seen in those with protein calorie malnutrition.[12] A number of nutritional factors, however, can also influence the total lymphocyte count, limiting its effectiveness in nutritional assessment.

In most investigations of stable malnourished COPD patients, evidence for significant reductions in parameters of subcutaneous fat stores (TSF) and lean body mass (AMC) are present.[17, 41, 78, 106, 135, 205] A decreased creatinine-height index and depressed delayed hypersensitivity assessed by skin testing are also frequent findings.[78, 205] Biochemical indicators of visceral protein status, though, are generally preserved. This combination of findings, as suggested by Blackburn and colleagues,[14] is most consistent with protein calorie malnutrition of the marasmic type.[14]

TABLE 40–3. Nutritional Parameters for Evaluation of COPD Patients

PARAMETER	MEASUREMENT
Anthropometric	Percentage of ideal body weight; triceps skin fold (body fat stores); arm muscle circumference (body cell mass)
Biochemical evaluation (estimate of visceral protein stores)	Albumin, total protein; transferrin; prealbumin, retinal binding protein; skin testing, total lymphocyte count
Urinary indices	Nitrogen balance; creatinine-height index
Metabolic evaluation	Caloric intake; basal energy expenditure; resting metabolic equivalent

Metabolic Testing

The caloric requirements of patients can be estimated from standard reference equations or can be measured directly. The precise energy expenditure can be determined with direct calorimetry; but this method requires elaborate equipment and is impractical for most clinical situations. Analysis of gas exchange using the principles of indirect calorimetry has been shown to provide similar results to those of direct calorimetry. The basal metabolic rate (BMR) is determined in the postabsorptive state (approximately 14 hours after a meal) under conditions of complete physical and mental rest shortly after awakening. The resting metabolic equivalent (RME) is determined when indirect calorimetry is carried out at rest under fasting conditions. This value is approximately 10% above the BMR in normals and is believed to represent approximately 70% of an individual's daily energy expenditure.[84] The Harris-Benedict equation is often used to estimate the daily caloric requirements based on a patient's age, height, weight, and sex.[66] This baseline value is multiplied by various stress factors, depending on the patient's clinical condition. In normals, these values have been shown to closely approximate the measured RME obtained with indirect calorimetry.[154]

Results of indirect calorimetric testing in malnourished COPD patients[57, 205] have suggested that the RME in malnourished COPD patients is significantly higher than values predicted by the Harris-Benedict equation. Malnourished COPD patients appear to have resting metabolic requirements approximately 20% above predicted values. The caloric requirements of stable, malnourished COPD patients are best estimated by indirect calorimetry, or by the Harris-Benedict equation and a 20% stress factor when indirect calorimetry is unavailable.

REFERENCES

1. Albert RE, Arnett LC. Clearance of radioactive dust from the lung. Arch Ind Health 1955; 12:99–106.
2. American Thoracic Society. Definitions and classification of chronic bronchitis, asthma, and pulmonay emphysema. Am Rev Respir Dis 1962; 85:762–768.
3. Arnold LA, Spurbeck GH, Shelver WH, Henderson WM. Effect of an antacid on the gastrointestinal absorption of theophylline. Am J Hosp Pharm 1979; 36:1054–1062.
4. Aubier M, Murciano D, Lecocguic Y, et al. Effect of hypophosphatemia on diaphragmatic contractility in patients with acute respiratory failure. N Engl J Med 1985; 313:420–424.
5. Aubier M, Viires N, Piquet J, et al. Effects of hypocalcemia on diaphragmatic strength generation. J Appl Physiol 1985; 58:2054–2061.
6. Back DJ, Breckenridge AM, MacIver M, et al. Hypokalaemia due to salbutamol overdosage. Br Med J 1981; 282:1515–1516.
7. Banner AS, Berman E, Sunderrajan E, et al. Drug interferences with the spectrophotometric assay of theophylline (letter). N Engl J Med 1977; 297:170–171.
8. Barry AL. Clinical specimens for microbiologic examination. In: Hoeprich PD, ed. Infectious Diseases. 2nd ed. New York: Harper & Row, 1977, 91–105.
9. Bartmann K, Fooke-Achterrath M, Koch G, et al. Bacteriological and biochemical criteria for the diagnosis of bacterial infection in chronic obstructive pulmonary disease (COPD). Infection 1984; 12:58–63.
10. Baum GL, Dick MM, Blum A, et al. Total body exchangeable potassium and sodium and extracellular fluid in chronic pulmonary insufficiency. Am Heart J 1959; 58:53–58.
11. Berlin NI. Diagnosis and classification of the polycythemias. Semin Hematol 1975; 12:339–351.
12. Bistrian B, Blackburn GL, Scrimshaw NS, Flatt J. Cellular immunity in semistarved states in hospitalized adults. Am J Clin Nutr 1975; 28:1148–1155.
13. Bjerkestrand G, Digranes A, Schreiner A. Bacteriological findings in transtracheal aspirates from patients with chronic bronchitis and bronchiectasis: A preliminary report. Scand J Respir Dis 1975; 56:201–207.
14. Blackburn GL, Bistrian BR, Maini BS, et al. Nutritional and metabolic assessment of the hospitalized patient. J Parenter Enter Nutr 1977; 1:11–22.
15. Block AJ. Dangerous sleep: Oxygen therapy for nocturnal hypoxemia. N Engl J Med 1982; 306:166–167.
16. Brashear RE. Arrhythmias in patients with chronic obstructive pulmonary disease. Med Clin North Am 1984; 68:969–981.
17. Braun SR, Keim NL, Dixon RM, et al. The prevalence and determinants of nutritional changes in chronic obstructive pulmonary disease. Chest 1984; 86:558–563.
18. Brent BN, Mahler D, Matthay RA, et al. Noninvasive diagnosis of pulmonary arterial hypertension in chronic obstructive pulmonary disease: Right ventricular ejection fraction at rest. Am J Cardiol 1984; 53:1349–1353.
19. Brody JS, Cohum RF. Carbon monoxide-induced arterial hypoxemia. Science 1969; 164:1297–1298.
20. Bruce RM, Cohen BH, Diamond EL. Collaborative study to assess risk of lung disease in Pi MZ phenotype subjects. Am Rev Respir Dis 1984; 130:386–390.
21. Burgi H, Wiesmann U, Richterich R, et al. New objective criteria for inflammation in bronchial secretions. Br Med J 1968; 654–656.
22. Camner P, Mossberg B, Philipson K. Tracheobronchial clearance and chronic obstructive lung disease. Scand J Respir Dis 1973; 54:272–281.
23. Campbell EJM, Short DS. The cause of oedema in "cor pulmonale." Lancet 1960; i:1184–1186.
24. Calatayud JB, Abad JM, Khoi NB, et al. P-wave changes in chronic obstructive pulmonary disease. Am Heart J 1970; 79:444–453.
25. Chang KC, Lauer BA, Bell TD, Chai H. Altered theophylline pharmacokinetics during acute respiratory viral illness. Lancet 1978; i:1132–1133.
26. Chan SK, Luby J, Wu YC. Purification and chemical compositions of human α_1-antitrypsin of the MM type. FEBS Lett 1973; 35:79–82.
27. Chetty KG, Brown SE, Light RW. Improved exercise tolerance of the polycythemic lung patient following phlebotomy. Am J Med 1983; 74:415–420.
28. Chodosh S. Examination of sputum cells. N Engl J Med 1970; 282:854–857.
29. Chou TC. Chronic obstructive lung disease, pneumothorax, and pulmonary embolism. In: Chou TC, ed. Electrocardiography in Clinical Practice. 2nd ed. New York: Grune & Stratton, 1979, 300–319.
30. Conradson T, Eklundh G, Olofsson B, et al. Cardiac arrhythmias in patients with mild-to-moderate obstructive lung disease. Comparison of beta-agonist therapy alone and in combination with a xanthine derivative, enprofylline or theophylline. Chest 1985; 88:537–542.
31. Conci F, Procaccio F, Boselli L. Hypokalemia from beta-2 receptor stimulation by epinephrine. N Engl J Med 1984; 310:1329.
32. Cordova C, Musca A, Violi F, et al. Platelet hyperfunction in patients with chronic airways obstruction. Eur J Respir Dis 1985; 66:9–12.
33. Dal Negro R, Turco P, Pomari C, Monici-Preti P. Effect of various disease states on theophylline plasma levels and on pulmonary function in patients with chronic airway obstruction treated with a sustained release theophylline preparation. Int J Clin Pharmacol Ther Toxicol 1987; 25:401–405.
34. Dederich RA, Szefler SJ, Green ER. Intrasubject variation in sustained-release theophylline absorption. J Allergy Clin Immunol 1981; 67:465–471.
35. Dhingra S, Solven F, Wilson A, McCarthy DS. Hypomagnesemia and respiratory muscle power. Am Rev Respir Dis 1984; 129:497–498.
36. Doherty JE, Perkins WH. Tritiated digoxin turnover in pulmonary heart disease with congestive heart failure [abstract]. Clin Res 1967; 15:54.
37. Doll DC, Greenberg BR. Cerebral thrombosis in smokers' polycythemia. Ann Intern Med 1985; 102:786–788.
38. Dolovich MB, Sanchis J, Rossman C, Newhouse MT. Aerosol penetrance: A sensitive index of peripheral airways obstruction. J Appl Physiol 1976; 40:468–471.
39. Drost RH, Schultz HU, Maes RAA, van Rossum JM. A comparative study of a monoclonal immunoassay reagent strip test and high pressure liquid chromatography for theophylline. Clin Toxicol 1987; 25:231–241.
40. Dutt AK, De Soyza ND, Au WY, et al. The effect of aminophylline on cardiac rhythm in advanced chronic obstructive pulmonary disease: Correlation with serum theophylline levels. Eur J Respir Dis 1983; 64:264–270.
41. Efthimiou J, Fleming J, Gomes C, Spiro SG. The effect of supplementary oral nutrition in poorly nourished patients with

chronic obstructive pulmonary disease. Am Rev Respir Dis 1986; 137:1075–1082.
42. Eliasson O, Hoffman J, Trueb D, et al. Corticosteroids in COPD: A clinical trial and reassessment of the literature. Chest 1986; 89:484–490.
43. Epstein FH, Rosa RM. Adrenergic control of serum potassium. N Engl J Med 1983; 309:1450–1451.
44. Epstein RL. Constituents of sputum: A simple method. Ann Intern Med 1972; 77:259–265.
45. Erickson AD, Golden WA, Claunch BC, et al. Acute effects of phlebotomy on right ventricular size and performance in polycythemic patients with chronic obstructive pulmonary disease. Am J Cardiol 1983; 52:163–166.
46. Erikson S. Studies in α_1-antitrypsin deficiency. Acta Med Scand 1965; 177(Suppl 6):5–85.
47. Erlanger BF, Kokowsky N, Cohen W. The preparation and properties of two new chromogenic substrates of trypsin. Arch Biochem Biophys 1961; 95:271–278.
48. Farber MO, Weinberger MH, Roberston GL, Fineberg NS. The effects of angiotensin-converting enzyme inhibition on sodium handling in patients with advanced chronic obstructive pulmonary disease. Am Rev Respir Dis 1987; 136:862–866.
49. Farber MO, Kiblawi SSO, Strawbridge RA, et al. Studies on plasma vasopressin and the renin-angiotensin-aldosterone system in chronic obstructive lung disease. J Lab Clin Med 1977; 90:373–380.
50. Farber MO, Roberts LR, Weinberger MH, et al. Abnormalities of sodium and H_2O handling in chronic obstructive lung disease. Arch Intern Med 1982; 142:1326–1330.
51. Fisher J, Magid N, Kallman C, et al. Respiratory illness and hypophosphatemia. Chest 1983; 83:504–508.
52. Fisher M, Akhtar AJ, Calder MA, et al. Pilot study of factors associated with exacerbations in chronic bronchitis. Br Med J 1969; 4:187–192.
53. Friedman M, Scott FD, Poole DO, et al. A new method of estimating mucous velocity by a roentgenographic technique. Am Rev Respir Dis 1976; 113:A206.
54. Gaidulis L, Muensch HA, Maslow WC, Borer WZ. Optimizing reference values for the measurement of alpha$_1$-antitrypsin in serum: Comparison of three methods. Clin Chem 1983; 29:1838–1840.
55. Gallo RC, Fraimow W, Cathcart RT, Erslev AJ. Erythropoietic response in chronic pulmonary disease. Arch Intern Med 1964; 113:559–568.
56. Golde DW, Hocking WG, Koeffler HP, Adamson JW. Polycythemia: Mechanisms and management. Ann Intern Med 1981; 95:71–87.
57. Goldstein S, Askanazi J, Weissman C, et al. Energy expenditure in patients with chronic obstructive pulmonary disease. Chest 1987; 91:222–224.
58. Goodman RM, Yergin BM, Landa JF, et al. Relationship of smoking history and pulmonary function tests to tracheal mucous velocity in nonsmokers, young smokers, ex-smokers, and patients with chronic bronchitis. Am Rev Respir Dis 1978; 117:205–214.
59. Goodwin JF, Abdin ZH. The cardiogram of congenital and acquired right ventricular hypertrophy. Br Heart J 1959; 21:523–544.
60. Green LH, Smith TW. The use of digitalis in patients with pulmonary disease. Ann Intern Med 1977; 87:459–465.
61. Guidet B, Offenstadt G, Boffa G, et al. Polycythemia in chronic obstructive pulmonary disease: A study of serum and urine erythropoietin and medullary erythroid progenitors. Chest 1987; 92:867–870.
62. Haas H, Morris JF, Samson S, et al. Bacterial flora of the respiratory tract in chronic bronchitis: Comparison of transtracheal, fiberbronchoscopic, and oropharyngeal sampling methods. Am Rev Respir Dis 1977; 116:41–47.
63. Habib MP, Schifman RB, Shon BY, et al. Evaluation of whole blood theophylline enzyme immunochromatography assay. Chest 1987; 92:129–131.
64. Hammarsten JF, Whitcomb WH, Johnson PC, Lowell JR. The hematologic adaptation of patients with hypoxia due to pulmonary emphysema. Am Rev Tuberc 1958; 78:391–398.
65. Harding SM, Freedman S. A comparison of oral and inhaled steroids in patients with chronic airways obstruction: Features determining response. Thorax 1978; 33:214–218.
66. Harris JA, Benedict FG. A biometric study of basal metabolism in man. Carnegie Inst Wash Publ 1919; 279.
67. Harrison BDW, Davis J, Madgwick RG, Evans M. The effects of a therapeutic decrease in packed cell volume on the response to exercise of patients with polycythaemia secondary to lung disease. Clin Sci Mol Med 1973; 45:833–847.
68. Harrison BDW. Polycythaemia in a selected group of patients with chronic airways obstruction. Clin Sci 1973; 44:563–570.
69. Harrison BDW, Stokes TC. Secondary polycythemia: Its causes, effects and treatment. Br J Dis Chest 1982; 76:313–340.
70. Hendeles L, Weinberger M, Bighley L. Disposition of theophylline after a single intravenous infusion of aminophylline. Am Rev Respir Dis 1978; 118:97–103.
71. Holford FD. The electrocardiogram in pulmonary disease. In: Fishman AP, ed. Pulmonary Diseases and Disorders. New York: McGraw-Hill, 1988, 471–478.
72. Holford FD, Mithoefer JC. Cardiac arrhythmias in hospitalized patients with chronic obstructive pulmonary disease. Am Rev Respir Dis 1973; 108:879–885.
73. Hollifield JW. Potassium and magnesium abnormalities: Diuretics and arrhythmias in hypertension. Am J Med 1984; 77(Suppl5A):28–32.
74. Homer GM, Katchman BJ, Zipf RE. A spectrophotometric method for measuring serum trypsin inhibitor capacity. Clin Chem 1963; 9:428–437.
75. Horowitz LN, Spear JF, Moore EN, Rogers R. Effects of aminophylline on the threshold for initiating ventricular fibrillation during respiratory failure. Am J Cardiol 1975; 35:376–379.
76. Hudson LD, Kurt TL, Petty TL, Genton E. Arrhythmias associated with acute respiratory failure in patients with chronic airway obstruction. Chest 1973; 63:661–665.
77. Hume R. Blood volume changes in chronic bronchitis and emphysema. Br J Haematol 1968; 15:131–139.
78. Hunter AMB, Carey MA, Larsh HW. The nutritional status of patients with chronic obstructive pulmonary disease. Am Rev Respir Dis 1981; 124:376–381.
79. Hutchison DCS, Cook PJL, Barter CE, et al. Pulmonary emphysema and α_1-antitrypsin deficiency. Br Med J 1971; 1:689–694.
80. Ingenbleek Y, Vanden Schrieck HG, DeNayer P, DeVisscher M. Albumin, transferrin and thyroxine binding prealbumin/retinal binding protein (RBA/RBP) complex in assessment of malnutrition. Clin Chem Acta 1975; 63:61–67.
81. Jackson JE, Powell RJ, Wandell M, et al. Cimetidine decreases theophylline clearance. Am Rev Respir Dis 1981; 123:615–617.
82. Jacobs MH, Senior RM, Kessler G. Clinical experience with theophylline: Relationships between dosage, serum concentration and toxicity. JAMA 1976; 235:1983–1986.
83. Jenne JW, Wyze E, Rood BS, MacDonald FM. Pharmacokinetics of theophylline: Application to adjustment of the clinical dose of aminophylline. Clin Pharmacol Ther 1972; 13:349–360.
84. Jequin E. Long-term measurement of energy expenditure in man: Direct or indirect calorimetry. In: Bjorntorp P, Cairella M, eds. Recent Advances in Obesity Research, III: Proceedings of the Third International Congress on Obesity. London: John Libbey, 1981, 130–135.
85. Johnson TS, Ellis JH, Steele PP. Improvement of platelet survival time with oxygen in patients with chronic obstructive airway disease. Am Rev Respir Dis 1978; 117:255–257.
86. Kelly RC, Prentice DE, Hearne GM. Cephalosporin antibiotics interfere with the analysis of theophylline by high performance liquid chromatography. Clin Chem 1978; 24:838–839.
87. Kilburn KH, Dowell AR. Renal function in respiratory failure. Arch Anat Med 1971; 127:754–762.
88. Kilcoyne MM, Davis AC, Ferrer MI. A dynamic electrocardiographic concept useful in the diagnosis of cor pulmonale. Circulation 1970; 42:903.
89. Kleiger RE, Senior RM. Long-term electrocardiographic monitoring of ambulatory patients with chronic airways obstruction. Chest 1974; 65:483–487.
90. Knochel JP. The pathophysiology and clinical characteristics of severe hypophosphatemia. Arch Intern Med 1977; 137:203–220.
91. Knochel JP. Neuromuscular manifestations of electrolyte disorders. Am J Med 1982; 72:521–535.
92. Knochel JP. Diuretic-induced hypokalemia. Am J Med 1984; 77(Suppl5A):11–17.
93. Kok-Jensen A. Simple electrocardiographic features of importance for prognosis in severe chronic bronchial obstruction. Scand J Respir Dis 1975; 56:273–284.

94. Koo KW, San DS, Snider GL. Arterial blood gases and pH during sleep in chronic obstructive pulmonary disease. Am J Med 1975; 58:663.
95. Kueppers F. Genetically determined differences in the response of alpha-1-antitrypsin levels in human serum to typhoid vaccine. Humangenetik 1968; 6:207.
96. Kueppers F, Black LF. α_1-Antitrypsin and its deficiency. Am Rev Respir Dis 1974; 110:176–194.
97. Kueppers F, Briscoe WA, Bearn AG. Hereditary deficiency of α_1-antitrypsin. Science 1964; 146:1678–1679.
98. Landay RA, Gonzalez MA, Taylor JC. Effect of phenobarbital on theophylline disposition. J Allergy Clin Immunol 1978; 62:27–29.
99. Laurell CB. Antigen-antibody crossed electrophoresis. Anal Biochem 1965; 10:358.
100. Laurell CB, Eriksson S. The electrophoretic α_1-globulin pattern of serum in α_1-antitrypsin deficiency. Scand J Clin Lab Invest 1963; 15:132–140.
101. Lawrence JH, Berlin NI. Relative polycythemia—the polycythemia of stress. Yale J Biol Med 1952; 24:498–505.
102. Lees AW, McNaught W. Bacteriology of lower respiratory tract secretions, sputum and upper-respiratory-tract secretions in "normals" and chronic bronchitics. Lancet 1959; 1112–1115.
103. Leitch AG, Clancy LJ, Costello JF, Flenley DC. Effect of intravenous infusion of salbutamol on ventilatory response to carbon dioxide and hypoxia and on heart rate and plasma potassium in normal men. Br Med J 1976; 1:365–367.
104. Lertzman M, Israels LG, Cherniack RM. Erythropoiesis and ferrokinetics in chronic respiratory disease. Ann Intern Med 1962; 56:821–833.
105. Levine JH, Micheal JR, Guarnieri T. Treatment of multifocal atrial tachycardia with verapamil. N Engl J Med 1985; 312:21–25.
106. Lewis MI, Belman MJ, Dorr-Uyemura L. Nutritional supplementation in ambulatory patients with chronic obstructive pulmonary disease. Am Rev Respir Dis 1987; 135:1062–1068.
107. Lieberman J, Gaidulis L, Garoutte B, Mittman C. Identification and characteristics of the common alpha$_1$-antitrypsin phenotypes. Chest 1972; 62:557–594.
108. Lieberman J, Mittman C, Kent JR. Screening for heterozygous α_1-antitrypsin deficiency III. A provocative test with diethylstilbestrol and effect of oral contraceptives. JAMA 1971; 217:1198.
109. Lieberman J, Winter B, Sastre A. Alpha$_1$-antitrypsin pi-types in 965 COPD patients. Chest 1986; 89:370–373.
110. Lourenco RV, Loddenkemper R, Carton RW. Patterns of distribution and clearance of aerosols in patients with bronchiectasis. Am Rev Respir Dis 1972; 106:857–866.
111. Lowell FC. The total eosinophil count in obstructive pulmonary disease. N Engl J Med 1975; 292:1182–1183.
112. Mancini G, Carbonara AO, Heremans JF. Immunochemical quantification of antigens by single radial immunodiffusion. Immunol Chem 1965; 2:235–254.
113. Manfredi RL, Vesell ES. Inhibition of theophylline metabolism by long-term allopurinol administration. Clin Pharmacol Ther 1981; 29:224–229.
114. Mangione A, Imhoff TE, Lee RV, et al. Pharmacokinetics of theophylline in hepatic disease. Chest 1978; 73:616–622.
115. Marchandise B, De Bruyne B, Delaunois L, Kremer R. Noninvasive prediction of pulmonary hypertension in chronic obstructive pulmonary disease by Doppler echocardiography. Chest 1987; 91:361–365.
116. Marchlinski FE, Miller JD. Atrial arrhythmias exacerbated by theophylline. Response to verapamil and evidence for triggered activity in man. Chest 1985; 88:931–934.
117. Marquis JF, Carruthers SG, Spence JD, et al. Phenytoin-theophylline interaction. N Engl J Med 1982; 307:1189–1190.
118. Matheson LE, Bighley L, Hendeles L. Drug interference with the Schack and Waxler plasma theophylline assay. Am J Hosp Pharm 1977; 34:496–499.
119. May JR. Pathogenic bacteria in chronic bronchitis. Lancet 1954; ii:839–842.
120. May JR. The bacteriology of chronic bronchitis. Lancet 1953; ii:534–537.
121. McElnay JC, Smith GD, Helling DK. A practical guide to interactions involving theophylline kinetics. Drug Intell Clin Pharm 1982; 16:533–542.
122. Medici TC, Chodosh S. Sputum cell dynamics in bacterial exacerbations of chronic bronchial disease. Arch Intern Med 1972; 129:597–603.
123. Melethil S, Carlson J, Houg M. Predictability of theophylline levels. Drug Intell Clin Pharm 1982; 16:695–698.
124. Mendella LA, Manfreda J, Warren CPW, Anthonisen NR. Steroid response in stable chronic obstructive pulmonary disease. Ann Intern Med 1982; 96:17–21.
125. Metropolitan Life Insurance Company. New Weight Standards for Men and Women. New York: Metropolitan Life, 1983.
126. Miech RP, Stein MS. Methylxanthines. Clin Chest Med 1986; 7:331–340.
127. Miller DL. A study of techniques for the examination of sputum in a field survey of chronic bronchitis. Am Rev Respir Dis 1963; 88:473–483.
128. Miller DL, Jones R. The bacterial flora of the upper respiratory tract and sputum of working men. J Pathol Bacteriol 1964; 87:182–186.
129. Morse JO, Lebowitz MD, Knudson RJ, Burrows B. Relation of protease inhibitor phenotypes to obstructive lung diseases in a community. N Engl J Med 1977; 296:1190–1194.
130. Murray JF. Arterial studies in primary and secondary polycythemic disorders. Am Rev Respir Dis 1965; 92:435–449.
131. Murray PR, Washington JA II. Microscopic and bacteriologic analysis of expectorated sputum. Mayo Clin Proc 1975; 50:339–344.
132. Nenci GG, Berretini M, Todisco T, et al. Exhausted platelets in chronic obstructive pulmonary disease. Respiration 1983; 44:71–76.
133. Newman JH, Neff TA, Ziporin P. Acute respiratory failure associated with hypophosphatemia. N Engl J Med 1977; 296:1101–1103.
134. Nielsen-Kudsk F, Magnussen I, Jakobsen P. Pharmacokinetics of theophylline in ten elderly patients. Acta Pharmacol et Toxicol 1978; 42:226–234.
135. Openbrier DR, Irwin MM, Rogers RM, et al. Nutritional status and lung function in patients with emphysema and chronic bronchitis. Chest 1983; 83:17–22.
136. Owens GR, Rogers RM, Pennock BE, Levin D. The diffusing capacity as a predictor of arterial oxygen desaturation during exercise in patients with chronic obstructive pulmonary disease. N Engl J Med 1984; 310:1218–1221.
137. Patakas DA, Christaki PI, Louridas GE, Sproule BJ. Control of breathing in patients with chronic obstructive lung diseases and secondary polycythemia after venesection. Respiration 1986; 49:257–262.
138. Patel AK, Skatrud JB, Thomsen JH. Cardiac arrhythmias due to oral aminophylline in patients with chronic obstructive pulmonary disease. Chest 1981; 80:661–665.
139. Paterson IC, Petrie GR, Crompton GK, Robertson JR. Chronic bronchitis: Is bacteriological examination of sputum necessary? Br Med J 1978; 2:537–538.
140. Pecora DV, Brook R. A method of securing uncontaminated tracheal secretions for bacterial examination. J Thoracic Surg 1959; 37:653–654.
141. Philips RW. The electrocardiogram in cor pulmonale secondary to pulmonary emphysema: A study of 18 cases proved by autopsy. Am Heart J 1958; 56:352.
142. Phillips J, Spano J, Burch G. Chaotic atrial mechanism. Am Heart J 1969; 78:171–179.
143. Phillips PJ, Vedig AE, Jones PL, et al. Metabolic and cardiovascular side effects of the beta$_2$-adrenoceptor agonists salbutamol and rimiterol. Br J Clin Pharmacol 1980; 9:483–491.
144. Pierce AF, Jarrett CE, Werkle G, Miller WF. Respiratory function during sleep in patients with chronic obstructive lung disease. J Clin Invest 1966; 45:631–636.
145. Pines A, Raafat H, Greenfield JSB, et al. Antibiotic regimens in moderately ill patients with purulent exacerbations of chronic bronchitis. Br J Dis Chest 1972; 66:107–115.
146. Planas RF, McBrayer RH, Koen PA. Effects of hypophosphatemia on pulmonary muscle performance. Adv Exp Med Biol 1982; 151:283–290.
147. Powell JR, Thiercelin JF, Vozeh S, et al. The influence of cigarette smoking and sex on theophylline disposition. Am Rev Respir Dis 1977; 116:17–23.
148. Raoof S, Wollschlager C, Khan FA. Ciprofloxacin increases serum levels of theophylline. Am J Med 1987; 82(Suppl 4A): 115–118.

149. Reinecke T, Seger D, Wears R. Rapid assay of serum theophylline levels. Ann Emerg Med 1986; 15:147–151.
150. Renton KW, Gray JD, Hung OR. Depression of theophylline elimination by erythromycin. Clin Pharmacol Ther 1981; 30:422–426.
151. Renzetti AD, McClement JH, Litt BD. The Veterans Administration Cooperative study of pulmonary function. Mortality in relation to respiratory function in chronic obstructuve pulmonary disease. Am J Med 1966; 41:1115–1129.
152. Richens JM, Howard P. Oedema in cor pulmonale. Clin Sci 1982; 62:255–259.
153. Robinson CA, Dobbs J. Acetazolamide interference with theophylline analysis by high performance liquid chromatography. Clin Biol Chem 1978; 24:2208–2209.
154. Roza AM, Shizgal HM. The Harris Benedict equation reevaluated: Resting energy requirements and the body cell mass. Am J Clin Nutr 1984; 40:168–182.
155. Sachs FL. Chronic bronchitis. Clin Chest Med 1981; 2:79–89.
156. Sackner MA, Rosen MJ, Wanner A. Estimation of tracheal mucous velocity by bronchofibroscopy. J Appl Physiol 1973; 34:495–499.
157. Sagone AL, Balcerzak SP. Smoking as a cause of erythrocytosis. Ann Intern Med 1975; 82:512–515.
158. Santa Cruz R, Landa J, Hirsch J, Sackner MA. Tracheal mucous velocity in normal man and patients with obstructive lung disease; effects of terbutaline. Am Rev Respir Dis 1974; 109:458–463.
159. Schooley JC, Mahlamann LJ. Hypoxia and the initiation of erythropoietin production. Blood Cells 1975; 1:429–448.
160. Schreiner A, Bjerkestrand G, Digranes A, et al. Bacteriologic findings in the transtracheal aspirate from patients with acute exacerbations of chronic bronchitis. Infection 1978; 6:54–56.
161. Segal N, Bishop JM. The circulation in patients with chronic bronchitis and emphysema at rest and during exercise, with special reference to the influence of changes in blood viscosity and blood volume on the pulmonary circulation. J Clin Invest 1966; 45:1555–1568.
162. Shaw DB, Simpson T. Polycythaemia in emphysema. Q J Med, 1961; 118:135–152.
163. Shepard JW, Garrison MW, Grither DA, et al. Relationship of ventricular ectopy to nocturnal oxygen desaturation in patients with chronic obstructive pulmonary disease. Am J Med 1985; 78:28–34.
164. Shetty PS, Jung RT, Watrasiewicz KE, James WPT. Rapid-turnover transport proteins: An index of subclinical protein-energy malnutrition. Lancet 1979; ii:230–232.
165. Shim C, Stover DE, Williams MH. Response to corticosteroids in chronic bronchitis. J Allergy Clin Immunol 1978; 62:363–367.
166. Shine KI, Kastor JA, Yurchak PM. Multifocal atrial tachycardia: clinical and electrocardiographic features in 32 patients. N Engl J Med 1968; 7:344–349.
167. Short MD, Dowsett DJ, Heaf PJD, et al. A comparison between monodisperse Tc-99m-labeled aerosol particles and Kr-81m for the assessment of lung function. J Nucl Med 1979; 20:194–200.
168. Shuck JW, Walder J, Oetgen WJ, Thomas HM. Right ventricular visualization by thallium-201 myocardial scintigraphy in chronic obstructive pulmonary disease. South Med J 1985; 78:1435–1439.
169. Sideris DA, Katsadoros DP, Valianos G, et al. Type of cardiac dysrhythmias in respiratory failure. Am Heart J 1975; 89:32–35.
170. Smit JM, Burema J, May JF, et al. Prognosis in severe chronic obstructive pulmonary disease with regard to the electrocardiogram. J Electrocardiol 1983; 16:77–86.
171. Smith JR, Landaw SA. Smokers' polycythemia. N Engl J Med 1978; 298:6–10.
172. Soldrui SJ, Hill JG. A rapid micromethod for measuring theophylline in serum by reverse phase high performance liquid chromatography. Clin Biochem 1977; 10:74–77.
173. Soroldoni M, Ferrarini F, Biffi E, et al. M-mode subxiphoid echocardiography in assessing pulmonary hypertension. Its usefulness in chronic obstructive pulmonary disease. Respiration 1985; 47:164–170.
174. Spencer CD, Beaty HN. Complications of transtracheal aspiration. N Engl J Med 1972; 286:304–306.
175. Spodick DH, Hauger-Klevene JH, Tyler JM, et al. The electrocardiogram in pulmonary emphysema. Am Rev Respir Dis 1963; 88:14–19.
176. Steele P, Ellis JH, Weily HS, Genton E. Platelet survival time in patients with hypoxemia and pulmonary hypertension. Circulation 1977; 55:660–662.
177. Sternberg JC. A rate nephelometer for measuring specific proteins by immunoprecipitin reactions. Clin Chem 1977; 23:1456–1464.
178. Stockley RA, Afford SC, Burnett D. Assessment of 7S and 11S immunoglobulin A in sputum. Am Rev Respir Dis 1980; 122:959–964.
179. Stockley RA, Mistry M, Bradwell AR, Burnett D. A study of plasma proteins in the sol phase of sputum from patients with chronic bronchitis. Thorax 1979; 34:777–782.
180. Stradling JR, Lane DJ. Development of secondary polycythaemia in chronic airways obstruction. Thorax 1981; 36:321–325.
181. Tager I, Speizer FE. Role of infection in chronic bronchitis. N Engl J Med 1975; 292:563–571.
182. Talamo RC, Langley CE, Levine BW, Kazemi H. Genetic vs. quantitative analysis of serum $alpha_1$-antitrypsin. N Engl J Med 1972; 287:1067–1069.
183. Tavill AS, Kershenobick D. Regulation of transferrin synthesis. In: Peters M, ed. Protides of the Biological Fluids. Proceedings of the 19th Colloquium. Oxford: Pergamon Press, 1971, 489–493.
184. Thomson ML, Short MD. Mucociliary function in health, chronic obstructive airway disease, and asbestosis. J Appl Physiol 1969; 26:535–539.
185. Tirlapur VG, Mir MA. Nocturnal hypoxemia and associated electrocardiographic changes in patients with chronic obstructive airways disease. N Engl J Med 1982; 306:125–130.
186. Tobin MJ. Diagnosis of pneumonia: Techniques and problems. Clin Chest Med 1987; 8:513–527.
187. Tornatore KM, Kanarkowski R, McCarthy TL, et al. Effect of chronic oral contraceptive steroids on theophylline disposition. Eur J Clin Pharmacol 1982; 23:129–134.
188. Tremoli E, Bertoli L, Maderna P, et al. Platelet anti-aggregating therapy in chronic obstructive lung disease. Clin Respir Phys 1980; 16:84–90.
189. Trowbride FL, Hiner CD, Robertson AD. Arm muscle indicators and creatinine excretion in children. Am J Clin Nutr 1982; 36:691–696.
190. Tura S, Pollycove M, Gelpi AP. Erythrocyte and iron-kinetics in patients with chronic pulmonary emphysema. J Nucl Med 1962; 3:110–127.
191. Vandenburgh E, Van de Woestigne K, Gyselen A. Weight changes in the terminal stages of chronic obstructive pulmonary disease. Am Rev Respir Dis 1967; 96:536–565.
192. Vanier T, Dulfano MJ, Wu C, Desforges JF. Emphysema, hypoxia and the polycythemic response. N Engl J Med 1963; 269:169–178.
193. Vaughan LM, Milavetz G, Ellis E, et al. Multicentre evaluation of a disposable visual measuring device to assay theophylline from capillary blood sample. Lancet 1986; i:184–186.
194. Wald JA, Friedman BF, Farr RS. An improved protocol for the use of troleandomycin (TAO) in the treatment of steroid-requiring asthma. J Allergy Clin Immunol 1986; 78:36–43.
195. Wasserburger RH, Kelly JR, Rasmussen HK, Juhl JH. The electrocardiographic pentalogy of pulmonary emphysema. Circulation 1959; 20:831–841.
196. Wedzicha JA, Cotes PM, Empey DW, et al. Serum immunoreactive erythropoietin in hypoxic lung disease with and without polycythaemia. Clin Sci 1985; 69:413–422.
197. Weil JV, Jamieson G, Brown DW, et al. The red cell mass-arterial oxygen relationship in normal man. J Clin Invest 1968; 47:1627–1639.
198. Weinberger M, Hendeles L. Slow-release theophylline: Rationale and basis for product selection. N Engl J Med 1983; 308:760–764.
199. Weinberger MW, Ginchansky E. Dose-dependent kinetics of theophylline disposition in asthmatic children. J Pediatr 1977; 91:820–824.
200. Weinreb NJ, Shih CF. Spurious polycythemia. Seminar Hematol 1975; 12:397–407.
201. Weisse AB, Moschos CB, Frank MJ, et al. Hemodynamic effects of staged hematocrit reduction in patients with stable cor pulmonale and severely elevated hematocrit levels. Am J Med 1975; 58:92–98.
202. White RJ, Woodings DF. Impaired water handling in chronic obstructive airways disease. Br Med J 1971; 2:561–563.
203. Wiggins J, Hill SL, Stockley RA. Lung secretion sol-phase proteins: Comparison of sputum with secretions obtained by direct sampling. Thorax 1983; 38:102–107.

204. Wilson D, Wright E, Rogers R, Anthonisen N. Body weight in COPD. Am Rev Respir Dis 1987; 135:A144.
205. Wilson DO, Rogers RM, Sanders MH, et al. Nutritional intervention in malnourished patients with emphysema. Am Rev Respir Dis 1986; 134:672–677.
206. Wilson RH, Borden CW, Ebert RV. Adaptation to anoxia in chronic pulmonary emphysema. Arch Intern Med 1951; 88:581–590.
207. Wintrobe MM. Polycythemia: Erythrocytosis. In: Wintrobe MM, ed. Clinical Hematology. 8th ed. Philadelphia: Lea & Febiger, 1981, 991–1010.
208. Wong LK, Barry AL, Horgan SM. Comparison of six different criteria for judging the acceptability of sputum specimens. J Clin Microbiol 1982; 16:627–631.
209. Woodman TF, Canada AT, Seidman J. Interference of allopurinol and alloxanthine in ultraviolet theophylline assay. Am J Hosp Pharm 1977; 34:984–985.
210. Yamaoka S, Yonekura Y, Koide H, et al. Noninvasive method to assess cor pulmonale in patients with chronic obstructive pulmonary disease. Chest 1987; 92:10–17.
211. Yeates DB, Aspin N, Levison H, et al. Mucociliary tracheal transport rates in man. J Appl Physiol 1975; 39:487–495.
212. York EL, Jones RL, Menon D, Sproule BJ. Effects of secondary polycythemia on cerebral blood flow in chronic obstructive pulmonary disease. Am Rev Respir Dis 1980; 121:813–818.
213. Zenker G, Forche G, Harnoncourt K. Two-dimensional echocardiography using a subcostal approach in patients with COPD. Chest 1985; 88:722–725.

Chapter 41

IMAGING IN CHRONIC OBSTRUCTIVE PULMONARY DISEASE

Alan Cohen Floro Miraldi

RADIOGRAPHIC TECHNIQUES

Almost all patients with chronic obstructive pulmonary disease (COPD) receive at least one chest radiograph during their lifetime. Many are also studied by other imaging techniques. Thus, the role of radiographic evaluation in COPD is an important consideration. The limited sensitivity and cost of imaging techniques do not allow them to replace pulmonary function testing (PFT), which is both sensitive and inexpensive. In this chapter, after describing the specific findings present in COPD, the accuracy of the various imaging techniques will be addressed.

Emphysema

Plain film radiographic changes usually associated with emphysema include the following:[1]

1. Alterations in pulmonary parenchymal aeration, including bullae (Figs. 41–1*A* through *D*)
2. Alterations in the pulmonary vasculature (oligemia) and the cardiac contour (Figs. 41–1*B* and *D*)
3. Alterations in the configuration of the chest wall and diaphragm (Figs. 41–1*A* and *D*)

The lungs are typically hyperlucent and may contain blebs, bullae, and pneumatoceles (Fig. 41–1). These result from the destructive process present in the lung interstitium and blood vessels (decreased density), as well as from a generalized overexpansion of the thorax. Whereas hyperinflation was found to correlate reasonably with emphysema by Thurlbeck and colleagues,[2] others have found that hyperinflation alone is not a reliable indicator of significant emphysema.[3] At times significant bullae may occur in lungs that are otherwise normal. Conversely, bullae often may not be recognized by conventional radiography (Fig. 41–1*C*).

Changes in the configuration of the chest wall and diaphragm often occur with emphysema, helping to cause the hyperlucency present on the plain film. The most reliable sign of emphysema is flattening of the dome of the diaphragm.[4] When the superior aspect of the diaphragm has a concave configuration, emphysema is highly likely to be present (Fig. 41–2). Hyperinflation can cause the insertions of the intercostal muscles to be visualized as a serrated or step-like pattern to the top of the diaphragmatic surface. Tenting of the diaphragm may also result from invagination of the thickened visceral pleura between basal bullae.[5] These are certain signs of the presence of emphysema. Unfortunately, not all patients with emphysema manifest these signs, which indicate the presence of significant disease. In fact, the thorax may have a "normal" volume and still have significant disease pathologically.[6]

Other signs usually associated with emphysema are less reliable. A large lung volume cannot be equated with emphysema.[5] Complicating the diagnosis further, normal people can inflate their lungs so that the eleventh rib posteriorly is present at the dome of the diaphragm. This is particularly apparent in long, thin individuals. Depression of the dome of the diaphragm below this level is rarely exceeded in the patient with emphysema.[7]

An increased anterior-posterior diameter and increased retrosternal clear space may indicate an increased lung volume (Fig. 41–3*A* and *B*). Thomson and associates demonstrated that these are unreliable signs.[8] The retrosternal clear space

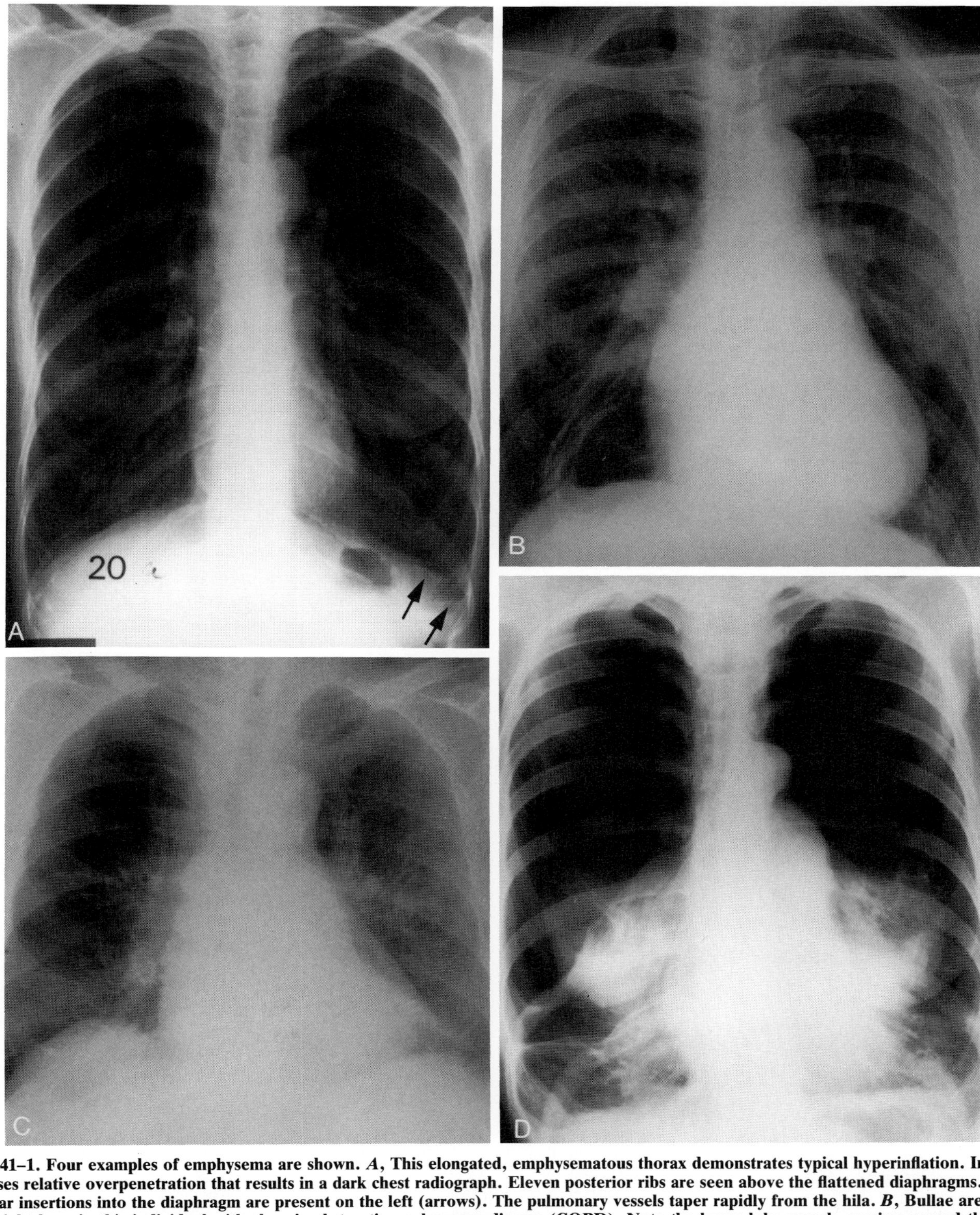

Figure 41–1. Four examples of emphysema are shown. *A*, This elongated, emphysematous thorax demonstrates typical hyperinflation. Increased air causes relative overpenetration that results in a dark chest radiograph. Eleven posterior ribs are seen above the flattened diaphragms. Several muscular insertions into the diaphragm are present on the left (arrows). The pulmonary vessels taper rapidly from the hila. *B*, Bullae are present at the right base in this individual with chronic obstructive pulmonary disease (COPD). Note the lower lobe vessels curving around the bullae and the prominence of the central pulmonary arteries. *C*, This more subtle example of emphysema also contains right lower lung bullae and demonstrates the difficulty in visualizing bullous disease by chest radiography. There are increased interstitial markings at the bases. *D*, Severe bullous disease is present in the upper lung zones. Regions of destroyed lung lack vascular markings. The more normal lung is compressed at the bases causing increased densities. Also note the flattened diaphragms and the large pulmonary trunk above the left heart margin denoting the presence of pulmonary hypertension.

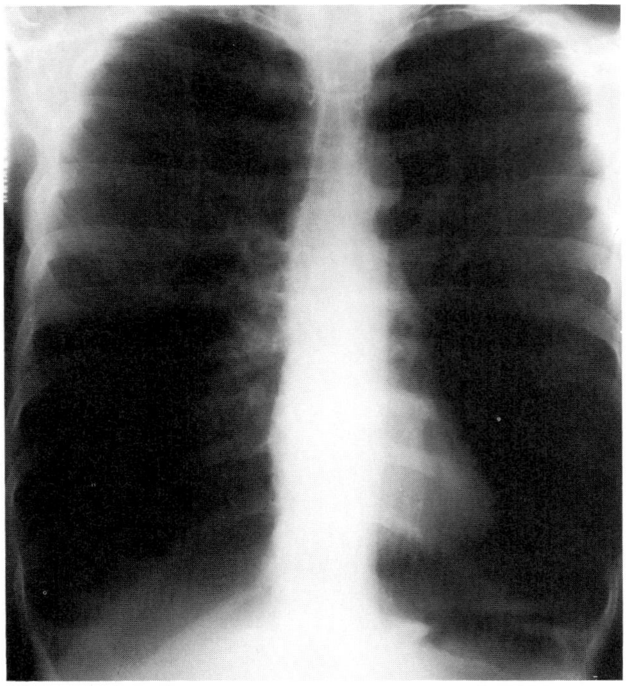

Figure 41–2. Severe flattening of the diaphragms resulting in a concave configuration to their pulmonary margins is present in this patient with alpha$_1$-antitrypsin deficiency. Basilar disease predominates in this condition, which is the classic pathologic example for panlobular emphysema. Note the bilaterally serrated pattern of the diaphragms, which are the intercostal muscular insertions into the diaphragms. The central vessels taper rapidly to all lobes. This is known as pruning.

must measure more than 4.5 cm to be considered an accurate finding. By this time the diaphragm is always flat and the lungs oligemic.[6] Many healthy individuals have a build with a long anterior-posterior dimension. Older individuals develop kyphosis from compression fractures caused by osteoporotic vertebrae. These may mimic hyperinflation.[9, 10]

Fluoroscopic visualization of diaphragmatic excursion can provide a real-time measure of overinflation. The normal diaphragm moves two to three interspaces from full inspiration to full expiration. Motion restricted to one interspace (or less) is pathologic. Special imaging techniques, including kymography or comparison of inspiration-expiration films, have been tried (Fig. 41–4).[1, 11] These techniques never were widely used, because they were less than adequate replacements for pulmonary function testing. Currently they have no role in the evaluation of patients with emphysema.

Computed tomography (CT) scanning can assess the severity of emphysema. Mean lung density can be determined by CT and focal loss of tissue can be imaged clearly.[12–18] The need for determining mean lung density is small and does not represent a study we currently use. CT imaging of emphysema is discussed subsequently.

The heart appears to be small and vertical in position in those with emphysema (Fig. 41–5).[19] This may partly represent a relative cardiac change in size as compared to the enlarged thorax. Some studies have suggested that the heart actually weighs less because of thinning of the left ventricular wall from atrophy.[20] Right ventricular hypertrophy occurs with severe emphysema, but this is difficult to evaluate. The large retrosternal space complicates the determination of right ventricular size. Thus, measurements are usually made of the right atrium, because it is generally easier to analyze than the right ventricle. The normal right atrium makes almost a 180°

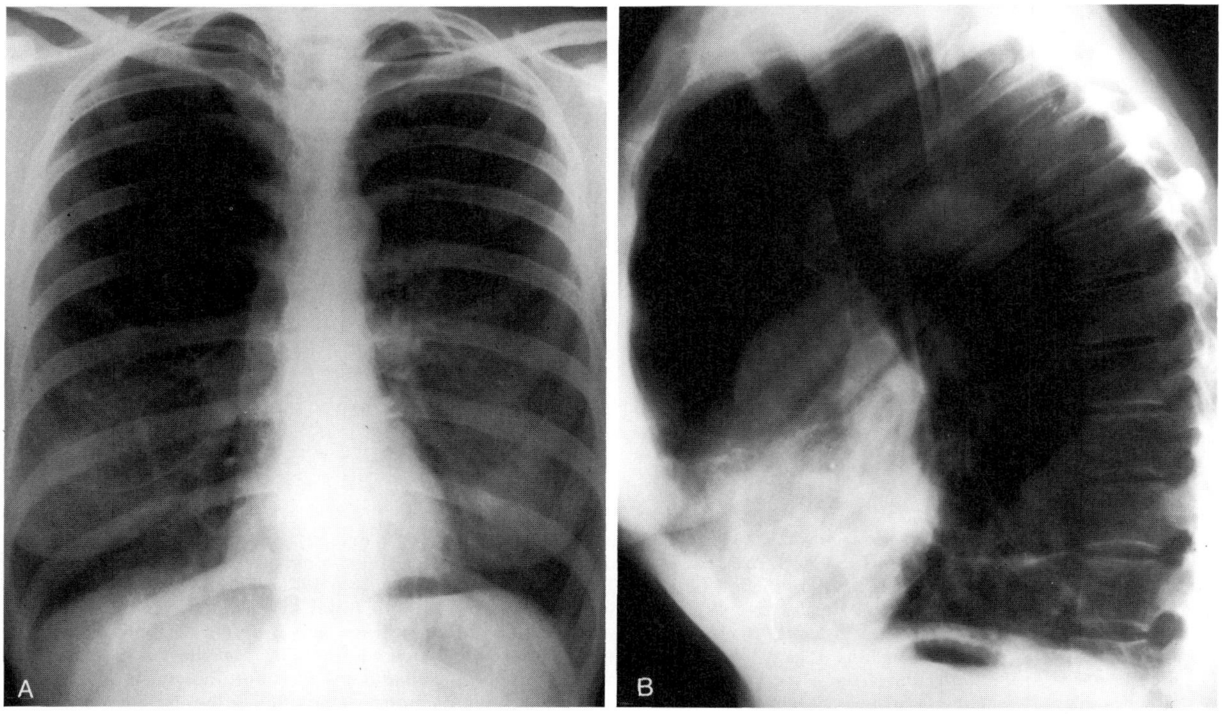

Figure 41–3. Posteroanterior (PA) and lateral chest radiographs in a patient with bullous emphysema. *A*, The posteroanterior (PA) film demonstrates vessels depressed and splayed around the bullae of the large right upper lobe. Pruning of the vessels to the periphery accompanies the lung destruction. Note the marker vessel of the right lower lobe carrying blood diverted from destroyed segments. *B*, The lateral view demonstrates the marked increase in anteroposterior (AP) diameter, increased anterior clear space, and flattened diaphragms.

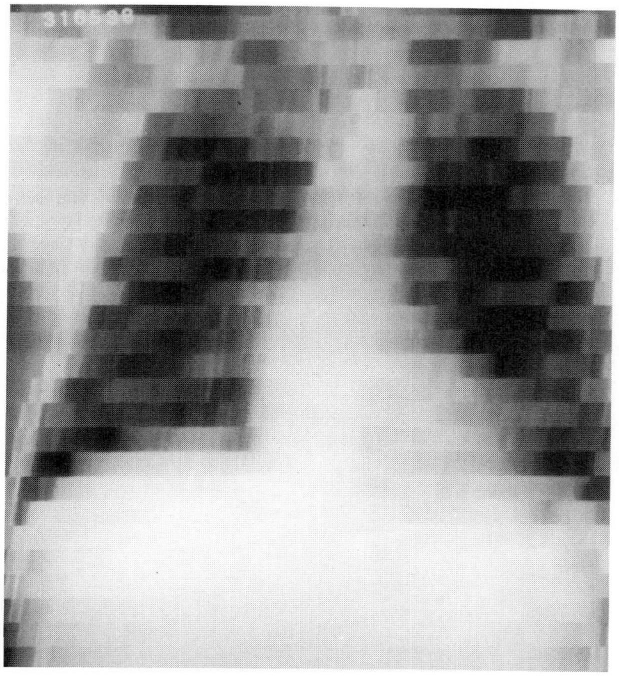

Figure 41–4. This kymogram depicts respiratory motion between inspiration and expiration.

angle with the superior vena cava in the left anterior oblique projection. A significant decrease in that angle implies right heart enlargement.

Prominence of the central pulmonary arteries occurs frequently in those with emphysema (Fig. 41–1*B*). Central vessel enlargement is accompanied by peripheral vessel dropout, which may explain this observation. Part of the central prominence may be illusory, however, caused by the vertical position of the heart.[1] Central vessel prominence may occur without pulmonary hypertension.

A decrease in the caliber of the parenchymal pulmonary vessels accompanied by rapid tapering peripherally (a decrease in the number of vessels) can occur and this is considered a reliable sign of the presence of emphysema by some authors (Figs. 41–1*A*, 41–2, 41–5).[5, 21–24] Sutinen and coworkers[25] demonstrated that the number and caliber of pulmonary vessels often decrease with mild centrilobular emphysema. Vessel changes were always present with moderate or severe disease and correlated with areas of lung destruction. Thurlbeck and Simon[26] have suggested the arterial deficiency pattern is the most reliable sign for the confident diagnosis of emphysema, better than overinflation. The diagnosis of emphysema is often missed, however, when this radiographic criteria is used alone. Nicklaus and colleagues[4] found that vessel attenuation was recognized in a small percentage of patients with moderate or severe emphysema by pulmonary function studies. They also had false positive results and poor interobserver and intraobserver consistency.

Emphysema is a diffuse pulmonary process, but the distribution of the disease is usually nonuniform. This asymmetry results in more local forms, a not unusual finding.[27] Asymmetric pulmonary involvement from nonuniform destruction of the lung allows some regions to retain more intact vessels. Consequently, blood is diverted to the more normal lung so that these vessels enlarge. These have been called "marker vessels" by Simon,[28] and they help to distinguish emphysema from other causes of hyperinflation (Fig. 41–3*A*).

A second recognized pulmonary parenchymal pattern in emphysema is the presence of increased bronchovascular markings.[2, 7, 29] This corresponds to the "dirty chest" (Figs. 41–1*C* and 41–6). The pulmonary vessels are more prominent than normal and have irregular, ill-defined edges. Pulmonary artery enlargement contributes to the increase in markings, at least in some patients.[30, 31] An increase of interstitial markings also occurs, and an increase in small irregular shadows would represent a further extreme in this process. Fraser and Pare[7] noted an element of chronic bronchitis in all their patients with this variant. Thoracic cavity enlargement is less pro-

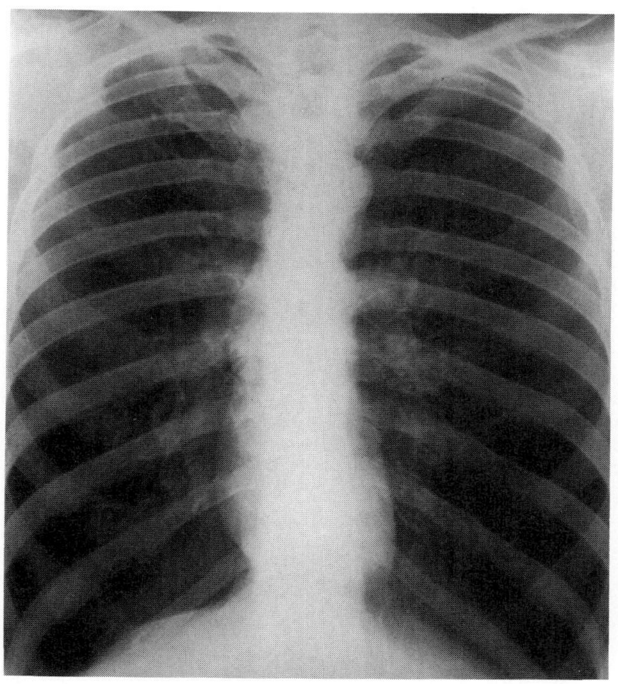

Figure 41–5. A small vertical heart is present in this individual with emphysema. Note severe peripheral pruning of the pulmonary arteries.

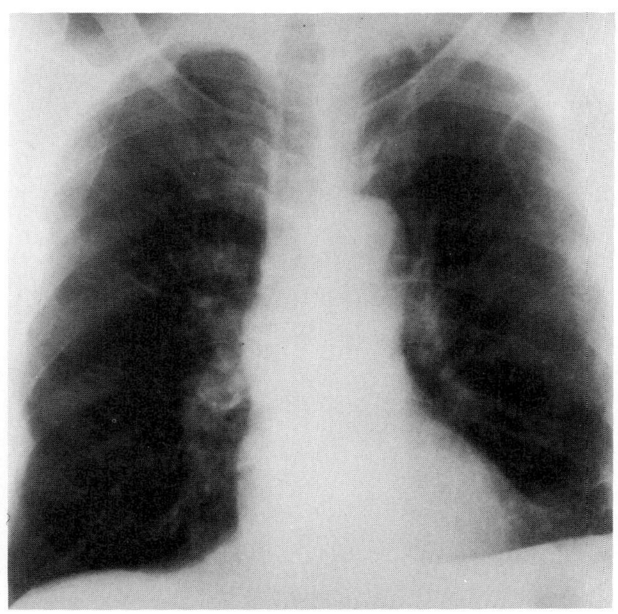

Figure 41–6. An increase in small lines is present, with peripheral accentuation. The vessels are fuzzy in the left lower lung. Some midlung arteries are stretched, possibly curving around regions of destroyed lung.

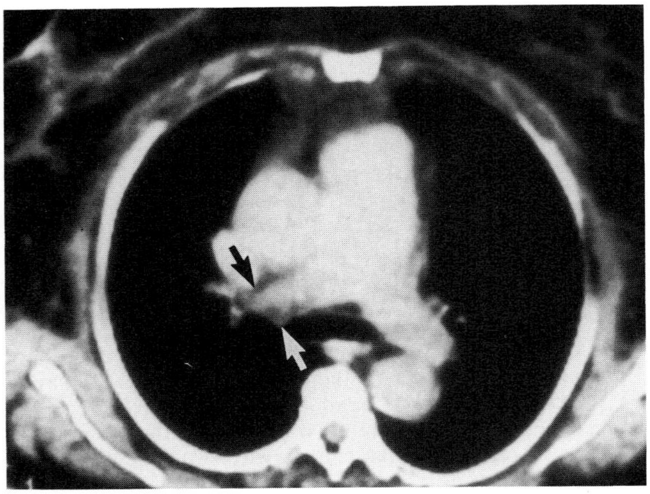

Figure 41–7. Large left and right pulmonary arteries on this computed tomographic (CT) scan allow diagnosis of pulmonary hypertension. Pulmonary artery size measurements are made at the region where the pulmonary artery lies behind the superior vena cava and in front of the trachea or right main stem bronchus (arrows).

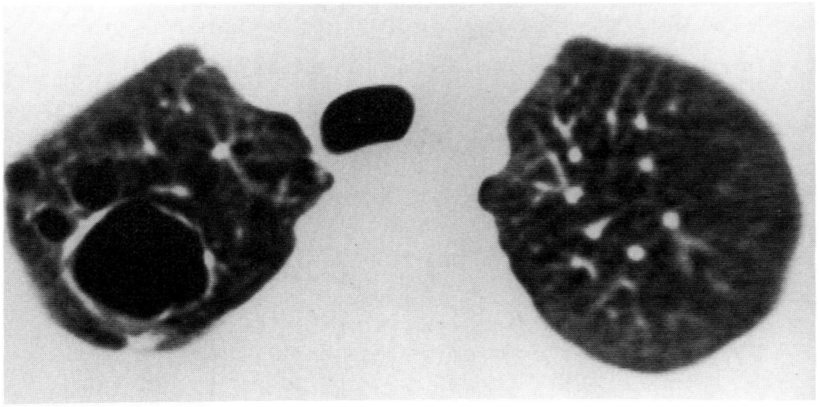

Figure 41–8. Multiple thin-walled holes, bullae, are present in the right upper lobe on this 1 cm thick computed tomographic (CT) slice through the upper thorax. Some splayed vessels are also present.

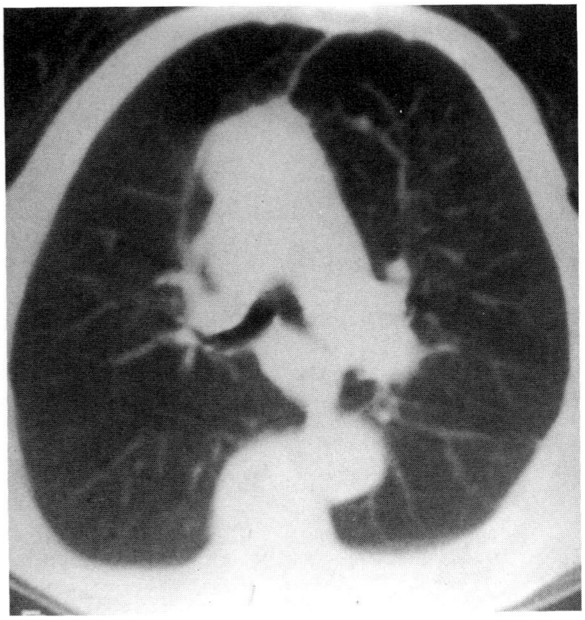

Figure 41–9. Long or accentuated anterior and posterior junction lines are present in this patient with emphysema. Note the absence of posterior, gravity-dependent density changes. An increased anteroposterior (AP) diameter is easily appreciated.

nounced in this subgroup and pulmonary hypertension is more frequent and severe.

Pulmonary hypertension develops late in the disease course. The normal pulmonary circulation has considerable reserve compliance, so that it easily dilates to accommodate changes in regional flow. Development of pulmonary hypertension is generally noted when the main pulmonary arteries become enlarged (Fig. 41–1*D*). This determination is often difficult on the chest radiograph.

CT scanning allows a more accurate determination of the presence of pulmonary hypertension. The normal intrapericardial portion of the right pulmonary artery has a reproducible diameter of 13.3 ± 1.5 mm, giving a 95% confidence level (two standard deviations) of 16.3 mm as the upper limits of normal. Patients with pulmonary hypertension have a mean diameter of 22.4 mm (range, 16.6 to 26.6 mm),[32] making these patients easily separable from the normal population (Fig. 41–7). Pulmonary artery flow as well as pressure determine pulmonary artery size; therefore, exact pulmonary artery pressures cannot be calculated by this technique.

Many attempts have been made to correlate the radiographic findings with the presence of panlobular or centrilobular emphysema. Using standard radiographs, Thurlbeck and associates[29] found that the pattern of increased markings and the pattern of decreased markings or arterial deficiency occur with equal frequency. Although patients with the arterial deficiency pattern more often had panlobular emphysema and those with the increased markings pattern more often had centrilobular emphysema, there was considerable overlap.[7, 29] The specific diagnosis could not be made by plain radiography. In fact, many patients had a mixture of the two patterns, both radiographically and pathologically. Additionally, chronic bronchitis was present in all patients manifesting the increased markings pattern.[29]

CT scanning has added a new dimension to the evaluation of emphysema. In addition to the usual findings, described previously, the use of CT scanning represents a noninvasive method for viewing the lung interstitium with good spatial and density resolution. The imaging parameters employed with CT are important when evaluating COPD patients. Routine, 1-cm thick CT slices suffice for imaging bullous disease, blebs and pneumatoceles; determining lung densities; and obtaining an overall picture of lung structure and destruction. Bullae, blebs, and pneumatoceles present as thin-walled, low-density (air-containing) structures (Fig. 41–8). The normal gravity-dependent density gradient in the lung diminishes or disappears in any diffuse interstitial disease, including emphysema (Fig. 41–9).[13, 33–35] The degree of focal destruction correlates well with the pathologic findings and severity of disease (Fig. 41–10).[12] An increased anteroposterior diameter, accentuated long junction lines, and low diaphragms indicative of pulmonary overexpansion are present on the CT scan (Figs. 41–9 and 41–11 *A* and *B*). Prominent long anterior and posterior junction lines correspond to the enlarged anterior and posterior clear spaces seen on the chest radiograph.

Vascular pruning with or without large, central pulmonary arteries is apparent on CT scan, as are the stretched vessels that curve around bullae. The lung parenchymal density becomes nonhomogeneous from patchy lung destruction and redistribution of blood to the more normal regions.[36]

Thin-section CT—using a CT slice thickness of 1 to 2 mm—allows visualization of all parameters discussed for routine CT, while adding greater morphologic detail (Fig. 41–12*A*, *B*, and *C*). The destroyed, low-density lung parenchyma, with rims of tissue surrounding air spaces, are exquisitely imaged.[15, 37] Thin-section CT has been best characterized for centrilobular emphysema (CLE). In CLE, earlier and more subtle changes of emphysema can be seen; but the earliest changes are still missed.[14] Two pathologic series scanning inflated post-mortem lungs demonstrated low-density focal structures, often in contiguity with the accompanying small arteries.[15, 18] In each series, the degree of CT-imaged lung destruction correlated significantly with the clinical severity of emphysema. The correlation was relative, however, and some cases of CLE could not be correctly separated from normal lung or panlobular emphysema (PLE) in each series. This suggests that CT sometimes aids in the diagnosis of CLE in vivo. Both types of emphysema commonly coexist. Further complicating this distinction may be chronic bronchitis, which is present in a significant percentage of patients with CLE (Fig. 41–13*A*, *B*, and *C*).[15, 18]

The use of CT is not infallible and does not replace pulmonary function testing. Although it is important to recognize emphysema by CT imaging, the use of CT is rarely indicated in the primary evaluation of emphysema. More commonly, emphysema is a disease that is imaged when a CT scan has been obtained for unrelated thoracic pathology.

Emphysema is often complicated by the imposition of another disease process, most commonly pulmonary edema or pneumonia. Radiolucency of the pulmonary parenchyma decreases with the presence of infiltrate. Pulmonary edema also causes the compliance of the lung to decrease, so that the degree of inspiration may decrease[38] and affect the radiolucency.

Conversely, the radiographic appearance of disease can be

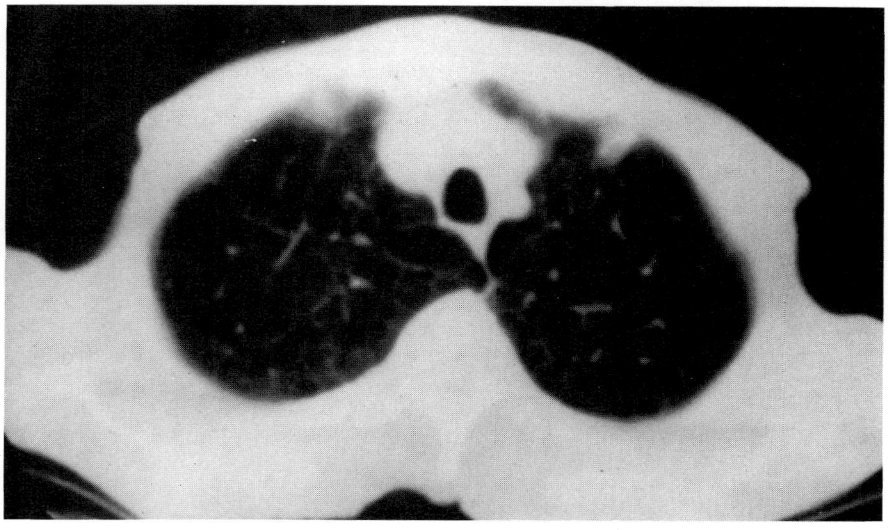

Figure 41–10. Marked emphysema is present, with multiple geographic areas of destroyed lung. Both upper lobes have multiple, large, air-containing structures devoid of vessels demarcated by polygonal remnants of interstitial tissues.

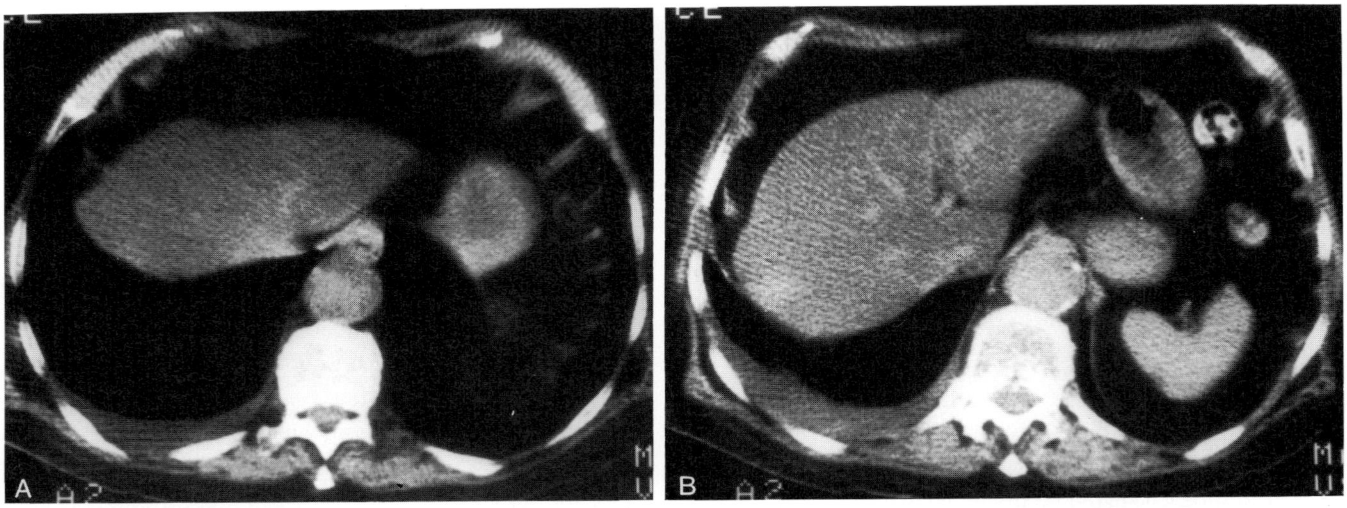

Figure 41–11. Computed tomographic (CT) scan depicts an overexpanded thorax. *A*, The insertions of the intercostal muscles into the diaphragm are present in this over-expanded thorax. Multiple lines (white) outlined by fat (gray) jut into the diaphragm perpendicular to its interface with the lung. *B*, A lower slice on the same patient shows the diaphragmatic point of entry of many of the muscular insertions. These correspond to the serrated appearance of the diaphragm on the chest radiograph.

altered by the presence of emphysema. Unusual patterns of pulmonary edema result from patchy destruction of the interstitial space, which also contains the vasculature. Classic pulmonary vascular redistribution may become impossible when upper lobe vessels are primarily involved (Fig. 41–14).[39] Similarly, changes caused by pneumonia can assume unusual patterns.[40]

Arteriography has been used to demonstrate the vascular and parenchymal findings discussed previously (Fig. 41–15). It is rarely indicated or performed for the diagnosis of emphysema, but the findings of emphysema are often present in patients undergoing pulmonary angiography for other reasons. A few proponents of angiography in emphysema have noted merit in its ability to evaluate patients prior to surgery to predict the outcome of emphysematous lung resections. Lung compressed by bullae has a marked vascular blush, whereas fibrotic, end-stage lung has a decreased vascular pattern.[41–44]

CT scanning has replaced angiography for predicting outcome in the few patients in whom resection of bullae is contemplated. Morgan and coworkers[45] examined 43 patients with emphysema, finding 12 with focal bullous disease. All 12 had improved pulmonary function studies following bullectomy, although the surgical and nonsurgical groups of patients could not be separated by pulmonary function testing before surgery. CT scanning can identify some patients for whom surgical intervention is warranted.[46–48]

Magnetic resonance imaging (MRI), the most recent adjunct to body imaging, has had minimal impact on the imaging of the lung to date. MRI can visualize infiltrates and other pathologic pulmonary processes, but the information gained is inferior in spatial resolution to that obtained by CT.[49–51] Imaging interstitial disease requires high spatial resolution, which is not practicable at this time and may not become realistic in the future. Of greater interest are attempts at monitoring lung physiology using MRI. Determination of tissue relaxation times can provide an estimation of lung water or other metabolites.[52–54] The role this assumes in the future for the diagnosis of emphysema or the monitoring of progression of disease is unknown.

Bronchography is an excellent but outdated means of evaluating the presence and extent of emphysema. Bronchographic findings are listed here for completeness:[55]

1. Small, round, berry-like pools of contrast are seen in those with centrilobular emphysema.
2. Blind-ending airways are present. When several of these airways radiate from a single point, the term "spider" is used.
3. Larger collections of contrast with irregular, flared margins are seen in those with panlobular and centrilobular emphysema.

Chronic Bronchitis

There have been no large radiographic studies of chronic bronchitis; this is probably related to a lack of diagnostic radiographic pulmonary changes. In one study of patients meeting clinical criteria for chronic bronchitis, 50% had no radiographic abnormalities. Hyperinflation was the most common finding in the group with abnormal radiographs.[56] Many patients have concomitant emphysema and chronic bronchitis—thus, hyperinflation is not a diagnostic finding.

Tram lines may be present in the midlung zones, usually at the lower hilar level (Fig. 41–16*A* and *B*). Some have suggested that these represent thickened bronchial walls imaged in a plane parallel with the bronchus. Fraser and coworkers, examining bronchi for wall thickness in a plane perpendicular to the x-ray beam, demonstrated that thickened bronchi correlate with chronic bronchitis to a limited degree. The absence of bronchial wall thickening did not exclude the diagnosis of chronic bronchitis, and many normal subjects had thick bronchial walls.[57]

Accentuated bronchovascular markings (the "dirty chest") is a described finding without adequate explanation.[7] This may represent thickened bronchi and prominent pulmonary arteries (Fig. 41–16*A* and *B*). The margins of the markings are usually fuzzy, suggesting the presence of peribronchiolar and periarterial edema.[55] The main pulmonary arteries are not enlarged, but pulmonary hypertension is often present.

Bronchography was formerly used for diagnosis, although it was never performed solely to diagnose chronic bronchitis. Filling of the mucous glands was considered to be pathognomonic.[56] A later study, in which normal subjects had mucous gland filling, cast doubt on this conclusion.[58] Sharp, square truncation of bronchi at the fifth to eighth branch points may suggest the presence of chronic bronchitis during bronchography.[56]

In summary, the diagnosis of chronic bronchitis is not based on radiographic criteria. It is a clinical and pathologic diagnosis

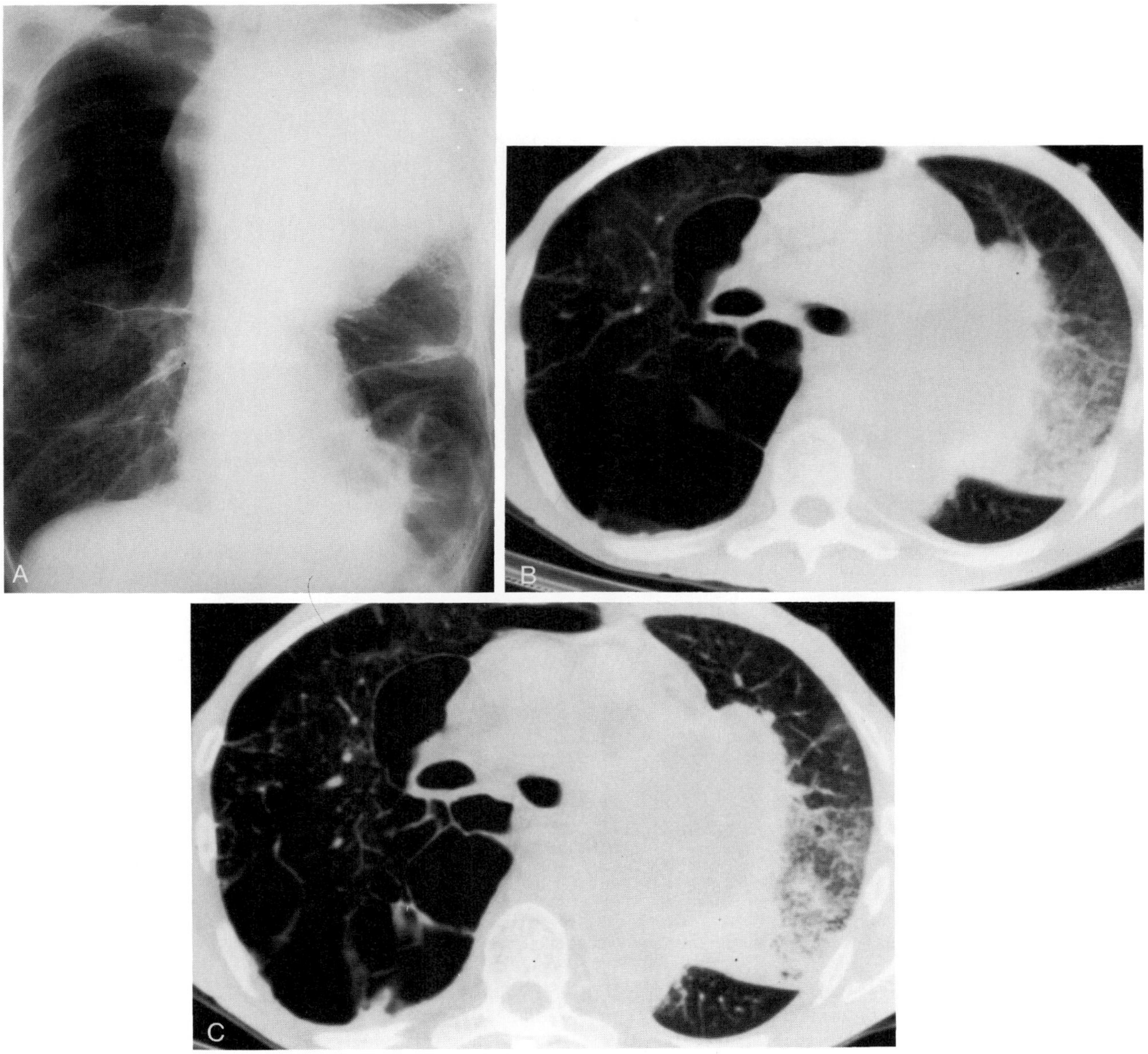

Figure 41–12. This patient has severe emphysema and a left upper lobe bronchogenic carcinoma. This series compares the anatomic detail present on a chest radiograph, a routine 1 cm-computed tomographic (CT) slice, and a thin-section 2 mm-thick CT slice. *A*, A large left upper lobe mass and multiple bilateral bullae are seen on this posteroanterior (PA) chest radiograph. The trachea deviates to the right from the mass. *B*, A 1-cm thick computed tomographic (CT) slice shows the left upper lobe mass with postobstructive pneumonitis. Large bullae are present in the right upper lobe, and the bronchi deviate to the right pushed by the left upper lobe mass. *C*, A 2-mm thick computed tomographic (CT) slice at the same level as *B* has identical findings; however, they are much better shown. Less image averaging allows sharper details. More bullae and tissue structure are seen. Note that many blebs and bullae are subpleural.

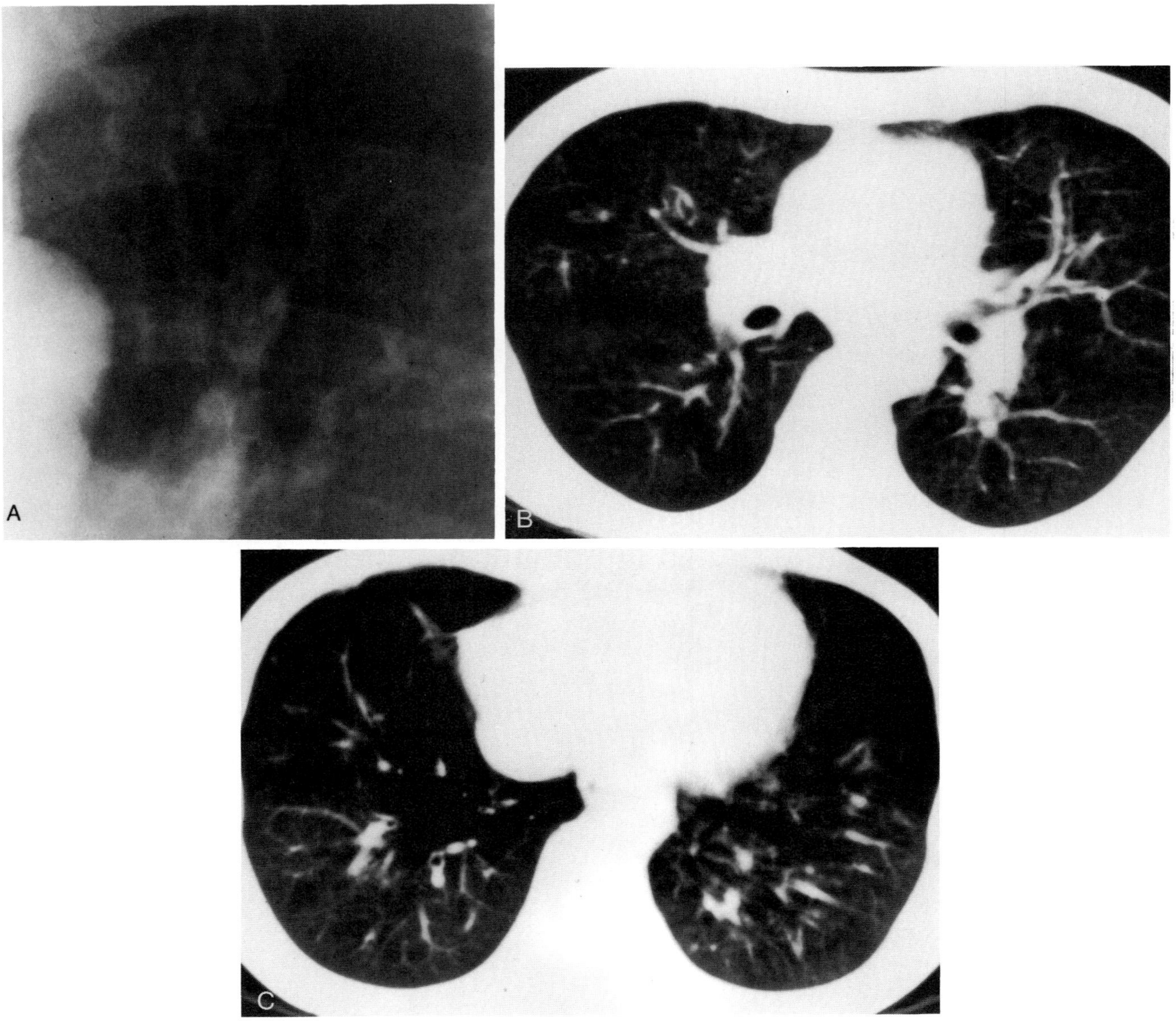

Figure 41–13. Three images are shown of a patient with emphysema and chronic bronchitis. *A*, The left upper lobe is hyperlucent and contains pruned vessels. However, two parallel lines heading cephalad represent peribronchiolar thickening, probably from chronic bronchitis. This finding is also termed "railroad tracking" or "tram lines." *B*, Areas of hyperlucency are seen bilaterally on this computed tomographic (CT) scan. Other areas of increased markings exist. *C*, A lower CT slice shows railroad tracking representing thickened bronchial wall in both posterior lungs. Geographic regions containing hyperlucency and decreased vessels are present in the anterior of both lungs.

that appears, in some cases, to have radiographic abnormalities. Usually it is impossible to determine whether the radiographic findings are caused by chronic bronchitis or other concomitant processes, such as emphysema.

Diagnostic Accuracy of Radiologic Findings in Emphysema

When matched for severity of disease, centrilobular and panlobular emphysema have similar clinical findings.[59] This underlines the difficulty in reaching a specific diagnosis in emphysema. The guidelines presented here may be useful.

Centrilobular emphysema, which causes destruction of the central portion of the pulmonary lobule, presents on CT scan as focal holes, often near an identifiable pulmonary artery. An upper lobe distribution predominates.[14, 15, 60] Panlobular emphysema, which causes uniform destruction of the pulmonary lobule, typically involves the lower lobes, with widespread areas of low attenuation.[26, 60] Severe CLE has a similar appearance to PLE on CT scan, and both have pruned vessels in severe cases.

Paraseptal emphysema involves the distal acinus and therefore is most apparent adjacent to the pleura, where it produces subpleural holes. These are known as blebs and bullae as they enlarge.[60] Only a few cases have been studied by CT scanning, hardly allowing firm conclusions. Furthermore, blebs and bullae can occur in any type of emphysema or in isolation. A fourth category, irregular emphysema, is associated with fibrosis. Localized zones of lucency or bulla are present in regions of pulmonary scarring.

Much of the literature discussing emphysema predates the advent of CT scanning. Some authors have suggested that the various types of emphysema can be distinguished radiographically,[26, 60] but the distinction always rests primarily on the

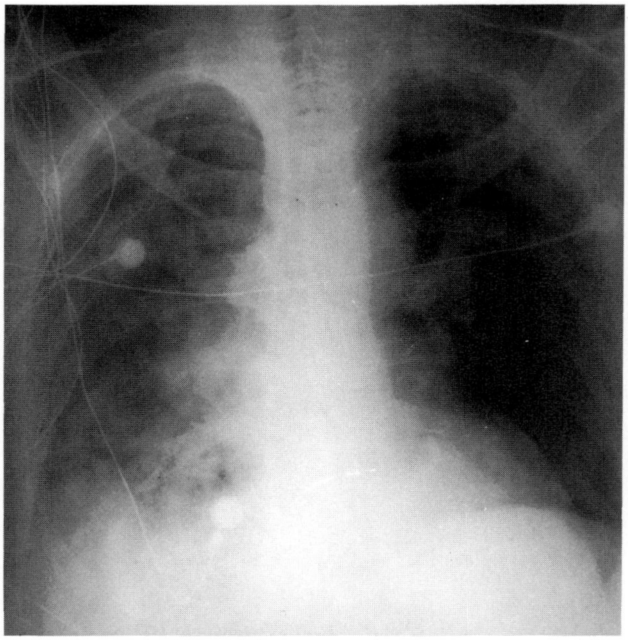

Figure 41–14. This patient with chronic obstructive pulmonary disease (COPD) developed congestive heart failure. Note the alveolar infiltrates are only right sided. Unilateral pulmonary edema resulted from the inability of severely destroyed left lung to respond normally to changes in the intravascular pressure.

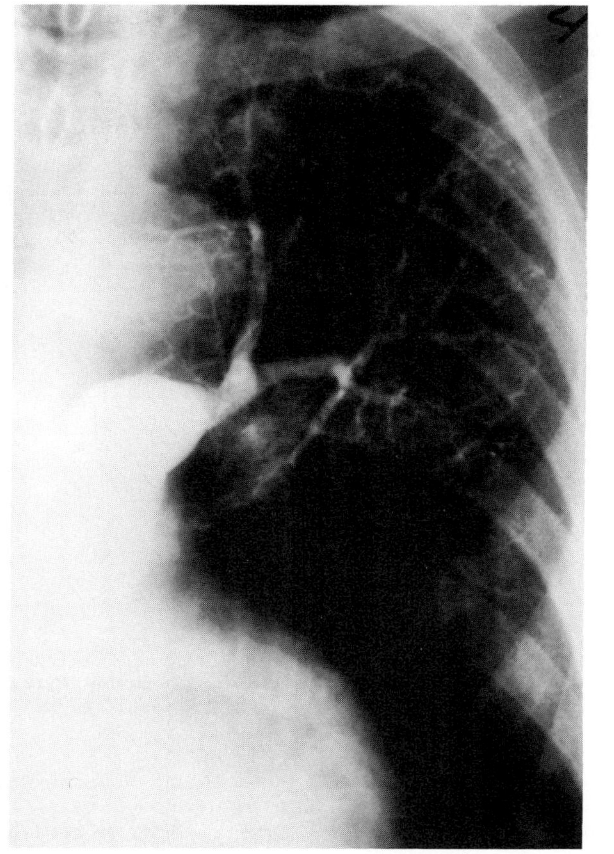

Figure 41–15. This selective pulmonary arteriogram in a patient with emphysema has splayed vessels curving around bullae and marked vascular pruning. Virtually no vessels are noted going into the severely involved left lower lobe.

distribution of the disease process rather than on unique radiographic criteria. There is considerable radiographic and pathologic overlap, particularly as the disease becomes more severe. Complicating the issue is the presence of chronic bronchitis in many individuals having CLE or, more unusually, PLE.

Debate also surrounds the morphologic staging of emphysema by radiographic methods. Some have firmly believed that the chest radiograph allows a reasonable estimation of the extent of disease.[7, 14, 18, 24, 61, 62] Others have emphasized the difficulty in making exact comparisons to the results of pulmonary function testing.[5, 55] The plain film usually underestimates the extent of disease. Chest radiographic and CT findings do correlate with the extent of disease in a general way, and become more accurate as the severity of emphysema increases. Computed tomography is more sensitive in less severe emphysema, allowing more accurate early diagnosis and staging. PFT and proper clinical evaluation, however, cannot be replaced by imaging modalities.

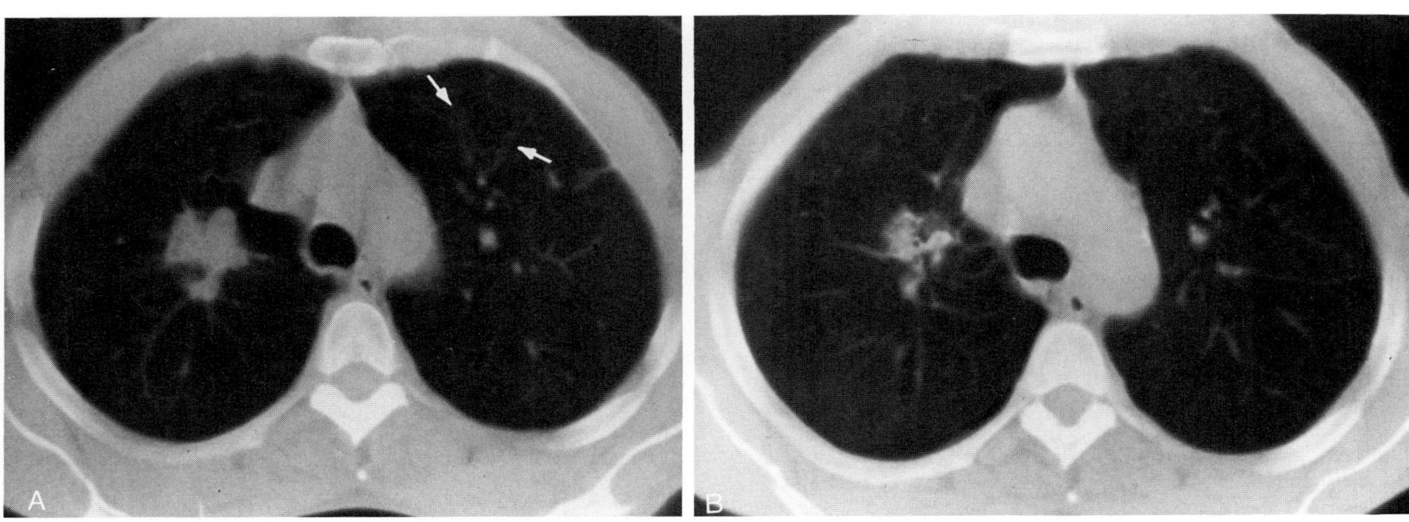

Figure 41–16. This long-time smoker has bronchogenic carcinoma and chronic bronchitis. *A*, The lobulated right upper lobe mass is an adenocarcinoma. There are "tram lines" in the left anterior chest (arrows) and a generalized increase in small markings corresponding to the "dirty chest." This patient had chronic bronchitis. *B*, An adjacent computed tomographic (CT) slice better demonstrates multiple circular shadows consistent with airway wall thickening. The right upper lobe carcinoma is seen as is the generalized increase in interstitial markings.

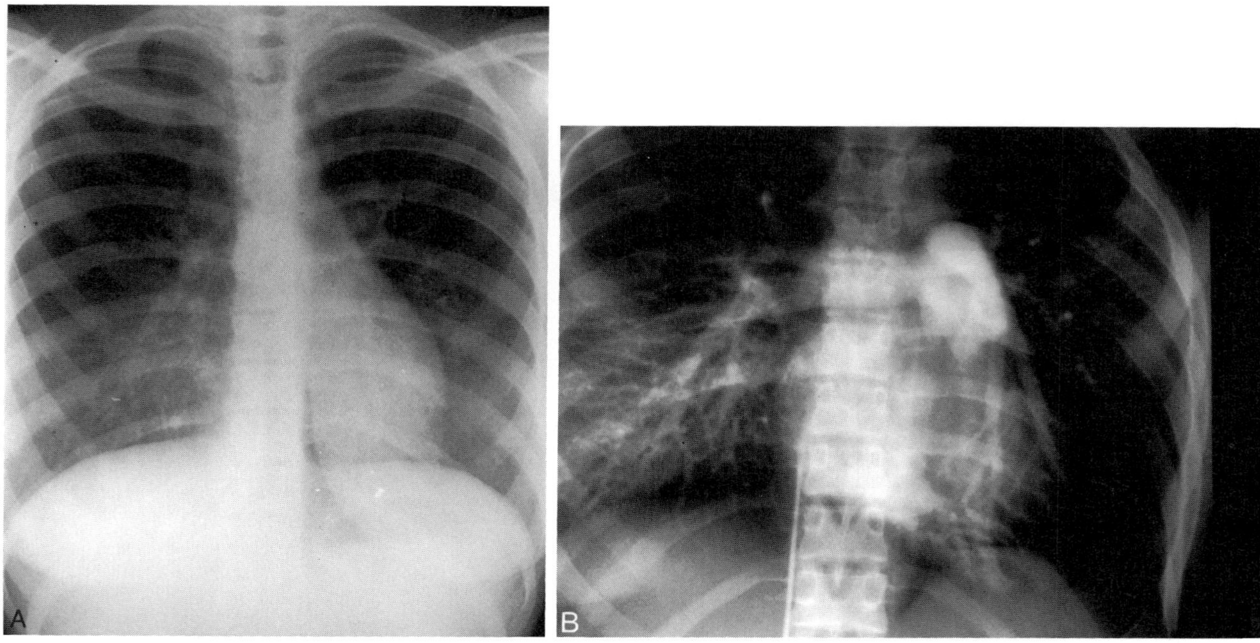

Figure 41–17. Findings in a patient with asthma. *A*, Posteroanterior (PA) chest radiograph in a patient undergoing acute asthmatic attack is overinflated, with slightly large central pulmonary arteries. *B*, A pulmonary arteriogram in the same patient shows the large central arteries with some pruning. Significant distal flow remains in contrast to the severe distal pruning present in emphysema.

Finally, the issue of "pink puffers" and "blue bloaters" requires comment. Few patients fit neatly into either category.[2] Most pink puffers have CLE or PLE, whereas most blue bloaters have chronic bronchitis or mixed chronic bronchitis and CLE. The arterial deficiency pattern is most common in pink puffers. The dirty chest is associated with blue bloaters. In neither case is the radiographic correlation absolute.[55]

Asthma

The chest radiograph may be normal during an acute attack of asthma. Depending on the severity of the attack, the age of onset of symptoms, and other factors, air trapping occurs, causing hyperinflation of the chest.[63, 64] Younger patients exhibit more frequent and severe air trapping than adults.[65–68] Approximately 25% of asthmatic patients have some radiographic abnormality during an acute attack. Hyperinflation, including an increased retrosternal space, bowed sternum, flat diaphragms, and wide intercostal rib spaces, represents the most common constellation of radiographic abnormalities (Fig. 41–17*A*). Another morphologic change, thickened bronchial walls, causes peribronchial cuffing and tram lines. These may disappear with remission of acute symptoms or may persist in the presence of chronic infection. Mucous plugging may develop in dilated bronchi. Transient pulmonary hypertension with large central arteries occurs during the acute attack. Although the central pulmonary arteries are large, they do not taper rapidly, as in emphysema (Fig. 41–17*B*).[68]

The chest radiograph reverts to normal when the bout of asthma terminates. The major usefulness of the chest radiograph is in the diagnosis of superimposed problems, such as pneumonia, exacerbating or triggering an attack, or discovering other complications of asthma that require therapy (Fig. 41–18), such as atelectasis, pneumomediastinum, and pneumothorax.[68] The chest radiograph also helps to exclude other causes of wheezing, such as foreign bodies or congestive heart failure. Other diagnostic radiographic studies are usually not indicated. One exception is the association of asthma and gastroesophageal reflux.[69] A ^{99m}-Tc-sulfur colloid scan, a noninvasive and sensitive method for measuring physiologic gastroesophageal reflux, is indicated in these instances.[70, 71]

Bronchiectasis

There are three types of bronchiectasis generally described in the literature: cylindric, varicose, and saccular.[72] Differentiation is artificial, because they are all variants of the same

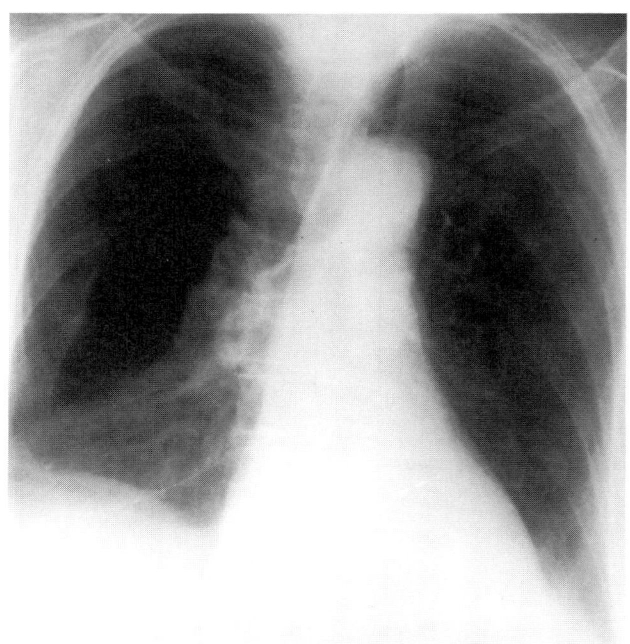

Figure 41–18. A right lower lobe pneumonia triggered this patient's acute asthmatic episode. Note the right lower lobe infiltrate.

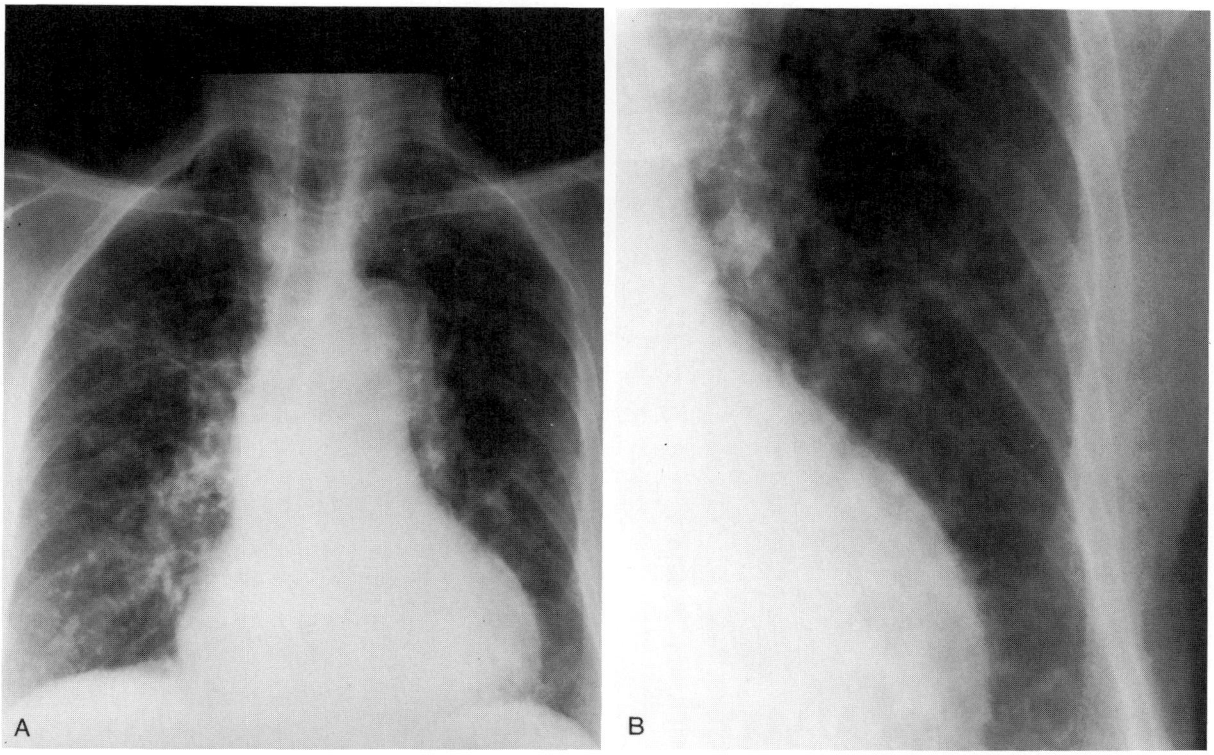

Figure 41–19. Bronchiectasis from infection with atypical mycobacteria is diagnosable from the chest radiograph in this individual. *A*, A generalized increase in small irregular shadows is seen. This is a nonspecific finding. However, the circular markings present represent dilated bronchi in all lung zones. *B*, Cone down view of the left lung better demonstrates some of the circular, ectatic bronchi. These are diagnostic for bronchiectasis.

process—chronic inflammation. The recognition of bronchiectasis is important for making appropriate therapeutic decisions involving antibiotic therapy or surgical intervention.

Abnormalities are often present on the chest radiograph. Nondiagnostic findings include increased markings, atelectasis, localized hyperlucencies, and pleural thickening.[73] In some instances the dilated bronchi can be identified, allowing a positive diagnosis to be made (Fig. 41–19*A* and *B*). Dilated bronchi have a varied appearance related to the amount of fluid inside the dilated, thick-walled bronchial space. Cystic spaces, demilunes inside cystic spaces, air-fluid levels, or fluid-filled ovoid structures describe this continuum. Fibrosis is a late finding in the presence of severe disease.

Diffuse bronchiectasis may be difficult to recognize on the chest radiograph. The thick bronchial walls may be indistinguishable from those seen with interstitial fibrosis. Whereas interstitial fibrosis is usually most severe in the subpleural regions of the lung, bronchiectasis is most severe in the central regions, because it involves bronchi. This distributional distinction may sometimes aid in the recognition of bronchiectasis.

Because the chest radiograph usually does not contain pathognomonic findings, bronchography was formerly used routinely to reach a diagnosis. Bronchographic findings include the following:

1. Dilated airways, identified by the fact that the bronchus becomes larger as it branches (cylindric or varicose forms of bronchiectasis)
2. Cystic puddles of contrast (cystic bronchiectasis)
3. Generalized reduction in the number of bronchial divisions

CT scanning allows more accurate diagnosis of bronchiectasis than chest radiography. Thin-section CT, using 1- to 2-mm thick sections, is mandatory to make maximal use of this modality. Thick-walled, dilated bronchi are identified near the lung periphery on CT scans. An accompanying pulmonary artery forms the signet ring sign. When bronchi are visualized running in plane they form tram lines, with thick walls (Fig. 41–20*A* and *B*).

Early reports suggested that CT scanning could replace bronchography for the diagnosis of bronchiectasis (Fig. 41–21 *A* and *B*);[74, 75] however, subsequent studies found that CT could diagnose or exclude bronchiectasis in approximately 80% of patients.[76, 77] CT scanning is less sensitive than bronchography, underestimating the number of positive patients and the extent of disease (Fig. 41–22*A*, *B*, and *C*).[77] Computed tomographic scanning should be used as a screening procedure for low-risk patients and should be the definitive procedure when bronchiectasis is identified and surgery is not contemplated. Bronchography is needed for high-risk patients having a negative CT scan for bronchiectasis, or when surgery may be indicated.

Bronchiectasis should not be diagnosed on CT scans when dilated bronchi are surrounded by infiltrate, because infection can cause reversible bronchiectasis. End-stage fibrosis can also cause bronchiectasis unrelated to inflammatory processes.[78]

NUCLEAR SCANNING METHODS

Radionuclide techniques for imaging of the lungs (scintigraphy) have gained wide acceptance because they enable the nuclear medicine specialist to determine both regional blood flow and regional ventilation of the lungs.[79] Thus, nuclear techniques provide regional functional information in contrast

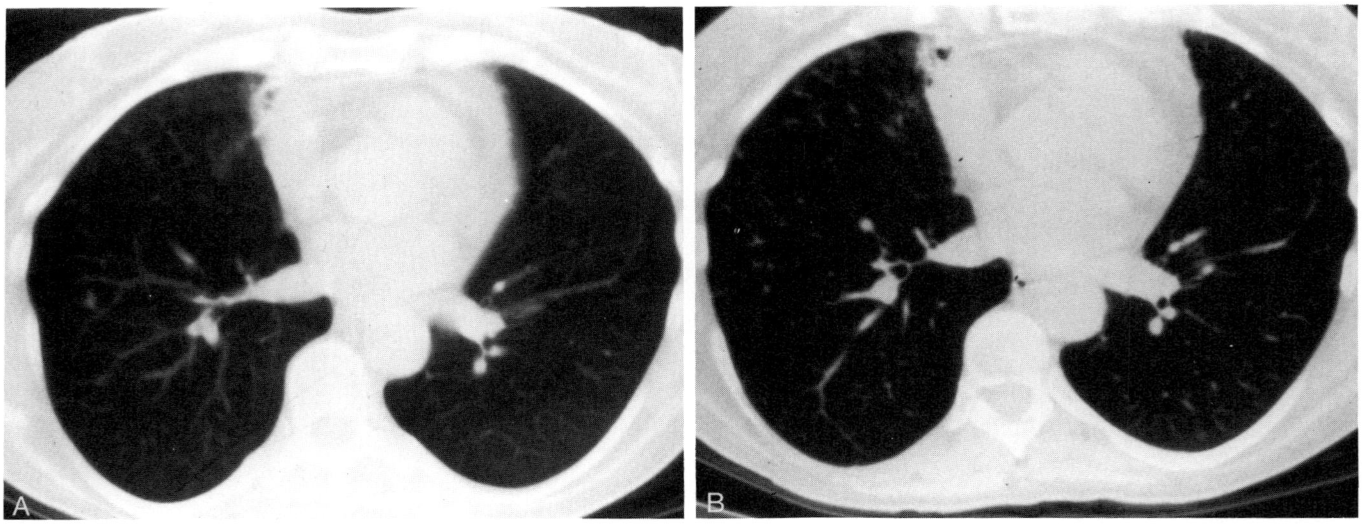

Figure 41–20. Two computed tomographic (CT) slices in a patient with bronchiectasis demonstrate the value of thin-section CT. *A*, The 1-cm thick CT slice shows circular lucencies in the right upper lobe adjacent to the heart with associated volume loss. This is bronchiectasis. *B*, The findings are far sharper and better seen on this 2-mm thick CT slice at a similar level. This patient had three episodes of right upper lobe pneumonia.

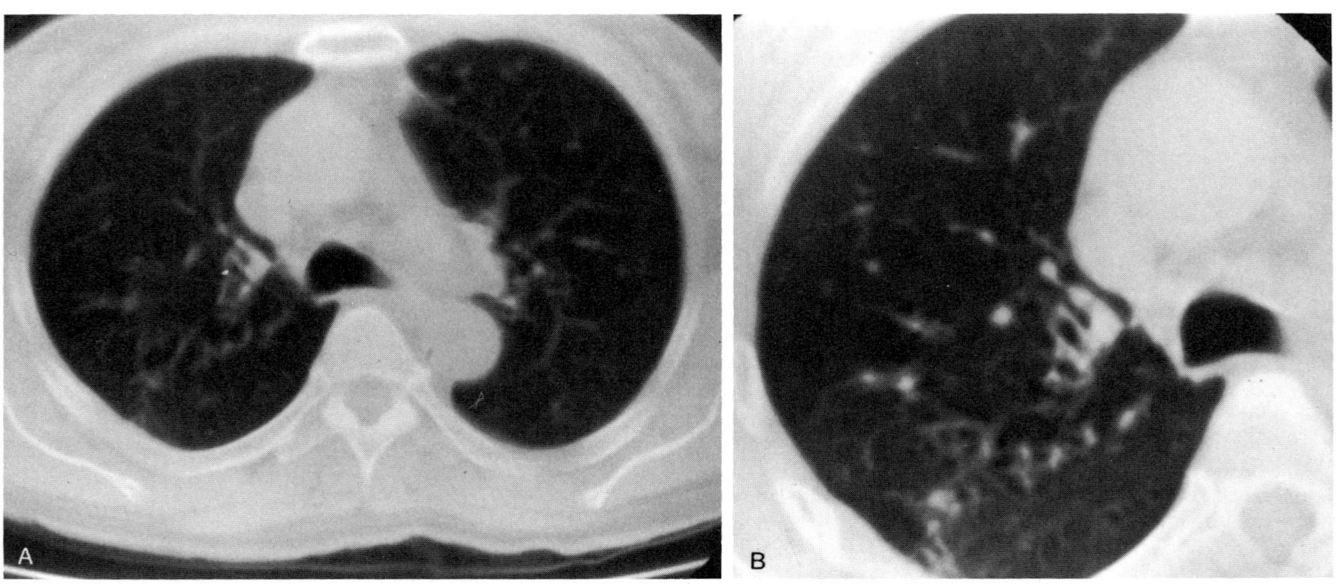

Figure 41–21. This patient had a history of prior infection with *Mycobacterium avium*. Clinical management required proof of the presence and location of suspected bronchiectasis. The chest radiograph was not helpful. *A*, The 1-cm thick computed tomographic (CT) scan shows increased small irregular shadows in the right posterior chest. These were not considered diagnostic for bronchiectasis. *B*, The 2-mm thick CT slice demonstrates posterior circular structures, allowing a definite diagnosis of bronchiectasis without the need for bronchography.

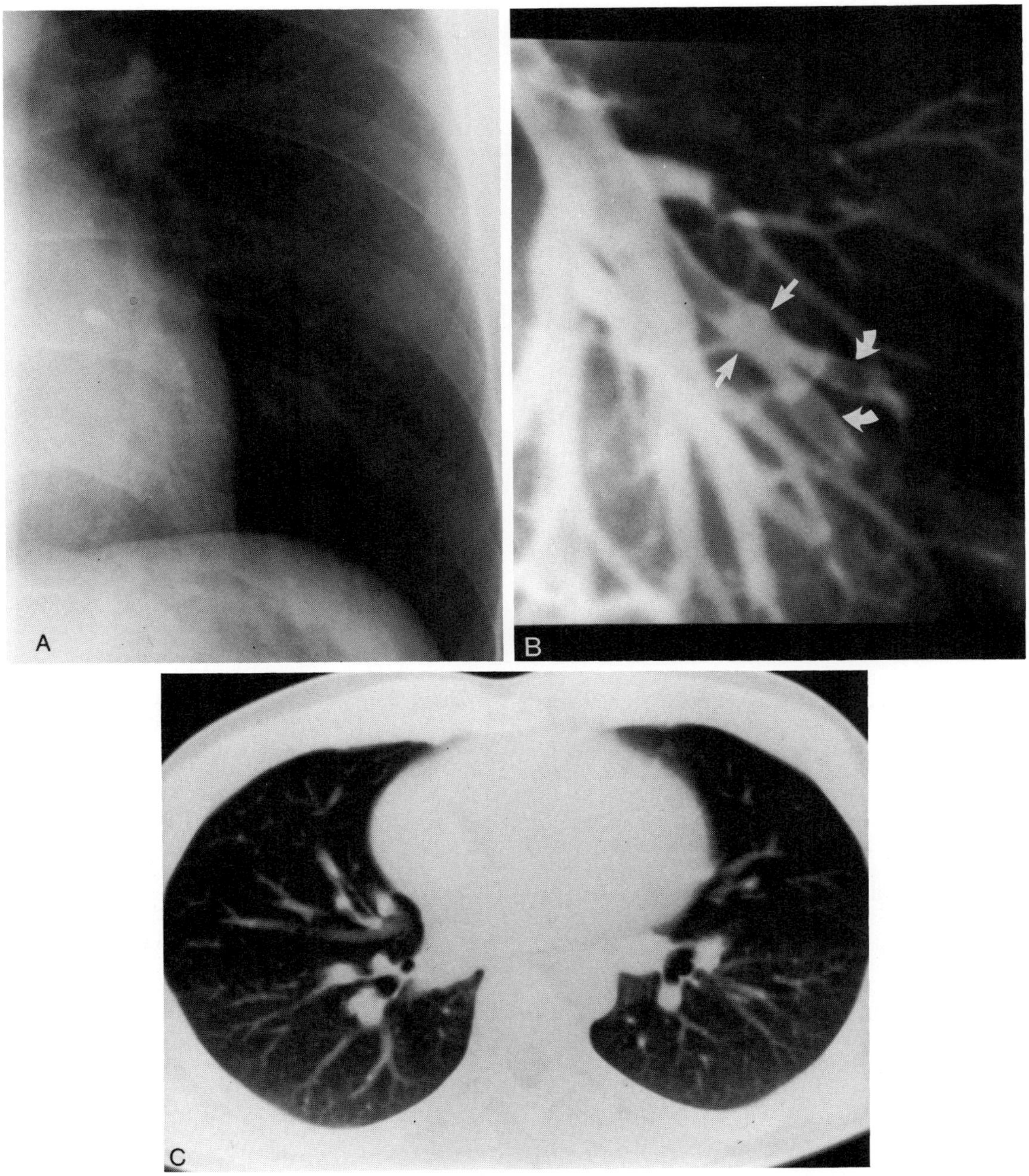

Figure 41–22. This patient had symptoms suggesting bronchiectasis. Chest radiography, computed tomographic (CT) scanning, and bronchography are compared. *A*, Cone down of a chest radiograph is normal. *B*, The bronchogram demonstrates cylindric bronchiectasis in the anterior segment of the left lower lobe. Note that the bronchus dilates slightly before it branches (arrows) and that both branches contain proximal bulges (curved arrows). *C*, Representative thin-section computed tomographic (CT) slice through a region shown by bronchography to contain bronchiectasis is also normal (see *B*).

to the radiographic methods described in the previous section, which provide information on regional anatomy. Ventilation imaging is also necessary to detect ventilatory abnormalities that may be the cause of perfusion defects seen in airway disorders, such as chronic bronchitis, emphysema, asthma, and bronchiectasis. Assessment of regional blood flow and ventilation enhances sensitivity and offers the possibility that functional information can lead to more specific diagnoses.

Imaging Agents and Techniques

Pulmonary perfusion scintigraphy involves the intravenous injection of radiolabeled particles that are trapped in the pulmonary vascular bed. Following the intravenous injection of particles, there is nearly complete extraction by the pulmonary bed in a distribution that reflects the relative regional pulmonary blood flow at the time of tracer injection.[80, 81] The most commonly employed agent is technetium-99m–labeled macroaggregated albumin (MAA). Approximately 90% of the MAA particles have diameters ranging from 10 to 90 μ, and usually 300,000 to 500,000 particles are administered. There is a wide margin of safety with this number of particles because the MAA particles are metabolized[83] and because normal persons have approximately 350 million precapillary arterioles, with diameters ranging from 10 to 30 μ.[80, 83, 84] Thus, there is temporary occlusion only of about 0.1% of the pulmonary vascular bed, and such occlusion has not been shown to cause any significant adverse cardiovascular effects.[80, 83, 84] The technique is also safe to use because hypersensitivity reactions are rare[85] and radiation exposure is very low, with the lungs receiving about 0.5 rad and the whole body less than 0.1 rad per examination.[86] Right-to-left shunts should be used with caution as a result of the rapid entry of MAA into the systemic circulation, but the small number of particles used has apparently obviated the problem because clinically recognizable difficulties with MAA injection of patients with such shunts have not arisen.

Imaging of the patient can begin almost immediately after the injection of the particles, because they are essentially all removed from the blood on the first pass through the lungs. The trapped MAA is cleared from the lungs by enzymatic hydrolysis, with a biologic half-life of 4 to 8 hours in normal persons.[80] As the particles are broken down into smaller sizes, they pass through the capillary bed and are phagocytized by the reticuloendothelial system. A normal perfusion study is shown in Figure 41–23.

The safety, simplicity, and remarkable sensitivity of perfusion scintigraphy has promoted widespread use. Soon after the introduction of the procedure, however, it became apparent that the high sensitivity of this technique was associated with a lack of specificity.[87–90] Initially, the chest film was used to sort out causes of perfusion defects, but it was soon realized that methods were needed for assessing regional ventilation. Consequently, a large variety of ventilation imaging techniques and radiopharmaceuticals were developed.[91] Commonly used radiopharmaceuticals were xenon-133, xenon-127, krypton-81m, and technetium-99m aerosols. Because xenon-127 and krypton-81m are not readily available to most laboratories and therefore are not widely used today, they are not discussed further here.

The most commonly used radioactive gas for ventilation imaging is xenon-133(^{133}Xe). In the usual technique, an image is obtained with breath holding at a near-total lung capacity inhalation following a single breath of a xenon-oxygen mixture. Subsequently, images are obtained at 30- to 60-second intervals while the patient rebreathes the xenon-oxygen mixture through a closed system for 3 to 5 minutes in an attempt to achieve equilibrium. In many patients with obstructive airway disease, true equilibrium is not reached during such a relatively short rebreathing period. As equilibrium is approached, the images acquired reflect the volume of the aerated lung rather than the distribution of regional ventilation. At the end of the wash-in period the patient breathes room air, and sequential 30- to 60-second images are obtained for 5 to 6 minutes during this "washout" phase.

In the erect position, the normal washout rate is highest in the lung bases and slowest in the apices. Normally, all xenon activity is cleared from the lungs in 3 to 4 minutes. Images obtained during the washout phase are the most sensitive for the detection of regional airway disease, whereas the equilibrium images are the least sensitive. In patients with obstructive airway disease from any cause, one or more zones of slow washout are demonstrated, which reflects retention. In such patients, however, the single breath image is sometimes normal. This difference is probably a result of the opening of some obstructive airways during the deep inspiration required for the single breath image.

The xenon generally ventilates freely, with a small amount entering the blood stream. Most of the xenon that enters the circulation is returned to the lungs and exhaled, but a small amount concentrates in body fat because of its high fat solubility.

Because ^{133}Xe has a physical half-life of 5.3 days, it cannot

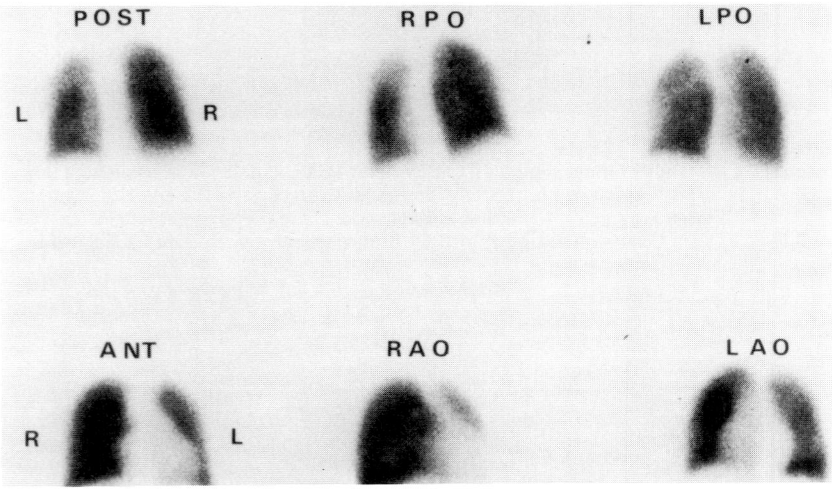

Figure 41–23. Normal perfusion study in six views. The uptake is relatively uniform throughout both lung fields except for cardiac shadows and the apices. The apical decrease is secondary to the normal lower perfusion. The edges of the lung fields are well delineated and are smooth. The costophrenic angles are not as sharp in lung scans as they are in chest radiographs because of the small volume of tissue combined with the coarser resolution in nuclear scans (POST = posterior; ANT = anterior; RPO = right posterior oblique; LPO = left posterior oblique; RAO = right anterior oblique; LAO = left anterior oblique).

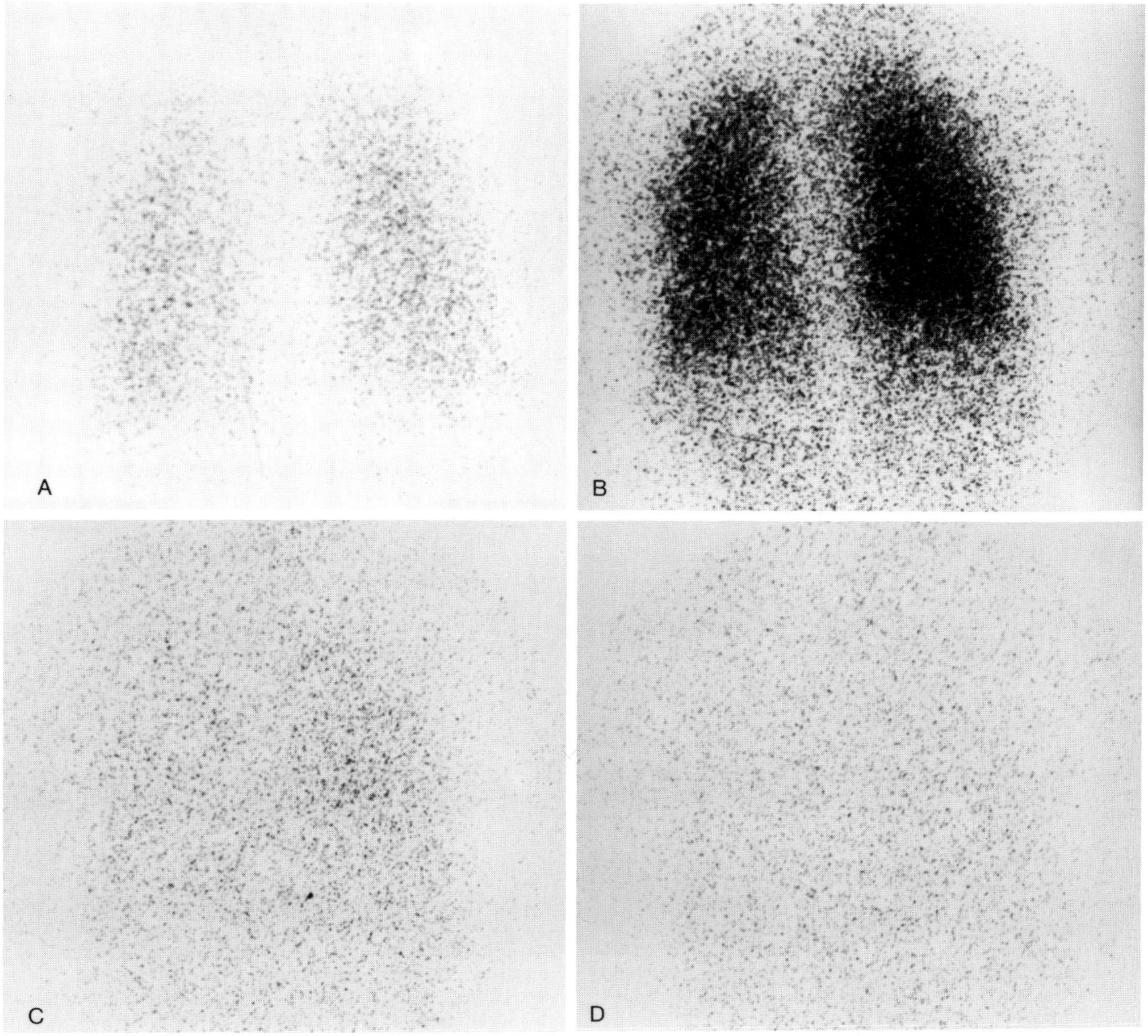

Figure 41–24. Normal xenon ventilation study performed in the posterior views. *A*, Single breath view. *B*, Equilibrium view. *C*, Early washout view (minute 0 to 0.5). *D*, Late washout view (minute 1.5 to 2.0).

be vented or exhaled into the examination room and must be collected and vented after adequate dilution to meet Nuclear Regulatory Commission requirements. The complexity of handling, therefore, is a major disadvantage in the use of this agent. On the other hand, patient safety is very good with radiation doses very low. The lungs receive 0.1 to 0.2 rad and the remainder of the body less than 2 to 4 mrad per examination.[86] A normal ^{133}Xe ventilation study is shown in Figure 41–24.

Radioaerosol inhalation lung imaging was introduced more than 20 years ago[92] but did not achieve clinical acceptance until fairly recently because the early aerosols contained many large particles, which provided low-quality images. Presently, commercially available disposable ultrasonic nebulizers produce aerosols with droplets that are nearly monodispersed, having mean diameters smaller than 1 μ. The patient breathes the aerosol through a mouthpiece in the normal fashion. Exhaled air is passed automatically to a negative pressure hood or collection bag. The airways become labeled in a few minutes with about 10% of the smaller particles (smaller than 1 μ in diameter) depositing in the alveoli. The remaining 90% remain airborne and are exhaled.[93] For particle sizes larger than 1 μ, radioaerosol deposition in the tracheobronchial tree is high because of inertial impaction. In patients with airway obstruction, however, the narrowing of the airways increases the velocity of airflow, so that the probability of particle impaction increases. This results in excessive central deposition, which destroys image quality and interpretation.

The radioaerosol most commonly used in the U.S. is labeled with technetium-99m (^{99m}Tc)—it is ^{99m}Tc-diethylenetriamine pentaacetic acid (DTPA). After deposition in the lung, the aerosol is cleared across the alveolar-capillary membrane into the blood, with a normal half-life of about 1 to 2 hours. Imaging is performed promptly to minimize changes in the images secondary to aerosol clearance. The resultant images are directly comparable to those obtained with the perfusion views, if acquired in similar projections. This is the main advantage over radioactive gas imaging with ^{133}Xe, in which

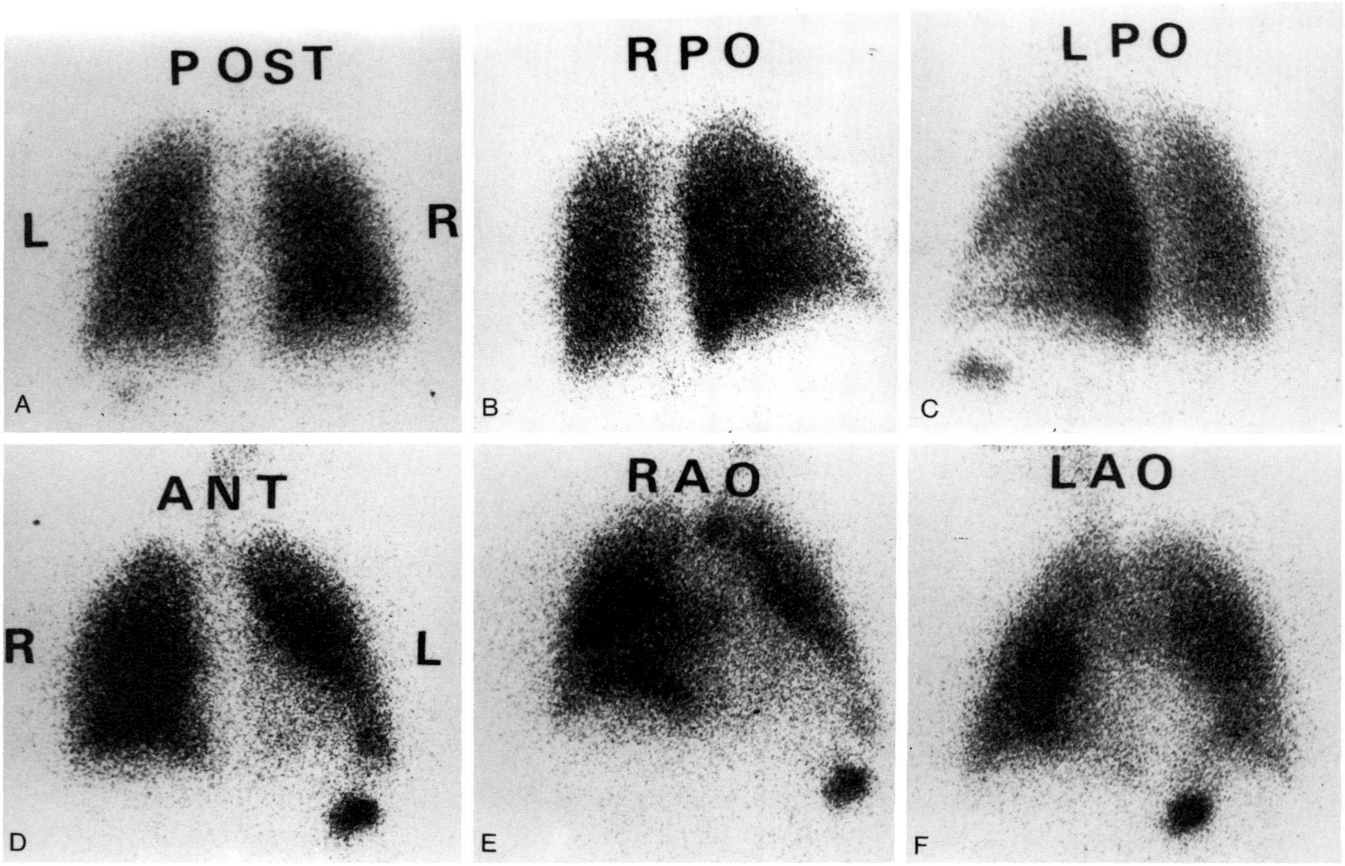

Figure 41–25. ***A* to *F*, Normal technetium-99m DTPA aerosol ventilation study in six views. The views are similar to those taken in perfusion studies and comparison should be made with Figure 41–23. Material is noted in the trachea and in the stomach. Stomach activity results from the swallowing of lung secretions.**

obtaining multiple projections is difficult. Generally, the results obtained with ventilation imaging using radioaerosols have been comparable to results of radioimaging with xenon gas in studies in which there was a wide mix of patients and critically ill patients were few. In some centers, in which critically ill patients constitute a large fraction of the studied population, many of the radioaerosol ventilation studies are of poor quality and the results are difficult to interpret.[94] Despite the difficulties with aerosol imaging, particularly in patients with obstructive lung disease, it is frequently used because it is the most practical means for evaluating ventilation as part of a portable examination. When portability is not a factor, xenon gas ventilation imaging appears to be the superior technique. Figure 41–25 shows a normal aerosol ventilation study.

A fairly recent innovation in aerosol ventilation imaging is the use of a technetium-99m pseudogas, which is an ultrafine, nearly monodispersed aerosol with particles about 0.1 μ in diameter.[95] The aerosol is generated when a spray of ^{99m}Tc-pertechnetate in ethanol solution is burned. Good quality is obtained after only a few breaths of the aerosol by most patients and in less than 1 minute of breathing by severely ill patients. Comparison studies have shown that less bronchial deposition occurs in patients with obstructive pulmonary disease with this agent than with conventional aerosols. Unfortunately, this radiopharmaceutical is not yet commercially available in the U.S.

In most modern laboratories today, radionuclide imaging is performed with scintillation cameras. This instrument is necessary for most ventilation imaging, although perfusion imaging can be accomplished with moving devices, such as rectilinear scanners. With the scintillation camera, perfusion images are usually obtained in multiple projections, including the anterior, posterior, both lateral, and four oblique. In many laboratories, the oblique or lateral views are omitted to reduce the scanning time and to increase the comfort of the patient. This becomes especially important for the severely ill or elderly. Aerosol images are usually obtained in the same projections as the perfusion images to obtain a one-to-one correspondence. Radioactive gas imaging is generally performed only in the posterior projection, because the largest volume of lung is viewed in this projection. Both posterior oblique projections are obtained for one frame during the equilibrium and sometimes during the washout phases to obtain better coverage of the lungs. Rarely is gas imaging performed in both anterior and posterior projections because of the necessity for repeating the inhalation procedure, equilibrium breathing, and washout phases.

Results in Chronic Lung Disease

Recognition of emphysema presents no problems in those with advanced disease, but early diagnosis is difficult. Pulmonary ventilation imaging is particularly helpful in the early stages of emphysema when the chest radiograph and other tests are normal. It has been shown that studies of regional ventilation using ^{133}Xe are nearly twice as sensitive as chest radiographs in detecting emphysema.[96] In addition, ventilation imaging enables the area and extent of the emphysematous process to be determined. In patients who develop large bullae, ventilation imaging is useful in documenting the integrity of the remaining lung tissue and the physiologic effects of the bullae on the surrounding lung.[97, 98]

Pulmonary perfusion imaging is usually abnormal in emphysema, but not as often as with ventilation imaging.[97–99] Usually the lung volume is increased and the lungs appear elongated, reflecting the generalized hyperinflation. In those with advanced disease focal defects are present, predominantly in the upper lungs, except for emphysema associated with alpha$_1$-antitrypsin deficiency, in which the perfusion abnormalities involve the lower parts of the lung bilaterally and symmetrically.[100] Perfusion defects in emphysema do not follow an anatomic distribution, but cross anatomic lines. In patients with pulmonary emphysema, the reduction in pulmonary vasculature, as visualized on angiograms, correlates well with the regions of impaired perfusion.[101] Pulmonary perfusion images in patients with emphysema are presented in Figures 41–26 and 41–27.

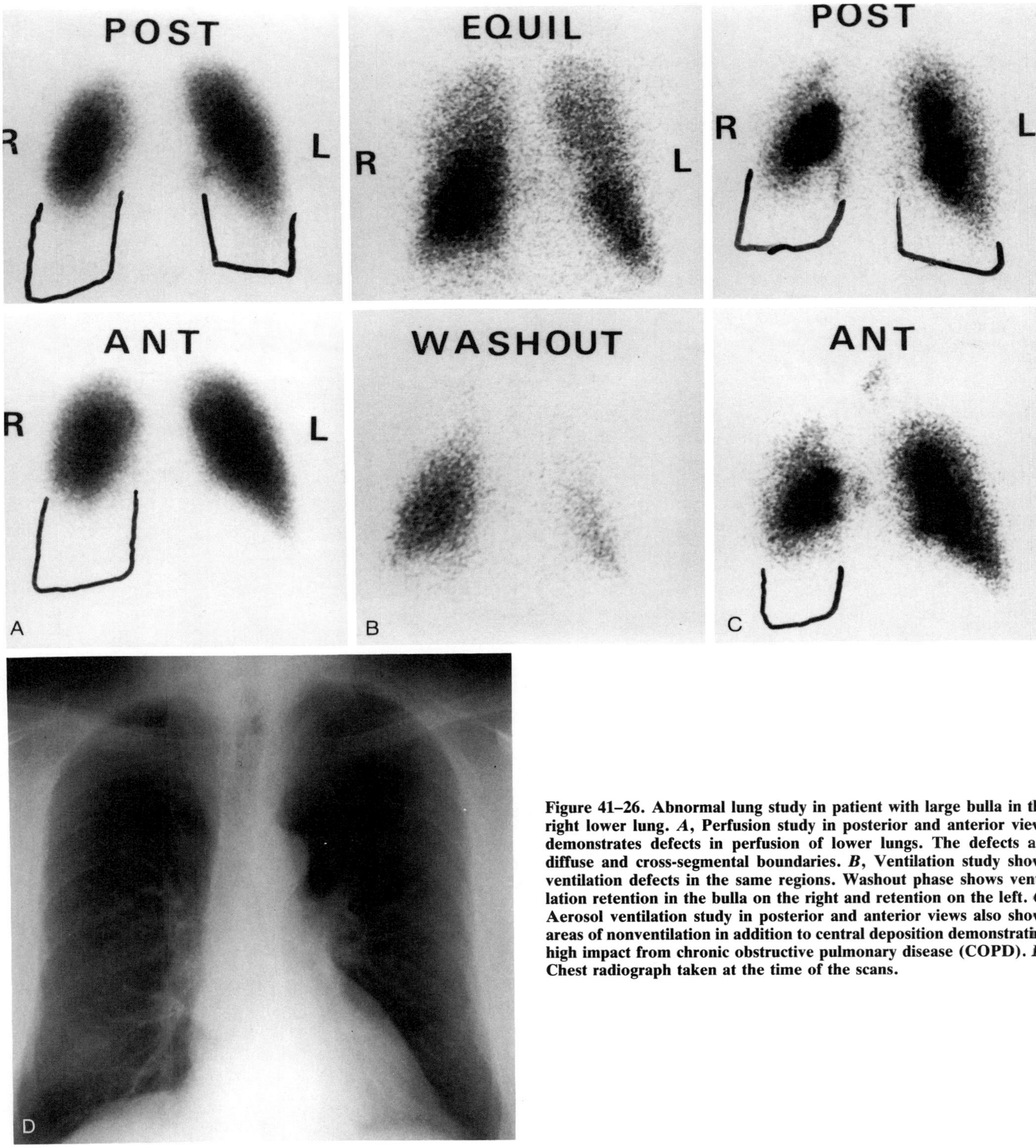

Figure 41–26. Abnormal lung study in patient with large bulla in the right lower lung. *A*, Perfusion study in posterior and anterior views demonstrates defects in perfusion of lower lungs. The defects are diffuse and cross-segmental boundaries. *B*, Ventilation study shows ventilation defects in the same regions. Washout phase shows ventilation retention in the bulla on the right and retention on the left. *C*, Aerosol ventilation study in posterior and anterior views also shows areas of nonventilation in addition to central deposition demonstrating high impact from chronic obstructive pulmonary disease (COPD). *D*, Chest radiograph taken at the time of the scans.

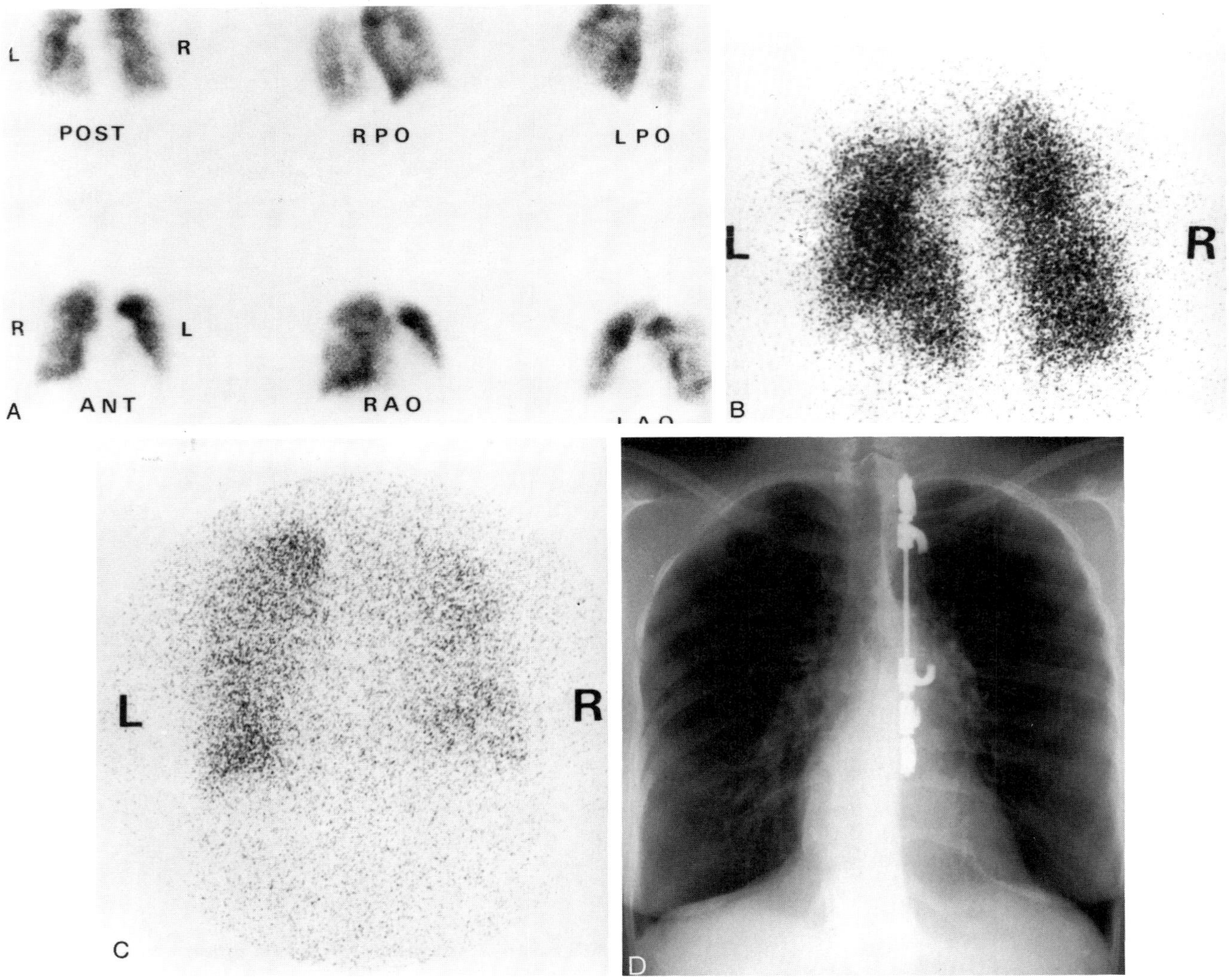

Figure 41–27. Abnormal lung studies in patient with respiratory distress. Note the close correspondence of the perfusion defects in *A*, with the equilibrium ventilation defects in *B*, and retention in the washout study *C*. Chest radiograph *D*, does not show changes of chronic obstructive pulmonary disease (COPD) as seen in scintiphotos (POST = posterior; ANT = anterior; RPO = right posterior oblique; LPO = left posterior oblique; RAO = right anterior oblique; LAO = left anterior oblique).

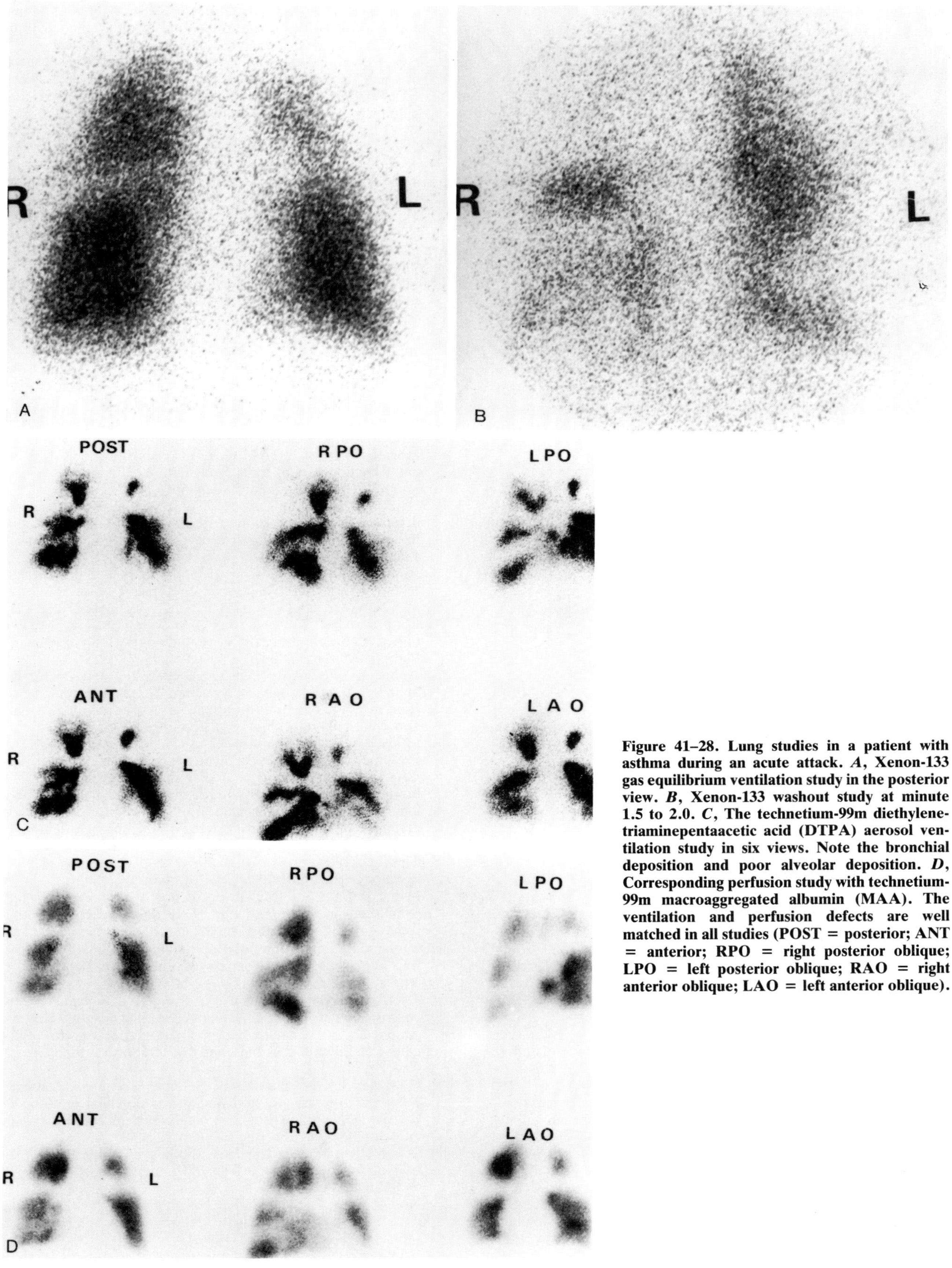

Figure 41–28. Lung studies in a patient with asthma during an acute attack. *A*, Xenon-133 gas equilibrium ventilation study in the posterior view. *B*, Xenon-133 washout study at minute 1.5 to 2.0. *C*, The technetium-99m diethylenetriaminepentaacetic acid (DTPA) aerosol ventilation study in six views. Note the bronchial deposition and poor alveolar deposition. *D*, Corresponding perfusion study with technetium-99m macroaggregated albumin (MAA). The ventilation and perfusion defects are well matched in all studies (POST = posterior; ANT = anterior; RPO = right posterior oblique; LPO = left posterior oblique; RAO = right anterior oblique; LAO = left anterior oblique).

In alpha$_1$-antitrypsin deficiency there is mainly an association with basal and lobar emphysema. Delayed basilar clearance of radioxenon (^{133}Xe) from the lungs of both homozygous and symptomless heterozygous individuals for this condition has been shown in patients with no other evidence of COPD. This suggests that ventilation imaging is a sensitive screening procedure.[102]

Chronic bronchitis, bronchiectasis, and bronchial asthma are disease states characterized by intermittent acute episodes. The major advantages of scintigraphy in these diseases of the airways include earlier detection, precise localization of abnormalities, and evaluation of treatment by serial studies. Scintigraphy can reveal abnormal ventilation and perfusion patterns in patients with chronic bronchitis, even when their overall spirometry tests are scarely abnormal. Abnormalities in chronic bronchitis have also been found by scintigraphy in patients without associated chest radiographic changes or measurable abnormalities of airway resistance.[101] During acute attacks, regional defects of pulmonary perfusion are found in most patients with any of these conditions, and these defects are associated with extensive abnormalites of regional ventilation. Ventilation abnormalities in particular may be present in asymptomatic asthmatics, but often in association with normal perfusion.[101] In those with chronic bronchitis and asthma, the sites of regional perfusion and ventilation abnormalities vary during different episodes and even during the same episode.[103–105] This constitutes evidence that the changes are partially a result of temporary alterations, such as bronchospasm and mucous impaction. The abnormalities of pulmonary imaging that occur in bronchiectasis are more central in location, are well defined, and persist during intervals of clinical remission. Studies have shown that such defects correspond well to bronchographic abnormalities.[101]

Scintigraphy of an asthmatic patient is presented in Figure 41–28. It shows the dramatic changes that can be seen in these diseases.

Although various characteristics have been described for different chronic states, ventilation perfusion scintigraphy is nonspecific, and generally a definitive diagnosis cannot be made from the image alone. As with most imaging procedures, the clinical history and results of other studies must be used in conjunction with scintigraphy to reach the final diagnosis.

REFERENCES

1. Simon G. Principles of Chest X-Ray Diagnosis. 2nd ed. London: Butterworth & Company, 1962, 110.
2. Thurlbeck WM, Henderson JA, Fraser RG, Bates DV. Chronic obstructive lung disease: A comparison between clinical, roentgenologic, functional and morphologic criteria in chronic bronchitis, emphysema, asthma, and bronchiectasis. Medicine 1970; 49:82–145.
3. Boushy SF, Aboumrad MH, North LB, Helagason AH. Lung recoil pressure, airway resistance and forced flows related to morphologic emphysema. Am Rev Respir Dis 1971; 104:551–561.
4. Nicklaus TM, Stowell DW, Chrisiansen WR, Renzetti AD Jr. The accuracy of the roentgenologic diagnosis of chronic pulmonary emphysema. Am Rev Respir Dis 1966; 93:889–899.
5. Laws JW, Heard BE. Emphysema and the chest film: A retrospective radiological and pathological study. Br J Radiol 1962; 35:750–761.
6. Simon G, Pride NB, Jones NL, Raimondi AC. Relation between abnormalities in the chest radiograph and changes in pulmonary function in chronic bronchitis and emphysema. Thorax 1973; 28:15.
7. Fraser RG, Pare JA. Pulmonary emphysema. Diagn Dis Chest 1979; 3:11.
8. Thomson KR, Eyssen GE, Fraser RG. Discrimination of normal and overinflated lungs and prediction of total lung cavity based on chest film measurements. Radiology 1976; 119:721.
9. Mori PA, Anderson AE Jr, Eckert P. The radiological spectrum of aging and emphysematous lungs. Radiology 1964; 83:48.
10. Jarvinen KAJ, Thomander K. The diagnosis of obstructive pulmonary emphysema in mass radiology. Ann Med Interne (Paris) 1959; 48:151.
11. Goldenthal S, Armstrong BW, Lowman RM. Roentgen studies of ventilatory dysfunction: An analysis of diaphragmatic movement in obstructive emphysema. Am J Roentgenol 1958; 79:279.
12. Goddard DR, Nicholson EM, Lazlo G, Watt I. Computed tomography in pulmonary emphysema. Clin Radiol 1982; 33:379–387.
13. Rosenblum LJ, Maucer RA, Wellenstein DE, et al. Computed tomography of the lung. Radiology 1978; 129:521–524.
14. Foster WL Jr, Pratt PC, Roggli VL, et al. Centrilobular emphysema: CT-pathologic correlation. Radiology 1986; 159:27–32.
15. Webb WR, Stein MG, Finkbeiner WE, et al. Normal and diseased isolated lungs: High-resolution CT. Radiology 1988; 166:81–87.
16. Meziane MA, Hruban RH, Zerhouni EA, et al. High-resolution CT of the lung parenchyma with pathologic correlation. Radiographics 1988; 8:27–54.
17. Bergin CJ, Muller NL. CT of interstitial lung disease: A diagnostic approach. AJR 1987; 148:9–15.
18. Murata K, Itoh H, Todo G, et al. Centrilobular lesions of the lung: Demonstration by high-resolution CT and pathologic correlation. Radiology 1986; 161:641–655.
19. Barnhard HJ, Pierce JA, Joyce JW, Bates JH. Roentgenographic determination of total lung capacity: A new method evaluated in health, emphysema, and congestive heart failure. Am J Med 1960; 28:51–60.
20. Reid L, Millard FGC. Correlation between radiologic diagnosis and structural lung changes in emphysema. Clin Radiol 1964; 15:307–311.
21. Foraker AG, Bedrossian CW, Anderson AE Jr. Myocardial dimensions and proportions in pulmonary emphysema. Arch Pathol 1970; 90:344–347.
22. Abbott OA, Hopkins WA, Van Fleit WE, Robinson JS. A new approach to pulmonary emphysema. Thorax 1953; 8:116.
23. Barden RP. The interpretation of some radiologic signs of abnormal pulmonary function. Radiology 1952; 59:481.
24. Milne ENC. The plain film versus CT in the diagnosis of COPD. Presented at the Society for Thoracic Radiology. Newport Beach, CA, February 1986.
25. Sutinen S, Christoforidis AJ, Kliegh GA, Pratt PC. Roentgenologic criteria for the recognition of nonsymptomatic pulmonary emphysema: Correlation between roentgenologic findings and pulmonary pathology. Am Rev Respir Dis 1965; 91:69–75.
26. Thurlbeck WM, Simon G. Radiographic appearance of the chest in emphysema. AJR 1978; 130:429–440.
27. Fraser RG, Bates DV. Body section roentgenography in the evaluation and differentiation of chronic hypertrophic emphysema and asthma. AJR 1959; 82:39.
28. Simon G. Complexities of emphysema. In: Simon M, Potchen EJ, Lemay M, eds. Frontiers of Pulmonary Radiology. New York: Grune & Stratton, 1969, 142–153.
29. Thurlbeck WM, Henderson JA, Fraser RG, Bates DV. Chronic obstructive lung disease. A comparison between clinical, roentgenologic, functional and morphological criteria in chronic bronchitis, emphysema, asthma and bronchiectasis. Medicine 1970; 49:81.
30. Heitzman EK, Markarian B, Soloman J. Chronic obstructive pulmonary disease. Radiol Clin North Am 1973; 11:49–75.
31. Scarrow GN. The pulmonary angiogram in chronic bronchitis and emphysema. Clin Radiol 1966; 17:54–67.
32. O'Callaghan JP, Heitzman ER, Somogyi JW, et al. CT evaluation of the pulmonary artery. J Comput Assist Tomogr 1982; 6:101–104.
33. Rosenblum CJ, Mauceri RA, Wellenstein DE, et al. Density patterns in the normal lung as determined by computed tomography. Radiology 1980; 137:409–416.
34. Robinson PJ, Kreel L. Pulmonary tissue attenuation with computed tomography: comparison of inspiration and expiration scans. J Comput Assist Tomogr 1979; 3:740–748.

35. Kreel L. Computed tomography of the lung and pleura. Semin Roentgenol 1978; 13:213–225.
36. Cohen AM, Haaga JR. The lungs. In: Haaga JR, Alfidi RJ, eds. Computed Tomography of the Whole Body. Vol. 2. 2nd ed. St. Louis: CV Mosby Co, 1988, 513–574.
37. Zerhouni EA, Naidich DP, Stitik FP, et al. Computed tomography of the pulmonary parenchyma. Part 2: Interstitial disease. J Thorac Imaging 1985; 1:54–64.
38. Milne ENC, Bass H. Roentgenologic and functional analysis of combined chronic obstructive pulmonary disease and congestive cardiac failure. Invest Radiol 1969; 4:129–147.
39. Hublitz VF, Shapiro JH. Atypical patterns of congestive failure in chronic lung disease: Influence of pre-existing disease on appearance and distribution of pulmonary edema. Radiology 1969; 93:995–1006.
40. Ziskind MM, George RB, Herbert SJ. Incomplete consolidation in pneumococcic lobar pneumonia complicating pulmonary emphysema. Ann Intern Med 1970; 72:835–839.
41. Chavez CM, Fain WR, Conn HJ. Angiography in giant cystic disease of the lung. J Thorac Cardiovasc Surg 1968; 55:638–641.
42. Parker FB. Surgery in chronic lung disease. Surg Clin North Am 1974; 54:1193–1202.
43. Potgieter PD, Benetar SR, Hewitson RP, Ferguson AD. Surgical treatment of bullous lung disease. Thorax 1981; 36:885–889.
44. Miscall L, Duffy RW. Surgical treatment of bullous emphysema. Contributions of angiography. Dis Chest 1953; 24:489–499.
45. Morgan MDL, Denison DM, Strickland B. Value of computed tomography for selecting patients with bullous lung disease for surgery. Thorax 1986; 41:855–862.
46. Fiore DW, Biondetti PR, Sartori F, et al. The role of computed tomography in the evaluation of bullous lung disease. J Comput Assist Tomogr 1982; 6:105–108.
47. Gaensler EA, Jederlinic PJ, Muiris MX. Patient work-up for bullectomy. J Thorac Imaging 1986; 1:75–93.
48. Carr DH, Pride NB. Computed tomography in pre-operative assessment of bullous emphysema. Clin Radiol 1984; 35:43–45.
49. Cohen AM. Magnetic resonance imaging of the thorax. Radiol Clin North Am 1984; 22:829–846.
50. O'Donovan PB, Ross JS. Magnetic resonance of the pulmonary parenchyma: Initial experience at 0.6 tesla. Cardiovasc Intervent Radiol 1986; 8:300.
51. Moore EH, Webb WR, Muller N, Sollito R. MRI of pulmonary air space disease: Experimental model and preliminary clinical results. AJR 1986; 146:1123–1128.
52. Cutillo AG, Morris AH, Ailion DC, et al. Determination of lung water content and distribution by nuclear magnetic resonance imaging. J Thorac Imaging 1986; 1:39–51.
53. Cutillo AG, Morris AH, Ailion DC, et al. Quantitative assessment of pulmonary edema by nuclear magnetic resonance methods. J Thorac Imaging 1988; 3:51–58.
54. Kveder M, Zupancic I, Lahajna G, et al. Water proton NMR relaxation mechanisms in lung tissue. Magnetic Resonance Med 1988; 7:432–441.
55. Heitzman ER. The Lung: Radiologic-Pathologic Correlations. 2nd ed. St. Louis: C.V. Mosby, 1984.
56. Simon G. Chronic bronchitis and emphysema—a symposium. Br J Radiol 1959; 32:292–294.
57. Fraser RG, Fraser RS, Renner JW, et al. The roentgenologic diagnosis of chronic bronchitis: A reassessment with emphasis on parahilar bronchi seen end-on. Radiology 1976; 120:1.
58. Gamsu G, Forbes AR, Ovenfors CO. Bronchographic features of chronic bronchitis in normal men. AJR 1981; 36:317–322.
59. Mitchell RS, Silvers GW, Goodman N, et al. Are centrilobular emphysema and panolobular emphysema two different diseases? Hum Pathol 1970; 1:433–441.
60. Bergin CJ, Muller NL, Miller RR. CT in the qualitative assessment of emphysema. J Thorac Imaging 1986; 1:94–103.
61. Milne ENC, Bass H. The roentgenologic diagnosis of early chronic obstructive pulmonary disease. J Can Assoc Radiol 1969; 20:3–15.
62. Nicklaus TM, Watanabe S, Mitchell MM, Renzetti AD Jr. Roentgenologic, physiologic, and structural estimations of the total lung capacity in normal and emphysematous subjects. Am J Med 1967; 42:547–553.
63. Simon G, Connolly N, Littlejohns DW, McAllen M. Radiological abnormalities in children with asthma and their relation to the clinical findings and some respiratory function tests. Thorax 1973; 28:115.
64. Rebuck AS. Radiological aspects of severe asthma. Australas Radiol 1970; 14:264.
65. Hodson ME, Simon G, Batten JC. Radiology of uncomplicated asthma. Thorax 1974; 29:296.
66. Gershel JC, Goldman HS, Stein REK, et al. The usefulness of chest radiographs in first asthma attacks. N Engl J Med 1983; 309:336–339.
67. Gilles JD, Reed MH, Simons FER. Radiographic findings in acute childhood asthma. J Can Assoc Radiol 1978; 29:28–33.
68. Blair DN, Coppage L, Shaw C. Medical imaging in asthma. J Thorac Imaging 1986; 1:23–35.
69. Landay MJ, Christensen EE, Bynum LJ. Pulmonary manifestations of acute aspiration of gastric contents. AJR 1978; 131:587–592.
70. Reich SB, Earley WC, Ravin TH, et al. Evaluation of gastropulmonary aspiration by a radioactive technique, concise communication. J Nucl Med 1977; 18:1079–1081.
71. Boonyaprapa S, Anderson PO, Garfinkel DJ, et al. Detection of pulmonary aspiration in infants and children with respiratory diseases, concise communication. J Nucl Med 1980; 21:314–318.
72. Reid L. Reduction in bronchial subdivision by bronchiectasis. Thorax 1955; 5:233–247.
73. Gudjberg CE. Roentgenologic diagnosis of bronchiectasis: An analysis of 112 cases. Acta Radiol 1955; 3:209–226.
74. Naidech DP, McCuley DI, Kouri NF. Computer tomography of bronchiectasis. J Comput Assist Tomogr 1982; 6:437–444.
75. Muller NL, Bergin CJ, Ostrow DN, et al. Role of computed tomography in the recognition of bronchiectasis. AJR 1987; 131:981–984.
76. Grenier PG, Maurice FM, Musset D, et al. Bronchiectasis: Assessment by thin section CT. Radiology 1986; 161:95–99.
77. Silverman PM, Godwin JD. CT/bronchographic correlations in bronchiectasis. J Comput Assist Tomogr 1987; 11:52–56.
78. Wescott JL, Cole SR. Traction bronchiectasis in end stage pulmonary fibrosis. Radiology 1986; 161:665–669.
79. Bates DV. Studies of regional lung function using radioisotopes. Presented at the IAFA Symposium on Dynamic Studies with Radioisotopes in Clinical Medicine and Research. Rotterdam, The Netherlands, August 31–September 4, 1970.
80. Taplin GV, MacDonald NS. Radiochemistry of macroaggregated albumin and newer lung scanning agents. Semin Nucl Med 1971; 1:132.
81. Tow DE, Wagner HN Jr, Lopez-Majaro V, et al. Validity of measuring regional pulmonary arterial blood with macroaggregates of human serum albumin. AJR 1966; 96:664.
82. Benacerraf B, Biozzi G, Halpern G, et al. A study of phagocytic activity of the reticuloendothelial system toward heat-denatured human serum albumin tagged with I-131. Res Bull 1956; 2:19.
83. Gold WM, McCormack KR. Pulmonary function response to radioisotope scanning of the lungs. JAMA 1966; 197:146.
84. Weibel R. Morphometry of the Human Lungs. New York: Academic Press, 1963, 81.
85. Physicians Desk Reference for Radiology and Nuclear Medicine. Oradell, NJ: Medical Economics Company, 1979–1980.
86. Kereiakes JG, Rosenstein M. Handbook of Radiation Doses in Nuclear Medicine and Diagnostic X-Rays. Boca Raton, FL: CRC Press, 1980, 161.
87. Moser KM, Miale A Jr. Interpretative pitfalls in lung photoscanning. Am J Med 1968; 44:336.
88. Poe ND, Swanson LA, Taplin GV. Physiological factors affecting lung scan interpretations. Radiology 1967; 89:661.
89. Potchen EJ. Lung scintiscanning. JAMA 1968; 204:907.
90. Potchen EJ, Evens RG. The physiologic factors affecting regional ventilation and perfusion. Semin Nucl Med 1971; 1:153.
91. Alderson PO, Live BR. Scintigraphic evaluation of regional pulmonary ventilation. Semin Nucl Med 1980; 10:218–242.
92. Hayes M, Taplin GV. Lung imaging with radioaerosols for the assessment of airway disease. Semin Nucl Med 1980; 10:243–251.
93. Taplin GV, Poe ND, Isawa T, et al. Comparison of radioaerosol with radioxenon inhalation procedures in obstructive lung disease and pulmonary embolism. In: Croll MN, Brody LW, eds. Clinical Dynamic Function Studies With Radionuclides. Englewood Cliffs, NJ: Prentice Hall, 1972, 193.

94. Alderson PO, Biello DR, Gottschalk A, et al. Tc-99m-DTPA aerosol and radioactive gases compared as adjuncts to perfusion scintigraphy in patients with suspected pulmonary embolism. Radiology 1984; 153:515–521.
95. Burch WM, Sullivan PJ, Lomas FE, et al. Lung ventilation studies with technetium-99m-pseudogas. J Nucl Med 1986; 27:842–846.
96. Alderson PO, Secker-Walker RH, Forrest JV. Detection of obstructive pulmonary disease: Relative sensitivity of ventilation-perfusion studies and chest radiography. Radiology 1974; 112:643.
97. Lopez-Majaro V, Torv DE, Wagner AN Jr. Regional distribution of pulmonary arterial blood flow in emphysema. JAMA 1966; 197:81.
98. Quinn JL III. Perfusion scanning in chronic obstructive lung disease. Semin Nucl Med 1971; 1:185.
99. Dore EK, Poe ND, Ellested MH, et al. Lung perfusion and inhalation scanning in pulmonary emphysema. AJR 1968; 104:770.
100. Welch MH, Richardson RH, Whitcomb WH, et al. The lung scan in α-antitrypsin deficiency. J Nucl Med 1969; 10:687.
101. DeNardo GL, Denardo ST. The lungs. In: Freeman LM, ed. Freeman and Johnson's Clinical Radionuclide Imaging. 3rd ed. Orlando, FL: Grune & Stratton, 1984, 1107–1108.
102. Fallat RJ, Powell MR, Kueppers F, et al. Xenon-133 ventilatory studies in α-antitrypsin deficiency. J Nucl Med 1973; 14:5.
103. Bentivaglio LG, Beerel F, Bryan AC, et al. Regional pulmonary function studies with xenon-133 in patients with bronchial asthma. J Clin Invest 1963; 42:1193.
104. Heckscher T, Bass H, Oriol A, et al. Regional lung function in patients with bronchial asthma. Clin Invest 1968; 47:1063.
105. Surprenant EL, Wilson AF, Nancy HS. Significance of regional ventilation and perfusion abnormalities in bronchial asthma. J Nucl Med 1970; 11:366.

Chapter 42

INVASIVE DIAGNOSTIC PROCEDURES IN CHRONIC OBSTRUCTIVE PULMONARY DISEASE

Daniel M. Goodenberger Gary R. Epler

The number of invasive procedures that are useful in the diagnosis of chronic obstructive pulmonary disease (COPD) is limited, but many are helpful in determining the presence of diseases or complications associated with COPD. Moreover, the approach to other illnesses and the use of diagnostic procedures may be modified by the coexistence of COPD. This chapter focuses on invasive diagnostic procedures, their complications and contraindications, and special problems in the ambulatory patient with chronic obstructive lung disease.

ARTERIAL BLOOD GASES

Applications

Sampling of arterial blood allows the measurement of the partial pressures of oxygen ($Pa{O_2}$) and carbon dioxide ($Pa{CO_2}$), pH, and the measurement (or, more commonly, the calculation) of hemoglobin oxygen saturation ($Sa{O_2}$).

Management of COPD Exacerbations

Arterial blood gas determinations can help to detect hypoxemia and guide oxygen therapy in the management of exacerbations of COPD. They allow detection of worsening hypercapnia and acidosis and permit safer, more rational decisions to be made regarding increased oxygen supplementation, intensity of general therapeutic measures and, if needed, the institution of mechanical ventilation.[1] Although several studies have demonstrated that serial peak expiratory flow and forced expiratory volume in 1 second (FEV_1) may reduce the frequency of measuring arterial blood gases in patients with acute asthma, this practice is much less satisfactory for those with exacerbations of COPD. Similarly, studies of the clinical signs of ventilatory muscle fatigue have shown that abdominal paradox and respiratory alternans are insufficiently sensitive to be reliable for therapeutic decisions.[50] Mental status changes are also late manifestations of worsening gas exchange. Therefore, repeated blood gas measurements in acute, severe exacerbations are necessary until stability has been reached.

Preoperative Evaluation

Arterial blood gases should be obtained in the evaluation of patients whose preoperative pulmonary function tests show moderate to severe spirometric abnormalities prior to general anesthesia. This is especially true for those undergoing upper abdominal and thoracic procedures and is mandatory prior to resectional lung surgery. In general, lung tissue should not be removed if the patient's $Pa{CO_2}$ is $\geq$ 45 mm Hg at rest or increases during exercise, or if the Pa_{O_2} is lower than 50 mm Hg at rest and does not improve with exercise. Rarely, when preoperative ventilation-perfusion ($\dot{V}/\dot{Q}$) lung scanning reveals that the area of lung to be resected has a low $\dot{V}$ to $\dot{Q}$ ratio, resection of such tissue may result in improvement in arterial oxygenation.

Commercial Airline Travel

Commercial airline travel is undertaken by millions yearly in the U.S. Patients with COPD commonly ask their family physician or pulmonary internist about the safety of air travel. Commercial airliners vary widely in cabin pressurization; presures are generally equivalent to those at 5400 to 8000 feet of altitude. An accurate estimate of cabin pressure can be obtained by determining the manufacturer and type of plane.[2] The potential importance of the altitude effect in a patient with hypoxemia can be seen by considering the alveolar gas equation:

$$P_{A_{O_2}} = (P_B - P_{H_2O})\,F_{I_{O_2}} - (Pa_{CO_2}/R)$$

where $P_{A_{O_2}}$ = alveolar partial pressure of oxygen, P_B = barometric pressure, P_{H_2O} = vapor pressure of water (47 at 37° C), $F_{I_{O_2}}$ = fraction of inspired oxygen (0.21 in room air), Pa_{CO_2} = arterial partial pressure of carbon dioxide, and R = respiratory exchange ratio. For example, if a patient with COPD at sea level has a Pa_{O_2} of 70 mm Hg, a Pa_{CO_2} of 40 mm Hg, and an assumed R = 0.8, the $P_{A_{O_2}}$ will be 100 mm Hg and the alveolar-arterial oxygen difference is 30 mm Hg. Keeping the alveolar-arterial oxygen gradient and Pa_{CO_2} constant for the sake of demonstration, the following results might be expected:

For an altitude of 5280 feet, the predicted Pa_{O_2} is ≤ 41 mm Hg.

For an altitude of 6000 feet, the predicted Pa_{O_2} is ≤ 32 mm Hg.

For an altitude of 8000 feet, the predicted Pa_{O_2} is ≤ 28 mm Hg.

In fact, the situation is neither this simple nor this severe, probably because of changes in the alveolar-arterial gradient associated with changes in ventilation-perfusion matching, as well as an average 12% increase in minute ventilation. One published regression equation[3] for predicting Pa_{O_2} at altitude is

$$Pa_{O_2} = 22.8 - 2.74x + 0.68y$$

where x = predicted cabin altitude in thousands of feet and y = sea level Pa_{O_2} in mm Hg. Applying this equation allows the examining physician to make a decision about recommendations for supplemental oxygen. The predicted Pa_{O_2} that the physician judges to be safe for short periods of travel depends on the clinical situation—for example, a physician would be less willing to accept a predicted Pa_{O_2} lower than 55 mm Hg in a patient with significant concomitant cardiovascular disease.

In addition to the clinical status of the patient, recommendations are tempered by the anticipated duration of the flight. As a rough guide, patients with stable COPD will have a Pa_{O_2} more than 55 mm Hg at 5000 feet if the sea level Pa_{O_2} is more than 68 mm Hg, and a Pa_{O_2} more than 50 mm Hg at 8000 feet if the sea level Pa_{O_2} is more than 72 mm Hg. A more precise evaluation can be undertaken by having the prospective passenger breathe hypoxic gas mixtures, a procedure well within the capabilities of most respiratory physiology laboratories. In general, an $F_{I_{O_2}}$ of 17.1% corresponds to an altitude of 5000 feet and an $F_{I_{O_2}}$ of 15.1% to 8000 feet.[3]

After equilibration, blood gases are drawn and recommendations made about oxygen supplementation. These decisions need to be made in a timely fashion, because the patient must arrange for the purchase of oxygen and oxygen supplies to be provided by the airline well in advance of the proposed flight.

Long-Term Oxygen Therapy

Studies have shown that oxygen therapy for the patient with hypoxemia prolongs and improves the quality of life. Oxygen therapy is expensive, however, and oxygen therapy costs may be reimbursed by third-party payers only if certain criteria are met. The general requirement is that the Pa_{O_2} is 55 mm Hg or lower, or the oxygen saturation (Sa_{O_2}) is 85% or lower, in a clinically stable patient at rest. If the patient satisfies the criteria only during exercise or sleep, the costs of oxygen therapy for those periods are usually reimbursed. For those patients who have a Pa_{O_2} of 56 to 59 mm Hg or if the Sa_{O_2} is 86% to 89%, oxygen therapy may be prescribed and third-party payers will reimburse the patient for its cost if there is accompanying peripheral edema, electrocardiographic evidence of cor pulmonale, or polycythemia with a hematocrit $\geq 56\%$. If the Pa_{O_2} is ≥ 60 mm Hg and the Sa_{O_2} is $\geq 90\%$, reimbursement will be denied without other evidence of need. The physician can prescribe oxygen outside these guidelines, but prescription costs to the patient may range from \$3600 to \$10,000 yearly, depending on the locale, oxygen flow rate, and method of delivery.

We prefer measurement of arterial blood gases for making this determination; pulse oximetry, although an excellent method for monitoring oxygen saturation over time during sleep studies and in critically ill patients, has a range of accuracy of $\pm 3\%$ to 5%. This may inappropriately exclude patients who would qualify for oxygen therapy if their blood gases were measured. In addition, if the pH, Pa_{CO_2}, and temperature are normal, a Pa_{O_2} of 55 mm Hg is approximately equivalent to an Sa_{O_2} of 88%. Exercise evaluation of the dyspneic patient with COPD who does not meet the above criteria may reveal exercise-induced hypoxemia, especially if the diffusing capacity of the lungs for carbon monoxide (D_{LCO}) is <55% of predicted. Measuring the Sa_{O_2} by pulse oximetry can be done continuously during cycle ergometry or treadmill exercise testing. Arterial blood gases are obtained at baseline, during any decrease in oxygen saturation, and at peak exercise. Arterial line placement facilitates the collection of accurate data, particularly if more than two arterial blood gases are to be measured or if difficulty in arterial puncture during exercise appears likely.

If the patient is not hypoxemic according to these criteria during rest or exercise but still has clinical evidence of cor pulmonale, polycythemia, or neuropsychiatric dysfunction, or electrocardiographic evidence of right ventricular hypertrophy, a sleep study with continuous Sa_{O_2} monitoring should be performed. A proportion of such patients demonstrate significant hypoxemia during sleep—some have classic sleep apnea, whereas more have non-apnea–associated desaturation. Those demonstrating significant hypoxemia during sleep should receive nocturnal oxygen therapy.

Transtracheal Oxygen Therapy

Newer forms of oxygen delivery include transtracheal and transtracheostomy oxygen. Patients almost uniformly require less oxygen with these than with nasal cannulae. Monitoring these patients at rest and with exercise with various oxygen flow rates allows a rational prescription to be written. We find that this can be performed most accurately after placement of a radial arterial line.

Home Ventilator Management

Increasing numbers of patients who are ventilator-dependent are managed at home or in chronic care facilities. Many such patients are stable and do not require frequent ventilator changes. However, measurement of arterial blood gases is necessary to investigate new symptoms, monitor the patient periodically, and initiate ventilator changes.

Exercise Testing

Routine cardiac exercise testing is rarely performed with arterial blood gas monitoring, and often without continuous monitoring of oxygen saturation. Because patients are referred to a pulmonary exercise laboratory for different reasons, and because the patient population is dissimilar, most pulmonary exercise laboratories measure gas exchange and monitor for evidence of oxygen desaturation. Noninvasive oximetric methods are generally used with arterial blood gas analysis reserved for those patients who develop desaturation or in whom pulmonary vascular disease is suspected. Because of the inherent 3% to 5% inaccuracy of noninvasive measurement, however, and because of the observed tendency of oximetric measurements to become less accurate with exercise in some individuals, it is advisable to monitor the patient with arterial blood gas measurements during exercise studies. This allows detection not only of hypoxemia, but also of an undetected decrease in $Pa{O_2}$ on the flat part of the oxyhemoglobin dissociation curve, an inappropriate response of $Pa{CO_2}$, the onset of metabolic acidosis, and accurate calculation of the dead space to tidal volume ratio (V_D/V_T), which may be important in the detection of pulmonary vascular disease.

Technique and Complications

Single arterial blood gases are obtained with a previously heparinized syringe and a small, 22- to 25-gauge needle. The site is cleaned and anesthetized with 1% lidocaine. The site of choice is the radial artery, desirable because it is close to the surface, easy to tamponade after puncture, and its distal circulation most often receives a second supply of blood from the corresponding ulnar artery; this must be confirmed by an Allen test prior to puncture. The brachial artery is the second choice and is a preferred site by some for indwelling catheters during exercise studies. The femoral artery is a distant third choice because of problems with antisepsis and hemostasis. Studies requiring one or two samples may be performed by needle puncture, but many investigators prefer the placement of an indwelling arterial line for a short period in those patients for whom multiple samples are needed. In addition, precise timing of blood withdrawal during exercise testing is important, facilitated by an indwelling line.

After the Allen test, a 22-gauge angiocath is placed percutaneously in the radial artery and attached to heparinized extension tubing with stopcock. The initial 5 ml of each sample withdrawn should be discarded and the next aliquot placed on ice. Failure to expel air bubbles from the syringe results in an increase in the $Pa{O_2}$ and a decrease in the $Pa{CO_2}$ within 2 to 3 minutes. White blood cell counts greater than 100,000 result in a significant reduction in the $Pa{O_2}$ if measurement is not performed immediately; this can be averted by the prior addition of azide to the syringe. Excessive dilution with heparin usually results in a false elevation of the $Pa{O_2}$, a false decrease in the $Pa{CO_2}$, bicarbonate levels and base excess, and little change in pH. Complications of single puncture are rare except for hematoma in those with a hemorrhagic diathesis, or when appropriate pressure is not applied after the procedure. Complications of indwelling arterial catheters used briefly are uncommon but may include occlusion, dissection or, rarely, infection.[4] Care must be taken in flushing such lines, because inappropriate force or volume may result in systemic or cerebral embolism.

FIBEROPTIC BRONCHOSCOPY

The flexible fiberoptic bronchoscope was developed by Ikeda in cooperation with the Olympus and Machida companies in Japan in the 1960s to improve on rigid bronchoscopy in the detection and evaluation of lung cancer.[9] The results of initial evaluation were reported in 1968 and the first clinical experience in the U.S. was reported in 1971. Rigid bronchoscopy became available early in this century, but it is technically difficult, usually requires general anesthesia, and provides limited views of the airways, especially the upper lobes. By contrast, flexible fiberoptic bronchoscopy is easily performed by appropriately trained physicians, has great patient tolerance and acceptance, and extends the range of visualization. Although many bronchoscopists premedicate and sedate patients to a variable degree for fiberoptic bronchoscopy, the procedure can be performed in an awake, alert patient without endotracheal intubation and with only local anesthesia. The extent of visualization is greatly expanded over that of rigid bronchoscopy. Using the standard fiberoptic scope with an outer diameter of 6 mm, all segmental and most subsegmental bronchi can be entered; all segmental, subsegmental, and most subsubsegmental bronchi can be visualized.[5] The widespread availability of even smaller instruments, including pediatric bronchoscopes with external diameters of less than 4 mm, has further expanded visualization capability. The choice of bronchoscope is determined in part by the nature of the procedure. Bronchoscope models vary in size, suction capability, and number of instrument channels. The therapy of lobar atelectasis may require a large-channel scope, whereas small scopes may be indicated for visualization of more distal airways, or for a patient with a small endotracheal tube.

Indications

The indications for fiberoptic bronchoscopy are numerous (Table 42–1).[6–9] Many are important in patients with chronic obstructive pulmonary disease.

Hemoptysis

Hemoptysis is not an uncommon complaint in patients with COPD. Minor hemoptysis is often caused by chronic bronchitis. Because most COPD patients are current or ex-cigarette smokers, however, bronchoscopy is usually indicated to rule out carcinoma.

Lung Cancer Evaluations

Cigarette smoking is the major risk factor for the development of bronchogenic carcinoma; cigarette smokers with COPD appear to be at even greater risk. Bronchoscopy is commonly used for the diagnosis, staging and, occasionally, therapy of lung carcinoma. Bronchoscopy is indicated in the patient with a positive sputum cytology and a normal chest roentgenogram for the detection of intratracheal or bronchial carcinoma. The transnasal approach is preferred in such patients to detect a possible nasopharyngeal malignancy. The use of hematoporphyrin derivative (HPD) with laser stimula-

TABLE 42–1. Indications for Fiberoptic Bronchoscopy

Diagnostic	Therapeutic
Traumatic tracheobronchial disruption	Treatment of hemoptysis (occasional)
Hemoptysis	Foreign body removal
New persistent hoarseness	Bronchopleural fistula occlusion (rare)
Persistent and changing cough	Treatment of lung cancer
Localized wheeze	Carcinoma in situ—derivative and laser
Nonresponding lung abscess	Laser therapy of malignant airway obstruction
Persistent pneumonia or infiltrate	Brachytherapy of unresectable lung cancer
BAL for diagnosis of pneumonia	Endotracheal intubation
Diagnosis of tuberculosis	Therapy of lobar atelectasis
Transbronchial biopsy for specific disease	
Unexplained pleural effusion	
Unexplained chylothorax	
Endotracheal tube placement and evaluation of associated injury	
Acute inhalation injury	
Diagnosis of tracheoesophageal fistula	
Localization of bronchopleural fistula	
Localized bronchography	
Positive sputum cytology with negative chest radiograph	
Pulmonary nodules and masses	
Paralyzed diaphragm or vocal cord	
Superior vena cava syndrome	
Staging of lung cancer—including Wang needle aspiration	
Postoperative bronchial stump inspection	
Follow-up of neoplastic therapy	

tion can aid in the detection of occult carcinoma.[10, 11] HPD accumulates in malignant cells and may be detected by fluorescence. Bronchoscopy is also indicated for the evaluation of patients with new vocal cord and hemidiaphragm paralysis, as well as for those with superior vena cava syndrome. Another indication is the evaluation and biopsy of a mass or solitary pulmonary nodule discovered on an incidental chest radiograph. Diagnostic success is determined by the location and size of the lesion. Cancer staging may be aided by transbronchial needle aspiration of mediastinal adenopathy. Malignant unresectable endobronchial disease can be palliated with laser resection or localized brachytherapy.

Bronchiectasis

Thin-section CT scanning appears to be the best initial diagnostic procedure for bronchiectasis. Occasionally, however, bronchography is still indicated. Lobar or segmental evaluations may cause fewer side effects in patients with COPD. The examination is performed by placing a guide wire bronchoscopically into the appropriate bronchus, threading a catheter over the guide wire, injecting Dionosil, and taking the appropriate radiographs.

Infectious Pneumonia

Lower respiratory tract infection is common in the patient with COPD. Most pneumonias can be successfully managed with antibiotic therapy guided by sputum Gram's staining, sputum culture, and blood cultures. Bronchoscopy is useful in the evaluation of persistent infiltrates, however, particularly with volume loss, to rule out malignancy. Persistent infiltrates also may be caused by mycobacterial or fungal infections. When diagnosis is not achieved noninvasively, bronchoscopy with brushing and transbronchial biopsy may be useful. Bronchoscopy may be helpful in the evaluation of acute severe pneumonia. The diagnostic material obtained through the bronchoscope channel is approximately equivalent to expectorated sputum in value. The Bartlett-Faling-Wimberley telescoping protected brush gives variable results. In the hands of experienced personnel who adhere to techniques that minimize the contamination of specimens with upper airway flora, organisms isolated in a concentration $\geq 10^5$ colony-forming units/ml correlate well with the actual pulmonary pathogen.[12, 13]

Bronchoalveolar Lavage

Bronchoalveolar lavage (BAL) has been used extensively in the last two decades as a research tool for sampling alveolar contents. A number of studies have shown that cells retrieved by lavage reflect those in the distal pulmonary interstitium.[14, 15]

BAL has no role in the actual diagnosis of COPD, but rarely eosinophilic granuloma of the lung can resemble COPD, presenting with dyspnea, airway obstruction, and radiographs in which cystic changes predominate. In this setting, lung lavage that identifies Langerhans' cells with their characteristic X bodies may be diagnostic. BAL shows considerable promise as an alternative method for the diagnosis of lower respiratory tract infections. It has been apparent for some time that BAL is highly sensitive in the diagnosis of pneumocystis pneumonia in those with acquired immunodeficiency syndrome (AIDS), primarily because of the huge number of organisms in such patients. Fairly recent reports have suggested that BAL may also be helpful in the diagnosis of bacterial pneumonia in non-AIDS patients.[16] There is a high correlation of the growth of $\geq 10^5$ colony forming units/ml of BAL fluid with the infecting organism, especially when Gram's staining is positive for bacteria, with fewer than 1% squamous epithelial cells. Thus, BAL may be indicated in the diagnosis of infection in patients with COPD in whom other procedures are dangerous (e.g., transbronchial biopsy in patients with a hemorrhagic diathesis or receiving mechanical ventilation), poorly tolerated, or refused (e.g., transtracheal aspiration or transthoracic needle aspiration biopsy).

BAL adds minimally to the risk of standard bronchoscopy by causing somewhat more postprocedure hypoxemia. The bronchoscope is wedged either in the right middle lobe or lingula when the disease is diffuse, or in the bronchus communicating with the infected region. A total of 200 to 250 ml of nonbacteriostatic saline is delivered to the distal airway and aliquots are removed by suction to undergo the appropriate tests.

Technique

Fiberoptic bronchoscopy may be performed safely on an ambulatory basis. It is our practice, however, to observe patients requiring transbronchial lung biopsy for a minimum of 6 hours and to admit them to the hospital if complications develop. Adequate preoperative evaluation includes history, physical examination, determination of the complete blood count, prothrombin time, partial thromboplastin time, platelet count, creatinine and electrolyte levels, and room air arterial blood gases, and an electrocardiogram. A bleeding time is indicated if the platelet count is less than 100,000, if the patient has a history of using salicylates or nonsteroidal anti-inflammatory agents within the preceding 2 weeks, or if the serum creatinine level is too high.

The patient receives nothing orally for at least 6 hours prior to the procedure and is premedicated 30 minutes before bronchoscopy. Although many bronchoscopists premedicate with moderate doses of meperidine (50 to 75 mg) and hydroxyzine (25 mg), and sedate with IV diazepam or midazolam during the procedure, many fiberoptic bronchoscopies have been performed in patients who receive only atropine 0.01 mg/kg IM. Atropine diminishes secretions and bronchorrhea and is vagolytic, helping to prevent hypotension and bradycardia during the procedure.

The local anesthesia technique depends on the route chosen for bronchoscopy. The transnasal approach is used in most stable patients in many institutions. Lidocaine 1% is sprayed in the most patent nostril, followed by instillation of 2 to 3 ml lidocaine jelly. Patients who have anatomically small nares or congested nasal passages may benefit from the topical application of phenylephrine or cocaine to shrink the mucous membranes. The oropharynx and hypopharynx are then sprayed with a 1% lidocaine solution using an air pressure-driven atomizer. Other protocols call for concentrations of lidocaine that vary from 2% to 4%. Lidocaine is used rather than tetracaine because it has a higher therapeutic-to-toxic ratio, and because toxicity typically results in observable central nervous system symptoms before the development of cardiovascular instability.

The choice of patient position for bronchoscopy is a matter of personal preference. Many studies are performed with the patient sitting in a dental chair with the bronchoscopist facing the patient and positioned to the patient's right. Other bronchoscopists perform the procedure from the head of the stretcher with the patient supine. This is particularly convenient for procedures using fluoroscopy and/or endotracheal intubation. The bronchoscope is guided under direct vision through the nose and into the hypopharynx.

When the vocal cords are visualized they are anesthetized with direct instillation of 2 ml of 4% lidocaine while the patient opposes the vocal cords by singing "E." The bronchoscope is then gently passed through the glottis and additional 1% lidocaine is given through the bronchoscope as necessary to treat or prevent coughing. The indicated examination and procedures are then performed. The use of video systems and video screens with the bronchoscope is helpful because it is more comfortable for the bronchoscopist, there is less likelihood of inhaling potentially dangerous aerosolized bronchial secretions from the patient, and photographs and videotapes can serve as a quality control record.

Occasionally the patient cannot tolerate transnasal bronchoscopy and the use of transoral bronchoscopy is preferable. The patient must have a bite block in place to prevent damage to the bronchoscope. The procedure is otherwise similar. Endotracheal intubation should be performed whenever there is concern about airway control. This is particularly useful in the patient with severe COPD and hypercapnia, which is otherwise a relative contraindication. It is also an important precaution for those patients requiring sedation. The airway should be secured with an endotracheal tube before transbronchial lung biopsy to aid in the management of serious complications.

Finally, the patient who is undergoing bronchoscopy for evaluation and possible therapy of major hemoptysis should be intubated. Ordinarily, the endotracheal tube is passed by mouth, using the bronchoscope as a guide. The prior administration of a laryngeal nerve block transcutaneously may facilitate passage and reduce the incidence of laryngospasm.

Patient Monitoring

Bronchoscopy is associated with a 15 to 20 mm Hg decrease in the Pa_{O_2}, which may last for several hours; therefore, it is important to monitor the patient with continuous pulse oximetry. A decrease in oxygen saturation may also be associated with hypoventilation, especially in patients with COPD who receive sedation. Oxygen is given as necessary to maintain oxygen saturation above 90%. Noninvasive blood pressure and continuous electrocardiographic monitoring allow early detection and treatment of cardiovascular complications. An intravenous line should be in place prior to the procedure and resuscitation equipment should be immediately available.

After bronchoscopy, the patient should be observed for a minimum of 2 hours. During this time the patient receives nothing orally until the gag reflex has returned. After transbronchial biopsy the patient is observed for 6 hours. A postprocedure chest film is necessary to rule out pneumothorax after transbronchial biopsy or vigorous brushing.

Complications

The complication rate for bronchoscopy is low.[17, 18] In nearly 25,000 bronchoscopy procedures, there was a reported mortality of 1 in 10,000, a morbidity of 0.2% (major, 0.08%), and hemorrhage ≥50 ml in 1.4%.[19] This study was retrospective and questionnaire-generated, and probably underestimated the frequency of complications. A prospective study of 908 patients by Pereira and colleagues showed a death rate of 1 in 10,000, a morbidity rate of 8.2% (1.7% major), and a procedure-related pneumonia rate of 0.6%.[17] Complications increased in the elderly, in patients with coronary artery disease, and in patients with COPD.

Complications include laryngospasm, which is uncommon if the vocal cords are anesthetized directly with 2 to 4 ml of lidocaine. Vasovagal reactions and syncope are also uncommon, particularly if the patient has been premedicated with atropine and if the dosage of meperidine was appropriate. Serious dysrhythmias from bronchoscopy are uncommon but are potentially lethal, and the means for detecting and treating them must be instantly available. Bleeding is uncommon from bronchoscopy alone. In general, patients with uremia should not be biopsied, because there is a high incidence of bleeding complications; the administration of cryoprecipitate or arginine vasopressin (DDAVP) may reduce hemorrhage if the bleeding time returns to normal. Postprocedure fever is relatively common, but pneumonia is not. Pneumothorax occurs almost exclusively with transbronchial lung biopsy. Lidocaine reactions are rarely seen if the total dose is lower than 300 mg and are rarely serious if the total dose is lower than 600 mg. They may be avoided if the cumulative dose of lidocaine is continuously recorded and monitored during the procedure.

Contraindications

Bronchoscopy may be performed with appropriate precautions, but the indications for bronchoscopy should be significant enough to justify the risk. Anticoagulation or an uncorrectable bleeding diathesis is a contraindication to biopsy, although bronchoscopy alone may be performed, preferably by an oral approach. Severe tracheal stenosis is a relative contraindication because procedure-related edema may precipitate total airway obstruction.

Increased intracranial pressure is a relative contraindication. Cerebral edema may be reduced by steroid administration before bronchoscopy, and evidence has shown that appropriate lidocaine prophylaxis topically and intravenously can blunt the increase in intracranial pressure associated with laryngeal manipulation.

Unstable angina or uncontrolled arrhythmia are significant contraindications. Recent myocardial infarction is a relative contraindication, and elective procedures are best delayed for 3 to 6 months. The indications for bronchoscopy are seldom truly elective, however, and the risk of bronchoscopy must be weighed against the risk of a delay in diagnosis and therapy.

Inability of the patient to cooperate with the procedure is a relative contraindication, although after appropriate consent the procedure may be performed with sedation and intubation or general anesthesia. Manipulation of an undrained lung abscess may cause spillage of the infected material and injury of previously uninvolved lung.

Uncontrolled asthma is a strong contraindication, because bronchoscopy before bronchospasm is brought under control may precipitate respiratory failure. Asthma is treated with theophylline and β-adrenergic agonists. If there is a history of severe bronchospasm, the patient may receive prednisone for several days at a dose of 0.5 mg/kg. It is helpful to anesthetize the airway in such patients by nebulization of 1% lidocaine mixed with a β-adrenergic agonist (e.g., 0.25 mg of albuterol). During passage of the bronchoscope the vocal cords should be anesthetized with lidocaine containing epinephrine in a 1 to 20,000 dilution.

The injudicious use of sedating premedication in hypercapnic patients may precipitate respiratory failure. Minimal sedation should be given to such patients and the airway controlled with endotracheal intubation. They must be carefully observed after the procedure, with oximetry monitoring for a minimum of 2 hours.

Hypoxemia is not a contraindication to bronchoscopy as long as the Po_2 can be increased to 70 mm Hg or more with oxygen. The Pao_2 routinely decreases by 15 to 20 mm Hg for 3 to 4 hours during and after the procedure, and both the intensity and duration of desaturation may be increased with bronchoalveolar lavage. Incipient respiratory failure, either hypoxic or hypercapnic, is a contraindication to bronchoscopy until the patient has been intubated and is receiving mechanical ventilation.

Table 42–2 summarizes the major contraindications to the use of bronchoscopy.

TRANSTRACHEAL ASPIRATION

The etiologic diagnosis of a lower respiratory tract infection is usually made by sputum culture and sensitivity testing, and occasionally by blood culture. Unfortunately, expectorated sputum specimens from patients with pneumonia provide an inadequate specimen in 20%, a misleading contaminant in 30% to 50%, and an appropriate pathogen in 30% to 50%. Diagnosis of infection by bronchoscopy and bronchoalveolar lavage has been discussed. Percutaneous lung aspiration for the diagnosis of pneumonia is used in children, but not in adults. To avoid problems with expectorated sputum samples, transtracheal aspiration has been popularized by Bartlett.[20, 21]

TABLE 42–2. Contraindications to Bronchoscopy and Transbronchial Biopsy

Tracheal stenosis
Increased intracranial pressure
Recent myocardial infarction
Unstable angina
Unstable cardiac dysrhythmia
Inability to cooperate
Acute lung abscess
Uncontrolled asthma
Respiratory failure prior to mechanical ventilation
Additional contraindications to transbronchial biopsy:
Anticoagulation
Uncorrectable bleeding diathesis
Positive-pressure ventilation
Pulmonary hypertension

Because the trachea is almost sterile in healthy individuals, transtracheal aspiration samples lower respiratory pathogen levels without contamination by upper airway flora. The diagnosis of lower airway infection is improved in a number of clinical settings but not for patients with COPD, because the lower airways are frequently colonized with *Streptococcus pneumoniae* and *Hemophilus influenzae*.

LUNG BIOPSY

Lung tissue is rarely required in the diagnosis of patients with airflow obstruction. A prominent exception is bronchiolitis obliterans and its variants, which may present with dyspnea and airflow obstruction.[22, 23] Lung biopsy is important in the diagnosis of pulmonary complications of COPD, however, including lung malignancy, bacterial pneumonias, and mycobacterial and fungal diseases. The use of the various techniques depends on the clinical situation; five basic approaches are possible.

Bronchial Biopsy

Endobronchial biopsy is indicated when lesions are visible. It is performed under direct visualization with bronchoscopic biopsy forceps. The best biopsy specimens are often obtained at the edge of the lesion, avoiding necrotic centers. Shure and Astarita have indicated that three or more biopsies maximize the diagnostic yield.[24] Cytologic samples are more likely to be positive when the lesion is brushed after the biopsy, rather than before. Endobronchial biopsy should not be undertaken in a patient with an uncontrolled bleeding diathesis, and hypervascular lesions should be biopsied with caution or not at all. Prior application of epinephrine diluted to 1 to 20,000 may decrease bleeding. When inspection of the lesion suggests the possibility of a carcinoid tumor, consideration should be given to needle aspiration rather than to cup forceps biopsy; simultaneous inspection of the lesion with a thoracic surgical consultant instead of biopsy is another possibility.

Transbronchial Needle Biopsy

Wang has popularized transbronchial needle aspiration biopsy and it is by his name that the procedure is most often known. Endobronchial biopsy provides tissue for histologic examination; Wang needle aspiration provides cytologic specimens only. It is indicated for the evaluation of infiltrating bronchial submucosal lesions and for mediastinal adenopathy.[25] It may confirm mediastinal spread of primary lung cancer and may yield the diagnosis of a malignancy when a peripheral primary tumor is inaccessible. Guided by prebiopsy CT scanning, the diagnostic yield in lung cancer may be as high as 75% when the mediastinum is abnormal on the chest radiograph. When a midlung or peripheral nodule cannot be biopsied by the transbronchial forceps, Wang needle aspiration with fluoroscopic guidance may be successful. The flexible catheter is tipped with a 1.3-cm, 23-gauge needle, with a syringe attachment at the proximal end for suction. It is passed through the channel of the bronchoscope, the needle is extended, and the area of interest is pierced. A small amount of saline solution is injected, the needle is agitated, and the lesion is aspirated. The catheter is withdrawn and the contents are smeared on glass slides and immediately fixed in 95% ethanol. If a pathologist is present for rapid review of the specimens during the procedure, the yield increases. Because infectious diseases such as tuberculosis may cause mediastinal adenopathy, at least one additional specimen should be obtained and given to the microbiology department for appropriate stains and cultures. Complications are unusual; pneumothorax occurs in less than 1% of patients.

Transbronchial Biopsy

Indications

Transbronchial biopsy provides small pieces of peripheral lung tissue, including alveoli, for histologic examination. The diagnostic accuracy is highest with diffuse infiltrative disease, wherein it should be the initial procedure of choice. It is also useful in the diagnosis of diffuse infections, including *Pneumocystis carinii*, cytomegalovirus, miliary tuberculosis, and certain fungal infections. Although transbronchial lung biopsy is not routinely indicated for the diagnosis of COPD, several interstitial lung diseases may present with airflow obstruction and may be diagnosed by transbronchial lung biopsy. Lymphangiomyomatosis is an infiltrative lung disease occurring in women of reproductive age who may present with chylothorax, pneumothorax, hemoptysis, dyspnea, and an obstructive pattern on pulmonary function testing (PFT). The characteristic histology may be seen on transbronchial lung biopsy. Sarcoid is a common interstitial granulomatous lung disease that may be associated with an obstructive PFT pattern. Transbronchial lung biopsy is frequently diagnostic, showing the characteristic noncaseating granulomata in a high proportion of patients. Eosinophilic granuloma is part of the spectrum of histiocytosis X. It produces interstitial lung disease with associated cystic lesions and may be associated with recurrent pneumothorax and an obstructive physiologic pattern. It can sometimes be diagnosed on transbronchial biopsy by characteristic histologic finding of Langerhans' cells that contain X bodies (Birbeck granules). Transbronchial lung biopsy is, unfortunately, inadequate for the diagnosis of bronchiolitis obliterans.

Transbronchial lung biopsy may be useful in the diagnosis of midlung or peripheral pulmonary nodules. Fluoroscopic guidance increases the yield and the chance of diagnosis increases with the number of biopsies; up to ten may be necessary to maximize the yield in a peripheral lesion. The likelihood of diagnosis also depends on the size of the lesion. Only 10% to 40% of peripheral lesions smaller than 2 cm in diameter can be diagnosed by transbronchial biopsy, whereas lesions larger than 3 cm in diameter can be diagnosed in up to 80%.[26]

Technique and Complications

Transbronchial biopsy performed with fluoroscopy facilitates forceps placement in a specific area or lesion and reduces the incidence of pneumothorax. The preoperative preparation, monitoring capabilities, and premedication are similar to those for bronchoscopy alone. Endotracheal intubation prior to transbronchial lung biopsy allows better control of a bleeding complication, and 2 to 3 ml of 1 to 20,000 epinephrine in the appropriate bronchus prior to the biopsy may reduce the amount of bleeding. The closed biopsy forceps are passed slowly and gently to a point of no further peripheral progress. If the patient perceives pleural pain, which is always asked for specifically, the forceps are withdrawn and redirected.

When the limits of extension have been reached the forceps are withdrawn approximately 5 cm and opened. The patient is instructed to breathe to total lung capacity and expire to residual volume while the biopsy forceps are held in position. At residual volume the biopsy forceps are closed and withdrawn. Typically, a characteristic tug is felt as the biopsy forceps are removed. The bronchoscope is left wedged in the segmental or subsegmental bronchus to maintain suction and control bleeding for several minutes; the procedure is then repeated three to nine times, depending on the expected disease process and the apparent adequacy of the biopsy specimens.[26] Because of the possibility of pneumothorax, biopsies are not taken from the contralateral lung on the same day. Blind biopsy is not performed in the upper or middle lobes, where it is easier to puncture the pleura without warning. Fluoroscopy is especially useful in the biopsy of diffuse lung disease, in which it reduces the danger of pleural injury. Biplane fluoroscopy is also helpful in ensuring that the biopsy forceps is in a nodule or localized infiltrate.

Complications and contraindications are the same as those for bronchoscopy, with several additions (Table 42–2). Pulmonary hypertension appears to increase bleeding. Particular attention should be paid to the presence of an uncorrected bleeding disorder. Mechanical ventilation, particularly with positive end-expiratory pressure, is a relative contraindication, although reports of performance with minimal adverse affects have appeared. Inability of the patient to cooperate fully is an indication for fluoroscopy and sedation. The complications are those of bronchoscopy, with the addition of major hemoptysis and pneumothorax. The latter occurs in 2% to 5% of patients but requires chest tube drainage in fewer than one-half of these cases. Air embolism is a rare complication.

Transthoracic Needle Aspiration Biopsy

Transthoracic needle aspiration biopsy is performed to obtain cytologic samples of peripheral lung lesions. Peripheral lung lesions that have eluded diagnosis after sputum sampling and bronchoscopy are often best managed by exploratory thoracotomy, but it is preferable to avoid thoracotomy for diagnosis in a patient with severe COPD. In the patient whose pulmonary function precludes lung resection, needle aspiration may allow distinction of a small cell from a non-small cell carcinoma. It may separate benign peripheral cavitary lesions from malignant and allow the identification of bacterial, fungal, or mycobacterial infections. Transthoracic needle aspiration is extremely effective in the diagnosis of peripheral lung cancer; cytologies are positive in more than 90% of carcinomas and in approximately 50% of pulmonary lymphomas. It is less effective in the diagnosis of peripheral benign granulomatous lung disease.[27–29]

Technique

The level of narcotic premedication is a matter of personal preference. Atropine should, however, be included in the premedication. Local preparation includes skin cleansing, local anesthesia, and sterile draping. Oxygen is administered to the patient. Biopsy needles range from thin (20-gauge) to ultrathin (24- to 25-gauge); the larger needles can be used without a guide needle. Although biopsy can be carried out under biplane fluoroscopic guidance, CT scanning has more recently supplanted fluoroscopy in many medical centers. Patients are instructed to hold their breath while the needle is passed through the pleura and then to breathe quietly. Needle localization is confirmed by CT scanning or fluoroscopy. Approximately 2 to 3 ml of saline solution are injected into the lesion. The needle is agitated and removed while constant suction is applied. The contents of the needle and syringe are smeared on glass slides, which are fixed immediately in 95% ethanol. A cytologist at the procedure can prepare and review the smears. The procedure can be repeated until a satisfactory specimen has been obtained. Several passes are usually made; the material obtained from at least one is hand-carried to the microbiology department for the appropriate studies. A post-procedure chest film is obtained and, in the absence of pneumothorax, the patient is observed for 4 hours.

Contraindications and Complications

Contraindications include severe bullous lung disease, because of the increased incidence of pneumothorax, an uncorrected bleeding disorder, the possibility that the lesion is an arteriovenous malformation, pulmonary hypertension, and the inability of the operator to insert a chest tube immediately. Complications include pneumothorax in 8% to 20% of procedures; up to one-half of these may require a chest tube. Tension pneumothorax is rare. Mild hemoptysis occurs in 4% to 10%, but major hemoptysis is rare. Other rare complications include air embolism, tumor seeding, and death.

Open Lung Biopsy

Open lung biopsy provides much larger samples of lung tissue. The need to resort to it in the diagnosis of COPD is rare, although it is required for the diagnosis of bronchiolitis obliterans. Open lung biopsy is superior to transbronchial biopsy in the diagnosis of most diffuse infiltrative lung disease.[30] CT-guided minithoracotomy may be appropriate for a localized peripheral infiltrate.

RIGHT-HEART AND PULMONARY ARTERY CATHETERIZATION

The introduction of the flow-directed pulmonary artery catheter in 1970[31] has had a profound impact on the practice of critical care medicine.[32–34] It allows the bedside or even ambulatory catheterization of the right heart and pulmonary circulation. It permits the routine measurement of cardiac output, pulmonary artery pressures, pulmonary artery occlusion pressure (often referred to as pulmonary capillary wedge pressure), mixed venous oxygen saturation (MVo_2), shunt fraction (Q_S/Q_T), and pulmonary vascular resistance (PVR). It also facilitates the direct delivery of vasoactive drugs to the pulmonary circulation. There are several uses for catheterization in the patient with COPD.

Preoperative Evaluation For Pneumonectomy

In the patient who has borderline spirometric values for pneumonectomy, a resting PVR of more than 190 dyne-sec-cm^{-5} suggests that the patient will probably not tolerate resection and will have unacceptable postresection pulmonary hypertension. This evaluation is rarely made. Occasionally, a patient for whom lobectomy was planned is found at operation to require a pneumonectomy. Preoperative pulmonary function tests may make it clear that this is possible; if not, the absence of pulmonary hypertension or significantly increased PVR (detected by a Swan-Ganz catheter in the contralateral pulmonary artery during hilar cross clamping) is reassuring.

Evaluation of Pulmonary Hypertension

The principal indication for elective pulmonary artery catheterization in COPD patients is the detection and quantitation of pulmonary hypertension and the subsequent determination of the effects of therapy. The clinical signs of pulmonary hypertension and cor pulmonale are late and insensitive, with the physical examination, the ECG, and the chest radiograph detecting only about 50% of those patients who could be diagnosed by echocardiography.[35, 36]

The normal physiologic response to exercise recorded by right-heart catheterization includes a small increase in mean pulmonary artery pressure, a greater increase in cardiac output, and a resultant decrease in PVR with levels approximately 10% of those of simultaneous systemic resistance.[37] Early in the development of pulmonary hypertension the pulmonary artery pressures and resistances are normal at rest but, during exercise, the mean pulmonary artery pressure rises disproportionately to cardiac output. As a result there is an elevation in pulmonary vascular resistance and an increase in right ventricular end-diastolic pressure. The response of these abnormalities to oxygen therapy can be evaluated by administering oxygen during the catheterization.

Persistent pulmonary hypertension at rest is a late occurrence in COPD and is eventually followed by right ventricular failure. In patients with COPD and pulmonary hypertension who are oxygen-unresponsive, vasodilator therapy may be beneficial. Many vasodilators have been tried in research protocols, including naloxone, isoproterenol, phentolamine, prazosin, verapamil, nifedipine, nitrendipine, felodopine, urapidil, nitroprusside, hydralazine, and prostacycline.[38, 39] If a trial of pulmonary vasodilators is to be attempted, it should be performed in a medical center with personnel experienced in their use and with the availability of right-heart monitoring equipment. Whereas a pulmonary vasodilator may decrease PVR and mean pulmonary artery pressure and increase cardiac output, it may also cause systemic vasodilation, diminished preload, decreased cardiac output, and diminished systemic oxygen transport. Moreover, if a beneficial effect is obtained, it may not be sustained, and responsive patients should be studied several days and months later. Because convincing evidence is still lacking that any pulmonary vasodilator except oxygen has long-term favorable effects on symptoms, exercise tolerance, pulmonary artery hemodynamics, and mortality in COPD, the use of pulmonary vasodilators and the invasive evaluation of pulmonary artery circulation in COPD should be considered an investigational procedure at present. Two-dimensional echocardiography, contrast-enhanced Doppler, and radionuclide angiography are more sensitive than the physical examination in making the early diagnosis of pulmonary hypertension and are less invasive than right-heart catheterization.

Exercise Evaluation of Dyspnea

Patients are frequently referred to pulmonary exercise laboratories for the assessment of exercise-induced dyspnea. It is possible to place a pulmonary artery flotation catheter prior to cycle ergometry or treadmill testing in an ambulatory setting. The pulmonary artery catheter allows a more precise diagnosis of exercise-related congestive heart failure and pulmonary hypertension, permits accurate cardiac output measurement, and allows determination of the MVo_2. However, such an invasive approach is rarely used. A noninvasive exercise study usually separates cardiovascular and pulmonary vascular causes of dyspnea from purely pulmonary causes. If the results are typical of coronary artery disease, the patient may be referred to a cardiologist for appropriate testing, such as a stress thallium study or exercise radionuclide ventriculography. If, on the other hand, the exercise study suggests pulmonary vascular disease (e.g., exercise oxygen desaturation with increased alveolar-arterial gradient, low maximum oxygen consumption, increased ratio of minute ventilation to carbon dioxide production (V_E/V_{CO_2}), increased V_D/V_T with exercise, low oxygen pulse, and early anaerobic threshold), the patient can be referred for noninvasive cardiovascular studies and a lung scan. A decision regarding the necessity of right-heart catheterization, pulmonary angiography, or even an open lung biopsy may then be made.

THORACENTESIS

Indications

Removal of pleural fluid for diagnostic purposes is indicated in the evaluation of any pleural effusion of unknown origin.[40] It has no particular application in the diagnosis of COPD, with the possible exception of lymphangiomyomatosis. In a reproductive-age woman with airway obstruction and diffuse linear opacities, the detection of a chylothorax provides strong evidence supporting the diagnosis. Given the common risk factors, pleural fluid accumulation in the COPD patient is often a result of congestive heart failure, carcinoma, or infection. Administration of a diuretic is occasionally acceptable as a substitute for thoracentesis when the most likely diagnosis is congestive heart failure, as long as infection or cancer is not suspected. Thoracentesis is also indicated for the improvement of dyspnea causd by a pleural effusion. Such an attempt should be determined by the patient's symptoms, and not by the results of pulmonary function tests, because the vital capacity may improve surprisingly little, even with removal of a large amount of fluid. Symptoms, however, may improve with removal of large effusions, especially when there is associated mediastinal shift. When pleural effusion is caused by malignancy and pleurodesis is not possible or desirable, serial thoracentesis may be useful, particularly if the effusion reaccumulates slowly.

Contraindications to thoracentesis include a bleeding diathesis, inability of the patient to cooperate, and local infection at the site of the proposed needle puncture.

Technique

Thoracentesis is usually performed with the patient sitting and leaning forward, with the arms resting comfortably on a bedside table. This facilitates the posterior collection of free-flowing fluid. Small effusions can occasionally be aspirated more easily when the patient leans backwards or lies supine, with the area to be tapped in the open space between two stretchers. The supine position may occasionally be required for thoracentesis in the severely weak and debilitated patient. In situations in which fluid is clearly present, as documented by chest radiography or ultrasonography, but is located in a single area of the pleural space, directed needle puncture is necessary.

No premedication is ordinarily needed. The skin is cleansed with iodophor and is anesthetized with lidocaine or a similar local anesthetic using a 25-gauge needle. The deeper tissues are subsequently anesthetized with a 22-gauge, 1½-inch needle passing directly over the top of the rib to avoid the intercostal vessels that course immediately below the ribs. The anesthesia needle is advanced with deposition of anesthetic alternating with suction until the pleural space has been entered, as documented by the return of fluid. The anesthesia syringe is then removed and diagnostic thoracentesis is performed. We prefer to use a 30-ml syringe connected to one side of a three-way stopcock, with an arterial blood gas syringe attached to the other side. The diagnostic syringe is lightly heparinized to prevent clotting of the pleural fluid if it is exudative.

Thirty ml of fluid for diagnostic tests are removed, the stopcock is turned, and pleural fluid is collected in the arterial blood gas syringe under anaerobic conditions. The syringe is placed immediately on ice and sent to the blood gas laboratory for pH analysis. The remainder of the fluid is sent for cell count and differential, total protein, glucose, lactose dehydrogenase (LDH), and amylase analyses. Determinations of each of the last four should be performed on a recently drawn serum specimen or the appropriate blood test should be ordered shortly after thoracentesis. In addition, the fluid is sent for Gram's staining, acid-fast staining, and appropriate cultures and sensitivities. An anaerobic specimen for culture may also be collected. Anticoagulated pleural fluid is also sent to the cytology laboratory. Additional fluid should be retained for tests that may subsequently be indicated after evaluation of the initial test results. These can include measurement of triglycerides and lipoproteins (by electrophoresis), antinuclear antibodies and rheumatoid factor, and lupus erythematosus (LE) cell preparation. The initial separation of the effusion into the categories of transudate or exudate may be decided on the basis of the LDH and protein levels.

Removal of fluid for therapeutic purposes must be performed carefully to avoid re-expansion pulmonary edema. Ordinarily, 1000 ml can be removed slowly without complications. Monitoring the intrapleural pressure during the procedure has been advocated to avoid this complication but may be necessary only if larger quantities of fluid are to be removed or if the patient has had a pneumonectomy. Generally, the removal of a large effusion by thoracentesis is limited to one or two episodes. Further recurrences are usually treated by chest tube placement and pleural sclerosis. Serial thoracenteses may be appropriate if the fluid reaccumulates slowly, however, or if the patient has a limited life expectancy.

Complications

The complications of thoracentesis are uncommon; the most serious is re-expansion pulmonary edema. Pneumothorax occurs occasionally but is rare with good technique. Other complications associated with needle puncture include introduction of pleural infection, parenchymal organ puncture, and, rarely, tumor seeding (although seeding may occur in as many as 25% of patients with mesothelioma). Organ puncture can be avoided by careful attention to the site of puncture. We have often observed that inexperienced operators perform an initial puncture at a level lower than that which is desirable or necessary. Finally, it is possible for the patient to have a reaction to local anesthesia, but most untoward reactions associated with the administration of anesthesia are probably vasovagal.

PLEURAL BIOPSY

Parietal pleural sampling is not part of the diagnosis of COPD, per se, but is indicated in the evaluation of an exudative effusion of unclear etiology. The differential diagnosis of effusion in COPD includes many disorders, but the most common are congestive heart failure, lung cancer and metastatic malignancy, parapneumonic effusion, and tuberculosis. It is reasonable to determine the nature of the pleural fluid before undertaking pleural biopsy, although biopsy has been advocated if visual inspection of the fluid suggests an exudate. Waiting for initial laboratory results may clarify the diagnosis, however, and obviate the need for further investigation, with little loss of time. An exception to this may be the patient in whom malignancy is strongly suspected and the initial fluid is bloody. It must be remembered that pleural biopsy changes the character of any subsequent thoracentesis.[41, 42]

Pleural biopsy is most useful in the diagnosis of tuberculosis and malignant effusion. Adequate tissue is obtained in approximately 90% of biopsies. The combination of pleural fluid cytology plus pleural biopsy results in the correct diagnosis of pleural malignancy in about 65% of patients.[43] The additive sensitivity of pleural biopsy histology and culture is considerably higher in those with tuberculosis (80% to 95%). When a single thoracentesis and pleural biopsy has been nondiagnostic, a second or even third biopsy may be productive.

Pleural biopsy requires a willing patient who can cooperate with the performance of the procedure. Lack of either is a contraindication. It should not be carried out if there is empyema or uncontrollable bleeding diathesis, or when the effusion is a transudate, because no condition causing a transudative effusion can be clarified by biopsy.

The initial preparation is the same as for thoracentesis. It is helpful to devote considerable attention to wider dispersal of anesthesia at the parietal pleural surface. For the pleural biopsy needle to enter the chest, it is necessary to make a small skin incision after sterile preparation and local anesthesia. Two biopsy needles are in common use. The Cope needle is easy to use but obtains only one piece of pleura with each pass and has a somewhat greater likelihood of causing pneumothorax, because it is an intrinsically open system. The Abrams' needle, which is preferred by many, is a closed system and therefore has less chance of producing pneumothorax. Moreover, it is often desirable to drain the residual pleural fluid following a biopsy and, because the outer cannula is blunt, there is less chance of pneumothorax with the end-of-procedure therapeutic thoracentesis. It is also possible to obtain three or more samples of pleural tissue with each pass and the pieces tend to be larger. Ultimately, the choice of instrument depends on training and personal preference.

Complications include hemothorax and pneumothorax. The latter requires a chest tube in fewer than 1% of procedures. Other puncture-dependent problems include splenic, renal, and hepatic biopsies. Malignant seeding may occur but is an unimportant complication, except in mesothelioma, in which the resultant skin involvement is extremely painful and may require local radiation therapy. Some clinicians have advocated prophylactic radiation to the biopsy sites if mesothelioma has been diagnosed.

PLEUROSCOPY

Pleuroscopy[44–46] was introduced in the early part of the 20th century by Jacobaeus to allow lysis of adhesions and successful collapse therapy of tuberculosis. Currently, the major indication is evaluation of effusions whose etiology remain unclear after thoracentesis, pleural fluid analysis, and pleural biopsy. It is also used in the sclerosis of malignant effusions and may be useful for pleurodesis of recurrent pneumothorax, particularly in a patient at high risk for thoracotomy. It has also been used to diagnose the chest wall extension of lung cancer in patients with limited pulmonary reserve to spare marginal resection candidates an unnecessary thoracotomy. Some investigators have even performed lung biopsies in selected patients. Contraindications include an uncontrollable clotting disorder and thick pleural adhesions.

General anesthesia has been used in most studies although, in one large series, all procedures were performed with local anesthesia, a rigid thoracoscope, and an intercostal incision.[44] This study included some elderly patients with respiratory insufficiency. Because the procedure involves the creation of a controlled pneumothorax, the ability to maintain an adequate airway is essential if the procedure is not performed with endotracheal anesthesia. Although the fiberoptic bronchoscope has been used, the field of vision is limited, and the biopsy specimens are small. Therefore, the rigid scope is preferred. A scope made specifically for thoracoscopy is available, although some prefer to use the mediastinoscope.

Complications include empyema in fewer than 4%, hemorrhage, and a chest tube for 1 to 3 days. A persistent air leak may occasionally occur, but this is rare.

The role of thoracoscopy in routine diagnosis remains somewhat unclear. It is most useful in the diagnosis of pleural malignancy. The diagnosis of pleural tuberculosis by pleuroscopy is less fruitful, with an approximate yield of 25%; the diagnosis is usually made with closed pleural biopsy. In one large study, when effusions were present for more than 4 weeks and undiagnosed after at least two thoracenteses and one pleural biopsy, thoracoscopy was successful in making the diagnosis of pleural malignancy in 87%.[45] It has been argued that this aggressive approach to the diagnosis of pleural malignancy is unnecessary given the prognosis and lack of effective therapy. The establishment of a firm diagnosis, however, allows rational planning for therapy on the part of the team of internist, oncologist, and radiotherapist, and additional time for coping and planning on the part of the patient.

BALLOON MANOMETRY AND ELECTROMYOGRAPHY

The measurement of intraesophageal pressure as a reflection of intrapleural pressure at different lung volumes and during various respiratory maneuvers has added greatly to the understanding of the mechanics of the respiratory system. Measurement of the transpulmonary pressure (intrapleural pressure, P_{pl} − airway pressure, P_{ao}) at different lung volumes defines lung compliance. Such studies have shown that emphysema is associated with increased pulmonary compliance and that pulmonary fibrosis is associated with diminished compliance. Considerable interest has focused on the possibility that disease in small airways precedes and predicts clinically significant COPD. Change in closing volume detected by nitrogen washout, increase in the lung volumes at which the flow rates for helium and oxygen are equivalent (volume of isoflow), and changes in pulmonary compliance with changes in respiratory rate (frequency dependence of compliance) are believed to reflect abnormalities in small airways. The latter test is performed using esophageal balloon manometry. Because studies have failed to reveal that abnormal tests of small airways function in smokers predict the development of COPD, however, none of these tests are performed routinely.

Balloon Manometry

Currently esophageal and gastric balloon manometry is used in the evaluation of diaphragmatic and other respiratory muscle function. The technique is not difficult but requires moderately expensive equipment. Esophageal balloons may be purchased commercially. They are attached to the end of long, thin polyethylene tubing. After local anesthesia, two balloons and tubes are passed through the nares. The proximal ends of the tubing are attached to pressure transducers, which in turn are connected to amplifiers and a calibrated strip chart recorder. Both tubes are passed into the stomach and the balloon position is confirmed by the presence of positive inspiratory pressures recorded on the strip chart recorder. One balloon is then withdrawn into the midesophagus, where inspiratory pressures are negative.

The following abbreviations are used: the gastric pressure is P_g; the intrapleural pressure is P_{pl} and is approximated by the esophageal pressure; the transdiaphragmatic pressure is P_{di}, which $= P_g - P_{pl}$ (ordinarily this is a positive number). The P_{di} that is generated with maximum inspiratory effort against a closed mouthpiece at functional residual capacity is the maximal transdiaphragmatic pressure, $P_{di\ max}$.

The measurement of transdiaphragmatic pressures and of the respiratory cycle duration and divisions allows the quantitation of respiratory muscle strength and the evaluation of diaphragmatic fatigue. The transdiaphragmatic pressure with quiet breathing (P_{di}) and maximum effort ($P_{di\ max}$) are measured using esophageal balloons. Phases of the respiratory cycle may be measured manometrically or by using respiratory inductive plethysmography. The relevant fractions are the inspiratory time (T_i), the total duration of inspiration plus expiration (T_{tot}), and the ratio of T_i to T_{tot} (T_i/T_{tot}, the duty cycle). The product of $P_{di}/P_{di\ max}$ and the duty cycle is the tension-time index (TT_{di}).

$$TT_{di} = (P_{di}/P_{di\ max}) \text{ X } (T_i/T_{tot})$$

With quiet breathing, the TT_{di} is approximately 0.015. Fatiguing respiratory work is associated with a product persistently ≥ 0.15. Partly because of hyperinflation and the resulting unfavorable diaphragmatic position, the $P_{di\ max}$ in the COPD patient is reduced. Thus, whereas a normal $P_{di\ max}$ is 150 ± 14 cm H_2O, in patients with COPD the value is often lower than 50 cm H_2O. A normal P_{di} with quiet breathing is 5 to 8 cm H_2O. The P_{di} in COPD may be greater. The increase in $P_{di}/P_{di\ max}$ increases the TT_{di}, which increases the likelihood of fatigue. Conditions associated with an increase in respiratory rate may increase T_i/T_{tot}, which also results in a TT_{di} that is more likely to be in the fatiguing range. The use of esophageal manometry allows the assessment of diaphragmatic strength and fatigue and it might be useful in ventilatory weaning. Use of this technique can also provide an objective measurement for the evaluation of therapeutic measures to improve respiratory muscle function, including medications, muscle training programs, and rehabilitation.[47, 48]

Electromyography

Respiratory muscle electromyography (EMG) is still a research tool but is the subject of considerable clinical interest. It has been observed that respiratory muscle fatigue is associated with the redistribution of EMG content from higher to lower frequencies. There is a decrease in the centroid frequency and a downward shift in the ratio of high to low frequencies (H to L), a comparison of the power content of a high-frequency band (150 to 350 Hz) and a low-frequency band (20 to 40 Hz). A number of studies have shown that changes in this ratio correlate with changes in the TT_{di}.[48] Although the cause of these changes in the EMG power spectrum remains unknown, the validity of this observation allows objective research regarding the efficacy of treatment of diaphragmatic fatigue, including the effects of methylxanthines and β_2-adrenergic agonists, to be carried out. Further development of the technique or of related procedures may allow objective evaluation of the need for mechanical ventilatory support and respiratory muscle rest. In addition, meaningful comparisons of ventilator weaning modes may finally be possible and the optimal timing for the cessation of ventilator support individualized.

Esophageal EMG requires expensive equipment, not commonly available in pulmonary physiology laboratories, and presently should be regarded as a research procedure. It requires a third transnasal tube. The electrode may be custom-made using a polyethylene tube and platinum wire, or a Swan-Ganz catheter with electrode incorporation may be used. The recording of electromyographic signals requires an EMG signal recorder; detection of changes in the power spectrum requires a band-pass filter adjusted to the frequencies selected, a rectifier, and an integrator.

Because diaphragmatic EMG measurement is moderately invasive, it would be advantageous if similar data could be obtained from surface measurements. Attempts to measure diaphragmatic EMG from surface electrodes have met with variable success, but generally the procedure is difficult and the data are poorly reproducible. Fatigue can be evaluated in accessory muscles of respiration by needle electrode EMG, particularly in the parasternal intercostals, but these measurements are not necessarily correlated with diaphragmatic fatigue.[49] Sternocleidomastoid and scalene skin surface recordings have usually been unreliable, partly because of contamination by electrical activity from the platysma.

A promising, recently reported technique correlates diaphragmatic EMG with inspiratory occlusion pressure, $P_{0.1}$—the pressure generated in the first 0.1 second following respiratory occlusion at functional residual capacity. $P_{0.1}$ is a measure of the drive to breathe and has been shown to be increased in patients early in the course of weaning from ventilator support. One report indicated that the success of weaning correlates with both the H to L ratio of the diaphragmatic EMG and the $P_{0.1}$. Success in weaning is associated with a progressive increase in the H to L ratio and a concomitant decrease in $P_{0.1}$.[50] If confirmed by other investigators, this observation will have considerable importance in the intensive care unit; the ability to measure respiratory occlusion pressure is widely available, and so this correlation promises to move evaluation of respiratory muscle fatigue from the laboratory to the bedside.

Bilateral diaphragm paralysis (BDP), most often idiopathic, is a rare cause of dyspnea, but it is sometimes confused with COPD. It is an occasional cause of weaning failure in the intensive care unit; BDP may occur in 1 in 500 cases of cardiac surgery in which cold cardioplegia has been employed.[51] Clues to its presence include increased dyspnea and paradoxic respiratory movement in a supine position. Pulmonary function tests show a vital capacity 30% to 65% of that predicted when upright, which declines by approximately 50% when supine; the flow volume loop shows a decrease in the FIF_{50} to FEF_{50} ratio and may resemble that seen in variable extrathoracic obstruction; and the maximal negative inspiratory force is weak. Traditional methods of evaluation include the so-called "sniff" test for diaphragmatic movement under fluoroscopy, which is often equivocal or uninterpretable in bilateral paralysis, and phrenic nerve conduction studies, which are useful only when conduction can be demonstrated. Definitive diagnosis requires demonstrating that the $P_{di\ max} - P_{di}$ (ΔP_{di}) is in the range of 0 to 6 cm of H_2O (normal >25).[52, 53] During this evaluation, if the technology is available, diaphragmatic EMG may be performed. No EMG activity is seen if BDP is present, but nerve conduction is present in patients with severe diaphragm weakness associated with hypothyroidism, acid maltase deficiency, and other myopathic processes.[54] These studies may be performed in patients who have failed to wean from mechanical ventilation and are particularly indicated when the patient has paradoxic respiration immediately on ventilator disconnection.

REFERENCES

Arterial Blood Gases

1. Raffin TA. Indications for arterial blood gas analysis. Ann Intern Med 1986; 105:390–398.
2. Cottrell J. Altitude exposures during aircraft flight. Chest 1988; 93:81–84.
3. Gong H, Tashkin DP, Lee EY, et al. Hypoxia-altitude stimulation test: The evaluation of patients with chronic airway obstruction. Am Rev Respir Dis 1984; 130:980–986.
4. Mangano DT, Hickey RF. Ischemic injury following uncomplicated radial artery catheterization. Anesth Analg 1979; 34:506–512.

Fiberoptic Bronchoscopy and Bronchoalveolar Lavage

5. Kovnat DM, Rath GS, Anderson WM, et al. Maximal extent of visualization of bronchial tree by flexible fiberoptic bronchoscopy. Am Rev Respir Dis 1974; 110:88–90.
6. Anderson HF, Faber LP. Diagnostic and therapeutic applications of the bronchoscope. Chest 1978; 73(Suppl):685–778.
7. Practice Committee, American Thoracic Society Council of Chapter Representatives. Guidelines for fiberoptic bronchoscopy. ATS News 1986; Spring, 14–15.
8. Fulkerson WJ. Current concepts: Fiberoptic bronchoscopy. N Engl J Med 1984; 311:511–515.
9. Sackner MA. State of the art: Bronchofiberoscopy. Am Rev Respir Dis 1975; 111:62–88.
10. Cortese DA, Kinsey JH, Woolner LB, et al. Clinical application of a new endoscopic technique for detection of in situ bronchial carcinoma. Mayo Clin Proc 1979; 54:635–641.
11. Cortese DA, Kinsey JH, Woolner LB, et al. Hematoporphyrin derivative in the detection and localization of radiographically occult lung cancer. Am Rev Respir Dis 1982; 126:1087–1088.
12. Wimberley N, Faling LJ, Bartlett JG. A fiberoptic bronchoscopy technique to obtain uncontaminated lower airway secretions for bacterial culture. Am Rev Respir Dis 1979; 119:337–343.
13. Wimberley NW, Bass JB, Boyd BW, et al. Use of a bronchoscopic protected catheter brush for the diagnosis of pulmonary infection. Chest 1982; 81:556–562.
14. Reynolds HY. State of the art: Bronchoalveolar lavage. Am Rev Respir Dis 1987; 135:250–263.
15. Daniele RP, Elias JA, Epstein PE, et al. Bronchoalveolar lavage: Role in the pathogenesis, diagnosis, and management of interstitial lung disease. Ann Intern Med 1985; 102:93–108.
16. Thorpe JE, Baughman RP, Frame PT, et al. Bronchoalveolar lavage for diagnosing acute bacterial pneumonia. J Infect Dis 1987; 155:858–861.
17. Pereira W, Kovnat DM, Snider GL. A prospective cooperative study of complications following flexible fiberoptic bronchoscopy. Chest 1978; 73:813–816.
18. Suratt PM, Smiddy JF, Graber B. Deaths and complications associated with fiberoptic bronchoscopy. Chest 1976; 69:747–751.
19. Credle WF, Smiddy JF, Elliott RC. Complications of fiberoptic bronchoscopy. Am Rev Respir Dis 1974; 109:67–72.

Transtracheal Aspiration

20. Bartlett J. Diagnostic accuracy of transtracheal aspiration bacteriologic studies. Am Rev Respir Dis 1977; 115:777–782.
21. Bartlett J. The technique of transtracheal aspiration. J Crit Ill 1986; 1:43–49.

Lung Biopsy Techniques

22. Epler GR, Colby TV. The spectrum of bronchiolitis obliterans. Chest 1983; 83:161–162.
23. Epler GR, Colby TV, McLoud TC, et al. Bronchiolitis obliterans organizing pneumonia. N Engl J Med 1985; 312:152–158.
24. Shure D, Astarita RW. Bronchogenic carcinoma presenting as an endobronchial mass: Optimal number of biopsy specimens for diagnosis. Chest 1983; 83:865–867.
25. Schenk DA, Bryan CL, Bowen JH, et al. Transbronchial needle aspiration in the diagnosis of bronchogenic carcinoma. Chest 1987; 92:83–85.
26. Popovich J, Kvale PA, Eichenhorn MS, et al. Diagnostic accuracy of multiple biopsies from flexible fiberoptic bronchoscopy. Am Rev Respir Dis 1982; 125:521–523.
27. Zavala DC, Schoell JE. Ultrathin needle aspiration of the lung in infectious and malignant disease. Am Rev Respir Dis 1981; 123:125–131.
28. Poe RH, Tobin RE. Sensitivity and specificity of needle biopsy in lung malignancy. Am Rev Respir Dis 1980; 122:725–729.
29. Palmer DL, Davidson M, Lusk R. Needle aspiration of the lung in complex pneumonias. Chest 1980; 78:16–21.
30. Wall CP, Gaensler EA, Carrington CB, et al. Comparison of transbronchial and open lung biopsies in chronic infiltrative lung diseases. Am Rev Respir Dis 1981; 123:280–285.

Right Heart and Pulmonary Artery Catheterization

31. Swan HJC, Ganz W, Forrester J, et al. Catheterization of the heart in man with use of a flow-directed balloon-tipped catheter. N Engl J Med 1970; 283:447–451.
32. Robin E. The cult of the Swan-Ganz catheter. Ann Intern Med 1985; 103:445–449.
33. Moser KM, Spragg AG. Use of the balloon-tipped pulmonary artery catheter in pulmonary disease. Ann Intern Med 1983; 98:53–58.
34. Sprung CL. The Pulmonary Artery Catheter: Methodology and Applications. Baltimore: University Park Press, 1983.
35. Matthay RA, Berger HJ, Davies RA, et al. Right and left ventricular performance in chronic obstructive pulmonary disease: Radionuclide assessment. Ann Intern Med 1980; 93:234–239.
36. Himelman RB, Struve SN, Brown JK, et al. Improved recognition of cor pulmonale in patients with severe chronic obstructive pulmonary disease. Am J Med 1988; 84:891–898.
37. Weber KT, Janicki JS. Cardiopulmonary Exercise Testing. Philadelphia: W.B. Saunders Company, 1986, 160–167, 220–234, 272–289.
38. Rubin LJ, Moser K. Long-term effects of nitrendipine on hemodynamics and oxygen transport in patients with cor pulmonale. Chest 1986; 89:141–145.
39. Adnot S, Defouilly C, Brun-Buisson C, et al. Hemodynamic effects of urapadil in patients with pulmonary hypertension. Am Rev Respir Dis 1987; 135:288–293.

Thoracentesis

40. Light RW. Pleural Diseases. Philadelphia: Lea & Febiger, 1983, 229–237.

Pleural Biopsy

41. Health and Public Policy Committee, American College of Physicians. Diagnostic thoracentesis and pleural biopsy in pleural effusions. Ann Intern Med 1985; 103:799–802.
42. Light RW. Pleural Diseases. Philadelphia: Lea & Febiger, 1983, 238–242.
43. Prakash UBS, Reiman HM. Comparison of needle biopsy with cytologic analysis for the evaluation of pleural effusion: Analysis of 414 cases. Mayo Clin Proc 1985; 60:158–164.

Pleuroscopy

44. Oldenburg FA, Newhouse MT. Thoracoscopy: A safe, accurate procedure using the rigid thoracoscope and local anesthesia. Chest 1979; 75:45–50.
45. Weissberg D, Kaufman M. Diagnostic and therapeutic pleuroscopy: Experience with 127 patients. Chest 1980; 78:732–735.
46. Light RW. Pleural Diseases. Philadelphia: Lea & Febiger, 1983, 56.

Balloon Manometry and Diaphragm Evaluation

47. Druz WS, Danon J, Fishman HC, et al. Approaches to assessing respiratory muscle function in respiratory disease. Am Rev Respir Dis 1979; 119:145–149.
48. Bellemarre F, Grassino A. Evaluation of human diaphragmatic fatigue. J Appl Physiol 1982; 53:1196–1206.
49. Fitting JW, Bradley TD, Easton PA, et al. Dissociation between diaphragmatic and rib cage muscle fatigue. J Appl Physiol 1988; 64:959–965.
50. Murciano D, Boczkowski J, Lecocguic Y, et al. Tracheal occlusion pressure: A simple index to monitor respiratory muscle fatigue during acute respiratory failure in patients with chronic obstructive pulmonary disease. Ann Intern Med 1988; 108:800–805.
51. Chandler KW, Rozas CJ, Kory RL, et al. Bilateral diaphragmatic paralysis complicating local cardiac hypothermia during open-heart surgery. Am J Med 1984; 77:243–249.
52. Newsom-Davis J, Goldman M, Loh L, et al. Diaphragm function evaluation and alveolar hypoventilation. Q J Med 1976; 177:87–100.
53. Loh L, Goldman M, Newsom-Davis J. The assessment of diaphragm function. Medicine 1977; 56:165–168.
54. Rosenow EA, Engel AG. Acid maltase deficiency in adults presenting as respiratory failure. Am J Med 1978; 64:485–491.

Chapter 43

PRECLINICAL COPD: DESCRIPTION, RECOGNITION, AND THERAPY

Richard E. Kanner

DESCRIPTION AND DIAGNOSTIC FEATURES

In any discussion of the preclinical or early stages of a disease, we must first define what is meant by "early." COPD is a complex disease process but what constitutes its preclinical or early stages? For our purposes here it is considered to be when COPD is present but the subject is asymptomatic and routine spirometric testing indicates values in the "normal range." Ideally, the physician should be able to identify those individuals with the initial features of COPD and to predict who is most likely to progress to the symptomatic state, and even to disability and death. In the subject with preclinical COPD, however, this is not possible at present. Currently, the best measurements for determining who is likely to develop the signs and symptoms of COPD are the forced expiratory volume in 1 second (FEV_1) and the ratio of the FEV_1 to the FVC (functional vital capacity) because abnormalities in these parameters in a relatively young cigarette smoker constitute evidence for future morbidity. This makes our definition awkward, because when these values become abnormal, COPD has passed from the preclinical to the clinical stage. As will be discussed subsequently, the more "sensitive" tests of small airways function popularized in the 1970s have not proven to be very specific. Other methods that are more sensitive than spirometry and more specific than tests of small airways function may be developed in the future. For the present, however, we must use the method that is available and has proven to be of value—spirometry. Despite its shortcomings, it is the best method available for detecting COPD, even if it cannot recognize early or preclinical disease in an individual subject.

Small Airways Disease

The concept of "small airways disease" was introduced in the late 1960s and came into popular usage during the 1970s. Although the term has been used rather loosely, it is meant to include abnormalities in the more peripheral airways. These airways are smaller than 2 mm in diameter and consist of the membranous and respiratory bronchioles. Despite the small size of each respiratory bronchiole, the total cross-sectional diameter of these airways is large relative to the more central airways, and so they normally make only a small contribution to the total airway resistance. Thus, there must be a considerable amount of disease present in these peripheral airways before abnormalities can be detected by routine tests such as spirometry or even by airway resistance measurements in the body plethysmograph. These peripheral airways have therefore been termed the "silent zone of the lung." The pathology of this area of the bronchial tree of smokers has been defined and physiologic tests have been developed that enable the investigator and clinician to detect changes by noninvasive means. Correlations between these physiologic tests of small airways function and pathologic findings have been established.[1–3] In the early 1970s, it was anticipated that by detecting abnormalities in these small airways, we would be able to identify smokers who were destined to progress to clinically significant COPD. This will be discussed in more detail, because subsequent follow-up studies did not confirm this hypothesis.

Pathologic Features of Early COPD

Respiratory bronchiolitis was noted by Niewoehner and colleagues in the lungs of 19 young smokers who died suddenly outside of the hospital.[4] In a matched group of nonsmokers, this was seen in only 5 of 20 subjects. The lesion consisted of clusters of brown pigmented macrophages in the first- and second-order respiratory bronchioles and was often associated with edema, fibrosis, and epithelial hyperplasia in the adjacent bronchiolar and alveolar walls.[4]

Two reports by Wright and associates have described increased goblet cell metaplasia in the membranous bronchioles of smokers and ex-smokers.[1, 2] There were increases in the intraluminal and airway wall inflammatory cells, wall fibrosis, and pigment deposition in the respiratory bronchioles. In membranous bronchioles smaller than 0.4 mm in internal diameter the walls were increased in thickness by about 50%, and the wall thickness in the respiratory bronchioles was doubled when compared to that of never-smokers. The findings correlated with abnormalities found on physiologic tests of small airways function, although the FEV_1 and FEV_1 to FVC ratio were usually normal in these subjects.[1, 2] Cosio and coworkers have made similar observations.[3]

Tests of Small Airways Function

Because the earliest changes of COPD are noted in the small membranous and respiratory bronchioles, tests were developed to evaluate these distal segments of the airway. It was thought that by detecting early small airway abnormalities it would be possible to convince the cigarette smoker to abstain from the habit and thus avoid disease progression to symptomatic stages. It should be pointed out that most smokers do not suffer a significant loss of FEV_1. In males only a minority of moderate smokers, about 12% (up to 15 cigarettes/day) and 26% of heavy smokers (more than 15 cigarettes/day) develop significant airway obstruction, as defined as an FEV_1 to FVC less than 0.67.[5] These percentages are lower for females. Thus, we must identify those cigarette smokers most likely to develop COPD, although for many other reasons all cigarette smokers should break this habit.

Several tests of small airway function have been developed. The "gold standard" is considered to be the frequency dependence of compliance, in which the compliance of the lung when measured under dynamic conditions decreases with an increasing respiratory frequency.[6] Unfortunately, this method is impractical for clinical use. Using first air and then a mixture of helium-oxygen allows for a comparison of instantaneous flow rates on the maximal expiratory flow volume curve. Also, the point at which the flow rate with these different gas mixtures coincides—the volume of isoflow—can be determined.[7, 8] This is an easier test to use than frequency dependence of compliance. The maximum midexpiratory flow rate from the spirogram has also been proposed as an indicator of small airways disease.[9] One of the easiest of these tests to perform, and the one that has been the most tried and studied, is the single-breath nitrogen washout test. The subject inhales 100% oxygen and, on expiration, the slope of the washout of nitrogen (slope of phase III) and the closing volume or closing capacity (the point at which a sudden rise in expired nitrogen concentration occurs) are measured.[10] Caution is advised before these tests of small airway function are applied as routine screening tools.[11] The high intersubject and intrasubject variability of these tests, as compared to the FEV_1, was and remains a problem.[12, 13]

Knudson and colleagues, in a preliminary report, showed that after 4.2 years of follow-up the slope of phase III of the nitrogen washout curve could not predict an accelerated decrease in the FEV_1.[14] In 1984 Buist concluded that tests of small airways function have a high sensitivity for detecting disease in the small airways but are not specific in predicting who will progress to the point of having clinically significant COPD.[13]

Olofsson and coworkers, in Goteborg, Sweden, followed 460 men over a 7-year period and found that the single-breath nitrogen test did predict the rate of decline of the FEV_1.[15] They found that this test, subject age, smoking habits, and FEV_1 at the onset of the observation period proved to be statistically significant predictors of population trends but were actually not helpful in predicting what happened to an individual subject. The r^2 for their multiple regression analysis, including the four significant variables (single-breath nitrogen test, subject age, smoking habits, and initial FEV_1) was only 0.13. Thus, the variability of the rate of change of the FEV_1 is not well explained by these four variables, let alone by the slope of phase III.[15]

Stanescu and associates have presented the results of a 6-year study of 105 steel workers in Belgium. They also found that the measurements made from the single-breath nitrogen washout could not accurately predict changes in the FEV_1. Only those who already had a low FEV_1 and FEV_1 to FVC ratio showed a strong correlation between the slope of phase III and a further decline in the FEV_1. In smokers with a normal FEV_1 and FEV_1 to FVC ratio the initial value of the slope of phase III was not significant, because the mean FEV_1 in these subjects varied little over the 6-year period. It was concluded that repeated determinations of the FEV_1 are the best means of detecting rapid decreases in this measurement.[16]

Buist and coworkers have reported on the predictive value of the single-breath nitrogen test in smokers after 9 to 11 years of follow-up. An abnormal single-breath nitrogen test was present at the beginning of the study in 80% to 90% of smokers who developed a low FEV_1 during the follow-up period. However, the predictive power of an abnormal single-breath nitrogen washout was poor, because a high proportion of smokers who were initially abnormal using this parameter did not go on to develop an abnormal FEV_1 during the next 9 to 11 years.[17]

In summary, the single-breath nitrogen washout test is the best studied of the tests of small airways function. It apparently can be used to detect disease in peripheral airways smaller than 2 mm in diameter, but it cannot predict who will go on to develop clinically significant airways obstruction. With waning enthusiasm for these tests, it is unlikely that the other tests of small airways function will be evaluated extensively, and the role for these measurements of small airways function is limited in the foreseeable future. Spirometry, with measurements of the FEV_1 and FEV_1 to FVC ratio, continues to be the most clinically important method for assessing patients with COPD, and it is still the best means of detecting who will develop accelerated declines in pulmonary function even though declines must first occur before the method can become predictive.

Spirometric Changes in Young Smokers

Changes in the peripheral airways probably begin in the first few years after an individual starts smoking cigarettes regularly. Although only a minority of these people progress to clinically significant airway obstruction, there is ample evidence that young smokers have some diminution in their spirometric measurements when compared to those of nonsmokers. More than 20 years ago Peters and Ferris demonstrated this in students attending Harvard University.[18] Although smoking students had expiratory flow rates within the range of normal, their mean values were statistically significantly lower than those of their nonsmoking classmates.[18]

Tashkin and coworkers followed young (ages 13 to 23)

residents in the Los Angeles basin for a 5-year period, during which time some of them started smoking. Among the men it was noted that those who started smoking had initial mean values (adjusted for height and age) for the FVC, FEV_1, peak expiratory flow, and $\dot{V}_{max\,75}$* that were higher than those noted in subjects who remained nonsmokers. When they were all restudied 5 years later these differences were no longer significant, except for the FVC. (This was not noted among the women, however.) The data suggest that young men with better lung function are more apt to start smoking but that, over only a 5-year period, cigarette smoking prevented them from maintaining the same rate of increase in their values as compared to those who remained nonsmokers. In other words, the better than average spirometric values noted prior to their starting smoking declined to average levels over the 5-year period.[19]

Burrows and colleagues, in their comprehensive ongoing epidemiologic study of the nonhispanic caucasian population of Tucson also noted that, in 15- to 29-year-olds, those smoking over 20 cigarettes per day had a lower mean FEV_1 than former smokers and nonsmokers.[20] Bosse and associates, in the Normative Aging Study of men in the Boston area, noted that the annual rate of decline of the FEV_1 in those in the 25- to 36-year-old group was much higher in smokers of high-tar cigarettes when compared to nonsmokers.[21] When they analyzed their data according to never, former, and current smoking groups, in those 20 to 34 years of age the annual rate of decline of the FEV_1 was a loss of 38, 30, and 60 ml per year, respectively, again showing the effects of cigarette smoking in young subjects. In this age group it is surprising that they found such large declines in never-smokers and former smokers but they did not discuss this finding.[22] Others confirming an early decline in FEV_1, even in young smokers, include Beck and coworkers[23, 24] and Van der Lende and colleagues.[25] In the latter study, lung function in two communities in Holland was compared. One community enjoyed clean air, whereas the other had chronic air pollution problems. The study not only demonstrated the adverse effects of smoking on lung function in young subjects, but also indicated that air pollution contributes an additional negative effect.[25]

A report by Dockery and associates[26] from the Six Cities Study demonstrated a linear relationship between pack-years of smoking and FEV_1 that confirmed the findings of other workers.[20] In the Six Cities Study, a "typical" male 173 cm in height had a loss of FEV_1 of 7.4 ml for each pack-year smoked, plus an added loss of 123 ml if they were still smoking. The "typical" female 161 cm tall suffered a loss of FEV_1 of 4.4 ml per pack-year, with an additional loss of 107 ml if they were current smokers.[26] Finally, in another report, Tager and coworkers noted that in neversmokers the FEV_1 in men does not start declining until about the age of 35, and then between the ages of 35 to 40 decreases at a rate of about 20 ml/year. In smokers, however, the decline begins sooner, with a mean loss of 25 ml/year in those 21 to 32 years old and 40 ml/year from 33 to 43. In women, nonsmokers had a mean decrease in FEV_1 from the ages of 18 to 42 of about 10 ml/year; but if they are smokers this loss is 20 ml/year from the ages of 19 to 29 and 30 ml/year starting at the age of 30.[27]

These findings indicate that clinically insignificant but quantifiable changes in spirometric function begin soon after a person starts smoking cigarettes, but this does not identify who will progress to clinically significant airway obstruction. Only repeated spirometric measurements determine which smokers have a more marked loss in their FEV_1 and thus are more apt to develop clinically significant COPD.

*$\dot{V}_{max\,75}$ = Instantaneous flow rate at the point where 75% of the forced vital capacity has been exhaled during a forced expiratory maneuver.

Mucosal Permeability and Bronchial Reactivity in Young Smokers

The early changes noted in cigarette smokers include bronchial hyperreactivity and increased bronchial mucosal permeability; Hogg summarized these findings in 1981.[28] The increased mucosal permeability is attributed to changes in the tight junctions that join epithelial cells. The loosening of these junctions exposes nerve endings and possibly cellular elements. Irritants can thus reach the nerve endings and antigens can reach the immune system for processing.[28] These changes can cause bronchial hyperreactivity. Studies using aerosols containing radioactive chelates, which diffuse slowly through intact epithelia, have demonstrated an accelerated clearance of the tracer from the lungs to the blood in asymptomatic smokers.[29] In a follow-up study by this same group of investigators, it was shown that stopping smoking slows the clearance rate but that after 21 days of smoking cessation the subjects still have more rapid clearance rates than neversmokers.[30]

Many studies have shown increased nonspecific bronchial reactivity to methacholine and histamine in asymptomatic cigarette smokers whose spirometric function is within the limits of normal.[31-33] In the study with the largest number of subjects, 35% of otherwise normal smokers had bronchial hyperreactivity.[33] This same group, however, wisely studied 50 normal nonsmokers in their laboratory and found that 28% had a positive response to methacholine, although the mean dose necessary to produce the finding was higher in the nonsmokers.[34] This creates problems in interpreting what a positive response means.

In an interesting study from the Netherlands, Postma and colleagues reported that among subjects with established COPD (FEV_1 to FVC ratio lower than 0.60), bronchial hyperresponsiveness correlated with polymorphonuclear leukocyte production of oxygen radicals. This suggests a role for airway inflammation in producing the hyperreactivity and is consistent with the inflammatory changes noted in the small airways of young smokers with normal lung function.[35] More studies of bronchial hyperreactivity in normal nonatopic nonsmokers, as well as in smokers, are needed to determine the significance of these findings.

Other Possible Predisposing Factors in the Development of COPD

Subjects who enroll in epidemiologic studies of COPD may participate because they are aware, subconsciously or otherwise, that there has been a change in their respiratory status. Despite this selection bias, however, the data collected are still valuable. Initial spirometric measurements appear to be predictors of long-term events. Burrows and coworkers have noted that among their male smokers who continued to smoke, a low FEV_1 to FVC ratio on entry was almost always associated with a rapid decline in FEV_1 during the follow-up period.[36] Thus, spirometry appears to be able to identify these individuals before clinically significant disease develops. In their study a low initial FEV_1 by itself was not as predictive of disease progression as has been noted by others.[36] Higgins and associates, in the Tecumseh (Michigan) Community Health Study, developed an index of risk for developing clinical COPD.[37] In their subjects initially low pulmonary function, as measured by spirometry, including a low FEV_1, predicted significant worsening of lung function, especially in those who continued to smoke.[37] Krzyzanowski and coworkers, in Cracow, Poland, also found that the rate of decline of the FEV_1 was greater in those smokers with a low initial FEV_1.[38]

Airway hyperreactivity has been associated with more rapid

declines when assessed by bronchoprovocation challenge[39] and by bronchodilator response.[40, 41] In these studies, however, clinical COPD was already present and, as previously discussed, the frequency of bronchial hyperreactivity among all smokers makes this observation less meaningful.

Although the frequency of nonspecific respiratory illness correlates with a more rapid decline in FEV_1 in subjects with established COPD, investigators have been unable to implicate any specific infections to explain this finding. This suggests that the nonspecific illnesses might be the result, rather than the cause, of the decline.[40, 42]

The Z phenotype of alpha$_1$-antiprotease also identifies those at high risk for COPD.[43, 44] One report has described a greater risk for COPD in former alcoholics that was independent of their smoking habits.[45] Thus, there are many indicators that can help to detect the subject with subclinical COPD who may subsequently develop clinically significant disease.

TREATMENT

The Benefits of Smoking Cessation in Early COPD

Cigarette smoking is the major cause of COPD. Smoking cessation is essential in preventing disease progression. The largest prospective study demonstrating this has been the UCLA population study of chronic obstructive respiratory disease.[46] Over a 5-year period 106 men and 62 women stopped smoking (quitters); they were compared to larger numbers of neversmokers, ex-smokers, and continuing smokers. Symptoms of cough, sputum, and wheeze decreased in the quitters, and their indices of "small airways function" did better than what was noted in those who continued to smoke. The most significant improvement in FEV_1 was seen in male quitters who had an initial FEV_1 to FVC ratio of 0.75 or better for those under the age of 50, or 0.70 or better for those aged 50 and older. For the women quitters the improvement in FEV_1 was marginal. The ex-smokers, who had given up the habit before the beginning of the observation period, had fewer pack-years of smoking and better spirometric values than the quitters and were comparable to the neversmokers. The authors concluded that, although improvement is seen relatively soon after stopping smoking, it takes at least 5 years and/or fewer pack-years of smoking for spirometric function to normalize completely.[46]

Camilli and coworkers in Tucson also reported on large numbers of smokers, ex-smokers (stopped before the period of observation), quitters (stopped during the period of observation), and neversmokers.[47] In men under the age of 35 the mean FEV_1 continued to increase in all but those continuing to smoke, in whom a decline was seen. In women similar findings were noted but in the current smokers the mean FEV_1 still increased slightly, although less so than in the others. Overall, those men and women who stopped smoking before the age of 35 had the greatest increases in FEV_1. In subjects over the age of 35, the FEV_1 declined in all groups, with the most rapid declines seen in current smokers, followed by the quitters, and then the ex-smokers, and the slowest rate of decline seen in the neversmokers (Fig. 43–1). It was calculated that, if at the age of 20, a neversmoker and a smoker had an FEV_1 of 4 L, then 50 years later the neversmoker's FEV_1 would be approximately 3.50 L whereas the smoker's FEV_1 would be about 2.83 L, a difference of almost 700 ml. If the smoker quit at the age of 50, however, by the age of 70 the FEV_1 would be about 3.18 L, a difference of only 350 ml less than the neversmoker. If a smoker gave up the habit early enough, before the age of 35, he or she would have spirometric function equivalent to that of neversmokers.[47]

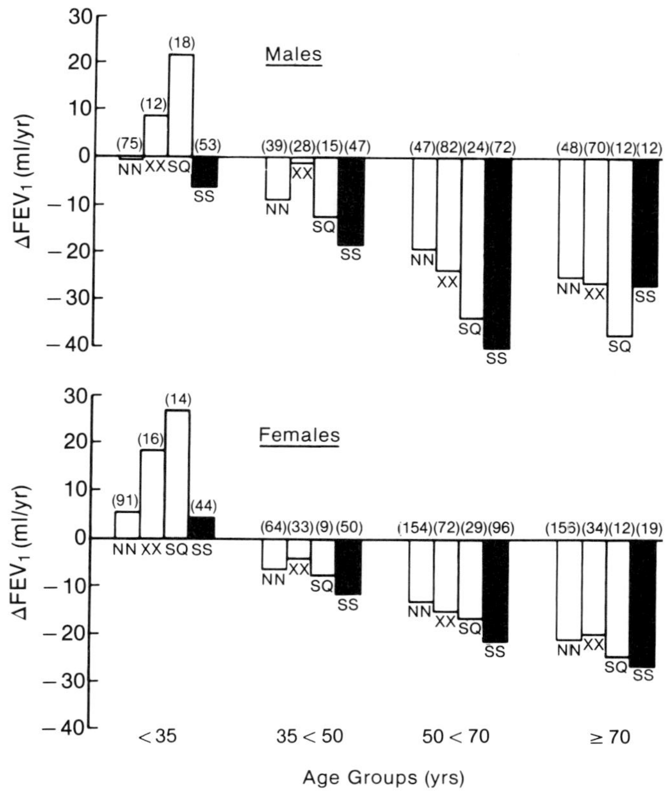

Figure 43–1. Mean change in FEV_1 in neversmokers (NN), ex-smokers who stopped prior to the onset of the study (XX), subjects who stopped smoking during the follow-up period (SQ), and consistent smokers (SS) according to age group and gender. Numbers of subjects in each category are shown in parentheses. (Reproduced with permission from Camilli et al. Am Rev Respir Dis 1987; 135:794–799.)

McCarthy and coworkers studied a group of smokers, of whom 59 gave up the habit for 6 to 24 weeks and 33 others decreased their consumption by 25%. They all had normal values for the FVC, FEV_1, FEV_1 to FVC ratio and peak expiratory flow rate. The *FEF_{25-75} was decreased and the values measured on the single-breath nitrogen washout test were abnormally elevated. There was improvement in those who stopped smoking in the slope of phase III of the nitrogen washout tracing after 6 to 12 weeks of abstinence. At 13 to 24 weeks the FVC and FEV_1 had risen and the single-breath nitrogen washout values all decreased toward normal. In those who decreased their cigarette consumption by 25% or more some improvement was noted, but it was not as great as in those who stopped smoking.[48] Other prospective studies with smaller numbers of quitters showed similar findings.[9, 22, 24, 49–53] Cross-sectional studies have also indicated improvement in lung function and a decrease in respiratory symptoms when smokers give up the habit.[23, 54] In the Six Cities Study it was noted that, for any given number of pack-years of smoking, ex-smokers have a higher FEV_1 than current smokers (Fig. 43–2).[26]

Other Possible Therapies

Any therapy for early COPD, other than smoking cessation, must be considered to be secondary and speculative. Mc-

*FEF_{25-75} = The mean flow rate from the point where the first 25% of the FVC is exhaled to the point where 75% of the FVC has been exhaled. It has also been called the maximal n.d.—expiratory flow rate.

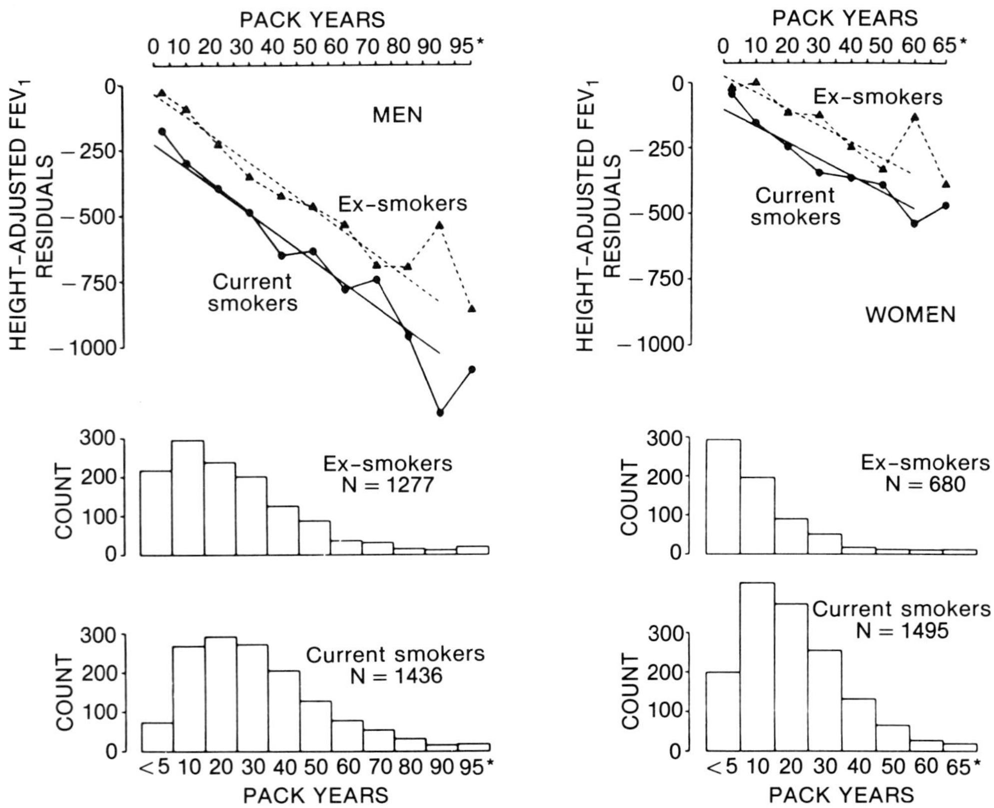

Figure 43–2. Sex-specific mean height-adjusted FEV_1 residuals (difference between subjects' values and the value predicted using only asymptomatic neversmokers) versus pack-years of smoking for current and ex-smokers. Distributions of number of subjects by pack-years are also presented. (Reproduced by permission from Dockery DW, et al. Am Rev Respir Dis 1988; 137:286–292.)

Fadden and Linden noted that bronchodilators enhance the positive effect of stopping smoking in four subjects.[9] Greenspon and Parrish, in a report of subjects with clinically significant COPD and bronchial hyperreactivity, also noted some benefits from the use of a bronchodilator, presumably because of its effect on inhibiting the contribution of the increased airways reactivity to the overall obstructive process.[55] Removal of subjects from polluted environments may also be helpful, because air pollution may be a factor in the development of COPD.[25] Finally, in those relatively few subjects with a severe deficiency of $alpha_1$-antiprotease, replacement therapy may be beneficial. This has not been demonstrated in clinical studies, however, even though such treatment is now commercially available.

In summary, preclinical or early COPD exists in cigarette smokers who still have spirometric measurements within the normal range but who usually have abnormal small airways function. Although inflammatory changes in the membranous and respiratory bronchioles can be detected, identification of these abnormalities does not predict which cigarette smoker has disease that will progress to clinically significant COPD. Young smokers begin to show declines in spirometric function earlier than their nonsmoking counterparts. Also, at any age, smokers have lower mean pulmonary function values than nonsmokers, as measured by spirometry, even though these results are still in the somewhat artificially determined range of normal. Spirometry is the best method for following people with early COPD and can detect subjects who are apt to develop accelerated losses in pulmonary function when these individuals begin to demonstrate abnormalities in the FEV_1 and FEV_1 to FVC ratio. Changes in mucosal permeability may be present in cigarette smokers and there is a high incidence of bronchial hyperreactivity. The significance of these findings is uncertain at this time. The best therapy for COPD, at any level of severity, is to convince the patient to stop smoking. The sooner this occurs, the less the degree of permanent lung damage. In those with early COPD, smoking cessation can even result in improvement in and normalization of lung function.

REFERENCES

1. Wright JL, Lawson LM, Pare PD, et al. Morphology of peripheral airways in current smokers and exsmokers. Am Rev Respir Dis 1983; 127:474–477.
2. Wright JL, Hobson J, Wiggs BR, et al. Effect of cigarette smoking on structure of the small airways. Lung 1987; 165:91–100.
3. Cosio M, Ghezzo H, Hogg JC, et al. The relations between structural changes in small airways and pulmonary function tests. N Engl J Med 1978; 298:1277–1281.
4. Niewoehner DE, Kleinerman J, Rice DB. Pathologic changes in the peripheral airways of young cigarette smokers. N Engl J Med 1974; 291:755–758.
5. Fletcher CM, Peto R, Tinker C, Speizer F. The natural history of chronic bronchitis and emphysema. Oxford: Oxford University Press, 1976, 83.
6. Woolcock AJ, Vincent NJ, Macklem PT. Frequency dependence of compliance as a test for obstruction in the small airways. J Clin Invest 1969; 48:1097–1106.
7. Despas RJ, Leroux M, Macklem PT. Site of airway obstruction in asthma as determined by measuring maximal expiratory flow breathing air and a helium-oxygen mixture. J Clin Invest 1972; 51:3235–3243.
8. Hutcheon M, Griffin P, Levison H, Zamel N. Volume of isoflow. A new test in detection of mild abnormalities of lung mechanics. Am Rev Respir Dis 1974; 110:458–465.
9. McFadden ER, Linden DA. A reduction in maximum mid-expiratory flow rate. A spirographic manifestation of small airway disease. Am J Med 1972; 52:725–737.
10. Buist AS, Ross BB. Quantitative analysis of the alveolar plateau in the diagnosis of early airway obstruction. Am Rev Respir Dis 1973; 108:1078–1087.

11. Macklem PT. Conference report. Workshop on screening programs for early diagnosis of airway obstruction. Am Rev Respir Dis 1974; 109:567–571.
12. Becklake MR, Permutt S. Evaluation of tests of lung function for "screening" for early detection of chronic obstructive lung disease. In: Macklem PT, Permutt S, eds. The Lung in the Transition Between Health and Disease. New York: Marcel Dekker, 1979, 345–387.
13. Buist AS. Current status of small airways disease. Chest 1984; 86:100–105.
14. Knudson RJ, Armet DB, Lebowitz MD. Reevaluation of tests of small airways function. Chest 1980; 77(Suppl):284–285.
15. Olofsson J, Bake B, Svardsudd K, Skoogh BE. The single-breath N_2 test predicts the rate of decline in FEV_1. Eur J Respir Dis 1986; 69:46–56.
16. Stanescu DC, Rodenstein DO, Hoeven C, Robert A. "Sensitive tests" are poor predictors of the decline in forced expiratory volume in one second in middle-aged smokers. Am Rev Respir Dis 1987; 135:585–590.
17. Buist AS, Vollmer WM, Johnson LR, McCamant LE. Does the single-breath N_2 test identify the smoker who will develop chronic airflow limitation? Am Rev Respir Dis 1988; 137:293–301.
18. Peters JM, Ferris BG Jr. Smoking, pulmonary function, and respiratory symptoms in a college-age group. Am Rev Respir Dis 1967; 95:774–782.
19. Tashkin DP, Clark VA, Coulson AH, et al. Comparison of lung function in young nonsmokers and smokers before and after initiation of the smoking habit. Am Rev Respir Dis 1983; 128:12–16.
20. Burrows B, Knudson RJ, Cline MG, Lebowitz MD. Quantitative relationships between cigarette smoking and ventilatory function. Am Rev Respir Dis 1977; 115:195–205.
21. Bosse R, Sparrow D, Garvey AJ, et al. Cigarette smoking, aging, and decline in pulmonary function: A longitudinal study. Arch Environ Health 1980; 35:247–252.
22. Bosse R, Sparrow D, Rose CL, Weiss ST. Longitudinal effect of age and smoking cessation on pulmonary function. Am Rev Respir Dis 1981; 123:378–381.
23. Beck GJ, Doyle CA, Schachter EN. Smoking and lung function. Am Rev Respir Dis 1981; 123:149–155.
24. Beck GJ, Doyle CA, Schachter EN. A longitudinal study of respiratory health in a rural community. Am Rev Respir Dis 1982; 125:375–381.
25. Van der Lende R, Kok TJ, Peset Reig R, et al. Decreases in VC and FEV_1 with time: Indicators for effects of smoking and air pollution. Bull Europ Physiopathol Resp 1981; 17:775–792.
26. Dockery DW, Speizer FE, Ferris BG Jr, et al. Cumulative and reversible effects of lifetime smoking on simple tests of lung function in adults. Am Rev Respir Dis 1988; 137:286–292.
27. Tager IB, Segal MR, Speizer FE, Weiss ST. The natural history of forced expiratory volumes—effect of cigarette smoking and respiratory symptoms. Am Rev Respir Dis 1988; 138:837–849.
28. Hogg JC. Bronchial mucosal permeability and its relationship to airways hyperreactivity. J Allergy Clin Immunol 1981; 67:421–425.
29. Jones JG, Lawler P, Crowley JCW, et al. Increased alveolar epithelial permeability in cigarette smokers. Lancet 1980; i:66–68.
30. Minty BD, Jordan C, Jones JG. Rapid improvement in abnormal pulmonary epithelial permeability after stopping cigarettes. Br Med J 1981; 282:1183–1186.
31. Gerrard JW, Cockcroft DW, Mink ST, et al. Increased nonspecific bronchial reactivity in cigarette smokers with normal lung function. Am Rev Respir Dis 1980; 122:577–581.
32. Malo JL, Filiatrault S, Martin RR. Bronchial responsiveness to inhaled methacholine in young asymptomatic smokers. J Appl Physiol 1982; 52:1464–1470.
33. Casale TB, Rhodes BJ, Donnelly AL, Weiler JM. Airway responses to methacholine in asymptomatic nonatopic cigarette smokers. J Appl Physiol 1987; 62:1888–1892.
34. Rhodes BJ, Casale TB, Donnelly AL, Weiler JM. Methacholine bronchial provocation challenge: A nondiagnostic test? (Abstract) J Allergy Clin Immunol 1986; 77:170.
35. Postma DS, Renkema TEJ, Noordhoek JA, et al. Association between nonspecific bronchial hyperreactivity and superoxide anion production by polymorphonuclear leukocytes in chronic airflow obstruction. Am Rev Respir Dis 1988; 137:57–61.
36. Burrows B, Knudson RJ, Camilli AE, et al. The "horse-racing effect" and predicting decline in forced expiratory volume in one second from screening spirometry. Am Rev Respir Dis 1987; 135:788–793.
37. Higgins MW, Keller JB, Becker M, et al. An index of risk for obstructive airways disease. Am Rev Respir Dis 1982; 125:144–151.
38. Krzyzanowski M, Jedrychowski W, Wysocki M. Factors associated with the change in ventilatory function and the development of chronic obstructive pulmonary disease in a 13-year followup of the Cracow Study. Am Rev Respir Dis 1986; 134:1011–1019.
39. Barter CE, Campbell AH. Relationship of constitutional factors and cigarette smoking to decrease in 1-second forced expiratory volume. Am Rev Respir Dis 1976; 113:305–314.
40. Kanner RE, Renzetti AD Jr, Klauber MR, et al. Variables associated with changes in spirometry in patients with obstructive lung diseases. Am J Med 1979; 67:44–50.
41. Campbell AH, Barter CE, O'Connell JM, Huggins R. Factors affecting the decline of ventilatory function in chronic bronchitis. Thorax 1985; 40:741–748.
42. Smith CB, Kanner RE, Golden CA, et al. Effect of viral infections on pulmonary function in patients with chronic obstructive pulmonary disease. J Infect Dis 1980; 141:271–280.
43. Laurell CB, Eriksson S. The electrophoretic alpha$_1$-globulin pattern of serum in alpha$_1$-antitrypsin deficiency. Scand J Clin Lab Invest 1963; 15:132–140.
44. Rawlings W Jr, Kreiss P, Levy D, et al. Clinical, epidemiologic, and pulmonary function studies in alpha$_1$-antitrypsin-deficient subjects of PiZ type. Am Rev Respir Dis 1976; 114:945–953.
45. Emirgil C, Sobol BJ. Pulmonary function in former alcoholics. Chest 1977; 72:45–51.
46. Tashkin DP, Clark VA, Coulson AH, et al. The UCLA population studies of chronic obstructive respiratory disease. VIII. Effects of smoking cessation on lung function: A prospective study of a free-living population. Am Rev Respir Dis 1984; 130:707–715.
47. Camilli AE, Burrows B, Knudson RJ, et al. Longitudinal changes in forced expiratory volume in one second in adults. Effects of smoking and smoking cessation. Am Rev Respir Dis 1987; 135:794–799.
48. McCarthy DS, Craig DB, Cherniack RM. Effect of modification of the smoking habit on lung function. Am Rev Respir Dis 1976; 114:103–113.
49. Bode FR, Dosman J, Martin RR, Macklem PT. Reversibility of pulmonary function abnormalities in smokers. Am J Med 1975; 59:43–52.
50. Buist AS, Sexton GJ, Nagy JM, Ross BB. The effect of smoking cessation and modification on lung function. Am Rev Respir Dis 1976; 114:115–122.
51. Bake B, Oxhoj H, Sixt R, Wilhelmsen L. Ventilatory lung function following two years of tobacco abstinence. Scand J Resp Dis 1977; 58:311–318.
52. Buist AS, Nagy JM, Sexton GJ. The effect of smoking cessation on pulmonary function: A 30-month follow-up of two smoking cessation clinics. Am Rev Respir Dis 1979; 120:953–957.
53. Zamel N, Leroux M, Ramcharan V. Decrease in lung recoil pressure after cessation of smoking. Am Rev Respir Dis 1979; 119:205–211.
54. Nemery B, Moavero NE, Brasseur L, et al. Changes in lung function after smoking cessation. An assessment from a cross-sectional survey. Am Rev Respir Dis 1982; 125:122–124.
55. Greenspon LW, Parrish B. Inhibition of methacholine-induced bronchoconstriction in patients with chronic obstructive pulmonary disease. Am Rev Respir Dis 1988; 137:281–285.

Section VIII

TREATMENT OF COPD

Chapter 44

TREATMENT OVERVIEW: CHRONIC HYPERCAPNIA AND COR PULMONALE

Herbert P. Wiedemann   Richard A. Matthay

Chronic obstructive pulmonary disease (COPD) is characterized by a gradually progressive clinical course that unfolds over years, or even decades. As COPD worsens, the homeostatic mechanisms that maintain normal ventilatory pump function and circulatory hemodynamics are stressed. The onset of either chronic hypercapnia or cor pulmonale generally heralds advanced COPD, with a poor prognosis for prolonged survival.

In this chapter we provide an overview of the available and potential treatments for advanced but stable COPD. The management of acute exacerbations of COPD is discussed in Chapter 45. Furthermore, because specific treatment measures for COPD (e.g., bronchodilators, oxygen, vasodilators) are discussed elsewhere in this book, we do not attempt to provide a comprehensive analysis of each available therapy. Rather, we emphasize therapeutic interventions as they relate specifically to the pathophysiology of cor pulmonale (updated and modified from our earlier reviews[1, 2]) and of chronic hypercapnia. For example, discussion of traditional bronchodilator therapy is deferred in favor of highlighting the potentially beneficial effects of theophylline and β-adrenergic agents on cardiac contractility, pulmonary vascular resistance, respiratory muscle function, and respiratory drives. Respiratory muscle rest therapy, nutritional manipulations, and respiratory stimulants are also discussed. Finally, other therapies, such as oxygen, vasodilators, almitrine, and phlebotomy, are reviewed in the context of pulmonary hypertension, cardiac output, and oxygen transport.

Overall, few definitive conclusions or recommendations can be made. Intriguing new treatment approaches have been proposed, but future studies are necessary to determine which patients are candidates for various therapies and the long-term efficacy of these therapies. Only in the case of oxygen therapy have these issues been fairly well resolved.

CHRONIC HYPERCAPNIA IN COPD

Pathophysiology

The arterial partial pressure of carbon dioxide (Pa_{CO_2}) depends on the ratio of metabolic CO_2 production (V_{CO_2}) to alveolar ventilation, as described by the following equation:

$$Pa_{CO_2} = \frac{V_{CO_2} \times K}{V_E(1 - V_D/V_T)}$$

where V_E is total pulmonary minute ventilation, V_D/V_T is the ratio of physiologic dead space to tidal volume, and K is a constant. Pa_{CO_2} is usually maintained within a very narrow range, but some patients lose their ability to sustain adequate alveolar ventilation and the Pa_{CO_2} increases. Chronic hypercapnia may have several different causes, including disturbances of central ventilatory drive, dysfunction of the respiratory muscles, neuromuscular disease, increased mechanical ventilatory load (e.g., chest wall deformity, obesity, airflow obstruction, severe lung fibrosis), and marked ventilation-perfusion mismatching (which leads to a large physiologic dead space).[3] In many patients with hypercapnia, including COPD patients, the interaction of several concurrent physiologic abnormalities is probably responsible.

Mechanical Impairment of Lung Function

Chronic CO_2 retention ($Pa_{CO_2} > 45$ mm Hg) occurs only in some patients with COPD, usually after severe mechanical impairment of lung function is present. In early studies, Burrows and coworkers[4] and Howell[5] found that when CO_2 retention exists in COPD patients, the forced expiratory volume in 1 second (FEV_1) is usually less than 1.0 L. More recently, Javaheri and colleagues[6] examined the charts of all COPD patients who received pulmonary function tests at Massachusetts General Hospital between 1968 and 1979. Fifteen patients were found who satisfied very strict criteria for stable, chronic, compensated hypercapnia without evidence of a superimposed primary metabolic acid-base abnormality; the mean FEV_1 was 0.59 L, with the highest value in the group equal to 1.09 L. Using less restrictive criteria for chronic hypercapnia, Glauser and coworkers[3] found 70 COPD patients with chronic hypercapnia in two Richmond, Virginia hospitals during 1985. The mean FEV_1 in these patients was 0.77 ± 0.2 L.

Although severe mechanical impairment of lung function is usually present in hypercapnic COPD patients, it is not by itself sufficient to explain chronic hypercapnia in most of these patients. A large group of patients with an FEV_1 less than 1.0 L is not hypercapnic, and there is no close relationship between the degree of mechanical impairment and the Pa_{CO_2}.[4, 5, 7] Factors other than mechanical limitation must often be present to explain why some patients develop hypercapnia and others do not.

Roussos[8] has proposed two alternative pathways, which are not mutually exclusive, to explain the gradual onset of hypercapnia in COPD as the degree of airflow obstruction worsens. As the disease progresses, the degree of respiratory muscle power output required to maintain eucapnia may exceed the threshold for the development of muscle fatigue. Faced with this predicament, two responses are possible. First, the central nervous system may accept a lower level of respiratory effort than that which would be required to maintain eucapnia to avoid respiratory muscle fatigue. Such hypercapnic patients could, in fact, still exhibit more respiratory effort than normal subjects, or as much as eucapnic COPD patients, but not as much as would be required to avoid hypercapnia in their particular circumstances. Alternatively, the central nervous system might drive the respiratory muscles to attempt to avoid hypercapnia at all costs, thereby pushing power output beyond the fatigue threshold. The development of chronic muscle fatigue could then lead to hypercapnia. In short, in these two different scenarios of chronic hypercapnia in COPD, respiratory muscle fatigue might be absent in one group of patients and present in a different group. Here we review what is known about ventilatory drives, inspiratory effort, and muscle function in hypercapnic COPD patients.

Ventilatory Drives

A reduced central ventilatory response to hypercapnia, perhaps as a result of a genetic predisposition, may contribute to CO_2 retention in some COPD patients. The "normal" family members of hypercapnic COPD patients often demonstrate blunted hypoxic and hypercapnic responses.[9] Furthermore, Light and colleagues[10] have evaluated 19 COPD patients (FEV_1 = 1.07 ± 0.5 L), seven of whom were hypercapnic, and found a strong linear correlation between Pa_{CO_2} and hypercapnic ventilatory responses. Although the resting Pa_{CO_2} also correlated with the FEV_1 ($r = -0.58$; $p < 0.01$), the closest single correlation was with the ventilation at P_{CO_2} = 60 mm Hg ($r = -0.74$; $p < 0.001$), as obtained from the hypercapnia response curve. Multiple regression analysis indicated that the greatest reduction in variance could be achieved by considering only two variables, the FEV_1 and the $\Delta P_{100}/\Delta P_{CO_2}$ (change in mouth pressure developed in the first 100 msec of inspiration plotted versus the change in P_{CO_2}). These results suggest that the resting Pa_{CO_2} depends on both the "ability to breathe," as indicated by the FEV_1, and on the "drive to breathe," as indicated by the $\Delta P_{100}/\Delta P_{CO_2}$. Other studies have supported an important role for depressed ventilatory drives in the development of hypercapnia in COPD. Altose and associates[11] found that five hypercapnic patients had lower $\Delta P_{100}/\Delta P_{CO_2}$ and P_{100} at P_{CO_2} = 60 mm Hg than did nine eucapnic patients with comparable FEV_1 values. Gelb and coworkers[12] and Lane and Howell[13] also found that the ventilatory response to hypercapnia is stronger in COPD patients without hypercapnia than in those patients with CO_2 retention. Lourenco and Miranda[14] demonstrated that hypercapnia causes a greater increase in diaphragmatic electrical activity in eucapnic COPD patients than in hypercapnic patients.

Breathing Pattern

Hypoventilation, a decrease in overall minute ventilation, is absent in most chronically hypercapnic COPD patients. Rather, several studies have suggested that COPD patients with hypercapnia have a different *pattern* of ventilation, characterized by a higher respiratory frequency and smaller tidal volume (and, therefore, an increased dead space ventilation, V_D/V_T), compared to eucapnic patients.[6, 15–20]

For example, in Javaheri's[6] study, the 15 hypercapnic patients were compared with 15 eucapnic patients with a similar FEV_1. In the CO_2 retainers, the mean Pa_{CO_2} was 52.5 ± 1.2 mm Hg, whereas in the eucapnic patients the mean Pa_{CO_2} was 40 ± 2 mm Hg. Minute ventilation was similar in both groups (7.63 L and 7.81 L, respectively), but the hypercapnic patients had a significantly higher respiratory rate per minute (22 versus 16.5) and a smaller tidal volume (355 versus 463 ml). This pattern of ventilation in the hypercapnic patients resulted in a larger dead space ventilation and lower alveolar ventilation, with subsequent CO_2 retention.

A shortened inspiratory time may contribute to the reduced tidal volume observed in hypercapnic patients. Sorli and colleagues[16] found that only the shortened inspiratory time and resultant low tidal volume separated CO_2 retainers from non-CO_2 retainers. A shortened inspiratory time in hypercapnic patients was also confirmed by Skatrud and colleagues.[19, 20] However, Javaheri and coworkers[6] found a shortened inspiratory time only when the hypercapnic patients were in the supine position.

The mechanisms responsible for the altered breathing pattern in hypercapnic patients remain undefined. Such respiratory cycle abnormalities might be a manifestation of respiratory muscle dysfunction, stimulation of irritant receptors in the airways or lung interstitium, or abnormalities of respiratory drives. Roussos,[8] however, has noted that large tidal breaths force the respiratory muscles to shorten more than small tidal breaths, and thereby increase the energy demand per breath (especially toward the end of the large tidal volume). Thus, adopting a breathing pattern of low tidal volume and increased respiratory frequency has some advantages (up to a point) for the fatiguing respiratory muscles (also see Fig. 44–2 and related discussion in text).

Respiratory drives are not depressed in hypercapnic patients with short inspiratory times. In fact, Skatrud and colleagues[19, 20] have shown that CO_2 retainers have a higher than normal respiratory effort response to hypercapnia (P_{100}). Furthermore, in a study that employed mean inspiratory flow (V_T/T_I) as a measure of resting respiratory drive, 75% of hypercapnic COPD patients and 65% of eucapnic COPD patients had mean inspiratory flow values above those of normal subjects (Fig. 44–1).[21, 22] Thus, this measure of respiratory drive was increased in both patient groups, but overall the hypercapnic patients had the same mean inspiratory flow

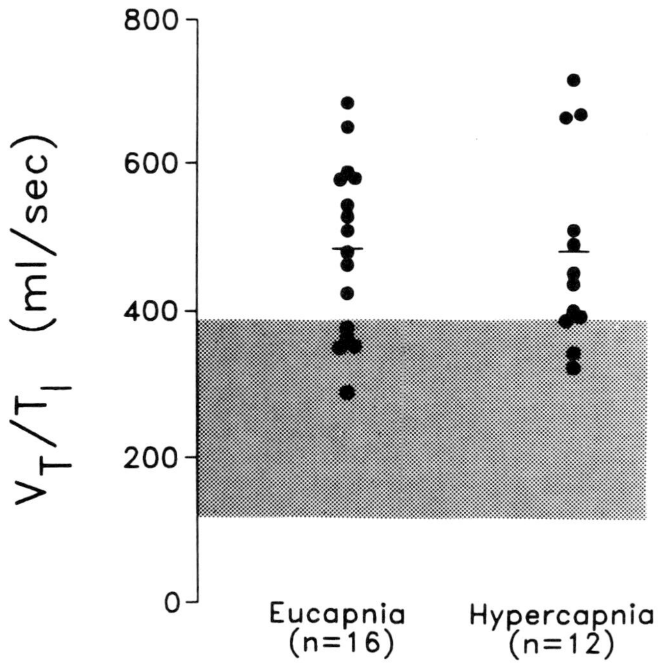

Figure 44–1. Mean inspiratory flow (V_T/T_I), an index of respiratory drive during resting breathing in patients with chronic obstructive pulmonary disease. The shaded area represents the 95% confidence limits of V_T/T_I in healthy subjects. (Reproduced with permission from Tobin MJ. Clin Chest Med 1988; 9:263–286.)

rate as the eucapnic patients. Therefore, even though respiratory drive was above normal in the hypercapnic patients, it could be interpreted as being deficient relative to the increased demands (e.g., airflow resistance, dead space) in these patients.

Respiratory Muscle Dysfunction

Although respiratory muscle fatigue or weakness is frequently cited as a cause of hypercapnia, the status of respiratory muscle function in stable chronic hypercapnic COPD patients is complex and controversial.[22] Peak inspiratory pressure ($P_{I\ max}$) is reduced in COPD patients and severe hypercapnia ($Paco_2 > 50$ mm Hg) is common in COPD patients whose $P_{I\ max}$ is less than 50% of normal.[23] However, a reduced $P_{I\ max}$ in COPD patients can be explained by hyperinflation, which causes the inspiratory muscles to shorten and operate at an unfavorable position on the length-tension curve. Nevertheless, Rochester and Brown[23] have proposed that hyperinflation accounts for only 41% of the observed reduction in $P_{I\ max}$ and that generalized muscle weakness also exists in many COPD patients. Furthermore, Oliven and coworkers[24] found that the degree of CO_2 retention caused by external resistive loading in COPD patients is inversely related to inspiratory muscle strength.

Ventilatory endurance, however, expressed as the *fraction* of the maximum voluntary ventilation (MVV) that can be sustained over several minutes, has been found to be normal in four different investigations of COPD patients.[22] In addition, Bellemare and Grassino[25] observed no relationship between $Paco_2$ and maximum transdiaphragmatic pressure ($P_{di\ max}$) or the diaphragmatic tension-time index (TT_{di}) in COPD patients. The TT_{di} helps assess the potential for diaphragm fatigue, which usually ensues when a critical value of 0.15 is reached.[22,26]

In contrast, hypercapnic patients might be distinguished from eucapnic patients based on the ratio of their peak transdiaphragmatic pressure (P_{di}) generated during normal tidal breathing to their $P_{di\ max}$. A report by Roussos[8] and results derived from the data of Bellemare and Grassino[25] show that hypercapnic patients develop a peak tidal P_{di} that is 25% to 30% of their $P_{di\ max}$, whereas the peak tidal P_{di} in eucapnic patients is only about 10% of the $P_{di\ max}$. Results from normal subjects breathing against high inspiratory resistance indicate that muscle fatigue is likely when pleural pressure (at functional residual capacity plus 50% of inspiratory capacity) is 25% to 30% of maximum. In Figure 44–2, the points representing these eucapnic and hypercapnic patients are superimposed on the "critical zone" for muscle fatigue as developed in normal subjects. These results suggest that hypercapnic COPD patients have respiratory muscle fatigue. However, as Roussos[8] has indicated, this remains speculative, because the critical zone was constructed from results obtained in normal subjects.

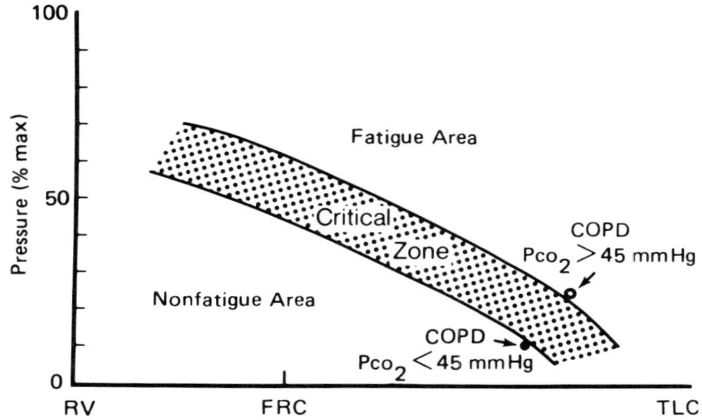

Figure 44–2. Diagram of the critical pressure at which normal subjects breathing against high inspiratory resistance develop respiratory muscle fatigue. The critical pressure depends on lung volume (as a result of the effect of lung volume on the length of the inspiratory msucles). Hypercapnic COPD patients ($Pco_2 > 45$ mm Hg) are at or above the critical zone, whereas eucapnic COPD patients are below the critical zone. RV = residual volume; FRC = functional residual capacity; TLC = total lung capacity. (Reproduced with permission from Roussus C, Macklem PT, eds. The Thorax, Part B. New York: Marcel Dekker, 1985, 1253–1279.)

Treatment

Stimulation of Respiration

Progesterone is a respiratory stimulant that presumably acts centrally in the nervous system and causes increased ventilation despite an increase in pH of the cerebral spinal fluid and arterial blood. Although progestins have been used therapeutically in central hypoventilation syndromes, clinical experience in hypercapnic COPD patients is limited. Skatrud and coworkers[19,20] evaluated the effect of 4 weeks of administration of medroxyprogesterone acetate, a synthetic progestin, on COPD patients with chronic CO_2 retention in placebo-controlled, single-blind crossover studies (Fig. 44–3). Of 16 patients, 10 responded with a decrease in $Paco_2$ (from 52 ± 1 to 45 ± 2 mm Hg). It is noteworthy that the inspiratory time remained short but the tidal volume increased, as did inspiratory effort (P_{100}). The authors concluded that a short inspiratory time, although frequently observed in hypercapnic patients, is not by itself the major determinant of chronic CO_2 retention. Rather, insufficient ventilatory effort in relation to the increased demands imposed by airflow limitation and increased dead space appear to be a more likely explanation.

In a similar study, Tatsumi and colleagues[27] evaluated the effect of 1 week of administration of chlormadinone acetate, a potent synthetic progesterone, in 12 COPD patients. As a group these patients were eucapnic ($Paco_2 = 42.5 \pm 1.7$ mm Hg), although five had CO_2 retention ($Paco_2 > 45$ mm Hg). Therapy was associated with a significant reduction in $Paco_2$ of 4.6 ± 0.6 mm Hg. This decrease was associated with an increase in tidal volume, mean inspiratory flow, and occlusion pressure response to CO_2, with and without inspiratory flow-resistive loading. The ratio of the loaded to unloaded slope in the occlusion pressure response also increased. The authors concluded that chlormadinone acetate augmented the respiratory neuromuscular response to hypercapnia, as well as the flow-resistive load compensation, in these COPD patients.

Although these short-term studies appear promising, little information is available regarding the efficacy and side-effects of long-term administration of progesterone agents. Decreased libido and impotence were reported by 3 of 15 patients after 4 weeks of therapy.[20] Furthermore, not all responders reported a decrease in dyspnea or overall subjective improvement. Finally, patients with severe mechanical limitation are unlikely to benefit. Skatrud and Dempsey excluded patients from the study with an FEV_1 less than 500 ml.[20] Even so, the nonresponders usually showed an inability to lower their $Paco_2$ (more than 5 mm Hg) with voluntary hyperventilation and had more severe obstructive airway disease (FEV_1, 24% predicted), hyperinflation, and lower diffusion capacity than the responders.

Acetazolamide, a carbonic anhydrase inhibitor, produces chronic hyperventilation in normal subjects and in some patients with COPD.[28,29] The increased ventilation appears to be mediated through the generation of a metabolic acidosis, with

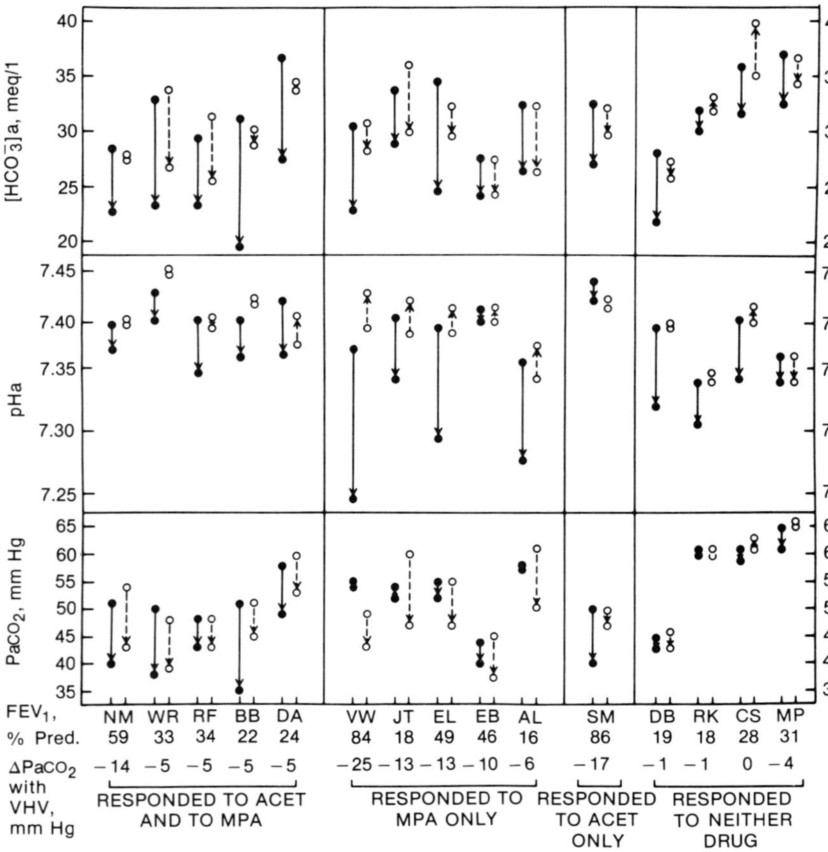

Figure 44–3. Effect of acetazolamide (ACET) and medroxyprogesterone acetate (MPA) on Pa_{CO_2} and acid-base status in 15 COPD patients with chronic CO_2 retention. Response to a drug is defined as a reduction of Pa_{CO_2} of at least 5 mm Hg. Each point represents the mean of four to six samples from the patient. The open circles represent testing of MPA; the closed circles represent testing of ACET. The arrow shows the directional change from placebo treatment to drug treatment. FEV_1 (% predicted) is shown for the placebo period. (VHV = voluntary hyperventilation.) (Reproduced with permission from Skatrud JB, Dempsey JA. Am Rev Respir Dis 1983; 127:405–412.)

a lower pH at the peripheral and medullary chemoreceptors. Skatrud and Dempsey compared the effect of acetazolamide with that of medroxyprogesterone as part of the study already described.[20] Only 6 of 15 hypercapnic patients responded to acetazolamide with a decrease in Pa_{CO_2} of 5 mmHg or more, and only 1 of these 6 patients responded only to acetazolamide (Fig. 44–3). As might be expected, several of the acetazolamide nonresponders developed a potentially clinically significant degree of uncompensated metabolic acidosis (pH = 7.25 to 7.35). The acetazolamide-produced acidification of the cerebrospinal fluid (CSF) and plasma did not cause a sustained augmentation of ventilation in these nonresponding patients, despite the fact that many could lower their Pa_{CO_2} with voluntary hyperventilation. The low number of responders, and the potentially significant acidosis in nonresponders, argues strongly against the clinical use of acetazolamide in hypercapnic COPD patients. It is not inconceivable, however, that future research may identify a carefully selected subgroup of CO_2 retainers who may benefit from long-term acetazolamide use.

Theophylline stimulates hypoxic and hypercapnic ventilatory drives in normal subjects.[30, 31] One report has indicated that aminophylline increases respiratory center sensitivity in emphysema patients.[32] The therapeutic implications of these findings are unclear.

Respiratory Muscle Rest Therapy

Although the precise role of respiratory muscle fatigue in the development of hypercapnia in COPD remains unclear, considerable interest has developed regarding the potential benefit of intermittent muscle rest therapy in hypercapnic COPD patients.[33, 34] Respiratory muscle rest has been achieved with a number of different devices. Negative pressure ventilation is the preferred method of achieving intermittent respiratory muscle rest in stable hypercapnic patients, because intubation is not required. Methods of achieving negative pressure ventilation include the tank respirator (or iron lung), cuirass device, and the poncho-type ventilator. Positive pressure ventilation techniques that do not require intubation can also be tried, but there is less experience in their use. Recently, however, the continuous positive airway pressure (CPAP) mask has been used successfully at night to treat chronic respiratory failure caused by neuromuscular disease.[35]

In an early study reported in 1959, Jameson and colleagues[36] treated several COPD patients with either negative or positive ventilation for 2 to 12 hours a day for 3 to 21 days. A decrease in Pa_{CO_2} from the usual baseline value could be found when arterial blood gases were sampled at least 12 hours after the most recent use of the ventilator.

More recently, in 1977, Rochester and associates[37] documented that negative pressure ventilation promptly abolished almost all diaphragmatic electrical activity in hypercapnic COPD patients as soon as the respirator developed a negative pressure of about −20 to −25 cm H_2O around the body. Their study provided important physiologic evidence that negative pressure ventilation could indeed "rest" the inspiratory muscles. These patients also reported an immediate relief of dyspnea that coincided with the decrease in electrical activity of the respiratory muscles, and that occurred before any acute change in arterial blood gas levels.

Braun and Marino[38, 39] have demonstrated beneficial effects of intermittent negative pressure ventilation in the treatment of hypercapnic COPD patients who had a history of recurrent episodes of respiratory failure requiring hospitalization. Eighteen such patients were treated with intermittent respiratory muscle rest therapy (14 patients received negative pressure ventilation using a poncho-type ventilator and 4 received positive pressure ventilation by tracheostomy) for 5 months at home. Respiratory muscle rest was used for 4 to 10 hours each night. At the end of 5 months, the Pa_{CO_2} decreased (54 ± 6 to 45 ± 2 mm Hg), the MVV increased (21 ± 7% to 28 ± 7% predicted), $P_{I\ max}$ increased (36 ± 17% to 58 ± 18% predicted), and maximum expiratory pressure increased (52 ± 29% to 70 ± 19% predicted). Furthermore, there was a decrease both in hospital admissions, from 2.8 ± 1.8 to 0.4 ± 1.0 per year, and in days of hospitalization, from 39 ± 30 to 4 ± 10 per year.

In a similar study, Cropp and DiMarco[40] demonstrated that the acute benefits of respiratory muscle rest could be achieved with a much shorter treatment period. They evaluated the effects of negative pressure ventilation for 3 to 6 hours daily for 3 consecutive days. Measurements obtained on the final day (about 2 to 3 hours after discontinuation of muscle rest) showed a reduction in the mean Pa_{CO_2} from 60 mm Hg before to 52 mm Hg after treatment. Significant improvements in MVV and maximum inspiratory and expiratory pressures were also observed. Patients also reported an improvement in their sensation of dyspnea.

Little published information is available regarding how long the salutary effects of muscle rest therapy are sustained following discontinuation of therapy. It appears, however, that patients return to their baseline status within a few days after cessation of intermittent rest therapy.[33] Thus, such therapy will probably have to be continued on a frequent and long-term basis. One encouraging report has suggested that rest therapy provided only once a week might lead to a sustained improvement in blood gas levels.[41]

Although respiratory muscle rest therapy remains investigational, there are enough indications of its efficacy and safety to suggest that such therapy be considered for severe COPD patients with chronic hypercapnia and frequent clinical decompensations. Firm guidelines for patient selection are not available, but Rochester and Martin have offered criteria.[34] They proposed that patients might benefit from intermittent rest therapy if several of the following variables are found: $P_{I\ max} < 50$ cm H_2O, $FEV_1 < 25\%$ predicted, $Pa_{CO_2} > 45$ mm Hg, and clinical evidence of muscle fatigue (tachypnea > 30/minute, chest-abdomen asynchrony).

Pharmacotherapy of Respiratory Muscles

The role of pharmacologic agents to treat or prevent respiratory muscle fatigue has been generating interest and controversy.[42–44] Most investigations have centered on the methylxanthines or the sympathomimetic amines, although some new information on digoxin is also available.

Theophylline has traditionally been used as a bronchodilator. The magnitude of this effect, however, is small or nonexistent in many COPD patients. Nevertheless, theophylline has been documented to reduce dyspnea, even in patients with nonreversible obstructive airway disease.[45] It has been argued that the salutary effect of theophylline in such patients may partly be a result of improvement in respiratory muscle function. Several experiments have indicated that theophylline has an inotropic effect on isolated skeletal or diaphragm muscle tissue.[42] Furthermore, the results of many animal studies suggest that theophylline increases diaphragm contractility and improves diaphragm force after fatigue is induced by electrophrenic stimulation[46] or by resistive loaded breathing.[47] In 1981, theophylline in usual therapeutic doses was reported to enhance diaphragm contractility in normal human subjects.[48] This was followed by evidence that similar effects are seen in patients with severe COPD.[49] In this study, 15 stable patients with hypoxia (Pa_{O_2} 57 ± 8 mm Hg) and hypercapnia (Pa_{CO_2} 53 ± 3 mm Hg) demonstrated an increased baseline $P_{di\ max}$ that persisted for at least 30 days of treatment and a resistance to diaphragm fatigue induced by resistive loaded breathing. A preliminary follow-up report from the same laboratory found that 2 months of oral theophylline therapy produces an increase in minute ventilation (caused entirely by an increase in tidal volume) and a significant decrease in hypercapnia (Pa_{CO_2} declined by 6 mm Hg on average).[42, 50] Dyspnea also improved and respiratory muscle reserve was enhanced. No significant improvement in lung function was reported, suggesting that these beneficial effects are a result of improved performance of the respiratory muscles.

However, several other investigators could not confirm a clinically important effect of theophylline on respiratory muscle function in COPD patients.[43, 51] Differences in methodology, patient selection, and interpretation of data account for much of the controversy.[42, 43] At this time, the role of theophylline in the treatment of respiratory muscle dysfunction in hypercapnic COPD patients remains uncertain.

Similarly, sympathomimetic agents may improve muscle function in vitro, but the clinical significance of these findings is unclear. Isoproterenol[46] and terbutaline[52] exert positive inotropic effects on the fatigued diaphragm of the dog in vivo, but no effect of oral albuterol on diaphragm fatigue was found in normal humans breathing against an inspiratory resistance.[53] Oral terbutaline did not enhance baseline diaphragm strength in patients with stable COPD.[54]

The diaphragm and myocardium appear to be similarly affected by extracellular calcium in the contractile process.[55] In this regard, the diaphragm may resemble myocardium more than skeletal muscle. Aubier and colleagues have tested the effect of digoxin in eight COPD patients receiving mechanical ventilation for acute respiratory failure.[55] Diaphragm strength following electrical stimulation of the phrenic nerves was improved markedly with digoxin administration, even though cardiac output was unchanged. Further research is necessary to confirm this effect and, especially, to define what role digoxin might have in the therapeutics of respiratory muscle fatigue. Nevertheless, this finding is likely to rekindle some interest in the use of digoxin in COPD patients, because this medication is not recommended in these patients for treatment of isolated right ventricular dysfunction (see subsequent discussion).

Nutrition and Diet

Nutritional deficiencies may contribute to respiratory muscle dysfunction in COPD patients.[56] Furthermore, large carbohydrate loads lead to increases in CO_2 production.[57] Therefore, nutritional considerations can be important in the prevention or treatment of chronic hypercapnia in patients with severe COPD.

At least two studies[58, 59] have suggested that protein and calorie repletion improves respiratory muscle function in patients with severe COPD. Apparently no studies have shown, however, that such nutritional repletion and improved inspiratory muscle strength lead to a lower Pa_{CO_2} in chronic, stable, hypercapnic COPD patients.[56]

Attempts at nutritional repletion in COPD patients need to take into account the potential adverse impact of large carbohydrate loads. Brown and coworkers have found that a large, single carbohydrate load causes an acute decrease in 12-minute walking distance and maximal exercise capacity in several COPD patients.[60, 61]

In stable ambulatory patients with COPD and chronic hypercapnia, a low-carbohydrate, high-fat diet (28% carbohydrate calories, 55% fat calories) resulted in significantly lower CO_2 production and lower Pa_{CO_2} compared to either the baseline (prestudy) values or to other study diets higher in carbohydrates.[62] The overall total calories given surpassed the daily requirements, eliminating any concern with malnutrition, but the decrease in Pa_{CO_2} was very small (49.24 ± 1.55 versus 47.50 ± 1.44 mm Hg) and the overall functional significance of these findings is unclear. In a different study, Tirlapur and Mir[63] achieved a reduction of Pa_{CO_2} from 59.9 ± 9.6 to 52.4 ± 5.4 mm Hg in COPD patients with a very low-calorie diet (600 kcal per day) for about 4 weeks, but a significant weight loss (8.5 ± 3.6 kg) also occurred. The usefulness and safety of such a drastic approach remains to be determined and clearly such caloric restriction cannot be maintained on a long-term basis.

Correction of significant deficiencies of phosphorus, magnesium, and potassium may acutely improve respiratory muscle function.[64, 65] It is uncertain to what degree deficiencies of these substances contribute to chronic hypercapnia.

COR PULMONALE

Definition, Incidence, and Etiology

Cor pulmonale is the alteration of right ventricular structure or function caused by pulmonary hypertension, when the latter has resulted from disease that affects the lung or its vasculature.[1, 2, 66] Primary disease of the left side of the heart and congenital heart disease are excluded.

COPD is the major cause of chronic cor pulmonale. At least 50,000 deaths in the U.S. each year are attributed to chronic obstructive bronchitis and emphysema. About 50% of these patients demonstrate anatomic evidence of right ventricular hypertrophy if examined at autopsy.[67] The percentage of COPD patients who exhibit clinically measurable dysfunction of the right ventricle during life, however, is probably even higher.

Noninvasive radionuclide techniques have provided evidence for a high incidence of right ventricular dysfunction in COPD patients.[68] Berger and colleagues[69] have determined the right ventricular ejection fraction using first-pass radionuclide angiocardiography in 36 randomly selected COPD patients. Nineteen patients had a depressed right ventricular ejection fraction, including all ten patients with clinical cor pulmonale. Among the 26 patients without clinical cor pulmonale, nine had a reduced right ventricular ejection fraction. Within 2 years of the original study, cor pulmonale developed in four of these nine patients. In contrast, within 2 years, cor pulmonale developed in none of the patients with a normal initial right ventricular ejection fraction. Abnormal right ventricular function in COPD patients is often demonstrable during exercise,[68, 70, 74] even if function at rest appears to be normal.

Pulmonary hypertension may occur in COPD patients from various causes.[71] Anatomic reduction in the cross-sectional area of the pulmonary vascular bed can result either from chronic hypoxia-induced structural narrowing of vessels or from direct destruction of vessels, as in emphysema. Active pulmonary vasoconstriction is induced by hypoxia and acidosis. Pulmonary hypertension in COPD patients may be exacerbated by other factors, including increased blood volume, increased blood viscosity, and elevated cardiac output. Also, expiratory airflow limitation may lead to a greater increase in alveolar pressure than pleural pressure, thereby contributing to pulmonary hypertension during hyperventilation or exercise.[72–74] Finally, left ventricular dysfunction is present in some COPD patients and contributes to pulmonary hypertension through an elevated pulmonary venous pressure.

Natural History of Untreated Pulmonary Hypertension in COPD

The resting pulmonary artery pressure increases relatively slowly in patients with emphysema or chronic obstructive bronchitis who have mild or moderate arterial hypoxemia.[75–78] In one study, 93 patients with severe COPD were followed for at least 5 years and for a mean of about 8 years.[78] Vasodilator medications and long-term oxygen therapy were not used. The patients were divided into two groups based on their initial mean pulmonary artery pressure ($\bar{P}ap$). Group 1 patients ($n = 61$) had no pulmonary hypertension when the study began ($\bar{P}ap < 20$ mm Hg); patients in group 2 had pulmonary hypertension initially ($\bar{P}ap > 20$ mm Hg). For those in group 1, the beginning FEV_1 was 1.42 ± 0.42 L and the beginning Pa_{O_2} was 67 ± 7.4 mm Hg. In those in group 2, the initial FEV_1 was 1.17 ± 0.39 L and the initial Pa_{O_2} was 62 ± 7 mm Hg. Changes in $\bar{P}ap$ were minor during the study. In group 1, the $\bar{P}ap$ increased from 15.5 ± 2.4 to 19.6 ± 7.0 mm Hg ($p < 0.001$). In group 2, the $\bar{P}ap$ rose from 25.8 ± 5.6 to 27.8 ± 9.5 mm Hg (not significant). No significant changes in cardiac output and right ventricular filling pressures were observed in either group.

Although the overall increase in pulmonary artery pressure was slow, a subgroup of 27 patients demonstrated progression of their pulmonary hypertension (defined as an increase of $\bar{P}ap \geq 5$ mm Hg). These patients did not differ from the others at the onset of the study with respect to blood gas levels, spirometry, pulmonary hemodynamic profile, age, or other identifiable characteristics. The evolution of blood gases was the primary difference. Patients in the subgroup with progression of pulmonary hypertension showed a deterioration of Pa_{O_2} (66.0 ± 8.0 to 59.1 ± 9.2 mm Hg) and an elevation of Pa_{CO_2} (37.2 ± 3 to 46.0 ± 6.8 mm Hg) during the study, whereas arterial blood gas levels remained constant in the group with stable $\bar{P}ap$. A weak correlation between changes in FEV_1 and $\bar{P}ap$ was also found. Weitzenblum's findings[78] suggest that hypoxemia is an important factor in the progression of pulmonary artery hypertension. In this regard, it is noteworthy that the untreated patients in the British Medical Research Council controlled oxygen study demonstrated a rapid rise in $\bar{P}ap$; these individuals were markedly hypoxemic (Pa_{O_2} = 40 to 60 mm Hg).[79]

Because hypoxic pulmonary vasoconstriction and subsequent pulmonary artery hypertension and cor pulmonale are generally accepted risk factors in the prognosis of COPD, a study by Kawakami and colleagues proved to be provocative.[80] Fifty COPD patients underwent a right-heart catheterization and mortality was assessed 4 years later. Twenty-three survivors were compared with the 27 patients who had died during the 4 years. The nonsurvivors had a significantly lower initial Pa_{O_2} and mixed venous P_{O_2} at the start of the study. However, initial $\bar{P}ap$, right ventricular work, oxygen transport, and coefficient of oxygen delivery (ratio of oxygen transport to oxygen consumption) were not signficantly different in survivors and nonsurvivors. The authors concluded that tissue oxygenation in nonsurvivors was disturbed because of unspecified diffusion abnormalities, rather than a primary defect of oxygen transport and delivery secondary to pulmonary hypertension.[80] In summary, arterial hypoxia and low mixed venous oxygen tension were associated with decreased survival, but apparently not through the generally accepted mechanism of cor pulmonale.

The conclusions of this study have been challenged on statistical grounds by Tockman and colleagues.[81] Because only a small number of patients were evaluated, the investigation may have failed to detect significant differences between survivors and nonsurvivors (e.g., pulmonary pressures), if they existed (type II error). Furthermore, because longitudinal hemodynamic data were not assessed, a significant progression of pulmonary hypertension or changes in oxygen transport subsequent to the initial evaluation may have occurred in the nonsurvivors and remained undetected. Therefore, the investigation by Kawakami and coworkers[80] does not necessarily reject the hypoxia-pulmonary hypertension-cor pulmonale mechanism as an important cause of death in COPD, but their findings relative to the apparent prognostic importance of mixed venous oxygenation do warrant further discussion.

Cardiac Output Response and the Successful Adaptation to COPD

Although cor pulmonale is generally viewed as a form of "heart failure," in reality the cardiac output often remains normal or slightly elevated in COPD patients until shortly prior to death.[82–84] In this regard, it is of interest that both survivors and nonsurvivors in the Kawakami study[80] initially had high cardiac indices (4.4 ± 0.8 and 4.1 ± 0.7 L/minute/m^2 of body surface area, respectively).

Tenney and Mithoefer[85] have studied the relationship between mixed venous oxygen saturation and coefficient of oxygen delivery in 68 COPD patients at rest breathing room air. Although there was a close correlation between oxygen delivery and mixed venous oxygenation ($r = 0.84$), there was a wide variation among individual patients. The difference related partly to whether a given value for oxygen delivery was achieved with a higher cardiac output and lower oxygen content (saturation multiplied by hemoglobin concentration), or vice versa. The latter type of patients (polycythemia and relatively lower cardiac output) had a lower mixed venous Po_2 than patients who had identical total oxygen delivery, but who achieved such delivery with a higher cardiac output and a lesser degree of polycythemia.

As discussed previously, Kawakami and associates[80] demonstrated that a lower mixed venous oxygen saturation is a marker for poor prognosis when comparing two untreated patients who otherwise have the same pulmonary hemodynamics and coefficient of oxygen delivery. Applying the findings of Tenney and Mithoefer,[85] one might hypothesize that the development of polycythemia in response to hypoxic COPD is not necessarily a successful long-term adaptation by itself, even though systemic oxygen transport is maintained. Instead, cardiac output should increase, allowing for the maintenance of mixed venous oxygenation. Thus, although the Kawakami study seems to refute the importance of cardiac output, an alternative interpretation is that the failure to increase cardiac output in the face of significant venous hypoxemia is the crucial maladaptation that adversely affects survival. Although unproven, this hypothesis advances a central role for cardiac output in the successful physiologic adaptation to COPD.[82, 83, 86]

Further support for this hypothesis comes from studies of the relationship between systemic oxygen transport and oxygen consumption in COPD patients.[87, 88] Results of these investigations have suggested that some COPD patients may have an abnormal "supply dependency" of oxygen consumption on oxygen delivery. In normal subjects, oxygen consumption does not change with variations in oxygen transport unless the latter becomes severely reduced.[89] In contrast, when Brent and coworkers[87] acutely altered the cardiac index in COPD patients by increasing it with hydralazine or decreasing it with nitroprusside, oxygen consumption varied so as to suggest that it was directly related to oxygen transport. Because vasodilators were used to produce the changes in the cardiac output, the possibility that these agents affected tissue metabolism or peripheral vasoregulation could not be excluded. To avoid this problem, Albert and colleagues[88] investigated the relationship between oxygen transport and oxygen consumption in stable COPD patients using a nonpharmacologic method (passive leg elevation) of altering cardiac output. Oxygen consumption appeared to depend on oxygen transport in this study, a result consistent with the earlier finding of Brent and associates.[87] Chappell and coworkers,[90] however, have found that changes in oxygen transport are not associated with predictable alterations in oxygen consumption in similar patients, indicating the need for additional studies to clarify this issue.

From the perspective of the previous discussions, interventions that defend or enhance the cardiac output in COPD patients could be assumed to have therapeutic importance. In the following discussion of the treatment of chronic cor pulmonale, further attention is paid to the theme of cardiac output and oxygen delivery.

Therapy for Chronic Cor Pulmonale

Theophylline and Cardiovascular Performance in COPD

Theophylline may have beneficial cardiovascular effects in COPD patients with and without cor pulmonale.[68, 91] An early study by Parker and colleagues[92] evaluated the acute hemodynamic effects of intravenous aminophylline in nine patients with cor pulmonale secondary to COPD. The mean pulmonary artery pressure decreased (from 39 to 25 mm Hg), as did right and left ventricular stroke work, but the cardiac index, arterial oxygen saturation, and oxygen consumption did not change significantly. More recently, Matthay and coworkers[93] investigated the acute effects of intravenous aminophylline on right and left ventricular ejection fraction in 15 patients with COPD, four of whom had cor pulmonale (Fig. 44–4). The right ventricular ejection fraction normalized in six of eight patients with initially depressed right ventricular performance, and the left ventricular ejection fraction also improved. The improvement in biventricular function was accompanied only by a minimal improvement in FEV_1, and the arterial oxygen tension remained unchanged.

Chronic therapy with oral theophylline also enhances right ventricular function in COPD patients. In a study by Matthay and associates,[94] 11 patients treated for an average of 4 months exhibited a sustained improvement in right ventricular ejection fraction (Fig. 44–5). The left ventricular ejection fraction showed a modest increase.

The improved biventricular pump function observed with theophylline therapy is apparently a result of a combination of reduced afterload (lowered pulmonary and systemic vascular resistance) and enhanced myocardial contractility.[91] In isolated papillary muscle preparations, theophylline causes a shift upward and to the right in the force-velocity relationship.[95] In vivo canine studies have also documented an increase in cardiac contractility from aminophylline.[96] Theophylline probably also acts directly to lower vascular resistance.[91, 97, 98] In dogs, however, aminophylline does not inhibit acute hypoxic pulmonary vasoconstriction.[99]

Clinical studies with aminophylline have not yielded uniformly positive results, however. Canny and coworkers[100] found no significant increase in the mean right or left ventricular ejection fraction, either at rest or exercise, following aminophylline infusion in cystic fibrosis patients.

β-Adrenergic Agents

Brent and colleagues[101] have evaluated the acute hemodynamic effects of 0.25 mg of subcutaneous terbutaline in eight patients with severe COPD. All patients had mild to moderate pulmonary hypertension and abnormal right ventricular function. Terbutaline administration reduced pulmonary vascular resistance in all patients; the right ventricular end-diastolic volume index and mean pulmonary artery pressure remained the same (Fig. 44–6). The right and left ventricular ejection fractions rose with terbutaline (Fig. 44–7). The cardiac index improved significantly (2.5 ± 0.7 to 3.7 ± 0.8 L/minute/m^2) and the PaO_2 remained stable, resulting in an increase in systemic oxygen delivery (45 ± 16 to 63 ± 19 ml/minute/m^2) and mixed venous oxygen tension (from 33 ± 8 to 37 ± 6 mm Hg) (Fig. 44–8). These findings are similar to observations in two other studies on COPD patients.[102, 103] In both investigations, intravenous terbutaline caused an increase in cardiac output and a reduction of pulmonary vascular resistance at rest, and in one study[103] these benefits were also found during exercise.

Pirbuterol, another β agonist, produced similar favorable hemodynamic changes that persisted during the 6 weeks of oral therapy.[104]

The observed cardiovascular effects of the β agonists probably derive from pulmonary vasodilation caused by stimulation of β-adrenergic receptors[101, 104, 105] or from improved myocardial performance through direct inotropic action.[104]

Digitalis

In patients with cor pulmonale, digitalis does not improve right ventricular function at rest or during exercise, except in

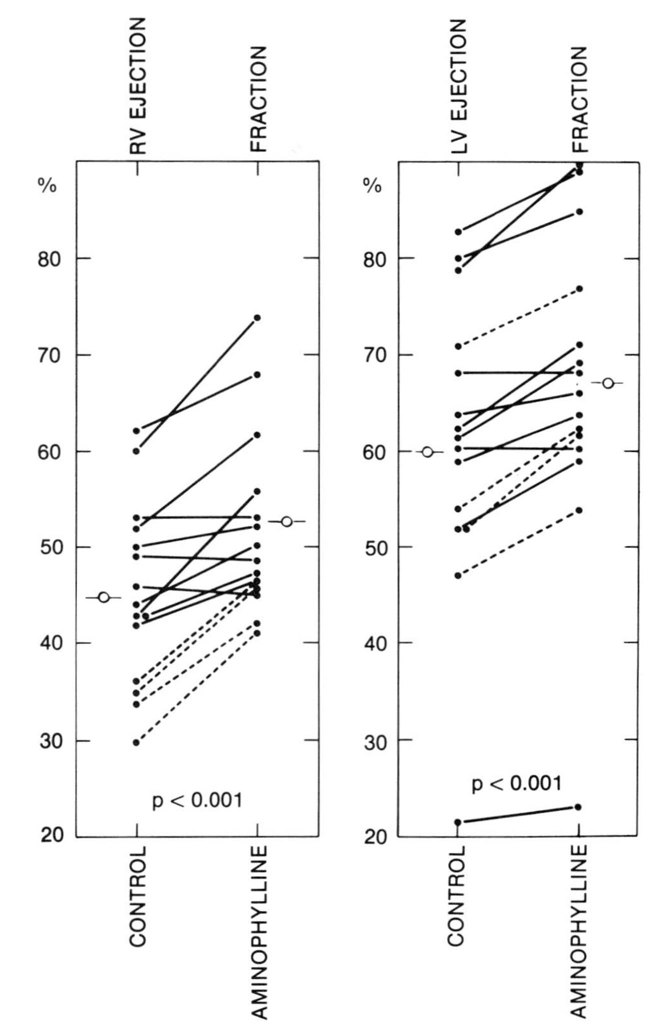

Figure 44–4. Effect of aminophylline on right ventricular (RV) and left ventricular (LV) performance in 15 patients with chronic obstructive pulmonary disease. The four dotted lines indicate patients with cor pulmonale. Right and left ventricular ejection fractions increased significantly with aminophylline. (Reproduced with permission from Matthay RA, et al. Am J Med 1978; 65:903–910.)

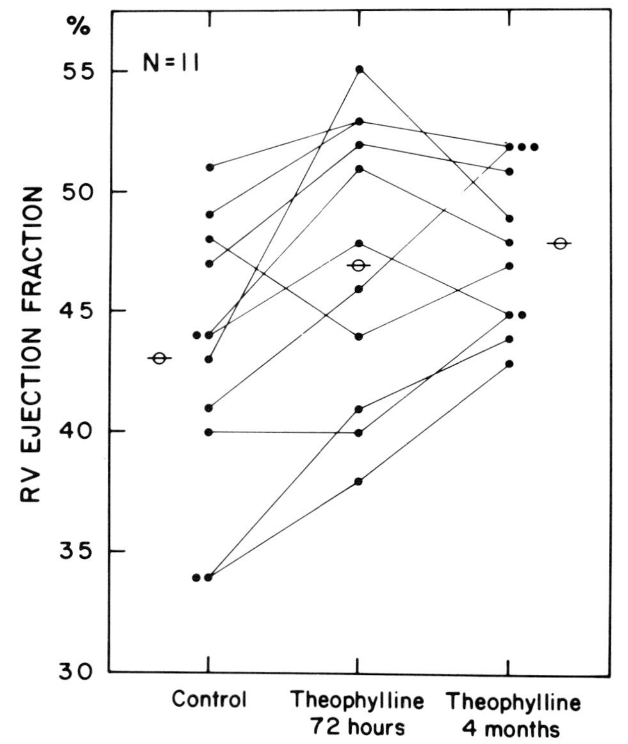

Figure 44–5. Oral long-acting theophylline (Theo-Dur) significantly increased right ventricular ejection fraction after 72 hours and after an average of 4 months of therapy in 11 patients with COPD. (Reproduced with permission from Matthay RA, et al. Clin Chest Med 1983; 4:269–295.)

cases of coexisting left ventricular failure or a supraventricular tachyarrhythmia for which digitalis is effective.[106–111]

The lack of efficacy of digitalis in COPD patients might be a result of at least two factors that could offset the beneficial effect of enhanced myocardial contractility. First, the cardiac glycosides may produce pulmonary vasoconstriction,[112] resulting in an increased right ventricular afterload. In addition, Sylvester and coworkers[113] have observed that in dogs digitalis increases the "unstressed reservoir volume" of the circulation through an action on the peripheral vasculature. This causes a shift in the venous return curve to the left, resulting in a lower right ventricular preload. If this effect also occurs in patients, it could adversely affect cardiac output.

The use of digitalis in cor pulmonale patients is associated with an increased incidence of adverse side effects, such as cardiac arrhythmias.[107] The reason for this is uncertain but appears to include the effect of hypoxia.

Although digoxin does not enhance cardiac function or exercise performance in those with cor pulmonale, except in the presence of concurrent left ventricular dysfunction, the possibility that digoxin may have favorable effects when used in combination with other medications, including theophylline, vasodilators, selective β_2-adrenergic agents, and oxygen, has not been excluded fully. Nevertheless, current evidence indicates that the routine use of digoxin in the treatment of cor pulmonale should be avoided.

Vasodilator Agents

GENERAL CONSIDERATIONS. Systemic vasodilating agents have a well-established role in the management of left ventricular failure. Success in this area has stimulated much interest in the potential role of vasodilators in treating COPD char-

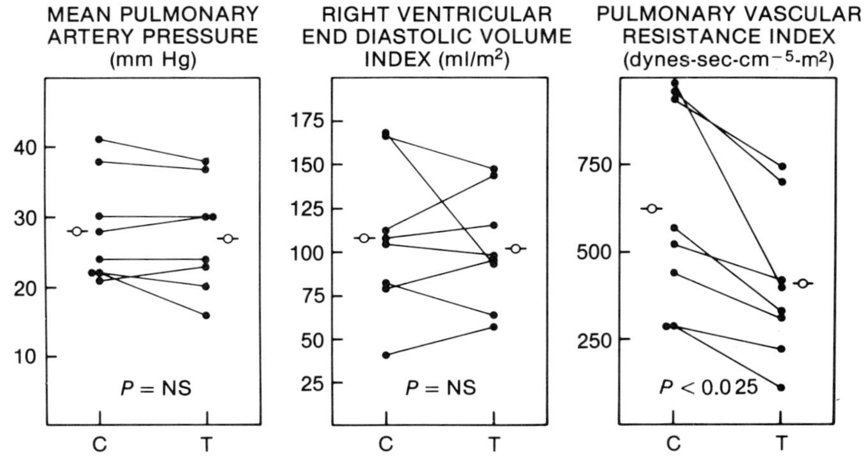

Figure 44–6. Acute effects of terbutaline on right ventricular preload and afterload. Mean pulmonary arterial pressure and right ventricular end-diastolic volume index are unaffected by terbutaline. In contrast, pulmonary vascular resistance index is decreased significantly. C = control state; P = NS; T = 30 minutes after adminstration of terbutaline. (Reproduced with permission from Brent BN, et al. Am J Cardiol 1982; 50:313–319.)

acterized by pulmonary hypertension and chronic cor pulmonale.

Assessing studies of vasodilator agents in COPD patients is difficult because the hemodynamic alterations are complex, and it has not been established which changes are desirable or undesirable. Although a reduction in pulmonary hypertension is a frequently stated goal of vasodilator therapy, a decrease in vascular resistance may be offset by an increase in cardiac output, leaving the pulmonary artery pressure unchanged. Perhaps this is a beneficial effect (e.g., increased oxygen transport), despite the unrelieved pulmonary hypertension. Conversely, a medication that reduces venous return (nitroglycerin) or depresses right ventricular function (nifedipine) may ameliorate pulmonary hypertension, partly by lowering cardiac output. Despite the reduction in pulmonary artery pressures, however, this might not be beneficial. Determining what constitutes a desirable hemodynamic response to vasodilators may ultimately require long-term studies to assess the overall survival effect of various vasodilators. Unlike the case with oxygen therapy, such information is not available.

HYDRALAZINE, NITRATES, AND NIFEDIPINE. Most investigations of vasodilator therapy in COPD patients have used hydralazine, nitrates (e.g., nitroprusside, nitroglycerin), or calcium channel blockers, such as nifedipine.

Results with hydralazine are mixed; some studies have claimed a beneficial hemodynamic effect[87, 114–118] and others have indicated limited or detrimental effects.[119–124] Lupi-Herrera and coworkers[122] have observed improved cardiac output and mixed venous oxygen saturation but found no change in pulmonary artery pressure and pulmonary vascular resistance. Rubin and colleagues[116, 117] have showed that hydralazine lowers mean pulmonary artery pressure and pulmonary vascular resistance during rest and exercise, and enhances cardiac output and mixed venous P_{O_2}. Some investigators have reported that hydralazine usually produces an increase in minute ventilation during rest and exercise.[115–117] This effect on ventilation might also account for an undesirable increase in dyspnea experienced by some patients receiving hydralazine.[117, 124]

The hemodynamic effects of hydralazine in COPD patients appear to be generally superior to those of nitroprusside and nitroglycerin.[87, 118, 125] Brent and associates[118] found that nitroglycerin and nitroprusside reduce preload, cardiac index, and Pa_{O_2}. In contrast, hydralazine decreased pulmonary vascular resistance and increased the right ventricular ejection fraction and cardiac index. Additional studies from the same investigators evaluated the effect of hydralazine and nitroprusside on oxygen transport and oxygen consumption.[87] Hydralazine increased oxygen delivery, whereas nitroprusside decreased it slightly.

The use of nifedipine in COPD patients is receiving much interest.[126–131] Nifedipine often produces an acute decrease in pulmonary vascular resistance and an increase in cardiac output. Pulmonary artery pressure often decreases, but this effect of nifedipine is inconsistent and sometimes relatively modest in magnitude. Limited information is available regarding the chronic administration of nifedipine, but Sturani and

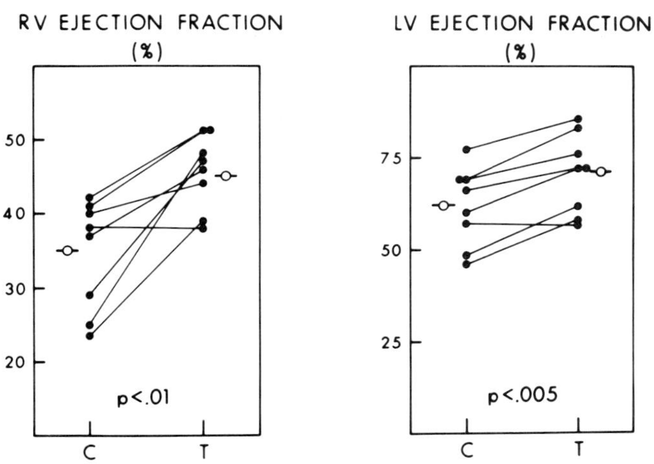

Figure 44–7. Acute effects of subcutaneously administered terbutaline on right ventricular (RV) and left ventricular (LV) ejection fraction. Both right and left ventricular ejection fractions increased significantly with terbutaline. C = control state; T = 30 minutes after administration of terbutaline. (Reproduced with permission from Brent BN, et al. Am J Cardiol 1982; 50:313–319.)

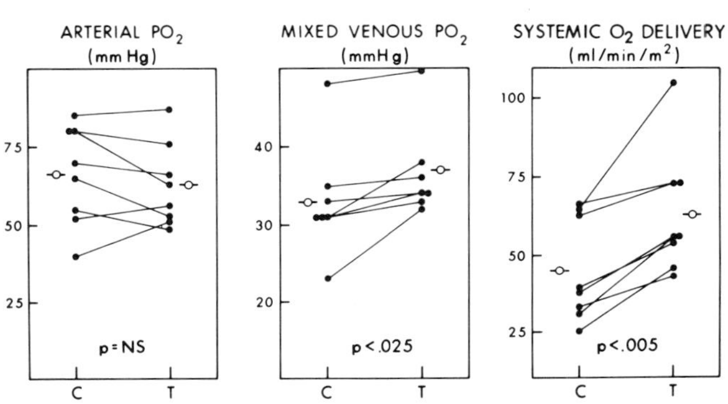

Figure 44–8. Acute effects of subcutaneously administered terbutaline on Pa_{O_2}, mixed venous P_{O_2}, and systemic O_2 delivery. Terbutaline caused an increase in oxygen transport and mixed venous P_{O_2}. (Reproduced with permission from Brent BN, et al. Am J Cardiol 1982; 50:313–319.)

coworkers[127] have demonstrated that acute hemodynamic effects are maintained after 2 months of therapy. Exercise studies indicate that nifedipine generally reduces pulmonary vascular resistance and pulmonary artery pressure while improving cardiac output and oxygen delivery.[129–131] Although a major action of nifedipine is inhibition of hypoxic vasoconstriction,[126] Kennedy and colleagues[130] have demonstrated that nifedipine further reduces pulmonary vascular resistance when administered to patients who are already receiving supplemental oxygen. This suggests that nifedipine may be a useful adjunct to oxygen therapy.

Nitrendipine is a calcium channel blocker with cardiovascular effects similar to those of nifedipine. Because of its long duration of action, nitrendipine can be administered orally bid. Rubin and Moser[132] have found that nitrendipine lowers pulmonary vascular resistance and pulmonary artery pressure and increases cardiac index after 6 weeks of therapy. Although the Pa_{O_2} decreased (53.1 ± 18.7 to 45.5 ± 11.3 mm Hg), systemic oxygen transport increased by over 30%. Together with the results of Sturani and associates[127] (previously discussed), these data indicate that long-term therapy with calcium channel antagonists may result in persistent hemodynamic improvement in COPD patients.

CAPTOPRIL. Only limited information is available regarding the use of captopril in COPD patients.[133–135] Captopril given at a dose of 25 mg tid for 3 days reduced pulmonary artery pressure and pulmonary vascular resistance while improving cardiac output, oxygen delivery, and mixed venous oxygenation in five COPD patients.[134] However, adverse effects, probably related to pronounced systemic vasodilatation, were observed in one of three patients given captopril by Kastanos and coworkers.[133] In another study, ten patients recovering from right heart failure resulting from COPD showed no change in pulmonary artery pressure or pulmonary vascular resistance after a single oral dose of captopril (25 mg).[135]

PROSTAGLANDINS. Prostaglandins (PGs) are involved in the normal physiologic regulation of pulmonary blood flow. Two prostaglandins, PGI_2 (prostacyclin) and PGE_1, have strong vasodilator action on the pulmonary circulation. Following intravenous administration of PGE_1 to 26 patients with decompensated COPD, Naeije and colleagues[136] found a decrease in pulmonary artery pressures while cardiac output and oxygen delivery increased. Ishizaki and associates[137] have studied the oral administration of an experimental PGE_1 derivative in five COPD patients. The hemodynamic effects were similar to those of the PGE_1 infusion and lasted for up to 8 hours after one dose. Adverse side effects, however (e.g., diarrhea, hypotension, flushing), were found in both studies.

RECOMMENDATIONS FOR SELECTION OF VASODILATORS. The administration of vasodilators to COPD patients should be considered only when conventional therapy and oxygen have failed to ameliorate signs of right-heart failure or pulmonary hypertension. Because of the potentially adverse consequences of these medications, careful assessment of their impact on hemodynamics and oxygenation must be undertaken; this usually requires invasive right-heart catheterization.

Rubin[138] has offered the following guidelines to help determine what constitutes a beneficial hemodynamic response to a vasodilator: (1) pulmonary vascular resistance is reduced by at least 20% *and* cardiac output is increased or unchanged; and (2) pulmonary arterial pressure is decreased or unchanged *and* systemic blood pressure is not significantly reduced (e.g., no side effects). If these benefits are realized and the patient is started on a particular medication, repeat right-heart catheterization after 4 to 6 months of chronic therapy is desirable to assess whether the hemodynamic benefits are persistent.

Oxygen

SURVIVAL BENEFIT. In clinical trials sponsored by the National Institutes of Health in the U.S.[139] and by the British Medical Research Council,[79] long-term oxygen therapy was found to improve the survival of hypoxemic COPD patients. The British study compared the effects of treatment with oxygen for about 15 hours per day, including sleep, with the effects of no oxygen therapy. The U.S. study compared nocturnal oxygen therapy (about 12 hours per day) with "continuous" oxygen therapy (at least 19 hours per day). The two studies used similar entry criteria—patients with COPD and a Pa_{O_2} lower than 60 mm Hg and no other major diseases. In the NIH study, individuals with Pa_{O_2} between 55 and 60 mm Hg were accepted only if they also had polycythemia edema or electrocardiographic evidence of cor pulmonale. Only clinically stable patients with persistent hypoxemia observed over a 3-week period were enrolled. Oxygen was administered at a rate of 2 L/minute through nasal prongs in most of the British patients. The oxygen dose used in the NIH study was that which raised the Pa_{O_2} to at least 65 mm Hg, and an additional 1 L/minute was administered at night. At entry, the mean Pa_{O_2} breathing ambient air was 51.0 mm Hg and the mean FEV_1 was about 0.7 to 0.8 L in both studies. However, the British patients had higher Pa_{CO_2} values (54.0 versus 43.7 mm Hg), higher hematocrits (53.0% versus 47.5%), higher mean pulmonary artery pressures (34.4 versus 29.5 mm Hg), and higher cardiac outputs (6.01 versus 5.07 L/minute).

Oxygen therapy was beneficial in both studies. In the British study, only 19 of 42 (45%) oxygen-treated patients died within 5 years, whereas 30 out of 45 (67%) untreated patients died. In the NIH study, the mortality rate after 1 year was 20.6% in the group receiving nocturnal oxygen and only 11.9% in the group receiving continuous oxygen therapy. After 2 years, the mortality rates was 40.8% and 22.4%, respectively. The relative risk of death for nocturnal oxygen therapy compared with continuous oxygen was 1.94. In brief, "no oxygen is bad, oxygen for some of the time is better, but oxygen for most of the time is best."[140]

HEMODYNAMIC EFFECTS OF LONG-TERM OXYGEN THERAPY AND POSSIBLE RELATIONSHIP TO SURVIVAL. In the British trial, pulmonary artery pressure increased significantly in the group receiving no oxygen and remained stable in the half-day oxygen group.[79] In the NIH trial, after 6 months of oxygen therapy, pulmonary vascular resistance decreased slightly in the continuous oxygen group and increased slightly in the nocturnal oxygen group.[139] Weitzenblum and colleagues[141] subsequently reported a decrease in the $\bar{P}ap$ of 2.15 mm Hg/year in 16 severely hypoxemic COPD patients undergoing oxygen therapy (15 to 18 hours/day) for 1 to 6 years, a longer follow-up period than in the NIH and British studies. Prior to initiation of oxygen therapy, $\bar{P}ap$ had been increasing by 1.47 mm Hg/year in these patients. The combined results of those three studies indicate that oxygen therapy ameliorates the progressive pulmonary hypertension of untreated COPD.

Statistical analysis of the data from the NIH trial indicates that changes in the mean pulmonary artery pressure within the first 6 months of therapy are related to subsequent survival, after adjustment for association with the baseline mean pulmonary artery pressure.[142] Similarly, the continuous treatment group's improvement in pulmonary vascular resistance is associated with improved cardiac function, as shown by increased stroke volume index. Ashutosh and associates[143] have added further support to the hypothesis that oxygen-related hemodynamic changes are associated with and predictive of survival. They divided 28 stable patients with COPD and cor pulmonale into two groups based on the response of the mean pulmonary artery pressure to breathing 28% oxygen for 1 day. They considered patients whose $\bar{P}ap$ decreased at least 5 mm Hg after acute oxygen breathing to be "responders." All patients subsequently received long-term continuous oxygen therapy (2 L/minute). Two years later, 85% of the responders were alive, whereas only 11% of the nonresponders survived.

RECOMMENDATIONS REGARDING OXYGEN THERAPY. These American and British clinical trials have clearly established that long-term oxygen therapy improves survival in hypoxic COPD patients. Based on these results, patients with COPD should be started on long-term "continuous" nasal oxygen therapy if the resting PaO_2 remains lower than 55 mm Hg after a 3-week stabilization period on maximal medical therapy (e.g., bronchodilating agents, antimicrobials, diuretics). In addition, patients with a PaO_2 above 55 mm Hg should be considered for oxygen therapy if there is polycythemia or clinical evidence (e.g., ECG, physical examination) of pulmonary hypertension and cor pulmonale. The requirement that hypoxemia be documented after a stabilization period is important to avoid the commitment of long-term oxygen therapy in patients who do not require it. In the Nocturnal Oxygen Therapy Trial, 45% of hypoxic patients initially selected for study improved enough during 3 to 4 weeks of observation and treatment to suspend plans for long-term oxygen therapy.[144] Another study has confirmed this finding, and it is suggested that an even longer period of 2 to 3 months may be necessary to exclude patients who eventually achieve an acceptable PaO_2 level on medical therapy alone.[145]

Almitrine

A rather recently introduced drug, almitrine bismesylate, causes an increase in PaO_2 and a decrease in $PaCO_2$ in COPD patients.[146, 147] Oral administration of almitrine is effective.

The precise mechanism underlying the beneficial effect of almitrine on arterial blood gas levels is uncertain. In humans, almitrine increases the responsiveness of the peripheral arterial chemoreceptors to hypoxia, but not hypercapnia. Nevertheless, the principal reason for the improvement in arterial blood gases may be related to a reduction in ventilation-perfusion mismatching within the lung. The improvement of ventilation-perfusion matching might be a result of enhancement of hypoxic pulmonary vasoconstriction by almitrine, although other mechanisms such as alterations in breathing pattern may be involved.

A placebo-controlled, double-blind study has evaluated the long-term (8-week) effect of oral almitrine in COPD patients.[146] Almitrine produced a sustained and dose-related improvement in arterial blood gas levels. The PaO_2 rose by 11.2 mm Hg in 21 patients receiving 100 mg bid and by 6.0 mm Hg in 22 patients receiving 50 mg bid. Those in the high-dose group also experienced a significant decline in $PaCO_2$, 3.8 mm Hg. Lung function was unchanged except for a slight improvement in midexpiratory flow in both treated groups. The only major side effect of almitrine was worsening of dyspnea. This problem occurred more frequently in the high-dose patients (19%) than in the low-dose patients (9%) or in those in the placebo group (4%).

If almitrine does enhance hypoxic pulmonary vasoconstriction, perhaps improved arterial blood gas levels result at the expense of worsening pulmonary hypertension. This possibility has been investigated by MacNee and coworkers.[147] They compared the acute effects of almitrine (100 mg) with those of oxygen (3 L/minute by nasal prongs) on arterial blood gas tensions, mean pulmonary artery pressure, and right ventricular ejection fraction, both at rest and during exercise in hypoxic COPD patients. Despite improving PaO_2, almitrine increased the mean pulmonary artery pressure at rest from 22 $\pm$ 4 to 38 $\pm$ 5 mm Hg and increased the mean pulmonary artery pressure during exercise from 38 $\pm$ 5 mm Hg before almitrine to 49 $\pm$ 7 mm Hg after almitrine. In contrast, oxygen breathing did not change pulmonary artery pressure at rest, but reduced the amount of increase during exercise. Whereas almitrine resulted in no change in the right ventricular ejection fraction at rest or exercise, oxygen therapy improved the right ventricular ejection fraction at exercise. These results strongly suggest that almitrine is associated with undesirable and probably detrimental acute hemodynamic effects, despite enhanced arterial oxygenation. The same study suggested that the adverse effects of almitrine on pulmonary artery pressure persist with chronic therapy. Five patients received 50 mg almitrine bid for 103 to 168 days; there was a small but significant increase in the mean pulmonary artery pressure after treatment at both rest and exercise. Furthermore, five other patients did not tolerate chronic therapy and dropped out of this phase of the study. These patients all complained of dyspnea.

Thus, almitrine increases PaO_2 in hypoxic COPD patients during rest and exercise, but it may also be associated with worsening of pulmonary hypertension. The side effect of dyspnea experienced by some patients may be related to this adverse effect on the pulmonary circulation. Further studies on the acute and chronic effects of almitrine are necessary to elucidate fully the role of this drug in the management of COPD. Until the long-term consequences of almitrine on pulmonary hypertension have been defined, use of this medication cannot be advocated.

Phlebotomy

The use of phlebotomy in polycythemic patients with cor pulmonale remains controversial. Despite several investigations of this subject over the last two decades, there is no consensus regarding the indications, if any, for phlebotomy.

In the resting COPD patient, phlebotomy usually causes a decrease in the mean pulmonary artery pressure and pulmonary vascular resistance, no significant change in cardiac output, and a decrease in systemic oxygen transport.[148–150] Despite the decrease in systemic oxygen transport, resting oxygen consumption remained unchanged in most investigations.[149, 150] Segal and Bishop,[148] however, have reported finding a decrease of resting oxygen consumption after phlebotomy, whereas Rakita and coworkers[151] found an increase in oxygen consumption 1 hour after phlebotomy.

The effect of phlebotomy on hemodynamic events during exercise may be more important than the changes observed at rest. Researchers have found a significant improvement in exercise performance when markedly polycythemic patients were subjected to phlebotomy. Chetty and colleagues[150] have studied 15 patients with moderate to severe COPD and marked polycythemia (hematocrit higher than 55%). Phlebotomy was performed until the hematocrit fell below 52% and was at least 5 percentage points below the initial value. The mean workload, duration of exercise, and maximal oxygen consumption all increased significantly after phlebotomy. Weisse and associates conducted their experiments on 12 patients with stable cor pulmonale and hematocrit values about 55%. Patients were studied three times: at baseline (mean hematocrit, 61%); after initial phlebotomy (mean hematocrit, 50%); and after a second phlebotomy (mean hematocrit, 44%). After the first reduction of hematocrit there was an improvement in exercise performance, but no significant changes occurred with the further reduction in hematocrit to normal levels.

Overall, current evidence suggests that the reduction of markedly elevated hematocrit values to more moderate degrees of elevation (about 50%) produces clearly beneficial effects on circulatory hemodynamics, especially during exercise, but it is not clear that there are chronic benefits of repeated phlebotomy. Furthermore, the application of continuous oxygen therapy in appropriately selected patients should reduce the number of COPD patients who become severely polycythemic. Currently, it appears that phlebotomy should be reserved for use as an adjunctive therapy in the acute management of the markedly polycythemic patient who presents with an acute decompensation of cor pulmonale.

REFERENCES

1. Wiedemann HP, Matthay RA. Cor pulmonale in chronic obstructive pulmonary disease: Circulatory pathophysiology and new concepts of therapy. In: Simmons DH, ed. Current Pulmonology, Vol. 8. Chicago: Year Book Medical Publishers, 1987, 127–162.
2. Wiedemann HP, Matthay RA. The management of acute and chronic cor pulmonale. In: Scharf S, ed. Heart-Lung Interactions. New York: Marcel Dekker, 1989, 915–981.
3. Glauser FL, Fairman RP, Bechard D. The causes and evaluation of chronic hypercapnia. Chest 1987; 91:755–759.
4. Burrows B, Niden AH, Fletcher CM, et al. Clinical type of chronic obstructive lung disease in London and Chicago. Am Rev Respir Dis 1964; 90:14–27.
5. Howell JBL. Breathlessness in pulmonary disease. In: Howell JBL, Campbell EJM, eds. Breathlessness. Oxford: Blackwell Scientific Publications, 1966, 167.
6. Javaheri S, Blum J, Kazemi H. Pattern of breathing and carbon dioxide retention in chronic obstructive lung disease. Am J Med 1981; 71:228–234.
7. Lane DJ, Howell JBL, Giblin B. Relation between airway obstruction and CO_2 tension in chronic obstructive airway disease. Br Med J 1968; 3:707–709.
8. Roussos C. Ventilatory failure and respiratory muscles. In: Roussos C, Macklem PT, eds. The Thorax, Part B. New York: Marcel Dekker, 1985; 1253–1279.
9. Mountain R, Zwillich C, Weil J. Hypoventilation in obstructive disease; the role of familial factors. N Engl J Med 1978; 298:521–525.
10. Light RW, Mahutte CK, Brown SE. Etiology of carbon dioxide retention at rest and during exercise in chronic airflow obstruction. Chest 1988; 94:61–67.
11. Altose MD, McCauley WC, Kelsen SG, Cherniack NS. Effects of hypercapnia and inspiratory flow-resistive loading on respiratory activity in chronic airways obstruction. J Clin Invest 1977; 59:500–507.
12. Gelb AF, Klein E, Schiffman P, et al. Ventilatory response and drive in acute and chronic obstructive pulmonary disease. Am Rev Respir Dis 1977; 116:9–16.
13. Lane DJ, Howell JBL. Relationship between sensitivity to carbon dioxide and clinical features in patients with chronic airways obstruction. Thorax 1970, 25:150–159.
14. Lourenco RV, Miranda JM. Drive and performance of the ventilatory apparatus in chronic obstructive lung disease. N Engl J Med 1968; 279:53–59.
15. Burrows B, Saksena PB, Diener CF. Carbon dioxide tension and ventilatory mechanics in chronic obstructive lung disease. Ann Intern Med 1966; 65:685–700.
16. Sorli J, Grassino A, Lorange G, Milic-Emili J. Control of breathing in patients with chronic obstructive lung disease. Clin Sci Mol Med 1978; 54:295–304.
17. Parot S, Saunier C, Gautier H, et al. Breathing pattern and hypercapnia in patients with chronic obstructive pulmonary disease. Am Rev Respir Dis 1980; 121:985–991.
18. Aubier M, Muciano D, Fournier M, et al. Central respiratory drive in acute respiratory failure of patients with chronic obstructive pulmonary disease. Am Rev Respir Dis 1980; 122:191–199.
19. Skatrud JB, Dempsey JA, Bhansali P, Irvin C. Determinants of chronic carbon dioxide retention and its correction in humans. J Clin Invest 1980; 65:813–821.
20. Skatrud JB, Dempsey JA. Relative effectiveness of acetazolamide versus medroxyprogesterone acetate in correction of chronic carbon dioxide retention. Am Rev Respir Dis 1983; 127:405–412.
21. Tobin MJ, Chadha TS, Jenouri G, et al. Breathing patterns. 2. Diseased subjects. Chest 1983; 84:286–294.
22. Tobin MJ. Respiratory muscles in disease. Clin Chest Med 1988; 9:263–286.
23. Rochester DF, Braun NMT. Determinants of maximal inspiratory pressure in chronic obstructive pulmonary disease. Am Rev Respir Dis 1985; 132:42–47.
24. Oliven A, Kelsen SG, Deal EC, Cherniack NS. Mechanisms underlying CO_2 retention during flow-resistive loading in patients with COPD. J Clin Invest 1983; 71:1442–1449.
25. Bellemare F, Grassino A. Force reserve of the diaphragm in patients with chronic obstructive pulmonary disease. J Appl Physiol 1983; 55:8–15.
26. Bellemare F, Grassino A. Evaluation of human diaphragm fatigue. J Appl Physiol 1982; 53:1196–1206.
27. Tatsumi K, Kirura H, Kunitomo F, et al. Effect of chlormadinone acetate on ventilatory control in patients with chronic obstructive pulmonary disease. Am Rev Respir Dis 1986; 133:552–557.
28. Nadel J. The effects of carbonic anhydrase inhibitor "6063" on electrolytes and acid-base balance in two normal subjects and two patients with respiratory acidosis. J Clin Invest 1953; 32:622–629.
29. Galdston M. Respiratory and renal effects of a carbonic anhydrase inhibitor (Diamox) on acid-base balance in normal man and patients with respiratory acidosis. Am J Med 1955; 19:516–532.
30. Lakshminarayan S, Sahn SA, Weil JA. Effect of theophylline on ventilatory responses in normal man. Am Rev Respir Dis 1978; 117:33–38.
31. Sanders JS, Berman TM, Bartlett MM, Kronenberg RS. Increased hypoxic ventilatory drive due to administration of aminophylline in normal men. Chest 1980; 78:279–282.
32. Dowell AR, Heyman A, Siekev HD, Tripathy K. Effect of aminophylline on respiratory-center sensitivity in Cheynes-Stokes respiration and in pulmonary emphysema. N Engl J Med 1965; 273:1447–1453.
33. Levine S, Henson D, Levy S. Respiratory muscle rest therapy. Clin Chest Med 1988; 9:297–309.
34. Rochester DF, Martin LL. Respiratory muscle rest. In: Roussos C, Macklem PT, eds. The Thorax, Part B. New York: Marcel Dekker, 1985, 1303–1328.
35. Kerby GR, Mayer LS, Pingelton SK. Nocturnal positive pressure ventilation via nasal mask. Am Rev Respir Dis 1987; 135:738–740.
36. Jameson AG, Ferrer MI, Harvey RM. Some effects of mechanical respirators upon respiratory gas exchange and ventilation in chronic pulmonary emphysema. Am Rev Respir Dis 1959; 80:510–521.
37. Rochester D, Braun N, Laine S. Diaphragmatic energy expenditure in chronic respiratory failure; the effect of assisted ventilation with body respirators. Am J Med 1977; 63:223–232.
38. Marino W, Braun NMT. Reversal of the sequelae of respiratory muscle fatigue by intermittent mechanical ventilation (abstract). Am Rev Respir Dis 1982; 125(Part 2):85.
39. Braun NMT, Marino WD. Effect of daily intermittent rest of respiratory muscles in patients with severe chronic airflow limitation (CAL). Chest 1984; 85(Suppl):59S.
40. Cropp A, DiMarco AF. Effects of intermittent negative pressure ventilation on respiratory muscle function in patients with severe chronic obstructive pulmonary disease. Am Rev Respir Dis 1987; 135:1056–1061.
41. Gutierrez M, Beroiza MT, Contreras G, et al. Weekly cuirass ventilation improves blood gases in chronic airflow limitation (CAL) patients (abstract). Am Rev Respir Dis 1987; 135:A42.
42. Aubier M. Pharmacotherapy of respiratory muscles. Clin Chest Med 1988; 9:311–324.
43. Moxham J. Aminophylline and the respiratory muscles: An alternative view. Clin Chest Med 1988; 9:325–336.
44. Aubier M, Roussos C. Pharmacotherapy. In: Roussos C, Macklem PT, eds. The Thorax, Part B. New York: Marcel Dekker, 1985, 1373–1405.
45. Mahler DA, Matthay RA, Snyder PE, et al. Sustained-release theophylline reduces dyspnea in nonreversible obstructive airway disease. Am Rev Respir Dis 1985; 131:22–25.
46. Howell S, Roussos C. Isoproterenol and aminophylline improve contractility of fatigued canine diaphragm. Am Rev Respir Dis 1984; 129:118–124.
47. Viires N, Aubier M, Murciano D, et al. Effects of aminophylline on diaphragmatic fatigue during acute respiratory failure. Am Rev Respir Dis 1984; 129:396–402.
48. Aubier M, DeTroyer A, Sampson M, et al. Aminophylline improves diaphragmatic contractility. N Engl J Med 1981; 305:249–252.
49. Murciano D, Aubier M, Lecocguic Y, et al. Effects of theophylline on diaphragmatic strength and fatigue in patients with chronic obstructive pulmonary disease. N Engl J Med 1984; 311:349–353.
50. Murciano D, Aubier M, Auclair MH, et al. Effects of long-term aminophylline administration on dyspnea, arterial blood gases

and respiratory muscle performance in COPD patients (abstract). Am Rev Respir Dis 1986; 134:A150.
51. Kongragunta VR, Druz WS, Sharp JT. Dyspnea and diaphragm fatigue in patients with chronic obstructive pulmonary disease: Responses to theophylline. Am Rev Respir Dis 1988; 137:662–667.
52. Aubier M, Viires N, Murciano D, et al. Effects and mechanisms of action of terbutaline on diaphragmatic contractility and fatigue. J Appl Physiol 1984; 56:922–929.
53. Javaheri S, Smith JT, Thomas JP, et al. Albuterol has no effect on diaphragm fatigue in humans. Am Rev Respir Dis 1988; 137:197–201.
54. Stoller JK, Wiedemann HP, Loke J, et al. Terbutaline and diaphragm function in chronic obstructive pulmonary disease: A double-blind randomized clinical trial. Br J Dis Chest 1988; 82:242–250.
55. Aubier M, Murciano D, Viires N, et al. Effects of digoxin on diaphragm strength generation in patients with chronic obstructive pulmonary disease during acute respiratory failure. Am Rev Respir Dis 1987; 135:544–548.
56. Rochester DF. Body weight and respiratory muscle function in chronic obstructive pulmonary disease. Am Rev Respir Dis 1986; 134:646–648.
57. Askanazi J, Rosenbaum SH, Hyman AI, et al. Respiratory changes induced by the large glucose loads of total parenteral nutrition. JAMA 1980; 243:1444–1447.
58. Wilson DO, Rogers RM, Sanders MH, et al. Nutritional intervention in malnourished patients with emphysema. Am Rev Respir Dis 1986; 134:672–677.
59. Kelly SM, Rosa A, Field S, et al. Inspiratory muscle strength and body composition in patients receiving total parenteral nutrition therapy. Am Rev Respir Dis 1984; 130:33–37.
60. Brown SE, Nagendran RC, McHugh JW, et al. Effects of a large carbohydrate load on walking performance in chronic air-flow obstruction. Am Rev Respir Dis 1985; 132:960–962.
61. Brown SE, Wiener S, Brown BA, et al. Exercise performance following a carbohydrate load in chronic air-flow obstruction. J Appl Physiol 1985; 58:1340–1346.
62. Angelillo VA, Bedi S, Durfee D, et al. Effects of low and high carbohydrate feedings in ambulatory patients with chronic obstructive pulmonary disease and chronic hypercapnia. Ann Int Med 1985; 103:835–838.
63. Tirlapur VG, Mir MA. Effect of low calorie intake on abnormal pulmonary physiology in patients with chronic hypercapnic respiratory failure. Am J Med 1984; 77:987–994.
64. Aubier M, Murciano D, Lecocguic Y, et al. Effect of hypophosphatemia on diaphragmatic contractility in patients with acute respiratory failure. N Engl J Med 1985; 313:420–422.
65. Malloy DW, Dhingra S, Salven FS. Hypomagnesemia and respiratory muscle power. Am Rev Respir Dis 1984; 129:497–498.
66. McFadden ER Jr, Braunwald E. Cor pulmonale and pulmonary thromboembolism. In: Braunwald E, ed. Heart Disease: A Textbook of Cardiovascular Medicine. Philadelphia: W.B. Saunders, 1984; 1572–1598.
67. Fishman AP. Chronic cor pulmonale. Am Rev Respir Dis 1976; 114:775–794.
68. Matthay RA, Berger HJ. Cardiovascular function in cor pulmonale. Clin Chest Med 1983; 4:269–295.
69. Berger HJ, Matthay RA, Loke J, et al. Assessment of cardiac performance with quantitative radionuclide angiography: Right ventricular ejection fraction with reference to findings in chronic obstructive pulmonary disease. Am J Cardiol 1978; 41:897–905.
70. Matthay RA, Berger HJ, Davies RA, et al. Right and left ventricular exercise performance in chronic obstructive pulmonary disease: Radionuclide assessment. Ann Intern Med 1980; 93:234–239.
71. Reid LM. Structure and function in pulmonary hypertension: New perceptions. Chest 1986; 89:279–288.
72. Harris P, Segel N, Creen I, Housley E. The influence of the airways resistance and alveolar pressure on the pulmonary vascular resistance in chronic bronchitis. Cardiovasc Res 1968; 2:84–92.
73. Wright JL, Lawson L, Pare PD, et al. The structure and function of the pulmonary vasculature in mild chronic obstructive pulmonary disease: The effect of oxygen and exercise. Am Rev Respir Dis 1983; 128:702–707.
74. Mahler DA, Brent BN, Loke J, et al. Right ventricular performance and central circulatory hemodynamics during upright exercise in patients with chronic obstructive pulmonary disease. Am Rev Respir Dis 1984; 130:722–729.
75. Boushy JF, North LB. Hemodynamic changes in chronic obstructive pulmonary disease. Chest 1977; 72:565–570.
76. Schrijen F, Uffholtz H, Polu JM, Poincelot F. Pulmonary and systemic hemodynamic evaluation in chronic bronchitis. Am Rev Respir Dis 1978; 117:25–31.
77. Weitzenblum E, Loisceau A, Hirth C, et al. Course of pulmonary hemodynamics in patients with chronic obstructive pulmonary disease. Chest 1979; 75:656–662.
78. Weitzenblum E, Sautegeau A, Ehrhart M, et al. Long-term course of pulmonary arterial pressure in chronic obstructive pulmonary disease. Am Rev Respir Dis 1984; 130:993–998.
79. British Medical Research Council Working Party. Long-term domiciliary oxygen therapy in chronic hypoxic cor pulmonale complicating chronic bronchitis and emphysema. Lancet 1981; 1:681–685.
80. Kawakami Y, Kishi F, Yamamoto H, Miyamoto K. Relation of oxygen delivery, mixed venous oxygenation, and pulmonary hemodynamics to prognosis in chronic obstructive pulmonary disease. N Engl J Med 1983; 308:1045–1049.
81. Tockman MS, Permutt S, Kennedy T. Prognosis in chronic obstructive pulmonary disease (letter). N Engl J Med 1983; 308:992–993.
82. Burrows B, Kettel LJ, Niden AH, et al. Patterns of cardiovascular dysfunction in chronic obstructive lung disease. N Engl J Med 1972; 286:912–918.
83. Howard P. Drugs or oxygen for hypoxic cor pulmonale? Br Med J 1983; 287:1159–1160.
84. Finlay M, Middleton HC, Peake MD, Howard P. Cardiac output, pulmonary hypertension, hypoxemia and survival in patients with chronic obstructive airways disease. Eur J Respir Dis 1983; 64:252–263.
85. Tenney SM, Mithoefer JC. The relationship of mixed venous oxygenation to oxygen transport: With special reference to adaptations to high altitude and pulmonary disease. Am Rev Respir Dis 1982; 125:474–479.
86. Bergofsky EH. Tissue oxygen delivery and cor pulmonale in chronic obstructive pulmonary disease. N Engl J Med 1983; 308:1092–1094.
87. Brent BN, Matthay RA, Hahler DA, et al. Relationship between oxygen uptake and oxygen transport in stable patients with chronic obstructive pulmonary disease: Physiologic effects of nitroprusside and hydralazine. Am Rev Respir Dis 1984; 129:682–686.
88. Albert RK, Schrijen F, Poincelot F. Oxygen consumption and transport in stable patients with chronic obstructive pulmonary disease. Am Rev Respir Dis 1986; 134:678–682.
89. Finch CA, Lenfant C. Oxygen transport in man. N Engl J Med 1972; 286:407–415.
90. Chappell TR, Rubin LJ, Markham RV Jr, Firth BG. Independence of oxygen consumption and systemic oxygen transport in patients with either stable pulmonary hypertension or refractory left ventricular failure. Am Rev Respir Dis 1983; 128:30–33.
91. Matthay RA. Effects of theophylline on cardiovascular performance in chronic obstructive pulmonary disease. Chest 1985; 88(Suppl):112S–117S.
92. Parker JO, Kelkar K, West RO. Hemodynamic effects of aminophylline in cor pulmonale. Circulation 1966; 33:17–25.
93. Matthay RA, Berger HJ, Loke J, et al. Effects of aminophylline upon right and left ventricular performance in chronic obstructive pulmonary disease: Noninvasive assessment by radionuclide angiocardiography. Am J Med 1978; 65:903–910.
94. Matthay RA, Berger JH, Davies R, et al. Improvement in cardiac performance by oral long-acting theophylline in chronic obstructive pulmonary disease. Am Heart J 1982; 104:1022–1026.
95. Marcus ML, Skelton CL, Grauer LE, Epstein SE. Effects of theophylline on myocardial mechanics. Am J Physiol 1972; 222:1361–1365.
96. Rutherford JD, Vatner SE, Braunwald E. Effects and mechanisms of action of aminophylline on cardiac function and regional blood flow distribution in conscious dogs. Circulation 1981; 63:378–387.
97. Murphy GW, Schreiner BF, Yu PN. Effects of aminophylline on the pulmonary circulation and left ventricular performance in patients with valvular heart disease. Circulation 1968; 37:361–369.

98. Stein PA, Leu JD, Welch MH, Guenter CA. Pathology of the pulmonary circulation in emphysema associated with alpha-1-antitrypsin deficiency. Circulation 1971; 43:227–239.
99. Benumof JL, Trousdale FR. Aminophylline does not inhibit canine hypoxic pulmonary vasoconstriction. Am Rev Respir Dis 1982; 126:1017–1019.
100. Canny GJ, deSouza ME, Gilday DL, Newth CJL. Radionuclide assessment of cardiac performance in cystic fibrosis: Reproducibility and effect of theophylline on cardiac function. Am Rev Respir Dis 1984; 130:822–826.
101. Brent BN, Mohler D, Berger HJ, et al. Augmentation of right ventricular performance in chronic obstructive pulmonary disease by terbutaline: A combined radionuclide and hemodynamic study. Am J Cardiol 1982; 50:313–319.
102. Stockley RA, Finnegan P, Bishop JM. Effect of intravenous terbutaline on arterial blood gas tensions, ventilation, and pulmonary circulation in patients with chronic bronchitis and cor pulmonale. Thorax 1977; 32:601–605.
103. Teule GJJ, Majid PA. Hemodynamic effects of terbutaline in chronic obstructive airways disease. Thorax 1980; 35:536–542.
104. MacNee W, Wathen CG, Hannan WJ, et al. Effects of pirbuterol and sodium nitroprusside on pulmonary hemodynamics in hypoxic cor pulmonale. Br Med J 1983; 287:1169–1172.
105. Packer M. Vasodilator therapy for primary pulmonary hypertension. Ann Intern Med 1985; 103:258–270.
106. Berglund E, Widimsky J, Malmberg R. Lack of effect of digitalis in patients with pulmonary disease with and without heart failure. Am J Cardiol 1963; 11:477–482.
107. Green LH, Smith TW. The use of digitalis in patients with pulmonary disease. Ann Intern Med 1977; 87:459–465.
108. Jezek V, Schrijen F. Haemodynamic effect of deslanoside at rest and during exercise in patients with chronic bronchitis. Br Heart J 1973; 35:2–8.
109. Brown SE, Pakron FJ, Milne N, et al. Effects of digoxin on exercise capacity and right ventricular function during exercise in chronic airflow obstruction. Chest 1984; 85:187–191.
110. Mathus PN, Powles ACP, Pugsley SO, et al. Effect of digoxin on right ventricular function in severe chronic airflow obstruction. Ann Intern Med 1981; 95:283–288.
111. Mathur PN, Powles ACP, Pugsley SO, et al. Effect of long-term administration of digoxin on exercise performance in chronic airflow obstruction. Eur J Respir Dis 1985; 66:273–283.
112. Kim YS, Aviado DM. Digitalis and the pulmonary circulation. Am Heart J 1961; 62:680–686.
113. Sylvester JT, Goldberg HS, Permutt S. The role of the vasculature in the regulation of cardiac output. Clin Chest Med 1983; 4:111–126.
114. Keller CA, Shepard JW Jr, Chun DS, et al. Effects of hydralazine on hemodynamics, ventilation, and gas exchange in patients with chronic obstructive pulmonary disease and pulmonary hypertension. Am Rev Respir Dis 1984; 130:606–611.
115. Miller MJ, Chappell TR, Cook W, et al. Effects of oral hydralazine on gas exchange in patients with cor pulmonale. Am J Med 1983; 75:937–942.
116. Dal Nogare AR, Rubin LJ. The effects of hydralazine on exercise capacity in pulmonary hypertension secondary to chronic obstructive pulmonary disease. Am Rev Respir Dis 1986; 133:385–389.
117. Rubin LJ, Peter RH. Hemodynamics at rest and during exercise after oral hydralazine in patients with cor pulmonale. Am J Cardiol 1981; 47:116–122.
118. Brent BN, Berger HJ, Matthay RA, et al. Contrasting acute effects of vasodilators (nitroglycerin, nitroprusside, and hydralazine) on right ventricular performance in patients with chronic obstructive pulmonary disease and pulmonary hypertension: A combined radionuclide-hemodynamic study. Am J Cardiol 1983; 51:1682–1689.
119. Packer M, Greenberg B, Massie B, Dash H. Deleterious effects of hydralazine in patients with pulmonary hypertension. N Engl J Med 1982; 306:1326–1331.
120. Cerda E, Esteban A, de la Cal MA, et al. Hemodynamic effects of vasodilators on pulmonary hypertension in decompensated chronic obstructive pulmonary disease. Crit Care Med 1985; 13:221–223.
121. McGoon MD, Seward JB, Vlietstra RE, et al. Hemodynamic response to intravenous hydralazine in patients with pulmonary hypertension. Br Heart J 1983; 50:579–585.
122. Lupi-Herrera E, Seoane M, Verdejo J. Hemodynamic effect of hydralazine in advanced, stable chronic obstructive pulmonary disease with cor pulmonale: Immediate and short-term evaluation at rest and during exercise. Chest 1984; 85:156–163.
123. Lupi-Herrera E, Seoane M, Verdejo J, et al. Hemodynamic effect of hydralazine in interstitial lung disease patients with cor pulmonale: Immediate and short-term evaluation at rest and during exercise. Chest 1985; 87:564–573.
124. Tuxen DV, Powles ACP, Mathur PN, et al. Detrimental effects of hydralazine in patients with chronic air-flow obstruction and pulmonary hypertension: A combined hemodynamic and radionuclide study. Am Rev Respir Dis 1984; 129:388–395.
125. Pearl RG, Rosenthal MH, Schroeder JS, Ashton CPT. Acute hemodynamic effects of nitroglycerin in pulmonary hypertension. Ann Intern Med 1983; 99:9–13.
126. Simonneau G, Escourrou P, Duroux P, Lockhart A. Inhibition of hypoxic pulmonary vasoconstriction by nifedipine. N Engl J Med 1981; 304:1582–1585.
127. Sturani C, Bassein L, Schiavina M, Gunella G. Oral nifedipine in chronic cor pulmonale secondary to severe chronic obstructive pulmonary disease (COPD): Short- and long-term hemodynamic effects. Chest 1983; 84:135–142.
128. Melot C, Hallemans R, Naeije R, et al. Deleterious effect of nifedipine on pulmonary gas exchange in chronic obstructive pulmonary disease. Am Rev Respir Dis 1984; 130:612–616.
129. Muramoto A, Caldwell J, Albert RK, et al. Nifedipine dilates the pulmonary vasculature without producing symptomatic systemic hypotension in upright resting and exercising patients with pulmonary hypertension secondary to chronic obstructive pulmonary disease. Am Rev Respir Dis 1985; 132:963–966.
130. Kennedy TP, Michael JR, Huang CK, et al. Nifedipine inhibits hypoxic pulmonary vasoconstriction during rest and exercise in patients with chronic obstructive pulmonary disease. Am Rev Respir Dis 1984; 129:544–551.
131. Singh H, Ebejer MJ, Higgins DA, et al. Acute hemodynamic effects of nifedipine at rest and during maximal exercise in patients with chronic cor pulmonale. Thorax 1985; 40:910–914.
132. Rubin LJ, Moser K. Long-term effects of nitrendipine on hemodynamics and oxygen transport in patients with cor pulmonale. Chest 1986; 89:141–145.
133. Kastanos N, Miro RE, Agusti-Vidul A. Captopril in pulmonary hypertension. Br Heart J 1983; 49:512–514.
134. Burke CM, Harte M, Duncan J, et al. Captopril and domiciliary oxygen in chronic airflow obstruction. Br Med J 1985; 290:1251.
135. Zielinski J, Hawrylkiewicz I, Gorecka D, et al. Captopril effects on pulmonary and systemic hemodynamics in chronic cor pulmonale. Chest 1986; 96:562–565.
136. Naeije R, Melot C, Mols P, Hallemons R. Reduction in pulmonary hypertension by prostaglandin E_1 in decompensated chronic obstructive pulmonary disease. Am Rev Respir Dis 1982; 125:1–5.
137. Ishizaki T, Miyabo S, Mifune J, et al. OP-1206, a prostaglandin E_1 derivative: Effects of oral administration to patients with chronic lung disease. Chest 1984; 85:382–386.
138. Rubin LJ. Cardiovascular effects of vasodilator therapy for pulmonary arterial hypertension. Clin Chest Med 1983; 4:309–319.
139. Nocturnal Oxygen Therapy Trial Group. Continuous or nocturnal oxygen therapy in hypoxemic chronic obstructive lung disease. Ann Intern Med 1980; 93:391–398.
140. Flenley DC. Long-term home oxygen therapy. Chest 1985; 87:99–103.
141. Weitzenblum E, Sautegeau A, Ehrhart M, et al. Long-term oxygen therapy can reverse the progression of pulmonary hypertension in patients with chronic obstructive pulmonary disease. Am Rev Respir Dis 1985; 131:493–498.
142. Timms RM, Khaja FU, Williams GW. Hemodynamic responses to oxygen therapy in chronic obstructive pulmonary disease. Ann Intern Med 1985; 102:29–36.
143. Ashutosh K, Mead G, Dunsky M. Early effects of oxygen administration and prognosis in chronic obstructive pulmonary disease and cor pulmonale. Am Rev Respir Dis 1983; 127:399–404.
144. Timms RM, Kvale PA, Anthonisen MR, et al. Selection of patients with chronic obstructive pulmonary disease for long-term oxygen therapy. JAMA 1981; 245:2514–2515.
145. Levi-Valensi P, Weitzenblum E, Pedinielli JL, et al. Three-month follow-up of arterial blood gas determinations in candi-

dates for long-term oxygen therapy. Am Rev Respir Dis 1986; 133:547–551.
146. Bell RC, Mullins RC III, West LG, et al. The effect of almitrine bismesylate on hypoxemia in chronic obstructive pulmonary disease. Ann Intern Med 1986; 105:342–346.
147. MacNee W, Connaughton JJ, Rhind GB, et al. A comparison of the effects of almitrine or oxygen breathing on pulmonary arterial pressure and right ventricular ejection fraction in hypoxic chronic bronchitis and emphysema. Am Rev Respir Dis 1986; 134:559–565.
148. Segal N, Bishop JM. The circulation in patients with chronic bronchitis and emphysema at rest and during exercise, with special reference to the influence of changes in blood viscosity and blood volume on the pulmonary circulation. J Clin Invest 1966; 45:1555–1568.
149. Weisse AB, Moschos CB, Frank MJ, et al. Hemodynamic effects of staged hematocrit reduction in patients with stable cor pulmonale and severely elevated hematocrit levels. Am J Med 1975; 58:92–98.
150. Chetty KG, Brown SE, Light RW. Improved exercise tolerance of the polycythemic lung patient following phlebotomy, Am J Med 1983; 74:415–420.
151. Rakita L, Gillespie DG, Sancetta SM. The acute and chronic effects of phlebotomy on general hemodynamics and pulmonary functions of patients with secondary polycythemia associated with pulmonary emphysema. Am Heart J 1965; 70:466–475.

Chapter 45

ACUTE EXACERBATIONS IN COPD PATIENTS

Charles B. Sherman James P. Osmanski Leonard D. Hudson

The number of newly diagnosed cases of COPD has been increasing in the U.S.[1,2] As a result, the care of acute clinical worsening in COPD patients is a common problem and requires a working knowledge of the diagnosis and treatment of acute exacerbations. Generally, most exacerbations are relatively mild, requiring only outpatient care, but some are severe enough to result in respiratory failure and ICU intervention. Worsening of pulmonary function during an exacerbation may be caused by infections,[3] environmental triggers (e.g., humidity, pollution, primary or secondary smoke exposure, occupational irritants), cardiac dysfunction, or progression of the underlying disease. The first part of this chapter discusses the symptoms and signs of acute exacerbations. Next, a step-wise treatment plan for outpatient and inpatient management of mild exacerbations is presented. Finally, the remainder of the chapter focuses on the care of patients with severe exacerbations who require more aggressive and invasive therapy. The recommendations presented are meant only as guidelines, because the broad spectrum of underlying pathophysiology in patients with COPD[4] mandates an individual approach to treatment.

SYMPTOMS AND SIGNS

In the evaluation of patients with acute exacerbations, certain symptoms may suggest a responsible cause. Usually, however, most patients present with several symptoms, making exact causal identification difficult. Patients with an infectious trigger often complain of increased cough and excess sputum production. The sputum may be more voluminous and tenacious than at baseline and may change in color from white to yellow or green. At times, mobilization of excess phlegm is limited by ineffective cough and tracheal transport, obscuring this symptom. Exposure to environmental irritants can result in a nonproductive cough, chest tightness, or wheezing. In contrast, patients with natural progression of their underlying COPD or with left ventricular dysfunction usually present with worsening dyspnea. Shortness of breath, which may have been present only with exertion, may now occur at rest. Orthopnea and chest pain may accompany dyspnea in patients with left ventricular failure.

Clinical signs of an acute exacerbation are relatively nonspecific and might represent an exaggeration of signs normally found at baseline. The patient may be breathing with a more rapid respiratory rate and with shallow excursions. This pattern often makes conversing in full sentences impossible. With more severe exacerbations, the accessory muscles of respiration may be in use. Furthermore, muscle fatigue, as suggested by paradoxic abdominal breathing,[5] can be observed. Normally, the abdomen and chest wall both move outward during inhalation. With paradoxic abdominal breathing, the abdomen moves inward during inhalation as the chest moves outward. Respiratory alternans is a relatively unusual manifestation of respiratory muscle fatigue. It consists of periods of inspiratory muscle activity involving only chest wall muscles and alternating with periods of only diaphragmatic inspiratory muscle activity. Additionally, patients may purse their lips or grunt on exhalation, maneuvers that can lengthen expiratory time, increase lung volume, and prevent early airway collapse.[6] Fever is usually low grade but can be higher if pneumonia is present. New onset or worsening of cyanosis may be seen.

Central nervous system (CNS) signs are relatively common

during exacerbations and range from irritability to coma. Patients may present with disorientation, confusion, somnolence, combativeness, fine tremors, asterixis, myoclonic jerks, and seizures.[7] The level of consciousness correlates well with the cerebrospinal fluid pH, which in turn usually decreases proportionately to the blood pH.[8] CNS findings can precede clinical recognition of an acute worsening of COPD, because patients might not report a change in pulmonary complaints.

On chest auscultation, expiratory wheezes, diffuse rhonchi, or an absence of breath sounds can be heard; the last finding indicates more severe airflow obstruction. If left ventricular failure is present, bibasilar rales, jugular venous distention, an S_3 gallop, and peripheral edema may be appreciated. Heart sounds can be difficult to auscultate, however, given the presence of loud respiratory noises.

MANAGEMENT OF MILD ACUTE EXACERBATIONS

Overall Goals

As previously noted, patients with COPD vary in their underlying pathophysiology and in their response to treatment.[4] Furthermore, inherent weekly variations in airflow and symptoms have been documented.[9] Thus, heterogeneity among patients and varying baseline levels of airway resistance and symptoms force clinicians to take an individualized approach when managing a patient with an acute exacerbation.[10] Several common goals, however, can be defined and should be remembered as specific therapeutic options are considered: (1) decreasing airway resistance; (2) treating primary or secondary infections; (3) improving oxygen saturation; and (4) strengthening respiratory muscle function. Improving oxygenation is paramount but, in general, several of these principles must be addressed simultaneously. Interventions that allow these goals to be met are discussed here. Although the focus is on outpatient management of mild exacerbations, in-hospital management of more severe exacerbations not requiring intubation and mechanical ventilation is similar to that used in the outpatient setting, but with more intensive therapy.

Decreasing Airway Resistance

Increased airway resistance during acute exacerbations can lead to significant respiratory symptoms and gas exchange abnormalities. Most often, bronchoconstriction, airway inflammation, and increased mucous plugging are responsible. Appropriate therapy with β_2-adrenergic and anticholinergic agents, methylxanthines, corticosteroids, and chest physiotherapy are used to overcome these mechanisms.

BETA-2 ADRENERGIC AGENTS. Bronchodilators remain the mainstay of treating acute exacerbations of COPD[11] (Table 45–1). Of the several types of bronchodilators currently available, the β_2-adrenergic agonists are the most frequently prescribed. These agents act by binding to bronchial smooth muscle receptors and stimulating adenylcyclase, which results in the intracellular accumulation of cyclic AMP. In turn, cyclic AMP is responsible for smooth muscle relaxation and bronchodilation.[12] Parenteral, oral, and inhalational forms of these sympathomimetic agents are available. The inhalational route, however, is preferred in acute exacerbations because its use results in greater bronchodilation and fewer side effects at comparable doses.[13, 14]

The β_2-adrenergic agents can be inhaled through an updraft nebulizer or a metered-dose inhaler. The updraft nebulizer uses compressed air and a nebulizer to create an aerosol of the medication, which the patient breathes until the desired dose has been delivered (approximately 5 to 15 minutes). This technique requires minimal patient coordination and cooperation. Metaproterenol (Alupent) and albuterol (Proventil) are the two β_2 agonists that are available in premixed unit-dose vials for nebulizer use. Alternatively, a metered-dose inhaler can be used. A propellant carries the agent into the larger airways during a controlled inhalation. If proper technique is used, this system is as effective as the updraft nebulizer for patients with acute exacerbations.[15–17] Unfortunately, improper technique is often employed, which can significantly reduce the amount of medication the patient receives. To overcome this problem, spacer devices between the inhaler and the patient have been developed, which can aid in particle deposition within the larger airways.[18]

Several β_2-inhalational agents are currently marketed in the U.S. for the treatment of acute exacerbations. Historically, isoproterenol (Isuprel) was favored, but it has fallen into disuse because of its significant α-adrenergic and β_1-adrenergic side effects. Isoetharine (Bronkometer), a less selective but fast-acting agent (1–2 minutes), can be used early in an exacerbation. This agent is limited in its usefulness, however, by its short duration of action (1 to 3 hours), which makes frequent administration necessary. Metaproterenol (Alupent; Metaprel) is an ideal medication for acute exacerbations, because it has a fast onset time (2 to 5 minutes), few α-adrenergic and β_1-adrenergic side effects, and a longer duration of action (3 to 5 hours). Albuterol (Proventil) and terbutaline (Brethaire) have slightly slower onset times (5 to 10 minutes) and marginally longer durations of action (4 to 5 hours). Two recently released inhalers, pirbuterol (Maxair) and bitolterol (Tornalate) have longer half-lives (6 to 8 hours) and may be more selective. Further clinical experience is needed with the use of these agents.

Most clinicians advise their patients to use their metered-dose inhaler with a maximal frequency of two puffs every 2 to 4 hours and to use a spacer device to facilitate administration. Several authors have challenged this dosing interval, claiming that undermedication may result. Anthonisen has routinely encouraged patients to use their inhalers as often as two puffs every 15 to 30 minutes for a total of six puffs, if needed, for symptomatic relief.[9] Further studies are needed to determine appropriate drug administration guidelines.

Side effects may develop with use of all the β-adrenergic agents. Tachycardia, nervousness, tremor, and nausea are the most frequently reported adverse reactions. Some tolerance to these effects may occur with more prolonged use of the agents. A rare but possibly more serious complication of therapy has been described by Nino and colleagues.[19] The authors reported three patients with severe COPD who had "catecholamine myocarditis," documented by endomyocardial biopsy and thought by the authors to be caused by the use of β-adrenergic agonists and/or methylxanthines. Whether myocardial damage is caused by β-adrenergic agonists remains controversial.

ANTICHOLINERGIC AGENTS. Anticholinergic agents are another type of bronchodilator commonly used as part of the treatment armamentarium.[20–22] These drugs work by blocking the cholinergic receptors located in the larger airways, thereby causing bronchodilation. Atropine sulfate and glycopyrrolate have short durations of action (2 to 3 hours) and are available only in solution form. Their small molecular size allows for greater mucosal absorption and, as a result, they cause more systemic side effects. These adverse reactions include dry mouth, blurred vision, urinary retention, and tachycardia. Ipratropium bromide, available only as a metered-dose inhaler, is a quaternary ammonium compound with poor mucosal absorption. This property causes fewer systemic muscarinic side effects.[21] Two puffs or 36 μg of ipratropium achieves

TABLE 45–1. Characteristics of Selected β_2-Adrenergic Agonists and Anticholinergic Agents

AGENT	ROUTE OF ADMINISTRATION	DOSE	ONSET OF ACTION (min)	PEAK OF ACTION (min)	DURATION OF ACTION (hr)
β_2-Adrenergic Agonists					
Isoetharine	MDI*	340 μg/puff	1–2	5–20	1–3
	Nebulizer	5 mg	1–2	5–20	1–3
Metaproterenol	MDI	650 μg/puff	2–5	10–60	2–5
	Nebulizer	2.5 mg	3–5	10–60	3–5
	Oral	10–20 mg	10–20	15–60	3–4
Terbutaline	MDI	250 μg/puff	5–30	120	3–4
	Oral	2.5–5 mg	10–30	120–180	4–6
	Subcutaneous	0.25 mg	2–5	30–60	2–4
Albuteral	MDI	90 μg/puff	4–10	60–90	3–6
	Nebulizer	2.5 mg	5–10	60–120	4–6
	Oral	2–4 mg	10–30	120–180	4–6
Anticholinergic agents					
Atropine	Inhaled	0.8 mg	15–20	120–240	5–6
Ipratropium	MDI	18–20 μg/puff	10–15	90–120	4–6

(Modified with permission from Theodore AC, Beer DG. Clin Chest Med 1986; 7:657–671.)
*MDI, metered-dose inhaler.

maximal bronchodilation in 1.5 to 2 hours and lasts for 4 to 6 hours.[23] None of these anticholinergic agents has been clinically shown to cause drying of the airways or to precipitate inspissation of secretions.[24]

In patients with stable COPD, 40 μg of ipratropium have been shown to be as effective as 200 μg (two puffs) of salbutamol[25] or 400 μg (two puffs) of fenoterol hydrobromide, two sympathomimetic agents used in Europe.[26] At these doses an additive effect has been observed.[26] Easton and associates, however, have found that when higher doses of salbutamol (600 μg, or six puffs) or ipratropium (120 μg, or six puffs) were studied, both agents were equipotent and no additive effect was noted.[27] Similar results were found by Gross and Skorodin in patients with emphysema.[28] Anthonisen has concluded from these data that the sympathomimetic and anticholinergic agents are comparable in their bronchodilatory properties, but that patients given therapeutic doses of β-agonist rarely benefit from the addition of an anticholinergic agent.[9]

These findings in stable COPD patients may be generalized to patients with acute exacerbations of their disease. Rebuck and coworkers have compared the effects of nebulized solutions of 0.5 mg of ipratropium bromide, 1.25 mg of fenoterol hydrobromide, and 0.5 mg of ipratropium bromide plus 1.25 mg of fenoterol hydrobromide in a double-blind study of 199 patients with acute airway obstruction (148 patients with asthma and 51 patients with severe COPD)[29]. In patients with COPD (mean FEV_1 0.7 ± 0.29 L), all three regimens resulted in statistically improved spirometric function at 45 and 90 minutes, but no further benefit was achieved with combination therapy. Statistically significant spirometric differences of less than 167 ml could not be detected by the study and might account for the lack of demonstrable additive effect. In asthmatics, by contrast, the largest improvements in FEV_1 were found in those patients with severe obstruction (baseline FEV_1 values below 1 L) who were treated with a combination of ipratropium and fenoterol.

In summary, β-agonist and anticholinergic agents appear to be equally effective in the initial treatment of acute COPD exacerbations. In patients with severe COPD and baseline hypoxemia, however, the anticholinergic agents have a theoretic advantage. Gross and Bankwala[30] have compared the effect on gas exchange of atropine methonitrate (a quaternary form of atropine) and metaproterenol hydrochloride in 12 patients with chronic bronchitis and emphysema. They found no statistically significant decrease in Po_2 with atropine for as long as 60 minutes after inhalation but noted a mean decrease in Po_2 of 5.0 ± 2.5 mm Hg with metaproterenol (Fig. 45–1). Thus, use of anticholinergic agents may carry less risk of inducing hypoxemia than β agonists in selective patients with COPD.

CROMOLYN SODIUM. Cromolyn sodium (Intal) is a bronchodilator whose mechanism of action appears to be stabilization of mast cells, which prevents the release of bronchoconstricting mediators.[31] The drug is effective in the prophylactic treatment of patients with exercise-induced and allergen-triggered asthma[32] but has no role in the acute treatment of patients with COPD exacerbations.

METHYLXANTHINES. Parenteral and oral methylxanthine agents (e.g., theophylline, aminophylline) have been effectively used to treat exacerbations of asthma since the 1930s.[33–37]

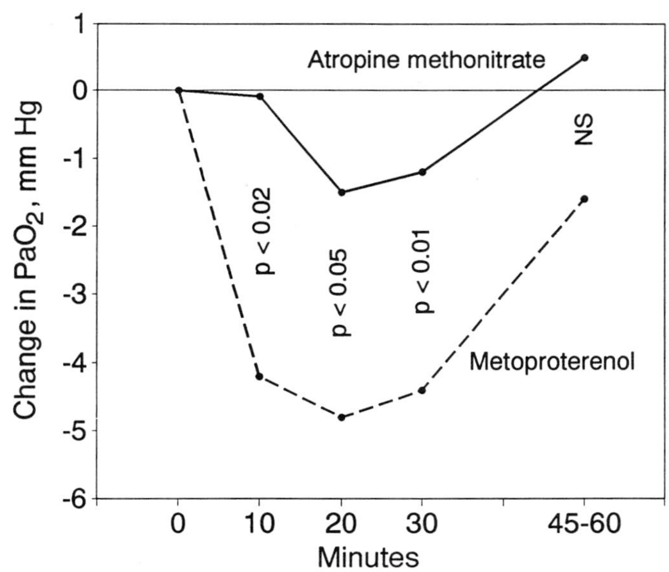

Figure 45–1. Changes in arterial oxygen pressure (Pa_{O_2}) following inhaled atropine or metaproterenol. Mean changes in Pa_{O_2} from prebronchodilator levels for each drug in 12 patients with COPD. Data at 45 or 60 minutes (eight patients) were pooled, p values between lines are the significances of the difference between the two agents (paired t test), NS = not significant. The intrasubject variability of Pa_{O_2}, at baseline (last determinations) was 1.1 mm Hg (SD). Asterisk indicates significantly different from baseline at $P < 0.01$, paired t tests; the difference from baseline was not significant unless indicated. (Modified from Gross NJ, Bankwala Z. Am Rev Respir Dis 1987; 136:1091–1094.)

Their exact mechanism of action is still unknown, but it is probably mediated through cyclic AMP.[38] Beneficial effects of the methylxanthines have been documented in patients with both asthma and COPD. These include bronchodilation,[39] improved contractility of respiratory muscles,[40–43] better mucociliary clearance,[44] enhanced right and left ventricular performance,[45] and more vigorous ventilatory response to hypoxia.[46] The level of benefit achieved with these agents is dose-related;[39] bronchodilation results in most patients at a serum level of 5 μg/ml.[47] There is no uniform relationship, however, between dose and serum blood level of theophylline because many factors affect metabolism, including age, smoking status, circulatory and hepatic function, and individual patient variation.[48] Significant side effects can be seen when serum blood levels increase above 20 μg/ml, including tachycardia, cardiac dysrhythmias,[49] convulsions, and even death.[50]

The role of the methylxanthines in treating patients with stable COPD or those with exacerbations of their disease remains controversial. Few studies of the methylxanthines have been performed in COPD patients and those that have been done usually included a small number of subjects and only evaluated single-dose therapy. In a study of ten patients with "irreversible" airflow obstruction off all sympathomimetic agents, Eaton and colleagues found greater improvement in spirometric function with high-dose theophylline (peak serum level, 17 to 22 μg/ml) than with low-dose theophylline (peak serum level, 9 to 12.5 μg/ml) or placebo.[39] Subjective relief of dyspnea was no different among both treatment regimens and placebo. Thus, a dose-response relationship with respect to ventilatory improvement was documented but subjective relief, the clinical end point, was not demonstrated. Filuk and associates[51] have studied the benefit of adding parenteral theophylline to large doses of inhaled salbutamol (800 μg or eight puffs) in patients with stable COPD. Salbutamol produced more bronchodilation than theophylline alone but a small additive effect was found when both agents were used. Whether the additional bronchodilation observed has any clinical relevance and justifies the increased risk of side effects is debatable. Again, comparable studies in patients with exacerbations are needed.

CORTICOSTEROIDS. The efficacy of corticosteroid use in both stable and unstable asthmatics has been well documented.[52–61] Studies of steroid responsiveness in patients with stable COPD have been less conclusive.[62–70] Little information is available about the use of corticosteroids in those with acute exacerbations of COPD.[71–73] The mechanisms of action, clinical usefulness in patients with acute exacerbations, appropriate routes of administration, and adverse effects are reviewed here.

The exact mechanisms of action of corticosteroids in obstructive airway disease are poorly understood. They appear to work by reducing airway inflammation and edema while also inhibiting the breakdown of epinephrine by catechol *o*-methyltransferase, thereby potentiating the bronchodilatory effect of the catecholamines.[52, 56]

Two studies have addressed the clinical usefulness of corticosteroids in the treatment of acute exacerbations of COPD. Emerman and coworkers have carried out a randomized, double-blind, placebo trial in 96 COPD patients treated in the emergency room for acute exacerbations.[71] All patients received standard bronchodilator therapy with β_2 agonists and theophylline. In addition, 52 patients were given 100 mg of intravenous methylprednisolone on admission. Both treatment groups were comparable with respect to age, theophylline level, white blood cell count, baseline spirometry, bronchodilator responsiveness, and arterial blood gas analysis. At the end of the 4-hour treatment period, patients treated with methylprednisolone had FEV_1 and functional vital capacity (FVC) values similar to those of the control subjects. Also, hospitalization rates were comparable in both groups. In patients treated with methylprednisolone, elevated eosinophils and increased bronchial responsiveness did not predict responsiveness to steroids.

In contrast, Albert and colleagues found significant improvement in airflow with corticosteroids in patients with chronic bronchitis admitted to the hospital with acute respiratory failure.[72] Forty-four patients were enrolled in the double-blind placebo controlled study, in which 22 patients received intravenous methylprednisolon, 0.5 mg/kg, every 6 hours over the 72-hour study period. All patients also received parenteral aminophylline, inhaled isoproterenol, supplemental oxygen, antibiotics, and chest physiotherapy. Spirometry was performed every 6 hours. Use of intravenous corticosteroids was associated with a significantly greater increase in prebronchodilator FEV_1 at 18 hours and thereafter and in postbronchodilator FEV_1 at 12 hours and thereafter throughout the 72-hour study period when compared to those in the placebo group (Fig. 45–2). Patient selection and length of follow-up may explain the discrepancies in the results of these two studies.[73] However, one possible interpretation of the results is that corticosteroids have little effect on pulmonary function in the first 4 hours after intravenous administration to COPD patients with acute exacerbations but have a significant effect by 12 to 24 hours.

If used, corticosteroids should be administered either orally or parenterally, depending on the severity of exacerbation. Additionally, they should be used early in the treatment course, because their effect is not apparent for several hours.[55, 59, 71] The only dosing regimen appropriately studied with positive results has been that of Albert and associates,[72] who

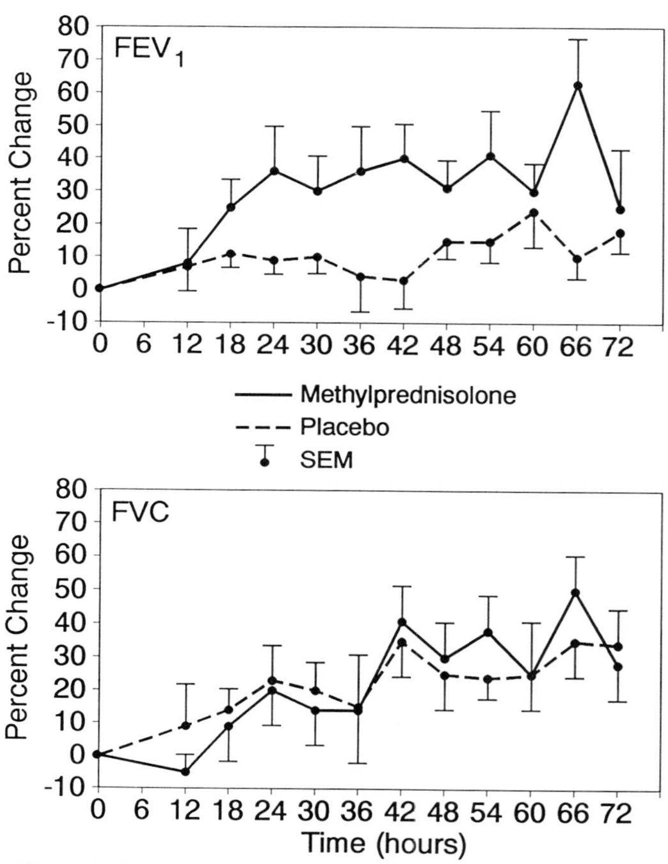

Figure 45–2. Improvement in airflow following methylprednisolone administration. FEV_1 = forced expiratory volume in 1 second; FVC = forced vital capacity. Patients receiving methylprednisolone had a greater improvement in airflow than did those receiving placebo. (Modified from Albert RK, et al. Ann Intern Med 1980; 92:753–758.)

administered methylprednisolone, 0.5 mg/kg, intravenously every 6 hours. Patients who show a rapid response to therapy with parenteral steroids can be switched to oral prednisone on the third or fourth day of treatment, followed by a 10- to 14-day tapering course. Albert's study was performed in hospitalized patients with severe exacerbations. It seems reasonable in less severely ill outpatients to use oral prednisone initially in a dose of 40 to 60 mg or more, with a taper over 1 to 2 weeks after initial clinical improvement has occurred, but no study has evaluated this regimen for this particular condition.

The most common side effects of both short-term and chronic corticosteroid administration are presented in Table 45–2. A short course of steroids (14 days) may result in few adverse effects, but chronic use may be associated with a 40% adverse reaction rate.[74, 75]

REMOVING EXCESS SECRETIONS. Coughing is the most effective way of clearing secretions from the tracheobronchial tree. Coughing is necessary to move secretions from the periphery of the lungs to the central airways and to expel these secretions from the central airways. Patients with airflow obstruction have impaired cough and must be taught or encouraged to cough properly. Patients should be in an upright position when coughing and instructed to take deep breaths and cough vigorously.

Even in patients with an effective cough, inspissated secretions or excessive viscous phlegm may be difficult to clear from the tracheobronchial airways. This difficulty in clearance can lead to increased airway resistance and worsening of ventilation-perfusion mismatch, and may prolong the reduction in pulmonary function seen during an acute exacerbation. Thus, thinning and mobilization of secretions constitute an important part of any treatment plan.

Increasing hydration may be all that is necessary to overcome mucous plugging in the airways, but little data are available to support this intervention.[76] Patients without heart or renal disease should probably be advised to increase their oral intake. There is little value, however, in forcing vigorous fluid intake in an already hydrated patient.[77] No objective data support the use of inhaled moisture, but patients have sometimes reported anecdotally that this intervention aids in raising secretions. Aerosolized mucolytic agents such as *N*-acetyl-L-cysteine (Mucomyst) can theoretically change the composition of mucus and thereby allow more expectoration. Clinically, however, these agents have not been shown to be effective and may, in fact, cause bronchospasm.[11] Improved mucociliary clearance may help in secretion mobilization. Both theophylline[44] and the β_2-adrenergic agents[78] have been shown to improve mucociliary function. Whether this is of clinical importance in patients with severe COPD is not known.

Chest physiotherapy may be helpful in improving secretion mobilization in patients who cannot cough effectively and expectorate excessive secretions. However, studies investigating the efficacy of chest percussion have either failed to show objective evidence of improved secretion clearance when controlled for cough[79–82] or have indicated only a mild improvement.[83, 84] Excess secretions can be removed through a series of maneuvers, including chest percussion and postural drainage. These can be carried out in the hospital by a trained respiratory therapist or in the home by educated family members. Chest physiotherapy is not without risks. Increased hypoxemia during chest percussion or postural drainage may occur;[84, 85] this is primarily related to the positioning of the patient.[85]

TABLE 15–2. Side Effects of Corticosteroid Administration

Short-term, high-dose corticosteroids	
	Hypokalemic alkalosis
	Diabetes mellitus
	Hyperosmolar nonketotic coma
	Hypertension
	Sodium and water retention
	Mood disorders
	Cerebral edema
	Proximal myopathy
	Glaucoma
	Pancreatitis
	Peptic ulceration and gastrointestinal hemorrhage
Long-term glucocorticoids	
	Osteoporosis
	Aseptic necrosis of bone
	Pseudotumor cerebri
	Mood disorders
	Seizure disorders
	Posterior subcapsular cataracts
	Hyperlipidemia
	Increased prevalence of gallstones (?)
	Centripetal obesity
	Growth failure
	Secondary ammenorrhea
	Suppression of hypothalamic-pituitary-adrenal axis
	Impaired wound healing
	Suppression of immune response

(Reproduced with permission from Skorodin MS. Am J Med 1986; 82:8–15.)

Treating Primary or Secondary Infections

Infections may be the most frequent cause of acute exacerbations in patients with COPD, although available data are inconclusive. The most common organisms implicated are *Streptococcus pneumoniae, Hemophilus influenzae, Mycoplasma pneumoniae,* and viruses such as influenza and adenovirus.[86] *Branhamella catarrhalis,* an anaerobic gram-negative diplococci, has been shown to be a pathogen capable of causing sinusitis, otitis media, laryngitis, meningitis, and endocarditis.[87] Additionally, *B. catarrhalis* has been isolated from both the sputum and transtracheal aspirates of COPD patients with stable disease, acute exacerbations, and pneumonia.[88–91]

Methods used to determine the presence of infection during an exacerbation include history and physical examination, white blood cell count, sputum Gram's staining and culture, and chest roentgenogram. Sputum for Gram's staining and culture must be of good quality to be clinically useful. Fewer than 25 squamous cells /high-powered field (100× magnification) are required to ensure that oral contamination is not responsible for the findings. Even then, most experts question the reliability of basing therapy on the results of the sputum Gram's staining test in COPD patients with acute bronchitis and without evidence of pneumonia. For example, Patterson has recommended that for patients without pneumonia, Gram's staining be done only if purulent sputum persists after starting empiric antibiotics.[92]

It is generally agreed that patients with exacerbations resulting from pneumonia require appropriate antibiotic therapy. Controversy exists, however, over whether patients with an exacerbation not caused by an obvious infectious source benefit from antibiotic therapy.[93–95] In 1975, Tager and Speizer[93] reviewed well-designed controlled studies that evaluated the short-term use of antibiotics in patients with exacerbations of chronic bronchitis. They concluded that little benefit from the use of antibiotics could be demonstrated.

In contrast, Anthonisen and colleagues,[94] in a more recent study, concluded that antibiotics lead to a quicker resolution of symptoms and a more rapid return of ventilatory function. In a double-blind placebo-controlled trial, 173 patients with 362 exacerbations were studied over a 3½-year period. Patients complaining of dyspnea, sputum purulence, and/or an increase in sputum production were treated with a 10-day course either of placebo or amoxicillin, doxycycline, or trimethoprim-sulfamethoxazole. Resolution of symptoms occurred in 68% of patients given an antibiotic, but in only 55% of patients receiving placebo. Similarly, peak flow rates improved more rapidly in patients treated with antibiotics. Deterioration of symptoms requiring hospitalization or further intervention was found twice as commonly in placebo-treated patients (19%) as compared to those treated with antibiotics. Furthermore, patients with all three symptoms (i.e., increased dyspnea, sputum volume, and sputum purulence) showed the most improvement with antibiotic therapy (Fig. 45–3).

Patient selection and differences in the definition of exacerbation and in the antibiotics used may explain the discordance in conclusions reached from these two patient populations. Also, Anthonisen and coworkers[94] found only modest differences between treatment groups, suggesting that previous negative studies with much smaller study populations may have suffered from a beta (type II) error.

Once the decision to treat with antibiotics has been made, the choice of antibiotic should be based on clinical findings, physician familiarity with the medication, and experience with previous infections in the same patient. A broad-spectrum antibiotic such as amoxicillin, doxycycline, erythromycin, and trimethoprim-sulfamethoxazole used in a 7- to 10-day course remains the recommended therapy. Parenteral antibiotics should be reserved for more seriously ill patients. Worsening of the clinical status should prompt the physician to re-evaluate the patient's therapy. For example, patients with *Branhamella catarralis* do not respond to ampicillin because of the organism's ability to produce β-lactamase,[89, 90] and purulent sputum may persist. Only after switching to a β-lactamase-resistant agent (e.g., erythromycin) or to a β-lactam antibiotic with a β-lactamase inhibitor (e.g., amoxicillin-clavulanate potassium) can resolution of symptoms occur.

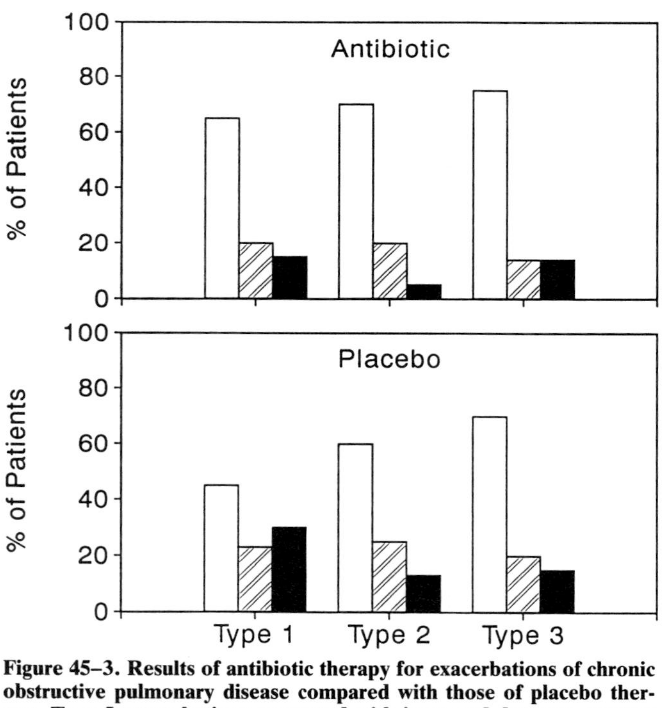

Figure 45–3. Results of antibiotic therapy for exacerbations of chronic obstructive pulmonary disease compared with those of placebo therapy. Type I exacerbations presented with increased dyspnea, sputum volume and sputum purulence, type II with two of those symptoms, and type III with one of those symptoms, as well as others such as coughing, wheezing, and signs of previous upper respiratory tract infections. White bars represent positive response to therapy, striped bars no response, and black bars deterioration. (Reproduced by permission from Anthonisen NR. Can Med Assoc J 1988; 138:503–510.)

Improving Oxygen Saturation

Hypoxemia (Pa_{O_2} < 55 mm Hg) may exist in some COPD patients presenting with clinical worsening of their disease; this often necessitates hospitalization. In most outpatients, however, hypoxemia is not detected and supplemental oxygen is not needed.

Signs and symptoms of hypoxemia resulting in hypoxia are nonspecific. They include hemodynamic changes such as increased blood pressure and tachyarrhythmias, alteration in mental status, and dyspnea.[96] Although pulse oximetry can be used to determine if oxygen desaturation is present, only arterial blood gas analysis can determine the exact degree of hypoxemia. The cause of a low P_{O_2} is usually multifactorial—hypoventilation, ventilation-perfusion mismatch, shunt, and physiologic dead space may contribute by varying degrees.

Regardless of the etiology, significant hypoxemia must be quickly treated with supplemental oxygen. The goal of correcting hypoxemia is to achieve a Pa_{O_2} of at least 55 mm Hg, which usually corresponds to an oxygen saturation of 87%. This saturation of hemoglobin ensures adequate oxygen delivery to tissue if the cardiac output is not compromised. In most COPD patients with hypoxemia there is little concern about precipitating respiratory acidosis and failure with supplemental oxygen.[97, 98] In a minority of patients, however, high concentrations of supplemental O_2 may worsen ventilation-perfusion mismatching and lead to significant hypoventilation.[99] Despite this risk hypoxemia must be corrected in these patients, usually with 1 to 2 L/minute of oxygen delivered through a nasal cannula.

Several delivery modes are available to achieve adequate oxygen saturation in patients with mild hypoxemia. Low-flow supplemental oxygen through a nasal cannula is well tolerated and does not have to be removed for eating, coughing, or expectorating excess phlegm. Supplemental oxygen with a fraction of inspired oxygen (FI_{O_2}) of 0.25 to 0.40 can be delivered. Another method of administering O_2 is with the Venturi mask. This device allows the administration of a set percentage of oxygen—24% to 40%—regardless of the patient's respiratory rate or oxygen flow setting. With both these systems, arterial blood gases or pulse oximetery must be monitored after initial settings to document adequate saturation and to make appropriate adjustments, if necessary.

Amelioration of hypoxemia by supplemental oxygen is only a supportive and temporizing measure. A more permanent improvement in oxygenation requires definitive treatment of the underlying exacerbation. Often, patients discharged from the hospital no longer need supplemental oxygen or require its use only for a short period of time on an outpatient basis.

Improving Respiratory Muscle Function

Respiratory muscle weakness and fatigue may develop during an acute exacerbation. Heightened airway resistance can cause an increased workload against which the respiratory muscles must contract with each breath. This acute strain can further compromise the already altered force-generating ability of the respiratory muscles. In a minority of severely impaired patients, respiratory muscle dysfunction may actually be the cause of the observed rapid deterioration in lung function.[100]

Few noninvasive therapies are available to improve respiratory muscle fatigue during an exacerbation. Specific metabolic causes of generalized muscle weakness that could affect respiratory muscle strength should be looked for and, if found, treated. These include hypokalemia, hypocalcemia, hypomagnesemia, and hypophosphatemia.[101–104] In several animal and human studies aminophylline has been shown to increase respiratory muscle contractility in a dose-related manner.[40–43] Murciano and associates, in a randomized trial, have found that theophylline improved respiratory function and dyspnea in 60 patients with severe COPD, probably by enhancing respiratory muscle function.[43] Again, the mechanism of action of theophylline is unknown but may result from the drug's direct effect on muscle, either through increasing intracellular calcium flux or by altering cyclic AMP within the cells. Support for the former mechanism is found in the observation that calcium channel blockers eliminate the effect of aminophylline on the diaphragm.[42] Furthermore, Aubier and coworkers showed that digoxin improved the contractile strength of the diaphragm in eight patients with severe COPD requiring mechanical ventilation.[105] They postulated that the inotropic action of digoxin on the diaphragm is similar to its action on the heart and is mediated by changes in intracellular calcium. Further evaluation is required, however, before widespread clinical use of aminophylline and digoxin can be recommended for respiratory muscle fatigue.

Stepwise Treatment Plan

The paucity of existing data does not permit formulation of a precise, stepwise treatment plan. Patients presenting with hypoxemia must be treated with supplemental oxygen until their gas exchange has improved. Also, patients with evidence of respiratory muscle fatigue must be evaluated for metabolic abnormalities, because correcting existing deficits can improve muscle function. During an exacerbation, sputum mobilization should be encouraged through cough and chest physiotherapy.

Medication type and amount should be matched to the severity of the exacerbation. In addition, the regular therapeutic regimen of the patient must be considered. During mild exacerbations, therapy should begin with the initiation or increase in dose of a β agonist delivered by a metered-dose inhaler using a spacer device. If the β agonist is ineffective, ipratropium bromide can be used in its place at a comparable dose, two puffs every 2 to 4 hours. Alternatively, if the patient improves on the β agonist alone but develops intolerable side effects, a lower dose of the β agonist can be supplemented with a lower dose of an anticholinergic agent (e.g., two puffs every 4 to 6 hours). A nebulized solution of these medications should be reserved for patients who cannot perform the appropriate inhalation maneuver because of eye-hand discoordination or respiratory distress.

For patients on maximal inhaled medication, with persistence of symptoms and airflow obstruction, corticosteroids should be administered (as previously discussed). Additionally, theophylline can be added to the regimen of patients not previously on the drug or can be increased in dose for patients at therapeutic levels. Intravenous administration of theophylline is not always necessary because, even with more significant exacerbations, orally delivered doses can achieve the same level of bronchodilation.[106]

MANAGEMENT OF EXACERBATIONS RESULTING IN ACUTE RESPIRATORY FAILURE

Acute respiratory failure is defined by a level of hypoxemia of relatively sudden onset that is a potential threat to life. The processes leading to this state are the same as described previously but the result is more serious clinically. Therefore, some differences in management often are indicated, including admission to hospital. This section reviews the presentation of acute respiratory failure in patients with COPD and discusses the management of such patients, emphasizing aspects of treatment that might differ from those in COPD patients with milder exacerbations.

Diagnosis

The COPD patient with acute respiratory failure often presents with symptoms or signs directly related to the respiratory system as emphasized previously. However, they might also present with signs or symptoms resulting from the effects of hypoxia and/or acidosis on the cardiovascular or central nervous system. Other nonpulmonary illnesses can stress the diseased pulmonary respiratory system—for example, by increasing CO_2 production. Therefore, the possibility of acute respiratory failure must be entertained in a patient with COPD who has any acute illness.

Cardiovascular symptoms and signs usually reflect the body's attempt to compensate for hypoxemia (e.g., by increasing heart rate in an attempt to increase oxygen delivery). They may also include arrhythmias that result from hypoxia or acidosis. Central nervous system symptoms are common, ranging from irritability to coma and including disorientation, confusion, somnolence, combativeness, fine tremors, asterixis, myoclonic jerks, and seizures.[7] The level of consciousness correlates well with the cerebrospinal fluid pH, which in turn usually decreases proportionately to the blood pH in respiratory acidosis.[8] It is important to consider acute respiratory failure when these findings occur, because the COPD patient may not report a change in pulmonary complaints.

Respiratory muscle fatigue can contribute significantly to the development of acute respiratory failure in COPD patients.[107] As previously discussed, clinical findings include rapid shallow respirations, paradoxic abdominal breathing, and respiratory alternans.[108] One series demonstrated that patients with paradoxic abdominal breathing were more apt to develop acute respiratory failure than patients without evidence of muscle fatigue, were more likely to fail on controlled oxygen therapy and need intubation and mechanical ventilation, and also had a higher mortality during acute respiratory failure.[109]

Once acute respiratory failure is suspected on the basis of these symptoms or signs, the diagnosis should be confirmed by arterial blood gas analysis. To qualify as having acute respiratory failure, a significant reduction in the PaO_2 from the patient's usual baseline and/or a rise in $PaCO_2$ with an accompanying acidosis must be present. The concept of defining acute respiratory failure as a functional disturbance of physiologic mechanisms rather than as a specific level of PaO_2 or $PaCO_2$ is particularly relevant for COPD patients because of their varying baseline values. Although the exact levels of abnormalities that qualify for acute respiratory failure are arbitrary, usual values include a PaO_2 of 55 mm Hg or lower and/or a $PaCO_2$ of 50 mm Hg or higher, with an accompanying respiratory acidosis. These values should be modified for individual patients. For example, a PaO_2 of lower than 50 mm Hg along with clinical worsening might be required for a patient whose usual PaO_2 is between 55 and 60 mm Hg.

Principles of Management

Once acute respiratory failure has been diagnosed in the COPD patient, certain principles of management can be applied. These encompass the same goals as management of the outpatient with a milder acute exacerbation, but the priorities are different in the patient with acute respiratory failure. These principles can be summarized as follows: (1) achieve adequate oxygenation; (2) begin to correct the acid-base abnormality, if present; (3) maintain an adequate cardiac output; (4) treat the underlying disease process; and (5) avoid complications.

These principles can be prioritized according to the most life-threatening abnormalities. In practice, several of these principles are addressed almost simultaneously. Because hypoxemia is usually the most life-threatening problem,[9] it should be dealt with immediately by administration of supplemental oxygen. The urgency of correcting respiratory acidosis depends on its severity and the time course over which it developed. Often, the management of this aspect is the same as treatment of the underlying disease process.

One goal of therapy in acute respiratory failure is maintenance of oxygen delivery to the tissues. It is important, therefore, to consider the adequacy of cardiac output, because this is an important determinant of tissue oxygen delivery. This may not require treatment in a COPD patient with acute respiratory failure, but adequacy of cardiac output and tissue oxygen delivery should always be assessed, and improvement of tissue oxygen delivery may be a critical aspect of management.

Other than achieving adequate oxygenation, treatment of the underlying disease process is probably the most important aspect of management. The other measures only provide supportive care and are temporizing. Definitive management depends on treatment of the processes that resulted in the physiologic abnormalities. This requires two separate diagnostic considerations in the patient with COPD. Obviously, the first is recognizing the chronic airflow obstruction as the underlying chronic disease process. The second, and equally important, is diagnosis of the acute precipitating illness. The precipitating etiology is not always obvious, but taking a careful history and performing a complete physical examination are important so that a treatable condition is not overlooked. Management of the underlying disease process in patients with acute respiratory failure is similar to that in patients with milder exacerbations (already described), although the same therapeutic measures may be intensified.

Measures to Correct Oxygenation

In addition to establishing that acute respiratory failure is present and diagnosing the disease(s) responsible for acute respiratory failure, the clinician should also evaluate which physiologic abnormalities have resulted in the hypoxemia. In the patient with COPD these might include hypoventilation, ventilation-perfusion mismatch, and shunt. The COPD patient usually presents with a combination of hypoventilation and ventilation-perfusion mismatch. Hypoventilation can be determined on the initial arterial blood gas by the presence of CO_2 retention. Whether hypoventilation explains all the hypoxemia can be determined by application of the alveolar air equation. If hypoxemia is not entirely explained by hypoventilation, the clinician should estimate whether the additional hypoxemia is primarily a result of ventilation-perfusion mismatch or intrapulmonary shunting. Diagnostic information on the underlying precipitating disease, including the history and chest roentgenogram interpretation, is useful in making this distinction. If shunting is present, usually there is an alveolar filling process or alveolar collapse, which results in an infiltrate on the chest roentgenogram caused by airless lung (lung that is filled with edema or purulent secretions, or is collapsed). Thus, if the history suggests pneumonia and the chest roentgenogram reveals evidence of this process, the possibility of intrapulmonary shunting should be suspected. In this case the clinician might choose a relatively higher FIO_2 for initial oxygen management. Conversely, if the history suggests exacerbation of bronchitis as the precipitating illness and the chest roentgenogram reveals no alveolar filling infiltrate, a ventilation-perfusion mismatch is most likely and only a small increase in the FIO_2 is indicated for initial management.

The goal of measures to correct the oxygenation abnormality are the same as previously described—essentially, to increase the arterial oxygen saturation and thus the arterial oxygen content. If possible, this should be accomplished while avoiding the risk of oxygen toxicity. Achieving a PaO_2 of 60 mm Hg or higher provides adequate arterial oxygen saturation. In the COPD patient with acute respiratory failure, this can usually be accomplished with a relatively small increase in the FIO_2 because hypoventilation and ventilation-perfusion mismatch are the predominant pathophysiologic abnormalities. Rarely is it necessary to use an FIO_2 in a range that could lead to parenchymal oxygen toxicity. Potential oxygen toxicity in the COPD patient involves worsening hypoventilation and respiratory acidosis. This was formerly assumed to be secondary to removal of the hypoxic drive to breathe in a patient with an already diminished CO_2 ventilatory drive. However, this mechanism has recently been questioned, and it has been suggested that the administration of oxygen may result in changes in ventilation and perfusion that cause the resultant increased $PaCO_2$.[99]

Whatever the mechanism, an increase in PaO_2 by oxygen administration can be associated with worsening respiratory acidosis in a minority of patients.[97] There are several relevant aspects of this phenomenon. First, this occurs only in a minority of COPD patients with acute respiratory failure and is usually associated with a PaO_2 that is considerably higher than that required for nearly complete oxygen saturation of hemoglobin. Second, the primary objective in the COPD patient with acute respiratory failure is still to oxygenate the arterial blood adequately; the potential risk of increasing $PaCO_2$ does not justify allowing the patient to remain significantly hypoxemic. Third, a significant improvement in oxygenation without a clinically important reduction in pH can be achieved in almost all patients by careful administration of oxygen and close monitoring, together with other forms of therapy aimed at the underlying disease process.[97, 98, 110–113]

Adequate oxygen saturation of hemoglobin can usually be achieved by the administration of 1 to 2 L/minute of oxygen by nasal prongs.[110, 111, 113] The flow rate is then adjusted according to the resulting arterial blood gas levels. Another method of administration is with a Venturi mask.[97, 112, 113] The Venturi mask allows the administration of a set percentage of oxygen, usually 24% or 28%. However, on an individual basis, the exact percentage of oxygen that is necessary to improve the PaO_2 is not clear. Therefore, nasal prongs represent an acceptable way of delivering oxygen to these patients. If the nasal passages are open, the oxygen delivered to the nasopharynx is entrained when the patient breathes through the mouth, so nasal oxygen is still effective even in mouth breathers. We prefer using nasal prongs for two reasons. First, they are usually better tolerated by the patient and are removed less often. Second, they do not have to be removed to cough out secretions or to eat or drink. On the other hand, some authors prefer to use a Venturi mask in the early stages of treatment of the COPD patient with acute respiratory failure. Occasionally, a COPD patient has pulmonary edema or severe pneumonia as a cause of the hypoxemia, so intrapulmonary shunting is the predominant pathophysiologic mechanism. These patients require a further increase in the FIO_2. This can usually be achieved by oxygen administered through a face mask, although occasionally endotracheal intubation might be required to allow delivery of a higher FIO_2.

Bone and coworkers have found an increased risk of an increase in the $PaCO_2$ with controlled O_2 therapy if hypoxemia is severe (PaO_2 < 40 mm Hg) and acidemia (pH < 7.35) is also present.[112] Warren and colleagues failed to confirm that severe hypoxemia is a significant predictor and found that severe acidemia is the best prognostic factor.[113] They also found that a pH < 7.26 is associated with a significant increase in mortality.

Correction of hypoxemia by supplemental oxygen is only a supportive and temporizing measure. A permanent improvement in oxygenation without continuation of supplemental oxygen requires definitive therapy of the underlying disease process.

Measures to Correct Respiratory Acidosis

The urgency for correction of the acidosis and the type of therapy indicated depend on the degree of acidosis, the time over which the acidosis has developed (often correlating with the degree of acidosis and whether partial compensation has taken place), and the specific cause of the respiratory acidosis. Often no specific therapy is required, other than aggressive treatment aimed at the underlying disease process to improve airflow obstruction. If the initial acidosis does not present a threat to life or does not interfere with other treatment, such as effective bronchodilation, specific treatment is usually not indicated. Even when the acidosis is life-threatening, it does not have to be totally corrected to normal immediately.

Administration of bicarbonate partially compensates for the respiratory acidosis.[114, 115] If the acidosis is severe and an acute threat to life, bicarbonate administration can provide rapid improvement. It has the additional benefit of allowing other medications that have been administered, such as bronchodilators, to work in a more optimal pH range. The major drawback of bicarbonate administration is that when the underlying cause of the respiratory acidosis has been corrected, the increased bicarbonate level can lead to metabolic alkalosis. Also, bicarbonate administration results in more CO_2 production. Therefore, bicarbonate administration is generally reserved for severe abnormalities (usually, pH lower than 7.2) and even then relatively small amounts are given as a temporizing measure.[114, 115]

Mechanical ventilation usually corrects the respiratory acidosis rapidly. The risk-to-benefit ratio must be carefully considered, however, because mechanical ventilation involves more detrimental effects in the COPD patient than in patients with other types of acute respiratory failure. Generally most COPD patients with acute respiratory failure can be managed without mechanical ventilation, but occasionally mechanical ventilation can be lifesaving. Indications for using mechanical ventilation in the COPD patient are discussed subsequently.

The use of respiratory stimulants to correct respiratory acidosis in COPD patients is controversial.[116, 117] Doxapram has been studied in clinical trials, with patients receiving doxapram having less of an increase in the $Pa{CO_2}$ during oxygen therapy.[118, 119] Despite this apparent benefit, however, in the best-controlled study there was no difference in the incidence of patients being intubated and mechanically ventilated between the treatment and control groups.[119]

Treatment of the Acute Precipitating Illness

A discussion of the specific treatment of the many possible acute illnesses that could tip the balance in the COPD patient and result in acute respiratory failure is beyond the scope of this chapter. The most common precipitating event underlying acute respiratory failure in the COPD patient is acute bronchitis (or exacerbation of chronic bronchitis). Other illnesses to be considered include pneumonia, congestive heart failure, pulmonary embolism, and oversedation. Considerations for the use of antibiotics in the treatment of acute bronchitis are the same as those described for outpatients with acute exacerbations. We recommend treatment with antibiotics when the acute bronchitis is severe enough to precipitate acute respiratory failure. This is based on the consideration that the risk of antibiotic therapy is relatively low and is more than balanced by the possibility of missing the occasional bacterial infection that might respond to antibiotics.

Treatment of the Chronic Disease Process

Measures aimed at treatment of COPD are similar to those reviewed previously for patients with milder exacerbations, but are applied more intensively. Only aspects that may differ are covered here. The frequency of inhaled bronchodilator administration should be adjusted to its effect in the individual patient. It may be necessary to repeat the inhalation every 2 hours if the therapeutic response is short-lived. The dosage recommendations for theophylline based on studies in relatively healthy subjects do not apply to acutely ill patients, especially those with COPD and pneumonia.[120] Therefore, the recommended loading and maintenance doses should be considered only as a reasonable starting point and should be adjusted according to known clinical factors that affect theophylline levels, to measured theophylline levels once therapy has been initiated, or to clinical response. Because of individual variability, in the patient with acute respiratory failure it is recommended that theophylline therapy be directed by measurement of serum theophylline concentrations. The desired goals of therapy are blood levels in the range of 10 to 20 μg/ml. This range is chosen because a therapeutic effect is usually present with 10 μg/ml; above 20 μg/ml the incidence of toxicity markedly increases and becomes prohibitive.

Corticosteroids are indicated for the COPD patient with acute respiratory failure and acute bronchitis as the precipitating illness. A controlled study of COPD patients with acute respiratory failure caused by exacerbation by acute bronchitis, comparing corticosteroids to placebo (previously discussed in greater detail), demonstrated significant improvement in airflow obstruction at any time over the 3 days that the corticosteroids were administered.[72] No adverse effects were recognized when those in the treatment group were compared to patients receiving placebo. Corticosteroids were administered as methylprednisolone sodium succinate, 0.5 mg/kg body weight, intravenously every 6 hours for 3 days. Because the effect of corticosteroids is not apparent for a few hours,[71] and peak effect takes 9 to 12 hours, they should be administered at the time of admission. Their use should be considered in patients who have precipitating illnesses other than acute bronchitis, with the possible risks weighed against the potential benefits.

Secretion removal is an important aspect of treatment of the COPD patient with acute respiratory failure. Most COPD patients have increased airway secretions when in acute respiratory failure. The principles and methods of secretion removal in patients with acute respiratory failure are the same as previously described for patients with milder exacerbations, including inhalation of heated moisture following inhalation of a bronchodilator aerosol, chest percussion, postural drainage, and encouraging the patient to cough. Unfortunately, it has not been well established which of these measures are effective. Therefore, at present the approach to this aspect of management is empiric.

Because the patient with airflow obstruction severe enough to result in acute respiratory failure has an impairment of the cough mechanism, it is reasonable to try chest physiotherapy to enhance the clearance of secretions from the peripheral to the more central airways. Chest percussion and postural drainage also should be given a therapeutic trial, and the results of these maneuvers plus coughing compared to coughing alone. There is a possibility of increased hypoxemia during the chest percussion or postural drainage treatment.[84, 85] This appears to be primarily related to the positioning of the patient.[85]

If the patient has pneumonia it can be reliably predicted that oxygenation worsens when the affected side is in the dependent position. (It is often recommended that chest percussion and postural drainage treatment be carried out on the opposite side of the initial treatment to remove any secretions that may have drained into the lung that is not involved with pneumonia.) This is a result of the adverse ventilation-perfusion matching with blood flow, which is gravity-dependent, increasing to the area of pneumonia and thus increasing shunt.

Even in the patient without pneumonia or with bilateral infiltrates, however, oxygenation can worsen in one lateral decubitus position or the other, but this cannot be reliably predicted.[85] It is prudent, therefore, to monitor the patient for desaturation with a pulse oximeter or to increase the oxygen flow during treatment, being careful to return it to its usual flow rate once the treatment has been completed. One study found that the risk of oxygen desaturation was inversely related to the amount of sputum produced during the treatment.[84] Patients who produced moderate to large amounts of mucopurulent secretions had no decrease in Pa_{O_2}, whereas those who produced little or no sputum had a significant reduction in Pa_{O_2}. It was concluded that the use of chest percussion and postural drainage in patients without sputum production is not indicated and potentially dangerous. Accordingly, if there is no evidence of efficacy after two treatments, chest physical therapy should be discontinued.

Coughing is the most effective way of clearing secretions from the tracheal bronchial tree. It is difficult to cough effectively when lying supine. The patient should be put in an upright sitting position and encouraged to take a deep breath and cough vigorously. This encouragement on a regular basis is one of the most important aspects of the early management of these patients. If the patient cannot cough, nasal tracheal suctioning should be carried out. The frequency of suctioning or encouraging coughing should be decided according to individual needs.

Treatment of Respiratory Muscle Fatigue

It is particularly important in patients with acute respiratory failure to seek specific metabolic causes of generalized muscle weakness that could affect respiratory muscle strength, including hypophosphatemia, hypokalemia, and hypomagnesemia. As previously discussed, the clinical importance of the use of theophylline and digoxin has not yet been established. The role of muscle training during acute respiratory failure is controversial. It is not clear whether a training effect on respiratory muscles can be achieved during acute respiratory failure, or which mode of training should be used. In fact, there is some evidence that total rest of the respiratory muscles is helpful and allows recovery from fatigue.[121] The mode of mechanical ventilation has also been debated. Some believe that intermittent mandatory ventilation is self-defeating when respiratory muscle fatigue is present and favor controlled mechanical ventilation, because active work throughout inspiration has been demonstrated with some patients in the assist-control mode.[123] A preliminary study of inspiratory muscle resistive training for short periods, with muscle resting by mechanical ventilation between the training periods, has shown promise in aiding the weaning process from mechanical ventilation.[124] More clinical studies are necessary to allow firm recommendations on both mechanical ventilatory modes and weaning and training techniques.

Mechanical Ventilation

Most COPD patients in acute respiratory failure can be managed without mechanical ventilation and, whenever clinically possible, management without mechanical ventilation is preferable. Endotracheal intubation further impairs the COPD patient's cough mechanism by preventing closure of the glottis. Also, COPD patients are at particular risk for complications of mechanical ventilation, including the possibility of pneumothorax,[125] air trapping with so-called auto-PEEP (positive end-expiratory pressure) or intrinsic PEEP developing, and subsequent hemodynamic compromise from impaired venous return,[126, 127] and development of nosocomial infections.[125, 128] Despite these risks, there are situations in which endotracheal intubation with mechanical ventilatory support is lifesaving.

The decision to ventilate the patient mechanically is primarily a clinical one.[129] The major determinant is the patient's mental status. If the patient is obtunded or cannot cooperate with other types of respiratory therapy, endotracheal intubation and mechanical ventilation are usually necessary. Worsening respiratory acidosis is usually the cause of the obtundation, but the abnormal mental status is the limiting clinical factor. No absolute value of pH can be selected as a criterion for mechanical ventilation. Even with fairly severe respiratory acidosis, if the patient is awake and alert aggressive respiratory therapy without mechanical ventilatory support should be tried initially.

The decision to withhold mechanical ventilatory support is complex.[130] Factors affecting this decision in the COPD patient include the quality of the patient's life when stable (from the patient's point of view) and whether potentially reversible elements are present during the acute bout of respiratory failure. The patient's views or wishes should be ascertained when the patient is clinically stable, prior to an episode of acute respiratory failure. This discussion between patient and physician is useful, even when no definite decision can be reached. Often the patient may wish to leave part of the decision up to the physician during the acute episode, wishing to be ventilated if a probable reversible element is present but receiving no ventilatory support if no such reversible element can be identified. The physician's role is mainly to provide information so that the patient can make an informed decision. If this subject has not been previously discussed with the patient, the patient's family may have to be a surrogate in the decision-making process. It is wise for the patient, while in a clinically stable state, to give power of attorney to a trusted friend or relative who can be involved in making decisions during the bout of acute respiratory failure.

Specific techniques of mechanical ventilation are beyond our discussion here, but a few aspects of mechanical ventilation pertinent to the COPD patient are important to mention. An initial tidal volume (V_T) of approximately 10 ml/kg body weight or lower is a reasonable starting point. It is rare for the COPD patient to require a larger V_T than this. The goal of ventilatory support is to return the pH toward normal, not to return the Pa_{CO_2} to normal. If a compensated respiratory acidosis was present prior to the acute further increase in the Pa_{CO_2}, returning the Pa_{CO_2} to "normal" could result in a significant metabolic alkalosis with serious clinical consequences, including arrhythmias and seizures.[131, 132] The inspiratory flow rate is of particular importance in the COPD patient. Formerly, it was popular to use a slow inspiratory flow rate, with the desired goal being a more uniform distribution of the inhaled gas. By prolonging inspiratory time, however, this has the adverse effect of shortening the expiratory time for any given respiratory rate. Because airflow obstruction is more severe on exhalation in the COPD patient, any manipulation that prolongs expiratory time, allowing more complete air emptying, is beneficial. Slow as opposed to fast inspiratory flow rates in the COPD patient are associated with a lower Pa_{O_2} and a higher V_D/V_T (ratio of physiologic dead space to tidal volume), and both these factors are related to shortening of expiratory time.[133] Therefore, a relatively fast inspiratory flow rate should be used in the COPD patient.

Any COPD patient receiving mechanical ventilation should be checked specifically for the development of auto-PEEP or intrinsic PEEP. Auto-PEEP, a positive alveolar pressure at the end of exhalation, results from incomplete emptying of the mechanically delivered breath, with subsequent air trapping.[126, 127] In COPD patients with high lung compliance, the alveolar pressure is more readily transmitted to the pleural space, resulting in impairment of venous return to the right heart. Although the possibility of air trapping during mechanical ventilation has been known for some time, this phenomenon often went unrecognized until a simple method for measuring the level of end-expiratory alveolar pressure was described.[126] Auto-PEEP is a frequent accompaniment of mechanical ventilation, especially in COPD patients.[134] Factors other than COPD that are associated with an increased incidence of auto-PEEP include age over 60 years, high minute ventilation (> 20 L/minute), and small endotracheal tube size.[134, 135] The best means of preventing auto-PEEP clearly is to attack the airflow obstruction itself. Any manipulation of mechanical ventilation that allows a longer expiratory emptying time is also helpful and should be considered. A rapid inspiratory flow has already been mentioned.[133, 136] Using a low compressible volume circuit is recommended.[136] Also, intermittent mandatory ventilation should be considered when auto-PEEP is recognized, because the lower mechanical ventilation rate minimizes air trapping, and any air trapping that does occur can often be dissipated during the spontaneous breaths.[126]

Tension pneumothorax should be considered in the COPD patient on mechanical ventilation who suddenly deteriorates. Pneumothorax appears to be particularly prevalent in patients with underlying necrotizing pulmonary infections.[125] The physician should alert all medical personnel to this possibility so that rapid treatment can be carried out if tension pneumothorax does develop.

If a COPD patient with acute respiratory failure is mechanically ventilated, particular attention must be paid to sitting patients up, getting them out of bed into a chair and, if possible, even having them walk. These aspects of care are often overlooked once mechanical ventilatory support has been started and the patient is kept in a supine position. This is potentially harmful, because the sitting position and physical activity bring important physiologic and psychologic benefits, including improved ventilation-perfusion matching, enhanced removal of secretions, and continued use of muscles, with maintenance of muscle strength.

Avoiding Complications

Development of complications during the course of acute respiratory failure often has a major effect on outcome. Many of these complications can be anticipated and prevented or identified early by appropriate monitoring to allow more effective treatment. The complications related to mechanical ventilation have already been mentioned. In such a case, prevention is achieved by avoiding this form of treatment unless it is clearly necessary. Complications in COPD patients with acute respiratory failure have been reviewed in detail elsewhere.[137] These include nosocomial pneumonia, pulmonary emboli, gastrointestinal bleeding, and arrhythmias. Administration of sucralfate has been shown to reduce the risk of nosocomial pneumonia as well as to prevent stress ulceration, and gastrointestinal bleeding.[138, 139]

Nutrition

The proper role of nutrition in the management of the acute respiratory failure patient with COPD is controversial. Clinical judgment of the risks and benefits must be used since few controlled clinical studies have been done. Clearly, specific nutritional deficiencies such as hypophosphatemia should be considered and treated, if present.[101, 102] Other considerations include the demonstration of blunted ventilatory drives in normal subjects with acute protein-calorie starvation[140] and the lower incidence of gastrointestinal bleeding with enteral feeding.[141] Factors favoring early feeding of the COPD patient with acute respiratory failure include the fact that the patient with COPD often has a chronic element of malnutrition and a high incidence of respiratory muscle fatigue and weakness. The potential of aspiration can be reduced by the use of small-bore flexible feeding tubes.[142] Feeding can increase ventilatory requirements by increasing CO_2 production.[143] This can be a problem, particularly in the weaning phase of mechanical ventilatory supports. It can be minimized, however, by manipulation of the carbohydrate and protein content (higher carbohydrate content is associated with an increase in respiratory quotient value and increased CO_2 production) or, more practically, by reducing the total caloric dose.[144] In the ventilated patient, increasing the ventilatory support compensates for this potential problem until the patient can be weaned from mechanical ventilation. As a general rule, the COPD patient should be encouraged to eat as soon as practically feasible. If a patient requires mechanical ventilatory support for longer than 1 day, internal feeding through a small-bore nasogastric or nasojejunal feeding tube should be started.

Patient Monitoring

COPD patients with acute respiratory failure should be treated initially in an intensive care unit, at least for the first day. This facilitates delivery of care, particularly aggressive respiratory therapy, and allows proper monitoring. Most aspects of therapy that have been mentioned include potential complications that can be monitored by careful and continuous observation. Monitoring should be individualized for each patient. Initial monitoring should include pulse oximetry, ECG, observation of mental status, and measurement of intake, output, and daily weight. Pulmonary artery catheterization should only be performed for specific indications and is usually not needed in most patients.

REFERENCES

1. Feinlieb M, Rosenberg HM, Collins JG, et al. Trends in COPD morbidity and mortality in the United States. Am Rev Respir Dis 1989; 140(Suppl):9–18.
2. Higgins M. Epidemiology of COPD. Chest 1984; 85(Suppl):35–85.
3. Burk RH, George RB. Acute respiratory failure in chronic obstructive pulmonary disease. Arch Intern Med 1973; 132:865–868. 1973.
4. Burrows B, Bloom JW, Traver GA, Cline MG. The course and prognosis of different forms of chronic airways obstruction in a sample from the general population. N Engl J Med 1987; 317:1309–1314.
5. Gilbert R, Ashutosh K, Anchincloss JH. Clinical value of observation of chest and abdominal motion in patients with pulmonary emphysema. Am Rev Respir Dis 1978; 119:155–158.
6. Loudon RG. The lung exam. Clin Chest Med 1987; 8:265–272.
7. Kilburn KH. Neurologic manifestations of respiratory failure. Arch Intern Med 1965; 115:155–160.
8. Posner JB, Plum F. Spinal-fluid pH and neurologic symptoms in systemic acidosis. N Engl J Med 1967; 277:605–606.
9. Anthonisen NR. Chronic obstructive pulmonary disease. Can Med Assoc J 1988; 138:503–510.
10. Guyatt GH. Additional comments on chronic obstructive pulmonary disease. Can Med Assoc J 1988; 138:503–510.

11. Snider GL. Control of bronchospasm in patients with chronic obstructive pulmonary diseases. Chest 1978; 73:927–935.
12. West JW. Update on drug therapy for your COPD patient. J Respir Dis 1985; 9:44–58.
13. Larsson S, Svedmyr N. Bronchodilating effect and side effects of β_2-adrenoceptor stimulants by different modes of administration. Am Rev Respir Dis 1977; 116:861–869.
14. Williams S, Seaton A. Intravenous or inhaled salbutamol in severe acute asthma? Thorax 1977; 32:555–558.
15. Jasper AC, Mohsenifar Z, Kahan S, et al. Cost-benefit comparison of aerosol bronchodilator delivery methods in hospitalized patients. Chest 1987; 91:614–618.
16. Turner JR, Corkery KJ, Eckman D, et al. Equivalence of continuous flow nebulizer and metered-dose inhaler with reservoir bag for treatment of acute airflow obstruction. Chest 1987; 93:476–481.
17. Gervais A, Begin P. Bronchodilation with a metered-dose inhaler plus an extension, using tidal breathing vs. jet nebulization. Chest 1987; 92:822–824.
18. Godden DJ, Crompton GK. An objective assessment of the tube spacer in patients unable to use a conventional pressurized aerosol effectively. Br J Dis Chest 1981; 75:165–168.
19. Nino AF, Berman MM, Gluck EH, et al. Drug-induced left ventricular failure in patients with pulmonary disease. Chest 1987; 92:732–736.
20. Gross NJ. Ipratropium bromide. N Engl J Med 1988; 319:486–492.
21. Pakes GE, Brofden RN, Heel RC, et al. Ipratropium bromide: A review of its pharmacological properties and therapeutic efficacy in asthma and chronic bronchitis. Drugs 1980; 20:237–266.
22. Gross NJ, Skorodin MS. Anticholinergic antimuscarinic bronchodilators. Am Rev Respir Dis 1984; 129:856–870.
23. Chapman KR. Anticholinergics: New uses in respiratory diseases. J Respir Dis 1985; 3:113–121.
24. Sackner MA, Chapman GA, Dougherty RD. Effects of nebulized ipratropium bromide and atropine sulfate on tracheal mucous velocity and lung mechanics in anesthetized dogs. Respiration 1977; 34:181–185.
25. Poppins H, Salorinne Y. Comparative trial of a new anticholinergic bronchodilator, Sch 1000, and salbutamol in chronic bronchitis. Br Med J 1973; 4:134–136.
26. Hughs JA, Tobin MJ, Bellamy D, et al. Effects of ipratropium bromide and fenoterol aerosols in pulmonary emphysema. Thorax 1982; 37:667–670.
27. Easton PA, Jadue C, Dhingra S, et al. A comparison of the bronchodilating effects of a beta–2-adrenergic agent (albuterol) and an anticholinergic agent (ipratropium bromide), given by aerosol alone or in sequence. N Engl J Med 1973; 315:735–739.
28. Gross NJ, Skorodin MS. Role of the parasympathetic system in airway obstruction due to emphysema. N Engl J Med 1984; 311:421–425.
29. Rebuck AS, Chapman KR, Abboud R, et al. Nebulized anticholinergic and sympathomimetic treatment of asthma and chronic obstructive airways disease in the emergency room. Am J Med 1987; 82:59–64.
30. Gross NJ, Bankwala Z. Effects of an anticholinergic bronchodilator on arterial blood gases of hypoxemic patients with chronic obstructive pulmonary disease. Am Rev Respir Dis 1987; 136:1091–1094.
31. Falliers CJ, Tinkelman DG. Alternative drug therapy in asthma. Clin Chest Med 1986; 7:383–391.
32. Bernstein IL. Cromolyn sodium. Chest 1985; 87(Suppl):68–73.
33. Jenne JW, Wyze E, Rood FS, MacDonald FM. Pharmacokinetics of theophylline application to adjustment of the clinical dose of aminophylline. Clin Pharmacol Ther 1972; 13:349–360.
34. Piafsky KM, Ogilvie RI. Dosage of theophylline in bronchial asthma. N Engl J Med 1975; 292:1218–1222.
35. Pierson WE, Bierman CW, Stamm SJ, VanArsdel PP. Double-blind trial of aminophylline in status asthmaticus. Pediatrics 1971; 48:642–646.
36. Weinberger MM, Bronsky EA. Evaluation of oral bronchodilator therapy in asthmatic children. J Pediatr 1974; 84:421–427.
37. McFadden ER. Introduction: Methylxanthine therapy and reversible airway obstruction. Am J Med 1985; 79(Suppl):1.
38. Sutherland EW, Robison CA, Butcher RW. Some aspects of the biological role of adenosine 3′,5′-monophosphate (cyclic AMP). Circulation 1968; 37:279–306.
39. Eaton ML, Green BA, Church TR, et al. Efficacy of theophylline in "irreversible" airflow obstruction. Ann Intern Med 1980; 92:758–761.
40. Sigrist S, Thomas D, Howell S, Roussos C. The effect of aminophylline on inspiratory muscle contractility. Am Rev Respir Dis 1982; 126:46–50.
41. Aubier M, DeTroyer A, Sampson M, et al. Aminophylline improves diaphragmatic contractility. N Engl J Med 1981; 305:249–252.
42. Aubier M, Murciano D, Viires N, et al. Diaphragmatic contractility enhanced by aminophylline: Role of extracellular calcium. J Appl Phys 1983; 54:460–464.
43. Murciano D, Auclair MH, Pariente R, Aubier M. A randomized, controlled trial of theophylline in patients with severe chronic obstructive pulmonary disease. N Engl J Med 1989; 320:1521–1525.
44. Sutton PP, Pavia D, Bateman JR, Clarke SW. The effect of oral aminophylline on lung mucociliary clearance in man. Chest 1981; 80:889–892.
45. Matthay RA, Berger HJ, Gottschalk A, Zaret BL. Effects of aminophylline upon right and left ventricular performance in chronic obstructive pulmonary disease. Am J Med 1978; 65:903–910.
46. Lakshminarayan S, Sahn SA, Weil JV. Effect of aminophylline on ventilatory responses in normal man. Am Rev Respir Dis 1978;117:38–43.
47. Mitenko PA, Ogilvie RI. Rational intravenous doses of theophylline. N Engl J Med 1973; 289:600–603.
48. Bone RC. Treatment of respiratory failure due to advanced chronic obstructive lung disease. Arch Intern Med 1980; 140:1018–1021.
49. Eiriksson CE, Writer SL, Vestal RE. Theophylline-induced alterations in cardiac electrophysiology in patients with chronic obstructive pulmonary disease. Am Rev Respir Dis 1975; 135:322–326.
50. Zwillich CW, Sutton FD, Neff TA, et al. Theophylline-induced seizures in adults. Ann Intern Med 1975; 82:784–787.
51. Filuk RB, Easton PA, Anthonisen NR. Responses to large doses of salbutamol and theophylline in patients with chronic obstructive pulmonary disease. Am Rev Respir Dis 1985; 132:871–874.
52. Theodore AC, Beer DS. Pharmacotherapy of chronic obstructive pulmonary disease. Clin Chest Med 1986; 7:657–671.
53. Skorodin MS. Pharmacologic management of obstructive lung disease: Current perspectives. Am J Med 1986; 82:8–15.
54. Pierson WE, Bierman CW, Kelley VC. A double-blind trial of corticosteroid therapy in status asthmaticus. Pediatrics 1974; 54:282–288.
55. Ramsdell SW, Berry CC, Clausen JL. The immediate effects of cortisol on pulmonary function in normals and asthmatics. J Allergy Clin Immunol 1985; 72:69–74.
56. Littenberg B, Gluck EH. A controlled trial of methylprednisolone in the emergency treatment of acute asthma. N Engl J Med 1986; 314:150–152.
57. Loren ML, Chai H, Leung P, et al. Corticosteroids in the treatment of acute exacerbations of asthma. Ann Allergy 1980; 45:67–71.
58. McNamara RM, Spivey WH, Greenspan LE, Mangione S. Early treatment of acute asthma with methylprednisolone. Ann Emerg Med 1987; 16:518.
59. McFadden ER, Kiser R, Degroot WJ, et al. A controlled study of the effects of single doses of hydrocortisone on the resolution of acute attacks of asthma. Am J Med 1976; 60:52–59.
60. Fanta CH, Rossing TH, McFadden ER. Glucocorticoids in acute asthma: A critical controlled trial. Am J Med 1983; 74:845–851.
61. Haskel RJ, Hansen JE. A double-blind, randomized clinical trial of methylprednisolone in status asthmaticus. Chest 1981; 80:377.
62. Alberts WM, Corrigan KC. Corticosteriod therapy for chronic obstructive pulmonary disease: Is it worth the risks? Postgrad Med 1987; 81:131–137.
63. James AL, Finucane KE, Ryan G, Musk AW. Bronchial responsiveness, lung mechanics, gas transfer, and corticosteroid response in patients with chronic airflow obstruction. Thorax 1988; 45:916–922.
64. Stoller JK. Systemic corticosteroids in stable chronic obstructive pulmonary disease: Do they work? Chest 1987; 91:155–156.
65. Blair GP, Light RW. Treatment of chronic obstructive pulmo-

nary disease with corticosteroids: Comparison of daily vs. alternate-day therapy. Chest 1984; 86:524–528.
66. Harding SM, Freedman S. A comparison of oral and inhaled steriods in patients with chronic airway obstruction: Features determining response. Thorax 1978; 33:214–218.
67. Shim CS, Williams MH. Aerosol beclomethasone in patients with steroid responsive chronic obstructive pulmonary disease. Am J Med 1985; 78:655–658.
68. Stoller JK, Gerbarg ZB, Feinstein AR. Corticosteroids in stable chronic obstructive pulmonary disease: Reappraisal of efficacy. Gen Intern Med 1987; 2:29–35.
69. Shim C, Stover DE, Williams MH. Response to corticosteroids in chronic bronchitis. J Allergy Clin Immunol 1978; 62:363–367.
70. Eliasson O, Hoffman J, Trueb D, et al. Corticosteroids in COPD: A clinical trial and reassessment of the literature. Chest 1986; 89:484–490.
71. Emerman CL, Connors AE, Lukens TW, et al. A randomized controlled trial of methylprednisolone in the emergency treatment of acute exacerbations of COPD. Chest 1989; 95:563–567.
72. Albert RK, Martin TR, Lewis SW. Controlled clinical trial of methylprednisolone in patients with chronic bronchitis and acute respiratory insufficiency. Ann Intern Med 1980; 92:753–758.
73. Glenny RW. Steroids in COPD: The scripture according to Albert. Chest 1987; 91:289–290.
74. Thomas TPL. The complications of systemic corticosteroid therapy in the elderly: A retrospective study. Gerontology 1984; 30:60–65.
75. Reid DM, Nicoll JJ, Smith MA, et al. Corticosteroids and bone mass in asthma: Comparisons with rheumatoid arthritis and polymyalgia rheumatica. Br Med J 1986; 293:1463–1466.
76. Chopra SK, Taplin GV, Simmons DH. Effects of hydration and physical therapy on tracheal transport velocity. Am Rev Respir Dis 1977; 115:1009–1014.
77. Francis PB. Acute respiratory failure in obstructive lung disease. Med Clin North Am 1983; 67:657–668.
78. Foster WM, Bergofsky EH, Bohning DE, et al. Effect of adrenergic agents and their mode of action on mucociliary clearance in man. J Appl Physiol 1976; 41:146–152.
79. Oldenburg FA, Dolovich MB, Montgomery JM, Newhouse M T. Effects of postural drainage, exercise, and cough on mucus clearance in chronic bronchitis. Am Rev Respir Dis 1979; 120:739–745.
80. Rossman CM, Waldes R, Sampson D, Newhouse MT. Effect of chest physiotherapy on the removal of mucus in patients with cystic fibrosis. Am Rev Respir Dis 1982; 126:131–135.
81. DeBoeck C, Zinman R. Cough versus chest physiotherapy: A comparison of the acute effects on pulmonary function in patients with cystic fibrosis. Am Rev Respir Dis 1984; 129:182–184.
82. Wollmer P, Ursing K, Midgren B, Eriksson L. Insufficiency of chest percussion in the physical therapy of chronic bronchitis. Eur J Respir Dis 1985; 66:233–239.
83. May DB, Munt PW. Physiologic effects of chest percussion and postural drainage in patients with stable chronic bronchitis. Chest 1979; 75:29–32.
84. Connors AF, Hammon WE, Martin RJ, Rogers RM. Chest physical therapy: The immediate effect on oxygenation in acutely ill patients. Chest 1980; 78:559–564.
85. Tyler ML. Complications of positioning and chest physiotherapy. Respir Care 1982; 27:458–466.
86. Wenk M. Successful treatment of respiratory tract infections in patients with chronic respiratory disease—how to make objective conclusions. J Antimicrobial Chemother 1982; 9:165–169.
87. Wardle JK, Freeman R, Ingham HR. Branhamella catarrhalis. Lancet 1982; i:1244.
88. Thornley PE, Aitken J, Drennan CS, et al. Branhamella catarrhalis infection of the lower respiratory tract: Reliable diagnosis by sputum examination. Br Med J 1982; 285:1537–1538.
89. McLeod DT, Ahmad F, Power JT, et al. Bronchopulmonary infection due to branhamella catarrhalis. Br Med J 1983; 287:1446–1447.
90. Nicotra B, Rivera M, Luman JI, Wallace RJ. Branhamella catarrhalis as a lower respiratory tract pathogen in patients with chronic lung disease. Arch Intern Med 1986; 146:890–893.
91. Slevin NJ, Aitken J, Thornley PE. Clinical and microbiological features of Branhamella catarrhalis bronchopulmonary infections. Lancet 1984; i:782–783.
92. Paterson IC, Petrie GR, Crompton GK, Robertson JR. Chronic bronchitis: Is bacteriological examination of sputum necessary? Br Med J 1978; 2:537–538.
93. Tager I, Speizer FE. Role of infection in chronic bronchitis. N Engl J Med 1975; 292:563–571.
94. Anthonisen NR, Manfreda J, Warren CPW, et al. Antibiotic therapy in exacerbations of chronic obstructive pulmonary disease. Ann Intern Med 1987; 106:196–203.
95. Nicotra MS, Rivera M, Awe RS. Antibiotic therapy of acute exacerbations of chronic bronchitis: A controlled study using tetracycline. Ann Intern Med 1982; 97:18–21.
96. Daniele RP, Rogers RM. Oxygen and nonventilatory therapy of respiratory failure in COPD. Postgrad Med 1973; 54:145–154.
97. Campbell EJM. The J Burns Amberson lecture: The management of acute respiratory failure in chronic bronchitis and emphysema. Am Rev Respir Dis 1967; 96:626–639.
98. Pierson DJ. The toxicity of low-flow oxygen therapy. Respir Care 1983; 28:889–897.
99. Aubier M, Murciano D, Milic-Emili J, et al. Effects of the administration of O_2 on ventilation and blood gases in patients with chronic obstructive pulmonary disease during acute respiratory failure. Am Rev Respir Dis 1980; 122:747–754.
100. Cropp A, DiMarco AF. Effects of intermittent negative pressure ventilation on respiratory muscle function in patients with severe chronic obstructive pulmonary disease. Am Rev Respir Dis 1987; 135:1056–1061.
101. Newman JH, Neff TA, Ziporin P. Acute respiratory failure associated with hypophosphatemia. N Engl J Med 1977; 296:1101–1103.
102. Varsano S, Shapiro M, Taragan R, et al. Hypophosphatemia as a reversible cause of refractory ventilatory failure. Crit Care Med 1983; 11:908–909.
103. Aubier M, Murciano D, Lecocguic Y, et al. Effect of hypophosphatemia on diaphragmatic contractility in patients with acute respiratory failure. N Engl J Med 1985; 313:420–424.
104. Aubier M, Viires N, Piquet J, et al. Effects of hypocalcemia on diaphragmatic strength generation. J Appl Physiol 1985; 58:922–929.
105. Aubier M, Murciano D, Viires N, et al. Effects of digoxin on diaphragmatic strength generation in patients with chronic obstructive pulmonary disease during acute respiratory failure. Am Rev Respir Dis 1987; 135:544–548.
106. Fanta CH, Rossing TH, McFadden ER. Emergency room treatment of asthma. Am J Med 1987; 82:59–64.
107. Newman SL, Roussos CS. Function and failure of the ventilatory muscles. In: Simmons DH, ed. Current Pulmonology, Vol 7. Chicago: Year Book Medical Publishers, 1986, 273.
108. Cohen CA, Zagelbaum G, Gross D, et al. Clinical manifestations of inspiratory muscle fatigue. Am J Med 1982; 73:308.
109. Gilbert R, Ashutosh K, Auchincloss JH Jr, et al. Prospective study of controlled oxygen therapy: Poor prognosis of patients with asynchronous breathing. Chest 1977; 71:456.
110. Cherniack RM, Hakimpour K. The rational use of oxygen in respiratory insufficiency. JAMA 1967; 199:178.
111. Bigelow BD, Petty TL, Levine BE, et al. The effect of oxygen breathing on arterial blood gases in patients with chronic airway obstruction living at 5,200 feet. Am Rev Respir Dis 1967; 96:28.
112. Bone RC, Pierce AK, Johnson RL. Controlled oxygen administration in acute respiratory failure in chronic obstructive pulmonary disease: A reappraisal. Am J Med 1978; 65:896.
113. Warren PM, Flenley DC, Millar JS, Avery A. Respiratory failure revisited: Acute exacerbations of chronic bronchitis between 1961–1968 and 1970–1976. Lancet 1980; i:467.
114. Addis GJ. Bicarbonate buffering in acute exacerbations of chronic respiratory failure. Thorax 1965; 20:337.
115. Kettle LJ, Diener CF, Morse JO, et al. Treatment of acute respiratory acidosis in chronic obstructive lung disease. JAMA 1971; 217:1503.
116. Bickerman HA, Chusid EL. The case against the use of respiratory stimulants. Chest 1970; 58:53.
117. Woolf CR. The use of "respiratory stimulant" drugs. Chest 1970; 58:49.
118. Riordan JF, Sillett RW, McNicol MW. A controlled trial of doxapram in acute respiratory failure. Br J Dis Chest 1975; 69:57.
119. Moser KM, Luchsinger PC, Adamson JS, et al. Respiratory stimulation with intravenous doxapram in respiratory failure. N Engl J Med 1973; 288:427.

120. Powell JR, Vozah S, Hopewell P, et al. Theophylline disposition in acutely ill hospitalized patients. Am Rev Respir Dis 1978; 118:229.
121. Rochester DF, Braun NMT, Laine S. Diaphragmatic energy expenditure in chronic respiratory failure: The effect of assisted ventilation with body respirators. Am J Med 1977; 63:223.
122. Pardy RL, Rivington R, Despas PJ, et al. The effects of inspiratory muscle training on exercise performance in chronic airflow limitation. Am Rev Respir Dis 1981; 123:426.
123. Marini JJ, Capps JS, Culver BH. The inspiratory work of breathing during assisted mechanical ventilation. Chest 1985; 87:612.
124. Aldrich TK, Karpel JP. Inspiratory muscle resistive training in respiratory failure. Am Rev Respir Dis 1985; 131:461.
125. Asmundsson T, Kilburn KH. Complications of acute respiratory failure. Ann Intern Med 1969; 70:487.
126. Pepe PE, Marini JJ. Occult positive end-expiratory pressure in mechanically ventilated patients with airflow obstruction. Am Rev Respir Dis 1982; 126:166.
127. Rossi A, Gottfried SB, Zocchi L, et al. Measurement of static compliance of the total respiratory system in patients with acute respiratory failure during mechanical ventilation: The effect of intrinsic positive end-expiratory pressure. Am Rev Respir Dis 1985; 131:672.
128. Johanson WG Jr, Pierce AK, Sanford JP, et al. Nosocomial respiratory infections with gram-negative bacilli. Ann Intern Med 1972; 77:701.
129. Pierson DJ. Indications for mechanical ventilation in acute respiratory failure. Respir Care 1983; 28:570.
130. Hyers TM, Briggs DD, Hudson LD, et al. NIH workshop summary: Withholding and withdrawing mechanical ventilation. Am Rev Respir Dis 1986; 134:1327.
131. Rotheram EB Jr, Safar P, Robin ED. CNS disorders during mechanical ventilation in chronic pulmonary disease. JAMA 1964; 189:993.
132. Kilburn KH. Shock, seizures, and coma with alkalosis during mechanical ventilation. Ann Intern Med 1966; 65:977.
133. Connors AF Jr, McCaffree DR, Gray BA. Effect of inspiratory flow rate on gas exchange during mechanical ventilation. Am Rev Respir Dis 1981; 124:537.
134. Brown DG, Pierson DJ. Auto-PEEP is common in mechanically ventilated patients: A study of incidence, severity, and detection. Respir Care 1986; 31:1069.
135. Scott LR, Benson MS, Bishop MJ. Relationship of endotracheal tube size to auto-PEEP at high minute ventilation. Respir Care 1986; 31:1080.
136. Scott LR, Benson MS, Pierson DJ. Effect of inspiratory flow rate and circuit-compressible volume on auto-PEEP during mechanical ventilation. Respir Care 1986; 31:1075.
137. Sherman C, Hudson LD. Complications of acute respiratory failure. In: Bone RC, Geroge RB, Hudson LD, eds. Acute Respiratory Failure. New York: Churchill Livingstone, 1987, 317–334.
138. Tryba M. Risk of acute stress bleeding and nosocomial pneumonia in ventilated intensive care patients: Sucralfate versus antacids. Am J Med 1987; 83(Suppl 3B):117.
139. Driks MR, Craven DE, Celli B, et al. Nosocomial pneumonia in intubated patients given sucralfate as compared with antacids or histamine type 2 blockers. N Engl J Med 1987; 317:1376–1380.
140. Doekel RC, Zwillich CW, Scoggin CH, et al. Clinical semistarvation: Depression of hypoxic ventilatory response. N Engl J Med 1976; 295:358.
141. Pingleton SK, Hadizman S. Enteral alimentation and gastrointestinal bleeding in mechanically ventilated patients. Crit Care Med 1983; 11:13.
142. Heymsfield SB, Bethel RA, Ansley JD, et al. Enteral hyperalimentation: An alternative to central venous hyperalimentation. Ann Intern Med 1979; 90:63.
143. Askanazi J, Carpenter YA, Elwyn DH, et al. Influence of total parenteral nutrition on fuel utilization in injury and sepsis. Ann Surg 1980; 191:40.
144. Grossman GD. Nutritional assessment of critically ill patients. Respir Care 1985; 30:463.

Chapter 46

ANTIBIOTIC TREATMENT OF BRONCHITIS AND CHRONIC LUNG DISEASE

Herbert Y. Reynolds

PATHOGENIC CONSIDERATIONS

Before discussing the selection of antibiotics for treating infectious exacerbations of bronchitis in chronic obstructive pulmonary disease (COPD) patients, it is appropriate to review the normal microbial flora that inhabits the oronasopharynx and major conducting airways of the lungs and to consider alterations in this flora when chronic illness is present. Because microbial cultures of expectorated secretions from COPD patients may yield mixtures of bacteria, and perhaps not reveal the causative agent, antibiotic therapy is often empiric. Thus, an educated guess about the most probable microbe(s) responsible is required. This is predicated on knowledge of which pathogens are colonizing the respiratory mucosa and which exogenous microbes must be suspected from current epidemiologic surveys (i.e., the status of influenza strains and other such pathogens in the community). With this background, a more rational choice of an antibiotic can be made.

Normal Microbial Flora

In the upper respiratory tract, or naso-oropharynx, various aerobic and anaerobic bacteria inhabit the mucosal surfaces.[1] Common isolates in cultures from surface swabs of the nose and throat include *Neisseria* sp., *Branhamella catarrhalis*, a variety of *Streptococcus* sp., and often, in people with chronic airway disease, *Streptococcus pneumoniae* and *Hemophilus* sp.; fungi and protozoa may also be recovered. Anaerobic bacteria around the teeth and gum crevices are numerous, reaching 10^8 micro-organisms/ml of oral secretions, and contain many varied species (but usually not *Bacteroides fragilis*). The prevalence of aerobic gram-negative bacilli, however, such as Enterobacteriaceae and *Pseudomonas* sp. is low; these are isolated from 15% of area swab cultures taken from normal subjects.[2]

It remains unclear whether micro-organisms inhabit the major bronchi and smaller conducting airways in normal lungs. Conflicting reports about the relative sterility of the lower airways probably reflect differences in sampling procedures. Cultures of bronchoalveolar lavage obtained during fiberoptic bronchoscopy reveal a mixture of upper airway microbes that are collected as the bronchoscope is passed through the nose and/or oropharynx into a bronchus, in which it is wedged;[3] these cultures do not represent airway flora. Whether a few colonies of bacteria can be cultured from a healthy airway mucosa seems of little consequence, though, because presumably active mucociliary clearance mechanisms and cough reflexes are efficient in removing any bacteria that are aerosolized or aspirated with oropharyngeal secretions.

In a careful study of 25 normal subjects,[4] a sterile brush was protected within a telescoping double catheter to obtain bronchial samples during fiberoptic bronchoscopy. Most cultures from multiple sites in the lower respiratory tract contained bacteria (38 of 52 specimens, or 73%) similar to those found in the nasopharynx. Because the colony counts were often so low (0 to 5 colonies/culture plate), especially when the volunteers were bronchoscoped in a supine or Trendelenburg position rather than a sitting position, the question was raised of whether these positive cultures always indicated upper respiratory tract contamination or whether they denoted true lower respiratory tract colonization.

Only bacterial cultures have been discussed, not viruses or other agents such as *Pneumocystis carinii* and *Mycoplasma* sp. Viruses are not normally present in lung secretions and, if cultured, should be considered to represent infection. Moreover, some organisms are inhaled and deposited directly onto the alveolar surfaces (with aerodynamic dimensions of 0.5 to 3 μ in diameter) and may not be cultured from the airways. Some microbes might exist selectively in the alveoli, perhaps residing in macrophages or in alveolar lining cells (possibly *Pneumocystis* organisms), so that the alveolar milieu might have a discernible flora.[5]

Thus, there is an extensive microbial flora in the nose and orpharynx, but the peripheral bronchi in normal humans are relatively sterile, perhaps completely. Nasopharyngeal bacteria may be transiently deposited but are then removed by mucociliary or cough mechanisms, so bacterial persistence or colonization does not usually occur. Certain pathogenic aerobic gram-negative rods are not often carried on the mucosa of the upper airways in normal persons, but with almost any alteration in health status (e.g., alcoholism, diabetes, dependent living in a health care facility),[6,7] an increase of these gram-negative rods in the nose and throat occurs. Subconscious aspiration of oropharyngeal secretions, such as during sleeping, is the most probable route for microbes to enter the lower airways and alveoli and then become a nidus for subsequent infection.

Airway Colonization in Chronic Bronchitis

Causes of chronic bronchitis have not been elucidated completely but three factors seem to be important in contributing to airway inflammation: cigarette smoking, atmospheric pollution, and infection.

An important issue in chronic bronchitis is the role of microbial infection.[8–12] Infection does not appear to initiate the disease but is probably important in perpetuating the illness and is responsible for many of the acute exacerbations. As mentioned previously, normal bronchi are almost always sterile. In contrast, pathogenic bacteria can be cultured from bronchial washings of some 82% of chronic bronchitics[3] but many of these organisms may represent oral flora if the specimen was not a transtracheal aspirate or was not obtained with a protected catheter technique.

Routine sputum cultures from patients with chronic bronchitis commonly contain nonencapsulated *Hemophilus influenzae* and *Streptococcus pneumoniae*. Other oropharyngeal commensal flora also can be recovered. In most clinical series, one or both of these species have been recovered from approximately 30% to 50% of sputum specimens and can be considered to be the baseline microbial flora of many patients with chronic bronchitis. Anaerobic bacteria are infrequent inhabitants and are recovered in only 17% of transtracheal aspirate specimens.[13]

Sputum carriage of *Hemophilus influenzae* and pneumococci, however, is of uncertain significance. These bacteria tend to persist in sputum during quiescent intervals and the frequency of recovery is not greatly increased during acute infectious episodes. Development of purulent sputum is not specifically correlated with the presence of one or the other of these bacteria in quantitative cultures. *Mycoplasma pneumoniae* does not seem to be of real importance, and some studies have attributed only 1% to 10% of acute infections to this organism.[12] Other bacteria, such as hemolytic streptococci, *Staphylococcus aureus,* and enteric gram-negative bacilli are infrequent causes of acute bronchitis. However, viruses may be a more frequent cause of acute infection than is suspected—about 25% of acute exacerbations are caused by viruses. These include influenza, parainfluenza, respiratory syncytial virus, rhinovirus, and coronavirus.[12] Viral infections are seasonal and usually occur more frequently in winter.

Thus, the affected COPD patient suffers from an exacerbation or worsening of cough, expectoration (often with an increase in the amount and altered coloration of sputum), variable constitutional symptoms (discernible fever may not occur), and perhaps few, if any, changes in laboratory values (leukocytosis can vary). The episode might go unnoticed and remain subclinical or be acute and require evaluation and therapy, including the use of an antibiotic. Although presumed to be caused by a bacterial pathogen colonizing the airways *(Hemophilus* sp. or a *Pneumococcus),* the infectious flare-up may be caused by a viral agent in a surprisingly large percentage of cases. An initial Gram's stain of the sputum and routine microbial culture might not determine the causative agent with certainty. Moreover, if this is an established pattern of repeated exacerbations in a patient well known to the physician, the sputum and culture analysis can be dispensed with for every episode and an antibiotic can be ordered by telephone to commence empiric treatment. The physician might not even be notified if patients have their own supply of antibiotics and have been instructed to begin therapy when the symptoms suggest acute infection, or if the patient is on a rotational plan of antibiotics for prophylactic suppression of airway bacteria.

SELECTION OF APPROPRIATE ANTIBIOTICS

Oral antibiotics are reviewed first in this section and then parenteral choices are discussed (if the infection warrants hospitalization and more intensive treatment).

Oral Antibiotics

Before prescribing an oral antibiotic for suppressing the microbial flora in the airways or for treating a flare-up of bronchitis, it should be mentioned that an antibiotic is only part of the treatment for irritated, hyperactive airways that may be causing wheezing, cough, and increased expectoration of phlegm or purulent sputum.[14] Supportive therapy with antibronchospastic medications, including β-agonist bronchodilators (inhaled aerosol or oral form), oral theophylline, corticosteroids, a cough suppressant, and judicious use of a sedative may be required. During a period of increased coughing and mucosal irritation, aerosol administration of a topical steroid in the airways or the use of drugs that inhibit mediator release by mast cells (i.e., cromolyn) are not advocated for acute use. Finally, if sinusitis, otitis media, or postnasal secretions reflecting rhinitis coexist with an exacerbation of bronchitis, special attention should be given to the nose and sinuses. Because postnasal secretions can stimulate coughing and generally complicate control of the lower airway irritation, a decongestant and topical nasal spray should be used.

For the person with COPD, productive cough, and susceptibility to flare-ups of bronchitis, it is reasonable to use an oral antibiotic with broad antimicrobial activity to suppress bacteria in the sputum or those colonizing the airways. Preventing an exacerbation of the bronchitis can be attempted. Various common antibiotics (Table 46–1) can be tried, rotating therapy using several different agents. For example, an antibiotic such as ampicillin is given for 5 to 7 days, discontinued for several days, and then restarted for another 5- to 7-day period. After several cycles of ampicillin a switch to tetracycline or amoxicillin can be made and given a similar trial. Because erythromycin can cause more gastrointestinal symptoms, it might not be tolerated as well as the others. With any of these antibiotics, especially tetracycline, oral thrush or vaginal candidiasis in women can be induced. As an alternative, this regular cycling can be replaced by a longer trial of one of the antibiotics for a 4- to 6-week period and then a week or so reprieve without any drug. In my experience this suppresses bacterial pathogens more thoroughly. It can be accompanied by a noticeable diminution in daily sputum production by some patients with chronic bronchitis. This can result in a longer period of less daily expectoration and of greater well-being.

The more intensive course of antibiotics for a longer period can be helpful for some patients in whom the shorter cycles are not as beneficial. The combination agent trimethoprim-sulfamethoxazole can be an effective antibiotic for this prolonged use, given as one double-strength tablet twice daily. Not only is the antimicrobial spectrum of this drug well suited for the probable bacterial pathogens in chronic bronchitis, but it is concentrated in acinar and glandular tissue such as the lung, so that high drug levels are reached. If bronchiectasis complicates the chronic airway disease, trimethoprim-sulfamethoxazole seems to be particularly effective.

Antibiotics Effective Against β-Lactamase-Producing Bacteria

A great variety of bacteria, both gram-positive and gram-negative species, secrete β-lactamase enzymes that hydrolyze a portion of the β-lactam ring (cyclic amide bond) found in the β-lactam antibiotics (e.g., penicillins, cephalosporins, monobactams, carbapenems), thus creating microbial resistance to this important group of antibiotics.[15] β-Lactam antibiotics are bactericidal—they inhibit bacterial cell wall synthesis by interrupting the linking of peptidoglycans. Various penicillin-binding proteins on the inner surface of the bacterial cell membrane are involved in assembling the cell wall and providing shape to it during growth and division.[15]

Because *Streptococcus pneumoniae* and *Hemophilus influenzae* are considered to be frequent causes of bronchitis in COPD patients, antibiotic therapy is often directed toward them. These bacteria can produce β-lactamases and their resistance to ampicillin is to be anticipated.

To counter the inactivation of β-lactam antibiotics by bacterial lactamase enzymes, inhibitors can be combined with an antibiotic that binds to and inactivates the lactamases. In effect the inhibitors, clavulanic acid and sulbactam, which resemble penicillin structurally, combine with the secreted β-lactamases and allow the other antibiotic to be active against the microbes. These "suicide inhibitors" are consumed and destroyed.[15] Thus, common penicillins have been combined in fixed amounts with β-lactamase inhibitors to create a useful group of antibiotic preparations. Most helpful for the bronchitis patient requiring oral therapy is the combination of clavulanic acid (125 mg) and amoxicillin (250 or 500 mg), known as Augmentin. This provides added activity against *Hemophilus influenzae,* Staphylococcus and *Neisseria* sp. and *Branhamella catarrhalis,* which may be a cause of respiratory infection. Parenteral combinations of ticarcillin and clavulanic acid (Timentin) or ampicillin and clavulanic acid (Unasyn) are also available.

Treatment of More Serious Infection

Initial Parenteral Antibiotic Therapy

When the usual flare-up of infective bronchitis does not respond to a few days of an oral antibiotic plus other supportive drug therapy, and the patient has fever, more systemic complaints, an elevated white blood cell count, and auscultatory or radiographic signs suggesting pneumonitis, a more intensive course of treatment is required and hospitalization is necessary. The patient may present acutely without having had the prodromal upper respiratory infection or flare-up previously described. A baseline sputum specimen for Gram's staining and microbial culture and several blood cultures should be obtained. These results can help to select and guide antibiotic administration; formerly, with a flare-up of bronchitis, an empiric choice was usually made. Again, the same bacteria or virus may be the causative agent, and antibiotics are directed against the major bacterial colonizers in the airways and sputum—*Hemophilus* sp., *Streptococcus pneumoniae,* and possibly mycoplasma, staphylococci, and *Legionella pneumophila.* The background of the patient (i.e., living or support environment, associated chronic disease(s), epidemiologic considerations about microbes going around the community) determines how seriously a possible community-acquired or nosocomial pneumonia might be with an aerobic gram-negative rod bacterium (e.g., *Klebsiella pneumoniae, Pseudomonas aeruginosa*). Recent antibiotic use by the patient could make it more likely that superinfecting bacteria such as staphylococci or the

TABLE 46–1. Antimicrobial Spectrum Best Covered

ANTI-BIOTIC	DOSAGE	MECHANISM OF ACTIVITY	CAUSATIVE AGENT: *Streptococcus pneumoniae*	*Hemophilus influenzae* (Non-β Lactamase Producers)	*Staphylococcus sp.* (Nonpenicillinase-Producing) and Other Common Gram-Positive Bacteria	β-Lactamase-Producing Bacteria	*Mycoplasma pneumoniae*	*Pseudomonas aeruginosa, Klebsiella pneumoniae*	Other Common Gram-Negative rods (*E. coli, Neisseria sp., Proteus mirabilis*)	Anaerobic Bacteria	*Legionella pneumophila*	Virus
Ampicillin	500 mg q6h	Penicillin, acts on cell wall	+	+	+	−	−	−	+	−	−	−
Amoxicillin	500 mg q8h	Semisynthetic penicillin and analogue of ampicillin; inhibits cell wall mucopeptide in multiplying bacteria	+	+	+	−	−	−	+	−	−	−
Tetracycline	500 mg q6h	Bacteriostatic; inhibits protein synthesis, binding 30-S ribosomal subunit blocking m-RNA	+	+/−	+/−	+	+	−	+/−	+/−	−	+/−
Erythromycin	250 mg q6h *or* 500 mg q12h	Bacteriostatic; macrolide group of antibiotics inhibiting RNA-dependent protein synthesis	+	+/−	+/−	+	+	−	+/−	−	+	+
Trimethoprim-sulfamethoxazole	Double-strength tablet (160/800 mg) q12h	Two-step block of protein and nucleic acid synthesis by inhibiting dihydrofolic acid and tetrahydrofolic acid through inhibition of dihydrofolate reductase	+	+	+	+	−	−	+	−	−	−
Clindamycin	150 to 300 mg q6h	Semisynthetic related to lincomycin; action similar to that of macrolides	+	−	+		−	−	−	+	−	−
Cefaclor	250 to 500 mg q8h	Second-generation cephalosporin	+	+	+	+	−	−	+	−	−	−
Cefuroxime axetil	250 mg q12h	Second-generation cephalosporin	+	+	+	+	−	−	+	±	−	−
Cephalexin	250 to 500 mg q6h	First-generation cephalosporin	+	−	+	+	−	+/−	+	−	−	−
Amoxacillin-clavulanic acid	250 to 500 mg q8h	Combined with β-lactamase inhibitor	+	+	+	+	−	−	+	−	−	−
Ciprofloxacin	500 mg q8h	Inhibits DNA gyrase synthesis, quinolone	+	+	+	+	−	+	+	−	+	−
Amantadine	200 mg daily	Inhibits viral replication										+

previously mentioned gram negative rods are inhabiting the respiratory tract.

Many antibiotic options exist for parenteral therapy. Some oral drugs can be used intravenously, and ampicillin or erythromycin are given often by this route. When given intravenously, the dosage of ampicillin used is 1 g q 6h. Also, a higher dosage of erythromycin is used, 1 g every 6 to 8 hours; this is recommended if *Legionella pneumophila* infection is suspected. However, for the serious exacerbation of bronchitis, many physicians rely on second-generation cephalosporins. These retain effective gram-positive coverage but are more active against some gram-negative bacteria, especially *Hemophilus influenzae*, which is a major bacterial pathogen. First-generation cephalosporins (e.g., cephalothin), which have relatively lower gram-negative activity and are not reliably active against penicillin-resistant strains of *Streptococcus pneumoniae,* are of little use. On the other hand, it is unusual to need a third-generation cephalosporin, which has special activity against troublesome gram-negative bacilli, including *Pseudomonas aeruginosa.* Only in a specific situation in which an acquired *Pseudomonas* pneumonia were likely would ceftazidime or cefoperazone be recommended. It is often the practice, however, to initiate therapy for a community-acquired pneumonia in an elderly patient with underlying chronic lung disease with a third-generation cephalosporin, because of the broad spectrum of bacteria covered and because a single antibiotic with little renal toxicity can be given. What antibiotic is preferable for the bronchitic patient without a community-acquired or nosocomial pneumonia? Cefamandole and cefuroxime are used extensively in this situation, with the presumption that *Hemophilus influenzae* is often the etiologic agent and could be an ampicillin-resistant strain. The dosage of these respective antibiotics is 2 g q4h and 1.5 g q8h.

The cephalosporin antibiotics represent a large and diverse group; they can be confusing to prescribe and use. Some of those mentioned previously might not be favored in the future as newer compounds are developed. Their efficacy can be excellent, but whether they will always suffice as a single agent for treating a serious respiratory infection needs more clinical verification. Bacteria that can produce β-lactamase enzymes (cephalosporinases) can disrupt the β-lactam ring and render the cephalosporins inactive. The presence of β-lactamase-secreting bacteria seems to be an increasing problem in treating respiratory infections. If the patient is quite ill and is significantly immunocompromised in any way, it may still be prudent to include an aminoglycoside with the cephalosporin, at least for initial therapy. In this situation, an aminoglycoside plus an extended-spectrum penicillin is also favored for initial treatment.[16]

Follow-Up Oral Antibiotic Therapy

After a few days of intravenous therapy with ampicillin or one of the cephalosporins, it may be appropriate to continue therapy at home or in an extended care facility, in which maintaining an intravenous line or heparin-lock site for drug administration is not feasible or permitted. Further treatment against a pathogen, possibly a gram-negative rod bacterium, is desirable. An oral cephalosporin antibiotic (e.g., cefaclor—Ceclor) may be considered. It is effective against staphylococci, *Streptococcus pneumoniae,* and *Hemophilus influenzae,* some β-lactamase-producing ampicillin-resistant strains, and *Klebsiella* sp. (but not *Pseudomonas* or *Serratia* sp. or enterococci). The usual adult dosage is 250 to 500 mg q8h.

A recently developed oral antibiotic, with much potential, is ciprofloxacin, an improved derivative of the quinolone nalidixic acid that has a broad spectrum of antibacterial activity. Ciprofloxacin is active against gram-positive bacteria (e.g., *Streptococcus pneumoniae, Staphylococcus aureus*), many important gram-negative rods (e.g., *Hemophilus influenzae, Pseudomonas aeruginosa, Klebsiella pneumoniae*), *Legionella pneumophila*, and *Chlamydia* sp., which can be causative agents in bronchitis. Ciprofloxacin can be used as initial oral therapy for serious bronchitis (and gave slightly better clinical results than ampicillin when the two antibiotics were compared[17]), but it seems prudent not to prescribe this drug indiscriminately as a first choice when others will suffice.

Microbial resistance develops quickly to ciprofloxacin when given for more than a few days. Such resistance of *Pseudomonas aeruginosa*, for example, can disappear in several weeks, after the antibiotic has been discontinued. The bacterium may become susceptible again, but it is not known whether this will continue to be the pattern in the future. Ciprofloxacin seemed to have great promise for suppressing *Pseudomonas aeruginosa* in cystic fibrosis patients who had smoldering bronchitis with this organism but, distressingly, after a few weeks of oral therapy microbial resistance may develop. Thus, intermittent use of ciprofloxacin seems best in this disease.

To preclude the development of more widespread microbial resistance to ciprofloxacin, and to continue to use it as an oral antibiotic effective against important gram-negative rods, judicious use is advised. It is proposed that it be reserved for the COPD patient discussed in this chapter as an oral antibiotic to finish up a course of intravenous antibiotic against particular gram-negative rods, if dictated by the patient's situation (i.e., home care or nursing care facility) after hospitalization.

PROPHYLAXIS AGAINST INFLUENZA

Patients with COPD and bronchitis should receive the currently recommended influenza vaccination annually. If they do not, or are perceived to be subjects who will produce poor antibody titers because of advanced age or concomitant illness that impairs antibody responses, amantadine can be given. It can be useful if an outbreak of influenza occurs before or in less than 2 weeks after vaccination, before peak titers of serum antibodies have been produced. Therefore, oral amantadine, given 200 mg once daily or 100 mg twice daily, starting before exposure to influenza A and continuing throughout the period (a 6- to 8-week interval), can prevent illness in 70% to 90% of adults.[18] Amantadine does not, however, prevent infection by influenza B strains. When the drug is given up to 48 hours after the onset of influenza A illness, it can help to decrease some symptoms and shorten the period of fever. Those over 65 years of age should take a reduced dose of 100 mg/day, as should those with renal disease.

REFERENCES

1. Mackowiak PA. The normal microbial flora. N Engl J Med 1982; 307:83–93.
2. Rosenthal S, Tager I. Prevalence of gram-negative rods in the normal pharyngeal flora. Ann Intern Med 1975; 83:355–357.
3. Reynolds HY, Newball HH. Analysis of proteins and respiratory cells obtained from human lungs by bronchial lavage. J Lab Clin Med 1974; 84:559–573.
4. Halperin SA, Suratt PM, Gwaltney JM, et al. Bacterial cultures from the lower respiratory tract in normal volunteers with and without experimental rhinovirus infection using a plugged double catheter system. Am Rev Respir Dis 1982; 125:678–680.
5. Reynolds HY. Lung immunology and its contribution to the immunopathogenesis of certain respiratory diseases. J Allergy Clin Immunol 1986; 78:833–847.
6. Johanson WG, Pierce AK, Sanford JP. Changing pharyngeal bacterial flora of hospitalized patients: emergence of gram-negative bacilli. N Engl J Med 1969; 281:1137–1140.

7. Valenti WM, Trudell RG, Bentley BW. Factors predisposing to oropharyngeal colonization with gram-negative bacilli in the aged. N Engl J Med 1978; 298:1108–1111.
8. Leeder SR. Role of infection in the cause of chronic bronchitis and emphysema. J Infect Dis 1975; 131:731–742.
9. Tager I, Speizer FE. Role of infection in chronic bronchitis. N Engl J Med 1975; 292:563–571.
10. Ellis DA, Anderson ME, Stewart SM. Exacerbations of chronic bronchitis: Exogenous or endogenous infection? Br J Dis Chest 1978; 721:115–121.
11. Bates JH. The role of the infection during exacerbation of chronic bronchitis. Ann Intern Med 1982; 97:130–131.
12. Gump DW, Phillips CA, Forsyth BR, et al. Role of infection in chronic bronchitis. Am Rev Respir Dis 1976; 113:465–474.
13. Haas H, Morris JF, Samson S, et al. Bacterial flora of the respiratory tract in chronic bronchitis: Comparison of transtracheal, fiber-bronchoscopic and oropharyngeal sampling methods. Am Rev Respir Dis 1977; 16:41–47.
14. Reynolds HY. Outpatient management of the bronchitic surgical patient. Infect Surg 1983; 2:897–906.
15. Donowitz GR, Mandell GL. Beta-lactam antibiotics. N Engl J Med 1988; 318:419–426, 490–500.
16. Reynolds HY. Aerobic gram-negative pneumonia. In: Bayless TM, Brain MC, Cherniack RM, eds. Current Therapy in Internal Medicine, 2. Philadelphia: B. C. Decker, 1987, 752–758.
17. Wollschlager CM, Raoof S, Khan FA, et al. Controlled, comparative study of ciprofloxacin versus ampicillin in treatment of bacterial respiratory tract infections. Am J Med 1987; 82(Suppl 4A):164–168.
18. Influenza prevention, 1987–88. Med Lett 1987; 29:81–82.

Chapter 47

MUCOLYTICS AND EXPECTORANTS IN THE TREATMENT OF COPD

Christopher S. Garrard

Mucolytic agents can, by one or several means, alter the physicochemical nature of mucus.[1–4] Although the term "mucolytic" is not entirely appropriate, because lysis is not the universal mechanism of action of these agents, it is used here for convenience, although more suitable descriptions have been proposed.[5, 6] Despite the relative lack of objective evidence to support the use of mucolytic agents in the treatment of airways disease, these agents continue to be used regularly in clinical practice. This chapter first considers aspects of mucous rheology and the proposed mechanisms of action of mucolytics, and then examines evidence supporting their therapeutic efficacy.

RHEOLOGIC PROPERTIES AND CHEMICAL CHARACTERISTICS OF MUCUS

Miller and Jones[7] have classified sputum according to the relative predominance of mucoid and purulent components, which serves to highlight the variability of the gross macroscopic properties of sputum. In more objective terms, sputum can be characterized according to its rheologic properties—that is, its deformation and flow characteristics.

The chemical nature of mucus is complex. It consists of a variable mixture of glycoproteins, proteoglycans, lipids,[8] and deoxyribonucleic acids. The dry weight of these compounds comprises about 6 mg/ml of healthy mucus, and often greater amounts with chronic bronchitis, asthma, and cystic fibrosis.[9] The glycoproteins and proteoglycans associate closely together to provide the mucus with most of its viscoelastic characteristics, with a smaller contribution from lipids.[8] Several proteins also play an important antibacterial role, including secretory IgA, lactoferrin, and lysozyme.[9, 10]

The various studies of mucous rheology are often difficult to interpret and compare because of inconsistencies in methodology. Delays in analysis following sputum collection and the effects of storage and preparation dramatically influence the final results.[11] The technical problems in studying the rheologic and chemical composition of sputum are considerable and have been comprehensively reviewed.[9]

The mucous gels formed from glycoproteins are propelled by airway epithelial cilia, and the rheologic behavior of the mucus appears to be critical in the interaction or coupling of cilia to the mucous blanket.[12, 13] It has been shown that with constant elasticity, changes in the viscosity have little effect on the rate of mucous transport in frog palate preparations.[14] In contrast, there appears to be an optimal concentration of mucous macromolecules for maximal ciliary transport rate in the same preparation, and mucus transport is greatest within a relatively narrow range of elastic behavior.[15] Elasticity appears to be the major rheologic property of mucus with regard to mucociliary transport, whereas viscosity influences the ability of mucus to trap and retain foreign particulate material.

Our understanding of the interactions between mucous rheology and airway cilia would be greatly simplified if mucus exhibited purely Newtonian behavior. Mucus is non-Newtonian, however; its viscosity decreases with increasing propelling force generated by cilia. In addition, the elastic modulus of mucus increases with increasing shear rate. Thus, at low rates of shear (slow ciliary beat) viscous properties predominate, whereas at a high rate of shear the elastic properties of mucus are enhanced. Within the airways cilia beat at a frequency estimated to be between 10 to 20 Hz, and the overlying mucus exhibits several combinations of viscosity and elasticity over that frequency range. To characterize mucous rheology adequately, the shear rates applied to the mucus should be defined; ideally, these should fall within the range of shear rates generated by beating cilia.

Several devices are available to measure the viscoelastic properties of mucus, and some of these are summarized in Table 47–1.[3, 9, 16–29] Techniques based on the pourability or the adhesive characteristics of mucus have the appeal of simplicity,[21, 22] whereas more complex devices such as the magnetic rheometer or the Weissenberg rheogoniometer facilitate the measurement of viscosity and elasticity over a range of shear rates. The ability of mucus to form stable threads, or mucous spinability,[30] has been shown to correlate with the mucous transport rate (frog palate) even when elasticity or viscosity are no longer within the normal range. Spinability can incorporate additional measures of the physical properties of mucus, such as cohesiveness, which enhances its use as an index of mucous rheology. In time, other rheologic indices may be introduced and gain popularity.

INTERACTIONS OF MUCUS WITH CILIATED EPITHELIUM

In health, the rheologic properties of mucus are closely integrated with the ciliary propulsion mechanism. In the presence of airway disease, changes in mucous elasticity, viscosity, and cohesiveness are likely to have an adverse effect on mucociliary transport, which in turn contributes to the pathophysiology of that disease.

The frog palate preparation provides a convenient and widely accepted laboratory method of determining mucociliary transport; if properly maintained, this preparation sustains active cilia for several hours.[30] Samples of the mucus under investigation are placed on the ciliated surface of the frog palate and the movement of markers added to the surface mucus indicates the mucous transport velocity. In fresh frog palate preparations (1 to 3 hours old), mucous transport rates are similar to those measured in vivo in both animals and humans.[31] It appears that for maximal mucous transport, mucus needs to fall within a specific range of elastic moduli. This range depends on the source of the mucus. For example, maximal transport with human bronchitic sputum is seen at 18 dynes/cm^2 but is seen at a lower level of 10 dynes/cm^2 with dog tracheal mucus. Irrespective of the source of the mucus, the range of optimal transport rates has a characteristic shape (Fig. 47–1). At elastic moduli below the maximal transport levels transport rates fall off rapidly; above the maximal level, transport rates decrease more gradually.

Whereas enzymes and mucolytic agents can lower elasticity and viscosity profoundly, the effects on mucociliary transport velocity can be equivocal. It is clear that to optimize mucociliary clearance, mucus rheology must be altered so as to have it lie within a relatively narrow range of elastic moduli. When mucus is highly elastic and viscous, a benefit of enzymes and mucolytics can be seen in terms of transport velocity. If airway mucus, prior to treatment, is near the optimal range for elasticity and viscosity, there actually may be a deleterious effect of mucolytics.[20] This could explain the apparent discrepancy between studies of rheology indicating the efficacy of acetylcysteine and in vivo studies, which largely have failed to demonstrate a significant therapeutic response in patients with airways disease.[32–35] Indeed, viscosity and elasticity can be low in patients with chronic bronchitis caused by decreased levels of secretory IgA.[36] In such patients it would be illogical to administer mucolytics.

In situations in which mucus is thinner (i.e., less viscous and less elastic than normal), the addition of an agent to increase viscosity and elasticity would seem to be a rational approach. Davis and Deverell[5] have termed such agents "mucospissic." Several antibiotics, including tetracycline, have such mucospissic activity.[37] Even if the appropriate agent can be selected (i.e., mucolytic or mucospissic), it might be unrealistic to expect the rheologic properties of airway mucus to be modified so as to maximize mucous transport consistently. Coughing may promote removal of airway secretions modified by mucolytics, even when mucous rheology would not be considered optimal for mucociliary clearance, and could explain some of the clinical benefit reported with the use of mucolytics.

In view of the complex interactions between cilia and mucous rheology, a methodology allowing in situ measurement of mucous rheology (i.e., while the mucus lies on the ciliated epithelium) would offer distinct advantages. Such methods have been devised but are not easily applicable to clinical practice.[38]

Abnormalities in the structure and function of airway cilia can also contribute to impaired mucociliary clearance in those with chronic bronchitis and bronchiectasis and cystic fibrosis.[39–41] Some of the slowing of ciliary beat frequency in these diseases can be a result of the effects of bacterial infection, which can be reversed by treatment with antibiotics.[42] Mucolytic agents are unlikely to have a direct effect on ciliary beat frequency and therefore would be unable to reverse any defect in mucociliary clearance caused by ciliary dysfunction.

MODIFICATION OF MUCOUS RHEOLOGY

Effects of Disease

A change in the glycoprotein content of mucus[43] has a major effect on mucous rheology and may be the chief pathway

TABLE 47–1. Devices Used to Measure Mucous Rheology

PARAMETER	APPARATUS	SOURCE (REF. NO.)
Pourability	Mucus container	Keal[21]
Adhesiveness	Inclined tube	Chodosh et al.[22]
Viscosity, elasticity	Capillary viscometer	Dulfano[23]; Kim et al.[24]
Viscosity, elasticity, creep	Magnetic rheometer	Denton et al.[25]
Viscosity	Ferranti-Shirley cone and plate viscometer	Lieberman[3]; Davis and Dippy[26]; Palmer et al.[27]; Sturgess et al.[19]; Keal[28]
Viscosity, elasticity	Chemical balance rheometer	Davis et al.[29]
Viscosity, elasticity, yield	Concentric cylinder rheometer	Benis et al.[16]
Viscosity, elasticity	Weissenberg rheogoniometer	Sturgess et al.[19]; Davis and Dippy[26]
Spinability	Filancemeter	Puchelle et al.[30]

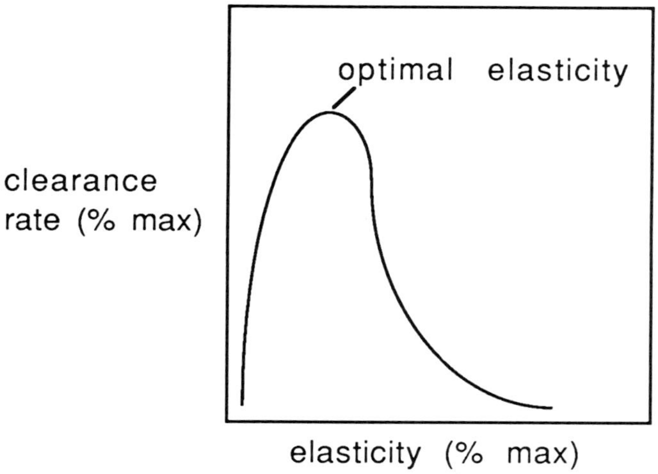

Figure 47–1. Graphic relationship of elasticity and rate of mucociliary clearance as might be seen when adding mucous samples of various elastic moduli to a frog palate preparation.

whereby mucus is modified in disease. The dry weight of macromolecules in those with chronic bronchitis and asthma is on average about 22 mg/ml, or about four times the level seen in health. Even greater concentrations may be found in those with cystic fibrosis.[44] There is considerable patient-to-patient variability, however, with asthmatics showing as much as a tenfold difference in macromolecular dry weight among patients. The macromolecular content in an individual patient with chronic bronchitis seems to remain relatively unchanged over a relatively long period (1 or 2 years), provided the patient's clinical condition remains stable.[45] However, there may be discernible seasonal changes in some components of mucus.[46]

When sputum of cystic fibrosis and chronic bronchitis patients are of similar degrees of purulence, viscosities are not significantly different.[47] The greater dry weight content of the sputum of cystic fibrosis patients is mainly the result of a greater DNA content. The elasticity of sputum in those with chronic bronchitis has been shown by Puchelle and associates[48] to be proportional to the secretory IgA, hexosamine, and neuraminic acid concentrations.

Effects of Medication

Although it has been difficult to confirm the clinical benefit of mucolytic agents, it has been relatively easy to demonstrate the modification of mucous rheology in vitro by several groups of agents. Results from in vitro studies evaluating the effects of drugs on mucous rheology are influenced greatly by the methodology. Most instruments used to determine mucous rheology measure viscosity, and some also measure elasticity (Table 47–1). Several mucolytic agents and enzymes have readily demonstrable effects on mucous rheology in vitro[1–4] whereas detergents appear to have little effect on the viscoelastic properties of sputum.[2]

Iodides

Iodides not only influence mucous secretion[6] but also reduce the viscosity of mucus when applied directly in vitro.[49, 50] The final therapeutic effect in vivo probably represents a combination of effects on mucous secretion and on mucous rheology directly.

Acetylcysteine

N-acetylcysteine, L-cysteine, cysteamine, and methylcysteine exert their activity by breaking the disulfide bonds that link glycoproteins, which in turn leads to a reduction in both viscosity and elasticity.[3, 5, 50] Acetylcysteine is generally used as an aerosol or as a topically applied solution (through an endoscope).[51] Oral administration, however, also appears to have an effect on mucous rheology.[52]

Glyceryl Guaiacolate

In contrast to acetylcysteine, glyceryl guaiacolate, a derivative of guaiacol, has been shown to be no more effective in altering sputum viscosity than water.[53]

Bromhexine

Bromhexine [*N*-cyclohexyl-*N*-methyl-2-(2-amino-3,5-dibromo)benzyl-ammonium hydrochloride] may be considered to be a mucolytic, although its mode of action is probably by direct stimulation of mucus-producing glands.[54] The mucus produced by chronic bronchitics receiving bromhexine therapy is of reduced viscosity and decreased DNA and glycoprotein fiber content.[55]

Sulfhydryl Bond-Disrupting Agents

A wide range of agents are known to disrupt sulfhydryl bonds, including dithiothreitol, glutathione, *N*-acetylpenicillamine, and sodium metabisulfite.[2, 3, 5, 56] Some of these are extremely potent mucolytic agents (e.g., dithiothreitol), but their irritant effects on the airways limit clinical applications.[56, 57]

Enzymes

Several enzymes directed at the constituent components of mucus can primarily reduce viscosity, with less effect on elasticity. These enzymes include trypsin, chymotrypsin, streptokinase, elastase, papain and, particularly, desoxyribonuclease.[3]

Mucus Thickening Agents

Oxytetracycline and progesterone, administered orally, are among a group of agents recognized to thicken mucus.[41, 58] Clinical application of these agents would require the recognition of those patients with low-viscosity mucus.[5]

EFFECTS OF MUCOLYTICS ON MUCOCILIARY TRANSPORT

Mucociliary clearance is measured by the rate of removal of inhaled markers (usually radiolabeled aerosol particles) from the lungs. Mucous transport velocity measures the absolute velocity of marker particles visualized endoscopically or detected externally using gamma emission detection or cinefluoroscopy. Such techniques have been extensively applied to studies of mucous transport in both health and disease.[59–63]

Acetylcysteine has not been shown to have a significant effect on mucociliary clearance or tracheal mucous velocity in smoking and nonsmoking healthy humans, chronic bronchitics, or in dogs.[64–66] Glyceryl guaiacolate (guaifenesin), although used extensively as an expectorant, also appears to have little short-term effect on mucociliary clearance in patients with chronic bronchitis.[67] In contrast, bromhexine, used widely in the United Kingdom and Europe, reduces the viscosity of sputum[68] and, following long-term administration, has been shown to enhance mucociliary clearance.[69]

EFFICACY OF MUCOLYTICS AND EXPECTORANTS

The obstruction of small airways by mucus is a major contributor to the pathophysiology of chronic bronchitis,[70] and attempts to mobilize mucus have produced improvements in vital capacity in those with chronic bronchitis[71] and cystic fibrosis.[72] Several studies have shown significant relationships among the viscosity of sputum in asthma, chronic bronchitis, and cystic fibrosis and tests of pulmonary function.[71–73] The higher the viscosity of sputum, the lower the values of various parameters, such as the forced expiratory volume in 1 second (FEV_1). Logically, it would be expected that the administration of a mucolytic would improve the FEV_1 in such patients.

Unfortunately, in asthmatics, the inhalation of acetylcysteine produces rapid onset of bronchoconstriction, which can persist for more than 30 minutes.[74, 75] In patients with chronic bronchitis the effects on airway function seem to be less consistent, with both improvement and deterioration being reported.[76, 77] In health, the administration of a 20% solution of *N*-acetylcysteine appears to have little effect on measures of airways obstruction.[74, 75] Bronchospasm has also been reported following the administration of pancreatic dornase and trypsin.[78, 79] Because mucolytics induce bronchospasm they are usually administered in combination with a bronchodilator, which can effectively prevent the bronchoconstrictor side effects.[80, 81]

The most effective mucolytic agents available are sulfhydryl compounds, such as acetylcysteine, which liquefy both mucoid and purulent bronchial secretions.[2, 3] Although there is a thinning of the sputum with in vitro application of acetylcysteine, pulmonary function does not improve substantially with in vivo administration. Studies have shown no change in the volume of sputum of patients with stable chronic bronchitis who were administered aerosolized acetylcysteine, although their sputum was thinned by this treatment.[82] In other studies, the subjective improvement in certain patients with COPD was attributed to the simultaneous use of a bronchodilator with the aerosolized acetylcysteine. In the presence of very thick bronchial secretions, acetylcysteine may disrupt the gel structure and loosen a mucous plug obstructing an airway.[83, 84] Direct instillation of acetylcysteine in the liquid form is more effective for this purpose than aerosol inhalation.[85]

Acetylcysteine has been studied in patients with chronic bronchitis and asthma over the short term (less than 1 month) and longer term (6 months), administered by the inhaled and oral routes.[76, 77, 86] Oral acetylcysteine binds to serum proteins and is released as an active agent to be widely distributed throughout the body. Detectable levels of active drug have been demonstrated in the lung tissues of experimental animals.[86]

In a multicenter study[88] involving 500 patients with chronic bronchitis in a double-blind, parallel study, acetylcysteine was evaluated over a 6-month period. The outcome was assessed by a number of clinical criteria, including quantity, thickness, and purulence of sputum, difficulty of expectoration, severity of cough, and number of acute exacerbations of bronchitis. Significant reductions in acute exacerbations, and in the quantity, thickness, and purulence of sputum were seen by the end of the 6-month study period. Spirometric assessment revealed an increase in the FEV_1 and forced vital capacity (FVC) of less than 100 ml following acetylcysteine. Although this was a statistically significant effect, the clinical significance of this small change is uncertain.

In a similar study[89] evaluating the effects of oral acetylcysteine over 6 months in those with chronic bronchitis, a reduction in the number of acute exacerbations of bronchitis was observed. However, the decrease in FEV_1 over the trial period was the same in both the active drug and placebo groups. Over a shorter period of 4 weeks, Aylward and colleagues showed marginal improvements in group forced expiratory peak flow and FEV_1, changes that were associated with increases in the "pourability" of the expectorated sputum.[90]

Thus, the evidence supporting a therapeutic benefit of acetylcysteine in those with chronic bronchitis is often subjective and largely unsupported by major improvements in spirometric measures.[54, 90, 91] However, it may be unreasonable to expect dramatic physiologic changes in a disease that is chronic in nature when treatment is evaluated over a relatively short period. Ambroxol [*trans*-4-(2-amino-3,5-dibromobenzylamino)cyclohexanolhydrochloride], a metabolite of bromhexine, has been shown to have inconsistent effects on mucociliary clearance.[92, 93] Although ambroxol has been widely used in chronic bronchitics in Europe as a secretolytic, a double-blind study showed no effect on peak flow, FEV_1, or chest symptoms over a 4-week period.[94] Although the treatment period was relatively short, the benefits reported by others were not confirmed.[95]

There have been conflicting reports of the effect of bromhexine used orally or intravenously on sputum volume, ease of expectoration, and ventilatory capacity.[96–98] Early uncontrolled studies suggested symptomatic and lung function improvement,[99] but controlled clinical evaluation has failed to demonstrate therapeutic benefit.[100, 101] Generally, in most of these studies, medication was administered for a relatively short period (less than 1 month), and the number of patients studied was small.

Pancreatic dornase contains deoxyribonuclease, which degrades deoxyribonucleoprotein and DNA. Deoxyribonuclease depolymerizes DNA in vitro, with a substantial reduction in viscosity and thickness of purulent sputum. It has been suggested that part of this action is a result of a protein in the sputum that becomes active when DNA is depolymerized.[102, 103] Because DNA is released from the breakdown of pus cells and is therefore present only in purulent sputum, deoxyribonuclease is an agent to be used with frankly purulent secretions.

Aerosolized dornase has been reported to improve the elimination of viscous bronchial secretions and may facilitate local antimicrobial treatment; by depolymerizing DNA, it may prevent the inactivation of antimicrobial drugs that results from their binding to DNA.[104, 105] Dornase is degraded by metals and so it must be used with a plastic or glass nebulizer. In several cases, bronchoconstriction, fever, and pharyngeal irritation have been reported with the use of dornase;[78] its use is not advisable in patients with asthma. Although dornase may be beneficial in the treatment of viscid, purulent secretions, acetylcysteine is regarded as the preferred aerosolized mucolytic agent. Dornase is not currently dispensed in the U.S. for use as an aerosolized mucolytic.

Proteolytic enzymes such as trypsin, chymotrypsin, and streptokinase have been proposed as mucolytic agents based on their efficacy in vitro. Like other mucolytic agents, however, the results of clinical trials have not fulfilled expectations. Trypsin, for example, is highly irritating, and can lead to sensitization and epithelial dysplasia.[106, 107]

Buffered L-arginine has been reported to produce beneficial effects in patients with cystic fibrosis.[108] It is believed that L-arginine disrupts hydrogen bonds, binds calcium, and has detergent activity. The detergent tyloxapol, in combination with bicarbonate and glycerin (Alevaire), is one of the more commonly adopted inhalational agents. Apart from its mucolytic and expectorant activity, Alevaire can enhance the deposition of other active agents, such as bronchodilators, by stabilizing aerosol droplets.[109]

CYSTIC FIBROSIS

The suppression of infection by antibiotics and the enhancement of sputum expectoration by physical therapy and coughing are important mainstays of the treatment of cystic fibrosis. Mucolytics are frequently added to this regimen in an attempt to improve the clearance of airway mucus. Clinical trials, however, have been inconclusive following administration of acetylcysteine by inhalation and the oral route.[111, 112] Results from studies of both routes of administration appear to be similar in terms of clinical response over the short term.[112, 113] After treatment for 3 months, Mitchell and Elliott[110] could not demonstrate a significant response in terms of clinical parameters or peak flow to oral acetylcysteine in a controlled trial. In a controlled trial comparing acetylcysteine and ambroxol to placebo over 3 months, Ratjen and colleagues[114] could not demonstrate clinical improvement and found only a small difference in the FEV_1, which deteriorated more within the placebo group.

If a rational approach to therapy is to be made, only those cystic fibrosis patients with mucus of increased viscosity and elasticity should be selected for treatment with mucolytics. Surprisingly, the viscosity of mucus in cystic fibrosis appears to be little different from that in non-cystic fibrosis patients.[115-117] By applying several measures of mucous rheology, Puchelle and associates[118] showed sputum viscosity to be increased only in those patients with superinfection or a low clinical Schwachman score.[119] Studies of mucociliary transport in cystic fibrosis have demonstrated impaired and even retrograde movement of mucus compared to that in chronic bronchitis patients or healthy subjects.[120] Retrograde movement of mucus, against the prevailing direction of the mucociliary escalator, is much more likely to respond to postural drainage than to the administration of mucolytics, which might even exaggerate retrograde mucous flow and further impair mucociliary clearance.

The popularity and widespread use of mucolytic and related agents is understandable in view of the pathophysiologic and clinical features of chronic bronchitis and the in vitro efficacy of mucolytics in modifying the rheologic properties of sputum. Early uncontrolled clinical trials supported the clinical impression of benefit but were largely unconfirmed by subsequent controlled experiments. Although it is possible that the pharmacologic modification of sputum has no significant short-term or lasting benefit, even the best-designed studies might be criticized on the basis of inadequate mucolytic dosage, relatively short duration of therapy, or the use of too few objective criteria (i.e., use of spirometric parameters alone without measures of ventilation distribution or gas exchange). Chronic bronchitics remain a heterogeneous group of patients, with varying degrees of airways obstruction, mucous hypersecretion, and mucous rheology. Before the therapeutic efficacy of mucolytics can be finally established or refuted, the effects of such agents should be studied in a more homogeneous group of patients characterized prospectively by their sputum rheology. Therapy would need to be extended for periods of up to 1 year or longer, and studies should use multiple objective outcome criteria.

REFERENCES

1. Sheffner A. The reduction in vitro in viscosity of mucoprotein solutions by a new mucolytic agent, *N*-acetylcysteine. Ann NY Acad Sci 1963; 106:298–310.
2. Hirsch SR, Zastrow JE, Kory RC. Sputum liquefying agents: A comparative in vitro evaluation. J Lab Clin Med 1969; 74:346–353.
3. Lieberman J. Measurement of sputum viscosity in a cone-plate viscometer. II. An evaluation of mucolytic agents in vitro. Am Rev Respir Dis 1968; 97:662–672.
4. Limber CR, Reiser HG, Roettig LC, Curtis GM. Enzymatic lysis of respiratory secretions by aerosol trypsin. JAMA 1952; 149:816–821.
5. Davis SS, Deverell LC. Rheological factors in mucociliary clearance. Mod Probl Paediatr 1977;19:207–217.
6. Ziment I. Respiratory Pharmacology and Therapeutics. Philadelphia: W. B. Saunders, 1978.
7. Miller DL, Jones R. A study of techniques for the examination of sputum in a field study of chronic bronchitis. Am Rev Respir Dis 1963; 88:473–483.
8. Sturgess JM, Palfrey AJ, Reid L. Rheological properties of sputum. Rheol Acta 1971; 10:36–43.
9. Lopes-Vidriero MT, Das I, Reid LM. Airway secretion: Source, biochemical and rheological properties. In: Brain JD, Proctor DF, Reid LM, eds. Respiratory Defense Mechanisms, Part I. New York: Marcel Dekker, 1977; 289–356.
10. Coles SJ, Hbaskar KR, O'Sullivan DD, et al. Airway mucus: Composition and regulation of its secretion by neuropeptides in vitro. Ciba Found Symp 1984; 109:40–60.
11. Clamp JR, Creeth FM. Some non-mucin components of mucus and their possible biological roles. Ciba Found Symp 1984; 109:121–136.
12. Litt M. Mucous rheology: Relevance to mucociliary clearance. Arch Intern Med 1970; 126:417–423.
13. Litt M. Flow behavior of mucus. Ann Otol Rhinol Laryngol 1971; 80:330–335.
14. Gelman RA, Meyer FA. Mucociliary transference rate and mucous viscoelasticity. Dependence on dynamic storage and loss modulus. Am Rev Respir Dis 197; 120:553–557.
15. Litt M. Physicochemical determinants of mucociliary flow. Chest 1981; 80(Suppl):846–849.
16. Benis AM, Puchelle E, Sadoul P. Adaption of a concentric cylinder viscometer to the routine measurement of the viscoelastic properties of sputum. In: Gabelnick HL, ed. Rheology of Biological Systems. U.S.A.: CC Thomas, 1973, 173–191.
17. Atassi MZ, Baker SA, Houghton LE, Mullard KG. Mucoproteins of bronchial mucins. Nature 1961; 192:1269–1270.
18. Atassi MZ, Barker SA, Stacey M. Neuraminic acid and its relation to chronic bronchitis. V. Glass-column electrophoresis of sputum. Clin Chem Acta 1962; 7:706–709.
19. Sturgess JM, Palfrey AJ, Reid L. Rheological properties of sputum. Rheol Acta 1971; 10:36–43.
20. Puchelle E, Azhm J, Polu J, Sadoul P. Drug effects on viscoelasticity of mucus. Eur J Respir Dis 1980; 61(Suppl):195–203.
21. Keal E. Methodes d'étude des modification de la secretion bronchique et de la viscosité. Poumun Coeur 1970; 26:52–58.
22. Chodosh S, Medici TC, Enslein K. Comparison of five methods for measuring sputum physical characteristics. Bull Physiopathol Respir 1973; 9:127–139.
23. Dulfano MJ. Viscoelastic studies using capillary methods. Bull Physiopathol Respir 1973; 9:91–101.
24. Kim CS, Berly BB, Abraham WM, Wanner A. A micro double capillary method for rheologic measurements of lower airway secretions. Bull Physiopathol Respir 1982; 18:915–927.
25. Denton R, Forsman W, Hwang SH, et al. Viscoelasticity of mucus. Rev Respir Dis 1968; 98:380–391.
26. Davis SS, Dippy JE. Rheological properties of sputum. Biorheology 1969; 6:11–21.
27. Palmer KNV, Ballabtyre D, Diament ML, Hamilton WFD. The rheology of bronchitic sputum. Br J Dis Chest 1970; 64:185–191.
28. Keal EE. Biochemistry and rheology of sputum in asthma. Postgrad Med J 1971; 47:171–177.
29. Davis SS, Warburton B, Dippy JE. The chemical balance as a rheometer for biological fluids. J Pharm Sci 1970; 59:1764–1769.
30. Puchelle E, Zahm JM, Duvivier C. Spinability of bronchial mucus. Relationship with viscoelasticity and mucous transport properties. Biorheology 1983; 20:239–249.
31. Wanner A. Clinical aspects of mucociliary transport. Am Rev Respir Dis 1977; 116:73–125.
32. Chodosh S, Baigelman W, Medici TC, Enslein K. Long-term home use of acetylcysteine in chronic bronchitis. Curr Ther Res 1975; 17:319–344.

33. Davis SS, Scobie S, Inglis A. The effect of sulfhydryl compounds and cross-linking agents on the viscous and viscoelastic properties of mucus. Biorheology 1975; 13:225.
34. Hirsch SR, Viernes PF, Korey RC. Clinical and physiological evaluation of mucolytic agents nebulized with isoproterenol: 10 percent 2-mercaptoethanol sulfonate. Thorax 1970; 25:737–743.
35. Sheffner AL. The reduction in vitro in viscosity of mucoprotein solutions by a new mucolytic agent *N*-acetyl-L-cysteine. Ann NY Acad Sci 1963; 106:298–302.
36. Sadoul P, Puchelle E, Girard F. Criteria for evaluating mucous functions and their disorders in chronic bronchitis. Respiratory tract mucus. Ciba Found Symp 1978; 54:277–295.
37. Marriott C, Kellaway IW. The effect of tetracyclines on the viscoelastic properties of bronchial mucus. Biorheology 1975; 12:391–395.
38. Gilboa A, Silberberg A. In-situ rheological characterization of epithelial mucus. Biorheology 1976; 13:59–65.
39. Afzelius BA. "Immotile-cilia" syndrome and ciliary abnormalities induced by infection and injury. Am Rev Respir Dis 1981; 124:107–109.
40. Rossman CM, Forrest JB, Ruffin RE, Newhouse MT. The dyskinetic cilia syndrome: Ciliary motility in persons with and without Kartegener's syndrome. Am Rev Respir Dis 1980; 121:1011–1016.
41. Miskovitz G, Appel J, Szule P. Ultrastructural changes of ciliated columnar epithelium and goblet cells in chronic bronchitis biopsy material. Acta Morphol Acad Sci Hung 1974; 22:91–98.
42. Pedersen M, Neilsen OH. Ciliary motility in cystic fibrosis. Proceedings of the 11th Annual Meeting of the European Working Group on Cystic Fibrosis. Brussels: Belgium Cystic Fibrosis Association, 1982, 108–109.
43. Barton AD, Weiss SGT, Lourenco RV, et al. Mucous glycoprotein content of chronic bronchitis sputum. Proc Soc Exp Biol Med 1977; 156:8–13.
44. Havez R, Roussel P, Degand P, et al. Biochemical exploration of bronchial hypersecretion. Protides Biol Fluids 1968; 16:343–360.
45. Lopez-Vidriero MT. Variation in neuraminic acid and fucose content of sputum in disease and during treatment. London University, Ph.D. thesis, 1976.
46. Keal EE, Reid L. Neuraminic acid content of sputum in chronic bronchitis. Thorax 1972; 27:643–653.
47. Sturgess JM, Palfrey AJ, Reid L. The viscosity of bronchial secretion. Clin Sci 1970; 38:145–156.
48. Puchelle E, Zahm JM, Havez R. Relation des proteines et mucines bronchique avec les properties rheologiques. Bull Physiopathol Respir 1973; 9:237–256.
49. Marriott C, Richards JH. The effects of storage and of potassium iodide, urea, *N*-acetylcysteine and Triton X-100 on the viscosity of bronchial mucus. Br J Dis Chest 1974; 68:171–182.
50. Martin R, Litt M, Marriott C. The effect of mucolytic agents on the rheologic and transport properties of canine tracheal mucus. Am Rev Respir Dis 1980; 121:495–500.
51. Chodosh S. Acetylcysteine in chronic bronchitis. Eur J Respir Dis 1980; 61(S111):90–92.
52. Verstraeten JM. Mucolytic treatment in chronic airways obstruction. Double-blind clinical trial with acetylcysteine, bromhexine and placebo. Eur J Respir Dis 1980; 61(S111):77.
53. Hirsch SR, Viernes PF, Kory RC. The expectorant effect of glyceryl guaiacolate in patients with chronic bronchitis. A controlled in vitro and in vivo study. Chest 1973; 63:9–14.
54. Boyd Em, Sheppard P. On the expectorant activity of Bisolvon. Arch Int Pharmacodyn Ther 1966; 163:284–290.
55. Burgi H. Change in the fibre system and viscosity of the sputum of bronchitics during treatment with bromhexine and guaiprenesin (guaicin glyceryl ether). Scand J Respir Dis [Suppl]1974; 90:81–84.
56. Lightowler JE, Lightowler NM. Comparative mucolytic studies on dithiothreitol, *N*-acetylcysteine and L-cysteine on human respiratory mucus in vitro and their effects on the flow of mucus in the exposed trachea of the rat on topical application. Arch Int Pharmacodyn Ther 1971; 189:53–58.
57. Hirsch SR. In vitro evaluation of expectorant and mucolytic agents. Bull Physiopathol Respir 1973; 9:435–438.
58. Brown DT. The interactions of some drugs with purified bronchial mucous glycoproteins. University of Nottingham, Ph.D. thesis, 1980.
59. Yeates DB, Aspin N, Levinson H, et al. Mucociliary tracheal transport rates in man. J Appl Physiol 1975; 39:487–495.
60. Goodman RM, Yergin BM, Landa JF, et al. Tracheal mucous velocity in non-smokers, smokers, and patients with obstructive lung disease. Fed Proc 1977; 36:607.
61. Wilkey DD, Lee PS, Hass FJ, et al. Mucociliary clearance of deposited particles from the lung: Intra- and intersubject reproducibility, total and regional clearance, and model comparison. Arch Environ Health 1980; 35:294–302.
62. Garrard CS, Levandowsky R, Gerrity TR, et al. The effects of acute respiratory viral infection upon tracheal mucous velocity in man. Arch Environ Health 1985; 40:322–325.
63. Garrard CS, Gerrity TR, Yeates DB. The relationships of aerosol deposition, lung size, and the rate of mucociliary clearance. Arch Environ Health 1986; 41:11–15.
64. Goodman RM, Yergin BM, Sackner MA. Effects of *S*-carboxymethylcysteine on tracheal mucous velocity. Chest 1978; 74:615–618.
65. Martin R, Litt M, Marriott C. The effect of mucolytic agents on the rheologic and transport properties of canine tracheal mucus. Am Rev Respir Dis 1980; 121:495–500.
66. Thomson ML, Pavia D, Jones CJ, McQuiston TAC. No demonstrable effect of *S*-carboxymethylcysteine on clearance of secretions from the human lung. Thorax 1975; 30:669–673.
67. Yeates DB, Cohen VR, Davis AL, et al. Effect of glyceryl guaiacolate in bronchial clearance in patients with chronic bronchitis (abstract). Am Rev Respir Dis 1977; 115:182.
68. Bruce RA, Kuman V. The effect of a derivative of vassicine on bronchial mucus. Br J Clin Pract 1968; 22:289–292.
69. Thomson ML, Pavia D, Gregg I, Stark JE. Bromhexine and mucociliary clearance in chronic bronchitics. Br J Dis Chest 1974; 68:21–27.
70. Hogg JC, Macklem PT, Thurlbeck WM. Site and nature of airway obstruction in obstructive lung disease. N Engl J Med 1968; 278:1355–1366.
71. Pham QT, Peslin R, Puchelle E, et al. Respiratory function and the rheological status of bronchial secretions collected by spontaneous expectoration and after physiotherapy. Bull Physiopathol Respir 1973; 9:293–314.
72. Polgar G, Denton R. Cystic fibrosis in adults. Studies of pulmonary function and some physical properties of bronchial mucus. Am Rev Respir Dis 1972; 85:319–327.
73. Chodosh S, Medici TC, Ishikawa S, Enslein K. Relationship of physical sputum characteristics and ventilatory capacity in chronic bronchial disease. Chest 1973; 63(Suppl):56–58.
74. Rao S, Wilson DB, Brooks RC, Sproule BJ. Acute effects of nebulization of *N*-acetylcysteine on pulmonary mechanics and gas exchange. Am Rev Respir Dis 1970; 102:17–22.
75. Bernstein IL, Ausdenmoore RW. Iatrogenic bronchospasm occurring during clinical trials of a new mucolytic agent, acetylcysteine. Dis Chest 1964; 46:469–473.
76. Hirsch SR, Kory RC. An evaluation of the effect of nebulized *N*-acetylcysteine on sputum consistency. J Allergy 1967; 39:265–273.
77. Sabath LD, Sasahara AA, Burlesen VA. Evaluation of a new mucolytic agent. Dis Chest 1966; 50:47–56.
78. Raskin P. Bronchospasm after inhalation of pancreatic dornase. Am Rev Respir Dis 1968; 98:697–698.
79. Unger L, Unger AH. Trypsin inhalation in respiratory conditions with thick sputum. JAMA 1953; 152:1109–1113.
80. Kory RC, Hirsch SR, Giraldo J. Nebulization of *N*-acetylcysteine combined with a bronchodilator in patients with chronic bronchitis: A controlled study. Dis Chest 1968; 54:504–509.
81. Pulle DF, Glass P, Dulfano MJ. A controlled study of the safety and efficacy of acetylcysteine-isoproterenol combination. Curr Ther Res 1970; 12:485–492.
82. Barton AD. Aerosolized detergents and mucolytic agents in the treatment of stable chronic obstructive pulmonary disease. Am Rev Respir Dis 1974; 110:104–110.
83. Lieberman J. The appropriate use of mucolytic agents. Am J Med 1970; 49:1–4.
84. Urschel HC, Paulson DL, Shaw RR. Mucoid impaction of the bronchi. Ann Thorac Surg 1966; 2:1–16.
85. Irwin RS, Thomas HM. Mucoid impactions of the bronchus: Diagnosis and treatment. Am Rev Respir Dis 1973; 108:955–999.
86. Grater WC, Cato A. Double-blind study of acetylcysteine-iso-

proterenol and saline-isoproterenol in non-hospitalized patients with asthma. Curr Ther Res 1973; 15:660–671.
87. Rodenstein D, De Coster A, Gazzaniga A. Pharmacokinetics of oral acetylcysteine. Absorption, binding and metabolism in patients with respiratory disorders. Clin Pharmacokinet 1978; 3:247–254.
88. Multicenter Study Group. Long-term oral acetylcysteine in chronic bronchitis, a double-blind controlled study. Eur J Respir Dis 1980; 61(Suppl 111):93–108.
89. Boman G, Backer U, Larsson S, et al. Oral acetylcysteine reduces exacerbation rate in chronic bronchitis: Report of a trial organized by the Swedish Society for Pulmonary Diseases. Eur J Respir Dis 1983; 64:405–415.
90. Aylward M, Maddock J, Dewland P. Clinical evaluation of acetylcysteine in the treatment of patients with chronic obstructive bronchitis. A balanced double-blind trial with placebo control. Eur J Respir Dis 1980; 61(Suppl 111):81–89.
91. Grassi C, Morandini GC. A controlled trial of intermittent oral acetylcysteine in the long-term treatment of chronic bronchitis. Eur J Clin Pharmacol 1976; 9:393–396.
92. Allegra L, Bossi R, Braga P. Influence of surfactant on mucociliary transport. Eur J Respir Dis 1985; 142:71–76.
93. Weiss T, Dorow P, Felix B. Effects of a beta-adrenergic drug and a secretolytic agent on regional mucociliary clearance in patients with COLD. Chest 1981; 80:881–885.
94. Guyatt GTH, Townsend M, Kazin F, Newhouse MT. A controlled trial of ambroxol in chronic bronchitis. Chest 1987; 92:618–620.
95. Ericsson CH, Juhasz J, Jonsson E, Mossberg B. Ambroxol therapy in simple chronic bronchitis: Effects on subjective symptoms and pulmonary functions. Eur J Respir Dis 1986; 69:248–255.
96. Hamilton WFD, Palmer KNV, Gent M. Expectorant action of bromhexine in chronic obstructive bronchitis. Br Med J 1970; 3:260–261.
97. Lal S, Bhalla KK. A controlled trial of bromhexine (Bisolvon) in outpatients with chronic bronchitis. Curr Med Res Opin 1975; 3:63–67.
98. Armstrong ML. Double-blind crossover trial of bromhexine (Bisolvon) in the treatment of chronic bronchitis. Med J Aust 1976; 1:612–617.
99. Matts SGF. Clinical experience of "Bisolvon" in 220 cases of chest disease. Br J Clin Pract 1969; 23:501–502.
100. Larglands JHM. Double-blind clinical trial of bromhexine as a mucolytic drug in chronic bronchitics. Lancet 1971; i:448–450.
101. Thompson KJ. A clinical trial of bromhexine. NZ Med J 1972; 70:73–76.
102. Lieberman J, Kurnick NB. Influence of deoxyribonucleic acid content on the proteolysis of sputum and pus. Nature 1962; 196:988–990.
103. Lieberman J, Kurnick NB. Proteolytic enzyme activity and the role of deoxyribonucleic acid in cystic fibrosis sputum. Pediatrics 1963; 31:1028–1032.
104. Salomon A, Herchfus JA, Segal MS. Aerosols of pancreatic dornase and antibiotics in bronchopulmonary disease. Ann Allergy 1954; 12:71–79.
105. Spier R, Witebsky E, Paine JR. Aerosolized pancreatic dornase and antibiotics in pulmonary infections: Use in patients with post-operative and non-operative infections. JAMA 1961; 178:878–886.
106. Unger L, Unger AH. The use of Tryptar (trypsin) in bronchial asthma and other respiratory conditions. Ann Allergy 1953; 11:494–501.
107. Farber SM, Pharr SL, Traut HF, et al. Metaplasia and dyskeratosis of bronchial epithelial cells following inhalation of trypsin and deoxyribonuclease. Lab Invest 1954; 3:33–38.
108. Solomons CC, Cotton EK, DuBois R. The use of buffered L-arginine in the treatment of cystic fibrosis. Pediatrics 1971; 47:384–390.
109. Walkenhorst W, Dautrebande L. New studies on aerosols 23. Arch Int Pharmacodyn Ther 1964; 150:264–294.
110. Mitchell EA, Elliott RB. Controlled trial of oral *N*-acetylcysteine in cystic fibrosis. Aust Paediatr J 1982; 18:40–42.
111. Reas HW. The use of *N*-acetylcysteine in the treatment of cystic fibrosis. J Pediatr 1964; 65:542–557.
112. Stephan U, Bowin B, Goering U, et al. Acetylcysteine in the oral mucolytic treatment of cystic fibrosis. Eur J Respir Dis 1980; 61(Suppl 111):127–131.
113. Crotz M, Kraemer R, Kerrebijn KR, Popow C. Oral acetylcysteine in cystic fibrosis. A co-operative study. Eur J Respir Dis 1980; 61(Suppl 111):122–126.
114. Ratjen F, Wonne R, Posselt HG, et al. A double-blind placebo-controlled trial with oral ambroxol, *N*-acetylcysteine for mucolytic treatment in cystic fibrosis. Eur J Pediatr 1985; 144:374–378.
115. Charman J, Ried L. Sputum viscosity in chronic bronchitis, bronchiectasis, asthma and cystic fibrosis. Biorheology 1972; 9:185–195.
116. Picot R, Pas I, Ried L. Pus, deoxyribonucleic acid, and sputum viscosity. Thorax 1978; 33:235–242.
117. King M. Is cystic fibrosis mucus abnormal? Pediatr Res 1981; 15:120–123.
118. Puchelle E, Jacquist J, Beck G, et al. Rheological and transport properties of airway secretions in cystic fibrosis—relationships with the degree of infection and severity of the disease. Eur J Clin Invest 1985; 15:389–394.
119. Schwachman H, Kulczycki LL. Long-term study of a hundred and five patients with cystic fibrosis; studies made over a five- to fourteen-year period. Am J Dis Child 1958; 96:6–15.
120. Garrard CS, Lourenco RV. Mucociliary clearance. In: Montenegro HD, ed. Chronic Obstructive Pulmonary Disease. New York: Churchill Livingstone, 1984, 29–48.

Chapter 48

OXYGEN THERAPY IN THE TREATMENT OF COPD

David C. Flenley

Joseph Priestley, who discovered oxygen in 1774, suggested that it might be "peculiarly salutary to the lungs in certain morbid cases." This notion was put into practice by Dr. Thomas Beddoes, who used oxygen therapeutically in his Pneumatic Institution in Clifton, Bristol (as described in his book *The Medicinal Uses of Factitious Airs,* published in 1798).

Oxygen is the final acceptor of the electron transfer system in the cellular mitochondria. Metabolism in the presence of oxygen generates 30 molecules of high-energy adenosine triphosphate (ATP) from each molecule of glucose. Without oxygen, however, glycolysis only yields three molecules of ATP for each glucose molecule, along with the formation of lactic acid. Oxygen reaches the mitochondria by diffusion from a neighboring capillary, in which oxygen is in combination with hemoglobin in the red cell. Oxygen delivery to the mitochondria thus depends on alveolar ventilation, the distribution of ventilation-perfusion relationships within lung alveoli, the circulating hemoglobin concentration, the affinity of the hemoglobin molecule for oxygen, and the concentration of other ligands of hemoglobin (e.g., pH, diphosphoglycerate, CO, CO_2 etc). In addition, the cardiac output and distribution of capillary blood flow within the tissues are also important. The only way in which oxygen therapy, which can only raise the inspired oxygen concentration, can improve delivery of oxygen is to restore the saturation of the circulating hemoglobin within the arterial blood toward normal.

MECHANISMS AND CONSEQUENCES OF HYPOXEMIA IN COPD

Mechanisms of Hypoxemia

Mechanisms include alveolar hypoventilation (in which hypoxia is combined with a raised Pa_{CO_2}) and ventilation-perfusion ($\dot{V}/\dot{Q}$) imbalance, in which underventilation of some alveoli (with a consequent low P_{O_2} in the blood draining from them) cannot be compensated for by overventilation of similarly perfused alveoli because of the sigmoid shape of the oxygen-hemoglobin dissociation curve. Such ventilation-perfusion imbalance is the most common cause of hypoxemia in COPD but an element of alveolar hypoventilation may also be present, particularly in acute exacerbations of chronic respiratory failure (see subsequent discussion). A true shunt, in which some desaturated blood from the right side of the heart entirely bypasses the ventilated alveoli, but still flows into the arterial blood, is relatively uncommon in COPD patients unless there are also areas of pneumonic consolidation, or atelectasis. A marked increase in the pulmonary arterial pressure (PAP) during an acute exacerbation of COPD, with CO_2 retention and respiratory acidosis,[1] however, may allow a patent foramen ovale to form a transient right-to-left shunt. This adds a degree of shunt hypoxemia to the marked $\dot{V}/\dot{Q}$ imbalance and alveolar hypoventilation as a mechanism of arterial hypoxemia in these patients. True diffusion hypoxemia, in which thickening of the alveolar capillary membrane prevents equilibration of P_{O_2} between alveoli and the end-pulmonary capillary blood, is probably uncommon in COPD.

The final mechanism causing arterial hypoxemia, a low inspired oxygen P_{O_2} (PI_{O_2}) occurs in patients who are connected to inadequate respiratory therapy or anesthetic devices. It can also occur as altitude hypoxemia, such as in commercial aircraft that are pressurized to an equivalent altitude up to about 9,000 feet (PI_{O_2} 113 mm Hg).[2]

Physiologic Consequences of Hypoxemia

The physiologic consequences of hypoxemia differ for acute and chronic exposures. In most COPD patients hypoxemia is chronic and also involves more severe acute hypoxemia in acute exacerbations (e.g., as with respiratory infection). There are two classic clinical patterns of patients with COPD: "pink puffers" and "blue bloaters." The pink puffers are characterized by relatively modest arterial hypoxemia (at least when at rest and awake), with a low or normal arterial Pa_{CO_2}, no secondary polycythemia, no elevation of pulmonary arterial pressure (at least when at rest), and no cor pulmonale. In contrast, patients with a similar degree of chronic airflow obstruction (i.e., forced expiratory volume in 1 second, or $FEV_1 < 1.5$ L) may present as blue bloaters, with central cyanosis indicating their definite arterial hypoxemia (even when at rest), associated with CO_2 retention, compensated respiratory acidosis, a modest elevation of the PAP, a history of cor pulmonale, and a greater or lesser degree of secondary polycythemia.[3–6]

Earlier notions that blue bloaters had only bronchitis whereas pink puffers had mainly emphysema, although lingering in some textbooks,[7] cannot be sustained either by physiopathologic correlation at autopsy[8] or by the newer method of quantitating emphysema in vivo, which uses the CT scan to measure regional lung density and can determine the increase in size of distal air spaces. This is the defining characteristic of emphysema.[9] The elegant demonstrations of differences in the pattern of gas exchange and ventilation-perfusion relationships in patients with the blue and bloated or pink and puffing pattern[10] were not related to the pathologic extent of emphysema in the lungs in these patients. Therefore, the simple and attractive notion that pink puffers have a high dead space ventilation, whereas blue bloaters tend to have more hypoxemic shunt, because of these alleged (but unproven) differences in lung structure, are regrettably not sustained. Despite this lack of physiopathologic correlation between blue bloaters and pink puffers and underlying lung structure, these descriptions nonetheless remain valid bedside observations, with important therapeutic implications.

Hypoxemia on exercise, even in COPD patients who are normoxic when at rest, is well recognized, although earlier notions that pink puffers tended to become more hypoxemic and blue bloaters became less hypoxemic with exercise[11] have not been widely confirmed. It now seems to be common experience that hypoxemia present when at rest worsens during exercise (i.e., in the blue bloater),[12, 13] and that the increase in cardiac output with exercise is associated with a worsening of pulmonary hypertension in these patients.[14] The long-recognized physiologic association between arterial hypoxemia and pulmonary hypertension, both in animals[15] and in humans during chronic high-altitude hypoxemia,[16] has been particularly observed in the chronic hypoxemia of COPD,[17] in which the mean level of PAP was best correlated with resting arterial oxygen saturation in over 600 patients.

Although altitude studies have long identified secondary polycythemia as a physiologic adaptation to chronic hypoxemia,[18, 19] controversy still surrounds the mechanism of this relationship in patients with hypoxemia caused by COPD. High carboxyhemoglobin (HbCO) levels as a result of chronic cigarette smoking seem to play a more important part in this hematopoietic response than does the level of arterial hypoxemia alone,[20] and persistence of these high HbCO levels in patients allegedly receiving long-term oxygen therapy appears to prevent a reduction in red cell mass with this treatment. In contrast, in others in whom the HbCO levels decreased during long-term oxygen therapy, the red cell mass was restored to more normal values.

Hypoxemia in Sleep in COPD

It is now widely recognized that hypoxemia, often of profound degree, occurs commonly in the rapid eye movement (REM) phase of sleep in patients with chronic bronchitis and emphysema (i.e., COPD) (Fig. 48–1).[21–23] This appears to be related principally to hypoventilation during the REM phase of sleep,[24] rather than to apneic episodes,[25] with an additional component from an increase in ventilation-perfusion mismatch in the lungs during REM sleep.[26] These hypoxemic episodes can be associated with a further increase in pulmonary arterial pressure,[27] leading to the hypothesis that the right ventricular hypertrophy and sustained pulmonary hypertension of the blue and bloated pattern of hypoxemic COPD is related to these recurrent episodes of pulmonary hypertension during recurrent hypoxemia in REM sleep.[28] The recognition of nocturnal oxygen hemoglobin desaturation in COPD patients with a Pa_{O_2} above 60 mm Hg when awake[29] raises the important possibility that this may also contribute to subsequent cor pulmonale, with the development of the blue and bloated syndrome. This theory, however, will take many years to prove or disprove.

The Need for Oxygen in COPD

In COPD chronic hypoxemia is characteristic of the blue and bloated pattern of patients with fixed airways obstruction. Such hypoxemia may be exaggerated during exercise, and this

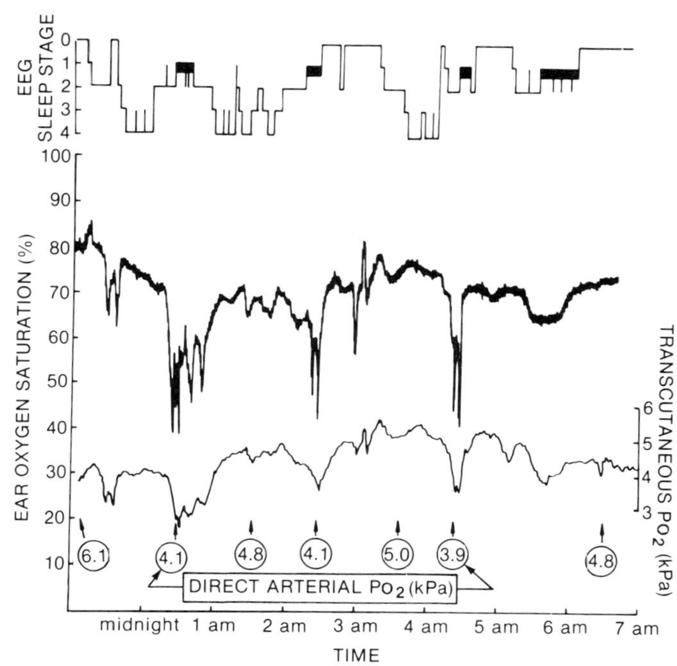

Figure 48–1. Sleep stage, continuous recorded ear oxygen saturation, and continuous transcutaneous P_{O_2} measurements, in a blue bloater throughout a normal night's sleep, breathing air. The EEG scoring (0 = wakefulness, 4 = deep sleep, ■ = rapid eye movement sleep) reveals that the patient did sleep and had periods of profound nocturnal hypoxemia (ear oxygen saturation, transcutaneous P_{O_2}, and directly measured arterial Pa_{O_2}, *bottom line*) during REM sleep.

may also occur in patients who are normoxic when at rest (i.e. pink puffers). Further exacerbation of hypoxemia, to life-threatening levels, is frequently seen in those with acute exacerbations of COPD, in whom CO_2 retention and acute on chronic respiratory acidosis is combined with the hypoxemia. It is now recognized that hypoxemia during REM sleep is common in COPD patients, and that this might be related to the pulmonary hypertension that characterizes blue bloaters. Earlier studies,[30] which related the poor prognosis of these patients to their hypoxemia, implied that correction of the hypoxemia could improve life expectancy. This has now been validated by the two important long-term trials of continuous domiciliary oxygen therapy,[31, 32] which have lent great impetus to the use of oxygen therapy in COPD.

OXYGEN THERAPY IN ACUTE EXACERBATIONS OF COPD

Increasing breathlessness, with cough and expectoration of purulent sputum, possibly with wheeze but rarely accompanied by chest pain, are common hallmarks of the acute exacerbation of COPD. These patients, with chronic airflow limitation and who are already breathless when at rest, have varying degrees of arterial hypoxemia—mild in the pink puffers and more severe in the blue bloater—but a clinical spectrum between these two extremes is frequently encountered. Such acute exacerbations are precipitated most frequently by lower respiratory tract infection, commonly with *Haemophilus influenzae* in combination with *Streptococcus pneumoniae,* but any (or none) of the common respiratory pathogens may be recovered from the sputum in the untreated patient. Although pneumonic consolidation can occur, chest radiographs in these patients are often unrevealing, except possibly for the increase in heart size and dilatation of pulmonary arteries suggesting the increased pulmonary arterial pressure that so frequently accompanies the acute exacerbation with hypoxemia.

It is important to realize that these patients are not invariably very breathless, but that the most important clinical clue is the recognition of central cyanosis. This is confirmed to indicate arterial hypoxemia by arterial blood gas analysis, which usually also reveals a raised Pa_{CO_2} and a greater or lesser degree of respiratory acidosis (Fig. 48–2). In many patients, particularly blue bloaters, CO_2 retention is present even when they are relatively well. This chronic elevation in the P_{CO_2} leads to renal tubular reabsorption of bicarbonate with the result that the arterial pH is characteristically within the normal range, despite the chronic elevated P_{CO_2}, when they are in a chronic stable state.[33, 34]

The problem posed in the management of these patients has been clearly recognized for over 25 years:[35, 36] correction of hypoxemia can be associated with further CO_2 retention, with death from respiratory acidosis[37] (the classic "CO_2 narcosis"). These patients are hypoxic, however, and face the alternative risk of death from hypoxia unless it is corrected. The dilemma is how to guide oxygen therapy so as to prevent death from hypoxia, but not to depress ventilation, with resultant respiratory acidosis and possibly death.

Two alternatives can be suggested:

1. Supervision of controlled oxygen therapy, using guidelines based on arterial blood gas analysis to achieve the above aims; or
2. Mechanical ventilation of the patient, to control respiratory acidosis and CO_2 retention, providing additional oxygen to whatever level is necessary to maintain adequate arterial oxygenation.

Both have advantages and disadvantages, and are discussed here in turn.

Controlled Oxygen Therapy

Respiratory failure can be defined as hypoxemia caused by lung disease (i.e., $P_{O_2} < 60$ mm Hg in a patient at rest, breathing air at sea level). If this hypoxemia is associated with a normal P_{CO_2} it is known as type I respiratory failure, whereas if CO_2 retention is associated with a $P_{CO_2} > 50$ mm Hg it is type II respiratory failure.[36] It is this latter condition, acute on chronic respiratory failure, that is of concern here. Thus, it would be helpful to determine the minimum level of oxygen required and the maximal level of P_{CO_2} (or respiratory acidosis) that can be tolerated. Obviously, the end point of such studies is death—it is clearly unethical to determine a direct experimental answer in humans, and animal studies have failed to provide a definitive answer. Nonetheless, over the years, a consensus has developed that Pa_{O_2} over 50 mm Hg is unlikely to be associated with an immediate risk of hypoxic death provided the patient has an adequate cardiac output, thereby ensuring a reasonable supply of oxygen to the mitochondria. A combination of arterial hypoxemia with a low cardiac output (the shock syndrome) is well recognized as carrying a high mortality and may be revealed by an increased arterial blood lactate level,[38] whereas the lactate level is not raised in hypoxemia, in which the cardiac output is maintained.[39] High lactate levels in shock are associated with a poor prognosis.[40] In acute exacerbations of COPD, however, the cardiac output, although not reaching the high levels formerly seen in the so-called "high-output failure" state, remains normal.[41] The question thus arises of whether a Pa_{O_2} of 50 mm Hg or above be obtained in patients with an acute exacerbation of COPD without a further severe rise in the P_{CO_2} and the development of lethal respiratory acidosis.

Early detailed studies in only ten patients using controlled oxygen therapy have led to the formulation of guidelines to help avoid the two dangers of respiratory acidosis and hypoxia—Pa_{O_2} maintained above 50 mm Hg without the pH falling below 7.25:[42]

Guidelines for controlled O_2 therapy in acute exacerbations of COPD:

1. Blood gas on air, *then,*
2. 2 L/minute O_2 by nasal prongs.
3. Repeat Pa_{O_2}, Pa_{CO_2}, pH in 2 hours.
4. *Aim:* $Pa_{O_2} > 50$ mm Hg and pH > 7.25. If not, administer doxapram or ventilate.

More recently, we have extended these observations to a further series of 157 admissions in 135 patients with acute exacerbations of chronic bronchitis and emphysema causing hypoxemia and CO_2 retention.[43] Patients were selected if,

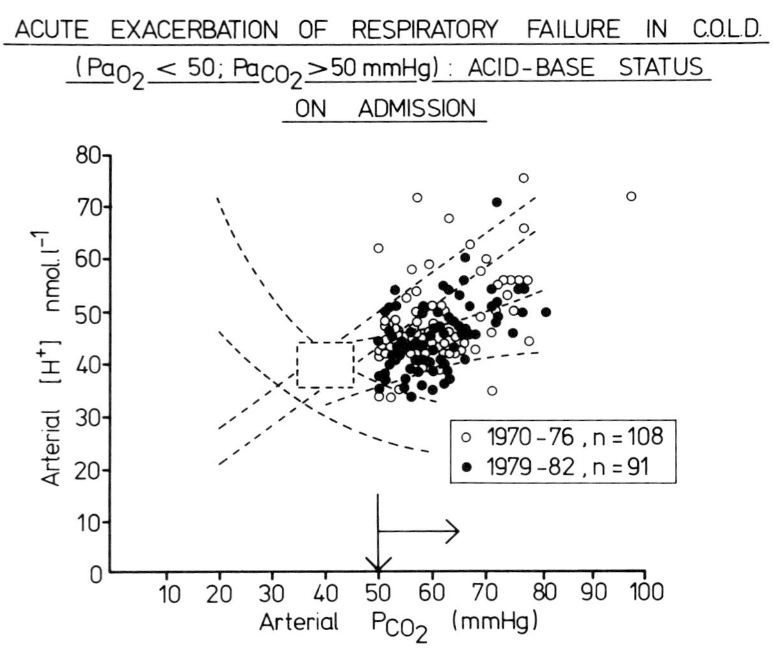

Figure 48–2. Acid-base status in terms of arterial acidity ([H^+]), as nmol/L, plotted against simultaneously determined Pa_{CO_2}, in patients with acute exacerbations of COPD. The patients were admitted to the study if the P_{O_2} was below 50 mm Hg and the P_{CO_2} was above 50 mm Hg. In most patients these measurements were made on admission to hospital when breathing air, and showed acid-base variables lying between the acute and chronic respiratory bands on the [H^+]-P_{CO_2} diagram.

during the acute exacerbation, their Pa_{O_2} (when breathing air on hospital admission) was below 50 mm Hg and/or their Pa_{CO_2} was more than 50 mm Hg. All were treated with controlled oxygen therapy. The risk of death in that episode of acute on chronic respiratory failure increased with the age of the patient, but did not correlate with the severity of hypoxemia on admission. However, those patients in whom the arterial pH fell below 7.26 during the controlled oxygen therapy had a higher death risk than did those in whom acidosis of this severity did not develop. Indeed, the probability of death was best predicted from an equation combining age and the most severe degree of acidosis (lowest arterial pH) that developed during treatment.

Bone and colleagues,[44] in a prospective study of 50 patients treated with controlled oxygen therapy, have also found that the severity of acidosis is a useful guide to prognosis in these patients during an acute exacerbation. They noted that the combination of the degree of arterial hypoxemia and acidosis when breathing air on admission could separate out those patients who ultimately needed mechanical ventilation. This "need" for mechanical ventilation, however, must remain a subjective judgment. It is notable that 26% of their patients "needed" ventilation, including some who had Pa_{O_2} values above 50 mm Hg on admission, in contrast to only 10% of our 135 patients in 157 admissions who were ventilated, although all had a Pa_{O_2} below 50 mm Hg on admission.[43]

A prospective study has been carried out to test the value of these guidelines, which aimed to maintain the Pa_{O_2} above 50 mm Hg without the arterial pH falling below 7.26.[43] If these guidelines could not be met within the first 2 to 4 hours of treatment using controlled oxygen therapy, the ventilatory stimulant drug doxapram (Dopram) was given by continued intravenous infusion. If the guidelines could still not be attained, despite continuance of controlled oxygen therapy, mechanical ventilation was considered. We studied 139 episodes in 95 patients with COPD aged 64 ± 8 years. On admission their Pa_{O_2} when breathing air averaged 37 ± 6.8 mm Hg and their Pa_{CO_2} averaged 60 ± 9 mm Hg. Using the scheme outlined previously, controlled oxygen therapy was started immediately after the initial blood gas measurement when breathing air, as 2 L/minute oxygen administered by nasal prongs, and arterial blood gas levels were measured again 2 hours later. If controlled oxygen therapy alone failed to achieve a $Pa_{O_2} > 50$ mm Hg and the pH was > 7.25, doxapram was used ("needed" in almost 25% of patients); mechanical ventilation was "needed" in only 3% because the guidelines could not be attained. The overall mortality was 13%, which compares with a 7% mortality in 50 episodes when 26% were ventilated,[44] and a 10% mortality in 187 patients when 40% were ventilated artificially.[45]

It seems that following the guidelines for controlled oxygen therapy can result in a low mortality without recourse to mechanical ventilation in most of these patients, thus reducing hazards and costs[46] and helping to prevent complications.[47]

Mechanical Ventilation

Mechanical ventilation of patients with severe airflow obstruction to relieve the hypoxemia and CO_2 retention of respiratory failure in acute exacerbations of COPD is not easy to accomplish. The increase in airways resistance and low respiratory compliance of these patients indicate that high inspiratory pressures are needed to generate adequate tidal volumes. The severe disturbance of the alveolar ventilation-perfusion relationship, however, means that inspired oxygen concentrations may need to be raised above 50% to provide adequate arterial oxygenation. Furthermore, rapid lowering of the Pa_{CO_2} to "normal" physiologic values (i.e., 38 to 40 mm Hg) in these patients, who have chronic pre-existing hypercapnia, and in whom renal tubular reabsorption of bicarbonate has raised plasma bicarbonate levels over many years, must inevitably result in some degree of respiratory alkalosis. This has potentially serious effects on cardiac, gastrointestinal, and neurologic function. Thus, the aim must be to lower the Pa_{CO_2} gradually. It is probably better to aim for a normal arterial pH value (7.42 to 7.38) than for a normal Pa_{CO_2}, provided that oxygenation is adequate (as can be easily arranged by an increase of inspired oxygen concentration) and that there is no gross shunt.

Controversy exists as to the ventilator pattern (e.g., tidal volume, inspiratory pause, flow rate, and respiratory rate). An increase in inspiratory flow has been claimed to improve gas exchange and increase respiratory system compliance in patients with severe airway obstruction.[48] Others,[49] however, have proposed a low minute ventilation but with a high inspiratory flow rate to minimize pulmonary hyperinflation. In contrast, Darioli and Perret[50] obtained 100% survival in 26 severe asthmatics who received mechanical ventilation using a low respiratory frequency (6 to 10 cycles/minute) with a tidal volume of 8 to 12 ml/kg. The Pa_{CO_2} was frequently not corrected to normal by these ventilator settings but the peak maximal airway pressure did not exceed 50 cm H_2O, thereby avoiding the risk of barotrauma.

Others[51] have shown that the slow expiratory flow rate, which is a consequence of the high airflow resistance in patients with either severe asthma or severe COPD, can indicate that progressive hyperinflation might occur and be complicated by pulmonary barotrauma and circulatory depression. They[51] have suggested that the volume exhaled during apnea is a sensitive and reproducible measurement of the extent of pulmonary hyperinflation. Furthermore, they suggested that this is more important than the airway pressures, which largely depend on the severity of airway obstruction. Again, the implication is that hypercapnia can be well tolerated in these patients even during mechanical ventilation and hyperinflation reduced to a minimum by reducing the tidal volume, with a constant minute ventilation, or by increasing the expiratory time.

LONG-TERM HOME OXYGEN THERAPY

The modern era of long-term oxygen therapy began in Denver, where Neff and Petty[52] showed that long-term home oxygen could improve survival in patients who suffered from severe hypoxic COPD despite living in the mile-high city. Similar uncontrolled studies[53, 54] have supported this idea, but formal testing of the proposal by two controlled clinical trials[32, 55] was required to show that long-term oxygen therapy is the only method for prolonging life in patients with the blue and bloated pattern of chronic bronchitis and emphysema (COPD). These two important studies, when combined, reported data on just under 300 patients (Table 48–1) who had fixed airways obstruction, chronic hypoxemia, ($P_{O_2} < 55$ mm Hg when breathing air when awake), most with CO_2 retention (particularly in the British series[32]), and modest pulmonary hypertension. The results (Fig. 48–3) indicate that, without oxygen, only about 30% of patients survive for 3 years, that oxygen for *some of the time* (12 to 15 hours) during the 24-hour day produces a significant improvement in survival, and that the best survival is obtained with oxygen for *most of the time*—that is, more than 19 hours in the 24-hour day.

These studies have had a profound impact worldwide, revealing again the importance of controlled clinical trials as a basis for rational therapeutic decisions. It was originally proposed from earlier uncontrolled studies that pulmonary

TABLE 48–1. Controlled Trials of Long-Term Oxygen Therapy*

PARAMETER	MRC	(mean)†	NOTT	(pooled)†
Regimen	15/24	0/24	24/24	12/24
Age (years)	58	56	65	65
FEV_1 (L)	0.76	0.65	(0.8)	(0.8)
Po_2 (mm Hg)	50	52	51	52
Pco_2 (mm Hg)	55	53	43	44
PAP (mm Hg)	34	35	30	29

*Measurement after 3/52 stabilization: at entry.

†Data taken from the Medical Research Council (MRC) Working Party (Lancet 1981; i:681–686); and from the Nocturnal Oxygen Therapy Trial Group (Ann Intern Med 1980; 93:391–398).

hypertension would be reversed by continuous oxygen therapy,[1, 56] but this effect could not be consistently confirmed, at least not in the Medical Research Council (MRC) study.[32] Reanalysis of the Nocturnal Oxygen Therapy Trial (NOTT) study showed that survival was best in those who showed a small but statistically significant improvement in pulmonary hemodynamics with oxygen.[57] Earlier expectations that oxygen therapy would reverse pulmonary polycythemia have also been partially fulfilled, because it appears that secondary polycythemia in blue bloaters is related more to elevation of carboxyhemoglobin levels as a result of chronic cigarette smoking rather than to arterial oxygen desaturation alone.[20] Secondary polycythemia, however, was corrected in those patients who received long-term oxygen therapy and who also had a decrease in HbCO levels as they stopped smoking cigarettes. The quality of life with oxygen also appeared to be improved, although clearly such an assessment must remain subjective, but few physicians experienced in treating such patients with oxygen over several years would disagree with this important result. Formal study, using neuropsychiatric assessments (e.g., intelligence quotient, brain age quotient, and average impairment rating), has shown improvement in re-evaluations after 6 months of oxygen therapy.[58]

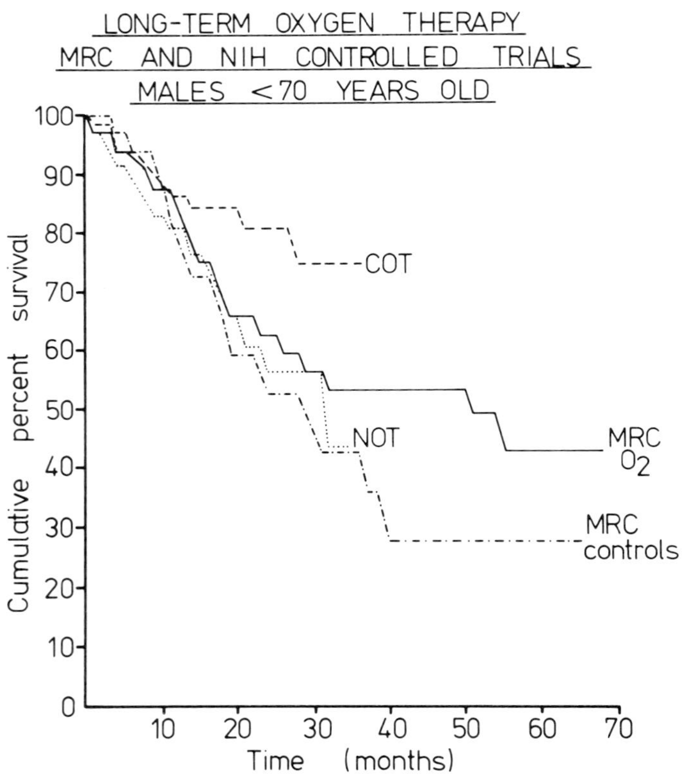

Figure 48–3. Survival with long-term oxygen therapy and control subjects—the MRC (Medical Research Council) and NOTT (Nocturnal Oxygen Therapy Trials). Survival of those in the MRC control group who received no oxygen was clearly the worst, but survival of those in the NOTT group who received oxygen for 12 hours in the 24-hour day was similar to that in the MRC group who received 15 hours of oxygen in the 24-hour day (MRC O_2). However, clearly the best survival was that in the continuous oxygen therapy (COT) group, who received oxygen for more than 19 hours in the 24-hour day.

Selection Criteria

Oxygen therapy does not benefit all patients, and much effort has been expended into trying to find predictors of prolonged survival with oxygen. In the MRC trial, a combination of a high arterial Pco_2 and high red cell mass appeared to define those patients who derived most benefit in terms of survival from long-term oxygen therapy.[32] Patients with COPD in whom pulmonary arterial pressures fell by more than 5 mm Hg when breathing 28% oxygen for 24 hours, at the start of therapy, also claimed to have a better 2-year survival than similar COPD patients whose pulmonary arterial pressure did not decrease by this amount.[59] A prospective study has shown that the survival benefit with long-term oxygen therapy lasts for at least 8 years, as compared to that of similar COPD patients treated without long-term oxygen. It was found that excess ventilation on exercise prior to the study, seemed to predict poor survival. Thus, if the ratio of the minute ventilation (V_E) to carbon dioxide output (Vco_2) was more than 31, this predicted those patients who were likely to die within 3 years (despite oxygen therapy), whereas a value of the V_E to Vco_2 ratio below 31 indicated those patients who were more likely to survive longer with long-term oxygen treatment. These preliminary results need to be tested by further prospective studies of many years' duration.

Current Recommendations

Current recommendations for therapy include patients suffering from COPD who are shown to have a stable course of disease on optimum medical therapy (i.e., bronchodilators, antibiotics, corticosteroids, if indicated) and in whom the Pao_2 is persistently below 55 mm Hg when breathing air for at least 20 minutes in two measurements made 3 weeks apart. Other criteria include a Pao_2 on air between 55 and 59 mm Hg, if associated with clinically diagnosed cor pulmonale and/or hematocrit > 55%. Current recommendations include continuous O_2 flow by double or single nasal cannula to yield arterial oxygen saturation in the 88% to 94% range when on therapy. Most patients require 2 L/minute oxygen to achieve this, but it is recommended that the flow rate of oxygen be increased to 1 L more at night. Again, the oxygen flow rate can often be usefully increased by 1 L/minute during exercise in these patients.

Although oxygen can also be considered for patients who do not meet these criteria (including those with restrictive lung disease, or as an attempt to relieve distressing symptoms in those with such conditions as terminal lung cancer), it must be emphasized that no controlled trial data have yet proven the benefit of oxygen in these circumstances. Oxygen therapy in hypoxemic patients with cystic fibrosis appears rational, but once more no controlled trials are available.

Methods of Administration

Nasal prongs are preferred to any form of oxygen mask, because experience has shown that masks are occasionally removed, and it is essential for domiciliary long-term oxygen therapy to be as continuous as possible. Nasal prongs are usually well tolerated and rarely require that the oxygen supply be humidified, unless used in very dry climates. These devices are undoubtedly obtrusive, however, which has led to a search for alternatives.

The use of transtracheal oxygen, originally introduced by Heimlich,[60] has received much attention. An impressive study by Christopher and coworkers[61] evaluated a new transtracheal catheter in 100 patients over a 2-year period. In the first phase of this program the patients were oriented to the regime, evaluated, and selected, with great emphasis on educating the patient about the benefits and problems associated with the treatment. In the second phase a needle-wire guide dilator technique was used to insert a nonfunctioning stent into the trachea, which remained in place for 1 week. This was followed by replacement with a functioning transtracheal catheter but, because the tract remained immature, over the next 5 to 7 weeks the catheter was cleaned in place. When full maturation was achieved the tract permitted daily removal of the catheter for cleaning and subsequent reinsertion by the patient. Complications were few. The most frequent was the formation of mucous balls in about 10% of patients during phase 2 of the procedure—pea-shaped accumulations of mucus on the tip of the catheter. These were removed in the cleaning process. In addition to reducing hospitalization needs, this treatment was clearly acceptable cosmetically to most patients and allowed them to live a normal life without appearing to be using oxygen, and was of great value for ambulant patients. In addition, the use of the transtracheal oxygen method appears to allow a reduction in the volume of oxygen needed, while achieving the same level of arterial oxygen saturation. This is usually at least 50% oxygen, so that whereas 2 L/minute of oxygen was previously required by nasal prongs, with the transtracheal catheter this can be reduced to 1 L/minute. This is of great value with liquid systems by prolonging the patient's period of ambulation from a given amount of oxygen in a liquid source (see subsequent discussion). Similar regimens have been described by Leger and colleagues.[62]

Oxygen-saving devices have been introduced that use valve systems or reservoirs, either as a moustache device or as a pendant; all of these aim to deliver oxygen only during inspiration and thus reduce the oxygen demand.[63]

Source of Oxygen Supply

The source of oxygen supply is also important. Formerly, oxygen was supplied as a compressed gas in tanks or cylinders, but these are costly, extremely heavy, and rarely allow effective portable oxygen therapy. Furthermore, they require a delivery service to bring the oxygen to the patient's home. Alternatives include a liquid oxygen system.[64] This provides a reservoir, or "cow," installed in the home. It is used to provide oxygen when the patient is at home and also to fill a "walker" or "stroller" device, which is carried by the patient (or spouse or assistant) when away from home. This provides efficient oxygen therapy for the ambulant patient but is usually more expensive than use of the oxygen concentrator.

Oxygen concentrators involve the use of molecular sieves and a compressor system to remove nitrogen from the air, thus providing up to 93% to 95% oxygen.[65] State-of-the-art concentrators are quiet enough to be placed in the bedroom and still allow the patient to sleep. They are reliable and relatively small. They require a source of electricity (an outlet) and regular service and maintenance, usually at 3-month intervals. They have been found to be acceptable in practice and are the cheapest form of long-term oxygen therapy in the home. New developments include further reduction in size and provision of devices that can also operate off an automobile electrical circuit. The ultimate aim—a battery-operated patient-carried device—has yet to be achieved.

OXYGEN THERAPY DURING SLEEP

Correction of the hypoxemia that occurs in REM sleep in COPD patients can be achieved by administering oxygen at night by nasal prongs.[66] Furthermore, such treatment can also reduce the further increase in pulmonary arterial pressure that occurs during this REM sleep-induced hypoxemia (Fig. 48–4).[67] Oxygen at night probably also increases the quality of sleep (as assessed by EEG) in these patients with hypoxemia combined with CO_2 retention (i.e., blue bloaters),[68] although this effect might not be as obvious in patients without CO_2 retention.[69] Fears that CO_2 retention may be aggravated by oxygen therapy during sleep in blue bloaters have not appeared to be sustained in most patients, except in those who suffer from a combination of obstructive sleep apnea and COPD (the overlap syndrome).[70, 71] In these overlap patients, many of whom are obese, a low FEV_1 indicating COPD was combined with hypoxemia by day. Sleep recordings revealed recurrent apneic episodes associated with profound persistent hypoxemia that occurred often throughout the night. In these patients CO_2 retention certainly can be provoked by nocturnal oxygen therapy,[72] because oxygen can prolong the apneic episodes in such patients.[73] Rational treatment of these patients with the overlap syndrome would be to combine nasal continuous positive airway pressure (CPAP)[74, 75] with nocturnal oxygen.

Nocturnal Oxygen Therapy in Patients without Daytime Hypoxemia

In a study of 152 COPD patients whose daytime Pa_{O_2} was above 60 mm Hg, polysomnography (EEG, airflow, respiratory muscle movement, and ear oximeter) revealed that in 37 of these patients (27%), the arterial oxygen saturation fell below 90% for at least a 5-minute period during sleep, with a nadir saturation of at least 85% or less.[76] Although the awake Pa_{O_2} in these "desaturators" was significantly lower than in those who did not desaturate, this study was the first to demonstrate that nocturnal hypoxemia can occur in patients who are not hypoxemic when awake.[76] These results carry the important implication that nocturnal oxygen therapy may be indicated in such patients, in the expectation that this would prevent the development of pulmonary arterial hypertension, with a possibility of eventual cor pulmonale.[28] As yet, no long-term studies have proved or disproved this hypothesis. Indeed, the prevalence of this entity has yet to be established in confirmatory studies. This would tend to counter the experience of others that excessive nocturnal hypoxemia in patients with COPD is not associated with a worse prognosis for survival than in those without such hypoxemia.[77]

Is Oxygen Always Necessary in Hypoxic COPD Patients?

The respiratory stimulant drug almitrine, a triazine derivative that stimulates peripheral chemoreceptors, has been shown to improve arterial blood gas tensions in patients with COPD, even when awake.[78] These acute results were confirmed in a 1-year, double-blind, placebo-controlled study,[79]

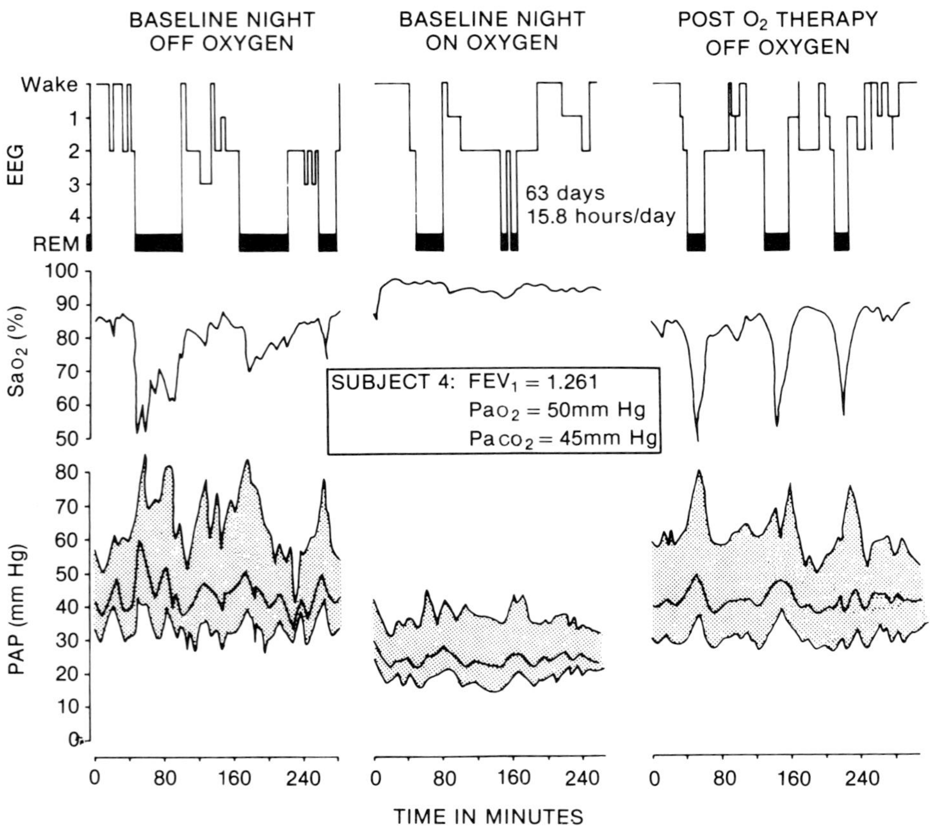

Figure 48–4. EEG sleep scoring (0 = wakefulness, 4 = deep sleep, ■ = rapid eye movement [REM] sleep); ear oxygen saturation, and continuous pulmonary arterial pressure (PAP) throughout the night in a blue bloater (i.e., FEV_1 = 1.26 L, Po_2 when breathing air = 50 mm Hg, $Paco_2$ when breathing air = 45 mm Hg). The scoring was done on one night (baseline) when the patient was not on oxygen therapy, on one night when receiving oxygen (as part of a long-term oxygen program of 63 days of oxygen at 15.8 hours of oxygen/24-hour day), and on a final night after this long-term oxygen therapy period, again when breathing air throughout the night. Note that the pulmonary arterial hypertension increased during REM periods and on the two nights when breathing air, but that the PAP was reduced when breathing oxygen throughout the night. Pulmonary arterial hypertension recurred when the patient again breathed air throughout the night following a period of long-term oxygen therapy. (Redrawn from Fletcher and Levin, Chest 1984; 85:6–14.)

and were confirmed in a more recent study.[80] Almitrine can also correct some of the nocturnal hypoxemic episodes occurring in REM sleep in patients with COPD.[81] Almitrine has been associated with peripheral neuropathy in these patients, however, particularly with long-term use, although the drug might merely exaggerate symptoms of a peripheral pre-existing neuropathy in these patients.[82, 83] Furthermore, almitrine potentiates hypoxic pulmonary vasoconstriction,[84] with a subsequent increase in pulmonary arterial pressure. This varies among patients, and can be noted especially when exercise reduces the hypoxia more profoundly.[85]

Hypoxemia in COPD patients largely arises from ventilation-perfusion mismatch in the lungs. It can be aggravated during exercise, particularly in blue bloaters in whom hypoxemia at rest is characteristic. The hypoxemia can also be aggravated during acute exacerbations of respiratory failure in these patients and during the REM sleep. Controlled oxygen therapy remains the mainstay of management of acute exacerbations, aiming to achieve an arterial $Po_2 > 50$ mm Hg without the arterial pH falling below 7.25. If these guidelines cannot be met by the administration of controlled oxygen alone, ventilatory stimulation by doxapram and eventually mechanical ventilation may be indicated. Long-term oxygen therapy has now achieved an established place in therapeutics, following the demonstration by two clinically controlled trials[32, 55] that this treatment can prolong life in blue bloaters. Such treatment is likely to achieve the most beneficial effect when given for as long as possible in the 24-hour day. The oxygen is usually given by nasal prongs, but administration by transtracheal catheter has been introduced and shown to be an acceptable method for reducing oxygen demand and improving patient compliance with treatment. Oxygen for long-term use is most economically provided by an oxygen concentrator, but liquid oxygen systems provide greatly increased mobility when patients are away from home. Hypoxemia at night, which can be associated with further pulmonary hypertension and potentially lethal cor pulmonale in the long term, can be prevented by oxygen given at night. This treatment is usually safe, without a further increase in the $Paco_2$, except in patients in whom COPD is combined with an obstructive sleep apnea syndrome (the overlap syndrome).

REFERENCES

1. Abraham AS, Cole RB, Bishop JM. Reversal of pulmonary hypertension by prolonged oxygen administration to patients with chronic bronchitis. Circ Res 1968; 23:147–157.
2. Cottrell JJ. Altitude exposure during aircraft flight. Chest 1988; 93:81–84.
3. Dornhorst AC. Respiratory insufficiency. Lancet 1955; i:1185–1187.
4. Filley GF, Beckwitt HJ, Reeves JT, Mitchell RS. Chronic obstructive bronchopulmonary disease: Oxygen transport in two clinical types. Am J Med 1968; 132:871–874.
5. Burrows B, Fletcher CM, Heard BE, et al. The emphysematous and bronchial types of chronic airways obstruction: A clinicopathological study of patients in London and Chicago. Lancet 1966; i:830–835.
6. Burrows B, Kettels LJ, Niden AH, et al. Patterns of cardiovascular dysfunction in chronic obstructive lung disease. N Engl J Med 1972; 286:912–918.
7. McFadden ER, Braunwald E. Cor pulmonale and pulmonary thromboembolism. In: Braunwald E, ed. Heart Disease. A Textbook of Cardiovascular Medicine. 2nd ed. Philadelphia: WB Saunders Company, 1984, 1572–1604.
8. Mitchell RS, Stanford RE, Johnson JM, et al. The morphologic features of the bronchi, bronchioles, and alveoli in chronic airway obstruction: A clinicopathologic study. Am Rev Respir Dis 1976; 114:137–145.
9. Gould GA, MacNee W, McLean A, et al. Measurements of lung

density in life can quantitate distal air space enlargement—an essential defining feature of human emphysema. Am Rev Respir Dis 1988; 137:380–392.
10. Wagner PD, Dantzker DR, Dueck R, et al. Ventilation-perfusion inequality in chronic obstructive pulmonary disease. J Clin Invest 1977; 59:203–216.
11. Jones NL. Pulmonary gas exchange during exercise in patients with chronic airway obstruction. Clin Sci 1966; 31:39–50.
12. Kay JM, Grover RF. Lung mast cells and hypoxic pulmonary hypertension. Prog Resp Res 1975; 9:157–164.
13. Ries AL, Farrow JT, Clausen JC. Pulmonary function tests cannot predict exercise hypoxemia in chronic obstructive pulmonary disease. Chest 1988; 93:454–460.
14. Burrows B, Kettels LJ, Niden AH, et al. Patterns of cardiovascular dysfunction in chronic obstructive lung disease. N Engl J Med 1972; 286:912–918.
15. Euler US von, Lilgestrand G. Observations on the pulmonary arterial blood pressure in the cat. Acta Physiol Scand 1946; 12:301.
16. Penaloza D, Sime F, Banchero N, Gamboa R. Pulmonary hypertension in healthy man born and living at high altitude. Med Thorac 1962; 19:449.
17. Bishop JM, Cross KW. Use of other physiological variables to predict pulmonary arterial pressure in patients with chronic respiratory disease. Multi-centre study. Eur Heart J 1981; 2:509–517.
18. Hurtado A, Mierino C, Delgado E. Influence of anoxemia on the haemopoietic activity. Arch Intern Med 1945; 75:284.
19. Weil JV, Jamieson G, Brown DW, et al. The red cell mass/arterial oxygen relationship in normal man. J Clin Invest 1968; 47:1627–1639.
20. Calverley PMA, Leggett RJ, McElderry L, Flenley DC. Cigarette smoking and secondary polycythaemia in hypoxic cor pulmonale. Am Rev Respir Dis 1982; 125:507–510.
21. Douglas NJ, Calverley PMA, Leggett RJE, et al. Transient hypoxemia during sleep in patients with cor pulmonale complicating chronic bronchitis and emphysema. Clin Sci Mol Med 1978; 55:31.
22. Wynne JW, Block AJ, Hemingway J, et al. Disordered breathing and oxygen desaturation during sleep in patients with chronic obstructive lung disease (COLD). Am J Med 1979; 56:573–579.
23. Coccagna G, Lugaresi E. Arterial blood gases and pulmonary and systemic arterial pressure during sleep in chronic obstructive pulmonary disease. Sleep 1978; 1:117–124.
24. Catterall JR, Calverley PMA, MacNee W, et al. The mechanism of transient nocturnal hypoxemia in hypoxic chronic bronchitis and emphysema. J Appl Physiol 1985; 59:1698–1703.
25. Catterall JR, Douglas NJ, Calverley PMA. Transient hypoxemia during sleep in chronic obstructive pulmonary disease is not a sleep apnea syndrome. Am Rev Respir Dis 1983; 128:24–29.
26. Fletcher EC, Gray BA, Levin DC. Nonapneic mechanisms of arterial oxygen desaturation during rapid-eye movement sleep. J Appl Physiol 1983; 54:632–639.
27. Fletcher EC, Levin DC. Cardiopulmonary hemodynamics during sleep in subjects with chronic obstructive pulmonary disease. Chest 1984; 85:6–14.
28. Flenley DC. Clinical hypoxia: Causes, consequences and correction. The Tudor Edwards Lecture to the Royal College of Physicians, London, 1977. Lancet 1977; i:542–546.
29. Fletcher EC, Miller JA, Divine GW, et al. Nocturnal oxyhemoglobin desaturation in COPD patients with arterial oxygen tensions above 60 mm Hg. Chest 1987; 92:604–608.
30. Renzetti AD, McClement JH, Litt BD. The Veterans Administration Co-Operative Study of Pulmonary Function, III. Mortality in relation to respiratory function in chronic obstructive pulmonary disease. Am J Med 1966; 41:115–129.
31. Niewoehner DE, Kleinerman J, Rice DB. Pathologic changes in the peripheral airways of young cigarette smokers. N Engl J Med 1974; 291:755–758.
32. Medical Research Council Working Party (Stuart-Harris C, Flenley DC, Bishop JM, et al.). Long-term domiciliary oxygen therapy in chronic hypoxic cor pulmonale complicating chronic bronchitis and emphysema. Lancet 1981; i:681–686.
33. Flenley DC. Another non-logarithmic acid-base diagram. Lancet 1971; i:961–965.
34. Flenley DC, Miller HC, King AJ, et al. Oxygen transport in acute pulmonary edema and in acute exacerbations of chronic bronchitis. Br Med J 1973; 1:78–81.
35. Campbell DB, Gordon B, Taylor A, et al. The biodisposition of almitrine bismesylate in man: A review. Eur J Respir Dis 1983; 64(Suppl 126):337–348.
36. Campbell EJM. The management of acute respiratory failure in chronic bronchitis and emphysema. Am Rev Respir Dis 1967; 96:626–639.
37. Donald KW. Neurological effects of oxygen. Lancet 1949; ii:1056–1057.
38. Cournand A, Riley RL, Bradley SE, et al. Studies of circulation in clinical shock. Surgery 1943; 13:965.
39. Eldridge F. Blood lactate and pyruvate in pulmonary insufficiency. New Engl J Med 1966; 274:878–883.
40. Peretz DI, Scott HM, Duff J, et al. The significance of lactic acidemia in the shock syndrome. Ann NY Acad Sci 1965; 119:1133–1141.
41. Abraham AS, Cole RB, Green ID, et al. Factors contributing to the reversible pulmonary hypertension of patients with acute respiratory failure: Studies by serial observations during recovery. Circ Res 1969; 24:51–60.
42. Hutchison DCS, Flenley DC, Donald KW. Controlled oxygen therapy in respiratory failure. Br Med J 1964; 2:1159–1166.
43. Warren PMA, Millar JS, Flenley DC, Avery A. Respiratory failure revisited: Acute exacerbations of chronic bronchitis between 1961–68 and 1970–76. Lancet 1980; i:467–471.
44. Bone RC, Pierce AK, Johnson TL. Controlled oxygen administration in acute respiratory failure in chronic obstructive pulmonary disease. Am J Med 1978; 65:896–902.
45. Hanson FN, Floreani AA, Pingleton SK, Bunce SB. Usefulness of APACHE II variables in predicting survival and death in COPD patients in the I.C.U. Am Rev Respir Dis 1987; 135:A144.
46. Bone RC, Balk RA. Non-invasive respiratory care unit, a cost-effective solution for the future. Chest 1988; 93:390–394.
47. Pierson DJ, Creagh CE, Sutton FD, et al. Complications of assisted ventilation. Am J Med 1974; 57:161–170.
48. Connors AF, McCaffree RD, Gray BA. Effect of inspiratory flow rate on gas exchange from a mechanical ventilation. Am Rev Respir Dis 1981; 124:537–543.
49. Pepe PE, Marini JJ. Occult positive end-expiratory pressure in mechanically ventilated patients with airflow obstruction. Am Rev Respir Dis 1982; 126:166–170.
50. Darioli R, Perret C. Mechanical control of hypoventilation in status asthmaticus. Am Rev Respir Dis 1984; 129:385–387.
51. Tuxen DV, Lane S. The effects of ventilatory pattern on hyperinflation, airway pressures and circulation, and mechanical ventilation in patients with severe airflow obstruction. Am Rev Respir Dis 1987; 136:872–879.
52. Neff TA, Petty TL. Long-term continuous oxygen therapy in chronic airway obstruction. Ann Intern Med 1970; 72:621–626.
53. Leggett RJE, Cooke NJ, Clancy LJ, et al. Long-term domiciliary oxygen therapy in cor pulmonale complicating chronic bronchitis and emphysema. Thorax 1976; 31:414–418.
54. Stark RD, Finnegan P, Bishop JM. Long-term domiciliary oxygen in chronic bronchitis with pulmonary hypertension. Br Med J 1973; 3:467–470.
55. Nocturnal Oxygen Therapy Trial Group. Continuous or nocturnal oxygen therapy in hypoxemic chronic obstructive lung disease: A clinical trial. Ann Intern Med 1980; 93:391–398.
56. Levine BE, Bigelow DB, Hamstra RD, et al. The role of long-term continuous oxygen administration in patients with chronic airways obstruction with hypoxemia. Ann Intern Med 1967; 66:639–650.
57. Timms RM, Khaja FU, Williams GW, et al. Hemodynamic response to oxygen therapy in chronic obstructive pulmonary disease. Ann Intern Med 1985; 102:29–36.
58. Heaton RK, Grant I, McSweeny AJ, et al. Psychological effects of continuous nocturnal oxygen therapy in hypoxemic chronic obstructive pulmonary disease. Arch Intern Med 1983; 143:1941–1947.
59. Ashutosh K, Mead G, Dunsky M. Early effects of oxygen administration and prognosis in chronic obstructive pulmonary disease and cor pulmonale. Am Rev Respir Dis 1983; 127:399–404.
60. Heimlich HJ. Respiratory rehabilitation with transtracheal oxygen system. Ann Otol Rhinol Laryngol 1982; 91:643–647.
61. Christopher KL, Spofford BT, Petrun MD, et al. Program for transtracheal oxygen delivery: Assessment of safety and efficacy. Ann Intern Med 1987; 107:802–808.
62. Leger P, Gerard M, Mercatello A, Robert D. Transtracheal

catheter for oxygen therapy of patients requiring high oxygen flow [abstract]. Respiration 1984; 46(Suppl 1):103.
63. Tiep BL, Nicotra B, Carter R, et al. Low-concentration oxygen therapy via a demand oxygen delivery system. Chest 1985; 87:636–638.
64. Petty TL, Flenley DC. Domiciliary and ambulatory oxygen in chronic respiratory insufficiency. In: Flenley DC, Petty TL, eds. Recent Advances in Respiratory Medicine, IV. Edinburgh: Churchill Livingstone, 1986, 217–229.
65. Gould GA, Scott W, Hayhurst MD, Flenley DC. Technical and clinical assessment of oxygen concentrators. Thorax 1985; 40:811–816.
66. Douglas NJ, Calverley PMA, Leggett RJE, et al. Transient hypoxemia during sleep in chronic bronchitis and emphysema. Lancet 1979; i:1–4.
67. Fletcher EC, Levin DC. Cardiopulmonary hemodynamics during sleep in subjects with chronic obstructive pulmonary disease. Chest 1984; 85:6–14.
68. Catterall JR, Douglas NJ, Calverley PMA. Transient hypoxemia during sleep in chronic obstructive pulmonary disease is not a sleep apnea syndrome. Am Rev Respir Dis 1983; 128:24–29.
69. Fleetham J, West P, Mezon B, et al. Sleep, arousals, and oxygen desaturation in chronic obstructive pulmonary disease. The effect of oxygen therapy. Am Rev Respir Dis 1982; 126:429–433.
70. Flenley DC. Disordered breathing during sleep in lung disease: Its importance to the clinician. In: Herzog H, Perruchoud AP, eds. Progress in Respiratory Research, Vol 19, Basel: S. Karger, 1985, 1–7.
71. Fletcher EC. Chronic lung disease in patients with sleep apnea. In: Fletcher EC, ed. Abnormalities of Respiration During Sleep. Orlando, FL: Grune & Stratton, 1986, 181–202.
72. Goldstein RS, Ramcharan V, Bowes F, et al. The effect of supplemental nocturnal oxygen on gas exchange in patients with severe obstructive lung disease. N Engl J Med 1984; 310:425–429.
73. Guilleminault C, Cummiskey J, Motta J. Chronic obstructive airflow disease in sleep studies. Am Rev Respir Dis 1980; 122:397–406.
74. Sullivan CE, Berthon-Jones M, Issa FG, Eaves L. Reversal of obstructive apnea by continuous positive airway pressure applied through the nares. Lancet 1981; i:862–865.
75. Martin RJ. Medical treatment for the sleep apnea syndrome. In: Fletcher EC, ed. Abnormalities of Respiration During Sleep. Orlando, FL: Grune & Stratton, 1986, 5:95–115.
76. Fletcher EC, Miller J, Devine GW, et al. Nocturnal oxygen hemoglobin desaturation in COPD patients with arterial oxygen tensions above 60 mm Hg. Chest 1987; 92:604–608.
77. Connaughton JJ, Catterall JR, Elton RA, et al. Do sleep studies contribute to the management of patients with severe chronic obstructive pulmonary disease? Am Rev Respir Dis 1988; 138:341–344.
78. Powles ACP, Tuxen DV, Mahood CB, et al. The effect of intravenously administered almitrine, a peripheral chemoreceptor agonist in patients with chronic airflow obstruction. Am Rev Respir Dis 1983; 127:284–289.
79. Arnaud F, Bertrand A, Charpin J, et al. Almitrine bismesylate in long-term treatment of patients with chronic bronchitis at the stage of chronic respiratory insufficiency. A multicentre, double-blind, placebo-controlled study. Bull Eur Physiopathol Respir 1982; 18(Suppl 4):373–382.
80. Voisin C, Howard P, Ansger JC. Almitrine bismesylate: A long-term placebo-controlled double-blind study in COAD—Vectarion International Multicentre Study Group. Bull Eur Physiopathol Respir, 1987; 23(Suppl 11):167S–182S.
81. Connaughton JJ, Douglas NJ, Morgan AD, et al. Almitrine improves oxygenation when both awake and asleep in patients with hypoxia and CO_2 retention due to chronic bronchitis and emphysema. Am Rev Respir Dis 1985; 132:206–210.
82. Gasnault J, Rondot P, Moore N. Peripheral neuropathies during hypoxemic chronic obstructive lung disease. Bull Eur Physiopathol Respir 1987; 23(Suppl 11):119S–202S.
83. Lerebours G, Senant J, Moore N, et al. Evolution of peripheral nerve function in hypoxemic COPD patients taking almitrine bismesylate: A prospective long-term study. Bull Eur Physiopathol Respir 1987; 23(Suppl 11):203S–206S.
84. Romaldini H, Rodriguez-Roisin R, Wagner PD, West JB. Enhancement of hypoxic pulmonary vasoconstriction by almitrine in the dog. Am Rev Respir Dis 1983; 128:288–293.
85. MacNee W, Connaughton JJ, Rhind GB, et al. A comparison of the effects of almitrine or oxygen breathing on pulmonary arterial pressure and right ventricular ejection fraction in hypoxic chronic bronchitis and emphysema. Am Rev Respir Dis 1986; 134:559–565.

Chapter 49

DIURETICS IN THE TREATMENT OF COPD

Vladimir Fencl

USE OF DIURETICS IN COPD

The main applications for diuretics, the agents that induce elimination of sodium, chloride, and water, in the management of patients with COPD, are summarized in Table 49–1. One indication is for the treatment of congestive heart failure, to correct the expansion of the extracellular (intravascular) volume. Diuretics are also prescribed for patients with COPD for the treatment of a coexistent systemic arterial hypertension. Finally, some less common indications for the use of diuretics are to alter purposefully the external balance of individual extracellular electrolytes and of water or to reduce the rate of formation of transcellular fluids (ocular and cerebrospinal).

An ideal diuretic would induce elimination of Na^+, Cl^-, and all other extracellular electrolytes, together with water, in

TABLE 49–1. Applications of Diuretics in Management of Patients with COPD

Reduction of excessive systemic extracellular volume
Treatment of systemic arterial hypertension
Miscellaneous:
Treatment of hypercalcemia or hyperkalemia (loop diuretics)
Reduction of renal water loss in diabetes insipidus (thiazides)
Hypochloremic alkalosis (acetazolamide)
Hyperchloremic acidosis (loop diuretics)
Reduction of rate of ocular and cerebrospinal fluid formation (treatment of glaucoma or hydrocephalus with acetazolamide)

the same proportion as all these constituents exist in the extracellular (interstitial) fluid. All diuretics typically act on the kidney and reduce the tubular reabsorption of water and electrolytes, either by a nonspecific osmotic effect (in the case of nonreabsorbable osmotic diuretics) or by interfering, in various segments of the nephrons, with specific transport processes for individual strong (i.e., fully dissociated) electrolytes: Na^+, K^+, Ca^{2+}, Mg^{2+}, and Cl^-. It is no surprise that the effect of all diuretics on electrolyte and water balance is far from the ideal, which would be to diminish the volume of the extracellular fluid without altering its chemical composition. This ideal is not achieved; hence the untoward effects of diuretic therapy manifest themselves as disturbances of electrolyte, water, and acid-base balance.

DIURETICS IN CLINICAL USE

Table 49–2 lists the diuretics in general use and gives a simplified overview of their main actions. For a detailed discussion of the specific renal effects of the various types of diuretic agents, the reader is referred to specialized texts (e.g., references 28, 35, and 42).

According to their potency, expressed as the highest fractional excretion of Na^+ ($FEmaxNa^+$, as per cent of the filtered load), the diuretic agents can be classified as weak ($FEmaxNa^+$ 2% to 4%: carbonic anhydrase inhibitors; K^+-sparing diuretics; osmotic diuretics), moderately potent ($FEmaxNa^+$ ~8%: thiazides and related compounds), and very potent ($FEmaxNa^+$ 20% to 25%: loop diuretics and the now abandoned mercurial compounds).

INHIBITORS OF CARBONIC ANHYDRASE. The renal effect of inhibiting the enzyme carbonic anhydrase can be characterized as a controlled induction of renal tubular (hyperchloremic) acidosis. The diuretic effect is limited, both in potency ($FEmaxNa^+$ ~4%) and in duration (because of the compensatory increase in distal Na^+ reabsorption). The main application of acetazolamide in the management of patients with COPD is in the correction of hypochloremic alkalosis and of the blunted hypercapnic respiratory drive[40] that accompanies this alkalosis.

LOOP ("HIGH CEILING") DIURETICS. In the thick ascending limb of the loop of Henle, these drugs inhibit the luminal transport system for strong electrolytes (coupled entry of Na^+, K^+, and Cl^-; this effectively blocks the active reabsorption of Na^+ and Cl^- at the basolateral membrane). Elimination of Cl^- increases more than that of Na^+, which results in depletion of Cl^- from the extracellular space and produces hypochloremic alkalosis. Secretion of K^+ in the distal nephron is increased, owing to increased distal delivery of Na^+ and Cl^-.[22, 44] By their action on the transport processes in the loop of Henle, these diuretics hamper the production of dilute or concentrated urine (by interfering with both the formation and reabsorption of "osmotically free water"). Thus, during the full diuretic effect of these agents, the osmolarity of the urine approaches that of plasma.[42] The great potency ($FEmaxNa^+$ 20% to 25%) and speed of action of these drugs frequently result in hypokalemia, hypochloremic alkalosis, and hypovolemia, often with a very sudden onset of these disturbances.

THIAZIDES AND RELATED COMPOUNDS. These agents inhibit the reabsorption of Na^+ and Cl^- mainly in the cortical diluting segment of the distal convoluted tubules; this impedes elimination of "osmotically free water" and the production of dilute urine. However, urine concentration (reabsorption of "free water") remains unimpaired since these drugs do not affect

TABLE 49–2. Properties and Effects of Diuretics

DIURETIC	DRUGS	MAIN SITE (or Mechanism) OF ACTION	DIURETIC EFFECT: Highest Na^+ Excretion*	DIURETIC EFFECT: Urinary Electrolytes	UNTOWARD EFFECTS: Plasma Electrolytes and Acid-Base Balance	UNTOWARD EFFECTS: Other
Inhibitors of carbonic anhydrase	acetazolamide	proximal tubules	4	↑ Na > ↑ Cl (↑ HCO_3), ↑ K	↓ K hyperchloremic acidosis	
Loop diuretics	furosemide, bumetanide, ethacrynic acid	loops of Henle	>20	↑ Na, ↑↑ Cl, ↑ K, ↑ Ca, ↑ Mg	↓ K, ↓ Ca, ↓ Mg, ↓ Cl hypochloremic alkalosis	hypovolemia, ototoxicity
Thiazides and related compounds	chloro- , hydro-chlorothiazide, trichlormethiazide, chlorthalidone, metolazone, indapamine	distal tubules	8	↑ Na, ↑↑ Cl, ↑ K, ↓ Ca, ↑ Mg	↓ K, ↓ Na, ↓ Cl, ↑ Ca, ↓ Mg hypochloremic alkalosis	↑ uric acid, ↑ plasma lipids, glucose intolerance
Potassium-sparing diuretics		collecting ducts	2			
	spironolactone	(aldosterone antagonist)		↑ Na > ↑ Cl, ↓ K	risk of ↑ K	gynecomastia
	amiloride, triamterene	(↓ Na conductance at apical membrane)		↑ Na > ↑ Cl, ↓ K	risk of ↑ K	
Osmotic diuretics	mannitol, urea, glycerol, (glucose)	whole nephron	2–3	↑ Na, ↑ Cl, ↑ K, ↑ water > ↑ NaCl		vascular overload, hyperosmolarity

*Per cent of the filtered load.

the transport in the loop of Henle. This is why (dilutional) hyponatremia is seen among the untoward effects of thiazides; on the other hand, this makes thiazides useful in curbing renal water loss in diabetes insipidus.

The diuretic potency of these agents is intermediate (FEmaxNa^+ 8% to 10%). Loss of Cl^- in proportion to that of Na^+ is excessive, which produces hypochloremic alkalosis. Increased elimination of K^+, with risk of hypokalemia, results from increased distal delivery of Na^+ and Cl^-.[22, 44]

POTASSIUM-SPARING DIURETICS. The three drugs in this group, spironolactone, triamterene, and amiloride, are unique among diuretic agents in conserving K^+ during diuretic action. The overall effect of all these agents is a mild natriuresis (FEmaxNa^+ ~2%) and a mild hyperchloremic acidosis.

Spironolactone blocks the effect of aldosterone on the cells in the collecting ducts by binding to the cytosolic receptors for the hormone. Response to aldosterone is eliminated, which suppresses in this segment of the nephron the reabsorption of Na^+ and secretion of K^+, but in addition augments the reabsorption of Cl^- (or, in the customary parlance, impairs H^+ secretion[49, 50]). Since the action of spironolactone is in the segment of the nephrons located beyond the sites of free water absorption or elimination, formation of diluted or concentrated urine is unimpaired. The usefulness of spironolactone as a diuretic is, of course, limited to conditions in which hyperaldosteronism contributes to Na^+ retention and edema formation.

The other two drugs in this group, amiloride and triamterene, inhibit Na^+ reabsorption in the distal portion of the distal tubule and in the cortical portion of the collecting ducts, by diminishing the conductance for Na^+ in the apical membrane of the epithelial cells. As a consequence, secretion of K^+ in these parts of the nephron is diminished, as is "H^+ secretion" (i.e., Cl^- elimination increases less than that of Na^+ [49, 50]). Triamterene and amiloride are used mainly in combination with other more potent diuretics, mainly thiazides, to reduce the obligatory losses of K^+.

OSMOTIC DIURETICS. Molecules that are not reabsorbed from the glomerular filtrate (e.g., mannitol, glycerol; also unreabsorbed glucose in uncontrolled diabetes mellitus) inhibit the tubular reabsorption of all electrolytes and water by their osmotic effect, predominantly in the proximal parts of the nephrons. Water is lost in excess of Na^+ and Cl^-. The main application of these drugs is in attempts to reverse oliguria and—since they are administered intravenously as hypertonic solutions—in the treatment of cerebral edema; the transfer of water from the cells into the extracellular space dilutes all plasma electrolytes.

BENEFITS OF DIURETIC THERAPY IN COPD

TREATMENT OF EDEMA. Chronic hypoxia and hypercapnia, together with destruction of the pulmonary vasculature in the course of COPD, eventually lead to right-sided cardiac failure,[9, 19] with retention of sodium and development of peripheral edema (see Chapters 18, 25, and 44). It is disputed whether the benefit of diuretic therapy in this condition goes beyond the mechanical removal of the peripheral edema and includes improvement in pulmonary hypertension and gas exchange.[21, 25, 39] However, healthy humans, when given a diuretic for 2 days to produce a weight loss of 4.5% of body weight, showed an increase in expiratory flow rates.[29]

Controversy also exists about whether left ventricular dysfunction in patients with COPD and cor pulmonale may simply result from the hypertrophy or failure of the right ventricle,[2, 25, 46] or whether such dysfunction always indicates a coexisting left ventricular disease (mainly coronary artery disease).[10, 34, 48] With pulmonary congestion in left ventricular failure, airway conductance may improve as a result of the increased elastic recoil of the pulmonary parenchyma with pulmonary edema.[12] However, the efficiency of the pulmonary gas exchange, especially the transfer of oxygen, is diminished owing to the increase in mismatch of ventilation and perfusion, which presumably results from a patchy perivascular edema that increases resistance in the extra-alveolar vessels.[54] The beneficial effect of diuretics in patients with COPD, like that of digitalis,[23, 38] probably is conditioned by the presence of left ventricular failure with pulmonary congestion.[39]

Thiazides or loop diuretics are usually used for the treatment of congestive heart failure, because of their diuretic potency. In isolated right ventricular failure, vigorous diuresis may drastically reduce venous return and the cardiac output. Furthermore, furosemide, when administered intravenously, increases the capacitance of the systemic venous reservoirs,[13] presumably by a direct vascular effect. Small doses of furosemide (less than 0.5 mg/kg of body weight) are claimed to improve alveolar ventilation and to increase the cardiac output; these changes appear to go with reduction of central blood volume and with lowering of pulmonary arterial pressure.[5, 52] These extrarenal effects of furosemide precede the diuretic effect of the drug.

TREATMENT OF SYSTEMIC ARTERIAL HYPERTENSION. Since diuretics do not induce bronchospasm,[37] in the treatment of hypertensive patients with COPD they are preferred over beta-adrenergic blocking agents, which are more commonly used for antihypertensive therapy in the general population of patients.[51]

The chloride- and potassium-wasting diuretics are commonly used[26, 51] rather than the potassium-sparing agents, because of their greater potency. Thiazides and related compounds are the drugs of choice. The loop diuretics, because of the short duration of their effect, are less suited for antihypertensive therapy and, because of their efficiency even with reduced glomerular filtration, are reserved for patients with renal or congestive heart failure.

Among the potassium-sparing diuretics only spironolactone, when used as a single agent and given in sufficient dose, produces a hypotensive effect comparable to that of the thiazides.[18] More commonly, the potassium-sparing diuretics are added to thiazides, mainly to prevent hypokalemia[45] and hypochloremic alkalosis.

ACETAZOLAMIDE IN THE TREATMENT OF DECREASED RESPIRATORY DRIVE. In the management of patients with COPD, this drug is now used mainly as an adjunct in correcting excessive hypochloremia (see later). In the 1950s, it was claimed that hypoventilation and chronic CO_2 retention can be reversed in some patients with COPD by a continuous administration of acetazolamide.[4, 43] Later studies suggested that when hyperchloremic acidosis was induced, the respiratory failure worsened, with excessive work of breathing that resulted from the high respiratory drive.[20] In retrospect, it appears that those patients with COPD in whom the treatment with acetazolamide did ameliorate the chronic hypercapnia and hypoxemia were those in whom the hypochloremia was "excessive" (see later), perhaps as a consequence of diuretic therapy (with mercurials, at that time) or other interventions.

COMPLICATIONS OF DIURETIC THERAPY IN PATIENTS WITH COPD

Interaction with Other Therapeutic Agents

All corticosteroids used for the treatment of patients with COPD exhibit some mineralocorticoid effect, which may significantly augment the urinary losses of K^+ and Cl^- produced by thiazides or loop diuretics. On the other hand, a potentially favorable effect may result when thiazides are combined with corticosteroids, improving the balance of Ca^{2+} and improving osteopenia.[1]

Administration of beta-adrenergic agonists to patients treated with thiazides or loop diuretics may transiently induce hypokalemia, reaching levels that could provoke arrhythmias: terbutaline given subcutaneously (0.25 mg) to asymptomatic asthmatics lowered serum K^+ by 0.6 mEq/L. The effect was apparent after 15 minutes, with a nadir at 30 minutes, and it lasted for over 60 minutes.[36] This effect is mediated by the $beta_2$-adrenergic receptors[7] and brought about by a shift of extracellular K^+ into the intracellular compartment.[53] The transient hypokalemia is thus a result of a redistribution, not of a loss, of K^+ between the extracellular and intracellular compartments of body fluids. Nonetheless, the potential for inducing cardiac arrhythmias is real, since the transmembrane gradients, not the total content, of K^+ are of importance in this respect. In patients with COPD, many of whom are hypoxic, have ischemic heart disease, and are treated with methylxanthines, this is even more worrisome.

Electrolyte, Acid-Base, and Water Imbalances

HYPOCHLOREMIC ALKALOSIS. With diuresis induced by thiazides or loop diuretics, the loss of Cl^- is greater than that of Na^+ (see Table 49–2), which produces hypochloremic ("metabolic") alkalosis.[17] Primary hypochloremia (or, alternatively, increase in plasma bicarbonate concentration) is accompanied by a compensatory retention of CO_2 (see reference 30 for review). From the compilation of data on the apparent dependence of Pa_{CO_2} on the bicarbonate concentration in arterial plasma[11, 31] or on base excess in blood,[15, 55] it can be estimated that the compensatory increase in Pa_{CO_2} is of the order of 0.9 to 1.0 torr for each mEq/L increase in the (positive) base excess,[15] or 0.8 to 0.9 torr with each mEq/L increase in (actual) bicarbonate concentration.[30] The compensation is never complete, and pH remains alkalemic (>7.40).[15, 55] Thus, in a primary hypochloremic alkalosis with a base excess of +10 mEq/L, the expected P_{CO_2} would be 40 + 10 = 50 torr ($[HCO_3^-]$ 24 + 9 = 33 mM, pH = 7.44). If ambient air is inhaled, the P_{O_2} in the alveolar gas would be about 86 torr (assuming a barometric pressure of 760 torr, a body temperature of 37°C, and a respiratory quotient of 0.8).

The mechanisms involved in this homeostatic lowering of respiratory drive in response to a primary hypochloremic alkalosis are believed to involve an adjustment in the ionic composition of cerebral extracellular fluids (an increase in their alkalinity[16]). The time course of the development of this respiratory adaptation in hypochloremic alkalosis (and the time of its disappearance after correction of the hypochloremia) corresponds to the turnover rate of the cerebral fluids[14]—about 24 hours for a full establishment or disappearance.

With chronic CO_2 retention, the renal compensation for the primary hypercapnia produces a positive base excess (or, in the customary parlance, increases the plasma bicarbonate concentration) by lowering plasma $[Cl^-]$. The appropriate degree of this homeostatic response, as empirically established[6, 15, 47, 55] in patients with uncomplicated chronic respiratory acidosis (range of Pa_{CO_2} values, 45 to 65 torr), is a base excess of +0.3 to +0.4 mEq/L for each torr of primary P_{CO_2} elevation.[15] This excess is produced by lowering plasma $[Cl^-]$ by that amount, which results in an increase in arterial $[HCO_3^-]$ by ~0.3 mM. The compensation is never complete, and pH in arterial plasma remains at acidemic values (< 7.40). According to this rule of thumb, for a primary hypercapnia with Pa_{CO_2} of 50 torr, the homeostatically appropriate base excess should be +3 to +4 mEq/L, chloride having been lowered by 3 to 4 mM, with $[HCO_3^-]$ in plasma 24 + 3 = 27 mM, pH = 7.36.[17]

When patients with COPD and chronic CO_2 retention are treated with the chloride-wasting diuretics, hypochloremia from diuretic-induced chloride losses will produce an additional "metabolic" alkalosis, beyond and above the homeostatically appropriate renal response to the primary hypercapnia. This will further reduce the chemical respiratory drive of the already hypercapnic patient and lead to further CO_2 retention.[3] These considerations are of particular importance in the management of those patients with chronic CO_2 retention who have to be weaned from mechanical ventilation. In addition to diuretics, many therapeutic interventions are routinely used in critically ill patients and produce hypochloremia, e.g., loss of gastric secretions by nasogastric suction, transfusion of citrated blood or blood products, and treatment with high doses of sodium penicillins.[17] For these reasons, primary hypochloremic alkalosis has become the most common acid-base disturbance in all critically ill patients.[27] If this metabolic alkalosis is superimposed on the homeostatically appropriate renal response to hypercapnia, the ventilatory drive is reduced to the point that attempts at weaning from the ventilatory support will fail.

In the treatment of such excessive hypochloremia in patients with chronic CO_2 retention, the principal aim is to restore a plasma chloride concentration to a value that is homeostatically appropriate for the established level of the patient's chronic CO_2 retention, as described earlier.

If, for some reason, expansion of the extracellular volume is desirable, infusion of isotonic solution of NaCl is the intervention of choice: adding saline ($[Na^+] = [Cl^-]$) to plasma ($[Na^+] > [Cl^-]$) increases plasma $[Cl^-]$, i.e., acidifies plasma (lowers plasma $[HCO_3^-]$). If expansion of the extracellular fluid volume must be avoided (which is the more common case), chloride has to be given without Na^+. Therapeutically useful sources of Cl^- unaccompanied by Na^+ are potassium chloride (KCl), calcium chloride ($CaCl_2$), and magnesium chloride ($MgCl_2$). Here Cl^- is given together with cations whose concentrations in the extracellular fluid are regulated within narrow limits, for purposes unrelated to acid-base balance. In patients receiving parenteral nutrition, a rapid correction of hypochloremic alkalosis can be achieved if all electrolytes (Na^+, K^+, Ca^{2+}, and Mg^{2+}) that are added to the solution of amino acids and dextrose are given as chlorides, rather than acetates.[17] Aside from this, KCl is most frequently used, because K^+ loss accompanies hypochloremia induced by diuresis (or by losses of gastric secretions). It is the Cl^- in KCl that corrects the metabolic alkalosis;[33] citrate or bicarbonate of potassium, although effective in correcting hypokalemia *per se,* are, of course, useless for the treatment of hypochloremia. Another therapeutically useful sodium-free source of Cl^- is NH_4Cl (1 gram provides 19 mEq of Cl^-). It has to be given by mouth; intravenous administration would produce hyperammonemia and encephalopathy. Arginine chloride given intravenously produces life-threatening hyperkalemia and therefore is no longer used for treatment of hypochloremia.[8] In acutely ill patients, intravenous administration of hydrochloric acid (sterile 0.1 N HCl in 5% dextrose solution, infused into a central vein) is a safe and efficient way of giving Cl^- without Na^+.

Acetazolamide, although weak as a diuretic produces a transient renal tubular acidosis by inhibiting carbonic anhydrase in the renal tubular cells. It is effective in correcting the hypochloremic alkalosis that results from vigorous therapy with the chloride-wasting thiazides and loop diuretics. However, the potassium losses induced by these diuretics are augmented by the administration of acetazolamide.

HYPOKALEMIA. In patients treated continuously with thiazides or loop diuretics, serum [K^+] falls, on the average by 0.67 mEq/L (as found in patients treated for hypertension).[41] There have been extensive discussions in the literature on when, or whether at all, to treat the diuretic-induced hypokalemia.[24, 32] Logically, prevention should be stressed;[32] this can be achieved by using the smallest effective dose of short-acting diuretics, by restricting both Na^+ intake and extrarenal losses of K^+ (laxatives), by increasing dietary intake of K^+, and by combining thiazides with potassium-sparing diuretics.[32] With the latter agents, supplements of K^+ definitely should not be given because of the danger of hyperkalemia.

The transient hypokalemia induced by treatment with beta-adrenergic agonists is of great concern (see earlier); random measurements of serum [K^+] will not detect it reliably. For this reason, treatment with K^+ supplements or the addition of potassium-sparing diuretics should be considered for those patients treated with beta-adrenergic agonists who are at increased risks of developing cardiac arrhythmias: those with (a) an increased susceptibility of the myocardium (ischemic heart disease, digitalis therapy, frequent ventricular ectopies), (b) severe respiratory acidosis or hypoxemia or both, and (c) potential sources of hypokalemia in addition to diuretic therapy (low K^+ intake or large extrarenal losses of K^+).[32] As a potassium supplement, KCl is preferable, since it will also correct an accompanying hypochloremic alkalosis.

HYPONATREMIA. This complication of diuretic therapy occurs in patients with congestive heart failure, mainly in those treated with thiazides. The pathogenesis includes a drug-induced defect in renal elimination of free water (see Table 49–2), increased secretion of vasopressin in response to volume reduction, and increased water intake in response to increased thirst from increased angiotensin levels. Restriction of fluid intake (below the urinary and insensible losses) is usually a sufficient treatment of mild hyponatremia. Severe hyponatremia ([Na^+] < 120 mEq/L) is treated with saline and loop diuretics; this usually requires careful hemodynamic monitoring.

REFERENCES

1. Adams JS, Wahl RO, Lukert BP. Effects of hydrochlorothiazide and dietary sodium restriction on calcium metabolism in corticosteroid-treated patients. Metabolism 1981; 30:217–221.
2. Baum GL, Schartz A, Llamas R, Castillo C. Left ventricular function in chronic obstructive lung disease. N Engl J Med 1971; 285:361–365.
3. Bear R, Goldstein M, Phillipson E, et al. Effect of metabolic alkalosis on respiratory function in patients with chronic obstructive lung disease. J Can Med Assoc 1977; 117:900–903.
4. Bell ALL Jr, Smith CN, Andreae E. Effects of the carbonic anhydrase inhibitor "6063" (Diamox) on respiration and electrolyte metabolism in patients with respiratory acidosis. Am J Med 1955; 18:536–546.
5. Bhatia ML, Singh I, Manchanda SC, et al. Effect of furosemide on pulmonary blood volume. Br Med J 1969; 2:551–552.
6. Brackett NC Jr, Wingo CF, Muren O, Solano JT. Acid-base response to chronic hypercapnia in man. N Engl J Med 1969; 280:124–130.
7. Brown MJ, Brown DL, Murphy MB. Hypokalemia from $beta_2$-receptor stimulation by circulating epinephrine. N Engl J Med 1983; 309:1414–1419.
8. Bushinski DA, Gennari FJ. Life-threatening hyperkalemia induced by arginine. Ann Intern Med 1978; 89:632–634.
9. Butler J. Cor pulmonale. In: Murray JF, Nadel JA, eds. Textbook of Respiratory Medicine. Philadelphia: WB Saunders, 1988, 1410–1433.
10. Christianson L, Shah A, Fisher V. Quantitative left-ventricular cineangiography in patients with chronic obstructive pulmonary disease. Am J Med 1979; 66:399–404.
11. Cohen JJ, Kassirer JP. Acid-Base. Boston: Little, Brown, 1982.
12. Cook CD, Mead J, Schreiner GL, et al. Pulmonary mechanics during induced edema in anesthetized dogs. J Appl Physiol 1959; 14:177–186.
13. Dikshit K, Vyden JK, Forrester JS , et al. Renal and extrarenal hemodynamic effects of furosemide in congestive heart failure after acute myocardial infarction. N Engl J Med 1973; 288:1087–1090.
14. Fencl V. Acid-base balance in cerebral fluids. In: Cherniack NS, Widdicombe JG, eds. Handbook of Physiology. Section 3: Respiratory System. Vol II. Control of Breathing. Bethesda, Md: American Physiological Society, 2nd ed. 1986, 115–140.
15. Fencl V, Gabel RA. Respiratory adaptations in acid-base disturbances: role of cerebral fluids. Contr Nephrol 1980; 21:145–149.
16. Fencl V, Miller TB, Pappenheimer JR. Studies on the respiratory response to disturbances of acid-base balance, with deductions concerning the ionic composition of cerebral interstitial fluid. Am J Physiol 1966; 210:459–472.
17. Fencl V, Rossing TH. Acid-base disorders in critical care medicine. Annu Rev Med 1989; 40:17–29.
18. Ferguson RK, Turek DM, Rovner DR. Spironolactone and hydrochlorothiazide in normal-renin and low-renin essential hypertension. Clin Pharmacol Ther 1977; 21:62–69.
19. Fishman AP. Chronic cor pulmonale. Am Rev Respir Dis 1976; 114:775–794.
20. Galdston M, Geller J. The effects of increased ventilation on the work of breathing in patients with pulmonary emphysema and in normals. J Clin Invest 1955; 34:935.
21. Gertz I, Henderstierna G, Wester PO. Improvement in pulmonary function with diuretic therapy in the hypervolemic and polycythemic patient with chronic obstructive pulmonary disease. Chest 1979; 75:146–151.
22. Good DW, Wright FS. Luminal influences on potassium secretion: sodium concentration and fluid flow rate. Am J Physiol 1979; 236:F192–F205.
23. Greene LH, Smith TH. The use of digitalis in patients with pulmonary disease. Ann Intern Med 1977; 87:459–465.
24. Harrington JT, Isner JM, Kassirer JP. Our national obsession with potassium. Am J Med 1982; 73:155–159.
25. Heinemann HO. Right-sided heart failure and the use of diuretics. Am J Med 1978; 64:367–370.
26. Hill NS. Fluid and electrolyte considerations in diuretic therapy for hypertensive patients with chronic obstructive pulmonary disease. Arch Intern Med 1986; 146:129–133.
27. Hodgkin JE, Soeprono FF, Chan DM. Incidence of metabolic alkalemia in hospitalized patients. Crit Care Med 1980; 8:725–728.
28. Hutcheon DE, Martinez JC. A decade of developments in diuretic drug therapy. J Clin Pharmacol 1986; 26:567–579.
29. Javaheri S, Bosken CH, Lim SH, et al. Effects of hypohydration on lung functions in humans. Am Rev Respir Dis 1987; 135:597–599.
30. Javaheri S, Kazemi H. Metabolic alkalosis and hypoventilation in humans. Am Rev Respir Dis 1987; 136:1011–1016.
31. Javaheri S, Shore NS, Rose B, Kazemi H. Compensatory hypoventilation in metabolic alkalosis. Chest 1982; 81:296–301.
32. Kaplan NM. Our appropriate concern about hypokalemia. Am J Med 1981; 77:1–4.
33. Kassirer JP, Berkman PM, Lawrenz DR, Schwartz WB. The critical role of chloride in the correction of hypokalemic alkalosis in man. Am J Med 1965; 38:172–189.
34. Kline LE, Crawford MH, MacDonald WF, et al. Noninvasive assessment of left ventricular performance in patients with chronic obstructive pulmonary disease. Chest 1977; 72:558–564.
35. Kokko JP. Site and mechanism of action of diuretics. Am J Med 1984; 77(Suppl 5A):11–17.
36. Küng M, White JR, Burki NK. The effect of subcutaneous administration of terbutaline on serum potassium in asymptomatic adult asthmatics. Am Rev Respir Dis 1984; 129:329–332.
37. Light RW, Chetty KG, Stansbury DW. Comparison of the effects of labetalol and hydrochlorothiazide on the ventilatory function of hypertensive patients with mild chronic obstructive pulmonary disease. Am J Med 1983; 75(Suppl 4A):109–114.
38. Mathur PN, Powles ACP, Pugsley SO, et al. Effect of digoxin on right ventricular function in severe chronic airflow obstruction. Ann Intern Med 1981; 95:283–288.
39. Mathur PN, Pugsley SO, Powles ACP, et al. Effect of diuretics

on cardiopulmonary performance in severe chronic airflow obstruction. Arch Intern Med 1981; 144:2154–2157.
40. Miller PD, Bens AS. Acute metabolic alkalosis perpetuating hypercarbia. A role for acetazolamide in chronic obstructive pulmonary disease. JAMA 1977; 238:2400–2401.
41. Morgan DB, Davidson C. Hypokalemia and diuretics: an analysis of publications. Br Med J 1980; 280:905–908.
42. Mudge GH, Wainer IM. Drugs affecting renal function and electrolyte metabolism. In: Gilman AG, Goodman LS, Gilman LS, Gilman A, eds. The Pharmacological Basis of Therapeutics. 7th ed. New York: Macmillan, 1985, 879–907.
43. Nadell J. The effects of the carbonic anhydrase inhibitor "6063" on electrolytes and acid-base balance in two normal subjects and two patients with respiratory acidosis. J Clin Invest 1953; 32:622–629.
44. Paterson LN, Wright FS. Effect of sodium intake on renal potassium excretion. Am J Physiol 1977; 233:F225–F234.
45. Ramsay LE, Hettiarachchi J, Fraser R, Morton JJ. Amiloride, spironolactone, and potassium chloride in thiazide-treated hypertensive patients. Clin Pharmacol Ther 1980; 27:533–543.
46. Rao BS, Cohn KE, Eldridge FL, Hancock EW. Left ventricular failure secondary to chronic pulmonary disease. Am J Med 1968; 45:229–241.
47. Refsum HE. Acid-base disturbances in chronic pulmonary disease. Ann NY Acad Sci 1966; 133:142–149.
48. Steele P, Ellis J, van Dyke D, et al. Left ventricular ejection function in severe chronic obstructive airway disease. Am J Med 1975; 59:21–28.
49. Stewart PA. How to Understand Acid-Base. New York: Elsevier, 1981.
50. Stewart PA. Modern quantitative acid-base chemistry. Can J Physiol Pharmacol 1983; 61:1444–1461.
51. The Joint National Committee on Detection, Evaluation, and Treatment of High Blood Pressure. The 1984 report of the Joint National Committee on Detection, Evaluation, and Treatment of High Blood Pressure. Arch Intern Med 1984; 144:1045–1057.
52. Turino GM, Goldring RM, Heinemann HO. Renal response to mechanical ventilation in patients with chronic hypercapnia. Am J Med 1974; 56:151–161.
53. Vick RL, Todd EP, Luedke DW. Epinephrine-induced hypokalemia: relation to liver and skeletal muscle. J Pharmacol Exp Ther 1972; 181:139–146.
54. West JB. Ventilation, blood flow, and gas exchange. In: Murray JF, Nadel JA, eds. Textbook of Respiratory Medicine. Philadelphia: WB Saunders, 1988, 47–84.
55. Winters RW, Engel K, Dell RB. Acid-Base Physiology in Medicine. Copenhagen: Munksgaard, 1967.

Chapter 50

PULMONARY VASODILATORS IN THE TREATMENT OF BRONCHITIS AND EMPHYSEMA

John R. Michael

Encouraged by the success of vasodilator therapy for systemic hypertension and congestive heart failure, in the past decade many investigators have aggressively explored the possibility that vasodilator therapy would be beneficial in COPD patients with pulmonary hypertension. The rationale for this approach in COPD patients springs from several sources: the belief that the degree of pulmonary hypertension influences survival,[1] the notion that increased afterload leads to the development of right ventricular failure, the concept that hypoxic pulmonary vasoconstriction causes the pulmonary hypertension, the finding that continuous oxygen therapy improves survival compared with intermittent oxygen use,[2] and the observation that eliminating hypoxia can reverse the pathologic and physiologic changes caused by alveolar hypoxia in experimental animals[3, 4] and in humans living at high altitude.[5] These concepts gave rise to the hypothesis that continuous inhibition of hypoxic pulmonary vasoconstriction by oxygen or oxygen combined with a vasodilator would produce hemodynamic benefits, such as reducing pulmonary vascular resistance and pulmonary hypertension and increasing cardiac output and systemic oxygen delivery. By analogy to the treatment of systemic hypertension, it has been hoped that these hemodynamic effects might eventually result in less right-sided heart failure and reduced morbidity and mortality. Because vasodilators might reduce right ventricular afterload and increase cardiac output and oxygen delivery during exercise, it was also anticipated that these drugs might improve ventricular function and perhaps even increase the severely limited exercise capacity in COPD patients.

This chapter reviews the published information about specific drugs and summarizes the current status of vasodilator therapy for pulmonary hypertension in patients with COPD.

SPECIFIC DRUGS

Nitroglycerin

All hemodynamic measurements with nitroglycerin have been made at rest. The intravenous infusion of nitroglycerin decreased pulmonary vascular resistance by 21%;[6] however, oral isosorbide dinitrate (30 mg)[7] or sublingual nitroglycerin (0.8 mg)[8] did not reduce pulmonary vascular resistance. Nitroglycerin primarily decreased preload, causing a fall in cardiac index, right ventricular end-diastolic volume, and right atrial, pulmonary capillary wedge, and pulmonary arterial pressures.[6–8] Nitroglycerin also may decrease oxygen delivery and arterial or mixed venous Po_2.[6–9] Although it did not reduce pulmonary vascular resistance, sublingual nitroglycerin (0.8 mg) increased resting right ventricular ejection fraction (RVEF) in COPD patients with depressed RVEF at baseline.[8]

Nitroprusside

All hemodynamic studies have been at rest. The intravenous infusion of nitroprusside decreased pulmonary vascular resistance by 16% to 21%.[8, 10] Its major effect appears to be on preload, decreasing right ventricular end-diastolic volume and right atrial, mean pulmonary arterial, and pulmonary capillary wedge pressures.[8, 10] Nitroprusside also may decrease cardiac index, oxygen delivery, and arterial and mixed venous Po_2.[8] In contrast to nitroglycerin or hydralazine, nitroprusside did not improve resting RVEF in COPD patients with depressed right ventricular function.[8, 10]

Beta-Adrenergic Agonists

PIRBUTEROL. All hemodynamic measurements with pirbuterol have been made at rest. Oral pirbuterol (15 or 22.5 mg) reduced pulmonary vascular resistance by 19% to 27%, did not affect mean pulmonary arterial pressure, and increased heart rate and stroke volume, resulting in a 21% to 24% increase in cardiac index.[10, 11] Pirbuterol may slightly decrease Pao_2, but the increase in cardiac index augments oxygen delivery.[10, 11] These doses also improved resting RVEF but not left ventricular ejection fraction (LVEF).[10] In one study, 9 of the 12 patients studied acutely were treated for 6 weeks with 15 mg bid.[10] Three of the 9 patients did not complete the 6-week trial: one because of acute respiratory failure and two because of an increase in premature ventricular contractions or the onset of atrial fibrillation. Both these patients had frequent ventricular and supraventricular ectopic beats before starting the drug. After 6 weeks of therapy, pirbuterol continued to decrease systolic but not mean pulmonary arterial pressure and increase RVEF but not LVEF. Cardiac index and pulmonary vascular resistance were not reported after 6 weeks of therapy. Despite the improvement in RVEF, chronic treatment did not improve exercise capacity, as measured by the distance walked in 12 minutes.[10]

SALBUTAMOL. Hemodynamic measurements have been made only with intravenous salbutamol. The intravenous infusion of 3 μg/kg over 3 minutes increased cardiac index and left ventricular dp/dt_{max} and decreased pulmonary arterial pressure and pulmonary vascular resistance.[12] These effects, however, were transient, lasting only 10 minutes.[12] During the intravenous infusion of salbutamol (0.2 μg/kg/min for 15 min), resting cardiac index increased by 31%, pulmonary arterial pressure was unchanged, and pulmonary vascular resistance decreased by 15%.[13] During exercise, intravenous salbutamol increased stroke volume, raised cardiac index by 32%, and did not affect pulmonary arterial pressure. The net effect was a 26% decrease in pulmonary vascular resistance during exercise.[13] Oral salbutamol (4 mg) increased RVEF and LVEF 60 and 90 minutes after a single dose.[14]

TERBUTALINE. The rapid intravenous infusion of up to 0.25 mg of terbutaline lowered resting pulmonary vascular resistance by 16% to 35% and increased the cardiac index by 11% to 26%, usually without affecting pulmonary arterial pressure.[15–17] During exercise, intravenous terbutaline (0.25 mg) increased the cardiac index by 24% and reduced pulmonary arterial pressure by 8 mm Hg, lowering pulmonary vascular resistance by 30%.[16] Subcutaneous terbutaline (0.25 mg) also decreased resting pulmonary vascular resistance by 35% and increased cardiac index (48%), heart rate, stroke volume, RVEF, and LVEF.[18] Terbutaline subcutaneously raised oxygen delivery without affecting Pao_2.

AMINOPHYLLINE. Intravenous aminophylline (1 g infused over 30 min) reduced pulmonary arterial pressure by 14 mm Hg without changing cardiac index, leading to a 27% decrease in pulmonary vascular resistance.[19] Intravenous infusion of aminophylline (9 mg/kg over 30 min) acutely increased RVEF and LVEF in normal subjects and COPD patients.[20] A single oral dose of theophylline (600 mg) improved RVEF but not LVEF (average theophylline serum level of 11 μg/ml).[14] Oral theophylline (14 mg/kg/d) for 72 hours significantly increased resting RVEF and LVEF in COPD patients with depressed baseline right ventricular function.[21] The improvement in RVEF and LVEF persisted during 16 weeks of therapy.[21] The average serum theophylline level in these patients was 15 μg/ml. All measurements were made at rest.

Alpha-Adrenergic Antagonists

The continuous intravenous infusion of phentolamine for 3 days decreased resting pulmonary vascular resistance by 36% and pulmonary arterial pressure by 8 mm Hg, and increased cardiac index by 25%.[21] Intravenous urapidil (0.75 mg/kg over 15 min) increased stroke volume, raised cardiac index by 18%, and lowered pulmonary arterial pressure by 7 mm Hg, resulting in a 32% decrease in pulmonary vascular resistance.[23]

The effects of oral prazosin (average of 5.5 mg/d) for 1 week and 2 months have been reported in eight patients.[24] One week of therapy increased resting cardiac index (11%) and stroke volume and decreased right ventricular end-diastolic pressure and pulmonary arterial pressure (4 mm Hg). The net effect was a 32% decrease in pulmonary vascular resistance.[24] After 1 week, prazosin increased cardiac index during exercise by 17% and decreased pulmonary arterial pressure by 3 mm Hg, leading to a 30% decrease in pulmonary vascular resistance.[24] These hemodynamic changes persisted after 2 months of chronic therapy. The hemodynamic response after 2 months of prazosin was similar to the response after 1 week of therapy, except that therapy for 1 week did not affect Pao_2, whereas chronic therapy significantly decreased Pao_2 during rest and exercise. In this uncontrolled study, one of the eight patients had subjective clinical improvement, but six complained of increased breathlessness.[24]

Angiotensin-Converting Enzyme Inhibitors

Two studies have evaluated the acute effects of a single dose of captopril on pulmonary hemodynamics in COPD patients.[25, 26] In a controlled clinical trial, a single dose of captopril (25 mg) did not affect cardiac index, pulmonary arterial pressure, pulmonary vascular resistance, or arterial blood gases.[25] In a separate report a single dose of captopril (50 mg orally) acutely increased oxygen delivery and cardiac index (22%) but did not change pulmonary arterial pressure or pulmonary vascular resistance.[26]

Prostaglandin E_1

Oral prostaglandin E_1 (20 μg) increased cardiac index by 24% and decreased pulmonary arterial pressure by 6 mm Hg, resulting in a 47% fall in pulmonary vascular resistance.[27] With this dose, the hemodynamic effects lasted for 8 hours but caused flushing in all patients.

TABLE 50–1. Studies with Oral Hydralazine

			REST						EXERCISE						
REF.	NO. OF PTS.	DOSE AND DURATION	PPA (mm Hg)	CI (%)	PVR (%)	SVR (%)	Pa_{O_2} (mm Hg)	Pa_{CO_2} (mm Hg)	PPA (mm Hg)	CI (%)	PVR (%)	SVR (%)	Pa_{O_2} (mm Hg)	Pa_{CO_2} (mm Hg)	COMMENTS
28	7	50 mg q6hr for 7 days	NS	+22	NS	−39	NS	NS	NS	+26	NS	−35	NS	NS	1 pt less dyspnea; 2 pts worsened
31	6	75 mg	NS	+37	−24	−35	+6	−7							
	10	50–75 mg q6hr for 48 hr	−5	+48	−42	−37	+4	−3							
32	10	50 mg q6hr for 24 hr	NS	+23	NS	NR	+4	−3	−3	NS	NS	NR	+5	−5	No change in exercise capacity
33	7	50 mg q6hr for 48 hr	NS	+60	−33	NR	NS	−8	−5	+25	−27	NR	NS	−8	No change in exercise tolerance at 48 hr or 2 mon
34	14	50 mg q6hr for 24 hr	NS	+35	NS	NR	+8	−7	−5	+15	−28	NR	+9	−8	3 pts could not tolerate drug because of marked tachycardia; 4 pts had increased exercise tolerance
35	5	50 mg q6hr for 48 hr	−5	+44	−48	−40	NS	NS	−10	NS	−24	−25	NS	NS	

The values are the average changes in hemodynamics and arterial blood gases caused by treatment with oral hydralazine. PPA, mean pulmonary arterial pressure; CI, cardiac index; PVR, pulmonary vascular resistance; SVR, systemic vascular resistance; Pa_{O_2}, arterial oxygen pressure; Pa_{CO_2}, arterial carbon dioxide pressure; NS, not statistically significant; NR, not reported.

Hydralazine

Intravenous hydralazine (0.33 mg/kg infused over 3 min) increased resting cardiac index by 15% and increased pulmonary arterial pressure by 4 mm Hg. Systemic vascular resistance was decreased, but pulmonary vascular resistance was not.[28] In a second report, intravenous hydralazine (30 to 40 mg) increased resting cardiac index by 71% without affecting pulmonary arterial pressure, decreasing pulmonary vascular resistance by 39%.[8] In this study, hydralazine increased oxygen delivery, mixed venous P_{O_2}, and resting RVEF.[8] In a third study, intravenous hydralazine (0.35 mg/kg infused over 15 minutes) did not change pulmonary arterial pressure, increased cardiac index by 51%, and consequently decreased pulmonary vascular resistance by 30%.[23] During exercise, intravenous hydralazine (0.33 mg/kg) increased cardiac index by 12% without affecting pulmonary arterial pressure, reducing pulmonary vascular resistance by 16%. Hydralazine also increased Pa_{O_2} during exercise.[28]

The effects of intravenous hydralazine (up to 40 mg) in COPD patients breathing room air or a hypoxic gas mixture also have been reported.[29] While the patients breathed room air (arterial oxygen saturation 90%), hydralazine increased cardiac index (22%), heart rate, and stroke volume but did not affect pulmonary arterial pressure or pulmonary vascular resistance.[29] Hydralazine also did not affect resting RVEF. Breathing a hypoxic gas mixture for 15 minutes reduced arterial O_2 saturation from 90% to 74% and increased pulmonary arterial pressure and pulmonary vascular resistance. Pretreatment with hydralazine did not prevent the increase in pulmonary arterial pressure or pulmonary vascular resistance caused by breathing the hypoxic gas mixture. In fact, the combination of hydralazine and hypoxia produced a significantly greater pulmonary arterial pressure and right ventricular stroke work index than occurred with either hydralazine or hypoxia alone.[29] The apparent lack of success of hydralazine in blocking hypoxic pulmonary vasoconstriction in patients corresponds with its failure to inhibit hypoxic vasoconstriction in experimental animals.[30] Seven of the nine patients in this uncontrolled study reported worsening dyspnea after receiving hydralazine.[29] In one patient the breathlessness was so severe that he was unable to continue in the study.

Studies with oral hydralazine are summarized in Table 50–1. Variable responses to hydralazine have been seen. Hydralazine generally does not lower pulmonary arterial pressure of patients at rest (four of six studies), consistently increases cardiac index, and has a variable effect on pulmonary vascular resistance (no change in three of six reports and a decrease in the other three) (Table 50–1). Hydralazine also frequently increases Pa_{O_2} and oxygen delivery and reduces Pa_{CO_2} of patients at rest. Oral hydralazine generally decreases pulmonary arterial pressure (four of five studies) of exercising subjects but has an inconsistent effect on cardiac output and pulmonary vascular resistance (Table 50–1). Hydralazine also may improve Pa_{O_2} and Pa_{CO_2} during exercise, although this varies (Table 50–1).

In the same patients, the acute hemodynamic response to intravenous hydralazine has been compared with the response to oral therapy for 1 week (50 mg q6hr).[28] The acute and chronic hemodynamic responses at rest were similar: hydralazine increased cardiac index by 15% when given intravenously and by 22% with oral therapy but did not reduce pulmonary arterial pressure or pulmonary vascular resistance.[28] The exercise responses, however, differed. Intravenous hydralazine lowered pulmonary vascular resistance during exercise by 16%, whereas 1 week of oral hydralazine did not reduce pulmonary vascular resistance.[28] During exercise, both intravenous or oral therapy increased cardiac index, but did not affect pulmonary arterial pressure. Intravenous hydralazine improved Pa_{O_2} and arterial and mixed venous oxygen saturation during rest and exercise. In contrast, after a week of therapy, Pa_{O_2} and arterial oxygen saturation were not improved during rest or exercise, although mixed venous saturation was increased. Upon restudy, only two of the seven patients treated for a week had improvement in both hemodynamics and Pa_{O_2}. One patient who had a 50% reduction in pulmonary vascular resistance during rest and exercise had relief of dyspnea with mild exertion. Two patients had an unfavorable hemodynamic response. Another patient had improved hemodynamics at rest, but pulmonary arterial pressure and vascular resistance were increased during exercise. An additional patient's Pa_{O_2} decreased from 55 to 45 mm Hg.

Another study investigated the hemodynamic response to hydralazine at 48 hours and the effect of therapy for 48 hours or 2 months on exercise capacity.[33] Three of the ten patients treated with hydralazine (50 mg q6hr) for 48 hours developed side effects that required discontinuing the drug. Two patients had increased dyspnea, and one patient had severe nausea. During exercise, hydralazine therapy for 48 hours improved oxygen delivery, increased cardiac index by 25%, and decreased pulmonary arterial pressure by 5 mm Hg, causing pulmonary vascular resistance to decrease by 27%. Despite these hemodynamic changes, hydralazine therapy for 48 hours or 2 months did not improve exercise capacity, as assessed by endurance time or symptom-limited maximal oxygen consumption.[33] Hemodynamics were not remeasured after 2 months of therapy.

In summary, hydralazine does not appear to inhibit hypoxic pulmonary vasoconstriction either in experimental animals or in hypoxic patients with COPD.[29, 30] Hydralazine generally lowers pulmonary vascular resistance at rest and during exercise, but this effect is variable (Table 50–1). In contrast with the calcium channel blockers, hydralazine frequently increases Pa_{O_2} and may decrease Pa_{CO_2} by 3 to 8 mm Hg. Enthusiasm for hydralazine has waned because of the relatively high rate of side effects that lead to stopping the drug (nausea, marked tachycardia, increased dyspnea, or hemodynamic worsening).[28, 29, 33, 34]

Calcium Channel Blockers

In animal studies, calcium channel blockers inhibit hypoxic pulmonary vasoconstriction.[36, 37] A number of different calcium channel blockers have been tried in humans to assess their effects on pulmonary hemodynamics. Nifedipine, a calcium channel blocker, also prevents hypoxic pulmonary vasoconstriction in hypoxic COPD patients.[38] Although verapamil and diltiazem inhibit hypoxic pulmonary vasoconstriction in experimental animals,[36, 37] these two drugs appear to be ineffective in hypoxic COPD patients.[39, 40] In contrast, numerous studies have found that the acute administration of nifedipine (20 to 40 mg) will reduce resting pulmonary vascular resistance in COPD patients.[6, 38, 41–46]

The clinical trials using oral nifedipine or nitrendipine are summarized in Table 50–2 (all used nifedipine except reference 47). Nifedipine frequently, but not always, lowers resting pulmonary arterial pressure, increases cardiac index, and reduces pulmonary and systemic vascular resistance by 20% to 30% (Table 50–2). In a controlled clinical trial, nifedipine also has been shown to augment significantly the vasodilation produced by low-flow oxygen.[38] Although nifedipine increases stroke volume,[38, 43] single doses of sublingual nifedipine (20 mg) did not increase resting RVEF or LVEF.[41] Nifedipine may either reduce or leave unchanged Pa_{O_2} and Pa_{CO_2}. Nitrendipine appears to produce similar hemodynamic changes at rest[47] (Table 50–2).

Only three studies have investigated the effect of nifedipine on the cardiovascular response to exercise (Table 50–2). In these studies, nifedipine produced an impressive decrease in pulmonary arterial pressure during exercise of 5 to 15 mm Hg, but had a variable effect on cardiac index. Two of the three studies found that nifedipine lowered pulmonary vascular resistance during exercise by 44% and 28%.[38, 42] Pulmonary vascular resistance was not significantly changed in the third study.[45] Despite an average decrease in pulmonary arterial pressure of 15 mm Hg during exercise, a single dose of nifedipine (20 mg) did not increase the duration of exercise.[42]

Three uncontrolled studies have compared the acute hemodynamic response to nifedipine with the response to longer-term therapy.[41, 43, 44] In the first study, measurements at baseline, after 24 hours of nifedipine therapy (20 mg q6hr), and after 6 weeks (20 mg q6hr) were made in three patients.[41] Nifedipine did not affect resting pulmonary hemodynamics at either time point. The second study assessed the acute response to nifedipine (20 mg sublingual) in 24 patients.[43] The investigators also measured the effects of nifedipine therapy (30 mg/day) for 15 days in a separate group of 10 patients. In both the acute and chronic therapy groups, nifedipine raised the resting cardiac index and oxygen delivery and decreased pulmonary arterial pressure, reducing pulmonary vascular resistance by 25% acutely and 23% chronically.[43] The acute response, however, differed in several respects from the chronic response. Acutely, nifedipine increased heart rate and decreased Pa_{O_2}. In the chronically treated patients, cardiac index was increased without a change in heart rate or Pa_{O_2}.[43] A third study determined the acute effects of nifedipine in 12 patients. The investigators also measured the response after an average of 55 days (10 to 20 mg q8hr) in 8 of the 12 patients. Acutely, nifedipine (20 mg sublingual) decreased resting pulmonary vascular resistance by 30%, increased cardiac index by 24%, increased oxygen delivery, and did not change Pa_{O_2} and pulmonary arterial pressure. None of the patients were receiving chronic oxygen therapy. Chronic therapy with nifedipine decreased resting pulmonary vascular resistance by 23%. In contrast to the acute effects in which there was an increase in cardiac index without an effect on pulmonary arterial pressure, chronic therapy did not increase the cardiac index but significantly reduced pulmonary arterial pressure by an average of 7 mm Hg.[44] Despite hemodynamic improvement, two of the eight patients had progressive clinical worsening. One patient had decreased dyspnea on exercise. One half of the patients receiving long-term therapy developed peripheral edema without other signs of right heart failure.

An uncontrolled trial of nitrendipine, a calcium channel blocker similar to nifedipine, has also been reported.[47] All patients studied were receiving supplemental oxygen. Measurements were made off oxygen. After 6 weeks of therapy (20 mg bid), nitrendipine decreased resting pulmonary arterial pressure by 9 mm Hg, increased cardiac index by 50%, and increased oxygen delivery and stroke volume. This resulted in a 56% decrease in pulmonary vascular resistance. Except for a mild headache, significant side effects were not present. Four of the seven patients receiving long-term therapy noted subjective improvement with increased activity tolerance, whereas three felt unchanged.

In summary, nifedipine, in contrast to hydralazine, inhibits hypoxic pulmonary vasoconstriction in COPD patients.[29, 38] Nifedipine or nitrendipine are the most promising of the currently available vasodilators. They frequently lower pulmonary arterial pressure and consistently reduce pulmonary vascular resistance both acutely and with chronic therapy. In addition, they produce relatively few side effects. The most common side effect is ankle edema unassociated with right ventricular failure.

GENERAL COMMENTS

The evaluation of vasodilator therapy may be considered from four viewpoints:

TABLE 50–2. Studies with Oral Nifedipine or Nitrendipine

REF.	NO. OF PTS.	DOSE AND DURATION	REST						EXERCISE						COMMENTS
			PPA (mm Hg)	CI (%)	PVR (%)	SVR (%)	Pa_{O_2} (mm Hg)	Pa_{CO_2} (mm Hg)	PPA (mm Hg)	CI (%)	PVR (%)	SVR (%)	Pa_{O_2} (mm Hg)	Pa_{CO_2} (mm Hg)	
6	11	20–40 mg SL	NS	+11	−21	−25	NS	−4							
38	6	40 mg PO	−3	+21	−27	−25	−4	NS	−12	+18	−44	−26	NS	NS	Controlled trial; additive effect of nifedipine and O_2
41	12	20 mg SL	NS	+25	NS	−35	NS	NS							
	10	20 mg q6hr for 24 hr	−6	NS	−11	−29	NS	−4							
42	8	20 mg SL	NS	+26	−32	−35	NS	NR	−15	NS	−28	−20	NS	NR	No change in exercise tolerance
43	24	20 mg SL	−4	+25	−25	−30	−2	NS							
	10	10 mg tid for 15 d	−4	+23	−23	−23	NS	NS							
44	12	20 mg SL	NS	+24	−30	NR	NS	NS							
	8	10–20 mg q8hr for 6–9 wk	−7	NS	−23	NR	NS	NS							
45	9	20 mg SL	NS	+30	−21	NR	NS	NS	−5	NS	NS	NR	NS	NS	
46	6	20 mg SL	NS	+29	−28	−36	−5	NS							
47*	8	20 mg bid for 6 wk	−9	+50	−56	NR	NS	NR							

*Only study with nitrendipine.

The values are the average changes in hemodynamics and arterial blood gases caused by treatment with oral nifedipine or nitrendipine. PPA, mean pulmonary arterial pressure; CI, cardiac index; PVR, pulmonary vascular resistance; SVR, systemic vascular resistance; Pa_{O_2}, arterial oxygen pressure; Pa_{CO_2}, arterial carbon dioxide pressure; SL = sublingual; NS, not statistically significant; NR, not reported.

- Does acute therapy produce potentially helpful effects?
- Do the potentially beneficial effects persist with ongoing therapy?
- Does therapy produce subjective or functional clinical improvement?
- Does therapy reduce morbidity or mortality?

As just reviewed, a number of vasodilators acutely cause potentially helpful changes in pulmonary vascular resistance, pulmonary arterial pressure, cardiac output, and oxygen delivery. Nitroglycerin,[8] pirbuterol,[10] salbutamol,[14] terbutaline,[18] aminophylline,[14, 21] and hydralazine[8] have also been reported to increase resting RVEF in COPD patients. Even though nifedipine increases stroke volume,[38, 43] it did not increase resting RVEF in the single study in which this was measured.[41] Although the great majority of these studies are uncontrolled, the few controlled clinical trials have found that placebo therapy does not affect pulmonary hemodynamics.[25, 38]

Acute effects have been shown to persist during ongoing therapy with pirbuterol,[10] aminophylline,[21] prazosin,[24] hydralazine,[33–35] nifedipine,[43, 44] and nitrendipine.[47] Although it is assumed in these uncontrolled trials that the drug is the only reason for the improvement, one cannot completely exclude the possibility that other factors contributed to the improvement, such as increased compliance with medical regimens or greater medical attention.

Even though therapy has been associated with clinical improvement in individual patients, most patients have not reported functional improvement. In fact, some patients have complained of increased breathlessness or significant side effects.[24, 28–30, 32–34] In addition, despite improving hemodynamics, hydralazine,[33] pirbuterol,[10] or nifedipine[42] does not improve exercise capacity. Based on the current evidence, vasodilator therapy does not generally produce subjective or functional improvement in COPD patients.

The important question of whether or not long-term vasodilator therapy alone or combined with oxygen would reduce morbidity or mortality has not been addressed and is unlikely to be directly tested. One could argue that the initial trials in systemic hypertension demonstrated hemodynamic changes, but patients did not notice clinical or functional improvement and frequently complained of unpleasant side effects. The protective effect of antihypertensive treatment on morbidity and mortality did not become apparent until long-term clinical trials were completed. Given the general lack of enthusiasm and the enormous effort and cost required, it is unlikely that a large-scale clinical trial will be done to determine whether or not vasodilator therapy will decrease morbidity or mortality in COPD patients.

The inital enthusiasm for vasodilator therapy in COPD patients with pulmonary hypertension has waned because of the difficulty in performing the studies, the variable hemodynamic effects, the minimal effect on pulmonary arterial pressure, the failure to document clinical or functional improvement, and the development of increased symptoms or side effects in some patients. In addition, as information has accumulated about specific vasodilators, they have suffered in comparison with oxygen therapy.

Oxygen therapy meets many of the criteria for an ideal pulmonary vasodilator.[48] It selectively dilates the pulmonary circulation,[49] inhibits hypoxic pulmonary vasoconstriction,[49] reduces pulmonary vascular resistance,[49–51] improves cardiac function,[49] enhances oxygen delivery,[49, 50] augments exercise capacity,[52, 53] improves quality of life,[2, 54] and increases survival.[2, 55] In contrast, no other vasodilator selectively dilates the pulmonary circulation or has been shown to improve exercise capacity, enhance quality of life, or increase survival.

Based upon the information gathered during the past decade, it is likely that the effort spent to study the effects of vasodilators in COPD patients with pulmonary hypertension will diminish. At the present time, vasodilator therapy for

COPD patients with pulmonary hypertension cannot be recommended. There are, however, two caveats. First, we should remember that the crucial question of whether vasodilator therapy will reduce morbidity and increase survival has not been answered. Perhaps in the future, armed with a better understanding of the mechanisms responsible for the pulmonary hypertension and with more potent and selective drugs, this question will be addressed. Second, the work of Ashutosh and his colleagues[56] suggests that hypoxic COPD patients can be divided into oxygen responders and nonresponders. They divided patients with COPD and cor pulmonale into these two groups, depending upon the fall in mean pulmonary arterial pressure that occurred while breathing 28% oxygen for 24 hours. Patients with a decrease in mean pulmonary arterial pressure of 5 mm Hg or more were defined as responders; nonresponders had a decrease of less than 5 mm Hg. Sixty-one percent of patients were responders. After 2 years of long-term oxygen therapy, 88% of responders were alive, whereas only 22% of nonresponders were still alive.[56] If generally applicable, these results suggest that therapy in addition to oxygen is needed in many hypoxic COPD patients. If the currently available vasodilators do not appear promising, this does not eliminate the need for additional therapy and should stimulate us to consider other potential approaches.

REFERENCES

1. Weitzenblum E, Hirth C, Ducolone A, et al. Prognostic value of pulmonary artery pressure in chronic obstructive pulmonary disease. Thorax 1981; 36:752–758.
2. Nocturnal Oxygen Therapy Trial Group. Continuous or nocturnal oxygen therapy in hypoxemic chronic obstructive lung disease. Ann Intern Med 1980; 93:391–398.
3. Rabinovitch M, Gamble W, Miettinen OS, Reid L. Age and sex influence on pulmonary hypertension of chronic hypoxia and on recovery. Am J Physiol 1981; 240:H62–H72.
4. Rabinovitch M, Gamble W, Nadas AS, et al. Rat pulmonary circulation after chronic hypoxia: hemodynamics and structural features. Am J Physiol 1979; 236:818–827.
5. Sime F, Penaloza O, Ruiz L. Bradycardia, increased cardiac output and reversal of pulmonary hypertension in altitude natives living at sea level. Br Heart J 1971; 33:647–657.
6. Morley TF, Zappasodi SJ, Belli A, Giudice JC. Pulmonary vasodilator therapy for chronic obstructive pulmonary disease and cor pulmonale: treatment with nifedipine, nitroglycerin, and oxygen. Chest 1987; 92:71–76.
7. Danahy DT, Tobis JM, Aronow WS, et al. Effects of isosorbide dinitrate on pulmonary hypertension in chronic obstructive pulmonary disease. Clin Pharmacol Ther 1979; 25:541–548.
8. Brent BN, Berger HJ, Matthay RA, et al. Contrasting acute effects of vasodilators (nitroglycerin, nitroprusside, and hydralazine) on right ventricular performance in patients with chronic obstructive pulmonary disease and pulmonary hypertension: a combined radionuclide-hemodynamic study. Am J Cardiol 1983; 51:1682–1689.
9. Kochukoshy KN, Chick TW, Jenne JW. The effect of nitroglycerin in gas exchange on chronic obstructive pulmonary disease. Am Rev Respir Dis 1975; 111:177–183.
10. MacNee W, Wathen CG, Hannan WJ, et al. Effects of pirbuterol and sodium nitroprusside on pulmonary haemodynamics in hypoxic cor pulmonale. Br Med J 1983; 287:1169–1172.
11. Peacock A, Busst C, Dawkins K, Denison DM. Response of pulmonary circulation to oral pirbuterol in chronic airflow obstruction. Br Med J 1983; 287:1178–1181.
12. Iodice F, Rufolo L, Piscione F, DeMichele G. Hemodynamic and ventilatory effects of intravenous salbutamol in patients affected by COLD. Respiration 1980; 40:272–277.
13. Vik-Mo H, Halvorsen FJ, Thorsen E, et al. Improved cardiac performance by salbutamol, a selective β2-agonist, in chronic cor pulmonale. J Cardiovasc Pharmacol 1987; 9:129–134.
14. Winter RJD, Langford JA, George RJD, et al. The effects of theophylline and salbutamol on right and left ventricular function in chronic bronchitis and emphysema. Br J Dis Chest 1984; 78:358–362.
15. Stockley RA, Finnegan P, Bishop JM. Effect of intravenous terbutaline on arterial blood gas tensions, ventilation, and pulmonary circulation in patients with chronic bronchitis and cor pulmonale. Thorax 1977; 32:601–605.
16. Teule GJJ, Majid PA. Haemodynamic effects of terbutaline in chronic obstructive lung disease. Thorax 1980; 35:536–542.
17. Jones RM, Stockley RA, Bishop JM. Early effects of intravenous terbutaline on arterial blood gas tensions, ventilation, and pulmonary circulation in patients with chronic bronchitis and cor pulmonale. Thorax 1977; 32:601–605.
18. Brent BN, Mahler D, Berger HJ, et al. Augmentation of right ventricular performance in chronic obstructive pulmonary disease by terbutaline: a combined radionuclide and hemodynamic study. Am J Cardiol 1982; 50:313–319.
19. Parker JO, Kelkar K, West RO. Hemodynamic effects of aminophylline in cor pulmonale. Circulation 1966; 33:17–25.
20. Matthay RA, Berger HJ, Loke J, et al. Effects of aminophylline upon right and left ventricular performance in chronic obstructive pulmonary disease: noninvasive assessment by radionuclide angiocardiography. Am J Med 1978; 65:903–910.
21. Matthay RA, Berger HJ, Davies R, et al. Improvement in cardiac performance by oral long-acting theophylline in chronic obstructive pulmonary disease. Am Heart J 1982; 104:1022–1026.
22. Van Mieghem W, DeBacker G, De Wispelaere B. Phentolamine infusion in cor pulmonale due to chronic obstructive pulmonary disease. Acta Cardiol 1978; 33:253–262.
23. Adnot S, Defouilloy C, Brun-Buisson C, et al. Hemodynamic effects of urapidil in patients with pulmonary hypertension: a comparative study with hydralazine. Am Rev Respir Dis 1987; 135:288–293.
24. Vik-Mo H, Walde N, Jentoft H, Halvorsen FJ. Improved haemodynamics but reduced arterial blood oxygenation, at rest and during exercise after long-term oral prazosin therapy in chronic cor pulmonale. Eur Heart J 1985; 6:1047–1053.
25. Zielinski J, Hawrylkiewicz I, Gorecka D, et al. Captopril effects on pulmonary and systemic hemodynamics in chronic cor pulmonale. Chest 1986; 90:562–565.
26. Richard C, Ricome JL, Rimailho A, et al. Effects of captopril on pulmonary haemodynamics. Eur J Clin Pharmacol 1984; 27:35–39.
27. Ishizaki T, Miyabo S, Mifune J, et al. OP–1206, a prostaglandin E_1 derivative: effects of oral administration to patients with chronic lung disease. Chest 1984; 85:382–386.
28. Lupi-Herrera E, Seoane M, Verdejo J. Hemodynamic effect of hydralazine in advanced, stable chronic obstructive pulmonary disease with cor pulmonale: immediate and short-term evaluation at rest and during exercise. Chest 1984; 85:156–163.
29. Tuxen DV, Powles ACP, Mathur PN, et al. Detrimental effects of hydralazine in patients with chronic air-flow obstruction and pulmonary hypertension: a combined hemodynamic and radionuclide study. Am Rev Respir Dis 1984; 129:388–395.
30. Bishop M, Kennard S, Artman L, Cheney F. Hydralazine does not inhibit canine hypoxic pulmonary vasoconstriction. Am Rev Respir Dis 1983; 128:998–1001.
31. Miller MJ, Chappell TR, Cook W, et al. Effects of oral hydralazine on gas exchange in patients with cor pulmonale. Am J Med 1983; 75:937–942.
32. Corriveau ML, Shepard JW Jr, Dolan GF. Effects of hydralazine on mouth occlusion pressure and ventilation response to hypercapnia in patients with chronic obstructive pulmonary disease and pulmonary hypertension. Am Rev Respir Dis 1987; 135:118–122.
33. Nogare ARD, Rubin LJ. The effects of hydralazine on exercise capacity in pulmonary hypertension secondary to chronic obstructive pulmonary disease. Am Rev Respir Dis 1986; 133:385–389.
34. Keller CA, Shepard JW Jr, Chun DS, et al. Effects of hydralazine on hemodynamics, ventilation, and gas exchange in patients with chronic obstructive pulmonary disease and pulmonary hypertension. Am Rev Respir Dis 1984; 130:606–611.
35. Rubin LJ, Peter RH. Hemodynamics at rest and during exercise after oral hydralazine in patients with cor pulmonale. Am J Cardiol 1981; 47:116–122.
36. McMurtry IF, Davidson AB, Reeves JT, Grover RF. Inhibition of hypoxic pulmonary vasoconstriction by calcium antagonists in isolated rat lungs. Circ Res 1976; 38:99–104.
37. Kennedy TK, Summer WR. Inhibition of hypoxic pulmonary vasoconstriction by nifedipine. Am J Cardiol 1982; 50:864–868.

38. Kennedy TP, Michael JR, Huang CK, et al. Nifedipine inhibits hypoxic pulmonary vasoconstriction during rest and exercise in patients with chronic obstructive pulmonary disease: a controlled double-blind study. Am Rev Respir Dis 1984; 129:544–551.
39. Clozel JP, Delorme N, Battistella P, et al. Hemodynamic effects of intravenous diltiazem in hypoxic pulmonary hypertension. Chest 1987; 91:171–175.
40. Brown SE, Linden GS, King RR, et al. Effects of verapamil on pulmonary haemodynamics during hypoxaemia, at rest, and during exercise in patients with chronic obstructive pulmonary disease. Thorax 1983; 38:840–844.
41. Mookherjee S, Ashutosh K, Dunsky M, et al. Nifedipine in chronic cor pulmonale: acute and relatively long-term effects. Clin Pharmacol Ther 1988; 44:289–296.
42. Singh H, Ebejer MJ, Higgins DA, et al. Acute haemodynamic effects of nifedipine at rest and during maximal exercise in patients with chronic cor pulmonale. Thorax 1985; 40:910–914.
43. Saadjian A, Philip-Joet F, Arnaud A. Hemodynamic and oxygen delivery responses to nifedipine in pulmonary hypertension secondary to chronic obstructive lung disease. Cardiology 1987; 74:196–204.
44. Sturani C, Bassein L, Schiavina M, Gunella G. Oral nifedipine in chronic cor pulmonale secondary to severe chronic obstructive pulmonary disease (COPD): short- and long-term hemodynamic effects. Chest 1983; 84:135–142.
45. Muramoto A, Caldwell J, Albert RK, Lakshminarayan S. Nifedipine dilates the pulmonary vasculature without producing symptomatic systemic hypotension in upright, resting and exercising patients with pulmonary hypertension secondary to chronic obstructive pulmonary disease. Am Rev Respir Dis 1985; 132:963—966.
46. Melot C, Hallemans R, Naeije R, et al. Deleterious effects of nifedipine on pulmonary gas exchange in chronic obstructive pulmonary disease. Am Rev Respir Dis 1984; 130:612–616.
47. Rubin LJ, Moser K. Long-term effects of nitrendipine on hemodynamics and oxygen transport in patients with cor pulmonale. Chest 1986; 89:141–145.
48. Michael JR, Selinger SR, Buescher PC, Kennedy TP. Pharmacologic therapy of cor pulmonale. In: Fisk RL, ed. The Right Heart: Cardiovascular Clinics. Philadelphia: FA Davis, 1987, 171–179.
49. Selinger S, Kennedy TP, Buescher P, et al. Effect of removing O_2 therapy in COPD patients receiving long-term O_2 therapy. Am Rev Respir Dis 1987; 136:85–91.
50. Timms RM, Khaja FU, Williams GW. Nocturnal Oxygen Therapy Trial Group. Hemodynamic response to oxygen therapy in chronic obstructive pulmonary disease. Ann Intern Med 1985; 102:29–36.
51. Weitzenblum E, Sautegeau A, Ehrhart M, et al. Long-term oxygen therapy can reverse the progression of pulmonary hypertension in patients with chronic obstructive pulmonary disease. Am Rev Respir Dis 1985; 131:493–498.
52. Levin BD, Bigelow DB, Hamstra RD, et al. The role of long-term continuous oxygen administration in patients with chronic airway obstruction with hypoxemia. Ann Intern Med 1967; 66:639–650.
53. Stein D, Bradley B, Miller W. Mechanisms of oxygen effects on exercise in patients with chronic obstructive pulmonary disease. Chest 1982; 81:6–10.
54. Krop HD, Block AJ, Cohen EC. Neuropsychologic effects of continuous oxygen therapy in chronic obstructive pulmonary disease. Chest 1973; 64:317–322.
55. Medical Research Council Working Party. Long-term domiciliary oxygen therapy in chronic hypoxic cor pulmonale complicating chronic bronchitis and emphysema. Lancet 1981; i:681–686.
56. Ashutosh K, Mead G, Dunsky M. Early effects of oxygen administration and prognosis in chronic obstructive pulmonary disease and cor pulmonale. Am Rev Respir Dis 1983; 127:399–404.

Chapter 51

BRONCHODILATORS IN THE TREATMENT OF BRONCHITIS AND EMPHYSEMA

Anthony S. Rebuck **Barbara M. Galko**

Appropriate medication, taken regularly, is the most effective treatment of asthma. Bronchodilators and corticosteroids raise the mean level of lung function and reduce the amplitude of variations in flow rates, both within the day and over time. Alternate forms of therapy play an uncertain and as yet untested role. By contrast, the standard therapeutic approach to chronic airways obstruction provides little symptomatic improvement in patients with emphysema, and alternate therapy such as smoking cessation or antibiotics may be of considerable importance in chronic bronchitis and its acute exacerbations. While the stated objective of this section is to describe the specific treatment modality of bronchodilators, it is necessary to place them in the context of their relatively unimportant role in patient management and of the limited expectations of their effectiveness in COPD.

PRIORITIES IN MANAGEMENT OF EMPHYSEMA AND BRONCHITIS

CIGARETTE SMOKING. The best way to treat emphysema is to prevent its development by avoiding or stopping cigarette smoking. The role of the physician should include setting a personal example, working toward creating smoke-free environments in the office, hospital, and recreational facilities, and urging patients not to smoke. Of the dozens of available approaches, the health care worker may wish to experiment with "wellness" programs at the community and fitness centers, self-help material, hypnosis, nicotine-containing gum, and educational activities at schools.[1]

INFECTIONS. If an ambulatory patient with chronic bronchitis has a change in sputum color, with an increase in sputum volume and an increase in dyspnea, a broad-spectrum antibiotic is given. Such an antibiotic is indicated even if there is no fever, no elevation in the white cell count, and no new infiltrate in the chest roentgenogram. If the chest film does show a pneumonic infiltrate, every effort is made to isolate a specific pathogen. If the infiltrate has developed during a patient's hospital stay, a gram-negative pneumonia is suspected and treated appropriately.

HYPOXEMIA. Supplemental oxygen administered to severely hypoxemic patients with COPD can reverse many of the adverse effects of chronic hypoxemia. In patients with acute exacerbations of their disease, in whom hypercapnia is a characteristic feature, oxygen enrichment of inspired air is mandatory. Our preference is for a high-flow, low-concentration oxygen delivery system with Venturi masks of 24% or 28% type, aiming to achieve an oxygen saturation of around 90%. Decisions regarding institution of long-term oxygen therapy with a low-flow system are made only after the patient is in a stable condition, while receiving optimal medical treatment and having quit smoking.

PULMONARY REHABILITATION. The goal of these multidisciplinary programs is to return patients to the highest possible physiologic and psychologic functional capacity allowed by their pulmonary handicap and overall life situation. Such programs subjectively help many patients and reduce hospitalization and the cost of medical care but have no effect on resting pulmonary function or arterial blood gases. The important elements are education, physical therapy, efficient functioning in the home, psychosocial counseling, and vocational training. Several of these elements can be incorporated into group practices and outpatient facilities.

BRONCHODILATORS. The foregoing aspects of management are directed toward treatment of complications and the provision of symptomatic relief.[2] The treatment of reversible airways obstruction, or the reversible component, is difficult. Some researchers[3] report that bronchodilator responsiveness of the FEV_1 in the laboratory is a poor predictor of clinical response. Others[8] have demonstrated that some patients with COPD have improved vital capacity and functional residual capacity despite no change in FEV_1 after inhaled bronchodilator. The laboratory evaluation is further complicated by the observation that theophylline used orally prior to pulmonary function testing masks the effects of test drugs such as isoproterenol.[4]

As a side-arm of their Intermittent Positive-Pressure Breathing clinical trial, Anthonisen and colleagues[2] have analyzed bronchodilator responses in nearly a thousand patients with COPD, studied repeatedly over a 3-year period. Patients with small bronchodilator responses tended to decline rapidly over the study period. Those with the largest bronchodilator responses declined less than half as fast as did others. It appears that in patients who are bronchodilator responsive the regular use of bronchodilators has a symptomatic benefit and also can change the course of the disease for the better. Anthonisen and colleagues concluded that unless there is repeated laboratory evidence of an absence of response to large doses of inhaled bronchodilator, all patients with COPD should receive these drugs.

Bronchodilator response shows some variability with time. Hence a decision made on the basis of acute bronchodilator responsiveness should not be made on the basis of a single testing session.[2] In general, hyperreactive subjects are those who smoke more, have severe small airway inflammation, and more baseline airway narrowing.[6]

RECOMMENDATIONS FOR BRONCHODILATOR THERAPY

In view of the limited usefulness of laboratory testing in predicting the clinical efficacy of bronchodilators in COPD, it seems reasonable to suggest a clinical trial in all such patients. The use of a patient diary and a questionnaire addressing dyspnea, exercise tolerance, and cough is important. Regular therapy should be continued if these features improve, or if lung function improves.

Three classes of bronchodilator are available and appropriate for the therapeutic trial: inhaled sympathomimetics ($beta_2$-agonists), inhaled anticholinergics, and oral sustained-release theophyllines. They should be used in a combination regimen: three drugs are better than two and any combination of two drugs is better than monotherapy.

INHALED SYMPATHOMIMETICS. The important $beta_2$-agonists, which have little effect on the $beta_1$-adrenergic receptors of the heart, are salbutamol, fenoterol, and terbutaline. In the oral form, they cause unpleasant side effects such as tremor; by inhalation, their side effects are minimal and their duration of action is 4 to 6 hours. Intravenous preparations offer little benefit and are seldom used. The generally recommended prescribing pattern is to suggest two puffs of a metered dose, to be taken every 6 hours. Some patients will not tolerate this dose; they complain of tremor or palpitations and may benefit from one puff three or four times a day; others may require and benefit from higher doses. More commonly, two puffs every six hours is not enough for symptom relief. In such patients, the standard dose may be repeated after quite a short interval (e.g., 30 to 60 minutes). When spacer devices are used, the coordination between actuation of the inhaler and inspiratory effort is improved.

ANTICHOLINERGICS. Inhaled $beta_2$-agonists are the first line of therapy for the treatment of asthma. There is, however, mounting evidence that anticholinergic therapy with atropinic drugs should be started prior to initiation of $beta_2$-agonists in COPD. These drugs exert their bronchodilator effects by competitive antagonism of muscarinic, cholinergic receptors, resulting in smooth muscle relaxation and decreases in bronchomotor tone. Ipratropium bromide is a quaternary ammonium derivative of atropine delivered by inhalation. It is very poorly absorbed; therefore inhalation virtually eliminates atropine-like side effects. It causes more prolonged bronchodilatation than atropine and does not result in tolerance.[10] The degree of bronchodilatation is at least equal to and usually superior to beta-agonists in COPD.[11]

METHYLXANTHINES. Still a mainstay in bronchodilator therapy, the mechanism of action of methylxanthines remains obscure. They are available in oral and intravenous forms; the intravenous form is used for acute exacerbations and the oral form, in sustained-release formulation, for maintenance therapy. The benefits of theophyllines are to an extent offset by their narrow therapeutic-toxic range, and serum levels are necessary to guide management. Bronchodilator effect is correlated with dose, at least within the therapeutic range of 55 to 100 μmol/L. Theophyllines have beneficial effects aside from bronchodilatation: augmentation of cardiac and diaphragmatic contractility, reduction of pulmonary vascular resistance, and enhancement of mucociliary clearance.

Anticholinergics appear to be more potent in COPD patients than do adrenergic agents or methylxanthines. If the patient has cardiovascular disease or some condition that is associated with poor tolerance of sympathomimetics and methylxanthines, monotherapy with an inhaled anticholinergic agent is appropriate. The suggested therapy is with ipratropium bromide, using a metered dose inhaler or a spacer device. Inhaled ipratropium may be combined with sustained-release theophylline in most patients. In those with particularly marked laboratory-documented responsiveness to sympathomimetics, combination therapy with a sympathomimetic and an anticholinergic, using a metered dose inhaler or a home nebulizer solution, is worthy of trial.

In severe acute exacerbations of chronic bronchitis, coughing of secretions is facilitated by inhaled bronchodilator treatment. Again, our recommendation is a combination of sympathomimetic and anticholinergic therapy. The regimen that we have found to be best tolerated is a 1.25-mg fenoterol or salbutamol respirator solution (2.5 mg), plus 0.5 mg of ipratropium in saline, nebulized and administered by mouthpiece over 10 to 15 minutes. We are in general cautious in our use of intravenous aminophylline, since the majority of presenting patients have been taking maintenance doses of slow-release theophylline preparations. Accordingly, bolus doses of aminophylline are not given unless it is known definitely that the patient has not been taking oral theophylline or until blood theophylline levels are available.

CORTICOSTEROIDS. Numerous studies have evaluated the efficacy of steroids in stable COPD. The gloomiest picture is that less than 10% of patients show a significant increase in FEV_1 after 2 weeks of 40 mg of prednisone daily. On the other hand, some believe that a significant response to steroids can be predicted from responsiveness to inhaled bronchodilator and from the presence of eosinophils in sputum. Inhaled steroids are less effective in COPD than they are in asthma, and they are associated with oropharyngeal candidiasis and dysphonia.

When symptoms of COPD are poorly controlled by standard medication with theophylline, anticholinergic agents, and $beta_2$-agonists, a trial of steroids is warranted.

Patients with a history of bronchial hyperreactivity or those who have previously required corticosteroids are given methylprednisolone, 50 mg intravenously, followed by prednisone, 30 to 40 mg per day in divided doses. Should all patients who have a trial of combination bronchodilator therapy also be given a trial of steroids before an acute exacerbation forces the decision? Steroids do appear to be beneficial in acute exacerbations of COPD. Sahn's[9] review of the literature suggests that corticosteroids are not useful in COPD, but the published trials were not controlled or blinded. On the other hand, Mendella and colleagues[6] showed that some patients had improved flow rates, but even in retrospect it was not possible to predict those likely to benefit. We feel that on the basis of the current literature no firm recommendation can be made with regard to a trial of steroids in stable COPD patients. Few, however, would quarrel with Make's[5] caution that steroids should be continued only in patients who have objective evidence of improved spirometry, in whom the questionable benefits may outweigh the considerable risk of side effects.

REFERENCES

1. Kottke TE, Battista RN, DeFriese GH, Brekke ML. Attributes of successful smoking cessation interventions in medical practice. JAMA 1988; 249:2883.
2. Anthonisen NR, Wright EC, IPPB Trial Group. Response to inhaled bronchodilators in COPD. Chest 1987; 19(5 Suppl):365.
3. Ayres SM, Griesbach SJ, Reimold F, et al. Bronchial component in chronic obstructive lung disease. Am J Med 1974; 57:183.
4. Dull WL, Alexander MR, Kasik JR. Isoproterenol challenge during placebo and oral theophylline therapy in chronic obstructive pulmonary disease. Am Rev Respir Dis 1987; 123:340.
5. Make B. Medical management of emphysema. Clin Chest Med 1983; 4:465.
6. Mendella LA, Manfreda J, Warren CPW, et al. Steroid response in stable chronic obstructive pulmonary disease. Ann Intern Med 1982; 96:17.
7. Pare PD, Armour C, Taylor S, et al. Airway hyperreactivity in COPD—cause or effect; an in vivo–in vitro comparison. Chest 1987; 19(5 Suppl):40S.
8. Ramsdell JW, Tisi GM. Determination of bronchodilatation in the clinical pulmonary function laboratory. Chest 1979; 76:622.
9. Sahn S. Corticosteroids in chronic bronchitis and pulmonary emphysema. Chest 1978; 73:389.
10. Gross NJ, Skorodin MS. Anticholinergic, antimuscarinic bronchodilators. Am Rev Respir Dis 1984; 129:856.
11. Rebuck AS, Chapman KR, Abboud R, et al. Nebulized anticholinergic and sympathomimetic treatment of asthma and chronic obstructive airways disease in the emergency room. Am J Med 1987; 82:59.

Chapter 52

ANTICHOLINERGIC AGENTS IN THE TREATMENT OF CHRONIC BRONCHITIS AND EMPHYSEMA

Nicholas J. Gross

RATIONALE OF ANTICHOLINERGIC USAGE IN AIRWAYS DISEASE

In humans, the cholinergic portion of the autonomic nervous system exerts control over the airways to an important extent. The principal features of its anatomy and physiology will be outlined here but are dealt with in more detail elsewhere.[1–4]

Autonomic Nerves and Receptors in the Lung

The predominant nerve supply to the human lungs consists of efferent branches of the vagal parasympathetic system.[4] A typical two-neuron system, the preganglionic fibers enter the lung at the hilum and travel along the walls of the airways and blood vessels in peribronchial and periarterial plexuses. The peribronchial nerves end at ganglia that are scattered along the walls of bronchi and bronchioles, rarely in smaller airways. The short postganglionic fibers, whose cell bodies form the peribronchial ganglia, travel into the airway wall and innervate smooth muscle bronchial vessels and submucosal glands. Acetylcholine liberated from varicosities along the postganglionic nerve is the transmitter, which is the agonist for muscarinic receptors on smooth muscle and submucosal gland cells. Its action is to cause contraction of smooth muscle cells and the release of preformed secretions from submucous glands. Bronchomotor tone, a low level of smooth muscle contraction presumed to be present in normal as well as abnormal human airways, is due to a basal level of cholinergic parasympathetic neural activity, which can be detected in animals.

Some afferent vagal fibers and efferent sympathetic fibers are also present in the lungs, but these are a minority of the fibers found in humans. The sympathetic fibers, all postganglionic, appear to end at submucous glands and on the (parasympathetic) ganglia, but few if any supply smooth muscle cells. Activation of sympathetic nerves stimulates submucous gland secretion and ciliary activity and may modulate parasympathetic activity by an inhibitory effect on ganglion cells, providing opposition to cholinergic bronchomotor tone. Sympathetic opposition to cholinergic tone also can be brought about pharmacologically by activation of beta-adrenergic receptors on smooth muscle cells. An additional important intrinsic means of opposition, however, is the third nervous system, the so-called nonadrenergic, noncholinergic system.[3, 5] Figure 52–1 is a simplified depiction of the relationships of these systems as they are currently conceived.

The location of receptors for transmitters of the various branches of the autonomic nervous system provides additional insight into their probable physiologic roles. Muscarinic receptors are found predominantly in the central airways, where they outnumber adrenergic receptors, but also are found in small airways.[6] This distribution coincides well with the distribution of cholinergic nerves. Beta-adrenergic receptors are found throughout the airways but outnumber muscarinic receptors in small airways. One may infer from this that bronchomotor tone acts predominantly on central airways and that adrenergic agonists might act on both central and peripheral airways.

The biology of the muscarinic receptor is currently a subject of intense study. A prolonged search for subtypes, by analogy with adrenergic receptor subtypes, has in recent years revealed at least two and possibly five subtypes, designated M1, M2, and so on. These appear to be encoded by separate genes, but the primary structure of the proteins is similar: a single glycosylated transmembrane polypeptide of molecular weight about 72,000. Terminology of the subtypes in the airways is at present confused so will not be enunciated here. At least three subtypes are postulated in the airway: those on the submucosal glands, on smooth muscle cells, and on postganglionic parasympathetic fibers (autoreceptors). The distinction between muscarinic receptor subtypes is at present only of theoretical interest, as the antagonists available for clinical use are not selective for any subtype.

From the foregoing, one would deduce that normal airway caliber is largely a function of the level of cholinergic bronchomotor tone. How this varies in airways disease is not known, but it is obvious that structural changes in and around the airways, which are not amenable to bronchodilator therapy, are likely to be of greater importance in determining airway obstruction in most patients with COPD (Chapter 9). Nevertheless, to the extent that these patients are able to respond to bronchodilators, they are likely to respond to anticholinergic agents because of the predominant role of cholinergic mechanisms in controlling bronchomotor tone.

The existence of such reflex pathways in humans as well as animals has been extensively documented by the work of Nadel,[1] Widdicombe,[2] and others. What is not known is the extent to which airflow in obstructive diseases is limited by tonic and reflex cholinergic activity, as opposed to irreversible structural changes in and around the airways. Nevertheless, the fact that anticholinergic agents do produce bronchodilatation in these patients suggests that cholinergic bronchoconstrictor mechanisms are present and that their ablation may improve airflow.

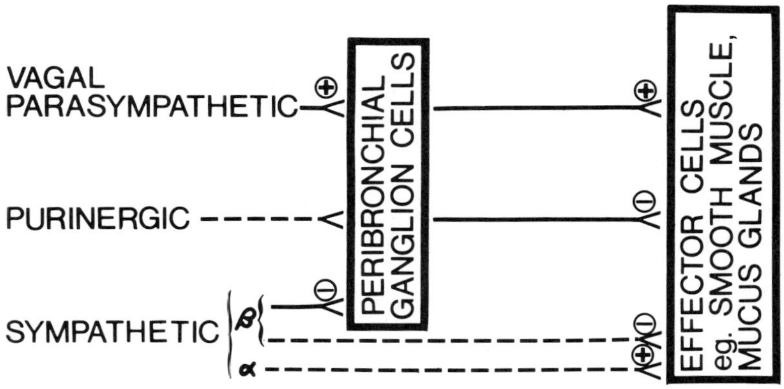

Figure 52–1. Diagrammatic representation of efferent autonomic innervation of the human airways. +, excitatory; −, inhibitory; dashed line, existence doubtful. (Reproduced with permission from Gross NJ, Skorodin MS. Am Rev Respir Dis 1984; 129:856–870.)

PHARMACOLOGY OF ANTICHOLINERGIC AGENTS

Anticholinergic agents fall broadly into two groups based on the valence of the nitrogen atom on the tropane ring (Fig. 52–2). Naturally occurring agents, of which atropine is the parent, are tertiary ammonium alkaloids and are well absorbed and distributed throughout the body. Quaternary ammonium congeners of atropine, such as atropine methonitrate and ipratropium bromide, have similar local anticholinergic actions but are poorly absorbed and, even if injected, do not cross the blood-brain barrier to a significant extent. Thus, when inhaled, they have anticholinergic effects on the airways but do not produce significant systemic effects. Details of this material are provided elsewhere.[7]

SPECIFICITY. Most of the differences between tertiary and quaternary ammonium congeners are due to the differences in their absorption, a fact that can be exploited in the treatment of airways disease. Neither atropine nor ipratropium is selective for muscarinic receptor subtypes. However, ipratropium, and possibly other quaternary agents, have less effect on inhibiting respiratory tract secretions than on relaxing airway smooth muscle. The reasons for this are unknown.

PHARMACOKINETICS. Following inhalation, atropine blood levels reach a peak at about 1 hour. The half-life in the blood is of the order of 3 hours but longer in children and older subjects. It is excreted in the urine largely unchanged within 24 hours. After patients inhale ipratropium bromide, blood levels are detectable only when the drug is isotopically labeled; peak levels are reached between 2 and 3 hours. Its half-life in the blood is again of the order of 3 hours. Much of the drug is excreted in the feces; some inactive metabolites are excreted in the urine. Its duration of action on the airways exceeds that of atropine, presumably because lack of absorption allows it to persist there longer.

DOSE RESPONSE. Nebulized atropine sulfate reaches optimal effects in a dose of 0.05 mg/kg in children and 0.025 to 0.04 mg/kg in adults. For nebulized ipratropium, the optimal dose is variably reported as 54 to 400 μg total dose. Administered by metered dose inhaler, ipratropium has its optimal effect at between 40 and 120 μg. The large discrepancy in optimal doses for ipratropium may be explained by technical differences between studies and, more important, the population of patients studied—more severely obstructed patients probably require a larger dose to reach optimal effect. Also, larger doses tend to produce bronchodilatation of greater duration rather than of greater magnitude.

TOXICITY. The toxicity of atropine is described in standard texts. In summary, a total dose of 0.5 to 1.0 mg of atropine may cause dryness of the mouth, warmth or flushing of the skin, and mild tachycardia. Between 2 and 5 mg, palpitations, blurred vision, urinary retention, slurred speech, and possibly restlessness may occur. Higher doses may result in ataxia and marked mental changes, such as excitement, confusion, hallucinations, and delirium. Death is uncommon even in massive overdosage. Idiosyncrasy occurs but is rare. These effects may be more common in patients with COPD, possibly because of their greater age, or possibly because they tend to be in poor general health, may be malnourished, and may have concomitant disease. Frank psychosis following usual therapeutic doses is rare but does occur in this population.

Quaternary agents lack these effects because of their poor absorbability. Some dryness of the mouth occurs, but systemic effects do not. Occasionally patients complain of a bad taste following ipratropium.

Of particular concern in the population of patients with COPD are effects on mucociliary clearance, the pupil, urinary sphincter, hemodynamics, and gas exchange. Atropine reduces the ciliary beat frequency and reduces mucous gland hypersecretion. It delays mucociliary clearance for both these reasons. This is a concern in patients with airways disease. For reasons that are not clear, ipratropium has been found not to have these effects in spite of intensive investigation. The effect of

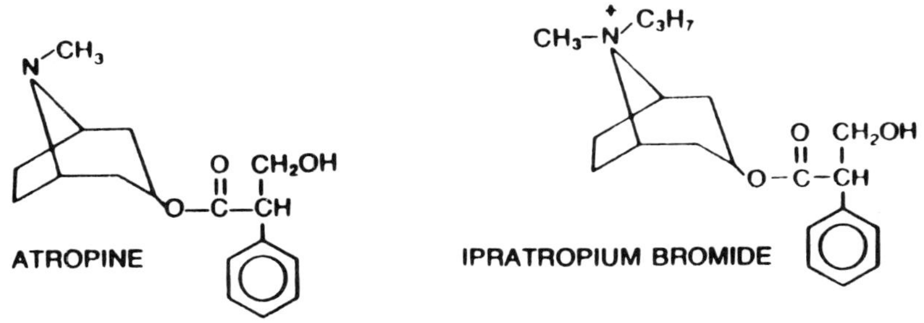

Figure 52–2. Structure of atropine, a tertiary ammonium alkaloid, and ipratropium bromide, a quaternary ammonium congener of atropine. The nitrogen atom responsible for differences in absorbability is shown at the top left corner of each molecule.

other quaternary agents on mucociliary clearance seems to be similar to that of ipratropium, but these have not been as extensively studied.

Inhaled atropine results in dilatation of the pupil. For this reason, it is contraindicated in patients with narrow-angle glaucoma. Inhaled ipratropium does not dilate the pupil or raise intraocular tension even in patients with narrow-angle glaucoma. However, it has marked and prolonged effects on the pupil when sprayed directly into the eye, which should be cautioned against.

Inhaled atropine can cause urinary retention by an effect on the urinary sphincter, particularly in patients with bladder neck obstruction. Ipratropium has, again, been found not to have such effects.

The hemodynamic effects of atropine are complex. Mild bradycardia at low doses is followed by tachycardia, peripheral vasodilatation, and increases in cardiac output, none of which are marked. It has small effects on the pulmonary circulation. Quaternary agents—ipratropium being the only one that has been extensively studied—have negligible effects on hemodynamics.

Effects of anticholinergic agents on gas exchange are relevant in that other bronchodilators have a tendency to increase ventilation-perfusion inequality and lower the Pa_{O_2}. Anticholinergic agents in general have rather small effects on gas exchange. Neither atropine nor its quaternary ammonium congeners lower the Pa_{O_2}, even in hypoxemic patients with COPD.[8]

Unfavorable interactions between anticholinergic agents and other drugs have not been reported.

CLINICAL EFFICACY IN COPD

GENERAL FEATURES. These have been reported in a large number of studies that have been extensively reviewed in recent publications.[9–11] Anticholinergic agents have a slower onset of action and longer time to peak effect than do adrenergic agents. Typically, peak effect following an anticholinergic agent occurs at 60 to 120 minutes, compared with 15 minutes following an adrenergic agent. Its effect at peak bronchodilatation tends to persist longer and declines more slowly, particularly following larger doses of a quaternary agent, when effective bronchodilatation is present for 6 to 12 hours, depending on the agent used. Anticholinergic agents have their predominant effect on large airways, even when given parenterally. This contrasts with the action of adrenergic agents that dilate both central and peripheral airways, particularly when given parenterally. The difference in the site of predominant effect of the two classes of agents corresponds well with the distribution of cholinergic and adrenergic receptors in the airways (see earlier). However, when given by inhalation, the preferred route in stable COPD, the site of effect of the two classes of agents is not measurably different, presumably because most of the dose of the inhaled agent that enters the lower respiratory tract is deposited in the central airways.

Like other agents, the bronchodilator effects of anticholinergic agents are reflected in decreases in lung volumes as well as increases in airflow and the forced vital capacity.

CLINICAL TRIALS IN STABLE COPD. A very large number of trials have compared anticholinergic drugs to other bronchodilators in stable COPD.[10] Trials that have employed conventional doses of each agent almost universally show that an anticholinergic agent results in more bronchodilatation than an adrenergic agent in this patient population. A result from the largest such study is shown in Figure 52–3. This finding is surprising and contrasts with studies in asthmatic patients which show that adrenergic agents are more effective bronchodilators. The different order of efficacy of the two classes of bronchodilators is confirmed by a number of studies in which asthmatic and bronchitic groups have been studied with both drugs.[10] Also, some patients with COPD are resistant to adrenergic agents but respond well to anticholinergic agents.[12]

Could the relative efficacy of anticholinergic agents in COPD simply be due to differences in the optimal dose of bronchodilator in the two diagnoses? To examine this question, a few studies have employed large or sequential doses of each class of agent to achieve optimal effect. The result of one such study is shown in Figure 52–4. In this study,[13] the plateau of effect from large sequential doses of an anticholinergic agent was significantly higher than that following the adrenergic agent. Moreover, administration of the anticholinergic was able to augment bronchodilatation achieved by maximal dosage of the adrenergic agent. Administration of both agents simultaneously resulted in an increase in the FEV_1 that was virtually identical to that of the anticholinergic agent alone. A previous study using a similar protocol gave similar results,[14] but a subsequent one showed that the two classes of agents were equivalent in potency.[15] If a difference in potency exists in COPD it is not great, amounting to differences in peak bronchodilatation of less than 100 ml, which is barely clinically significant. A reasonable conclusion might be that the two classes of agents, when given in optimal dosage, are equipotent at peak effect in patients with COPD. This conclusion contrasts with the relative efficacy of the two drugs in asthma, in which adrenergic agents are universally found to be more potent.

Despite the evidence from pulmonary function tests, there is no evidence that patients prefer anticholinergic agents to alternative bronchodilators, nor is there objective evidence that effort tolerance is greater following an anticholinergic agent.

In COPD, therefore, the choice between agents comes down to other factors, such as the speed of onset, duration of action, propensity to side effects, and logistic considerations. These are considered later.

TRIALS IN ACUTE EXACERBATIONS. Patients with acute exacerbations of COPD treated for 7 days with either class of agent had a greater bronchodilator response to nebulized solutions of ipratropium than to the $beta_2$ selective adrenergic agent fenoterol.[16] However, all other parameters, e.g., increase in baseline FEV_1 during the 7-day period, improvement in arterial blood gases, and duration of hospitalization, were not distinguishable on the basis of which drug the patient received. Over the first 90 minutes of treatment of acute exacerbations of COPD in the emergency room, Rebuck and coworkers found no difference in the improvement in FEV_1 between nebulized fenoterol, nebulized ipratropium, and the combination of both agents.[17]

COMBINATIONS OF ANTICHOLINERGIC AND OTHER BRONCHODILATOR AGENTS. It has been suggested that adrenergic agents and anticholinergic agents potentiate each other, but a greater body of evidence suggests they do not, but that they are additive. If sufficiently large doses are used, combinations do not result in greater peak increases in airflow, as discussed. However, when recommended doses are used, a combination may provide the speed of onset of the adrenergic with the prolonged duration of action of the anticholinergic, together with the additive potency of the two agents at intermediate times. In theory, both large and small airways would be affected, and side effects might be minimized. The evidence that these considerations are materially important in clinical practice is not strong.

If a combination is elected, a single metered dose inhaler containing both agents would be a convenience for patients. Although such inhalers are available elsewhere, and widely used (Berodual, Duovent), they are not available in the United

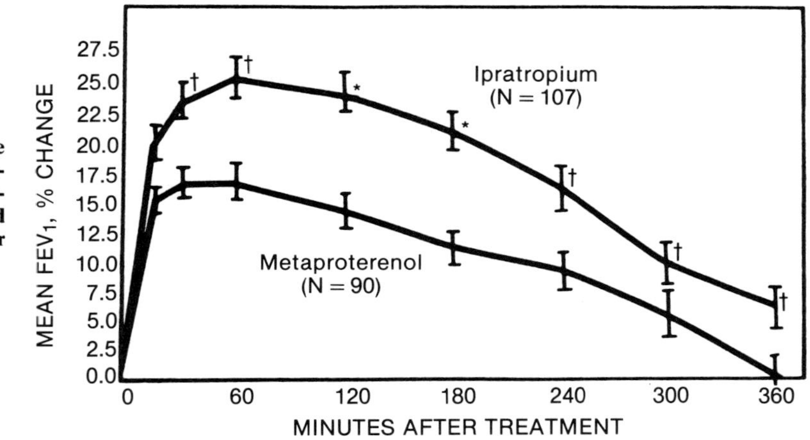

Figure 52–3. Mean changes in FEV_1 following metered-dose inhalation of ipratropium bromide (40 μg) or metaproterenol (1.5 mg) in patients with chronic bronchitis and emphysema. N, number of patients in each group. (Reproduced with permission from Tashkin DP, Ashutosh K, Bleecker ER, et al. Am J Med 1986; 81(Suppl 5A):81–89.)

States. If two inhalers are prescribed, it is debatable in which order they might best be used.

SIDE EFFECTS. The toxicity of anticholinergic agents was discussed. We consider here the side effects that the physician may see in typical practice. Atropine use is regularly followed by dryness of the mouth and sometimes warmth of the skin and palpitations. These effects are generally well tolerated by patients. Because of its effects on sphincters, atropine should not be used in patients with narrow-angle glaucoma or prostatism, not uncommon coexisting conditions in the COPD population. Rarely, patients become confused or frankly psychotic following usual doses, possibly because patients with COPD are often older and in poor general health.

When atropine-like effects are severe, they can be rapidly reversed by parenteral administration of physostigmine, 1 to 2 mg.

Some indication of the incidence of adverse effects of a quaternary agent such as ipratropium in routine use is provided by a recent large multicenter study in which patients received either ipratropium or metaproterenol in recommended dosage for 90 days (Table 52–1).[18] The only differences relate to tremor, which does not occur following anticholinergic agents, and cough, which was commoner, although not significantly so, in the patients who received ipratropium. A few patients experience a short paroxysm following the inhalation. This has not been found to require withdrawal of the drug, but patients may mention it.

A quite rare side effect deserves mention. A small number of asthmatic patients have been reported in the British literature who experienced paradoxic bronchoconstriction following ipratropium.[19] The mechanism is unknown. It is possible that similar idiosyncratic effects might occur in patients with COPD.

There is also, of course, the large experience from the general clinical use of ipratropium over the last decade in many patients in many countries other than the United States. This has revealed only the small number of adverse reactions mentioned in the preceding paragraph.

PRACTICAL CONSIDERATIONS

In stable COPD, a quaternary ammonium anticholinergic agent can be considered to be as effective as other bronchodilator modalities. Its principal advantage is that it has few side effects and a very wide therapeutic margin. As the metered-dose formulation is effective, economical, and convenient, it is likely to meet with greatest patient compliance as well as being the preferred modality. Ipratropium is the only quaternary agent available by metered-dose inhaler at present and can be regarded as appropriate initial therapy for patients with COPD. Because anticholinergic agents are relatively slow in onset of action, ipratropium is best used on a

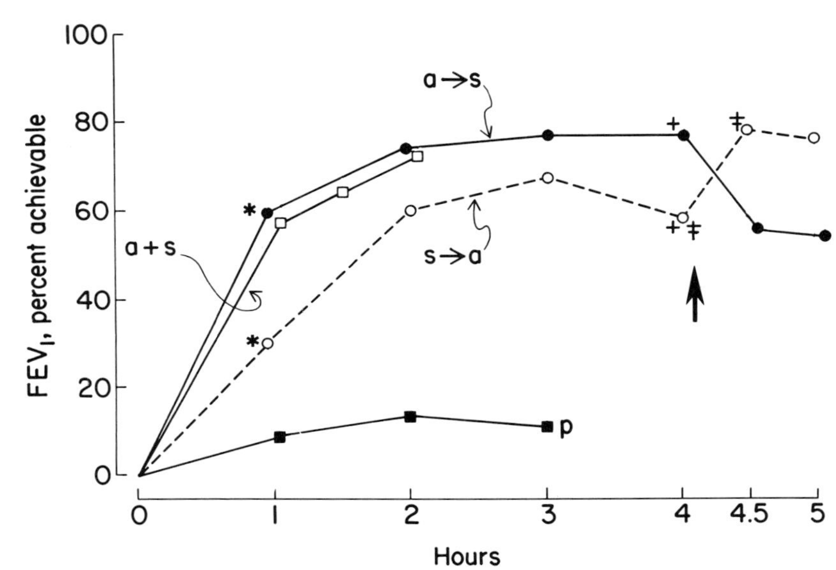

Figure 52–4. Responses of ten patients with emphysema to sequential doses of atropine methonitrate *(a)* and salbutamol *(s)* in various sequences. a→s, atropine methonitrate hourly followed by salbutamol at the large arrow; s→a, same agents in reverse order; a + s, both agents simultaneously; p, placebo. Pairs of symbols indicate significant differences between values. (Reproduced with permission from Gross NJ, Skorodin MS. N Engl J Med 1984; 311:421–425.)

TABLE 52–1. Numbers of Patients with Adverse Experience(s)* After Ipratropium or Metaproterenol

	IPRATROPIUM	METAPROTERENOL
Total number treated	132	129
Palpitations	4	1
Nervousness	2	3
Dizziness	1	3
Gastrointestinal distress	2	3
Nausea	5	2
Tremor	0	5
Dry mouth	3	2
Cough	6	3
Worsening of dyspnea	0	6
Number with more than 1 adverse experience	20	25

*Less than two patients in either group complained of headache, insomnia, drowsiness, rash, tinnitus, diarrhea, vomiting, difficulty in urinating, difficulty in accommodating, or irritation from the aerosol.

(Reproduced with permission from Tashkin DP, Ashutosh K, Bleecker GR, et al. Am J Med 1986; 81(Suppl SA):81–89.)

routine basis, three to four times daily, one of these times being at bedtime. Adrenergic agents can be used as adjunctive therapy, or in mild cases, as prn therapy when episodes of dyspnea occur. Long-acting methylxanthines also can be used on a routine basis in patients whose dyspnea is severe. Many patients with severe COPD are best managed with all three drugs given on a regular, maintenance basis.

Because quaternary agents such as ipratropium result in no somatic sensations other than bronchodilatation, patients who are used to the mild sympathetic stimulation of an adrenergic agent may be unaware of the bronchodilatation following ipratropium, particularly if they are not physically active.

In acute exacerbations of COPD, anticholinergic agents may be included in the regimen of bronchodilator therapy but probably are not more potent bronchodilators than other agents. Nebulized solutions are the most appropriate means of administering bronchodilators to these patients as they have difficulty with deep inspiration, breath-holding, and coordinating actuation of the inhaler with inspiration. The only forms of anticholinergic agents available for nebulization in the United States are tertiary ammonium compounds such as atropine sulfate and the quaternary ammonium compound glycopyrrolate bromide. Neither is approved by the Food and Drug Administration for respiratory use at present, nor is there much literature on their use in acute exacerbations of COPD. Both, however, are widely used for this purpose, and anecdotal experience suggests both are effective. Ipratropium bromide is not yet available as a solution for nebulization. Nevertheless, it can be used as a metered-dose inhaler, administered through an improvised spacer device, or delivered into the endotracheal tubing for patients on ventilators.

For all these uses, the recommended dose of ipratropium, two actuations (36 μg), is probably suboptimal. Many patients derive greater benefit from larger doses, to which there can be few objections in view of the large therapeutic margin. When patients do not derive clinical benefit from the recommended dose, four or six actuations can be recommended without additional risk.

REFERENCES

1. Nadel JA. Autonomic regulation of airway smooth muscle. In: Nadel JA, ed. Physiology and Pharmacology of the Airways. New York: Marcel Dekker, 1980, 217–257.
2. Widdicombe JG. Reflex control of tracheobronchial smooth muscle in experimental and human asthma. In: Lichtenstein LM, Austen KF, eds. Asthma: Physiology, Immunopharmacology and Treatment. New York: Academic Press, 1977, 225–231.
3. Barnes PJ. Neural control of human airways in health and disease. Am Rev Respir Dis 1986; 134:1289–1314.
4. Richardson JB. Innervation of the lung. Eur J Respir Dis 1982; 117(Suppl):13–31.
5. Barnes PJ. The third nervous system in the lung: physiology and clinical perspectives. Thorax 1984; 39:561–567.
6. Barnes PJ, Basbaum CB, Nadel JA. Autoradiographic localization of autonomic receptors in airway smooth muscle: marked differences between large and small airways. Am Rev Respir Dis 1983; 127:758–762.
7. Gross NJ, Skorodin MS. Anticholinergic agents. In: Jenne JW, Murphy S, eds. Drug Therapy for Asthma: Research and Clinical Practice. New York: Marcel Dekker, 1987, 615–668.
8. Gross NJ, Bankwala Z. Effects of an anticholinergic bronchodilator on arterial blood gases of hypoxemic patients with COPD: comparison with a beta-adrenergic agent. Am Rev Respir Dis 1987; 136:1091–1094.
9. Pakes GE, Brogden RN, Heel RC, et al. Ipratropium bromide: a review of its pharmacological properties and therapeutic efficacy in asthma and chronic bronchitis. Drugs 1980; 20:237–266.
10. Gross NJ, Skorodin MS. Anticholinergic, antimuscarinic bronchodilators. Am Rev Respir Dis 1984; 129:856–870.
11. Mann JS, George CF. Anticholinergic drugs in the treatment of airways disease. Br J Dis Chest 1985; 79:209–228.
12. Marini JJ, Lakshminarayan S. The effect of atropine inhalation in "irreversible" chronic bronchitis. Chest 1980; 77:591–596.
13. Gross NJ, Skorodin MS. Role of the parasympathetic system in airway obstruction due to emphysema. N Engl J Med 1984; 311:421–425.
14. Douglas NJ, Davidson I, Sudlow MF, Flenley DC. Bronchodilatation and the site of airway resistance in severe chronic bronchitis. Thorax 1979; 34:51–56.
15. Easton PA, Jadue C, Dhingra S, Anthonisen NR. A comparison of the bronchodilating effect of a beta-2 adrenergic agent (albuterol) and an anticholinergic agent (ipratropium bromide), given by aerosol alone or in sequence. N Engl J Med 1986; 315:735–739.
16. Backman R, Hellstrom P-E. Fenoterol and ipratropium bromide in respiratory treatment of patients with chronic bronchitis. Curr Ther Res 1985; 38:135–140.
17. Rebuck AS, Chapman KR, Abboud R, et al. Nebulized anticholinergic and sympathomimetic treatment of asthma and chronic obstructive airways disease in the emergency room. Am J Med 1987; 82:59–64.
18. Tashkin DP, Ashutosh K, Bleecker ER, et al. Comparison of the anticholinergic bronchodilator ipratropium bromide with metaproterenol in chronic obstructive pulmonary disease: a 90-day multicenter study. Am J Med 1986; 81(Suppl 5A):81–89.
19. Connolly CK. Adverse reaction to ipratropium bromide. Br Med J 1982; 285:934–935.

Chapter 53

VENTILATORY MANAGEMENT OF COPD

John J. Marini

Positive pressure ventilators have been in widespread clinical use for more than three decades. Our understanding of respiratory muscle function and ventilatory failure has recently undergone a major revision, however, helping to gear equipment and treatment strategies more effectively to patient requirements. These advances have contributed to the lower morbidity and mortality that now accompany exacerbations of COPD.

Some of the more important advances in this area concern the interaction of patients with chronic obstructive pulmonary disease (COPD) with the mechanical ventilator. Others concern physiologic principles important in withdrawing machine support from chronically ventilator-dependent patients, many of whom have COPD. With these advances in mind, the purpose of this chapter is to provide an updated physiologic background for understanding mechanical ventilation in patients with COPD, as well as to review selected aspects of this problem that, although noteworthy, may be unfamiliar to many practitioners.

By assuming a major portion of the ventilatory workload, mechanical ventilation affords the patient the opportunity to rest the respiratory muscles while maintaining pH homeostasis, thereby averting the consequences of progressive ventilatory failure and/or respiratory arrest. Maintained alveolar ventilation, large tidal volumes, oxygen supplementation, and modification of the end-expiratory and mean alveolar pressures also help to support the oxygen exchange process. Unfortunately, these benefits are not cost-free—mechanical ventilation is expensive, uncomfortable, and inherently hazardous. Few would dispute the desirability of avoiding the need for its implementation or of accelerating the process of machine withdrawal.

SPECIAL PROBLEMS OF PATIENTS WITH COPD

Although deceptively simple in concept, the management of patients with airflow obstruction who require machine support is an exceedingly complex clinical problem. To manage respiratory failure effectively in patients with severe airflow obstruction, it is important to understand their distinctive problems. Patients with COPD can be characterized by a number of salient clinical features (Table 53–1). Paramount among these are increased work of breathing and weakness of the ventilatory pump that must deal with it. Such patients are also distinguished by their susceptibility to the hazards of machine support.

TABLE 53–1. Features of COPD of Special Relevance to Mechanical Ventilation

Increased breathing workload	
Airway resistance	
Structure	fixed narrowing
Bronchospasm	collapse
Secretions	
Edema	
Air trapping	
Reduced thoracic compliance	
Lung	
Chest wall	
Inspiratory threshold effect of auto-PEEP	
Increased $\dot{V}_E$	
Ventilatory muscle activity	
$\dot{V}/\dot{Q}$ mismatching	
Compromise of the ventilatory pump	
Muscle wasting	
Hyperinflation	
Mechanical disadvantage	
Reduced precontractile fiber length	
Ineffective contraction sequence	
Impaired muscle blood supply	
Predisposition to ventilatory complications	
Gastrointestinal bleeding or ulceration	
Pneumonitis	
Barotrauma	

Increased Work of Breathing

Increased Impedance to Breathing

The mechanical breathing workload can be quantified by the product of mean inflation pressure and minute ventilation.[1,2] The mean inflation pressure ($\bar{P}$) is approximated by a modification of the equation of motion of Otis and Mead:[1]

Equation 53–1: $$\bar{P} = \dot{V}R_{aw} + (V_T/2C) + P_{ex}$$

where $\dot{V}$ = mean inspiratory flow rate, R_{aw} = airway resistance, C = compliance, V_T = tidal volume, and P_{ex} is end-expiratory alveolar pressure (Fig. 53–1).[1–3] As the term COPD suggests, increased resistance to airflow is responsible (directly or indirectly) for many of the physiologic disturbances that typify this disease. Flow resistance, an important determinant of $\bar{P}$, is increased by structural and functional narrowing of the airway. Structural changes include a reduced number of airway channels as well as a reduction in their cross-sectional caliber. In this already narrowed system of tubes, any additional reduction of airway caliber caused by mucosal edema, functional compression, increase of bronchomotor tone (bronchospasm), or secretion accumulation noticeably increases the work of breathing, because resistance relates linearly to the airway length but inversely to the fourth power of the airway radius.[4] For similar reasons, resistance within these critically narrowed airways is highly volume-dependent, so that loss of lung volume is accompanied by loss of elastic recoil tension, reduction of cross-sectional area, and major increases in the frictional workload.[5]

Although each factor just enumerated contributes to airflow obstruction, *functional* compression of the airway during exhalation is of overriding importance in many patients. Loss of elastic recoil encourages collapse of these narrowed bronchi as their distending gradients decline (or reverse) during the course of exhalation. In most patients who require mechanical ventilatory support, dynamic airway collapse occurs even during tidal breathing, so that the average expiratory resistance is often several-fold higher during the exhalation phase than during the inspiratory phase of ventilation.[6–8] This compressive mechanism underlies the phenomenon of air trapping and such hyperinflation-related consequences as loss of inspiratory power and reduced compliance of the respiratory system.

Dynamic Hyperinflation (Air Trapping)

Expiration is normally a passive process that uses elastic energy stored during inflation to drive expiratory airflow.[8] If the energy potential developed during inflation is insufficient to return the system to relaxed equilibrium before the next inspiration begins, flow continues throughout expiration and alveolar pressure remains positive at end-exhalation, at a greater pressure than that in the central airway. This positive distending pressure within the alveoli represents an increased driving pressure for expiratory airflow and increases lung volume, thereby improving airflow resistance. Unfortunately, such "hyperinflation" also places the inspiratory musculature at a mechanical disadvantage. Furthermore, because this end-expiratory alveolar pressure (auto-PEEP) is expiratory in nature, it must first be counterbalanced by positive pressure applied to the central airway or by negative pleural pressure before inspiration can begin.[9] Thus, P_{ex} adds to the other components of the equation of motion (Eq. 53–1) to elevate the mean inflation pressure and the work of breathing (Fig. 53–1).

The process of air trapping contributes to an increase in the

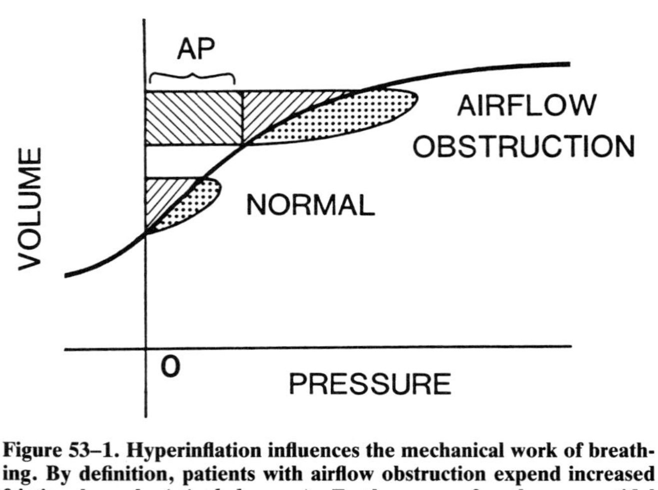

Figure 53–1. Hyperinflation influences the mechanical work of breathing. By definition, patients with airflow obstruction expend increased frictional work *(stippled areas)*. Furthermore, for the same tidal volume, moving higher on the pressure-volume curve of the respiratory system *(heavy line)* increases elastic work relative to the end-expiratory position *(cross-hatched areas)*. The process of hyperinflation requires inspiratory work to be done against the pressure needed to hold the chest dynamically distended at end-exhalation (AP = auto-PEEP).

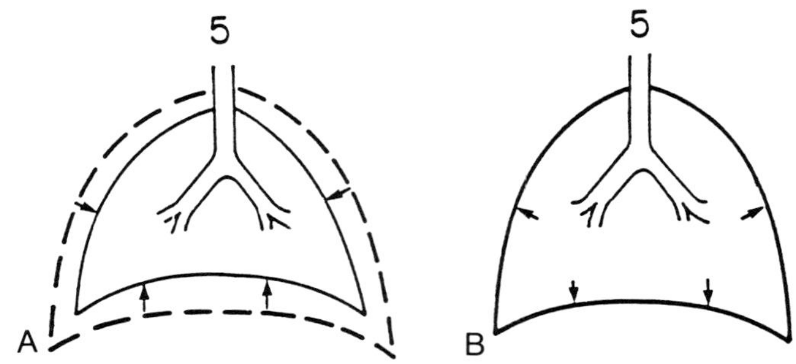

Figure 53–2. Mechanism of "inspiratory work sharing." By forcing the chest to a volume below the equilibrium position appropriate to the applied level of end-expiratory pressure (5 cm H_2O), the mechanical advantage of the inspiratory muscles is improved. Furthermore, the potential energy stored in the chest wall during expiration *(left panel)* can be released to aid inflation *(right panel)*.

inspiratory work of breathing in at least two other ways. Hyperinflation drives the respiratory system toward the least compliant portion of the pressure-volume relationship, so that increased elastic work is required per liter of ventilation (Fig. 53–1). At these higher volumes, the lung approaches its elastic limit and the recoil tension of the distended rib cage becomes expiratory rather than inspiratory in nature. Furthermore, hyperinflation tends to convert more of the lung into zones 1 and 2,[10] thereby increasing ventilatory dead space and the minute ventilation requirement.

It should be mentioned that dynamically positive end-expiratory alveolar pressure can also exist without hyperinflation, provided that airway collapse does not occur. In these instances, expiratory muscle contraction increases pleural pressure, alveolar pressure, and the speed of expiratory airflow, obviating the need for hyperinflation to complete exhalation in the obligate time. Such mechanisms are employed by normal subjects during heavy exercise or when faced with major expiratory loads.[11] Indeed, many uncoached and untrained normal subjects expire to a position *below* the equilibrium point of the chest when exposed to positive end-expiratory pressure.[12] In this way the inspiratory muscles can begin contraction from a mechanically advantageous position, and the expiratory muscles can share in the ventilatory burden. Using this strategy, positive end-expiratory pressure actually provides a boost to inspiration when the expiratory muscles relax (Fig. 53–2). This "work-sharing" strategy, although effective for a normal individual, cannot be implemented by patients with dynamic airway collapse during tidal breathing, because forceful expiratory efforts succeed not only in raising alveolar pressure but also in enhancing the intensity of dynamic airway collapse. In these circumstances, flow rate is determined strictly by lung volume and not accelerated by expiratory muscle activity. Thus, when dynamic collapse occurs during tidal breathing, there is little alternative to hyperinflation and/or CO_2 retention. At the chosen level of minute ventilation, maintenance of a lower lung volume may be either too energy costly or physically impossible. For this reason, many patients with severe obstruction do not or cannot decrease their lung volume in recumbency (Fig. 53–3).[13] Such considerations may help to explain the extreme dyspnea experienced by some COPD patients on assuming a recumbent position.

In some patients, especially those who passively receive ventilatory support, the problems presented by air trapping and dynamic hyperinflation are as much cardiovascular as pulmonary in nature.[14] A relatively high fraction of the positive alveolar pressure is transmitted to the pleural space, where it impedes venous return and confuses interpretation of hemodynamic pressure measurements (Fig. 53–4). Lung distention also adds to pulmonary vascular resistance, exacerbating the

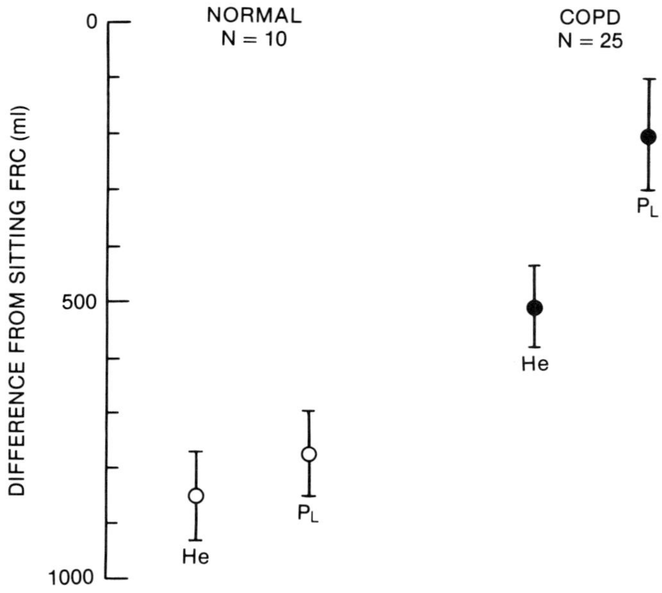

Figure 53–3. Position-related changes in FRC, as determined by plethysmography (P_L) and helium dilution (He) in normal subjects and in patients with COPD. Whereas normal subjects lose considerable volume in going from the upright to supine position, patients with COPD lose much less. The apparent positional loss in lung volume by He may be an artifact, reflecting airway closure and gas trapping. (Reproduced with permission from Pepe PE, Marini JJ. Am Rev Respir Dis 1984; 129:101–105.)

tendency of patients with cor pulmonale toward low cardiac output and hypotension.

Increased Minute Ventilation Requirement

Ventilation-perfusion mismatching is widespread in COPD, reducing the efficiency of carbon dioxide elimination. It is not uncommon for the resting minute ventilation requirement ($\dot{V}_E$)

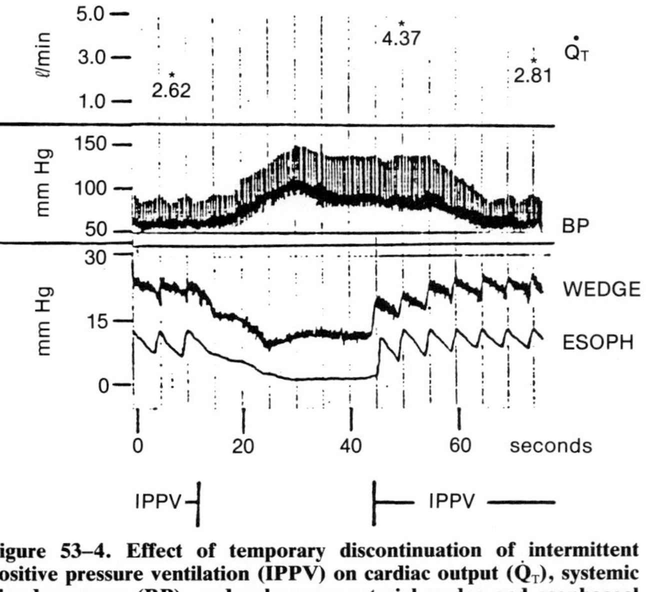

Figure 53–4. Effect of temporary discontinuation of intermittent positive pressure ventilation (IPPV) on cardiac output ($\dot{Q}_T$), systemic blood pressure (BP), and pulmonary arterial wedge and esophageal pressures in a patient with severe airflow obstruction and auto-PEEP. Note that wedge pressure during IPPV was elevated by the increase in intrathoracic pressure. (Reproduced with permission from Pepe PE, Marini JJ. Am Rev Respir Dis 1982; 126:167.)

to exceed 12 L/minute (twice the normal value) in patients with extensive emphysema and preserved chemical drives to breathe. Not only do such increases in ventilation requirement act as a linear cofactor in the total work of breathing equation ($W_B = \bar{P} \times \dot{V}_E$), but the high minute ventilation requirement itself increases most components of $\bar{P}$: flow, elastance (the reciprocal of compliance), tidal volume, and P_{ex} (see Eq. 53–1). It is not surprising, therefore, that enormous increases in the oxygen consumption rate of the ventilatory muscles have been observed in patients with obstructive lung disease.[15] During exacerbations, the oxygen consumed by ventilation can double the total body oxygen consumption observed during ventilator-supported breathing.

Reduced Mechanical Efficiency

In patients with exacerbated COPD, the oxygen consumption dedicated to the ventilatory task is disproportionate to the amount of mechanical work actually performed. The muscles of the hyperinflated ventilatory system are inefficiently aligned, force-length relationships of the shortened inspiratory fibers are suboptimal, and the normally efficient coordination among the various muscles of the ventilatory group is often disrupted (see subsequent discussion). The energy cost of breathing, therefore, is greatly increased for the pressure (and mechanical work) actually generated by the breathing effort.

Compromise of the Respiratory Pump

Faced with this extraordinary array of factors acting to increase the work of breathing, an ideal power generator would adapt itself to cope effectively. Unfortunately, the breathing stress placed on patients with chronic obstructive pulmonary disease is compounded by a seriously disadvantaged ventilatory pump.

For reasons that are not completely understood, patients with severe COPD and hyperinflation tend to be asthenic; in fact, overt malnutrition is not uncommon. Because the bulk of the respiratory musculature parallels lean body weight, muscle strength is significantly compromised in many such patients.[16–18] Furthermore, the process of hyperinflation impairs pump function in several important ways (Fig. 53–5).

DISTORTED GEOMETRY. The muscle fibers of the flattened diaphragm may contract powerfully, but produce no useful inspiratory force vector because of their abnormal (medial) orientation. In keeping with LaPlace's law, increasing the radius of curvature of the diaphragm (R_{di}) reduces the transdiaphragmatic pressure (P_{di}) that can be generated at any given tangential muscle tension (T_{di}): $P_{di} = T_{di}/R_{di}$. Complete flattening or inversion of the diaphragm converts it to an expiratory muscle. As another mechanical consequence of hyperinflation, the lower ribs become horizontally oriented, losing part of their "bucket handle" action. The diaphragmatic "zone of apposition" along the lower rib cage is also reduced or obliterated.

FIBER LOADING. The intrinsic loading properties of individual muscle fibers are detrimentally affected. When hyperinflation occurs acutely, individual muscle fibers foreshorten, so that precontractile length and force-generating capability are compromised.

FIBER ALIGNMENT. The muscle fibers of the hyperinflated thorax, particularly the diaphragm, change their alignment, converting from a parallel to a series arrangement—an exchange that sacrifices ventilatory force.[19] Over time, sarcomeres may be reabsorbed from chronically foreshortened muscle fibers, causing bulk and force to diminish.[20]

Not only are the muscle fibers themselves impaired during

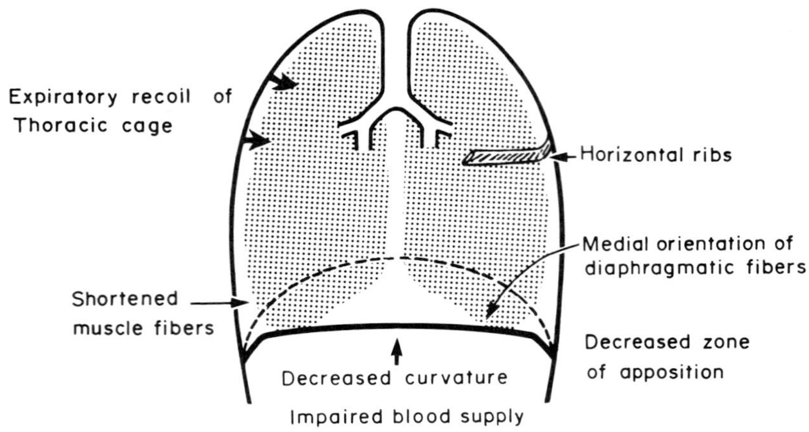

Figure 53–5. The detrimental effects of hyperinflation on respiratory muscle function. (Adapted with permission from Tobin MJ. Clin Chest Med 1988; 9:264.)

exacerbations of COPD, but their sequence of contraction may be inefficient. Discoordination among the various components of the ventilatory muscle group is often recognizable in patterns such as respiratory alternans, abdominal paradoxical motion, and predominant use of the accessory respiratory muscles.[21] Furthermore, fluctuations of respiratory rate, rhythm, and functional residual capacity (FRC) are sometimes extreme.[22] These patterns reflect the response of a system under serious stress,[23] and have been generally interpreted as an attempt to rest certain groups as others contract.[21–23] Such patterns may be maladaptive, however, in the sense that they are inefficient in generating the negative intrapleural pressure that drives inspiration.

The muscles of the ventilatory pump must receive an adequate supply of oxygen and nutrients, a demand that may go partially unmet during the stress of acute illness. Increased tissue tension may cause capillary compression and restrict perfusion to stressed inspiratory muscle fibers.[24] Attenuation of the pulmonary capillary bed, together with acidosis and hypoxemia, frequently cause sufficiently high pulmonary vascular resistance to impair the output of the stressed right ventricle. As a result, cor pulmonale frequently contributes to the inability of the patient to sustain the effort needed for spontaneous breathing during acute exacerbations. Furthermore, although cor pulmonale is characteristic, patients with COPD often suffer from left ventricular ischemia or failure as well; advanced age and cigarette smoking are common linking risk factors among these diseases.

Hazards of Positive Pressure Ventilation

Patients with COPD who require mechanical ventilation present special challenges to the clinician for yet another reason—an unusual predisposition to the adverse consequences of this mode of therapy. For reasons that are not entirely clear, patients with COPD have been reported to have an increased incidence of gastrointestinal ulceration and bleeding, especially during stress periods.[25] This tendency is abetted somewhat by poor nutrition, by the therapeutic use of corticosteroids, and perhaps by the administration of parenteral bronchodilators (e.g., theophylline, sympathomimetics). Even when able to cough with maximal force, COPD patients have difficulty in clearing contaminated secretions from their central and peripheral airways, predisposing them to bronchial and lung infections. This tendency is accentuated when the airway is intubated, an intervention that removes the patient's ability to generate high airway pressures and facilitates entry of contaminated secretions into the lower airway. In conjunction with mucous plugging, air trapping, and a tendency toward parenchymal infections, marked inhomogeneity of ventilation inclines the ventilated patient with COPD to the varied forms of barotrauma—pneumomediastinum, subcutaneous emphysema, and tension pneumothorax. Even a small pneumothorax in a ventilated patient with chronic obstructive pulmonary disease can rapidly develop a tension component, leading to ventilatory and circulatory compromise.

PRINCIPLES OF MANAGING THE VENTILATED PATIENT WITH COPD

Most patients hospitalized with exacerbations of COPD can be managed effectively by a regimen that incorporates aggressive secretion clearance techniques, antibiotics, corticosteroids, intensified bronchodilators, cardiovascular support, and supplemental oxygen.[26] Only a minority of patients so treated need translaryngeal intubation and institution of mechanical ventilatory support. When mechanical ventilation is required, however, the rationale underlying certain key management principles can be easily understood against the background of the physiologic derangements already described:

1. Provide adequate support for muscle rest at adequate Pa_{O_2} and pH.
2. Do not overventilate.
3. Minimize the minute ventilation requirement.
4. Minimize the risk of barotrauma.
5. Maintain adequate bronchial hygiene.
6. Prevent "panic" reactions.
7. Maintain appropriate nutrition.

Principle 1: Provide adequate support to rest the ventilatory muscles while avoiding hypoxemia and profound acidemia.

Poised on the edge of decompensation, the ventilatory muscles must be rested adequately before withdrawal of machine support can be considered. Rest may allow recovery of energy reserves and restore the balance between ventilatory capability and demand. Indeed, benefits may accrue to muscle rest, even when it occurs intermittently on a chronic basis (see subsequent discussion). Sufficient oxygen and mechanical support must be provided to achieve this goal and to avoid significant hypoxemia (arterial oxygen saturation, $Sa_{O_2} < 85\%$) and acidemia (pH < 7.25)—derangements that increase pulmonary vascular resistance and inhibit cardiac and skeletal muscle function.

Principle 2: Do not overventilate.

Although it is important to provide adequate ventilation, overventilation is detrimental on several counts. Rapid reduction in the alveolar CO_2 tension (Pa_{CO_2}) tends to cause bronchoconstriction and impairs neuromuscular and cardiovascular function. Furthermore, excessive ventilation exacerbates dynamic hyperinflation and auto-PEEP.[14, 27–29] It is generally a mistake to depress the Pa_{CO_2} below the chronically maintained level. Such a strategy may reset chemical drives and increase the respiratory workload intensity so that the patient cannot maintain unassisted breathing without intolerable effort.

Principle 3: Minimize minute ventilation requirement.

Because hyperinflation, mean inflation pressure, and the adverse cardiovascular consequences of mechanical ventilation are intimately linked to the minute ventilation requirement, ventilatory dead space and CO_2 output must be minimized while metabolic acidosis and spontaneous hyperventilation are avoided.

Principle 4: Minimize the risk of barotrauma.

The predisposition of patients with COPD to barotrauma must be combated by an intelligent choice of tidal volume, ventilatory frequency, positive end-expiratory pressure, and machine settings of trigger sensitivity and flow. Reduction of the $\dot{V}_E$ requirement decreases the mean and/or peak alveolar pressures, reducing the incidence of barotrauma. The relative contributions of mean alveolar pressure, peak dynamic cycling pressure, and peak static (plateau) ventilatory pressure to the risk of barotrauma are not clear.[30] Based on epidemiologic evidence, however, peak inflation pressures should be kept below 40 cm H_2O whenever possible.[30–31] It is probably best to select a tidal volume at the low end of the recommended range (7 to 9 ml/kg of ideal body weight). The question of optimal flow setting is of no small importance: auto-PEEP and mean alveolar pressure are reduced by the selection of rapid flow settings, and overall ventilation-perfusion ($\dot{V}/\dot{Q}$) matching may improve as well.[32–33] Higher peak dynamic pressures, however, may place certain units served by low-resistance pathways at jeopardy for overdistention. The risk of barotrauma can also be minimized by maintaining the lungs free of infection and the airways clear of secretions.

Principle 5: Maintain effective bronchial hygiene.

It is difficult to overemphasize the importance of maintaining adequate secretion clearance in patients with COPD. In such patients secretion retention may dramatically increase airflow resistance and/or effectively seal off distal parenchyma, preventing its participation in ventilation. Resulting dynamic hyperinflation can detrimentally affect cardiovascular function, work of breathing, and ventilatory capability. In addition to effective suctioning, bronchodilators, adequate hydration, and infection control, frequent repositioning, mobilization, and physiotherapy are fundamental to secretion management. Tracheostomies not only reduce resistance and provide improved access to the lower airway, but also eliminate the translaryngeal pathway between the oropharynx and trachea.

Principle 6: Prevent "panic" reactions.

In patients susceptible to dynamic airway collapse, an abrupt need to augment ventilation often precipitates a downward spiral in which the capability of the patient is overwhelmed by the imposed workload. Not only is minute ventilation increased during such episodes, but the resulting increase of dynamic hyperinflation impairs inspiratory muscle strength and endurance and impairs the mechanical efficiency of the system. Hyperinflation, in turn, may increase the mean pleural pressure and decrease venous return, leading to impaired nutrition of the muscles of the ventilatory pump, respiratory acidosis, dyspnea, and anxiety. The resulting imbalance in the demand-capability relationship may then create a need for aggressive intervention. It is my experience that many patients can be "talked through" what would otherwise prove to be an event that precipitates reinstitution of mechanical ventilation, augmentation of support, or the need for pharmacologic sedation.

Principle 7: Maintain appropriate nutrition.

In these stressed and often malnourished patients, the nature and quantity of nutritional support can make the difference between compensation and decompensation. Some studies have underscored the catabolic and often malnourished state of patients with COPD,[16–18, 34] whereas other reports have shown the hazards of aggressive refeeding.[35, 36] It is now clear that excessive caloric loads can increase the output of carbon dioxide, thereby adding to the ventilatory burden. Although best documented for carbohydrate loads, overfeeding of any type can cause this problem, particularly after a period of semistarvation.[35–37] Although reasonable caution is advisable, an adequate number of calories should be provided. It also must not be forgotten that many of these patients are in negative nitrogen balance and require an appropriate calorie-to-nitrogen ratio to rebuild their protein reserves. Withholding appropriate nutrition for fear of precipitating a ventilatory crisis is misguided.

Although the enteral route is preferred whenever possible, patients with COPD frequently develop breathing discomfort because of abdominal overdistention and its adverse effects on the function of the depressed diaphragm. Furthermore, enteral feedings can encourage the growth of pathogenic bacteria or pose the risk of aspiration when the infusion is initiated from a site proximal to the jejunum.[37]

PRACTICAL MANAGEMENT OF THE VENTILATED PATIENT

This section outlines key considerations in the practical management of the ventilated patient with COPD, based on the pathophysiology and principles of management just described.

Intubation

There is an understandable reluctance to initiate mechanical ventilation in patients with COPD, because many such individuals are so chronically disabled as to be miserable or despondent at home—even when everything is going as well as possible from a physiologic viewpoint. Nonetheless, it has been shown that some patients suffering repeated exacerbations of COPD recover uneventfully, even after several life-threatening episodes that require mechanical ventilation.[38] Very recently, there has been great enthusiasm for methods of ventilatory support that do not require airway intubation. Encouraging data are now available for "grid and wrap" negative pressure systems and nasal positive pressure ventilation. Considerably more evidence will be needed, however, before such "noninvasive" ventilatory support techniques can be recommended for patients undergoing acute exacerbations.

Although numerical criteria are sometimes given specifying the critical limits of pH, Pa_{O_2} or Pa_{CO_2} that warrant intubation,[39] the decision to undertake mechanical ventilation in patients with COPD remains a highly individual one that defies facile description. It seems clear that a patient whose mental status is deteriorating, one who experiences cardiovascular abnormalities (related to pH, CO_2 retention or hypoxemia), or one who experiences progressive fatigue, worsening respiratory acidosis, or advancing dyspnea in the face of aggressive treatment requires machine support. Other cases are less clear. A mounting secretion load audibly retained within the central airways generally indicates a patient too weak or breathless to expectorate, and often portends an imminent crisis. Hence, when this sign arises in a compatible clinical setting, most physicians consider it to be strong evidence favoring intubation for secretion management and ventilation support. Disorganization of the breathing rhythm—gasping or ataxic respirations, for example—strongly suggests approaching exhaustion.[40]

Selection of Endotracheal Tube

There is no consensus as to whether an oral (OT) or nasal (NT) endotracheal tube is most appropriate for an elective, semi-emergent intubation.[41] Although oral tubes are less comfortable in the initial phase, tend to prompt gagging or vomiting during insertion, and present problems with maintaining appropriate oral hygiene, they are generally of larger caliber than the largest NT tube that can be passed in the same patient, and somewhat less prone to kink or bend. Except when (unprotected) OT tubes are bitten, they maintain patency better than their nasal counterparts and provide better suctioning access. Pharyngeal pain and laryngeal trauma, however, may be greater problems because of increased tube mobility.[42]

The stability of NT tubes has been reported to give them some advantage with regard to laryngeal and tracheal trauma,[41, 42] but this is highly controversial. Furthermore, by allowing the patient to close the mouth, oral hygiene, comfort, and communication are improved. Unfortunately, small-diameter NT tubes tend to bend, kink, and narrow with accumulated secretions—important limitations in the management of patients with COPD. Bronchoscopy and suctioning are inhibited by the relatively small, angulated lumen these tubes present. Finally, nasal tubes frequently block sinus drainage pathways, encouraging purulent sinusitis, a common cause of occult fever in the ventilated patient.[41, 43] Blind nasal intubation can be difficult to perform, especially in an apneic patient. In my view, therefore, it should not be attempted under urgent or emergent circumstances.

Tracheostomy offers multiple advantages, particularly for patients who remain ventilator-dependent despite multiple attempts at weaning. Shorter and of larger caliber than either the nasal or oral tubes, tracheostomies present less resistance and facilitate airway suctioning. Swallowing, although impaired, is more effective than with nasal or oral intubation, and some patients with tracheostomies can eat a modified normal diet, despite machine support.

Initial Support

Postintubation Problems

The first 24-hour period following tracheal intubation and initiation of positive pressure ventilation is a highly dynamic one for the patient with COPD. Many of these individuals have decreased intravascular volume and impaired cardiovascular reflexes, features that prepare them poorly to compensate for the suddenly increased pleural pressure and impediment to venous return that usually accompany initiation of mechanical support. In this postintubation phase there is an understandable tendency for the physician to unintentionally overventilate the patient, and many patients cough vigorously or fight against the rhythm imposed by the machine.

One reason for the agitation that some patients experience is the sudden build-up of positive intrathoracic pressure through the process of dynamic hyperinflation. When these agitated patients are deeply sedated or paralyzed, inspiratory efforts cease and drug-related vasodilation occurs. The consequent rise of intrathoracic pressure, coupled with the fall of mean systemic pressure, can depress cardiac output. The physician, therefore, is well advised to remain alert to the abrupt development of cardiovascular depression and hypotension following intubation or sedation, and to be prepared to intervene to reduce ventilation and/or to support the circulation at the initially selected level. When sedation and paralysis are required, the drugs of choice are a benzodiazepine (e.g., midazolam), with or without a muscle relaxant (vecuronium or pancuronium). In patients with any suggestion of asthma, opiates, thiopental, succinylcholine, tubocurarine, metacurine, and atracurium should be used cautiously, if at all, because each has been linked with histamine release or bronchospasm.[44]

Shortly after intubation there may be agitation, coughing, and retching related to tube insertion. When this interferes with comfort or ventilation, many patients benefit from 3 to 5 ml of 1% to 2% lidocaine instilled through the endotracheal tube. Although lidocaine instillation may need to be repeated as often as every 10 minutes during the initial period, intolerance to tube placement gradually abates.

Machine Settings

As a general rule, ventilation should be fully supported during this initial phase, but it is better to underventilate cautiously than to overventilate the patient. In addition to the cardiovascular consequences just outlined, overventilation may precipitously reduce $Pa{CO_2}$, causing central nervous system alkalosis, obtundation, and even seizures.[45] Such consequences are not rare if there has been chronic CO_2 retention and theophylline usage. One approach is to use assisted mechanical ventilation delivered with a square or decelerating waveform, with a back-up rate set to provide about two-thirds the estimated minute ventilation requirement. Although the flow setting is adjusted empirically to coordinate the cycle lengths of the patient and ventilator, an initial peak flow setting of approximately five to six times the minute ventilation requirement usually suffices to meet inspiratory flow demands and minimize auto-PEEP, without imposing undue risks that attend extraordinarily high peak cycling pressures. (For example, if the $\dot{V}_E$ is 12 L/minute, a flow setting of 60 to 70 L/minute is usually sufficient.) The inspired oxygen fraction is usually set at 0.8 to 1.0, with oxygen saturation monitored by oximetry until a "postequilibration" blood gas level measurement can be obtained (about 15 to 20 minutes after stable ventilator settings have been accomplished). The triggering threshold of the ventilator is set to be as sensitive as possible and the auto-PEEP level is estimated. If auto-PEEP exceeds 5 cm H_2O and there is expiratory flow limitation during tidal breathing (which is almost invariably the case during this initial phase), the uncomfortable patient who makes spontaneous breathing efforts may benefit from the addition of a low level of end-expiratory pressure (3 to 5 cm H_2O). Machine adjustments are made as often as required, guided by arterial blood gas analysis, clinical signs and symptoms, and airway pressure characteristics (waveform, peak dynamic and static pressures, and auto-PEEP).

Monitoring Thoracic Mechanics

In addition to the indices of chest mechanics usually measured in the ventilated patient, the clinician should closely monitor end-expiratory lung pressure (auto-PEEP, intrinsic PEEP). This allows appropriate interpretation of chest compliance and pulmonary arterial pressure data and helps to monitor the progress of disease.[3, 14, 29] During passive ventilation, auto-PEEP can be measured by the end-expiratory port occlusion technique (Fig. 53–6) or by the "counterbalancing" method of Rossi and colleagues.[29]

In the latter method, the principle is to record the airway

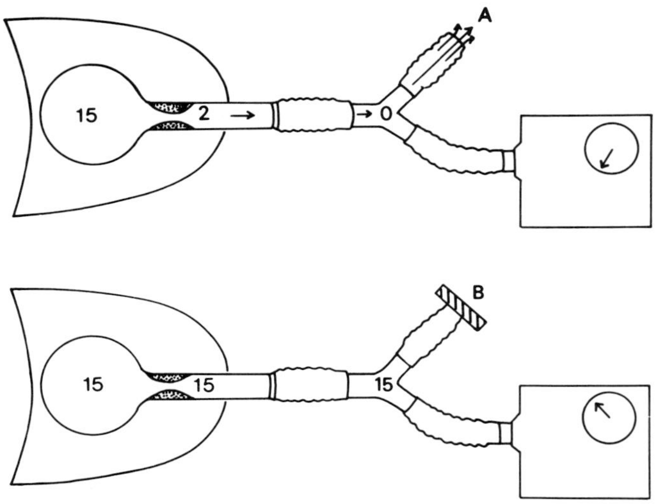

Figure 53–6. Measurement of auto-PEEP by expiratory port occlusion. During passive deflation very slow flow continues throughout exhalation and alveolar pressure remains positive until interrupted by the next inflation cycle (A). Occlusion of the exhalation port (for about 0.5 to 1.0 second) allows pressure to equilibrate throughout the circuitry and auto-PEEP to register on the ventilator's manometer (B). (A number of newer ventilators provide a button that automatically occludes the circuit at end-exhalation and delays delivery of the next machine cycle without the need for operator intervention or timing.) This technique is not applicable during active exhalation. (Reproduced with permission from Pepe PE, Marini JJ. Am Rev Respir Dis 1982; 126:167.)

pressure at which inspiratory flow begins during passive inflation. Theoretically, this pressure, the amount needed to counterbalance auto-PEEP and stop expiratory flow, should equal the end-expiratory alveolar pressure. In practice, however, its measurement requires simultaneous tracings of airway pressure and flow, very rapid recording speed, and a sensitive recording scale. Although such measurements are not routine in clinical practice, newer microprocessor-driven equipment promises to make them readily available in the near future.

Measuring auto-PEEP is more difficult when the patient initiates the inspiratory cycle. Qualitative detection of auto-PEEP is most easily accomplished by observing substantial residual flow at end-exhalation. Although some indication of the magnitude of end-expiratory alveolar pressure can be gleaned by end-expiratory port occlusion, timing is extremely difficult during spontaneous breathing. Precise measurement of auto-PEEP during spontaneous efforts requires insertion of an esophageal balloon and simultaneous recording of pleural pressure and flow (similar to the counterbalancing method).[45a]

Support Phase

Level of Support

After the first hours of ventilatory support, rational management focuses not only on reversal of the underlying problems of infection, bronchospasm, secretion retention, and heart failure, but also on replenishing spent nutritional reserves and building endurance. It makes sense to support ventilation fully in patients intubated for ventilatory failure while fundamental pathologic processes are being reversed, at least for the initial 24 to 48 hours. This is perhaps most appropriately done with volume-cycled assisted mechanical ventilation (AMV) adjusted to meet the patient's requirements (or, alternatively, with synchronized intermittent mandatory ventilation, SIMV) that provides a high proportion of the V_E requirement).

Choice of Ventilatory Mode

Because it is not known what intensity of ventilatory effort is best for the patient with COPD to undertake during the support phase of the illness, controversy exists as to the optimal mode of ventilation. During the support phase, the major objective should be to provide sufficient machine assistance to alleviate discomfort, yet not risk deconditioning the ventilatory muscles. To this end, it is reasonable to use AMV or SIMV applied at moderate to high levels, in keeping with the general principle of maintaining patient comfort. Usually, pressure-limited modes of ventilation (e.g., pressure support, intermittent positive pressure breathing, pressure control) are not appropriate in these patients during the most critical phase of their illness. Assisted machine cycles require patient work in direct proportion to levels of ventilatory drive. Thus, machine-aided cycles (in conjunction with the vigorous efforts that occur during episodic airway suctioning), usually provide sufficient exercise to forestall muscular atrophy, even during AMV. At night, it is my practice to increase the level of ventilatory support so that effective sleep and rest can be achieved. Complete control of ventilation (achieving a passive condition) is neither necessary nor desirable for effective resting.

Sedation and Paralysis

Deep sedation and paralysis (DSP), although very helpful in achieving therapeutic objectives early in the ventilatory process, may prove detrimental when their use is prolonged unnecessarily. On the positive side, DSP reduces carbon dioxide production related to the work of breathing. Establishing control of minute ventilation can also reduce mean alveolar pressures and diminish auto-PEEP. Reductions of peak ventilator cycling pressure are commonly observed as chest wall compliance improves and rhythm dysynchrony is eliminated. Finally, DSP enforces muscle rest and may improve the balance between cardiac output and demand.[46–47]

Unfortunately, secretions tend to pool in dependent airways when sedation and/or paralysis are continued for long periods. Stagnation occurs as forceful coughing efforts are eliminated and the breathing pattern becomes monotonous. Furthermore, unless the patient is turned at frequent intervals, DSP prevents the normal shifts of body position that help to maintain bronchial drainage and airway patency. Sedation and paralysis also inhibit inspiratory swings of pleural pressure and blunt the ability of the systemic circulation to return blood to the heart, amplifying the cardiovascular effects of auto-PEEP and/or volume depletion. Finally, muscle atrophy may accelerate after 3 days of complete immobilization. As a general rule, sedation and paralysis should not be continued for longer than 48 to 72 hours postinitiation.

Inspired Oxygen Fraction and Flow Setting

In the support phase of ventilation, the inspired oxygen fraction (FIO_2) should be adjusted to maintain arterial oxygen saturation above 85% to 90%. Oxygen-sensitive patients who make spontaneous efforts to breathe may retain additional CO_2 as the PaO_2 rises. When this occurs abruptly, ventilatory muscle strength may be transiently impaired.[48] These effects, however, are likely to abate with time. Furthermore, improvements in the PaO_2 tend to reduce right-heart afterload, and the higher CO_2 content of each exhalation improves the breathwise efficiency of CO_2 elimination. Taken together, these effects probably assist the patient in gaining independence from the ventilator.

Apart from improving expiratory resistance and reducing the minute ventilation requirement, increasing expiratory time (e.g., by increasing inspiratory flow rate) is the other major intervention aimed at reducing the mean alveolar pressure and auto-PEEP. As suggested previously, flow rate should initially be set at approximately 70 L/minute (or five to six times the $\dot{V}_E$ requirement) to achieve this end. Monitoring the central airway pressure waveform can prove invaluable in making machine adjustments. If not provided directly by the ventilator in use, such monitoring can be easily conducted using a standard disposable transducer commonly used for pulmonary arterial pressure measurement.[3, 49] An air-filled transducer is tapped into the central airway and connected to the bedside monitor and strip chart recorder. To avoid risking air embolism, such equipment should be dedicated to the purpose, and not shared with vascular catheters.

Pressure Support

Inspiratory pressure assist (pressure support) applies a clinician-set level of positive airway pressure above the end-expiratory pressure baseline to all spontaneous cycles, terminating when the flow rate falls to about 25% of the peak value.[50, 51] Although introduced primarily as a weaning modality, pressure support also helps during the support phase. I believe it makes sense to use approximately 3 to 5 cm H_2O of pressure support when SIMV or continuous positive airway pressure (CPAP) is used to help overcome the inherent resistance of the endotracheal tube.[50–52]

PEEP and CPAP in COPD

The deliberate use of positive end-expiratory pressure in patients with COPD has historically been considered undesirable, but there is now reason to believe that most of these patients benefit from the application of low levels (3 to 5 cm H_2O) of PEEP or CPAP. When applied downstream to airways that collapse dynamically during the exhalation phase of tidal breathing, this level of PEEP helps to improve the intrinsic trigger sensitivity of the machine without significantly increasing the alveolar pressure or hyperinflation (Fig. 53–7).[53, 53a] Most benefit is provided to patients who do not experience increases in peak static or peak dynamic cycling pressures after PEEP application. Applied PEEP may also help to keep airways more widely patent, and therefore improve secretion clearance.

When pressure support is used, there is another reason to use PEEP or CPAP in COPD patients. Because the difference between applied pressure and alveolar pressure drives inspiratory flow, end-expiratory alveolar pressure in excess of central airway pressure interferes with the ventilatory efficacy of the set level of pressure support.[54, 54a] In a sense, unsuspected auto-PEEP offsets the ventilatory action of the applied inspiratory pressure. (Conversely, pressure support can be used in an attempt to offset the inspiratory workload associated with auto-PEEP.) This same principle helps to explain why pressure cycled modes of mechanical ventilation have generally been unsuccessful or unreliable in ventilating patients with obstructive airway disease—to the extent that the patient develops auto-PEEP, the efficacy of a fixed pressure applied at the airway is negated.

Such considerations may also help to explain why pressure-supported patients who develop bronchospasm or secretion retention during the course of a weaning trial tend to decompensate abruptly. Newer modes of mechanical ventilation, currently available or planned for release in the near future, may be helpful in this regard. For example, minimum minute ventilation (also known as mandatory minute volume, or MMV) guarantees that a certain minute ventilation is achieved and (at least in theory) provides an acceptable back-up when pressure support is used as a primary ventilating mode.[55] A few ventilators recently introduced into clinical practice ensure that an adequate tidal volume as well as an adequate minute ventilation are maintained. Unfortunately, most earlier versions of MMV did not ensure that the guaranteed level of ventilation would be achieved at acceptable values for tidal volume and frequency.

Avoiding Complications

Pneumonitis, gastrointestinal bleeding, and barotrauma are extremely common complications of mechanical ventilation in patients with COPD, during the support phase.

GASTROINTESTINAL BLEEDING. Prophylaxis of gastrointestinal bleeding has been studied. Continuous enteral feeding, when delivered into the stomach or proximal duodenum, effectively buffers acid production and, more importantly, maintains mucosal nutrition.[56] Because proximal instillation risks aspiration, patients who receive enteral feedings should be nursed with their head inclined at least 30° from horizontal, and gastrointestinal motility should be closely monitored. Jejunal infusion poses the least risk of aspiration, but is relatively ineffective in ulcer prophylaxis. Therefore, many physicians add antacids or histamine (H_2) blockers to their medication regimen, sampling gastric contents intermittently to maintain a pH > 4.0. Although this strategy may help to avert ulceration of the gastrointestinal mucosa, it is not without hazard. Gastric acidity is a major natural defense employed to reduce colony counts of pathogenic bacteria in the upper gastrointestinal tract.[57] (Pneumonia or gastrointestinal motility

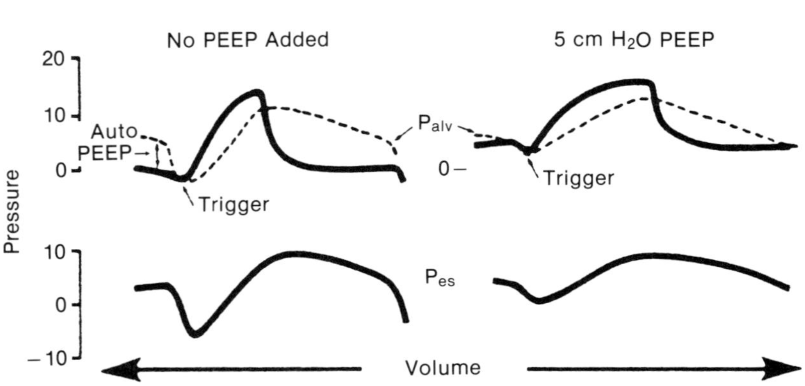

Figure 53–7. Effect of PEEP on auto-PEEP. As a positive end-expiratory alveolar pressure (P_{alv}), auto-PEEP presents an inspiratory threshold load to inspiration that must be overcome by inspiratory effort (negative esophageal pressure—P_{es}—deflection) before external airway pressure *(heavy dark line, upper tracing)* can begin to fall, triggering an inflation cycle. The addition of PEEP (less than the original auto-PEEP) to a patient with dynamic airway collapse reduces the effective triggering threshold and the work of breathing.

disturbances may follow pH neutralization. Pharyngeal and esophageal colonization may also seed the tracheobronchial tree.) Sucralfate, an alternative to antacids, histamine blockers, or gastric feeding for pH control, depends largely on acidity for its action (which is not to lower pH, but to bolster the vulnerable gastrointestinal mucosa against injury). Whether sucralfate offers a true advantage in ulceration and/or pneumonia prophylaxis in the critically ill patient remains to be determined.[58] The judicious use of sedatives may also help to reduce the ulceration tendency.

BAROTRAUMA. Minimizing barotrauma should be a major therapeutic objective. It is likely that the incidence of barotrauma relates not only to the height of peak dynamic and peak static (plateau) cycling pressures, but also to the mean airway pressure. Focusing on airway cycling pressures is certainly appropriate, but the important contribution of airway plugging (with ball valve action) and parenchymal necrosis must not be forgotten; infection control and secretion clearance are vitally important in the attempt to minimize barotrauma. It would seem reasonable to monitor peak static pressure carefully, reducing tidal volume and/or PEEP as necessary to keep this value within acceptable limits (<40 cm H_2O).[30, 59] Adequate hydration of the inspired air stream, intravascular volume repletion, reversal of bronchospasm, and treatment of secretion purulence are equally important. Mucolytics are not routinely helpful, and can irritate the airway if used alone, without prior bronchodilation.

ATELECTASIS. Segmental atelectasis is less a problem in patients with chronic airflow obstruction than in those recovering from abdominal surgery or in those with other acute restrictive lung disorders. Nonetheless, chest percussion, postural drainage, inhalation of bronchodilators, deep breathing and coughing, and (occasionally) bronchoscopy may be required when a large plug of mucus occludes a major lung segment.[60]

Pharmacotherapy

With regard to using bronchodilators in the ventilated patient with COPD, aerosols are perhaps of more consistent value than systemically administered medications. Although parenteral theophylline and adrenergic compounds have been shown to augment diaphragmatic contractile force and delay fatigue,[61] their clinical usefulness for this purpose remains to be convincingly proven. Indeed, theophylline preparations are notoriously difficult to titrate to maximum advantage without toxicity.[62] β_2-agonists are the mainstay of bronchodilator treatment, but quarternary ammonium compounds such as ipatropium bromide have been introduced as alternatives with particular efficacy for this disease.[63] In COPD, if not asthma, anticholinergic bronchodilators have been shown to be at least as effective as β_2 agonists in reversing bronchospasm.[64] Although this "newer" class of medications is welcome, it should be acknowledged that bronchodilators in COPD do not assume the same importance as they do in the treatment of asthma. Similarly, corticosteroids, a vital and even lifesaving intervention in the asthmatic patient, have more limited use in the setting of COPD. Initial doses of 0.5 mg/kg q6h may be used effectively to reduce intrabronchial inflammation and bronchospasm,[65] but should probably not be continued for longer than 24 to 48 hours. The detrimental effects of corticosteroids on glucose metabolism, protein wasting, and immune function produce serious consequences when these agents are used for protracted periods.[66]

Weaning Phase

Protracted ventilator dependence is perhaps the most feared consequence of intubating the patient with COPD. Not only are breathing workloads very high, but the ability of the patient to sustain them is compromised by muscle weakness, hyperinflation, disadvantageous thoracic geometry, blunted ventilatory drive and, often, by abnormal cardiovascular function. Rational management of the "weaning" patient with COPD includes provision of adequate rest and nutritional support, enhancement of neuromuscular and cardiovascular function, and minimization of the breathing workload. Maintenance of a positive mental attitude can greatly speed the weaning process.

Predicting the Outcome of the Weaning Trial

Patients may fail to wean from mechanical ventilation for a wide variety of reasons.[67] Among these are hypoxemia, cardiac arrhythmias or cardiovascular instability, and psychologic dependence (Table 53–2). However, imbalance between ventilatory capability and demand is perhaps the most common reason for failure to wean in patients with COPD.

In clinical practice a panel of indices are used to predict the outcome of the weaning trial.[68] Most of these can be classified as indicators either of ventilatory capability or demand, but not both. Thus, a maximal inspiratory pressure measurement that exceeds 30 cm H_2O, and a $\dot{V}_E$ requirement of less than 10 L/minute, are standard components of the predictive weaning battery. Other measures (such as the ability to double $\dot{V}_E$ or V_T on demand) attempt to assess the ventilatory reserve, but have generally been unsuccessful in the clinical setting when full patient cooperation cannot be secured.

Two integrative indices of capability and demand—the pressure-time index (inspiratory effort quotient, PTI) and the mouth occlusion pressure have been receiving increasing attention—partly because of their physiologic appeal and partly because they do not strictly require patient cooperation. The mean inflation pressure ($\bar{P}$) during a tidal breathing cycle can be estimated from the modified equation of motion of the respiratory system, as outlined previously. The ratio of $\bar{P}$ to P_{max} (the maximum pressure that can be generated by the patient during airway occlusion at FRC) fulfills the criterion of relating demand to capability. When $\bar{P}/P_{max}$ is multiplied by the inspiratory time fraction (T_i/T_{tot}, an involuntary measure easily determined from a tracing of flow or central airway pressure) the combined expression (the PTI) bears a strong resemblance to the tension-time or pressure-time index long used in cardiology and skeletal muscle physiology to assess the oxygen demand placed on the heart muscle.[69] If studies in normal subjects can be extrapolated to the clinical setting, the $\bar{P}/P_{max}$ ratio should not exceed 0.40, and the PTI should be < 0.20 in patients who successfully wean from support.[70] Of the PTI components, P_{max} still eludes reliable measurement in the poorly cooperative subject. Because all parts of the PTI can, in theory, be estimated or measured at the bedside, however, this index holds promise for future clinical use.

The same can be said of the mouth occlusion pressure (P_{100}, $P_{0.1}$), a pressure generated in the first 100 msec of a surreptitiously occluded breath.[71] The P_{100}, an indicator of the motor outflow of the respiratory neurons, tends to correlate with the intensity of demand placed on the system and is relatively insensitive to the status of lung and chest wall mechanics. It is, however, influenced by muscle strength and therefore by the lung volume at which it is measured. Because of its simplicity and integrative nature, the P_{100} holds special promise for bedside clinical use.

The P_{100} appears to relate to weaning outcome in patients with COPD. For example, Sassoon and colleagues have shown that patients with COPD who have P_{100} values > 6.0 cm H_2O seldom wean successfully.[72] Perhaps a better test of the venti-

TABLE 53–2. Therapeutic Measures for Factors that Limit Weaning Progress

HYPOXEMIA	↑ IMPEDANCE	CARDIOVASCULAR FUNCTION	↑ $\dot{V}_E$	↓ DRIVE	MUSCLE WEAKNESS	PSYCHOGENIC FACTORS
Positioning ↓ Secretions Bronchodilation Diuresis CPAP ↑ FIO_2	Positioning ↓ Secretions Bronchodilation CPAP Tracheostomy ↓ $\dot{V}_E$ ↓ Circuit resistance	Correct O_2, pH Adjust intravascular volume Diuresis Inotropics	Sedation ↓ Fever ↓ Pain ↓ V_D/V_T ↓ Work of breathing	↑ Nutrition ↓ Loading ↓ Alkalosis ↓ Sedatives ↑ Sleep ↓ Thyroid deficiency	Positioning Correct electrolytes Correct pH Steroids ↑ Calories ↓ or ↑ steroids ↓ Pain Ambulation, physical therapy Intermittent rest Muscle training Δ Ventilatory mode O_2 Therapy Sleep	Convey therapeutic plan Reassurance Anxiolytics Encourage normal activity Adequate sleep

latory reserve than the absolute value of the P_{100} itself is provided by the response of P_{100} to inspired CO_2. Some preliminary data obtained by Montgomery and colleagues[73] have suggested that patients who fail to wean from mechanical ventilation have exhausted their ventilatory reserve and have curtailed their response to carbon dioxide-enriched gas. Therefore, the ventilatory and P_{100} responses to this chemical stimulus are relatively flat, despite a rising $PaCO_2$. Conversely, patients with ample ventilatory reserve tend to respond to the CO_2 challenge by increasing both drive and work outputs. The eventual place of these P_{100} measures in clinical practice has yet to be determined. At present, an empiric trial of spontaneous breathing would appear to be the most satisfactory method of assessing the potential outcome of machine withdrawal, particularly since the limitation is often non-ventilatory in origin.

Preparations for Ventilator Withdrawal

Many patients with COPD who fail to wean from mechanical ventilation have been suboptimally prepared. Preparations should include attempts to restore electrolyte balance and hemoglobin saturation to near-normal levels, to adjust arterial blood gas levels to reflect appropriate spontaneous values for PaO_2 and $PaCO_2$, and to optimize thoracic mechanics by ensuring adequate bronchodilation, secretion clearance, relief of abdominal distention, and optimal positioning (preferably upright). The performance capability of the ventilatory system is enhanced by ensuring *adequate nocturnal rest* (with fully supported breathing), adequate nutrition, good circulatory reserve, and minimization of the minute ventilation requirement. Whether ventilatory muscle training has a place in this program is currently unknown.[74]

It should be emphasized that many patients with COPD who fail to wean from mechanical ventilation have occult congestive heart failure or coronary ischemia, elicited by the stresses of the imposed breathing workload and/or the "autotransfusion effect" that accompanies discontinuation of mechanical ventilation.[75–76] Careful cardiovascular assessment and support are prudent in puzzling cases.

Graded Ventilator Withdrawal

The patient must be fully involved in the weaning attempt and given a careful explanation of the overall plan. In short, the patient must be co-opted into therapeutic decision making and given as much control as feasible over the duration of each weaning trial. As a general rule, patients with COPD should not be re-exposed abruptly to the full breathing workload unless there are adequate breathing and cardiovascular reserves, as judged from the clinical setting and predictive indices outlined previously. Abrupt changes in workload are likely to cause dyspnea, initiating a cyclical process of increasing $\dot{V}_E$, air trapping and ultimately resulting in ventilatory failure.

On the other hand, the weaning process should not be unduly prolonged. In general, support should be gradually reduced over a period of several days. The optimal pace of withdrawing machine support is open to question. However, the duration of this weaning period should generally parallel the duration of ventilation that preceded it.[77] Whether it is best to use graded pressure support ventilation, SIMV, intermittent breathing on a T piece or blow-by circuit, or a newer mode of ventilation (such as MMV[55]) in the weaning attempt is not clear at present, and remains largely a matter of physician preference. It is my bias that T-piece trials are useful in assessing the likelihood of successful machine withdrawal, but intermittent (unmodified) T-piece breathing should not usually be used as the weaning technique of choice. When such trials are conducted, it is advisable to use low PEEP levels (3 to 5 cm H_2O) supplemented by 3 to 5 cm H_2O of pressure support (above the elevated end-expiratory pressure baseline). This recommendation is based on the knowledge that PEEP (CPAP) combats the work-augmenting tendency of auto-PEEP,[53, 78] whereas pressure support helps to overcome endotracheal tube resistance.[50, 51] This recommendation also applies to the spontaneous breathing cycles of SIMV.

Whatever level of machine support is chosen, the patient should be kept as comfortable as possible during the day and fully rested at night. Used alone, pressure support ventilation may be especially risky in these patients, for several reasons. First, as is true for almost all pressure-cycled modes of ventilation, the efficacy of a given level of pressure support in aiding ventilation relates directly to the impedance of the chest. Increased resistance, reduced thoracic compliance, and auto-PEEP blunt the effectiveness of pressure support. Thus, a patient who appears to be tolerating a certain level of pressure support with equanimity shortly after the airway has been suctioned free of secretions may demonstrate precipitious deterioration as minute ventilation increases, secretions accumulate, or bronchospasm and/or agitation develop. Such changes may abruptly force the patient to undertake a larger share of the ventilatory burden. Obtunded patients, those with impaired or unstable ventilatory drive, and those receiving intermittent sedatives or analgesics require some guaranteed form of minute ventilation back-up (apnea back-up, SIMV, MMV) when pressure support is used. Clinicians should be aware that a disproportionate fraction of the ventilatory workload is borne by the lowest range of pressure support. In other words, a high percentage of the ventilatory load is transferred to the patient as the last increments of pressure support are removed. Such consideration helps explain why a patient who progressed nicely through the initial stage of machine withdrawal fails to tolerate the final step. In particularly difficult cases, various different weaning modalities should be tried in an attempt to find the one that is best tolerated. It is not necessary or desirable to discontinue CPAP or pressure support completely before extubation. Furthermore, most patients should not have SIMV weaned lower than two to four breaths per minute before extubation is contemplated. Generally, at least 2 hours (and occasionally as long as 8 hours) of observation should be made on the lowest level of support before decannulation. In cases of extraordinarily difficult weaning, a biofeedback signal in the form of a capnography tracing or verbal coaching may help to achieve an optimally efficient breathing pattern.

Tracheostomy often proves to be invaluable in the difficult-to-wean patient, not only because it facilitates tracheal suctioning, secretion clearance, speech, and eating, but also because it enables the patient to ambulate with assistance, using a hand-actuated bag or pressure-cycled ventilator. Physical conditioning often plays a vital role in the physiologic capability and psychologic well-being of the patient. Important unanswered questions relate to the value of specific ventilatory muscle-conditioning exercises and to the most appropriate training regimen.[79, 80]

The postextubation period should be as carefully managed as the preextubation phase. The first few hours off the ventilator are often labile.[81] Coughing, deep breathing, maintenance of a mechanically efficient posture, and adequate oxygenation are crucial. Heart rate and rhythm, respiratory rate, and breathing pattern should be closely monitored. Oral refeeding must be undertaken with extreme caution, because swallowing difficulty and glottic dysfunction can persist days to weeks postextubation. Above all, the postextubated patient must be watched very closely for the first 48 to 72 hours, preferably under direct vision.

Chronic Intermittent Ventilatory Support

When unrelieved, excessive work of breathing leads to CO_2 retention, impairment of oxygen exchange, disordered sleep, and impaired physical and mental functioning. Exacerbations of disease may be distressingly frequent. Intermittent rest of the ventilatory musculature appears to hold some promise for helping to rehabilitate such patients. Studies of patients with neuromuscular disease, kyphoscoliosis, and COPD have convincingly shown improvement in muscle strength, endurance, sleep quality, and nutritional status.[82] Activity level and sense of well-being often improve as well. Although a well-accepted technique for the chronic management of neuromuscular disease, this modality cannot be considered proven for general use in patients with COPD, for whom the available scientific literature is too meager to support such recommendations. On the strength of current information, such an intervention, although a major commitment, should be considered in nonterminal patients with COPD who are disabled because of one or more of the following: severe irreversible disease, frequent rehospitalization, multiple failed attempts of prolonged ventilator independence, sleep disturbances consequent to ventilatory insufficiency, intolerable dyspnea, or refractory cor pulmonale.[83]

REFERENCES

1. Otis AB. The work of breathing. In: Fenn WO, Rahn H, eds. Handbook of Physiology, Sec 3, Vol 1. Bethesda, MD: American Physiological Society, 1964, 463–476.
2. Peters RM. The energy cost (work) of breathing. Ann Thorac Surg 1969; 7:51–67.
3. Marini JJ. Monitoring during mechanical ventilation. Clin Chest Med 1988; 9:73–100.
4. Nunn JF. Applied Respiratory Physiology. 3rd ed. London: Butterworths, 1987, 46–50.
5. Briscoe WA, DuBois AB. The relationship between airway resistance, airway conductance and lung volume in subjects of different age and body size. J Clin Invest 1958; 37:1279–1285.
6. Knudson RJ, Mead J, Knudson DE. Contribution of airway collapse to supramaximal expiratory flows. J Appl Physiol 1974; 36:653–667.
7. Hyatt RE. The interrelationships of pressure, flow and volume during respiratory maneuvers in normal and emphysematous subjects. Am Rev Respir Dis 1961; 83:676–683.
8. Rodarte JB, Rehder K. Dynamics of respiration. In: Fishman AP, Macklem PT, Mead J, eds. Handbook of Physiology, Sec 3: The Respiratory System. Mechanics of Breathing, Vol 3. Bethesda, MD: American Physiological Society, 1986, 131–144.
9. Fleury B, Murciano C, Talamo C, et al. Work of breathing in patients with chronic obstructive pulmonary disease in acute respiratory failure. Am Rev Respir Dis 1985; 131:822–827.
10. West JB, Dollery CT, Naimark A. Distribution of blood flow in isolated lung in relation to vascular and alveolar pressures. J Appl Physiol 1964; 19:713–724.
11. Grimby G, Bunn J, Mead J. Relative contribution of rib cage and abdomen to ventilation during exercise. J Appl Physiol 1968; 24:159–166.
12. Gherini S, Peters RM, Virgilio RW. Mechanical work on the lungs and work of breathing with positive end-expiratory pressure and continuous positive airway pressure. Chest 1979; 76:257–261.
13. Marini JJ, Tyler ML, Hudson LD, et al. Influence of head-dependent positions on lung volume and oxygen saturation in chronic airflow obstruction. Am Rev Respir Dis 1984; 129:101–105.
14. Pepe PE, Marini JJ. Occult positive end-expiratory pressure in mechanically ventilated patients with airflow obstruction: The auto-PEEP effect. Am Rev Respir Dis 1982; 126:166–170.
15. Field S, Kelley SM, Macklem PT. The oxygen cost of breathing in patients with cardiorespiratory disease. Am Rev Respir Dis 1982; 126:9–13.
16. Arora NS, Rochester DF. Respiratory muscle strength and maximal voluntary ventilation in undernourished patients. Am Rev Respir Dis 1982; 126:5–8.
17. Arora NS, Rochester DF. Effects of general nutritional muscular states on the human diaphragm. Am Rev Respir Dis 1977; 115:84–89.
18. Rochester DF, Arora NS, Braun NMT, et al. The respiratory muscles in chronic obstructive pulmonary disease (COPD). Bull Eur Physiopathol Respir 1979; 15:951–975.
19. Macklem PT, Macklem DM, DeTroyer A. A model of inspiratory muscle mechanics. J Appl Physiol 1983; 55:547–557.
20. Farkas GA, Roussos C. Diaphragm in emphysematous hamsters: Sarcomere adaptability. J Appl Physiol 1983; 54:1635–1640.
21. Cohen C, Zagelbaum D, Gross D, et al. Clinical manifestations of inspiratory muscle fatigue. Am J Med 1982; 73:308–316.
22. Tobin MJ, Chadha TS, Jenouri G, et al. Breathing patterns: 2. Diseased subjects. Chest 1983; 84:286–294.
23. Tobin MJ, Perez W, Guenther SM, et al. The pattern of breathing during successful and unsuccessful trials of weaning from mechanical ventilation. Am Rev Respir Dis 1986; 134:1111–1118.
24. Supinski GS. Respiratory muscle blood flow. Clin Chest Med 1988; 9:211–223.
25. Hastings PR, Skillman JJ, Bushnell LS, et al. Antacid titration in the prevention of acute gastrointestinal bleeding. A controlled randomized trial in 100 critically ill patients. N Engl J Med 1978; 298:1041–1045.
26. Pierson DJ. Exacerbation of chronic bronchitis and emphysema: Ventilatory management. In: Kacmarek RM, Stoller JK, eds. Current Respiratory Care. Philadelphia: BC Decker, 1988, 267–272.

27. Kimball WR, Leith DE, Robins AG. Dynamic hyperinflation and ventilator dependence in chronic obstructive pulmonary disease. Am Rev Respir Dis 1982; 126:991–995.
28. Bergman NA. Pulmonary gas trapping during mechanical ventilation at rapid frequencies. Anesthesiology 1972; 37:626–633.
29. Rossi A, Gottfried SB, Zocchi L, et al. Measurement of static compliance of the total respiratory system in patients with acute respiratory failure during mechanical ventilation. The effect of "intrinsic PEEP." Am Rev Respir Dis 1985; 131:672–677.
30. Peterson GW, Horst B. Incidence of pulmonary barotrauma in a medical ICU. Crit Care Med 1983; 11:67–69.
31. Strieter RM, Lynch JP. Complications in the ventilated patient. Clin Chest Med 1988; 9:127–139.
32. Connors AF Jr, McCaffree DR, Gray BA. Effect of inspiratory flow rate on gas exchange during mechanical ventilation. Am Rev Respir Dis 1981; 124:537–543.
33. Tuxen DV, Lane S. The effects of ventilatory pattern on hyperinflation, airway pressures, and circulation in mechanical ventilation of patients with severe air-flow obstruction. Am Rev Respir Dis 1987; 136:872–879.
34. Vandenberg E, Van de Woestijne KP, Gyselen A. Weight changes in the terminal stages of chronic obstructive pulmonary disease; relation to respiratory function and prognosis. Am Rev Respir Dis 1978; 95:556–566.
35. Covelli HD, Black JW, Olsen MS, et al. Respiratory failure precipitated by high carbohydrate loads. Ann Intern Med 1981; 95:579–581.
36. Askanazi J, Rosenbaum SM, Hyman AJ, et al. Respiratory changes induced by the large glucose loads of total parenteral nutrition. JAMA 1980; 243:1444–1447.
37. Heymsfeld SB, Erbland M, Casper K, et al. Enteral nutritional support. Clin Chest Med 1986; 7:41–67.
38. Martin TR, Lewis SW, Albert RK. The prognosis of patients with chronic obstructive pulmonary disease after hospitalization for acute respiratory failure. Chest 1982; 82:310–314.
39. Grum CM, Morganroth ML. Initiating mechanical ventilation. J Int Care Med 1988; 3:6–20.
40. Pardee NE, Winterbauer RH, Allen JD. Bedside evaluation of respiratory distress. Chest 1984; 85:203–206.
41. Heffner JE. Tracheal intubation in mechanically ventilated patients. Clin Chest Med 1988; 9:23–35.
42. Dubick MN, Wright BD. Comparison of laryngeal pathology following long-term oral and nasal endotracheal intubations. Anesth Analg 1978; 57:663–668.
43. O'Reilly MJ, Reddick EJ, Black W, et al. Sepsis from sinusitis in nasotracheally intubated patients. A diagnostic dilemma. Am J Surg 1984; 147:601–604.
44. Duncan SR, Raffin TA. Status asthmaticus: Ventilatory management. In: Kacmarek RM, Stoller JK, eds. Current Respiratory Care. Philadelphia: BC Decker, 1988, 285–293.
45. Kilburn KH. Shock, seizures and coma with alkalosis during mechanical ventilation. Ann Intern Med 1966; 65:977–984.
45a. Petrof BJ, Legaré M, Goldberg P, Milic-Emili J, Gottfried SB. Continuous positive airway pressure reduces work of breathing and dyspnea during weaning from mechanical ventilation in severe chronic obstructive pulmonary disease. Am Rev Respir Dis 1990; 141:281–289.
46. Viires N, Sillye G, Aubier M, et al. Regional blood flow distribution in dog during induced hypotension and low cardiac output. J Clin Invest 1983; 72:935–947.
47. Aubier M, Trippenbach T, Roussos C. Respiratory muscle fatigue during cardiogenic shock. J Appl Physiol 1981; 51:499–508.
48. Juan G, Calverley P, Talamo C, et al. Effect of carbon dioxide on diaphragmatic function in human beings. N Engl J Med 1984; 310:874–879.
49. Truwit JD, Marini JJ. Evaluation of thoracic mechanics in the ventilated patient. Part 1: Primary measurements. J Crit Care 1988; 3:133–150.
50. Kacmarek RM. The role of pressure support ventilation in reducing work of breathing. Respir Care 1988; 33:99–120.
51. MacIntyre NR. Respiratory function during pressure support ventilation. Chest 1986; 89:677–683.
52. Gottfried SB, Rossi A, Higgs BD, et al. Noninvasive determination of respiratory system mechanics during mechanical ventilation for acute respiratory failure. Am Rev Respir Dis 1985; 131:414–420.
53. Smith TC, Marini JJ. Impact of PEEP on lung mechanics and work of breathing in severe airflow obstruction. The effect of PEEP on auto-PEEP. J Appl Physiol 1988; 65:1488–1499.
53a. Marini JJ. Should PEEP be used in airflow obstruction? Am Rev Respir Dis 1989; 140(1):1–3.
54. Truwit JD, Marini JJ. Hyperinflation limits pressure control ventilation (abstract). Chest 1988; 94:2S.
54a. Marini JJ, Crooke PS III, Truwit JD. Determinants and limits of pressure present ventilation: A mathemetical model of pressure control. J Appl Physiol 1989; 67(3):1081–1092.
55. Hewlett AM, Platt AS, Terry VG. Mandatory minute volume. A new concept in weaning from mechanical ventilation. Anaesthesia 1977; 32:163–169.
56. Pingleton SK, Hadzima SK. Enteral alimentation and gastrointestinal bleeding in mechanically ventilated patients. Crit Care Med 1983; 11:13–16.
57. Palmer LC, Merrill WW, Neiderman MS, et al. Bacterial adherence to respiratory tract cells. Relationships between in vivo and in vitro pH and bacterial attachment. Am Rev Respir Dis 1986; 133:784–788.
58. DuMoulin GC, Hedley-Whyte J, Paterson DG, et al. Aspiration of gastric bacteria in antacid-treated patients: A frequent cause of postoperative colonization of the airways. Lancet 1982; i:242–245.
59. deLatorre F, Tomasa A, Klemburg J, et al. Incidence of pneumothorax and pneumomediastinum in patients with aspiration pneumonia during ventilatory support. Chest 1977; 72:141–144.
60. Marini JJ, Pierson DJ, Hudson LD. Acute lobar atelectasis: A prospective comparison of fiberoptic bronchoscopy and respiratory therapy. Am Rev Respir Dis 1979; 119:971–978.
61. Aubier M, DeTroyer A, Sampson M, et al. Aminophylline improves diaphragmatic contractility. N Engl J Med 1981; 305:249–252.
62. Miech RP, Stein M. Methylxanthines. Clin Chest Med 1986; 7:331–340.
63. Ashutosh K, Land H. Comparison between long-term treatment of chronic bronchitic airway obstruction with ipratropium bromide and metaproterenol. Ann Allergy 1984; 53:401–406.
64. Gross NJ, Skorodin MS. Anticholinergic, antimuscarinic bronchodilators. Am Rev Respir Dis 1984; 129:856–870.
65. Albert RK, Martin TR, Lewis SW. Controlled trial of methylprednisolone in patients with chronic bronchitis and acute respiratory insufficiency. Ann Intern Med 1980; 92:753–758.
66. Haynes RC Jr, Larner J. Adrenocorticotropic hormone; adenocortical steroids and their synthetic analogs. In: Goodman LL, Gilman A, eds. The Pharmacological Basis of Therapeutics. 5th ed. New York: MacMillan, 1975, 1472–1506.
67. Marini JJ. The physiologic determinants of ventilator dependence. Respir Care 1986; 31:271–282.
68. Sahn SA, Lakshminarayan S, Petty TL. Weaning from mechanical ventilation. JAMA 1986; 235:2208–2212.
69. Sarnoff SJ, Braunwald E, Welch GH, et al. Hemodynamic determinants of oxygen consumption of the heart, with special reference to the tension time index. Am J Physiol 1958; 192:148–156.
70. Milic-Emili J. Is weaning an art or a science? Am Rev Respir Dis 1986; 134:1107–1108.
71. Whitelaw WA, Derenne JP, Milic-Emili J. Occlusion pressure as a measure of respiratory center output in conscious man. Respir Physiol 1975; 23:181–199.
72. Sassoon CSH, Te TT, Mahutte CK, et al. Airway occlusion pressure. An important indicator for successful weaning in patients with chronic obstructive pulmonary disease. Am Rev Respir Dis 1987; 135:107–113.
73. Montgomery AB, Holle RHO, Neagley SR, et al. Prediction of successful ventilator weaning using airway occlusion pressure and hypercapnic challenge. Chest 1987; 4:496–499.
74. Pardy RL, Reid WD, Belman MJ. Respiratory muscle training. Clin Chest Med 1988; 9:287–296.
75. Kumar A, Falke KJ, Geffin B, et al. Continuous positive pressure ventilation in acute respiratory failure. Effects on hemodynamics and lung function. N Engl J Med 1970; 283:1430–1436.
76. Lemaire F, Teboul JL, Cinotti L, et al. Acute left ventricular dysfunction during unsuccessful weaning from mechanical ventilation. Anesthesiology 1988; 69:171–179.
77. Morganroth ML, Morganroth JL, Nett LM, et al. Criteria for weaning from prolonged mechanical ventilation. Arch Intern Med 1984; 144:1012–1016.
78. Smith TC, Marini JJ, Lamb VJ. The inspiratory threshold load

resulting from air trapping during mechanical ventilation (abstract). Am Rev Respir Dis 1987; 135:A52.
79. Belman MJ, Mittman C. Ventilatory muscle training improves exercise capacity in chronic obstructive pulmonary disease patients. Am Rev Respir Dis 1980; 121:273–280.
80. Aldrich T. Inspiratory muscle resistive training in respiratory failure. Am Rev Respir Dis 1985; 131:461–462.
81. Gilbert R, Auchincloss JH Jr, Peppi D, et al. The first few hours off a respirator. Chest 1974; 65:152–157.
82. Braun NMT, Marino WD. Effect of daily intermittent rest of respiratory muscles in patients with severe chronic airflow limitation (CAL). Chest 1984; 85:595–596.
83. Braun NMT. Intermittent mechanical ventilation. Clin Chest Med 1988; 9:153–162.

Chapter 54

TREATMENT OF ALPHA$_1$-ANTITRYPSIN DEFICIENCY AND OTHER FORMS OF EMPHYSEMA

Allen B. Cohen Steven Idell

Based on current knowledge of the pathogenesis of emphysema, new treatment strategies have been developed to treat the underlying cause of emphysema. Most of these strategies involve attempts to address the postulated imbalance of proteases and their natural inhibitors and to reduce the burden of proteolytic enzymes, mainly of neutrophilic origin. In particular, the replacement of alpha$_1$-protease inhibitor in patients with a genetically determined deficiency of this protein has become feasible. Other promising avenues of intervention include reduction of the neutrophil elastase load and the use of synthetic protease inhibitors. Although the efficacy of these modalities remains to be established in large-scale clinical trials, they are currently the best hope of addressing the causes of emphysema and offer the prospect of specific therapy. This chapter reviews the protease-antiprotease hypothesis, the evidence that supports it, and the role of other effectors of lung injury in the pathogenesis of emphysema. How these theories of the pathogenesis of emphysema have been used to develop the treatment strategies that have recently become available or are now being studied is then discussed. Lastly, the logistics of providing these treatments for clinical use and the assessment of their impact are considered.

THEORIES OF THE PATHOGENESIS OF EMPHYSEMA

The protease-antiprotease hypothesis was first proposed as a result of the observation, in 1963, of an association between homozygous alpha$_1$-protease inhibitor deficiency and emphysema.[1] These observations provided initial support for the protease-antiprotease hypothesis, which holds that pulmonary emphysema results from the digestion of lung elastin by proteolytic enzymes that exceed the ability of their natural inhibitors to contain their effects.

Alpha$_1$-protease inhibitor is a glycoprotein of molecular weight 52,000[2] that inhibits proteases in a 1 to 1 molar ratio.[3] Alpha$_1$-protease inhibitor appears to be an important modulator of inflammatory events. Neutrophil elastase, collagenases, kallikrein, plasmin, and thrombin[4–8] are inhibited by alpha$_1$-protease inhibitor. Alpha$_1$-protease inhibitor is distributed in almost every body compartment in which albumin is found and has been detected in alveolar lining fluids.[9] This inhibitor is also an acute phase reactant and serum levels have been found to rise in association with pregnancy, infections, and after severe burn injuries.[10–12] Serum concentrations may also be elevated by up to 20% in smokers.[13]

Clinical Manifestations of Alpha$_1$-Protease Inhibitor Deficiency

Genetic variants of alpha$_1$-protease inhibitor are classified based on the Pi (protease inhibitor) system.[14] The Pi^{MM} phenotype is normal and subjects with phenotype Pi^{Z} have a marked deficiency of alpha$_1$-protease inhibitor in serum. Available clinical studies suggest that these patients are prone to the development of pulmonary emphysema. Of 246 Pi^{Z} patients in Sweden, most showed signs of emphysema, and greatly reduced survival was shown in male and female patients.[15] In Pi^{Z} patients with emphysema, a rapid, progressive decline in pulmonary function has been observed. The rate of decline of the FEV_1 (forced expiratory volume in 1 second) was nearly double the average rate of decline observed in patients with "ordinary" chronic obstructive pulmonary disease (COPD).[16]

Other factors may significantly effect expression of clinically important lung disease in patients deficient in alpha$_1$-protease inhibitor. Not all patients who are deficient in alpha$_1$-protease inhibitor develop emphysema. Ganrot and colleagues reported five patients with no history of COPD who had normal pulmonary function tests and were over the age of 50.[17] In another study in which pulmonary function testing was not described, 26 patients with the Pi^Z phenotype were reported who clinically did not have emphysema.[18]

The onset of emphysema in patients with alpha$_1$-protease inhibitor deficiency appears to be hastened by smoking. The mean age of onset of dyspnea was found to be 44 years in Pi^Z nonsmokers versus 35 years in Pi^Z subjects who smoked.[19] Pulmonary function and radiographic changes suggestive of emphysema similarly occurred earlier in smoking versus nonsmoking Pi^Z subjects. Air pollution has also been implicated as a potentially important influence on mortality in patients with alpha$_1$-protease inhibitor deficiency,[20] suggesting that avoidance of respiratory irritants may be particularly beneficial to these patients.

Interaction of the Protease-Antiprotease Balance, Smoking, and Oxidants

The role of oxidants and other effector systems in the pathogenesis of COPD has been described elsewhere in this book (Section II). In this section, the effects of oxidants and smoking on the protease-antiprotease balance are reviewed. Oxidation of the methionine residue at the active site of alpha$_1$-protease inhibitor results in reduced interaction of the molecule with neutrophil and pancreatic elastase and trypsin.[21–24] The rate of association of alpha$_1$-protease inhibitor with neutrophil elastase is reduced by a factor of about 2000 compared to that of the native inhibitor, and the elastase-alpha$_1$-protease inhibitor complexes formed appear to be less stable than normal.[22] The relevance of these observations to the pathogenesis of emphysema is suggested by the development of changes compatible with the early stages of emphysema in animals treated experimentally with the oxidant chloramine-T.[25] Although cigarette smoke is an important source of oxidant stress, the lungs are also exposed to oxidizing agents from environmental pollution and from endogenous sources, such as alveolar macrophages and neutrophils.[26]

Some studies have suggested that oxidation is the mechanism responsible for the inactivation of alpha$_1$-protease inhibitor with cigarette smoking. The functional inhibitory activity of alpha$_1$-protease inhibitor was decreased in bronchoalveolar lavage from smokers compared to the lavage fluid of nonsmokers.[27, 28] Oxidation of alpha$_1$-protease inhibitor was shown to be the mechanism responsible for inactivation of the inhibitor in rats exposed to cigarette smoke inhalation.[29] Inactivation of alpha$_1$-protease inhibitor in lavage fluids of human smokers has also been demonstrated,[28] but this observation has not been uniformly repeated.[30] The oxidative capacity of cigarette smoke is enhanced by hydrogen peroxide.[3] Because alveolar macrophages secrete hydrogen peroxide, collections of these cells in small airways may serve to explain the development of central alveolar emphysema in smokers.

Experimental Evidence Supporting the Protease-Antiprotease Hypothesis

Support for the protease-antiprotease hypothesis is also derived from experimental observations. A critical experiment that supported this hypothesis was performed by Gross and colleagues, who showed that intratracheal administration of papain in rats was followed by destruction of the alveolar walls, with a resultant enlargement of the air spaces.[31] Figure 54–1 illustrates these pathologic changes, which were corroborated by the results of similar experiments carried out by Kimbel and Weinbaum (unpublished data, 1980).

Additional studies have supported the contribution of neutrophil proteases, and of neutrophil elastase in particular, to the proteolytic destruction of lung elastin in emphysema. As previously reviewed,[32] neutrophils gain access to the normal lungs. A small pool of neutrophils rapidly turns over in the air spaces.[33] Also, although few neutrophils are found in normal human bronchoalveolar lavage fluids, increased numbers are found in lavages of smokers.[34] These observations suggest that neutrophils are accessible to the alveoli in numbers sufficient to effect proteolytic or oxidant-related injury. Agents that attract neutrophils have also been demonstrated to be present within the lungs.[35–38] The flux of neutrophils into the normal lungs of rabbits and the putative events occurring in the alveoli relating macrophages, neutrophils, and lung tissues are represented in Figures 54–2 and 54–3.

Other cell types may influence the development of emphysema directly or indirectly. In particular, two chemotactic factors are secreted by alveolar macrophages that are responsible for the influx of neutrophils.[36, 38] One of these is probably leukotriene B4 (LTB4)[39] and the other is a peptide.[40] Whereas the LTB4 level increases quickly after the macrophages ingest a particulate load, the peptide appears to be constitutively secreted and its concentration does not increase when particulates are ingested.[41] Macrophages may therefore influence neutrophil traffic and secretion within the lung. Also, some investigators have found that macrophages from smokers secrete an elastase.[42, 43] It is currently uncertain whether the elastase is uniquely synthesized by the macrophages, is a neutrophil elastase earlier scavenged by the macrophages, or is a metalloprotease similar to that secreted by mouse macrophages.[44]

Morphologic evidence further supports a role of both neutrophils and macrophages in the pathogenesis of emphysema. Morphometric studies have shown the presence of these inflammatory cells in the small airways of smokers.[45] Clusters of pigmented alveolar macrophages are observed in respiratory bronchioles, a characteristic early lesion seen in the lungs of young smokers.[46] Additional support for the protease-antiprotease hypothesis and for the role of neutrophils in the pathogenesis of emphysema has been provided by an elegant morphologic study.[47] Elastase was immunochemically localized in neutrophils in the lung interstitium and extracellularly in association with interstitial elastic fibers in human lungs showing local emphysema of varying severity. The local distribution of neutrophil elastase in contact with alveolar interstitial elastin was quantitated and found to correlate with local emphysematous lesions.

The clinical observation of emphysema associated with alpha$_1$-protease inhibitor deficiency and experimental evidence that supports the protease-antiprotease hypothesis has led to the development of new therapeutic strategies. Largely predicated on technologic advances, restoration of the normal balance of proteases and their inhibitors within the lung has now become feasible. In the next section the development and application of specific interventions that are derived mainly from the protease-antiprotease hypothesis are presented. Strategies for addressing other possible causes of emphysema and the logistics of developing new interventions are also reviewed.

USING THE THEORIES TO DEVELOP TREATMENT

Replacement of Alpha$_1$-Protease Inhibitor

History

Eleven years after Eriksson's discovery that patients deficient in plasma alpha$_1$-protease inhibitor develop emphysema,[48]

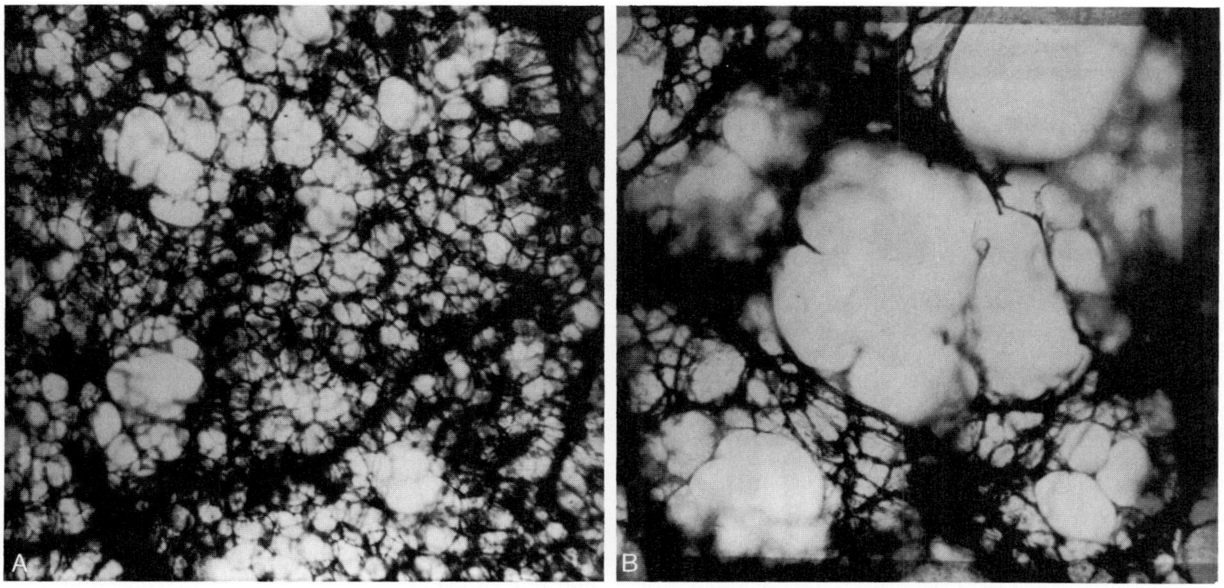

Figure 54–1. Thick sections of a dog's lungs. *A*, Normal. *B*, After treatment with elastase. (Reproduced with permission from Flenley DC, Petty TL, eds. Recent Advances in Respiratory Medicine, Vol 3. Edinburgh: Churchill Livingstone, 1983.)

the Lung Division of the National Heart, Lung, and Blood Institute (NHLBI) of the National Institutes of Health (NIH) convened the first of many workshops that facilitated the development of replacement therapy for alpha$_1$-protease inhibitor deficiency. The first meeting, in 1976, focused on the mechanisms of action of proteases and inhibitors. In 1977, the Blood Division of the NHLBI held another international workshop to investigate the feasibility of developing alpha$_1$-protease inhibitor as a therapeutic agent from plasma fractionation.[49] It was noted that enormously large amounts of plasma would have to be fractionated to supply all the alpha$_1$-protease inhibitor-deficient patients. However, it was also emphasized that there was already a large amount of plasma being fractionated and that the alpha$_1$-protease inhibitor was being destroyed or discarded. The kinetics of alpha$_1$-protease inhibitor in plasma were described and the feasibility of replacement therapy suggested. A workshop was convened in 1978 by the NHLBI to define the problems more specifically, and to discuss opportunities for treating the genetic form of emphysema. Based on a review of the available literature, the following postulates were presented:[49]

1. Alpha$_1$-protease inhibitor replacement in patients with pulmonary emphysema has a strong likelihood of preventing the progression of emphysema in patients with the Pi^{ZZ} phenotype for alpha$_1$-protease inhibitor.

2. If such replacement therapy appears to be successful, therapeutic trials of low-molecular-weight inhibitors could be undertaken.

3. If safe elastase inhibitors become available, they could be tried on patients with common forms of emphysema regardless of the results in patients with the Pi^{ZZ} phenotype for alpha$_1$-protease inhibitor.

The committee recognized that a series of formidable problems had to be solved before clinical trials of the specific agents could be carried out. Five problem areas for replacement therapy were identified:

1. Isolation of alpha$_1$-protease inhibitor on a clinical scale and proven safety for licensing

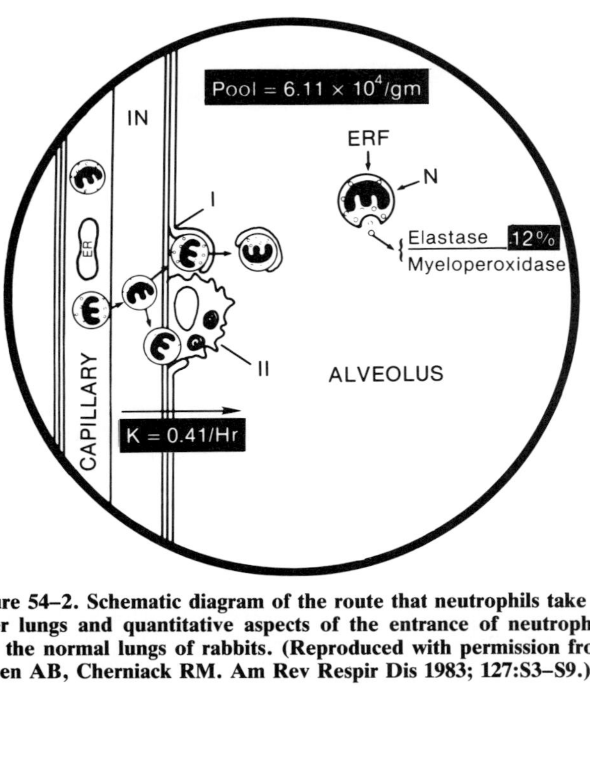

Figure 54–2. Schematic diagram of the route that neutrophils take to enter lungs and quantitative aspects of the entrance of neutrophils into the normal lungs of rabbits. (Reproduced with permission from Cohen AB, Cherniack RM. Am Rev Respir Dis 1983; 127:S3–S9.)

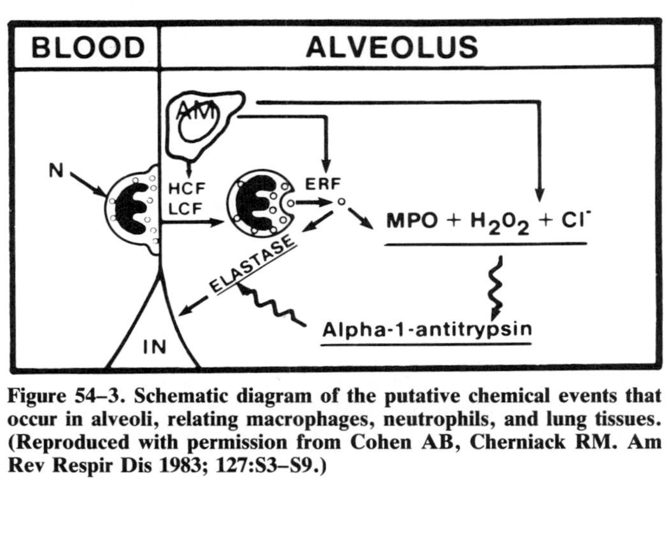

Figure 54–3. Schematic diagram of the putative chemical events that occur in alveoli, relating macrophages, neutrophils, and lung tissues. (Reproduced with permission from Cohen AB, Cherniack RM. Am Rev Respir Dis 1983; 127:S3–S9.)

2. Determination of the pharmacokinetics of alpha$_1$-protease inhibitor in humans
3. Development and testing of the safety of elastase inhibitors
4. Development of chemical markers of lung destruction
5. Determination of the natural history of emphysema in patients with the Pi^Z phenotype to determine if a study of replacement therapy is feasible

The progress toward these goals was reviewed in 1987,[50] but the review is already outdated. The following update is fairly current (as of January 1988).

ISOLATION OF ALPHA$_1$-PROTEASE INHIBITOR FROM BLOOD. Cutter Laboratories has developed a method for isolating alpha$_1$-protease inhibitor on a clinical scale. They applied for a license to sell the drug under the Orphan Drug Law. The status of this application is discussed subsequently.

PHARMACOKINETICS OF ALPHA$_1$-PROTEASE INHIBITOR. A definitive study of the pharmacokinetics of the Cutter alpha$_1$-protease inhibitor was carried out by Wewers and colleagues.[51] This study will become the standard by which alpha$_1$-protease inhibitor is administered to patients. It is described in more detail subsequently.

DEVELOPMENT OF SAFE ELASTASE INHIBITORS. A number of elastase inhibitors have been synthesized.[52] Classes of such compounds include alkylating agents (chloromethyl ketones), acylating agents (azapeptides), and beta-lactams and peptides. Some of these inhibitors exhibit a high reactivity and specificity for human leukocytic elastase, whereas others can inhibit a broad range of serine proteases. Generally, these agents are rapidly destroyed in aqueous environments or are poorly soluble in water. Studies of these compounds have been hampered by a lack of first-class animal models and of a rapid process for determining whether lung destruction is slowed.

DEVELOPMENT OF CHEMICAL MARKERS OF LUNG DESTRUCTION. Current tests of lung function are sufficiently insensitive that they fail to detect early disease. In addition, the variation among measurements in the same person is sufficiently great that large numbers of patients must be studied for a long time to determine whether a new treatment reduces the rate of deterioration of lung function. Therefore, chemical indicators of lung destruction that predict rapidly and accurately whether a drug has stopped the lung destruction would be extremely valuable. Three such markers have been proposed—plasma elastin peptides,[53] urinary desmosine,[54] and plasma fibrinopeptides created by the action of elastase on fibrinogen.[55] The concentrations of the first and third of these are higher in patients with emphysema and in cigarette smokers. The urinary desmosine level is not higher in patients with emphysema, but theoretically it could only come from elastin. Recent studies have suggested that prior assays did not discriminate desmosine from similar products (Starcher, personal communication, 1989). These tests are still being evaluated.

NATURAL HISTORY OF EMPHYSEMA IN Pi^{ZZ} SUBJECTS AND REPLACEMENT THERAPY. It is necessary to know the natural history of the emphysema in these patients to determine the size of treated and control groups and the duration of a clinical trial. This could help to determine whether a therapeutic agent can reduce the rate of decline of lung function and mortality. The natural history of emphysema has been examined by a retrospective longitudinal study of American and Swedish patients with alpha$_1$-protease inhibitor deficiency. The NHLBI sponsored a series of workshops that were used to collect data from major laboratories in the two countries that have studied this disease. Retrospective data on 298 Pi^Z individuals collected at several institutions in the United States and Sweden were reviewed.[56, 57] Baseline FEV$_1$ values were compared with follow-up measurements obtained after more than 12 months had elapsed. Linear regression analysis was carried out separately for each individual to determine the annual rate of change of the FEV$_1$. From these analyses, group mean rates of decline were calculated and the standard deviations of these rates determined. The proportion of nonsmoking Pi^Z patients in this cohort was 19.7%. This subpopulation is smaller than might be expected from the rate of smoking in the general population and may reflect a bias in case ascertainment—a large proportion of pulmonary patients whose clinical disease may have been potentiated by smoking were studied selectively. Pi^Z subjects, particularly nonsmokers, and those who escaped clinical disease sufficient to declare itself, were therefore under-represented. The resulting analysis was therefore skewed toward a description of the progression of disease in more severely affected Pi^Z individuals.

Although cases collected in this manner pose problems in regard to the interpretation of data, the rates of decline in FEV$_1$ observed in clinically significant but not end-stage Pi^Z disease are nearly twice the average rates of decline reported in smokers with COPD. Therefore, Pi^Z subjects who develop significant airflow obstruction enter a phase of relatively rapid functional decline.

These studies demonstrated that it would require about 800 patients per group studied for 5 years to determine whether the rate of decline of FEV$_1$ had been reduced by more than 50%. The implications of these numbers is discussed subsequently.

A second question of great interest to the consideration of therapy is whether heterozygotes for the Z gene develop emphysema. As reviewed elsewhere,[57] the literature is controversial. Whereas several studies failed to detect differences in lung function between Pi^{MZ} and Pi^M subjects,[58–61] others have demonstrated greater pulmonary dysfunction in Pi^{MZ} subjects.[62–64] Smoking in some studies appeared to be a significant determinant of the development of COPD in heterozygotes for alpha$_1$-protease inhibitor deficiency.[63] Studies of disease prevalence are strongly influenced by the means of ascertainment of the heterozygotes, the ages of the patients studied (if heterozygotes develop disease, they are likely to do so later than Pi^Z individuals), and the types of measurements used to detect the disease. These disparate data indicate that, if Pi^{MZ} individuals develop emphysema, the differences from normal populations must be small. Importantly, then, the blood concentrations of alpha$_1$-protease inhibitor in Pi^{MZ} individuals can serve as a useful minimum in patients undergoing replacement therapy.

Given these data, the FDA has considered two applications for alpha$_1$-protease inhibitor to be used as a drug for treating patients with Pi^Z phenotype and emphysema. One application was for a product derived from recombinant technology and the other for a product derived from blood fractionation. At the first meeting, in January 1985, a group of scientists and physicians reviewed the available data and reached several conclusions. The thorny issue of what should constitute proof of efficacy was addressed.[65] After consideration of the natural history of alpha$_1$-protease inhibitor-deficient patients and the scarcity of patients with the Pi^Z phenotype, it was concluded that a clinical trial would be extremely expensive, if it were possible at all. After reviewing many options, the participants decided that proof of efficacy would require a demonstration that the product could maintain blood concentrations of alpha$_1$-protease inhibitor, at least at the level seen in patients with the Pi^{MZ} phenotype, and that it would restore the protease-inhibitor balance in fluids obtained by lung washes.[65]

Current Status

In the months that followed, Wewers and colleagues[51] carried out an excellent trial of replacement therapy. The agent used for infusion was a sterile lyophilized preparation of partially purified human alpha$_1$-proteinase inhibitor obtained from pooled plasma from normal donors.[51] The preparation had been heat-treated in solution at 60° C for 10 hours to lower the risk of transmission of plasmaborne diseases. Patients received hepatitis vaccine prior to the initiation of therapy.

The Cutter blood fraction of alpha$_1$-protease inhibitor was administered to 21 patients who had been given 60 mg/kg of active alpha$_1$-proteinase inhibitor kg intravenously for up to 6 months. (It is important that clinicians not retitrate the preparation, either for total alpha$_1$-proteinase inhibitor or for activity. Standards for alpha$_1$-proteinase inhibitor concentration vary among manufacturers and vary from true concentrations.) After the preparation was reconstituted with sterile water to a concentration of 25 mg/ml of active alpha$_1$-proteinase inhibitor (dose calculated on the basis of the amount of alpha$_1$-protease inhibitor specified on the label), the preparation was filtered (0.22-μm filter, pharmacy transfer set, Millipore) and administered within 4 hours.[51] After a steady state had been reached, the lowest serum concentrations were 126±1 mg/dl (as compared with 30 ± 1 mg/dl before treatment), and the serum antineutrophil elastase capacities were 13.3 ± 0.54 μM (as compared with 5.4 ± 0.1 μM before treatment). The concentration in the epithelial-lining fluid of the lungs was 0.46 ± 0.16 μM before treatment, and the antineutrophil elastase capacity was 0.81 ± 0.13 μM. Six days after infusion, the alpha$_1$-proteinase inhibitor concentrations were still higher than those in patients with the Pi^{MZ} phenotype.

Administration of 507 infusions did not cause any severe adverse reactions. There were no acute reactions. One patient had low-grade fever lasting 48 hours that had begun 12 hours after an infusion of 90 mg/kg. Blood cultures were negative. This patient subsequently received therapy for 6 months without any reactions. The serum half-life of the material was similar at 3 and 6 months, and no antibodies developed to the preparation. Although no patients with Pi^{null} were reported in this group, some have been treated without adverse effects (Crystal, personal communication, 1987). However, adverse immunologic response in Pi^{null} patients must be considered as a possibility based on experience with other diseases.[66]

In January 1988 the blood fraction was released by the Cutter Biologicals Division of Miles Laboratories under the trade name Prolastin. The quoted price of the drug is $0.10/mg. For a 70-kg individual, the drug would cost $21,840 annually. The product is clearly labeled for use only in patients with Pi^{Z}, $Pi^{Z,\ null}$ or Pi^{null} phenotype for alpha$_1$-protease inhibitor. Since the initial distribution there have been 2 recalls for adverse reactions by particular lots.

Reduction of the Elastase Load

Because current theories of the mechanisms of lung destruction in emphysema involve the digestion of lung elastin by neutrophil elastase, and perhaps the oxidation of alpha$_1$-protease inhibitor by oxidants from smoke and from phagocytic cells, it is reasonable to suggest that the lung destruction might be stopped by drugs that prevent neutrophils from entering the lungs or from dumping their enzymes into the lungs. This goal might be a simplistic one, however. There are about 30 to 40 drugs now on the market that affect neutrophil function without increasing the patient's susceptibility to infection. Neutrophils enter the lungs in response to chemotaxins and degranulate in response to specific agents, as described previously. Agents that prevent neutrophil chemotaxis or degranulation, or that diminish signals emanating from the lungs, may reduce the elastase load in the lungs. Generally, investigations have divided the cells' machinery necessary for chemotaxis and degranulation into several categories. Cell-surface receptors initiate these processes, cyclic nucleotides translate the message, cellular serine proteases and divalent actions modulate the system, and cytoskeletal components achieve the movement of the cells or granules. Drugs do not necessarily fall into neat packages that affect only one of these functions, but some categories of drugs can be developed:

1. Drugs that affect microfilaments
2. Drugs that affect microtubules
3. Drugs that affect cyclic nucleotides
4. Drugs that affect calcium transport
5. Drugs that affect surface receptors
6. Antimicrobial drugs
7. Nonsteroidal antiinflammatory drugs
8. Corticosteroids
9. Antielastases

Colchicine is a drug that affects neutrophil function. When neutrophils that adhere to surfaces are exposed to such agents as chemotaxins[67] or to the alveolar macrophage enzyme-releasing factor,[68] they release granules containing enzymes, such as elastase and myeloperoxidase. The release depends on the function of a component of the neutrophil cytoskeleton, the microtubules. Colchicine prevents degranulation by interfering with the assembly of microtubules.[69, 70]

In our laboratory we are currently testing colchicine in a double-blind controlled trial in smokers with normal blood concentrations of alpha$_1$-proteinase inhibitor to determine whether the drug lowers the elastase load in the lungs and to measure various parameters of elastin degradation. If this drug or a subsequent drug can be found that alters the chemistries in these patients in a manner suggesting that the pathogenetic process can be favorably altered, a larger study will be carried out to determine if the mortality or rate of decline of lung function has been modified. Any alteration in the routine management of patients with emphysema awaits the results of a definitive study.

Protease Inhibitors

A number of reversible and irreversible inhibitors of leukocyte elastase have been developed, several of which have been shown to be effective in preventing emphysema in animal models.[52] Peptide chloromethyl ketones were the first class of selective inhibitors of human leukocyte elastase to be developed.[71, 72] Acylating agents, sulfonyl fluorides, alpha$_1$-protease inhibitor analogues, heterocyclic elastase inhibitors, and various other compounds serve as inhibitors of human leukocyte elastase.[52] Although inhibitors to date have had chemical problems that preclude their clinical use, it now appears that the overall prospects for the development of synthetic elastase inhibitors suitable for human use in the near future are good. If the major cause of emphysema in smokers is the inactivation of alpha$_1$-proteinase inhibitor, one would hope that these agents could be used in this larger group of patients.

Other Forms of Therapy

Because diethylstilbestrol, an anabolic steroid, can increase the release of alpha$_1$-protease inhibitor from the liver, Gadek and associates[73] attempted to achieve increased plasma concentrations of alpha$_1$-proteinase inhibitor with an anabolic steroid called danazol, which has fewer side effects. They achieved a mean increase of 37% in patients with the Pi^{Z} phenotype. The concentrations of alpha$_1$-proteinase inhibitor were still far below those thought to be safe (those seen in individuals with the Pi^{MZ} phenotype). It is unclear whether these concentrations affect morbidity or mortality in patients with the Pi^Z phenotype. However, one might be cautiously optimistic that other agents that can achieve a greater release of alpha$_1$-protease inhibitor from the livers of patients with the Pi^Z phenotype will be found.

LOGISTICS OF SEEKING SOLUTIONS

As noted previously, the demonstration that alpha$_1$-protease inhibitor could replace the missing inhibitor was judged by the FDA to be adequate proof of efficacy. No other form of therapy for emphysema will probably be brought into use without a clinical trial to determine whether the drug reduces the rate of clinical decline of lung function or mortality. Clinical trials of this nature would cost about $6 million and last 5 years, like the NIH Early Intervention Trial. Therefore, a means of testing possible therapeutic strategies must be developed. I would like to suggest such a strategy. The first step would be to develop methods in vitro or in animals to select drugs that might reduce the lung elastase load. For example, if one wishes to reduce the influx of neutrophils into the lungs, drugs might be screened for their antichemotactic ability for neutrophils or for their ability to prevent neutrophils from secreting their elastase. Drugs that might modify the clinical course of emphysema could be studied in smaller and less expensive clinical trials if adequate chemical predictors of lung destruction or of the pathogenic process could be developed. These chemical tests might include the measurement of fairly specific chemicals liberated by the eroding lung tissue, such as plasma elastin peptides or fibrinopeptides, or urinary desmosines (as noted previously). The elastin peptide and fibrinopeptide levels have been shown to be elevated in patients with emphysema. Although blood and urine tests are ideal for this purpose other tests could be used, such as bronchoalveolar lavage fluids in which neutrophils or neutrophil elastase concentrations could be measured.

Ideally, one would know in advance that the chemical test predicted the clinical course, but the strategy for these studies is complex. First, a correlation must be shown between the disease and the chemical measurement. Then, a minitrial should be carried out to determine whether promising antiemphysema drugs modify the chemical test of lung destruction in a beneficial manner. If the chemical marker is modified a large-scale clinical trial should be undertaken, with reduction in the rate of lung function decline and mortality as a goal. If the drug is successful in this trial the chemical marker would be judged to be a successful correlate of lung destruction, and the cycle could then be repeated with other drugs. If this approach is successful, a step-by-step approach could be used to find the most effective drugs for treating the underlying cause of emphysema.

REFERENCES

1. Laurell CB, Eriksson S. The electrophoretic α-1-globulin pattern of serum in α-1-antitrypsin deficiency. Scand J Clin Lab Invest 1963; 15:132–140.
2. Eriksson S. Studies in alpha-1-antitrypsin deficiency. Acta Med Scand 1965; 177(Suppl):1–85.
3. James HL, Cohen AB. Mechanism of inhibition of porcine elastase by human alpha-1-antitrypsin. J Clin Invest 1978; 62:1344–1353.
4. Ohlsson K, Ohlsson I. The neutral proteases of human granulocytes: Isolation and partial characterization of two granulocyte collagenases. Eur J Biochem 1973; 36:473–481.
5. Harris ED Jr, DiBona DR, Krane SM. Collagenases in human synovial fluid. J Clin Invest 1969; 48:2104–2113.
6. Tokoro Y, Eisen AZ, Jeffrey JJ. Characterization of a collagenase from rat skin. Biochim Biophys Acta 1972; 258:289–302.
7. Rimon A, Shamash Y, Shapiro B. The plasmin inhibitor of human plasma. IV. Its action on plasmin, trypsin, chymotrypsin and thrombin. J Biol Chem 1966; 241:5102–5107.
8. Fritz H, Wunderer G, Kummer K, et al. Antitrypsin and C1-Inactivator. Progresswinhibitgoren für Serumkallikreine von Mensch und Schwein Hoppe-Seylers. Z Physiol Chem 1972; 353:906–910.
9. Tuttle WC, Jones RF. Fluorescent antibody studies of alpha-1-antitrypsin in adult human lung. Am J Clin Pathol 1975; 64:477–482.
10. Ganrot PO, Bjerre B. Alpha-1-antitrypsin and alpha-2-macroglobulin concentration in serum during pregnancy. Acta Obstet Gynecol Scand 1967; 46:126–137.
11. Ascoli M, Bezola C. Das Verhalten des antitryptischen Vermogens dens Beautserums bei der Croupsosen Pneumonie. Berl Klin Wochenschr 1903; 40:391.
12. Busch R, Wilms K. Das Verhalten des α-1-antitrypsin bei Verbrennungen und Verbruhungen. Kinderartzl Prax 1974; 42:352–356.
13. Elson LA, Betts TE, Darcy DA. Alpha-1-antitrypsin in cigarette smokers. In: Maltoni C, Davis W, eds. Advances in Tumour Prevention, Detection, and Characterization. Vol 1, Proceedings of the Fifth International Symposium on the Biological Characterization of Human Tumors. International Congress No. 321. Amsterdam: Excerpta Medica, 1974, 151–153.
14. Fagerhol MK, Laurell CB. The polymorphism of "prealbumins" and alpha-1-antitrypsin in human sera. Clin Chim Acta 1967; 16:199–203.
15. Larsson C. Natural history and life expectancy in severe alpha-1-antitrypsin deficiency. PiZ. Acta Med Scand 1978; 204:345–351.
16. Burrows B, Earle RH. Course and prognosis of chronic obstructive lung disease. N Engl J Med 1969; 280:397–404.
17. Ganrot PO, Laurell CB, Eriksson S. Obstructive lung disease and trypsin inhibitors in alpha-1-antitrypsin deficiency. Scand J Clin Lab Invest 1967; 19:205–208.
18. Fagerhol MK, Laurell CB. The Pi system: Inherited variants of serum alpha-1-antitrypsin. Prog Med Genet 1970; 7:96–111.
19. Kueppers F, Black LF. Alpha-1-antitrypsin and its deficiency. Am Rev Respir Dis 1974; 110:176–194.
20. Black LF, Kueppers F. Alpha-1-antitrypsin deficiency in nonsmokers. Am Rev Respir Dis 1978; 117:421–428.
21. Abrams WR, Eliraz A, Kimbel P, et al. The effect of the oxidizing agents chloramine-T and cigarette smoke on dog serum proteinase inhibitors. Exp Lung Res 1980; 1:211–223.
22. Beatty K, Bieth J, Travis J. Kinetics of association of serine proteinases with native and oxidized alpha-1-proteinase inhibitor and alpha-1-antichymotrypsin. J Biol Chem 1980; 255:3931–3934.
23. Johnson D, Travis J. The oxidative inactivation of human alpha-1-antiproteinase inhibitor. J Biol Chem 1979; 254:4022–4026.
24. Satch S, Kurecki T, Kress LF, et al. The dual nature of the reaction between porcine elastase and human plasma alpha-1-proteinase inhibitor. Biochem Biophys Res Commun 1979; 86:130–137.
25. Abrams WR, Cohen AB, Damiano VV, et al. A model of decreased functional alpha-1-antiproteinase inhibitor. Pulmonary pathology of dogs exposed to chloramine T. J Clin Invest 1981; 68:1132–1139.
26. Janoff A, Carp H, Laurent P, et al. The role of oxidative processes in emphysema. Am Rev Respir Dis 1983; 127:S31–S38.
27. Carp H, Miller F, Hoidal R, et al. Potential mechanism of emphysema: Alpha-1-proteinase inhibitor recovered from lungs of cigarette smokers contain oxidized methionine and has decreased elastase inhibitory capacity. Proc Natl Acad Sci USA 1982; 79:2041–2045.
28. Gadek JE, Fells GA, Crystal RG. Cigarette smoking induces functional antiprotease deficiency in the lower respiratory tract of humans. Science 1979; 206:1315–1316.
29. Janoff A, Carp H. Cigarette smoke inhalation decreases alpha-1-antitrypsin activity in rat lung. Science 1979; 206:1313–1314.
30. Stone PJ, Calore JD, McGowan SE, et al. Functional alpha-1-protease inhibitor in the lower respiratory tract of cigarette smokers is not decreased. Science 1983; 221:1187–1189.
31. Gross P, Pfitzer EA, Toker E, et al. Experimental emphysema: Its production with papain in normal and silicotic rats. Arch Environ Health 1965; 11:50–58.

32. Cohen AB, Rossi M. Neutrophils in normal lungs. Am Rev Respir Dis 1983; 127:S3–S9.
33. Cohen AB, Rossi M, Geczy D, Knight L. Neutrophil turnover in normal rabbit lungs. J Clin Invest 1982; 69:794–798.
34. Hunninghake G, Gadek J, Kawanami O, et al. Inflammatory and immune processes in the human lung in health and disease: Evaluation by bronchoalveolar lavage. Am J Pathol 1979; 97:149–206.
35. Kazmierowski JA, Gallin JI, Reynolds HY. Mechanism for the inflammatory response in primate lungs. J Clin Invest 1977; 59:273–281.
36. Hunninghake G, Crystal RG. Cigarette smoking and lung destruction. Accumulation of neutrophils in the lungs of cigarette smokers. Am Rev Respir Dis 1983; 128:833–838.
37. Hunninghake G, Gadek J, Crystal RG. Human alveolar macrophage neutrophil chemotactic factor. J Clin Invest 1980; 66:473–483.
38. Merrill WW, Naegel GP, Matthay RA, Reynolds HY. Alveolar macrophage-derived chemotactic factor. Kinetics of in vitro production and partial characterization. J Clin Invest 1980; 65:268–276.
39. Fels AOS, Pawlowski NA, Cramer EB, et al. Human alveolar macrophages produce leukotriene B4. Proc Natl Acad Sci USA 1982; 79:7866–7870.
40. Cohen AB, Chenoweth DE, Hugli TE. The release of elastase and other enzymes from human alveolar macrophages. Am Rev Respir Dis 1982; 126:241–247.
41. McArthur S, Cohen AB. Secretion from human alveolar macrophages of a peptide which releases granules from neutrophils. Fed Proc 1985; 44:1276.
42. Rodriguez RJ, White RR, Senior RM, Levine EA. Elastase release from human alveolar macrophages: Comparison between smokers and nonsmokers. Science 1977; 198:313–314.
43. Chapman HA, Stone OL, Zdenek V. Degradation of fibrin and elastin in intact human alveolar macrophages in vitro. J Clin Invest 1984; 73:806–815.
44. Werb Z, Gordon S. Elastase secretion by stimulated macrophages: Characterization and regulation. J Exp Med 1975; 142:361–377.
45. Cosio MG, Hale KA, Niewoehner DE. Morphologic and morphometric effects of prolonged cigarette smoking on the small airways. Am Rev Respir Dis 1980; 122:265–271.
46. Niewoehner DE, Kleinerman J, Rice DB. Pathologic changes in the peripheral airways of young cigarette smokers. N Engl J Med 1974; 291:755–758.
47. Damiano VV, Tsang A, Kucich U, et al. Immunolocalization of elastase in human emphysematous lungs. J Clin Invest 1986; 78:482–493.
48. Eriksson S. Studies on alpha-1-antitrypsin deficiency. Acta Med Scand 1965; 177:1–85.
49. Cohen AB, James HL. Evaluation of alpha-1-antitrypsin as a potential therapeutic agent. In: Sandberg HE, ed. Proceedings of the First International Workshop on Technology for Protein Separation and Improvement of Blood Plasma Fractionation. Bethesda: US Department of Health, National Institutes of Health, Public Health Service, 1977, 326–338.
50. Cohen AB. Treatment of the underlying cause of emphysema. In: Cohen AB, ed. Seminars in Respiratory Medicine, Vol 8. New York: Thieme, 1986, 177–187.
51. Wewers MD, Casolaro MA, Sellers SE, et al. Replacement therapy for alpha-1-antitrypsin deficiency associated with emphysema. N Engl J Med 1987; 316:1055–1061.
52. Powers JC. Synthetic elastase inhibitors: Prospects for use in the treatment of emphysema. Am Rev Respir Dis 1983; 127:554–558.
53. Kucich U, Christner P, Lippman M, et al. Utilization of peroxidase-antiperoxidase complex in an enzyme-linked immunosorbent assay of elastin-derived peptides in human plasma. Am Rev Respir Dis 1985; 131:709–713.
54. Goldstein RA, Starcher BC. Urinary excretion of elastin peptides containing desmosine after intratracheal injection of elastase in hamsters. J Clin Invest 1978; 62:1286–1290.
55. Weitz JI, Crowley K, Landman SL, et al. Increased neutrophil and elastase activity in cigarette smokers. Ann Intern Med 1987; 107:680–682.
56. Buist AS, Burrows B, Eriksson S, et al. The natural history of PiZ emphysema. Am Rev Respir Dis 1983; 127(Suppl):S43–S44.
57. Idell S, Cohen AB. Bronchoalveolar lavage in patients with the adult respiratory distress syndrome. Clin Chest Med 1985; 6:459–471.
58. Buist AS, Sexton GJ, Azzan AM, et al. Pulmonary function in heterozygotes for alpha-1-antitrypsin deficiency: A case-control study. Am Rev Respir Dis 1979; 120:759–766.
59. Gelb AF, Klein E, Lieberman J. Pulmonary function in nonsmoking subjects with alpha-1-antitrypsin deficiency (M2 phenotype). Am J Med 1977; 62:93–98.
60. Larsson C, Eriksson S, Dirksen H. Smoking and intermediate alpha-1-antitrypsin deficiency and lung function in middle-aged men. Br Med J 1977; 2:922–925.
61. McDonagh DJ, Nathan SP, Kuudson RJ, et al. Assessment of alpha-1-antitrypsin deficiency heterozygosity as a risk factor in the etiology of emphysema. J Clin Invest 1979; 63:299–310.
62. Hall WJ, Hyde RW, Schwartz RH, et al. Pulmonary abnormalities in intermediate alpha-1-antitrypsin deficiency. J Clin Invest 1976; 58:1069–1077.
63. Klayton R, Fallat R, Cohen AB. Determinants of chronic obstructive pulmonary disease in patients with intermediate levels of alpha-1-antitrypsin. Am J Respir Dis 1975; 112:71–75.
64. Tattersall SF, Pereira RP, Hunter D, et al. Lung distensibility and airway function in intermediate alpha-1-antitrypsin deficiency (PiMZ). Thorax 1979; 34:637–646.
65. Cohen AB. Unraveling the mysteries of alpha-1-antitrypsin deficiency. N Engl J Med 1986; 314:778–779.
66. Boyer SH, Siggers DC, Krueger LJ. Caveat to protein replacement therapy for genetic disease: Immunological implications of accurate molecular diagnosis. Lancet 1973; ii:654–659.
67. Henson PM. The immunologic release of constituents from neutrophil leukocytes. 1. The role of antibody and complement on nonphagocytosable surfaces or phagocytosable particles. J Immunol 1971; 107:1535–1546.
68. MacArthur CK, Miller EJ, Cohen AB. A peptide secreted by human alveolar macrophages which releases neutrophil granule contents. J Immunol 1987; 139:3456–3462.
69. Malawista SE, Bensch KG. Human polymorphonuclear leukocytes: Demonstration of microtubules and effect of colchicine. Science 1967; 156:521–523.
70. Weissmann G, Zurier RB, Hoffstein S. Leukocytic proteases and the immunologic release of lysosomal enzymes. Am J Pathol 1972; 68:549–559.
71. Powers JC, Gupton BF, Harley AD, et al. Specificity of porcine pancreatic elastase, human leukocyte elastase and cathepsin G: Inhibition with peptide chloromethyl ketones. Biochim Biophys Acta 1977; 485:156–166.
72. Tuhy PN, Powers JC. Inhibition of human leukocyte elastase by peptide chloromethyl ketones. FEBS Lett 1975; 50:359–361.
73. Gadek JE, Fulmer JD, Gelfand JA, et al. Danazol-induced augmentation of serum alpha-1-antitrypsin levels in individuals with marked deficiency of this antiprotease. J Clin Invest 1980; 66:82–87.

Chapter 55

RESPIRATORY STIMULANTS IN THE TREATMENT OF COPD

Barbara M. Galko **Anthony S. Rebuck**

Many drugs have been noted to stimulate ventilation in humans but, because of the high incidence of unacceptable side effects, few have found a place in clinical practice. The currently acceptable categories of useful therapeutic agents include the methylated xanthines, analeptics, narcotic antagonists, progestins, carbonic anhydrase inhibitors, and the piperazine derivative almitrene. The recent interest in near-miss sudden infant death syndrome (SIDS) patients and the sleep apneas has provided impetus to research in respiratory stimulants. These agents have long been useful in the therapy of chronic respiratory insufficiency, primary alveolar hypoventilation, and narcotic and sedative overdose, but there is no universal agreement as to their clinical role. The objective of this chapter is to review the currently available respiratory stimulants and to examine trends in current research that might point to the physiologic properties required of the ideal agent.

METHYLATED XANTHINES

The methylated xanthines, commonly known as xanthine derivatives (e.g., caffeine, theobromine), can occur naturally and are found in such beverages as coffee, tea, and cola, and in chocolate. For decades this drug's major clinical role was that of a potent bronchodilator. Recently, interest has shifted to its properties of stimulating central respiratory neurons, enhancing the contractility of the diaphragm, and delaying fatigue in other respiratory muscles.

The mechanisms of action of xanthines include the competitive inhibition of cyclic nucleotide phosphodiesterase,[7] the translocation of intracellular Ca^{2+},[5] and the blockade of receptors for adenosine.[30] Xanthines are readily absorbed after oral or parenteral administration and less predictably as a rectal formulation. Although oral administration in large doses is especially apt to produce gastric irritation, rectal and parenteral administration do not eliminate these problems, the gastrointestinal symptoms apparently reflecting plasma theophylline concentration to some degree. Because the rate and extent of absorption differ among various slow-release formulations, as well as among subjects, trial and error may be required with various preparations to maximize patient tolerance and compliance to the regimen. Toxicity can be monitored by assays of serum concentration of the drug. This is of particular importance, because a wide range of illnesses and drugs affect clearance. For example, theophylline clearance decreases in the elderly, in those with hepatic cirrhosis, acute hepatitis, cholestasis, cardiac decompensation, cor pulmonale, or viral infections, and during concurrent administration of macrolide antibiotics, cimetidine, high-dose allopurinol, or oral contraceptives. Rapid clearance is enhanced by smoking tobacco or marijuana and by the use of phenytoin or phenobarbital.

Clinical Studies

Theophylline compounds play an important role as bronchodilators in the management of bronchospasm. In addition, methylxanthines have undergone clinical trials for the treatment of apnea of undetermined origin. Studies in premature infants have demonstrated that the oral or intravenous administration of aminophylline eliminates episodes of apnea that last more than 20 seconds and markedly reduces those of shorter duration.[61] Stroud and colleagues[63] examined the effect of aminophylline and meperidine on the ventilatory response to CO_2. The end-tidal P_{CO_2} was fixed at 46 mm Hg by the addition of CO_2 to the breathing circuit. Aminophylline (6 mg/kg) produced sufficient respiratory stimulation to counter the respiratory depressant effects of 100 mg of meperidine.

Murciano and associates[50] have studied the effects of theophylline on diaphragmatic strength and fatigue in patients with severe COPD. Maximal transdiaphragmatic pressure at functional residual capacity was increased by 16% after 7 days of administration of 13 mg/kg of theophylline; and this increase persisted after 30 days. Theophylline also suppressed diaphragmatic fatigue, as assessed by the high-low ratio of the electrical activity of the diaphragm under conditions of resistive loaded breathing. Despite these findings, more recent studies by Belman and coworkers[4] questioned whether these changes are likely to improve ventilatory endurance in the long term. They measured maximal sustained ventilatory levels during prolonged isocapnic hyperpnea as an index of ventilatory muscle function in seven controls and seven patients with COPD during intravenous infusion of saline and aminophylline in the usual therapeutic dose on two separate days. Although all showed slightly higher sustained ventilatory levels during aminophylline infusion, the magnitude of change was small and unlikely to have a significant clinical benefit in the setting of respiratory muscle fatigue.

Therapeutic Implications

Xanthine derivatives have been used since 1900 as therapy for reactive airways disease. Newly discovered actions of these

ACKNOWLEDGMENTS
We wish to thank Mr. J. White and Ms. L. Bagnulo for their assistance in the preparation of the manuscript.

drugs include dose-dependent improvement of diaphragmatic contractility, augmentation of ventilatory responses to hypoxia, and an effect on sleep disturbances. Although the role of xanthines as respiratory stimulants is still evolving, these drugs play an important role in the management of both acute and chronic airways obstruction. Because respiratory muscle fatigue may tip the balance between success and failure during prolonged periods of weaning from mechanical ventilator support, and because most such patients benefit from maximal bronchodilatation, the addition of xanthines to the usual pharmacologic regimen in such patients appears to be appropriate and justified.

ANALEPTICS

Central nervous system stimulation can be produced in animals and humans by a large number of natural and synthetic substances. Drugs that produce central stimulation as their most prominent action are classified as analeptics or convulsants. Many attempts have been made to find drugs to reverse ventilatory depression in drug overdose or to stimulate ventilation in patients in respiratory failure. The analeptics stimulate ventilation by direct effects on ventilatory control mechanisms, but they have stimulatory effects on other brain centers and may produce generalized convulsions when given in sufficient doses. Unfortunately, the margin of safety of doses that stimulate central ventilatory centers is small and unpredictable. This accounts for the overwhelming discreditation of these drugs, and patients who may have otherwise benefited from their use are more frequently helped by a period of mechanical ventilation.

Clinical Studies

Ethamivan

Ethamivan, or vanillic acid diethylamide, is a central respiratory stimulant that was synthesized in Vienna in 1950.[31] When administered to healthy volunteers at a rate of 9 mg/minute, it can induce hyperventilation and a decrease in the end-tidal P_{CO_2}.[1] However, if ventilation is first stimulated by hypercapnia (end-tidal P_{CO_2} = 47 to 50 mm Hg), the administration of ethamivan fails to increase ventilation further.

Miller and colleagues[45] have evaluated ethamivan in 119 patients with ventilatory depression associated with pulmonary disease, obesity, or drug overdose, and found that the tidal volume and respiratory rate increased in 95 of them.

Rodman and associates[57] have studied 22 patients under baseline conditions and 3 minutes after the intravenous infusion of 50 mg of ethamivan or 250 mg of aminophylline. Ethamivan increased minute ventilation by 0.8 L/m^2 body surface area, a 16% increase over baseline, primarily by an increase in tidal volume, without altering the P_{CO_2}. The effects were transient and disappeared within 5 minutes. Aminophylline, 250 mg, increased minute ventilation by 24% over baseline, was more uniform, and was associated with a reduction in P_{CO_2} from a mean of 46 to 43 mm Hg. The effects were more persistent and were still present 15 minutes after administration.

The lack of specific action of ethamivan and picrotoxin on respiratory and nonrespiratory neurons was examined by Hirsh and Wang.[28] Both groups of neurons were stimulated equally by both analeptics in a study of 33 decerebrate cats; severing the carotid nerve failed to alter the response.

Doxapram

Hirsh and Wang[28] found that the soluble crystalline powder doxapram selectively stimulated respiratory neurons, activating carotid chemoreceptors when administered intravenously at low doses. In higher doses (greater than 1 mg/kg) it stimulated both the respiratory and nonrespiratory neurons equally in the feline medulla oblongata.

Doxapram has been in clinical usage since 1964, when Canter and Luchsinger analyzed its effect on 22 patients in respiratory failure.[11] Doxapram in doses of 1 to 3 mg/minute was given for 2½ to 95 hours, with concurrent O_2 therapy at a rate of 1 to 4 L/minute. Clinical improvement was noted in 18 patients, with the mean P_{CO_2} falling from 66 to 60 mm Hg and the P_{O_2} rising from 42 to 73 mm Hg. Firm conclusions about the specific role of doxapram cannot be drawn from these observations, because other therapeutic modalities, such as antibiotics, bronchodilators, and tracheal suctioning, were administered concurrently.

A double-blind multicenter cooperative study involving 78 patients with COPD was undertaken in the U.S. and reported by Moser and coworkers.[47] The patients were admitted for management of acute respiratory failure and were considered to require O_2 administration. During the study period (2 hours) they received either 2 to 3 mg/kg of doxapram intravenously or a placebo. Supplemental oxygen was given to maintain the Pa_{O_2} between 60 and 70 mm Hg. During this period, O_2 administration was associated with an elevation in CO_2 tension beyond the desired range in 37% of patients receiving placebo, but in only 18% of those receiving doxapram. This short-term maintenance of oxygenation and ventilation was thought to be helpful in "buying" sufficient time to allow other therapeutic interventions to exert their salutary effects, and perhaps avoid mechanical ventilation.

The ventilatory effects of doxapram in normal humans were studied by Calverley and colleagues.[10] Doxapram, infused to maintain a constant plasma level, changed neither resting CO_2 uptake nor CO_2 production, but produced a substantial increase in resting ventilation. The mean ventilatory responses to isocapnic hypoxia and to progressive hypercapnia each doubled during doxapram infusion.

In addition to doxapram and ethamivan, nikethamide has been studied in patients with acute respiratory failure[17] and acute exacerbations of COPD.[43] In both studies there was an improvement in the level of consciousness of some of the patients, but many experienced anxiety and vomiting.

Five analeptic respiratory stimulants were compared by Edwards and Leszczynski in a double-blind trial involving 32 patients with acute respiratory failure.[19] The stimulants used were nikethamide (15 mg/kg), prethcamide (12 mg/kg), amiphenazole (3 mg/kg), ethamivan (12 mg/kg), and doxapram (3 mg/kg). The infusion was maintained for 4 hours and the use of concomitant therapy was allowed. Doxapram, on clinical and statistical analysis, was the most effective in reducing P_{CO_2}, increasing O_2 saturation, and increasing minute ventilation, whereas prethcamide and nikethamide were the least effective.

Therapeutic Implications

Side effects of analeptics occur frequently despite subconvulsive CNS stimulation. These include hypertension, tachycardia, arrhythmias, coughing, sneezing, vomiting, tremors, muscle rigidity, flushing, and hyperpyrexia. They may serve as temporary measures in the management of acute respiratory failure in those with COPD.

NARCOTIC ANTAGONISTS

Narcotics, derived from the juice of the poppy *Papaver somniferum*, have been used medicinally since the 3rd century B.C. Although the problems of addiction and ventilatory depression have been noted for centuries, it was not until the 20th century that compounds with opioid antagonist properties were studied. The narcotic antagonists either have pure antagonistic actions, such as naloxone,[22] or agonist-antagonist properties, such as nalorphine.[42] Because naloxone lacks any agonist properties it has become the choice agent for the reversal of ventilatory depression secondary to narcotic abuse.

Clinical Studies

Postoperative respiratory depression secondary to morphine sulfate is reversed with naloxone.[38] Although naloxone 5 μg/kg IV initially reverses the respiratory depression associated with morphine sulfate, 1.25 to 1.56 mg/kg, it may be necessary to give repeated doses of naloxone to maintain adequate ventilation. A similar study by Johnstone and colleagues[29] examined the results of naloxone infusion 5 hours after administration of 2 mg/kg morphine sulfate to seven healthy adults. An 8-hour infusion resulted in the gradual restoration of ventilatory parameters to control values.

Endogenous opioids (or endorphins) have been postulated to be involved in the responses to chronic pain,[66] neuroendocrine regulation[15] and, more recently, the control of breathing. Naloxone stimulates the output of central respiratory neurons in anesthetized and ventilated cats[35] and in fetal sheep.[48] Naloxone has no effect on ventilatory responses to hypoxia or hypercapnia in normal subjects,[21] however, or in anesthetized human subjects.[22] Similarly, the hypercapnia associated with pulmonary disease[8] or hypothalamic disturbance[18] is not altered by the administration of naloxone. Santiago and associates[59] studied 14 normocapnic patients with COPD and 8 normal controls, measuring ventilation, pulmonary function, ventilatory response to CO_2, and ventilatory response to flow-resistive loading, before and after the administration of naloxone. Before naloxone, increased resistance to breathing enhanced respiratory effort in all controls but in only 7 of 14 patients with COPD. After naloxone, these patients augmented their ventilatory response to loaded breathing, a pattern similar to that observed in healthy controls. These findings suggest that the elaboration of endorphins in patients with COPD minimizes the stress of their chronic airway obstruction. Restoration of respiratory drive by naloxone in decompensated patients with COPD may allow for conservative management and avoid mechanical ventilation, although the results in clinical trials of this aspect of narcotic antagonist therapy are still awaited.

Therapeutic Implications

Although naloxone has an established place in the resuscitation of otherwise healthy patients with narcotic overdose, the therapeutic role of narcotic antagonists as ventilatory stimulants is less certain in those with chronic respiratory acidosis. These drugs are, however, providing a useful tool for studying the mechanisms of the neuroendocrine regulation of breathing in research laboratories.

PROGESTINS

Clinical Studies

The hyperventilation now recognized to occur during pregnancy was originally described simultaneously by two groups over 70 years ago,[26,36] and was subsequently found to be caused by increased levels of endogenous progesterone,[16] although recent studies by Brodeur and coworkers[6] have indicated that progesterone receptor numbers contribute to the stimulatory effect. Exogenous progesterone, when administered to normal human subjects, increases minute ventilation,[27,39] and it is this property that has led to its therapeutic use. When Lyons and Huang[40] administered progesterone (100 mg daily) to eight pickwickian patients, a syndrome characterized by obesity, hypercarbia, hypoxia, and elevated pulmonary artery vascular resistance, a uniform improvement in alveolar ventilation of at least 30% was found. Laboratory studies of the ventilatory response to hypercapnia showed an increased sensitivity at all levels of CO_2. In these studies, however, only parenterally administered progesterone in hospitalized patients was studied. Sutton and colleagues[64] then treated ten ambulatory pickwickian male patients using medroxyprogesterone acetate, 20 mg sublingually, q8h. Within 1 month, the PaO_2 rose by approximately 13 mm Hg, from a mean of 49 mm Hg, whereas the $PaCO_2$ decreased by a similar amount, from a mean of 51 mm Hg. A marked diuresis was noted in four patients, and several possible mechanisms were postulated: relief of right ventricular failure associated with their chronic hypoxemia, increased glomerular filtration rate, and the antialdosterone diuretic effect associated with progesterone administration. During the course of the study progressive increases in the ventilatory responses to isocapnic hypoxia were noted. Adverse effects during therapy included impotence in two patients and the occurrence of diabetes mellitus in one.

These encouraging results prompted Orr and associates[53] to study seven morbidly obese patients with sleep-related upper airway obstruction who underwent physiologic measurements during sleep, before and during progesterone treatment (20 mg sublingually, tid). All subjects had severe daytime somnolence, and five of seven had congestive heart failure. There was no significant difference in the incidence, mean duration, or rate per minute of apneic episodes occurring before and with progesterone treatment. Both severe hypoxemia and cardiac arrhythmias during sleep persisted with treatment. Over the course of treatment with progesterone, however, all patients improved clinically, with a reduction in heart failure, peripheral edema, and daytime somnolence. The awake values of PaO_2 rose from a mean of 48 to 64 mm Hg ($p < 0.05$) during progesterone therapy, although the decrease in the $PaCO_2$, from a mean of 39 to 34 mm Hg, was not considered to be significant. These parameters, when measured during sleep, were unchanged before and during treatment. Therefore, in this group, the mechanisms of improvement of hypoxemia were probably related to increased glomerular filtration, diuresis, and improved cardiac function, whereas increased minute ventilation played a minor role.

Progesterone's effectiveness as a ventilatory stimulant has been studied in emphysematous patients in respiratory failure. Tyler[67] administered 50 mg progesterone intramuscularly daily to nine patients with emphysema and CO_2 retention. Alveolar ventilation increased by 0.75 L/minute and the $PaCO_2$ decreased by a mean of 8.4 mm Hg. In a study by Cullen and coworkers[14] of seven patients with emphysema and severe airflow obstruction, the administration of progesterone, 50 mg daily, resulted in a mean increase in alveolar ventilation of 0.53 L.

Therapeutic Implications

Progesterone administration leads to increased ventilation in normal subjects and in patients with central or pulmonary hypoventilation of any cause. It may have beneficial effects in patients with COPD and sleep apnea syndromes. Disturbing side effects decrease its role as a useful therapeutic agent. Despite apparent improvement in patient well-being and arterial blood gas levels (drawn while awake), potentially serious nocturnal arterial desaturations and arrhythmias may persist.

ACETAZOLAMIDE

Mobilization of edema fluid and production of a negative extracellular fluid balance can be achieved by many diuretics that act directly on the kidney. When mobilization of edema fluid is rapid (e.g., with drugs such as ethacrynic acid), metabolic alkalosis can result from the contraction of extracellular fluid volume.[49] With chronic therapy the combined effects of negative chloride balance and hypokalemia are also associated with metabolic alkalosis. In healthy subjects, a diuretic-induced (or for that matter, any metabolically induced) alkalosis is compensated to some extent by hypoventilation,[58] clearly an undesirable response in patients with impaired ventilatory drive. The induction of a diuresis in patients with chronic respiratory insufficiency is therefore undertaken with caution, taking into consideration the realistic concern that fluid balance might be improved at the expense of further impairment of respiratory failure. Whereas acetazolamide has limited usefulness as a diuretic, its action as a noncompetitive inhibitor of carbonic anhydrase results in an increased concentration of the bicarbonate anion in urine and a decrease in the urinary chloride level.[49] Consequently, the concentration of bicarbonate in the extracellular fluid decreases and metabolic acidosis results. It is this latter property of acetazolamide that has suggested its use as a therapeutic agent in patients with impaired central respiratory drive.

Clinical Studies

Acetazolamide produces chronic hyperventilation in awake, normal subjects[23, 51] by increasing the blood hydrogen ion concentration, which acts at both peripheral and medullary chemoreceptor sites.[32, 37] It has been used to improve hypoventilation in acute[46] and chronic[2] metabolic alkalosis in patients with COPD and decreases apneic awakenings and arousals in patients with central sleep apnea.[69]

Although acetazolamide appears to stimulate ventilation through its renal acid-base mechanism, there is now evidence that, like other respiratory stimulants, it might also have a direct (although nonspecific) effect on respiratory neurons. Cain[9] gave a 12-minute intravenous infusion of the drug and found that ventilation increased markedly, even before the infusion was completed. Carbonic anhydrase is a ubiquitous compound in the body. It appears that part of its respiratory stimulant action may be unrelated to the acidosis produced by the kidney but explained by increased cerebral blood flow. Despite limited understanding of its action, acetazolamide has found a therapeutic use in the prophylaxis of acute mountain sickness and in augmenting the ventilatory effects of hypoxia at high altitudes.[33]

Therapeutic Implications

Acetazolamide may be given orally or as an intravenous bolus to promote a bicarbonate diuresis and metabolic acidosis. It has an important clinical role in critically ill patients who have developed compensatory and drug-induced (steroids, diuretics) metabolic alkalosis during the course of their chronic hypercapnic ventilatory insufficiency. During the course of management of patients with acute exacerbations of COPD, when intensive therapy is being directed to avoidance of or weaning from mechanical ventilation, acetazolamide promotes a significant diuresis and, in so doing, acts as a respiratory stimulant by correcting the complicating alkalemia.

ALMITRENE

Clinical Studies

Almitrene bismesylate is a piperazine derivative that specifically stimulates peripheral chemoreceptors. It is pharmacologically unrelated to central-acting agents and is reported to be free of their side effects. The most convincing experimental evidence that almitrene has no effect on the central nervous system comes from the work of Laubie and Diot,[34] who have shown that after carotid denervation the action of the drug is abolished and no effect can be observed when the drug is injected directly into the cisterna. Its pharmacologic action lasts for at least 6 hours when administered intravenously and carbon-labeled isotope studies have suggested a half-life of 35 hours.[34] When almitrene is administered orally in a dose of 5 mg/kg in awake normal subjects,[25] both tidal volume and respiratory frequency increase, with ventilation returning to normal levels within 1 minute of administration of pure oxygen. When administered intravenously in a dose of 1 mg/kg, normal subjects increase their minute ventilation by approximately 12%, with oxygen suppressing the increase in ventilation within 20 to 40 seconds.[20]

Aside from its effects as a primary ventilatory stimulant, almitrene has been shown to improve arterial oxygen tension in patients with COPD to a degree that cannot be fully explained on the basis of a lowering of the Pa_{CO_2} tension. It appears that the drug improves ventilation-perfusion mismatching as a result of redistribution of blood flow away from poorly ventilated areas.[60, 65] In addition to improvements in blood gas levels with almitrene, the evidence that the drug affects the distribution of pulmonary blood flow includes increased pulmonary vascular resistance with minor changes in cardiac output[52] and an improvement in perfusion lung scans with an increase in blood flow to previously underperfused upper lung fields.[56] Continuous monitoring of regional ventilation-perfusion ($\dot{V}/\dot{Q}$) ratios by an inert gas method[68] has substantiated the finding of redistribution of perfusion toward zones with higher $\dot{V}/\dot{Q}$ in patients with severe COPD.[13] As shown by Castaing and colleagues,[12] almitrene improved the Pa_{O_2}, even in the absence of changes in ventilation in mechanically ventilated patients, with the increase occurring in parallel with a decrease in ventilation-perfusion inequality.

The reported changes in distribution of pulmonary blood flow and pulmonary vascular resistance have caused some concern that pulmonary hypertension might be caused or exacerbated by almitrene, but its significant effect on impaired peripheral chemoreceptor drive justifies extensive study in these compromised patients. In this context, Powles and associates[55] administered almitrene intravenously to 11 patients with severe chronic airflow obstruction and hypoxemia in a randomized double-blind study. They found a reduction in venous admixture and an improvement in blood gas levels in some, but not all, patients. The acute effects in most patients were improvement in the Pa_{O_2} and Pa_{CO_2}, either by increasing ventilation or improving ventilation-perfusion relationships. Oral administration (100 mg) in patients with a similar degree of impaired pulmonary function produced a significant improvement of arterial oxygen saturation with no change in pulmonary artery pressure or minute ventilation.[44] Because $\dot{V}/\dot{Q}$ mismatching is more marked in patients with COPD than in normal subjects, almitrene causes less improvement in blood gas tensions, with more noticeable changes in minute ventilation in healthy volunteers.[54]

Stradling and coworkers[62] concluded that in COPD the improvement in blood gas levels after a low oral dose of almitrene could be ascribed to an increase in minute ventilation and to subtle changes in the pattern of breathing, especially the speed and depth of inspiration.

The major side effect of almitrene reported by Bell and colleagues[3] was unexplained worsening of dyspnea, occurring in 4 of 21 patients (19%) receiving 200 mg/day, in 2 of 22 patients (9%) receiving 100 mg/day, and in 1 of 24 patients (4%) receiving a placebo. Sensory peripheral neuropathy has been reported, and discontinuation of the drug is recommended at the first suggestion of paresthesias. Gherardi and associates[24] reported sensory peripheral neuropathy developing in five patients treated with 60 to 100 mg/day for 7 to 25 months. The interval between the onset of symptoms and the first dose of almitrene ranged from 2 to 4 months.

Further investigation of its long-term usefulness is indicated because MacNee and coworkers[41] have shown that almitrene, when given orally to hypoxic patients with COPD, both acutely and over a period of 3 months, can cause a small increase in the mean pulmonary arterial pressure, associated with a mild impairment of right ventricular ejection fraction when at rest.

Therapeutic Implications

Almitrene increases tidal volume and respiratory frequency while simultaneously improving ventilation–blood flow mismatching by its effect on pulmonary blood flow distribution. The potential but unproven hazard of exacerbating pulmonary hypertension may be outweighed by its obvious advantages over other respiratory analeptic drugs.

Although ventilation may be increased acutely in COPD patients by various drugs, their clinical usefulness is hampered by significant side effects. Theophylline, an established bronchodilator, has an apparent beneficial action on diaphragmatic contractility and fatigue, and may be useful in acute deteriorations in COPD. A more promising agent, almitrene, can be used orally to increase ventilation and decrease ventilation-perfusion mismatching, but its clinical benefit in long-term studies remains to be evaluated.

REFERENCES

1. Anderton JL, Cowie JF, Harris EA, et al. Effect of ethamivan (vanillic acid diethylamide) on the respiratory response of healthy young men to carbon dioxide in the absence of hypoxia. Br J Pharmacol 1962; 19:142–152.
2. Bear R, Goldstein M, Philipson E, et al. Effect of metabolic alkalosis on respiratory function in patients with chronic obstructive lung disease. Can Med Assoc J 1977; 117:900–903.
3. Bell RC, Mullins RC, West LG, et al. The effect of almitrene bismesylate on hypoxemia in chronic obstructive pulmonary disease. Ann Intern Med 1986; 105:342–346.
4. Belman MJ, Sieck GC, Mazar A. Aminophylline and its influence on ventilatory endurance in humans. Am Rev Respir Dis 1985; 131:226–229.
5. Blinks JR, Olson CB, Jewell BR, et al. Influence of caffeine and other methylxanthines on mechanical properties of isolated mammalian heart muscle. Evidence for dual mechanism of action. Circ Res 1972; 30:367–392.
6. Brodeur P, Mockus M, McCullough R, et al. Progesterone receptors and ventilatory stimulation by progestin. J Appl Physiol 1986; 60:590–595.
7. Butcher RW, Sutherland EW. Adenosine 3',5'-phosphate in biological materials. J Biol Chem 1962; 237:1244–1250.
8. Butland RJ, Woodcock AA, Gross ER, et al. Endogenous opioids (endorphins) and the control of breathing. N Engl J Med 1981; 305:1096.
9. Cain SA. A ventilatory effect of carbonic anhydrase in man. Proc Soc Exp Biol Med 1961; 106:770.
10. Calverley PMA, Robson RH, Wraith PK, et al. The ventilatory effects of doxapram in normal man. Clin Sci 1983; 65:65–69.
11. Canter HG, Luchsinger PC. The treatment of respiratory failure without mechanical assistance. Am J Med Sci 1964; 248:206–211.
12. Castaing Y, Manier G, Guenard H. Improvement in ventilation-perfusion relationships by almitrene in patients with chronic obstructive pulmonary disease during mechanical ventilation. Am Rev Respir Dis 1986; 134:910–916.
13. Castaing Y, Manier G, Varene N, et al. Effets de l'almitrene orale sur la distribution continue des rapport V_A/Q dans les bronchopneumopathies chroniques obstructives. Bull Eur Physiopathol Respir 1981; 17:917–932.
14. Cullen JH, Brum VC, Reidt WU. The respiratory effects of progesterone in severe pulmonary emphysema. Am J Med 1959; 27:551–557.
15. Davis GC. Studies of the role of endorphins in normal subjects and psychiatric patients. In: Bunney WE Jr, moderator. Basic and clinical studies of endorphins. Ann Intern Med 1979; 91:246–248.
16. Doring GH, Loeschcke HH. Atmung und Saure-Basengleichgewigt in der Schwangerschaft. Pflugers Arch 1947; 249:437–451.
17. Dulfano MJ, Segal MS. Nikethamide as a respiratory analeptic. JAMA 1963; 185:69–74.
18. Dunger DB, Leonard JV, Wolfe OH, et al. Effect of naloxone in a previously undescribed hypothalamic syndrome. Lancet 1980; i:1277–1281.
19. Edwards G, Leszczynski SO. A double-blind trial of five respiratory stimulants in patients with acute ventilatory failure. Lancet 1967; ii:226–229.
20. Flandrois R, Guerin JC. Action de l'almitrene sur le controle chemoreflexe de la ventilation chez l'homme sain et l'insuffissant respiratoire chronique. Rev Fr Mal Respir 1980; 8:561–567.
21. Fleetham JA, Clarke H, Dhingra S, et al. Endogenous opiates and chemical control of breathing in humans. Am Rev Respir Dis 1980; 121:1045–1049.
22. Foldes FF, Duncalf D, Kuwabara S. The respiratory, circulatory and narcotic antagonistic effects of nalorphine, levallorphan and naloxone in anaesthetized subjects. Can Anaesth Soc J 1969; 16:151–162.
23. Galdston M. Respiratory and renal effects of a carbonic anhydrase inhibitor (Diamox) on acid-base balance in normal man and in patients with respiratory acidosis. Am J Med 1955; 19:516–532.
24. Gherardi R, Louarn F, Benvenuti C, et al. Peripheral neuropathy in patients treated with almitrene dimesylate. Lancet 1985; i:1247–1250.
25. Guillerm R, Radziszewski E. Effets ventilatoires chez l'homme sain d'un nouvel analeptique respiratoire, le S2620. Bull Eur Physiopathol Respir 1974; 10:776–791.
26. Hasselbalch KA. Ein Beirag zur Respirationphysiologie der Graviditaet. Scand Arch Physiol 1912; 27:1–12.
27. Heerhaber I, Loeschcke HH, Westphal U. Eine Wirkung des progesterons auf die Atmung. Pflugers Arch 1948; 250:42–55.
28. Hirsh WH, Wang SC. Selective respiratory stimulating action of doxapram compared with pentylenetetrazol. J Pharmacol Exp Ther 1974; 189:1–11.
29. Johnstone RE, Jobes DR, Kennell EM, et al. Reversal of morphine anesthesia with naloxone. Anesthesiology 1974; 41:361–367.
30. Kakiuchi S, Rall TW, McIlwain H. The effect of electrical stimulation upon the accumulation of adenosine 3',5'-phosphate in isolated cerebral tissue. J Neurochem 1969; 16:485–491.
31. Kratze K, Kvasnicka E. On chemistry of vanillin and its derivatives. Monatsschr Chem 1952; 83:18–23.
32. Lane DJ, Horwell JB, Stretton TB. The effect of dichlorphenamide on blood and cerebrospinal fluid acid-base state in chronic ventilatory failure. Clin Sci 1977; 39:391–406.
33. Larson EB, Roach RC, Schoene RB, et al. Acute mountain

sickness and acetazolamide. Clinical efficacy and effect on ventilation. JAMA 1982; 248:328–332.
34. Laubie M, Diot F. A pharmacological study of the respiratory stimulant action of S2620. J Pharmacol 1972; 3:363–374.
35. Lawson EE, Waldrop TG, Eldridge FL. Naloxone enhances respiratory output in cats. J Appl Physiol 1979; 47:1105–1111.
36. Leimdorfer A, Novak J, Porges O. Über die Kohlensaurespannung des Blutes in der Graviditat. Z Klin Med 1912; 75:301.
37. Lerche D, Katsaros B, Lerche G, et al. Vergleich der Wirkung verschiedener acidosen (NH_4Cl, $CaCl_2$, Acetazolamid) auf die Lungenbeluftung beim Menschen. Pflugers Arch 1960; 270:450–460.
38. Longnecker DE, Grazis PA, Eggers GWN Jr. Naloxone for antagonism of morphine-induced respiratory depression. Anesth Analg 1973; 52:447–453.
39. Lyons HA, Antonio R. The sensitivity of the respiratory center in pregnancy and after the administration of progesterone. Trans Assoc Am Physicians 1959; 72:173–180.
40. Lyons HA, Huang CT. Therapeutic use of progesterone in alveolar hypoventilation associated with obesity. Am J Med 1968; 44:881–888.
41. MacNee W, Connaughton JJ, Rhind GB, et al. A comparison of the effects of almitrene or oxygen breathing on pulmonary arterial pressure and right ventricular ejection fraction in hypoxic chronic bronchitis and emphysema. Am Rev Respir Dis 1986; 134:559–565.
42. Martin WR. Opioid antagonists. Pharmacol Rev 1967; 19:463–521.
43. McNicol MW, Pride NB, Reynolds EO, et al. Nikethamide for severe CO_2 retention in exacerbations of chronic bronchitis. Br Med J 1963; 5331:646–648.
44. Melot C, Naeije R, Hallemans R, et al. Beneficial effects of almitrene bismesylate on pulmonary gas exchange in COPD. Eur J Respir Dis 1983; 126(Suppl):249–254.
45. Miller WF, Archer RK, Taylor HF, Ossenfort WF. Severe respiratory depression. Role of a respiratory stimulant, ethamivan, in the treatment. JAMA 1962; 180:905–911.
46. Miller PD, Berne AS. Acute metabolic alkalosis perpetuating hypercarbia: A role for acetazolamide in chronic obstructive pulmonary disease. JAMA 1977; 238:2400–2401.
47. Moser KM, Luchsinger PC, Adamson JS, et al. Respiratory stimulation with intravenous doxapram in respiratory failure: A double-blind co-operative study. N Engl J Med 1973; 288:427–431.
48. Moss IR, Scarpelli EM: Generation and regulation of breathing in utero: Fetal CO_2 response test. J Appl Physiol 1979; 47:527–531.
49. Mudge GH. Diuretics and other agents employed in the mobilization of edema fluid. In: Goodman LS, Gilman A, eds. Pharmacological Basis of Therapeutics. 5th ed. New York: Macmillan Publishing Company, 1975, 817–821.
50. Murciano D, Aubier M, Lecocguic Y, et al. Effects of theophylline on diaphragmatic strength and fatigue in patients with chronic obstructive pulmonary disease. N Engl J Med 1984; 311:349–353.
51. Nadell J. The effects of carbonic anhydrase inhibitor "6063" on electrolytes and acid-base balance in two normal subjects and two patients with respiratory acidosis. J Clin Invest 1953; 32:622–629.
52. Naeije R, Melot C, Mols P, et al. Effects of almitrene in decompensated chronic respiratory insufficiency. Bull Eur Physiopathol Respir 1981; 17:153–161.
53. Orr WC, Imes NK, Martin RJ. Progesterone therapy in obese patients with sleep apnea. Arch Intern Med 1979; 139:109–111.
54. Pariente R. Clinical pharmacology of almitrene bismesylate. Eur J Respir Dis 1983; 126(Suppl):271–274.
55. Powles ACP, Tuxen DV, Mahood CB, et al. The effect of intravenously administered almitrene, a peripheral chemoreceptor agonist, on patients with chronic air-flow obstruction. Am Rev Respir Dis 1983; 127:284–289.
56. Rigaud D, Dubois F, Boutet J, et al. Effets de l'almitrene sur la distribution isotopique de la ventilation et de la perfusion regionales chez l'insuffissant respiratoire chronique. Rev Fr Mal Respir 1980; 8:605.
57. Rodman T, Fennelly JF, Kraft AJ, et al. Effect of ethamivan on alveolar ventilation in patients with chronic lung disease. N Engl J Med 1962; 267:1279–1285.
58. Sabatini S, Arruda JAL, Kurtzman NA. Disorders of acid-base balance. Med Clin North Am 1977; 62:1223–1255.
59. Santiago TV, Remolina C, Scoles V, et al. Endorphins and the control of breathing. Ability of naloxone to restore flow-resistive load compensation in chronic obstructive pulmonary disease. N Engl J Med 1981; 304:1190–1195.
60. Sergysels R, Etien JL, Schandevyl W, et al. Functional evaluation of a new analeptic drug in patients with chronic hypoxemia and hypercapnia (preliminary study). Acta Tuberc Pneumolog Belg 1978; 69:237–246.
61. Shannon DC, Gotay F, Stein IM, et al. Prevention of apnea and bradycardia in low-birthweight infants. Pediatrics 1975; 55:589–594.
62. Stradling JR, Nicholl CG, Cover D, et al. The effects of oral almitrene on pattern of breathing and gas exchange in patients with chronic obstructive pulmonary disease. Clin Sci 1984; 66:435–442.
63. Stroud MW, Lambertsen CJ, Ewing R, et al. Effects of aminophylline and meperidine alone and in combination on the respiratory response to carbon dioxide inhalation. J Pharmacol Exp Ther 1955; 114:461–469.
64. Sutton FD, Zwillich CW, Creagh CE, et al. Progesterone for outpatient treatment of Pickwickian syndrome. Ann Intern Med 1975; 83:476–479.
65. Tenaillon A, Labrouse J, Longchal J, et al. Effects of almitrene on blood gases in chronic obstructive lung disease (COPD) with acute respiratory failure (ARF) [abstract]. Intensive Care Med 1980; 6:64.
66. Terenius L. Endogenous peptides and analgesia. Annu Rev Pharmacol Toxicol 1978; 18:189–204.
67. Tyler JM. The effect of progesterone on the respiration of patients with emphysema and hypercapnia. J Clin Invest 1960; 39:34–41.
68. Wagner PD, Salzman HA, West JB. Measurement of continuous distributions of ventilation-perfusion ratio: theory. J Appl Physiol 1974; 36:588.
69. White DP, Zwillich CW, Pickett CK, et al. Central sleep apnea. Improvement with acetazolamide therapy. Arch Intern Med 1982; 142:1816–1819.

Chapter 56

REHABILITATION OF PATIENTS WITH COPD

Steven G. Kelsen Gerard Criner

Chronic obstructive pulmonary disease (COPD) alters the mechanical and gas exchange properties of the respiratory system and impairs the patient's ability to be physically active and participate in the activities of daily living. Elevations in lung volume and the resistance to airflow increase the work of breathing. Increases in the dead space volume of the lung require greater than normal levels of ventilation to maintain the P_{CO_2} within the normal range. These changes in lung function in COPD patients require them to expend greater efforts to breathe and impose an added stress on the respiratory muscles.

In addition, patients with advanced COPD who become dyspneic during exercise tend to shun physical activities. Patients who assume a sedentary existence for prolonged periods may become deconditioned with negative effects on the cardiovascular system and on limb muscles. Deconditioning in COPD patients may further worsen their ability to perform physical activities.

Avoidance of physical activity and a limited ability to perform the normal activities of daily living can be expected to lead to various psychosocial impairments. Patients with COPD, for example, have a high incidence of morbid anxiety and depression and preoccupation with bodily symptoms.[1, 3] Disturbances in psychosocial function may impair interpersonal relationships and isolate the patient emotionally and physically.

DEFINITION AND INDICATIONS

The treatment of patients with advanced COPD should focus on improvements in lung and airway function and on the prevention of further loss in lung performance. Many patients with COPD demonstrate some reversibility in airway obstruction and should receive bronchodilators. Patients who are hypoxemic at rest or with exercise demonstrate relief of dyspnea and improved exercise tolerance when given supplemental oxygen.[85, 86, 89, 91, 92] Patients with advanced COPD who have achieved maximal benefit from conventional medical treatment and are still physically incapacitated are candidates for entry into a rehabilitation program. A definition of pulmonary rehabilitation has been formulated by the American College of Chest Physicians (1974):[17]

> Pulmonary rehabilitation may be defined as an art of medical practice wherein an individually tailored, multi-disciplinary program is formulated which through accurate diagnosis, therapy, emotional support, and education, stabilizes or reverses both the physio- and psychopathology of pulmonary disease and attempts to return the patient to the highest possible functional capacity allowed by his pulmonary handicap and overall life situation.

This definition was subsequently endorsed by the American Thoracic Society in its 1981 official statement on pulmonary rehabilitation.[27]

The diverse processes that contribute to exercise impairment and incapacitation in the COPD patient lend themselves to a multidisciplinary treatment approach. In broad outline, the approaches of most rehabilitation programs designed for patients with COPD incorporate some form of physical reconditioning, attention to nutritional status, psychosocial assessment, education about the disease and its treatment, and attempts to achieve a smoke-free state.

EFFECTIVENESS OF REHABILITATION

In the past 20 to 25 years, a number of studies have demonstrated the effectiveness of multidisciplinary rehabilitation programs involving some form of arm and leg exercise reconditioning. Exercise reconditioning appears to be associated with diminished breathlessness, enhanced endurance during external work, an increased performance of the activities of daily living, and an improvement in psychosocial status and quality of life.[11, 18, 20–24, 28, 29, 31–35, 37] It has even been suggested that patients who participate in such programs have a lower rate of hospitalization than historical controls.[19]

The value of rehabilitation programs that include some form of exercise training on exercise performance, the activities of daily living, and the subjective feeling of well-being has been demonstrated in a number of controlled studies. Cockcroft and colleagues[32] have studied 39 patients with COPD caused by coal miner's pneumoconiosis who were short of breath on exercise. Subjects were given a 6-week period of exercise training in a rehabilitation center in the form of graduated exercise on a bicycle ergometer, swimming, rowing, and twice-daily walks of increasing distance. Subjects were also instructed in the performance of exercises (stair climbing and walking on level ground) in the home environment. The responses of these subjects were compared to those of a control group tested over the same period prior to entry into the rehabilitation program and retested after a 6-week period of exercise training. Subjects receiving training experienced significant improvements in the feeling of general well-being, diminution of breathlessness during exercise, and the ability to walk. The subjects receiving exercise training demonstrated significantly greater increases in distance walked during a 12-minute test as compared to control subjects. Trained subjects demonstrated increases of approximately 8% to 10% in maximum oxygen uptake and maximal ventilation during treadmill exercise. Control subjects demonstrated decreases in oxygen uptake and maximal ventilation. Control subjects who were subsequently enrolled in the program showed increases in function, similar to those achieved by those in the initially trained group. It is of considerable interest that the benefits derived appeared to persist throughout a 7-month follow-up period after formal training had ceased but home training continued.

Mungall and Hainsworth[33] reported on ten well-studied patients who were observed at 2-week intervals during three 12-week periods—control, exercise, and postexercise periods. They made six observations during each of the three periods, in which the exercise consisted of calisthenics using the Canadian Air Force program for women. Subjects showed no improvement during the 12-week control period, but it was reported that seven of the ten subjects demonstrated an increase in 12-minute walking distance with training. This improvement was maintained during the 12-week post-training period of observation. Two of the subjects were unchanged, however, and one became worse.

Sinclair and Ingram[37] compared the responses of 33 COPD patients enrolled in an exercise training program in the home setting to a group of control subjects. Training consisted of a daily 12-minute walk and stair climbing as rapidly as possible for 1.5 to 2 minutes twice a day. The period of training averaged 10.3 months. There was a reduction in symptoms in trainees, with a decrease in the sense of dyspnea, a heightened sense of well-being, and a greater ability to perform the activities of daily living. Improvements in those in the training group were statistically significant when compared to those in the control group. With most subjects, beneficial effects gradually reached a maximum at 8 to 10 months. In contrast, those in the control group demonstrated significant decreases in the 12-minute walking distance. This study demonstrated that a program largely geared toward home exercise can provide significant symptomatic and physical improvement.

Nicholas and associates[20] examined the effectiveness of exercise therapy in 13 COPD patients. A novel aspect of this study was the use of a 3-month observation period with no formal exercise training as a control to establish the baseline value. Subjects trained for 30 minutes three times a week on a treadmill for 3 months. The intensity of the training was described as being "sufficient to exhaust the subject initially in less than 10 but more than one minute."[20] Three of the eight subjects derived excellent increases in oxygen uptake at the break point of exercise and in the walking score during the control period. There was, however, a further significant increase in oxygen uptake at the break point and the walking score during the period of exercise training. These results[20] therefore indicate that there may be a slight increase in function, even during a control period of observation (perhaps related to learning or motivation); improvements were derived largely during the first several weeks of training; and the overall level of benefit for the entire group during training was modest.

The precise mechanisms underlying symptom reduction arising from exercise reconditioning remain unclear at present. Most studies, however, have suggested that physical reconditioning of the arms and legs is not associated with improved lung or airway function, cardiovascular performance, or the metabolism of the exercising limbs.[10, 11, 20–24, 30, 35] In the absence of obvious signs of improvement in lung or cardiovascular function, it has been suggested that the enhanced ability to perform external work is a result of greater neuromuscular efficiency (i.e., the ability to perform work at a lower metabolic cost), desensitization of a phobic attitude toward dyspnea, enhancements in ventilatory muscle strength and endurance, or nonspecific motivational or learning responses.[1, 3, 11] There is current support for each of these hypotheses, but the precise role of each factor in the overall improvement observed in COPD patients as a result of exercise rehabilitation remains the subject of active investigation. In particular, the role played by ventilatory muscle fatigue and/or dysfunction is being actively studied.

VENTILATORY MUSCLE TRAINING

Impairments in respiratory muscle strength and/or endurance can limit ventilation in COPD patients.[7, 9, 12, 62, 65, 80, 134, 135] In many subjects with advanced COPD, exercise limitation is secondary to an inability to increase ventilation further.[61] That is, at the point of exercise cessation, minute ventilation may equal or exceed the subject's ventilatory capacity as reflected by the maximal voluntary ventilation (MVV). Increases in the ability to ventilate, therefore, would be expected to allow more intense levels of exercise to be performed.

In COPD patients the respiratory muscles are under a high degree of stress. Respiratory muscle oxygen consumption is greater in COPD patients than in normal subjects, even at rest, and each increase in ventilation is associated with a disproportionate increase in respiratory muscle oxygen consumption.[62, 69] Hyperinflation of the thorax places the inspiratory muscles at a mechanical disadvantage by diminishing their precontraction length and altering their alignment, which thereby impairs their ability to reduce intrathoracic pressure.[131, 132] Thoracic configuration is altered in patients with COPD, resulting in a synchronous rib cage and abdominal movements during breathing at rest but discoordinate movements in most patients when ventilation is increased above resting levels.[167] In at least some subjects with COPD, electromyographic (EMG) evidence of inspiratory muscle fatigue and contractile dysfunction has been documented during the performance of arm and leg exercises.[16, 133, 168]

An additional complicating factor in some COPD patients may be the presence of respiratory muscle atrophy.[40] Several studies that have examined respiratory muscle structure in COPD patients noted diaphragm fiber atrophy.[153–156, 169] Development of atrophy *per se* would decrease the tension-generating ability of these muscles. Furthermore, the mass (weight) of the entire diaphragm is significantly lower in subjects with COPD than in age-matched normal subjects.[153] Currently, the precise mechanisms causing the development of respiratory skeletal muscle atrophy in subjects with COPD remain under investigation. A large percentage (approximately 40%) of stable outpatients with COPD, however, appear to be malnourished. Studies in the hamster[158] and rat[159] have indicated that a decrease in caloric intake that reduces body weight by 25%[158] is associated with preferential atrophy of fast-twitch fibers in the costal region of the diaphragm,[158] an impaired ability to generate tension at any given fiber length,[158] slowing in the rate of relaxation, and a leftward shift in the force-frequency relationship.[159] In fact, underweight subjects with COPD (i.e., <80% ideal body weight) develop significantly lower inspiratory and expiratory pressures as compared to normal-weight COPD subjects.[39] The assumption that ventilatory muscle fatigue and ventilatory muscle weakness are important in limiting exercise performance in COPD patients has led to the use of various approaches to train the ventilatory muscles specifically.[8, 134]

Hyperpneic Ventilatory Muscle Training

Studies by Leith and Bradley[48] in the late 1970s indicated that, in young normal subjects, the respiratory muscles can be trained to increase their endurance or strength, or both, by appropriate training regimens. They demonstrated that several weeks of daily hyperpnea at levels of ventilation close to the MVV, performed for 15-minute periods, can lead to an increase in the MVV and in the ability to sustain that ventilation for prolonged periods. In the technique of hyperpneic ventilatory muscle training, subjects breathe on a low-resistance circuit that allows them to generate extremely high levels of ventilation. Isocapnia is maintained by increasing the inspired CO_2 concentration. The circuit includes the capability of monitoring ventilation (real time) and of displaying a "target" level of ventilation. Training is achieved by progressively increasing the target level of ventilation that can be sustained for 12 to 15 minutes.

A training program consisting of repeated maximal static contractions of the inspiratory and expiratory muscles against an occluded airway can lead to increases in the maximum static inspiratory and expiratory pressures. Belman and Gaesser[137] have demonstrated that ventilatory muscle training performed by isocapnia-hyperpnea increases the sustainable ventilation and MVV in elderly (65- to 75-year-old) normal subjects.

Carrying out sustainable isocapnic hyperventilation training requires a significant amount of complex hardware and experienced personnel. At present, the technique is not suitable for routine clinical use. Leith[6] has described a relatively simple device that allows a range of ventilation targets to be displayed easily, and this approach may circumvent the problem.

These observations, which indicate the plasticity of function of the respiratory muscles in young and old normal subjects by specific training maneuvers, are the basis of approaches to improve respiratory muscle function in COPD patients to even greater than normal levels.

Keens and associates[168] have demonstrated, in children with cystic fibrosis, that strenuous training of the upper extremities achieved by 1.5-hour periods of rowing and other arm exercises with associated hyperventilation leads to increases in the MVV and maximal sustainable ventilatory capacity. Belman and Mittman,[12] in a small number of stable COPD patients, showed that daily 15-minute trials of isocapnic hyperventilation increased the MVV, sustainable ventilatory capacity, and maximum oxygen uptake of the respiratory muscles over a 6-week period. The increase in respiratory muscle oxygen uptake with ventilatory muscle training suggests that the increases in ventilatory capacity and endurance are not the result of greater efficiency or better neuromuscular coordination, but of an enhancement in the metabolic capacity of the exercising respiratory muscles to perform work. Interestingly, this regimen also enhanced the maximum oxygen uptake and maximal external work on a bicycle ergometer.

On the other hand, Belman and Kendregan[10] found that the daily performance of arm or leg exercises on a bicycle ergometer for 6 weeks did not increase the sustainable ventilatory capacity or maximum oxygen uptake of the respiratory muscles, but their studies did not include a control population. Other studies in normal subjects, however, have indicated that a 10- to 20-week period of strenuous running (40 minutes a day, three times a week, at 80% maximum heart rate) raises the MVV, maximal sustainable ventilation, and maximum static expiratory pressure.[2] Presumably, the intensity of arm and leg exercise in the Belman study[10] produced levels of ventilation too low to achieve a training effect on the respiratory muscles.

Levine and coworkers[11] in a carefully controlled prospective study have compared the effects of 6 weeks of sustained isocapnic hyperventilation training to intermittent positive-pressure breathing (IPPB) on exercise performance and ventilatory muscle endurance in 32 stable COPD subjects. Patients were entered into the study in pairs. The training regimen for both groups consisted of a 2-hour daily period in the hospital. The first hour involved the administration of a bronchodilator aerosol by IPPB. The second hour involved either a repeat IPPB treatment in those subjects randomized to the IPPB arm (control group) or two 15-minute periods of maximal isocapnic sustainable hyperventilation separated by an appropriate rest period (respiratory muscle endurance training group). Levine and colleagues[11] found that subjects who undergo isocapnic hyperventilation training demonstrate significant increases in maximal sustainable ventilation, whereas subjects receiving IPPB treatment do not. Both groups demonstrated significant increases in endurance time during submaximal bicycle and treadmill exercise at two thirds of maximum workload and in peak oxygen uptake during a progressive incremental work test to a symptom-limited maximum. The distance walked during a 12-minute period also increased significantly. Both groups also demonstrated significant improvements in several standard psychologic tests and in the ability to perform the activities of daily living. Noteworthy was the lack of any significant difference in the magnitude of improvement in any parameter observed between the group that received ventilatory muscle training and the group that received IPPB alone.

Because IPPB treatment can be considered to be a placebo, Levine and associates[11] concluded that increases in the ability to perform external work in subjects undergoing specific respiratory muscle training may not necessarily be a result of enhanced respiratory muscle endurance but might reflect nonspecific responses to the overall rehabilitation program, such as a learning phenomenon, increased motivation, or improved neuromuscular coordination. This latter possibility was supported by the observation that increases in endurance time during submaximal work are not associated with increases in oxygen uptake (Fig. 56–1).

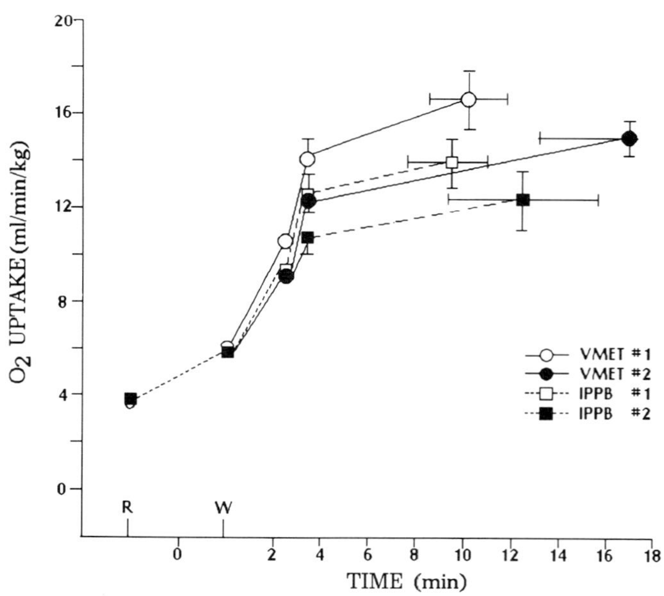

Figure 56–1. Endurance treadmill exercise tests in subjects given respiratory muscle endurance training *(circles)* and intermittent positive-pressure breathing (IPPB) treatment *(squares)*. Baseline data *(open symbols)* and following intervention *(solid symbols)* are shown. Both respiratory muscle–trained and IPPB-treated subjects demonstrate an increase in endurance time at any level of work. Oxygen uptake is unchanged, however, suggesting that external work performance increases as a result of improved neuromuscular efficiency. (Reproduced with permission from Levine S, et al. Am Rev Respir Dis 1986; 133:400–406.)

Inspiratory Resistance Training

Pardy and coworkers[16] first demonstrated that inspiring against an inspiratory resistance for two 15-minute periods a day increases the ability to sustain ventilation against high levels of external resistance. They studied 12 subjects with advanced COPD who inhaled against an alinear resistor of sufficient magnitude to produce EMG evidence of fatigue of the sternocleidomastoid, diaphragm, or intercostal muscles daily for 4 to 8 weeks. All subjects demonstrated an increase in the resistance that could be sustained without producing EMG changes of fatigue. A subgroup of seven subjects demonstrated an increase in endurance time for submaximal work performed on a bicycle ergometer, maximal power output, and maximum oxygen uptake. The subjects showing a greater endurance time for bicycle work were the ones who had previously manifested EMG evidence of fatigue during bicycle work. The five subjects in whom bicycle work was not associated with EMG evidence of fatigue did not increase work performance, despite improved respiratory muscle function.

In another study, Pardy and colleagues[71] found that subjects who performed inspiratory resistance breathing for 4 to 8 weeks walked farther in 12 minutes, whereas subjects who participated in a rehabilitation program involving arm and leg exercises did not. Unfortunately, the nature of the exercise training and its intensity in the latter group were not specified. Furthermore, neither of the studies by Pardy and colleagues[16, 71] incorporated a control group.

Studies by Chen and associates[13] and by Sonne and Davis[15] using a placebo (a circuit in which the resistance was not increased) have demonstrated, however, that increases in inspiratory muscle strength and endurance achieved by daily inspiratory resistance breathing reflect specific responses to increases in inspiratory pressure. Chen and coworkers[13] have suggested that increases in inspiratory muscle strength and the ability to tolerate increasing resistance may not be associated with an increased ability to perform external work on a bicycle or treadmill. The changes in exercise performance in COPD patients who received inspiratory resistance training and in those who received placebo were similar and insignificant over the study period. On the other hand, Sonne and Davis[15] have demonstrated increased exercise performance in patients receiving inspiratory resistance training. The reason for the discrepancy between these results is unknown.

None of these studies,[13, 15, 16, 71] however, involved monitoring or controlling the pattern of breathing of subjects during inspiratory resistance breathing, so the pressures generated during training sessions were not known. It seems probable that subjects breathing spontaneously on a given resistance may vary their inspiratory flow rate so as to minimize the sense of effort of breathing by decreasing the peak intrathoracic pressure or the pressure-time index of the inspiratory muscles. Patients may reduce inspiratory air flow sufficiently so that the peak intrathoracic pressure generated during resistance breathing may be similar to the pressure changes that occur in the absence of the external resistance. Patients may also reduce breathing frequency and ventilation.

The overall result of such changes in breathing pattern may be that the pressure-time index of the inspiratory muscles (i.e., the area under a curve of pressure versus time) may not be significantly different with or without the resistance.[42a] Jederlinic and coworkers,[14] in support of this hypothesis, have demonstrated reductions in ventilation and increases in end-tidal CO_2 during resistance breathing in COPD subjects. Belman and colleagues[42a] have also demonstrated that subjects coached to achieve a desired pressure-time index demonstrate a training effect, whereas those allowed to breathe spontaneously do not.

Jederlinic and colleagues[14] have shown that most COPD subjects, using a commercially available inspiratory resistor and breathing spontaneously, demonstrated significant decreases in minute ventilation, increases in end-tidal CO_2, and decreases in arterial oxygen saturation during the resistive breathing. In individual subjects, levels of hypoxia and hypercapnia were reached that may be associated with significant adverse clinical consequences. These alterations in ventilation and gas exchange persisted throughout the entire 6-week period of daily inspiratory resistance breathing.

Belman and colleagues[42a] have made an important contribution by emphasizing the role of "breathing strategy" as a determinant of the efficacy of inspiratory resistive training. Ten COPD subjects performed two 15-minute sessions of resistive breathing daily for 6 weeks using a commercially available inspiratory resistive device. After the training period the subjects were retested; no increases were noted over those of controls in maximal inspiratory pressure or the ability to sustain breathing through a higher resistive load. Subjects were then instructed to watch an oscilloscope display of mouth pressure versus time, and coached to breathe with a longer inspiratory time but lower peak mouth pressure and frequency. During coached breathing, five of the seven individuals exhibited an increase in the resistive load that they could endure for 15 minutes. Whereas peak mouth pressure was higher during spontaneous breathing, the pressure-time index of the inspiratory muscles (i.e., the area under the pressure-time curve) was appreciably greater during the "coached state."[42a]

Studies that monitor and control breathing pattern so as to achieve target levels of peak pressure and increase the pressure-time index of the inspiratory muscles need to be performed to assess the importance of this issue and their effects on inspiratory muscle training.

Zack and Palange[170] have utilized inspiratory resistance training in COPD subjects by using a circuit that allows inspiratory pressure and ventilation to be observed by the patient and maintained at target levels. Additionally, subjects underwent exercise training of the arms and legs. More than 50 patients were studied, and impressive improvements were seen in maximum static inspiratory pressure, maximum voluntary ventilation, and the ability to perform external work and the activities of daily living. No control group, however, was included in this study.

Conclusions About Respiratory Muscle Training

The studies described in this section suggest that, although specific respiratory muscle training can enhance the strength and endurance of the respiratory muscles in most subjects, improvements in respiratory muscle function may not result in enhanced exercise performance. The mechanisms by which individuals achieve significant improvements in their ability to ventilate and increase their exercise performance remain unclear. There remains, therefore, a need to identify discriminators to predict those subjects most likely to demonstrate improvements in exercise performance following specific respiratory muscle training. Furthermore, the nature of the respiratory training associated with maximal benefit in terms of respiratory muscle strength and endurance and the ability to perform external work remains unclear.

Given the nature of the two most prevalent forms of respiratory muscle training (inspiratory resistance breathing and isocapnic hyperventilation), and the highly specific nature of the biochemical and structural responses of the respiratory muscles to mechanical stress,[46–48, 180, 181] it seems likely that they have differing effects on respiratory muscle structure, biochemical properties, and contractile performance. Inspiratory resistance is associated with relatively high levels of pressure and low levels of airflow. Isocapnic hyperventilation, on the other hand, is associated with relatively rapid inspiratory muscle shortening and much lower levels of tension or pressure. These two different forms of training may make the respiratory muscles operate at different ends of the force-velocity relationship.[45] Isocapnic hyperventilation may train the respiratory muscles to perform high-velocity shortening at low levels of tension and to undergo a greater extent of overall shortening than that which occurs during resistance breathing, which generates a higher level of pressure and muscular tension.[45] Also, uncertainty exists about the precise intensity and duration of respiratory muscle training needed to achieve maximal clinical benefit. At present, no studies have examined the effect of inspiratory resistive training or isocapnic hyperventilation on the incidence of respiratory failure, hospitalization, or mortality in COPD patients.

In certain situations, respiratory muscle training might even worsen respiratory muscle function and adversely affect the subject's ability to ventilate.[8] For example, patients with pre-existing chronic stable respiratory muscle fatigue may become clinically worse as a result of inspiratory resistance breathing or isocapnic hyperventilation training. Worsening of a stable state of chronic fatigue, however, has not been described and, given the widespread use of inspiratory resistive breathing, the risk would appear to be largely theoretic.

Another important aspect of the rehabilitation process that has received little attention in COPD patients is the prevention of detraining. It is well understood that cessation of muscle training without a maintenance program is associated with a loss in training-related improvements in muscle function and work performance. Leith and Bradley have found that in young normal subjects ventilatory muscle detraining results in a loss of 50% in the gains achieved in approximately 15 weeks.[48] Whether a similar detraining time course occurs in elderly COPD patients remains to be seen. It is to be expected, however, that some time after complete discontinuation of training COPD subjects lose whatever benefits were previously derived. It would appear essential, therefore, that some form of physical activity be continued after the completion of a formal rehabilitation program, but the exact nature, frequency, duration, and intensity of the exercises best suited to prevent detraining are as yet unknown.

CARDIOVASCULAR RESPONSES TO EXERCISE IN COPD

Alterations in the mechanical properties of the lung, diminution in the volume of the pulmonary capillary bed as a result of emphysema, and alterations in arterial blood gas tensions produce various hemodynamic changes that stress the cardiovascular system and limit its ability to deliver oxygen to the exercising muscles and heart.[178] Inactivity and deconditioning are also associated with decreases in maximum oxygen uptake, cardiac output, stroke volume, and arteriovenous oxygen difference. There is considerable evidence that the heart rate and stroke volume responses of COPD patients to exercise differ from those of age-matched normal subjects.

Spiro and colleagues[31] have compared the cardiovascular responses to bicycle exercise in patients with COPD and age-matched normal sedentary males. They found that the heart rate at any given oxygen uptake was increased in COPD patients as compared to normals. Subjects with more severe airway obstruction demonstrated greater elevations in heart rate. The cardiac output response to exercise in COPD subjects was normal, but the stroke volume decreased at any given level of oxygen uptake or cardiac output. It was also demonstrated that lactate levels in the blood increase in the last minute of exercise in subjects with COPD, but not as much as in sedentary normal subjects. Interestingly, the increase in blood lactate level was not associated with an increase in ventilation in COPD subjects unlike the normal subjects. It appears that the use of ventilatory parameters to assess the anaerobic threshold, therefore, may not be as useful in COPD patients as in normals, because the patients with COPD may be unable to increase ventilation further in response to an acid stimulus.

Matthay and associates[179] have reported that the cardiac responses to exercise of COPD patients appear to be different than those of normal subjects. Specifically, the stroke volume response of both the right and left ventricles was impaired in COPD patients. In normal subjects, increases in the intensity of exercise were associated with increases in right and left ventricular stroke volumes. In contrast, it was observed[179] that right and left ventricular stroke volumes change variably during exercise, increasing in some patients with COPD but not in others. In fact, in some patients, stroke volume decreased with exercise. In the entire group there was no change in either right or left ventricular stroke volume during exercise. Some, but not all, of this discrepancy is explained by marked differences in the intensity of the exercise performed by COPD patients and normal subjects (i.e., patients with COPD were assessed at a lower intensity of exercise than normal subjects).

Effects of Training on Cardiovascular Performance

Exercise training of appropriate intensity in middle-aged sedentary men can elicit increases in maximum oxygen uptake, arteriovenous oxygen difference, and stroke volume, and, at submaximal work, decreases in heart rate and cardiac output. Davis and associates[174] demonstrated in middle-aged sedentary men (mean age, 43 years) that an intense program of bicycle exercise over 9 weeks improved their exercise performance and the aerobic capacity of the exercising muscle. Subjects trained for 45 minutes, five times each week, at a target heart rate associated with an oxygen uptake of 50% to 70% of the difference between their baseline anaerobic threshold and maximum oxygen uptake. That is, training intensity was associated with a heart rate at which oxygen uptake was about 80% to 85% of the initial maximum value. With this training approach, subjects demonstrated a significant increase in anaerobic threshold (assessed both in absolute terms and as a percentage of the maximum oxygen uptake) during a progressive incremental work test on a cycle ergometer. Maximum oxygen uptake and maximum ventilation also increased. Carbon dioxide production and the respiratory quotient (RQ) during submaximal exercise were reduced following the period of training. The changes in maximum oxygen uptake, CO_2 production, RQ, and anaerobic threshold in sedentary men suggest that the exercising limbs undergo alterations in intermediary metabolism so that less glycogen is used and less lactate is produced.

Adaptive responses of aerobic power and heart rate at a single intensity of training are extremely rapid. Hickson[175] reported that, during a vigorous 6-day-a-week period of training in young healthy subjects, increases in oxygen uptake and decreases in heart rate and lactate production at a given level of work are complete by 3 weeks. The half-time for the decrease in heart rate is approximately 5 days, whereas the half-time for the increase in oxygen uptake is approximately 10 days. It therefore appears that to achieve progressive increases in the effect achieved the regimen must be intensified at least every 3 weeks. Constancy of the exercise regimen beyond this 3-week period would therefore appear to represent only maintenance exercise.

Increases in anaerobic threshold in COPD patients (in those who manifest an anaerobic threshold) are potentially beneficial. An increase in anaerobic threshold may diminish the decrease in blood pH, lessen the acid stimulus to breathe, and thus diminish ventilation during submaximal exercise. Because exercise in most subjects with COPD is ventilation-limited, a reduction in the level of ventilation at any given level of exercise should diminish dyspnea and the tendency to develop respiratory muscle fatigue. Training that elevates the anaerobic threshold may therefore enhance endurance time for submaximal exercise. At present there is little information about the frequency with which COPD patients achieve an anaerobic threshold and about the effect of endurance training on the anaerobic threshold in COPD patients.

The effects of physical training on cardiopulmonary performance in patients with COPD have been examined by several investigators. Chester and coworkers[35] devised a 4-week program of daily exercise training on a treadmill along with graded-intensity pulley, bicycle, and rowing exercises for 1 to 2 hours/day at a heart rate of approximately 70% of maximum. Their subjects generally increased their ability to perform external work on the treadmill and bicycle. It was reported that in the group as a whole, however, exercise training did not alter the cardiac index, heart rate, pulmonary vascular resistance, or stroke volume index when assessed at comparable levels of submaximal work. It was concluded that there are no obvious consistent cardiovascular changes that explain the increased ability to perform external work. Rather, the increased work capacity was attributed to increases in efficiency, motivation, or a desensitization to the phobic responses to dyspnea.[35]

Conversely, Degre and colleagues[21] demonstrated in a smaller group of subjects that a 6-week period of exercise training on the bicycle ergometer was associated with a decrease in mean pulmonary artery pressure and an increase in maximum oxygen uptake (approximately 10%). Exercise consisted of three 25-minute sessions/week at an intensity equal to 75% of the maximal tolerated load. Increases in maximum oxygen uptake appeared to be the result of an increase in the maximum arteriovenous oxygen difference. There were no changes in maximum cardiac output, maximum heart rate, or maximum stroke volume. These changes were not apparent in the control group of subjects who were given breathing exercises only.

Alpert and associates[23] used what appears to be a more intensive form of exercise training than that usually reported. Their small group of five subjects trained at home on a bicycle ergometer for three 20-minute sessions daily for 18 weeks. The results included an increase in work capacity in all subjects, a decrease in resting heart rate, cardiac output, ventilation, and arteriovenous oxygen difference during submaximal work, and an increase in inspiratory capacity and maximum voluntary ventilation. The oxygen uptake on a standard submaximal load, however, did not change.

Paez and coworkers[22] also demonstrated beneficial cardiovascular effects of exercise training in a small group of COPD patients (n = 8). The subjects trained on a treadmill daily for 50 minutes for 3 weeks, and were found to increase their work performance on the treadmill. In part, the increase in work performance was related to a longer stride. Subjects were, however, able to walk faster and farther during submaximal exercise and demonstrated decreases in heart rate and ventilation. There appeared to be some transference of the training effect to exercise on a bicycle ergometer. Cardiac output decreased and the arteriovenous oxygen difference decreased during submaximal work on the bicycle after training.

Of interest is the finding by Belman and Kendregan[30] that the activity of several rate-limiting enzymes in the tricarboxylic acid pathway does not appear to be altered in the limb muscles of COPD patients following a 4- to 6-week period of bicycle training. Their data suggest that training-related changes in aerobic metabolism previously observed repeatedly in normal subjects may not occur in COPD patients, perhaps because the intensity of the training program is insufficient to induce adaptive biochemical responses.

ARM EXERCISE

Most investigators examining the factors responsible for exercise limitation in those with severe COPD have ignored arm exercise and have primarily focused on changes that occur during lower extremity exercise.[50–55] The reasons for this are unclear, because the arms are constantly involved in performing the essential tasks of daily living. Many patients with severe COPD complain of dyspnea when performing seemingly trivial tasks involving the upper extremities, such as shaving, brushing hair, bending over, or tying shoes. Often, the level of dyspnea experienced seems disproportionate to the degree of work performed. Several studies have suggested that respiratory muscle function is impaired in the presence of unsupported arm exercise and that respiratory muscle dysfunction may contribute to the development of dyspnea and impaired exercise performance in patients with severe COPD.[56–58]

Tangri and Woolf[59a] have examined the pattern of breathing in seven obstructed subjects while they performed several common daily activities (bending over and tying shoes, brushing teeth, or combing hair). An irregular and rapid pattern of breathing was observed in all subjects during arm exercise. At the conclusion of the exercise routine the subjects demonstrated a period of rapid and deep breathing. The authors reasoned that the period of hyperventilation after exercise is an attempt to restore normal gas exchange and is responsible for the dyspnea experienced by these subjects during the activities of daily living.

Celli and colleagues have studied the ventilatory response (as measured by the forced expiratory volume in 1 second, FEV_1) to unsupported arm exercise in greater detail in 12 subjects with severe COPD ($FEV_1 = 0.68 \pm 0.28$ L) and compared it to that of unloaded leg cycling.[56] In the five most severely obstructed subjects, arm exercise was associated with the onset of dyssynchronous breathing and was terminated because of severe dyspnea. Dyssynchronous breathing, or uncoordinated movements of the rib cage and abdomen, was not observed in these five subjects when performing leg cycling, even though it was associated with a higher heart rate and oxygen uptake and a shorter endurance time. Seven patients performed arm exercise for a mean of 6.1 ± 2.0 minutes without complaining of dyspnea, and stopped exercising only because of arm fatigue. It was postulated that those subjects with dyssynchronous breathing during arm exercise may become increasingly hyperinflated during exercise, thereby placing the diaphragm at a mechanical disadvantage.[56] Under conditions in which the function of the diaphragm is impaired, the contribution of the accessory inspiratory muscles to ventilation generally increases. If the inspiratory rib cage muscles reduce their ventilatory activity when the unsupported arm is extended, the diaphragm or expiratory muscles must assume a greater portion of the ventilatory burden. The investigators suggested that alterations in the pattern of upper extremity use may influence chest wall mechanics and the level of activity of the inspiratory and expiratory muscles, and therefore affect the susceptibility to respiratory muscle fatigue.[56]

To test this hypothesis, Criner and associates have compared the pattern of ventilatory muscle recruitment in 11 subjects with severe COPD during both unsupported and supported arm exercise.[57] Arm cycling was used for a trial of supported arm exercise while unsupported arm exercise was performed by asking subjects to shift lightweight plastic rings on a pegboard elevated to shoulder level. The latter routine mimicked activities found to provoke marked dyspnea in some COPD patients. Plots of the pleural and gastric pressures (i.e., Macklem plots[59]) were used to determine the mechanical activity of the diaphragm and of the accessory muscles at rest and during exercise.

Endurance time for unsupported arm exercise was shorter than that for supported arm exercise, even though the latter was more stressful (as reflected by the heart rate, minute ventilation, and oxygen uptake). The difference between end-inspiratory and end-expiratory transdiaphragmatic pressures was greatest during unsupported arm exercise. In eight subjects more positive end-inspiratory and end-expiratory pleural and gastric pressures occurred when they performed unsupported arm exercise (Fig. 56–2).[38] This pattern of pressures was interpreted to mean that unsupported arm exercise shifts a portion of the ventilatory load from the inspiratory muscles of the rib cage to the diaphragm and to the muscles of expiration.

Unsupported arm exercise, as compared to leg exercise, also appears to alter ventilatory muscle recruitment, even in normal subjects.[58] In eight of eleven normal subjects, pleural-gastric pressure plots during arm exercise demonstrated a decrease in mechanical activity of the inspiratory rib cage muscles and an increase in diaphragm and abdominal muscle activity. In three of these eight subjects, arm exercise precipitated dyspnea and the onset of dyssynchronous thorocoabdominal movement.

There are several possible reasons why the pattern of ventilatory muscle use may differ during unsupported and supported arm exercise, including the following: (1) an increase in thoracic impedance during unsupported arm exercise; (2) a decrease in the resting length of the inspiratory rib cage muscles during arm elevation; and (3) alterations in afferent input from the chest wall, with subsequent changes in the pattern of distribution of motor outflow to the inspiratory muscles.

Although the exact mechanism(s) for this shift in the pattern of respiratory muscle activity during arm exercise remain unclear, it is apparent that performance of certain arm activities may have important implications for the maintenance of ventilation. This is especially true for patients with severe COPD who have limited ventilatory reserve. Obviously, the respiratory effects of certain arm exercises need to be considered when planning pulmonary rehabilitation programs or determining the suitability of jobs for patients with severe lung disease. Additional studies need to be directed toward understanding the interaction of the respiratory and pectoral girdle and back muscles during postural and upper body activities.

RESPIRATORY MUSCLE REST

Patients with severe COPD are predisposed to the development of respiratory muscle fatigue.[60, 61] Respiratory muscle fatigue, like fatigue of any skeletal muscle, results in the inability of the muscle to maintain force output.[62] A critical factor in the development of skeletal muscle fatigue is the percentage of maximal muscle tension generated to perform a required task.[63] It has been suggested that the tension-time threshold for fatigue of the human diaphragm (TT_{di}) is determined by the product of the percentage of maximal transdiaphragmatic pressure generated ($P_{di}/P_{di\ max}$) during breathing multiplied by the portion of the respiratory cycle spent in inspiration (T_i/T_{tot}).[64] TT_{di} values greater than 15% of maximum appear to represent the threshold for fatigue in some patients with severe COPD.[60] More recent studies have indicated that respiratory muscle endurance at a given TT_{di} may also depend on the velocity of muscle shortening and muscle length.[138, 139, 159] Increases in the velocity of airflow during inspiration and increases in lung volume diminish inspiratory muscle endurance.

The force reserve of the diaphragm in COPD patients is markedly reduced because hyperinflation alters the length and shape of the diaphragm and reduces maximal transdiaphragmatic pressure (lower $P_{di\ max}$). In addition, hypoxemia, hypercapnia, and/or malnutrition further impair respiratory muscle function, both by increasing the demand for ventilation (hypoxia, hypercapnia) and by diminishing $P_{di\ max}$ (malnutrition, hypercapnia).[151, 152] Subjects with COPD, therefore, are predisposed to develop respiratory muscle fatigue with even small increases in ventilation or changes in breathing pattern.[60]

Most authorities now classify fatigue into central and peripheral components.[65] Central fatigue is believed to occur when there is a reduction in motor outflow to the contracting muscle.[173] Peripheral fatigue occurs with failure of neural transmission at the muscle cell or at the neuromuscular junction, or because of impaired coupling of excitation to contraction coupling. Peripheral fatigue is further divided into high- and low-frequency subtypes.[67, 68, 136] High-frequency fatigue is defined as a reduction in muscle forces during high-frequency stimulation (i.e., >75 Hz), and appears to arise from impaired propagation of an action potential along the sarcolemmal membrane or from failure of transmission at the neuromuscular junction. Low-frequency fatigue is manifested as a reduction in force during low-frequency stimulation (i.e., approximately 20 Hz), and is believed to be secondary to impairment in excitation-contraction coupling. Low-frequency fatigue is commonly observed following repeated submaximal contractions of a skeletal muscle, and recovery from this form of fatigue takes longer than recovery from the high-frequency

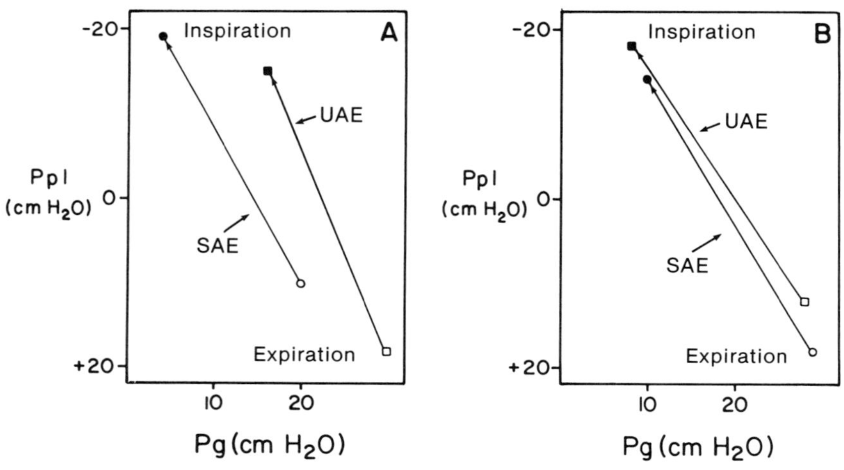

Figure 56–2. Plots of gastric (P_g) and pleural (P_{pl}) pressures at end-inspiration and end-expiration during supported arm exercise (SAE) and unsupported arm exercise (UAE). Shown are data from two subjects demonstrating the two patterns of breathing observed. *A*, During UAE, most subjects demonstrated more positive end-inspiratory pleural, gastric, and end-expiratory pleural pressures. *B*, Subject in whom no change in the pattern of pressures was observed in the two types of exercise. (Reproduced with permission from Criner GJ, Celli BR. Am Rev Respir Dis 1988; 138:856–861.)

subtype.[67, 68] These characteristics of low-frequency fatigue are important because of its long duration and the fact that the firing rate of phrenic motor neurons falls into this range.

Therapeutic regimens in COPD must be multifaceted and directed at reducing the mechanical load on the muscles, in addition to improving respiratory muscle contractility.[69] Mechanical demands can be reduced by alleviating airway obstruction and by controlling excessive secretions. Further reductions in respiratory muscle contractile activity can be achieved by correcting derangements in Pa_{O_2} and Pa_{CO_2} using supplemental oxygen, avoiding high-carbohydrate intake, and controlling fever. Respiratory muscle contractility can be enhanced pharmacologically (e.g., by methylxanthines, beta-agonists),[70, 160–167] by oxygen,[85–93] and by proper nutritional support.[72, 172] Once a respiratory muscle fatigues, however, rest is the preferred form of treatment.[62]

Intermittent mechanical ventilatory support has been demonstrated to be effective therapy in patients with chronic ventilatory failure caused by neuromuscular disease or restricted ventilatory defects.[73–78] Curran has found significantly better gas exchange after daily use of nocturnal negative-pressure ventilation in nine patients in ventilatory failure caused by advanced muscular dystrophy.[73] Garay and colleagues[74] have noted similar improvements in gas exchange using nocturnal negative-pressure ventilation in eight patients with alveolar hypoventilation. Furthermore, three patients who underwent right-heart catheterization before and after assisted ventilation showed a significant reduction in pulmonary artery pressure.

Marino and Braun treated 35 patients with ventilatory failure, 17 with neuromuscular disease, using ventilatory support for 4 to 10 hours daily for an average of 5.2 ± 3.8 months.[77] Post-treatment data for the group revealed a decrease in the Pa_{CO_2} (54 ± 9 versus 43 ± 5 mm Hg), an increase in respiratory muscle strength (PI_{max}, 28% ± 17% versus 45% ± 23% predicted), and an increase in ventilatory muscle endurance (maximum voluntary ventilation, 21% ± 10% versus 45% ± 20% predicted). Celli and associates[78] have reported similar results in three patients with bilateral idiopathic diaphragmatic paralysis who showed an improvement in the ability to perform the activities of daily living and in resting respiratory muscle strength several weeks after beginning daily periods of negative-pressure ventilation.

Studies of intermittent ventilatory support in patients with severe COPD have yielded conflicting results. Braun and Marino provided 4 to 10 hours of daily ventilatory support (uncontrolled) to 18 patients, 13 of whom suffered from hypercapnia and severe COPD.[79] Results following institution of mechanical ventilation were compared retrospectively to data obtained during the baseline period. Following 5 months of daily intermittent ventilation, increases were noted in vital capacity (from 3.6 ± 1.4 to 5.3 ± 1.8 L), maximum inspired pressures (from 36 ± 17 to 58 ± 18 cm H_2O), and MVV (from 21 ± 7 to 28 ± 7 L).[79] The Pa_{CO_2} decreased from 54 ± 6 to 45± 2 mm Hg. The number of hospital admissions and days of hospitalization after beginning partial ventilatory support were also reduced. Cropp and Dimarco[80] have reported similar improvements in the mean Pa_{CO_2} and resting maximal inspired and expired pressures after only 3 days of partial ventilatory support for periods of 3 hours daily in a smaller number of subjects with COPD. Improvement was observed after the initial 3-hour period of mechanical ventilation. Conversely, three other studies have failed to show any increase in respiratory muscle strength or exercise endurance with intermittent mechanical ventilation in patients with COPD.[81–83] Zibrak and coworkers[81] have treated 11 COPD patients with 2 to 7 hours of mechanical ventilation and found no difference in inspiratory muscle strength, exercise performance, gas exchange, or frequency of hospital admissions. Pluto and colleagues[82] have measured pulmonary function and lower leg cycle performance in five patients with COPD following 1 to 2 months of daily ventilatory support (4 to 7 hours daily). At the conclusion of the study period, they observed no improvement, either in exercise performance or inspiratory muscle function. Lee and associates[83] have prospectively randomized 12 COPD patients to pulmonary rehabilitation (five patients) or to daily negative-pressure ventilation plus pulmonary rehabilitation (seven patients). Similar degrees of severe airflow obstruction (FEV_1 0.59 ± 0.2 versus 0.66 ± 0.1 L) and hypercapnia (Pa_{CO_2} 46 ± 7 versus 42 ± 7 mm Hg) were present in both groups. After 3 weeks of inpatient therapy, no differences in respiratory muscle strength or exercise performance were found in the two groups.

There are many problems with evaluating the results of studies using intermittent mechanical ventilation to rest the respiratory muscles in patients with severe COPD. Most studies enrolled only small numbers of participants, lacked a proper control population, or were not conducted in a prospective or randomized fashion. Furthermore, there are major differences among these studies in terms of the length of ventilatory support and documentation that respiratory muscle rest actually occurred during mechanical ventilation.

A prospective randomized study is needed to determine the effects of intermittent respiratory muscle rest on respiratory muscle function in patients with severe COPD. Rochester and Martin[84] have proposed using clinical parameters of inspiratory muscle fatigue (e.g., decreased $P_{di\ max}$ or exercise endurance, elevated respiratory rate and Pa_{CO_2}, or paradoxical thoracoabdominal motion) to classify COPD patients.

THE EFFECT OF SUPPLEMENTAL OXYGEN ON EXERCISE PERFORMANCE

It is clear that the administration of supplemental oxygen can increase exercise performance in subjects with COPD.[85–93] Right ventricular function,[94] thoracoabdominal compliance,[95] and airway resistance[96] have been shown to improve during exercise with oxygen administration. The beneficial effects of breathing oxygen during exercise in subjects with severe COPD appear to be related to three factors: (1) a decrease in the work of breathing; (2) a delay in the onset of diaphragmatic fatigue; and (3) an alteration in the pattern of ventilatory muscle recruitment.

Inspiratory muscle fatigue appears to be a major factor limiting exercise performance in some patients with severe COPD.[55] Based on this information, attempts have been made to examine the relationship between the increase in exercise endurance observed with oxygen and its effects on respiratory muscle function. It has been suggested that breathing oxygen during exercise may have important effects on the respiratory muscles by reducing the mechanical load and improving contractile performance.[86–88]

Patients with severe COPD have a reduced exercise capability because of a limited ventilatory reserve, and may even breathe on the envelope of their maximum expiratory flow curve at rest.[97–99] To achieve the higher levels of ventilation demanded during exercise, these patients must increase inspiratory and expiratory flow. Some subjects with severe COPD increase end-expiratory lung volume during exercise, thereby allowing expiratory flow to increase.[55, 99, 100] Increases in end-expiratory lung volume, however, result in an increase in the inspiratory elastic work of breathing and in vigorous recruitment of the inspiratory intercostal-accessory muscles. This pattern of respiratory muscle recruitment results in higher positive end-expiratory gastric and pleural pressures than needed to produce maximal expiratory flow. Although the development of highly positive end-expiratory pressures was once considered to be "inefficient" in patients who breathe on the envelope of their flow-volume loop,[99, 101] several authors have suggested that this may be a mechanism to store elastic energy that can be used to assist or unload the inspiratory muscles during the next inspiration.[55, 86] Because the diaphragm appears to be flattened during hyperinflation, and its ability to generate force is severely impaired, a greater portion of the respiratory burden may be placed on the accessory inspiratory muscles and muscles of expiration.

Several studies have now shown that, at equivalent workloads, minute ventilation is significantly lower in subjects while breathing oxygen as compared to air.[85–87] It is believed that hyperoxia lowers the drive to breathe during exercise by minimizing the hypoxic stimulation to the peripheral chemoreceptors[94] and by delaying anaerobic metabolism with the development of lactic acidosis.[102–104] In addition, Scano and colleagues have shown that hyperoxia improves the mechanics of breathing in moderately severe COPD (FEV_1 = 1.45 ± 0.57 L).[95] They found that thoracoabdominal mechanics, as reflected by the $P_{0.1}/\dot{V}_E$ ratio and the $P_{0.1}/(V_T/T_I)$ ratio,* were significantly decreased while exercising with oxygen. They were uncertain whether the reductions in thoracic impedance were a result of a decrease in airway resistance or lung volume.

Bye and colleagues[86] have showed in a group of eight patients with moderate to severe airflow obstruction that endurance time during submaximal exercise doubled while breathing a 40% oxygen mixture. This increase in exercise performance was associated with a reduction both in minute ventilation (12%) and respiratory rate at equivalent points of time during exercise. Furthermore, while breathing oxygen, electromyographic signs of diaphragmatic fatigue (a fall in the high-to-low ratio) and paradoxical motion of the upper abdomen were delayed in five of eight patients. They concluded that endurance during submaximal exercise is increased by breathing oxygen because of decreased minute ventilation and delayed ventilatory muscle fatigue. Although the reduction in minute ventilation was small, large increases in endurance could result if the pressure-time index ($P_{di}/P_{di\ max} \times T_i/T_{tot}$) falls below the critical value necessary to cause respiratory muscle fatigue.

A reduction in the work of breathing with oxygen inhalation is not the sole factor contributing to improved exercise performance in COPD patients. For example, Bye and associates[87] studied six normal men breathing through an inspiratory resistor at a fixed minute ventilation and work of breathing while inspiring air or oxygen. The mean endurance time was 100% greater and the electromyographic pattern of diaphragmatic fatigue was delayed while subjects breathed with supplemental oxygen. Therefore, it appears that hyperoxia may also enhance diaphragmatic function by decreasing the production of metabolic products that have an adverse effect on skeletal muscle performance.

Hypoxia may also have significant detrimental effects on the accessory muscles of respiration. Criner and Celli[88] have studied six patients with severe COPD (FEV_1 = 0.66 ± 0.13 L) and mild hypoxemia (Pa_{O_2} 67 ± 2 mm Hg) and observed an increase in endurance time during leg cycling while inspiring 30% oxygen. Improvements in endurance were accompanied by a change in the pattern of ventilatory muscle recruitment.[88] Even though minute ventilation and breathing frequency were similar whether patients breathed air or 30% oxygen, the pattern of pleural and gastric pressures was significantly altered while breathing oxygen. The pattern of pleural and gastric pressures signified that the diaphragm was more active and that the accessory inspiratory muscles and muscles of expiration were less active (Fig. 56–3).

*Where $P_{0.1}$ is the change of mouth pressure in the first 0.1 second of inspiration, $\dot{V}_E$ is the resting minute ventilation requirement, and V_T/T_I is the mean inspiratory flow.

In conclusion, when COPD is severe, improved exercise performance can result from breathing oxygen. A portion of this improvement appears to be caused by effects of hyperoxia on the pattern of respiratory muscle activity and respiratory muscle endurance. More research is needed to determine whether the benefits of inspiring oxygen can be sustained on a chronic basis and to develop indices to predict which subjects with severe COPD will respond favorably to supplemental oxygen.

PHYSICAL THERAPY MODALITIES

Physical therapy modalities commonly used in treating patients with severe COPD can be divided into three major categories: (1) controlled breathing and postural exercises; (2) measures to enhance secretion mobilization; and (3) energy conservation techniques (i.e., educating patients to perform the activities of daily living in an energy-efficient fashion). These procedures improve the functional status of COPD patients and are an important part of a pulmonary rehabilitation program.

The importance of breathing pattern and its relationship to dyspnea has been recognized for well over a century. Several different modes of chest physiotherapy that alter breathing pattern have been found to reduce dyspnea in subjects with COPD, including the following: pursed-lip breathing; the assumption of a head-down or leaning-forward posture; abdominal strapping; and controlled slow or diaphragmatic breathing. Postulated mechanisms whereby these maneuvers cause a reduction in dyspnea include a decrease in minute ventilation, an improvement in gas exchange, and an increase in the mechanical advantage of the diaphragm.

Since the time of Laennec, subjects with severe COPD have been observed to reduce their respiratory effort during pursed-lip breathing.[106] Several studies have examined the physiologic basis for this effect. Thomas and colleagues compared respiratory rate, tidal volume, Pa_{CO_2}, and end-expiratory lung volume during eupneic breathing in subjects with severe COPD during pursed-lip breathing and slow breathing without pursed-lips.[107] Similar reductions in the respiratory rate and the Pa_{CO_2} and increases in tidal volume were observed during pursed-lip and slow breathing. Values for end-expiratory lung volume were similar during the different breathing patterns. The authors concluded that pursed-lip breathing improves gas exchange in poorly ventilated lung zones and that this mechanism causes a reduction in the Pa_{CO_2}.[107]

Mueller and coworkers[108] obtained similar results when they studied the effects of pursed-lip breathing at rest and during exercise in 12 subjects with severe COPD. Pursed-lip breathing was associated with tidal volume increases, slowing of respiratory rate, and reduction in minute ventilation and the ventilatory equivalent for oxygen uptake. Symptomatic relief of dyspnea correlated with the decrease in respiratory rate and increase in tidal volume. The ventilatory equivalent for O_2 uptake was reduced during pursed-lip breathing, but the total O_2 uptake was similar with and without pursed-lip breathing. It was concluded that the work of breathing is not significantly altered during pursed-lip breathing, because the total O_2 uptake remains unchanged.[108]

Barach[106] and others have challenged the assertion that pursed-lip breathing relieves dyspnea solely by reducing respiratory rate. Barach observed that patients experience a decrease in dyspnea at the onset of pursed-lip breathing, which is too rapid to be explained by better gas exchange or a reduction in respiratory rate. Furthermore, Paul and colleagues[109] have noted that voluntary reductions in respiratory rate in ten subjects with severe COPD made them more uncomfortable, even though total ventilation was reduced.

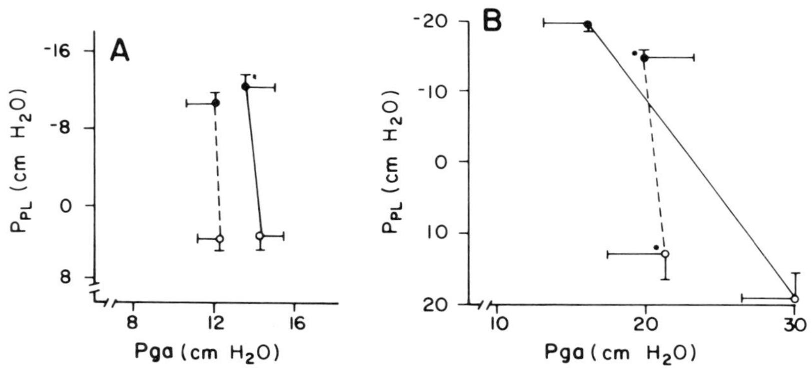

Figure 56–3. Pattern of pleural (P_{pl}) and gastric (P_{ga}) pressures with air and O_2 breathing at rest *(A)* and again during exercise *(B)*. Values at end-inspiration *(filled circles)* and end-exhalation *(open circles)* are shown breathing air *(solid line)* or 30% O_2 *(dashed line)*. Note that the pattern of P_{pl} and P_{ga} pressures remained similar during 30% O_2 and air breathing at rest, although the transdiaphragmatic pressure during inspiration was lower with inspiration of 30% O_2. During exercise, however, not only was the transdiaphragmatic pressure lower during O_2 breathing, but the pattern of end-inspiratory and end-expiratory P_{pl} and P_{ga} was different as compared with O_2-air breathing. With oxygen, at end-inspiration, the P_{ga} became more positive and the P_{pl} less negative than while breathing air. Moreover, P_{pl} and P_{ga} at end-expiration were significantly lower. (Reproduced with permission from Criner GJ, Celli BR. J Appl Physiol 1987; 63:195–200.)

Ingram and Schilder[110] have offered an alternative explanation for the relief of dyspnea during pursed-lip breathing. They found that five of eight patients who claimed relief of dyspnea during pursed-lip breathing had spirometric evidence suggesting tracheobronchial collapse. During pursed-lip breathing, these five patients had a greater decrease in pulmonary resistance than those who did not experience relief. The authors concluded that pursed-lip breathing, by preventing large airway collapse, causes symptomatic relief of dyspnea, and that alteration in the length-tension relationship of the respiratory muscles is an additional explanation for the reduction in dyspnea during pursed-lip breathing.[110] This latter hypothesis remains tenuous, however, because most investigators have failed to show alterations in end-expiratory lung volume during pursed-lip breathing.

Many dyspneic patients with COPD derive immediate relief on assuming a head-down or leaning-forward position. Barach and Beck[112] found that the minute ventilation for a group of 24 emphysematous patients was 22% less when the patients were tilted head-down in a slight Trendelenburg position at an angle between 12° and 20° as compared with the sitting position. In subjects who had blood gas tensions measured in both positions, the decrease in minute ventilation in the head-down position was associated with a 3% to 8% increase in oxygen saturation in six patients and an increase in the $Pa{CO_2}$ of 4 to 5 mm Hg in two of ten patients, respectively. Diaphragmatic excursions monitored by fluoroscopy in 15 of these patients were found to be 2 to 3.5 cm greater when patients were maintained in a head-down position. The authors concluded that the reduction in dyspnea and decrease in accessory inspiratory muscle activity that occur when patients are placed in a supine position are related to an increase in the effectiveness of diaphragmatic contraction.[112] They also suggested that cephalad displacement of the diaphragm by gravitational effects on the abdominal contents improves its contractile performance.

Further evidence that alterations in posture may reduce dyspnea in subjects with COPD by improving diaphragmatic function has been provided by Sharp and colleagues.[113, 114] They measured gastric, esophageal, and transdiaphragmatic pressures and carried out electromyography of the diaphragm and several accessory inspiratory muscles in 17 COPD patients during tidal breathing in the supine, standing, seated-erect, and leaning-forward positions.[113] Paradoxical motion of the upper abdomen during inspiration was observed when the seven most severely hyperinflated patients were standing or sitting erect. Resolution of the paradoxical breathing pattern occurred in all patients with assumption of a leaning-forward posture and in an additional three patients while in the supine position. Electromyographic activity and the pattern of pleural and gastric pressure changes suggested greater activity of the accessory inspiratory muscles when patients are erect or seated. Conversely, in these positions, the diaphragmatic contribution to breathing appeared to be less. On the other hand, in the supine or leaning-forward position, relief of dyspnea was associated with a greater transdiaphragmatic pressure but a reduction in diaphragm EMG activity and sternocleidomastoid EMG activity. These results suggest that assumption of the supine or leaning-forward position improves diaphragm length and its mechanical efficiency in transducing electrical activity into pressure, and thereby avoids overtaxing the accessory inspiratory muscles.

Posturally related improvements in diaphragmatic function have also been observed during exercise. Delgado and associates[52] have shown in two patients with severe COPD that treadmill exercise performed while they were flexed forward 45° at the waist alleviated paradoxical respiration. In addition, the sensation of dyspnea was reduced and exercise performance was improved in this posture. Only one of the two patients, however, showed an improvement in diaphragmatic function (i.e., higher peak inspiratory pressure and a greater peak inspiratory flow) while leaning forward. Therefore, there may be additional but as yet obscure benefits in relieving dyspnea and improving exercise performance by leaning forward.

Several investigators have attempted to improve the function of the diaphragm by using abdominal weights, abdominal strapping, or even pneumoperitoneum to displace that muscle mechanically toward the optimal portion of its length-tension curve.[115–118] Dodd and coworkers[115] have studied the effects of abdominal strapping on chest wall mechanics in seven COPD subjects with severe hyperinflation. They found that, although abdominal strapping resulted in a 40% increase in transdiaphragmatic pressure generation, it precipitated intense dyspnea and significantly reduced endurance during leg cycling. They suggested that abdominal strapping produces dyspnea by adversely affecting the ventilatory activity of the accessory inspiratory muscles and not by precipitating diaphragmatic fatigue. Because the resting volume of the thoracic cage was greater during abdominal strapping, the inspiratory muscles of the rib cage may have been forced to operate over a less effective portion of their length-tension curve. Furthermore, abdominal strapping prevented rapid relaxation of the abdominal muscles at end-expiration and consequently limited the potential of the abdominal muscles to assist the inspiratory muscles by rapidly relaxing and hence decreasing intra-abdominal pressure.

Celli and colleagues[116] have evaluated the effects of abdominal strapping on exercise performance in a subject with severe COPD (FEV_1 = 0.63 L) and a large ventral hernia. In this patient, reduction of the ventral hernia by an abdominal binder was associated with an approximately 100% increase in maximal transdiaphragmatic pressure, a decrease in thoracoabdominal paradox, and an increase in oxygen saturation. Furthermore, the sensation of dyspnea was less while the abdomen was bound and exercise performance as assessed by distance walked was enhanced.

Therefore, in selected individuals with severe COPD, abdominal strapping may improve diaphragmatic function, increase exercise endurance, and markedly reduce the sensation of dyspnea.

For many years abdominal-diaphragmatic breathing was thought to be an important adjunct in the rehabilitation of patients with severe COPD. Proposed benefits of this form of breathing have included more even distribution of inspired gas, an increase in ventilatory efficiency, and improved respiratory mechanics. Although some COPD patients claim a reduction in dyspnea during diaphragmatic breathing, there is generally a lack of objective evidence showing that ventilatory parameters improve following diaphragmatic breathing[119–122] or that diaphragmatic breathing improves the distribution of inspired gas.[123–127]

The only study demonstrating a favorable effect of diaphragmatic breathing was that of Miller.[119] The effects of diaphragmatic breathing on ventilatory mechanics, maximum expiratory pressure, oxygen saturation, and diaphragmatic excursion were examined in 24 patients with chronic bronchopulmonary disorders (13 patients had asthma or chronic asthmatic bronchitis).[119] Patients were studied at baseline and then after 6 to 8 weeks of daily diaphragmatic breathing (five or six training periods daily). All patients were first treated with bronchodilators, secretion control, and abstinence from smoking. After the period of diaphragmatic breathing training, significant increases in diaphragmatic excursion, vital capacity, tidal volume, maximum expiratory pressure, and oxygen saturation were observed and the respiratory rate and Pa_{CO_2} were decreased. Miller concluded that diaphragmatic breathing training increases diaphragmatic movement and produces a more efficient pattern of respiration.[119]

Miller's findings contrast with those of Becklake and colleagues,[120] who found no difference in vital capacity after a period of breathing exercises or breathing exercises supplemented with electrical stimulation of the chest and abdominal muscles. Results similar to those of Becklake and associates[120] were also reported by Sinclair[121] and by McNeill and McKenzie.[122] None of these investigators could demonstrate alterations in ventilation or in the pattern of breathing following an extended period of breathing exercises.

The regional distribution of ventilation in animals and normal subjects appears to correlate with regional changes in chest wall shape and the adjacent pleural pressure.[127] Minh and associates[128] have shown that electrophrenic stimulation of the diaphragm in supine dogs generates pleural pressures that are most negative over the lower lobes. Roussos and coworkers[129] have demonstrated that voluntary contraction of specific inspiratory muscles in normal human volunteers alters the distribution of inspired gas. In that study there were different distributions of inspired gas assessed by ^{133}Xe or by the helium bolus washout technique during three different breathing patterns—normal breathing, preferential contraction of the accessory inspiratory muscles, and abdominal-diaphragmatic breathing, when the tracer gas was inhaled from functional residual capacity. The distribution of boluses administered at residual volume, however, was not affected by changes in the pattern of muscle use.

Sackner and coworkers found similar results in five of eight normal subjects who could redirect a bolus of radioactive xenon to the lower lung zones during diaphragmatic breathing.[124] Additionally, they studied 11 subjects with COPD by analysis of nitrogen washout curves, but found no alteration in the distribution of ventilation during diaphragmatic breathing.[125] Furthermore, the inspiration of radioactive xenon in five of these COPD subjects failed to show any topographic variation in ventilatory distribution during diaphragmatic breathing. The observed difference in the distribution of ventilation between normal and COPD subjects was explained by the suggestion that the COPD patients had less voluntary control over diaphragmatic movement in the presence of severe hyperinflation.[124]

Two additional reports in subjects with COPD have confirmed the findings of Sackner and colleagues[124] by failing to show diaphragmatic breathing changes in the distribution of ventilation during diaphragmatic breathing.[126, 127] Therefore, at present, there is no objective evidence to support the hypothesis that diaphragmatic breathing improves ventilation-perfusion relationships in COPD by preferentially increasing ventilation of the lung bases.

Another proposed benefit of abdominal-diaphragmatic breathing in COPD is that it increases the mechanical efficiency of respiration, but results of studies of thoracoabdominal motion during diaphragmatic breathing suggest that this is not the case.[123, 124] Willeput and associates[123] used magnetometers to monitor thoracoabdominal movement in 11 subjects with COPD as a chest physiotherapist coached subjects to achieve various breathing patterns. Subjects were studied in the seated position while breathing spontaneously and during each of five imposed breathing patterns. These five breathing patterns were designed to alter the end-expiratory volume (three exercises) or to emphasize either the diaphragm or the thoracic inspiratory muscles. During imposed breathing patterns, as compared to spontaneous breathing, the respiratory rate was reduced and tidal volume increased. During diaphragmatic breathing, however, the reduction in respiratory rate was not always offset by an increase in tidal volume. Dyssynchronous and paradoxical movements of the rib cage were frequently observed during abdominal-diaphragmatic breathing. Nine of the 11 COPD subjects had outward movement of the rib cage during expiration, whereas the other two subjects had paradoxical inward motion.

Sackner and coworkers[124] have monitored thoracoabdominal motion during diaphragmatic breathing by the use of respiratory inductive plethysmography in ten normal subjects and in nine patients with severe COPD. Subjects were studied in the supine position and no effort was made to reduce their respiratory frequency. In both normal subjects and COPD patients, abdominal-diaphragmatic breathing was associated with asynchronous and paradoxical breathing movements.

Both Willeput and colleagues[123] and Sackner and associates[124] concluded that diaphragmatic breathing may actually cause a distortion of the rib cage and abdomen and produce a mechanically less efficient form of breathing. The role of diaphragmatic breathing in the pulmonary rehabilitation of COPD patients is not clear at present. Further study is needed to determine whether the subjective reduction in dyspnea noted by some patients during this breathing pattern is related to a placebo effect or to some as yet unidentified physiologic mechanism.

The results of most studies indicate that comprehensive rehabilitation programs incorporating some form of exercise reconditioning of the limbs produce beneficial effects on the quality of life, exercise performance, and, perhaps, even the prognosis of most subjects with advanced COPD. At present, it appears reasonable to offer these forms of treatment to those who have achieved maximal improvement in lung mechanics and gas exchange but in whom extreme dyspnea limits their ability to exercise or perform the activities of daily living. Studies of the effects of exercise training on respiratory and cardiac function have not elucidated the precise mechanism(s) that underlie the benefits derived. The involvement of the respiratory muscles in this process, however, has attracted great interest and is under intense investigation. In addition to ignorance about mechanisms, many questions related to practical issues remain, including uncertainty about the precise nature of the training program that might achieve maximal benefit, characteristics of patients most likely to achieve the greatest benefits, and the manner in which any benefits derived could be maintained after the program has ended.

REFERENCES

1. Morgan AD, Peck DF, Buchanan DR, McHardy GJR. Effect of attitudes and belief on exercise tolerance in chronic bronchitis. Br Med J 1983; 286:171–173.
2. Robinson EP, Kjeldgaard JM. Improvement in ventilatory muscle function with running. J Appl Physiol 1982; 52:1400–1406.
3. Agle DP, Baum GL, Chester EH, et al. Multidisciplinary treatment of chronic pulmonary insufficiency: Psychological aspects of rehabilitation. Psychosom Med 1973; 35:41–49.
4. Watt PW, Kelly FJ, Goldspink DF, Goldspink G. Exercise-induced morphological and biochemical changes in skeletal muscles of the rat. J Appl Physiol 1982; 53:1144–1151.
5. Make B, Gilmartin M, Brody JS, Snider GL. Rehabilitation of ventilator-dependent subjects with lung diseases: The concept and initial experience. Chest 1984; 86:358–365.
6. Leith DE. Target device for regulating ventilation during voluntary hyperpnea. J Appl Physiol 1983; 55:1932–1935.
7. Martin B, Heintzelman M, Chen H. Exercise performance after ventilatory work. J Appl Physiol 1982; 52:1581–1585.
8. Braun NMT, Faulkner J, Hughes RL, et al. When should respiratory muscles be exercised? Chest 1983; 84:76–84.
9. Martin BJ, Chen H, Kolka MA. Anaerobic metabolism of the respiratory muscles during exercise. Med Sci Sports Exerc 1984; 16:72–86.
10. Belman MJ, Kendregan BA. Physical training fails to improve ventilatory muscle endurance in patients with chronic obstructive pulmonary disease. Chest 1982; 81:440–443.
11. Levine S, Weiser P, Gillen J. Evaluation of a ventilatory muscle endurance training program in the rehabilitation of patients with chronic obstructive pulmonary disease. Am Rev Respir Dis 1986; 133:400–406.
12. Belman MJ, Mittman C. Ventilatory muscle training improves exercise capacity in chronic obstructive pulmonary disease patients. Am Rev Respir Dis 1980; 121:273–280.
13. Chen H, Dukes R, Martin BJ. Inspiratory muscle training in patients with chronic obstructive pulmonary disease. Am Rev Respir Dis 1985; 131:251–255.
14. Jederlinic P, Muspratt JA, Miller MJ. Physiologic conditioning or habituation to suffocation? Chest 1984; 86:870–873.
15. Sonne LJ, Davis JA. Increased exercise performance in patients with severe COPD following inspiratory resistive training. Chest 1982; 81:436–439.
16. Pardy RL, Rivington RN, Despas PJ, et al. The effects of inspiratory muscle training on exercise performance in chronic airflow limitation. Am Rev Respir Dis 1981; 123:426–433.
17. Petty TL. Pulmonary rehabilitation. Basics RD 1975; 4:1–6.
18. Cherniack RM, Handford RG, Svanhill E. Home care of chronic respiratory disease. JAMA 1969; 208:821–824.
19. Hudson LD, Tyler ML, Petty TL. Hospitalization needs during an outpatient rehabilitation program for severe chronic airway obstruction. Chest 1979; 70:606–610.
20. Nicholas JJ, Gilbert R, Gabe R, Auchincloss JH Jr. Evaluation of an exercise therapy program for patients with chronic obstructive pulmonary disease. Am Rev Respir Dis 1970; 102:1–9.
21. Degre S, Sergysels R, Messin R, et al. Hemodynamic responses to physical training in patients with chronic lung disease. Am Rev Respir Dis 1974; 110:395–402.
22. Paez PN, Phillipson EA, Masangkay M, Sproule BJ. The physiologic basis of training patients with emphysema. Am Rev Respir Dis 1967; 95:944–953.
23. Alpert JS, Bass H, Szucs MM, et al. Effects of physical training on hemodynamics and pulmonary function at rest and during exercise in patients with chronic obstructive pulmonary disease. Chest 1974; 66:647–651.
24. Casciari RJ, Fairshter RD, Harrison A, et al. Effects of breathing retraining in patients with chronic obstructive pulmonary disease. Chest 1981; 79:393–398.
25. McGavin CR, Gupta SP, McHardy GJR. Twelve-minute walking test for assessing disability in chronic bronchitis. Br Med J 1976; 1:822–823.
26. Lertzman MM, Cherniack RM. Rehabilitation of patients with chronic obstructive pulmonary disease. Am Rev Respir Dis 1976; 114:1145–1165.
27. Hodgkin JE, Farrell JE, Gipson MJ, et al. Pulmonary rehabilitation. Am Rev Respir Dis 1981; 124:663–668.
28. Tydeman DE, Chandler AR, Graveling BM, et al. An investigation into the effects of exercise tolerance training on patients with chronic airways obstruction. Physiotherapy 1984; 70:261–264.
29. Moser KM, Bokinsky GE, Savage RT, et al. Physiologic and functional effects of patients with chronic obstructive pulmonary disease. Arch Intern Med 1980; 140:1596–1601.
30. Belman MJ, Kendregan BA. Exercise training fails to increase skeletal muscle enzymes in patients with chronic obstructive pulmonary disease. Am Rev Respir Dis 1981; 123:256–261.
31. Spiro SG, Hahn HL, Edwards RHT, Pride NB. An analysis of the physiological strain of submaximal exercise in patients with chronic obstructive bronchitis. Thorax 1975; 30:415–425.
32. Cockcroft AE, Saunders MJ, Berry G. Randomized controlled trial of rehabilitation in chronic respiratory disability. Thorax 1981; 36:200–203.
33. Mungall IPF, Hainsworth R. An objective assessment of the value of exercise training to patients with chronic obstructive airways disease. Q J Med 1980; 193:77–85.
34. Vyas MN, Banister EW, Morton JW, Grzybowski S. Response to exercise in patients with chronic airway obstruction. Am Rev Respir Dis 1971; 103:390–399.
35. Chester EH, Belman MJ, Bahler RC, et al. The effect of physical training on cardiopulmonary performance in patients with chronic obstructive pulmonary disease. Chest 1977; 72:695–702.
36. Weil JV, McCullough RE, Cline JS, et al. Diminished ventilatory response to hypoxia and hypercapnia after morphine in normal man. N Engl J Med 1975; 292:1103–1106.
37. Sinclair DJM, Ingram CG. Controlled trial of supervised exercise training in chronic bronchitis. Br Med J 1980; 280:519–521.
38. Criner GJ, Celli BR. Effect of unsupported arm exercise on ventilatory muscle recruitment in patients with severe chronic airflow obstruction. Am Rev Respir Dis 1988; 138:856–861.
39. Arora NS, Rochester DF. Respiratory muscle strength and maximal voluntary ventilation in undernourished patients. Am Rev Respir Dis 1982; 126:5–8.
40. Arora NS, Rochester DF. Effect of body weight and muscularity on human diaphragm muscle mass, thickness and area. J Appl Physiol 1982; 52:64–70.
41. Aubier M, Trippenbach T, Roussos C. Respiratory muscle fatigue during cardiogenic shock. J Appl Physiol 1981; 51:499–508.
42. Santiago TV, Pugliesi AC, Edelman NH. Control of breathing during methadone addiction. Am J Med 1977; 62:347–354.

42a. Belman MJ, Thomas SF, Lewis MI. Resistive breathing training in patients with chronic obstructive pulmonary disease. Chest 1986; 90:663–670.

43. Bellemare F, Wight D, Lavigne CM, Grassino A. Effect of tension and timing of contraction on the blood flow of the diaphragm. J Appl Physiol 1983; 54:1597–1606.
44. Bye PTP, Esau SA, Walley KR, et al. Ventilatory muscles during exercise in air and oxygen in normal man. J Appl Physiol 1984; 56:464–471.
45. Duchateau J, Hainaut K. Isometric or dynamic training: Differential effects on mechanical properties of a human muscle. J Appl Physiol 1984; 56:296–301.
46. Farkas GA, Roussos C. Adaptability of the hamster diaphragm to exercise and/or emphysema. J Appl Physiol 1982; 53:1263–1272.
47. Keens TG, Chen V, Patel P, O'Brien P. Cellular adaptations of the ventilatory muscles to a chronic increased respiratory load. J Appl Physiol 1978; 44:905–908.
48. Leith DE, Bradley M. Ventilatory muscle strength and endurance training. J Appl Physiol 1976; 41:508–516.
49. Kryger MH, Yacoub O, Dosman J, et al. Effect of meperidine on occlusion pressure responses to hypercapnia and hypoxia with

and without external resistance. Am Rev Respir Dis 1976; 114:333–340.
50. Stubbing DG, Pengelly LD, Morse JLC, Jones NL. Pulmonary mechanics during exercise in subjects with chronic airflow obstruction. J Appl Physiol 1980; 49:511–515.
51. Loke J, Mahler DA, Paulman SF, et al. Exercise impairment in chronic obstructive pulmonary disease. Clin Chest Med 1984; 5:121–143.
52. Delgado HR, Braun SR, Skatrud JB, et al. Chest wall and abdominal motion during exercise in patients with chronic obstructive pulmonary disease. Am Rev Respir Dis 1982; 126:200–205.
53. Potter WA, Olafsson S, Hyatt RE. Ventilatory mechanisms and expiratory flow limitation during exercise in patients with obstructive lung disease. J Clin Invest 1971; 50:910–919.
54. Dodd DS, Brancatisano T, Engel LA. Chest wall mechanics during exercise in patients with severe chronic airflow obstruction. Am Rev Respir Dis 1984; 129:33–38.
55. Dodd DS, Brancatisano T, Engel LA. Chest wall mechanics during exercise in patients with severe chronic air-flow obstruction. Am Rev Respir Dis 1984; 129:33–38.
56. Celli BR, Rassulo J, Make BJ. Dyssynchronous breathing during arm but not leg exercise in patients with chronic airflow obstruction. N Engl J Med 1986; 314:1485–1490.
57. Criner GJ, Rassulo J, Celli BR. Respiratory muscle recruitment during unsupported and supported arm exercise in patients with severe chronic obstructive pulmonary disease (COPD). Chest 1985; 85:14S.
58. Celli BR, Criner GJ, Rassulo R. Ventilatory muscle recruitment during unsupported arm exercise in normal subjects. J Appl Physiol 1988; 64:1936–1941.
59. Macklem PT, Gross D, Grassino A. Partitioning of inspiratory pressure swings between the diaphragm and intercostal accessory muscles. J Appl Physiol 1978; 44:200–208.
59a. Tangri S, Woolf CR. The breathing pattern in chronic obstructive lung disease during the performance of some common daily activities. Chest 1973; 63:126–127.
60. Bellemare F, Grassino A. Force reserve of the diaphragm in patients with chronic obstructive pulmonary disease. J Appl Physiol 1983; 55:8–15.
61. Jones NL, Jones G, Edwards RHT. Exercise tolerance in chronic airways obstruction. Am Rev Respir Dis 1971; 103:477–491.
62. Roussos C, Macklem PT. The respiratory muscles. N Engl J Med 1982; 307:787–797.
63. Roussos CS, Macklem PT. Diaphragmatic fatigue in man. J Appl Physiol 1977; 43:189–197.
64. Bellemare F, Grassino A. Evaluation of human diaphragm fatigue. J Appl Physiol 1982; 53:1196–1206.
65. Bryant S, Edward RHT, Faulkner JA, et al. Respiratory muscle failure: Fatigue or weakness? The role of theophylline. Chest 1986; 89:116–124.
66. Jones DA, Bigland-Ritchie B, Edwards RHT. Excitation frequency and muscle fatigue: Mechanical responses during voluntary and stimulated contraction. Exp Neurol 1979; 64:401–413.
67. Edwards RHT, Mill DK, Jones DA, Merton PA. Fatigue of long duration in human skeletal muscle after exercise. J Physiol 1977; 272:769–778.
68. Aubier M, Farkas G, DeTroyer A, et al. Detection of diaphragmatic fatigue in man by phrenic stimulation. J Appl Physiol 1981; 50:538–544.
69. Sharp JT. Therapeutic considerations in respiratory muscle function. Chest 1985; 88:1185–1235.
70. Aubier M, DeTroyer A, Sampson M, et al. Aminophylline improves diaphragmatic contractility. N Engl J Med 1981; 305:249–252.
71. Pardy RL, Rivington RN, Depas PJ, Macklem PT. Respiratory muscle training compared with physiotherapy in patients with chronic airflow obstruction. Am Rev Respir Dis 1981; 123:421–425.
72. Wilson DO, Rogers RM, Sanders M, et al. Nutritional intervention in patients with emphysema. Am Rev Respir Dis 1986; 134:672–677.
73. Curran FJ. Night ventilation by body respirators for patients in chronic respiratory failure due to late stage Duchenne muscular dystrophy. Arch Phys Med Rehabil 1981; 62:270–274.
74. Garay SM, Turino GM, Goldring RM. Sustained reversal of chronic hypercapnia in patients with alveolar hypoventilation syndromes. Am J Med 1981; 70:269–274.
75. Stein DA, Bradley BL, Miller WC. Mechanisms of oxygen effects on exercise in patients with chronic obstructive pulmonary disease. Chest 1982; 81:6–10.
75a. Wiers PWJ, Lecoultre R, Dallinga OT, et al. Cuirass respiratory treatment of chronic respiratory failure in scoliotic patients. Thorax 1977; 32:221–228.
76. Splaingard ML, Frates RC, Jefferson LS, et al. Home negative pressure ventilation: Report of 20 years of experience in patients with neuromuscular disease. Arch Phys Med Rehabil 1985; 66:239–242.
77. Marino W, Braun NMT. Reversal of the clinical sequelae of respiratory muscle fatigue by intermittent mechanical ventilation. Am Rev Respir Dis 1982; 125(Suppl):85.
78. Celli BR, Rassulo J, Corral R. Ventilatory muscle dysfunction in patients with bilateral idiopathic diaphragmatic paralysis: Reversal by intermittent external negative pressure ventilation. Am Rev Respir Dis 1987; 136:1276–1278.
79. Braun NMT, Marino WD. Effect of daily intermittent rest of respiratory muscles in patients with severe airflow limitation (CAO). Chest 1984; 85(Suppl):59–60.
80. Cropp A, Dimarco AF. Effects of intermittent negative pressure ventilation on respiratory muscle function in patients with severe chronic obstructive pulmonary disease. Am Rev Respir Dis 1987; 135:1056–1061.
81. Zibrak JD, Federman EC, Jua SL, et al. Effects of negative pressure ventilatory assistance on pulmonary function in severe COPD. Chest 1986; 89(Suppl):515.
82. Pluto LA, Fahey PJ, Sorenson L, Chandrashekan AJ. Effect of eight weeks of intermittent negative pressure ventilation on exercise parameters in patients with severe chronic obstructive lung disease. Am Rev Respir Dis 1985; 131:A164.
83. Lee H, Criner G, Rassulo J, et al. A controlled study of rehabilitation vs. rehabilitation and respiratory muscle resting with negative external ventilation in patients with severe COPD. Am Rev Respir Dis 1985; 133:A168.
84. Rochester DF, Martin LL. Respiratory muscle rest. In: Roussos C, Macklem PT, eds. The Thorax. New York: Marcel Dekker, 1985, 1303–1328.
85. Bradley BL, Garner AE, Billiu J, et al. Oxygen-assisted exercise in chronic obstructive lung disease: The effect on exercise capacity and arterial blood gas tensions. Am Rev Respir Dis 1978; 118:239–243.
86. Bye PTP, Esau SA, Levy RD, et al. Ventilatory muscle function during exercise in air and oxygen in patients with chronic airflow limitation. Am Rev Respir Dis 1985; 132:236–240.
87. Bye PTP, Esau SA, Walley KR, et al. Ventilatory muscles during exercise in air and oxygen in normal men. J Appl Physiol 1984; 56:464–471.
88. Criner GJ, Celli BR. Ventilatory muscle recruitment in exercise with O_2 in obstructed patients with mild hypoxemia. J Appl Physiol 1987; 63:195–200.
89. Cotes JE, Gilson JC. Effect of oxygen on exercise ability in chronic respiratory insufficiency. Use of portable apparatus. Lancet 1956; i:872–876.
90. Pardy RL, Bye PTP. Diaphragmatic fatigue in normoxia and hyperoxia. J Appl Physiol 1985; 3:738–742.
91. Pierce AK, Paez PN, Miller WF. Exercise training with the aid of a portable oxygen supply in patients with emphysema. Am Rev Respir Dis 1965; 91:653–659.
92. Raimondi AC, Edwards RHT, Denison DM, et al. Exercise tolerance breathing a low-density gas mixture, 35% oxygen and air in patients with chronic obstructive bronchitis. Clin Sci 1970; 39:675–685.
93. Woodcock AA, Geddes DM, Gross ER. Oxygen relieves breathlessness in "pink puffers." Lancet 1981; i:907–909.
94. Olvey SK, Redutor LA, Stevens PM, et al. First-pass radionuclide assessment of right and left ventricular ejection fraction in chronic pulmonary disease. Chest 1980; 78:4–9.
95. Scano G, VanMeerhaeghe A, Willeput R, et al. Effect of oxygen on breathing during exercise in patients with chronic lung disease. Eur J Respir Dis 1982; 63:23–30.
96. Libby DM, Briscoe WA, King TKC. Relief of hypoxia-related bronchoconstriction by breathing 30% oxygen. Am Rev Respir Dis 1981; 123:171–175.
97. Hyatt RE. The interrelationships of pressure, flow and volume during various respiratory maneuvers in normal and emphysematous subjects. Am Rev Respir Dis 1961; 83:676–683.

98. Takishima T, Grimby G, Graham W, et al. Flow-volume curves during quiet breathing, maximum voluntary ventilation and forced vital capacities in patients with obstructive lung disease. Scand J Respir Dis 1967; 48:384–393.
99. Grimby G, Striksa J. Flow-volume curves and breathing patterns during exercise in patients with obstructive lung disease. Scand J Clin Lab Invest 1970; 25:303–313.
100. Stubbing DD, Pengelly LD, Morse JL, Jones NL. Pulmonary mechanics during exercise in subjects with chronic airflow limitation. J Appl Physiol 1980; 49:511–515.
101. Potter WA, Olafsson S, Hyatt RE. Ventilatory mechanisms and expiratory flow limitation during exercise in patients with obstructive lung disease. J Clin Invest 1971; 50:910–919.
102. Adams RP, Welch HG. Oxygen uptake, acid-base status and performance with varied inspired oxygen fractions. J Appl Physiol 1980; 49:863–868.
103. Jones NL, Sutton JR, Taylor R, Toews CJ. Effects of pH on cardiorespiratory and metabolic responses to exercise. J Appl Physiol 1977; 43:959–964.
104. Linnarsson D, Karlsson J, Fagraeus L, Saltin B. Muscle metabolites and oxygen deficit with exercise in hypoxia and hyperoxia. J Appl Physiol 1974; 36:399–402.
105. Santiago TV, Johnson J, Riley DJ, et al. Effects of morphine on ventilatory response to exercise. J Appl Physiol 1979; 47:112–118.
106. Barach AL. Physiologic advantages of grunting, groaning and pursed-lip breathing: Adaptive symptoms related to the development of continuous positive pressure breathing. Bull NY Acad Med 1973; 49:666–673.
107. Thomas RL, Stoker GL, Ross JC. The efficacy of pursed-lips breathing in patients with chronic obstructive pulmonary disease. Am Rev Respir Dis 1965; 93:103–106.
108. Mueller RE, Petty TL, Filley GF. Ventilation and arterial blood gas changes induced by pursed-lips breathing. J Appl Physiol 1970; 28:784–789.
109. Paul G, Eldridge F, Mitchell J, Feine T. Some effects of slowing respiration rate in chronic emphysema and bronchitis. J Appl Physiol 1966; 21:877–882.
110. Ingram RH, Schilder DP. Effect of pursed-lips expiration on the pulmonary pressure-flow relationship in obstructive lung disease. Am Rev Respir Dis 1967; 96:381–383.
111. Campbell EJM, Howell JB. The sensation of breathlessness. Br Med Bull 1963; 19:36–40.
112. Barach AL, Beck GJ. The ventilatory effects of the head-down position in pulmonary emphysema. Am J Med 1954; 16:55–60.
113. Sharp JT, Druz WS, Moisan T, et al. Postural relief of dyspnea in severe chronic obstructive pulmonary disease. Am Rev Respir Dis 1980; 122:201–211.
114. Druz WS, Sharp JT. Electrical and mechanical activity of the diaphragm accompanying body position in severe chronic obstructive pulmonary disease. Am Rev Respir Dis 1982; 125:275–280.
115. Dodd DS, Brancatisano TP, Engel LA. Effect of abdominal strapping on chest wall mechanics during exercise in patients with severe chronic airflow obstruction. Am Rev Respir Dis 1985; 131:816–821.
116. Celli BR, Rassulo J, Berman JS, Make B. Respiratory consequences of abdominal hernia in a patient with severe chronic obstructive pulmonary disease. Am Rev Respir Dis 1985; 131:178–180.
117. Gayrard P, Becker M, Bergofsky EM. The effect of abdominal weights on diaphragmatic position and excursion in man. Clin Sci 1968; 35:589–601.
118. Callaway JJ, McKusick VA. Carbon dioxide intoxication in emphysema: Emergency treatment by artificial pneumoperitoneum. N Engl J Med 1951; 245:9–13.
119. Miller WF. A physiologic evaluation of the effects of diaphragmatic breathing training in patients with chronic pulmonary emphysema. Am J Med 1954; 17:471–477.
120. Becklake MR, McGregor M, Goldman HI, Braudo JL. A study of the effects of physiotherapy in chronic hypertrophic emphysema using lung function tests. Dis Chest 1954; 16:180–191.
121. Sinclair JD. The effect of breathing exercise in pulmonary emphysema. Thorax 1955; 10:246–249.
122. McNeill RS, McKenzie JM. An assessment of the value of breathing exercise in pulmonary emphysema. Thorax 1955; 10:250–252.
123. Willeput R, Vachaudez JP, Lenders D, et al. Thoracoabdominal motion during chest physiotherapy in patients affected by chronic obstructive lung disease. Respiration 1983; 44:204–214.
124. Sackner MA, Gonzalez HF, Jenousi G, Rodriguez M. Effects of abdominal and thoracic breathing on breathing pattern components in normal subjects and in patients with chronic obstructive pulmonary disease. Am Rev Respir Dis 1984; 130:584–587.
125. Sackner MA, Silva G, Banks JM, et al. Distribution of ventilation during diaphragmatic breathing in obstructive lung disease. Am Rev Respir Dis 1974; 109:331–337.
126. Brach BB, Chao RP, Sgroi VL, et al. ^{133}Xenon washout patterns during diaphragmatic breathing. Chest 1977; 71:735–739.
127. Grimby G, Oxho JH, Bake B. Effects of abdominal breathing on distribution of ventilation in obstructive lung disease. Clin Sci Mol Med 1975; 48:193–199.
128. Minh VD, Kurihara N, Freidman PJ, Moser KM. Reversal of the pleural pressure gradient during electrophrenic stimulation. J Appl Physiol 1974; 37:496–504.
129. Roussos CS, Fixley M, Genest J, et al. Voluntary factors influencing the distribution of inspired gas. Am Rev Respir Dis 1977; 116:457–467.
130. Woodcock AA, Gross ER, Gellert A, et al. Effects of dihydrocodeine, alcohol, and caffeine on breathlessness and exercise tolerance in patients with chronic obstructive lung disease and normal blood gases. N Engl J Med 1981; 305:1611–1616.
131. Grassino A, Goldman MD, Mead J, Sears A. Mechanics of the human diaphragm during voluntary contractions; statics. J Appl Physiol 1978; 44:829–839.
132. Evanich MJ, Franco MJ, Lourenco RV. Force output of the diaphragm as a function of phrenic nerve firing rate and lung volume. J Appl Physiol 1973; 35:208–212.
133. Wilson SH, Cooke NT, Moxham J, Spiro SG. Sternomastoid muscle function and fatigue in normal subjects and in patients with chronic obstructive pulmonary disease. Am Rev Respir Dis 1984; 129:460–464.
134. Macklem PT, Roussos CS. Respiratory muscle fatigue: A cause of respiratory failure? Clin Sci Mol Med 1977; 53:419–422.
135. Bai TR, Rabinovitch BJ, Pardy RL. Near-maximal voluntary hyperpnea and ventilatory muscle function. J Appl Physiol 1984; 57:1742–1748.
136. Moxham J, Morris AJR, Spiro SG, et al. Contractile properties and fatigue of the diaphragm in man. Thorax 1981; 36:164–168.
137. Belman MJ, Gaesser GA. Ventilatory muscle training in the elderly. J Appl Physiol 1988; 64:899–905.
138. Clanton TL, Dixon GF, Drake J, Gadek JE. Effects of breathing pattern on inspiratory muscle endurance in humans. J Appl Physiol 1985; 59:1834–1841.
139. McCool FD, McCann DR, Leith DE, Hoppin FG Jr. Pressure-flow effects on endurance of inspiratory muscles. J Appl Physiol 1986; 60:299–303.
140. Criner GJ, Bartolome CR. Ventilatory muscle recruitment in exercise with O_2 in obstructed patients with mild hypoxemia. J Appl Physiol 1987; 63:195–200.
141. Bradley BL, Garner AE, Billiu D, et al. Oxygen-assisted exercise in chronic obstructive lung disease. The effect on exercise capacity and arterial blood gas tensions. Am Rev Respir Dis 1978; 118:239–243.
142. Bye PTP, Esau SA, Levy RD, et al. Ventilatory muscle function during exercise in air and oxygen in patients with chronic airflow limitation. Am Rev Respir Dis 1985; 132:236–240.
143. Cotes JE, Gilson JC. Effect of oxygen on exercise ability in chronic respiratory insufficiency. Use of portable apparatus. Lancet 1956; i:872–876.
144. Ekblom B, Huot R, Stein EM, Thorstensson T. Effect of changes in arterial oxygen content on circulation and physical performance. J Appl Physiol 1975; 39:71–75.
145. Jones NL, Jones G, Edwards RHT. Exercise tolerance in chronic airway obstruction. Am Rev Respir Dis 1971; 103:477–491.
146. Linnarsson D, Karlsson J, Fargaeus L, Saltin B. Muscle metabolites and oxygen deficit with exercise in hypoxia and hyperoxia. J Appl Physiol 1974; 36:399–402.
147. Olvey SK, Redutor LA, Stevens PM, et al. First pass radionuclide assessment of right and left ventricular ejection fraction in chronic pulmonary disease. Effect of oxygen upon exercise response. Chest 1980; 78:4–9.
148. Woodcock AA, Geddes DM, Gross ER. Oxygen relieves breathlessness in "pink puffers." Lancet 1981; i:907–909.

149. Foster S, Lopez D, Thomas HM. Pulmonary rehabilitation in COPD patients with elevated P_{CO_2}. Am Rev Respir Dis 1988; 138:1519–1523.
150. Collett PW, Perry C, Engel LA. Pressure-time product, flow, and oxygen cost of resistive breathing in humans. J Appl Physiol 1985; 58:1263–1272.
151. Schnader JY, Juan G, Howell S, et al. Arterial CO_2 partial pressure affects diaphragmatic function. J Appl Physiol 1985; 58:823–829.
152. Schnader J, Howell S, Fitzgerald RS, Roussos C. Interaction of fatigue and hypercapnia in the canine diaphragm. J Appl Physiol 1988; 64:1636–1643.
153. Arora NS, Rochester DF. COPD and human diaphragm muscle dimensions. Chest 1987, 91:719–724.
154. Butler C. Diaphragmatic changes in emphysema. Am Rev Respir Dis 1976; 114:155–159.
155. Ishikawa S, Hayes JA. Functional morphometry of the diaphragm in patients with chronic obstructive lung disease. Am Rev Respir Dis 1973; 198:135–138.
156. Steele RH, Heard BE. Size of the diaphragm in chronic bronchitis. Thorax 1973; 28:55–60.
157. Hunter AMB, Carey MA, Larsh HW. The nutritional status of patients with chronic obstructive pulmonary disease. Am Rev Respir Dis 1981; 124:376–381.
158. Kelsen SG, Ference M, Kapoor S. Effects of prolonged undernutrition on structure and function of the diaphragm. J Appl Physiol 1985; 58:1354–1359.
159. Lewis MI, Sieck GC, Fournier M, Belman MJ. Effect of nutritional deprivation on diaphragm contractility and muscle fiber size. J Appl Physiol 1986; 60:596–603.
160. Supinski GS, Deal EC Jr, Kelsen SG. The effects of caffeine and theophylline on diaphragm contractility. Am Rev Respir Dis 1984; 130:429–433.
161. Wittmann TA, Kelsen SG. The effect of caffeine on diaphragmatic muscle force in normal hamsters. Am Rev Respir Dis 1982; 126:499–504.
162. Esau S. Effect of theophylline on membrane potential and contractile force in hamster diaphragm muscle in vitro. J Clin Invest 1986; 77:638–640.
163. Jones DA, Howell S, Roussos C, Edwards RHT. Low-frequency fatigue in isolated skeletal muscles and the effects of methylxanthines. Clin Sci 1982; 63:161–167.
164. Esau SA. Interaction of theophylline, verapamil, and diltiazem on hamster diaphragm muscle force in vitro. Am J Physiol 1988; 254(Cell Physiol 23):C365–C371.
165. Viires N, Murciano D, Seta JP, et al. Effects of Ca^{2+} withdrawal on diaphragmatic fiber tension generation. J Appl Physiol 1988; 64:26–30.
166. Belman MJ, Sieck GC, Mazar A. Aminophylline and its influence on ventilatory performance in humans. Am Rev Respir Dis 1985; 131:226–229.
167. Supinski GS, Levin S, Kelsen SG. Caffeine effect on respiratory muscle endurance and sense of effort during loaded breathing. J Appl Physiol 1986; 60:1789–1796.
167a. Sharp JT, Goldberg NB, Druz WS, et al. Thoracoabdominal motion in chronic obstructive pulmonary disease. Am Rev Respir Dis 1977; 115:47–56.
168. Keens TG, Krastins IRB, Wanamaker EM, et al. Ventilatory muscle endurance training in normal subjects and patients with cystic fibrosis. Am Rev Respir Dis 1977; 116:853–860.
168a. Rochester DF, Braun NM, Caine S. Diaphragmatic energy expenditure in chronic respiratory failure: The effect of assisted ventilation with body respirators. Am J Med 1977; 63:223–231.
169. Thurlbeck WM. Diaphragm and body weight in emphysema. Thorax 1978; 33:483–487.
170. Zack M, Palange A. Oxygen-supplemented exercise of ventilatory and non-ventilatory muscles in pulmonary rehabilitation. Chest 1985; 58:669–675.
171. Sigrist S, Thomas D, Howell S, et al. The effect of aminophylline on inspiratory muscle contractility. Am Rev Respir Dis 1982; 126:46–50.
172. Openbrier DR, Irwin MM, Rogers RM, et al. Nutritional status and lung function in patients with emphysema and chronic bronchitis. Chest 1983; 83:17–22.
173. Bellemare F, Bigland-Ritchie B. Central components of diaphragmatic fatigue assessed by phrenic nerve stimulation. J Appl Physiol 62:1307–1316, 1987.
174. Davis JA, Frank MH, Whipp BJ, et al. Anaerobic threshold alterations caused by endurance training in middle-aged men. J Appl Physiol 1979; 46:1039–1046.
175. Hickson RL. Time course of adaptive responses of aerobic power and heart rate to training. Med Sci Sports Exerc 1981; 13:17–20.
176. Murciano D, Aubier M, Lecocguic Y, et al. Effects of theophylline on diaphragmatic strength and fatigue in patients with chronic obstructive pulmonary disease. N Engl J Med 1984; 311:349–353.
177. Aubier M, Murciano D, Viires N, et al. Diaphragmatic contractility enhanced by aminophylline: Role of extracellular calcium. J Appl Physiol 1983; 54:460–464.
178. Belman M. Exercise in chronic obstructive pulmonary disease. Clin Chest Med 1986; 7:585–597.
179. Matthay RA, Berger RA, Davies HJ, et al. Right and left ventricular exercise performance in chronic obstructive pulmonary disease: Radionuclide assessment. Ann Intern Med 1980; 93:234–239.
180. Supinski GS, Kelsen SG. Effect of elastase-induced emphysema on the force-generating ability of the diaphragm. J Clin Invest 1982; 70:978–988.
181. Kelsen SG, Wolanski T, Supinski GS, et al. The effect of elastase-induced emphysema on diaphragmatic muscle structure in hamsters. Am Rev Respir Dis 1983; 127:330–334.

Chapter 57

BEHAVIOR MODIFICATION IN COPD

Wylie L. McNabb　**Ellen H. Elpern**

The degree to which COPD patients take responsibility for their day-to-day care largely determines the effectiveness of medical management. Patients may follow a medically prescribed regimen, engage in adaptive behaviors of their own invention, or choose some combination of both. This chapter focuses primarily on the potential role of behavior modification in enhancing patient compliance with prescribed COPD regimens, although some consideration is given to patient-initiated adaptive behaviors.

We begin with a review of the principles of behavior modification as defined in social learning theory. Following that, we present research related to identifying and changing patient behaviors in COPD, discuss the issues related to efficacy and compliance in implementing therapeutic regimens in COPD, describe behavior modification techniques that can be used to enhance self-management in COPD patients, and conclude with recommendations for future research.

BEHAVIOR MODIFICATION THEORY

Behavior modification is not a single treatment but is comprised of various strategies that have been empirically proven to be effective in promoting voluntary adaptations in human behavior. Although there is no specific behavior modification theory, the strategies employed are all loosely based on the principles of social learning theory.[12] Social learning theory, as described by Bandura,[5–7] provides a description of the psychologic environment and situations in which behaviors are learned. Techniques to alter behaviors are also explained by the theory.[28, 43, 51]

Determinants of Behavior

According to social learning theory,[5, 6] individuals are motivated to perform in a particular way when two different beliefs exist: (1) the belief that performing the behavior leads to a desirable consequence *(outcome expectation)*; and (2) the belief that the behavior can actually be performed with enough precision to produce the desired outcome *(efficacy expectation)*. It is highly unlikely that people will learn and practice a behavior if they do not believe that the action will bring about some desirable consequence. For example, if dyspneic patients do not believe that pursed-lip breathing leads to a reduction in dyspnea, they are not likely to expend the effort needed to learn and practice it. Conversely, even if people believe that a certain course of action leads to a desirable outcome, that belief does not influence their behavior if they entertain serious doubts about their ability to perform the necessary actions.[5] For example, although some COPD patients may believe that daily exercise routines can improve functioning, their lack of confidence in their ability to walk two or three blocks without experiencing excessive fatigue or acute dyspnea may prevent them from attempting even mild forms of exercise.

Factors Influencing Personal Efficacy Expectations

According to Bandura,[6] there are four major ways that personal efficacy expectations can be influenced: performance accomplishment, vicarious experience, verbal persuasion, and emotional arousal (Fig. 57–1).

PERFORMANCE ACCOMPLISHMENT. Learning to perform a behavior and actually practicing it is especially influential, because it is based on personal mastery experiences. Success in walking two blocks without undue fatigue, for example, increases a person's confidence in walking; conversely, the inability to do so decreases confidence.

VICARIOUS EXPERIENCE. Seeing others perform an activity can generate expectations in observers that they also can perform the activity. Thus, self-help groups, such as a "better breathers club," may be effective in motivating COPD patients to increase their physical activities if they can interact with others who have successfully done so. This is a less dependable source of information about one's capabilities than performance accomplishment, but it can promote behavior change.

VERBAL PERSUASION. It is possible to persuade people that they can perform certain behaviors or cope successfully with what has overwhelmed them in the past. Caregivers can provide such verbal encouragement to COPD patients, but to raise expectations of personal competence without facilitating effective performance through some form of skills training will most likely lead to failure.

EMOTIONAL AROUSAL. Intense emotional reactions can accompany physical sensations such as pain or extreme dyspnea; fear of these unpleasant sensations can lead to anxiety reactions that inhibit behavior. Therapies such as relaxation training can be used to help patients relax and overcome their fear of a stressful stimulus (e.g., dyspnea), thereby increasing self-efficacy and promoting behavior change.

Performance accomplishment is the most effective method. If a person can actually learn to perform a behavior successfully, self-efficacy is enhanced. Self-efficacy is greater when less effort is required to be successful and when successful performance is perceived as resulting from a person's own skill rather than from fortuitous or external aids.[6] It has been shown that efficacy expectations are task-specific rather than general. If people learn and practice a specific behavior (e.g., walking on a treadmill), they increase their efficacy expectation

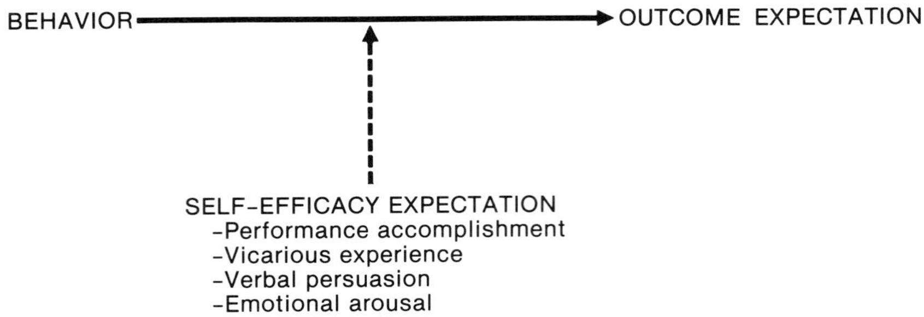

Figure 57–1. Determinants of behavior and ways to increase personal self-efficacy. Behavior is determined by an individual's belief that the behavior will lead to beneficial results (outcome expectation), but this is mediated by the individual's belief that he or she can actually perform the behavior (self-efficacy).

for walking but not for a dissimilar behavior, such as playing golf.[20, 28]

BEHAVIORAL ISSUES IN COPD

One of the tenets of effective behavior modification in health care is identifying behaviors that are related to improvement in health status. In COPD, this link between behavior and outcome is far from straightforward and is complicated by several issues. First, health status of COPD patients can be assessed by several parameters that are conceptually different—these include pulmonary function, symptom control, and quality of life. A particular treatment may change one parameter (e.g., pulmonary function) but not another (e.g., control over symptoms).

Second, assessments of health status may be objective (e.g., measurements of functional ability) or subjective (e.g., reported "sense of well-being"). An example is the Quality of Well-Being Scale,[29] which provides an *objective* score on well-being that is based on mobility, physical activity level, and social activities. The scale does not measure a patient's *subjective* feelings about satisfaction with life. It is possible, therefore, for patients to score moderately high on "well-being" while not necessarily feeling satisfied with their quality of life.

Third, caregivers and patients may not share the same perceptions on how the efficacy of treatments should be determined. For example, a particular treatment may be judged by physicians to be effective because of improvement in physiologic measurements but may be considered ineffective by patients because its benefit may not be directly verifiable by daily experiences.

Finally, the therapeutic consequence of a particular behavior may be variable with respect to its clinical significance or its generalizability from patient to patient.

The importance of these issues can best be illustrated by describing specific patient behaviors indicated for common COPD therapies and then discussing the efficacy and degree of patient compliance with each intervention strategy.

Patient Behaviors in COPD

The general categories of interventions used in the management of COPD are medication (including supplemental oxygen); breathing retraining; physical exercise training; and other therapies, such as smoking cessation, chest physiotherapy, and nutritional therapy. The various behaviors required of patients in following each of these regimens effectively are briefly described here.

MEDICATION AND SUPPLEMENTAL OXYGEN. Bronchodilators are routinely prescribed for patients with COPD; antibiotics, diuretics, and vasodilators are also employed in certain conditions.[32] A typical COPD patient takes five different medications each day.[55] Most regimens require administration of medicines at least four times per day. Patients must learn to administer drugs by the inhaled route, a process that usually takes considerable coordination and practice. Supplemental oxygen may be prescribed for use continually, during sleep, or with physical exertion. When prescribed for patients who are hypoxemic at rest, the maximal benefit of oxygen therapy depends on a pattern of continuous rather than intermittent use.[23]

BREATHING RETRAINING. Patients may be advised to use "controlled breathing" to limit dyspnea. They receive instruction to relax, to inhale by using the diaphragm, and to exhale slowly through pursed lips. They are told to exhale during exertion (e.g., lifting objects) and to interrupt activity during inhalation. This breathing pattern is practiced several times daily.

PHYSICAL EXERCISE. Exercise programs designed to increase activity tolerance are frequently advocated for COPD patients. Although various training protocols are recommended, patients are typically instructed to exercise daily until some predetermined level of tolerance has been reached. Patients are expected to maintain a regular training schedule if they wish to sustain any gains in exercise capability that are achieved.[56]

The potential benefits of selective inspiratory muscle training programs for COPD patients have been studied.[1, 44] Such regimens usually involve repetitive daily use of resistive breathing devices for 10 to 30 minutes. Improved inspiratory muscle performance is expected to increase one's ability to carry out general activities. Once training has been completed, a maintenance program is usually recommended. Generalized exercise training and inspiratory muscle training programs may be prescribed concurrently, but training sessions are not performed simultaneously.

OTHER THERAPIES. Smoking cessation is almost always prescribed. Frequently the patient is referred to group or individual smoking cessation programs. Patients who produce large amounts of sputum may require chest physiotherapies, including postural drainage, chest percussion, chest vibration, and cough, which are prescribed as a daily routine or only during exacerbations of COPD. With postural drainage, each prescribed position is maintained for 10 minutes and is followed by percussion or vibration when secretions are difficult to mobilize.[22] Weight loss is often observed in those with advanced COPD. Programs of nutritional repletion may be instituted with the hope of reversing malnutrition and increasing muscle strength and performance.[54] Refeeding programs may not be well tolerated by patients with advanced disease and cor pulmonale.[24]

Compliance with COPD Regimens

A number of studies have reported high levels of noncompliance with prescribed medical regimens by COPD patients.

In the multicenter Intermittent Positive Pressure Breathing (IPPB) Trial sponsored by the National Heart, Lung, and Blood Institute, only half the patients used their IPPB machines as instructed.[26] Similarly, in a study evaluating the effects of bronchodilators, only three of 18 COPD patients used an inhaled agent as prescribed.[25] Zack and Palange[56] have studied 53 COPD patients before and after a 12-week outpatient program of exercise and inspiratory muscle training with supplemental oxygen. Despite improvement in inspiratory force and walking ability, the investigators noted that many patients failed to continue exercise after the program ended. Mertens and colleagues[36] have described the effects of an exercise training program for 13 patients with COPD. Only five conscientiously adhered to the program. Efthimiou and associates[16] have tested a 3-month program of nutritional repletion for poorly nourished patients with COPD. As the patients' nutritional intake increased, they gained weight. Improvements were then observed in hand grip, respiratory muscle strength, general well-being, and control of dyspnea. When patients were allowed to resume a diet of their own choice, however, daily calorie and protein intakes fell back to preintervention levels.

Causes of Noncompliance

There are several possible explanations for noncompliance with COPD regimens. These may be grouped into three areas:

1. Treatment efficacy (physiologic function versus symptomatic improvements).
2. Patient characteristics (age, anxiety and depression, disturbance in cognition).
3. Education (lack of motivation and/or skills to implement treatment regimen).

TREATMENT EFFICACY. Patients and caregivers may have differences in opinion with respect to treatment efficacy. If a physician recommends a treatment that the patient does not perceive to be effective, the patient may be noncompliant. Whereas many physicians define efficacy in terms of changes in physiologic function, patients may judge efficacy in terms of symptomatic improvements. Some therapies may produce improvements in airflow as measured by spirometry, but these improvements may have no perceivable symptomatic benefit to the patient. On the other hand, some therapies may produce physiologic or symptomatic benefits but may still not be perceived by patients as efficacious, because the benefit is too delayed or may not be worth the degree of energy required to produce it. Although a detailed critique of the efficacy of each of the various therapies is beyond the scope of this chapter, the following summarizes some problems inherent in determining the treatment efficacies of COPD regimens.

Many COPD patients have a degree of reversibility in their airway obstruction as measured by an increase in the forced expiratory volume in 1 second (FEV_1) after bronchodilator administration. This increase, however, is generally only about 5% to 6% of the predicted normal value,[3] which may be too small to be noticed by most patients. The chronic use of bronchodilators has not yet been shown to affect the clinical course of COPD. In hypoxemic patients, long-term supplemental oxygen has improved survival rates; the more prolonged the therapy, the greater the benefit.[42] When using supplemental oxygen, patients have reported improvement in intellectual function and an enhanced sense of well-being.[30] Oxygen does not improve pulmonary function at rest, but can increase the duration of exercise. Both pursed-lip breathing and paced, slow breathing can increase tidal volume at rest in COPD patients, but this improvement is not related to symptomatic relief. In fact, a significant number of patients have reported that slow-rate breathing actually increases discomfort and dyspnea.[40, 46]

Consistently demonstrated outcomes of exercise training are increased exercise performance, symptomatic improvement, and an increased sense of well-being,[4, 10, 31, 39, 53] but improvements in exercise tolerance are variable.[36] Although some improvements in exercise tolerance may be noted by patients soon after the start of training, maximum benefits are generally not reached until after 8 to 12 months.[49] There are few data on the long-term effects of exercise. Training of the inspiratory muscles reportedly improves exercise tolerance in some but not all COPD patients.[1, 44]

Research in smoking cessation specifically directed to effects on COPD patients is largely nonexistent. Whereas it has been observed that some COPD patients with severe disability often continue to smoke, it is not known whether COPD patients differ from other smokers in their response to certain types of smoking cessation strategies. Certainly, strategies such as aversive smoking may be unsuitable for COPD patients, who have an already compromised cardiopulmonary system.[52]

Even if there is no improvement in spirometry, gas exchange, or sputum production, many patients report feeling better after chest physiotherapy.[37] The actual effects of chest physiotherapies on functional abilities, sense of well-being, or natural history of the disease have not been well investigated.[14] For patients who do not produce large volumes of sputum, there is no evidence that chest physiotherapies are beneficial in improving airflow or oxygenation during acute exacerbations.[2, 41] Nutrition therapy has been reported to bring about improvements in muscle function on a short-term basis, but long-term benefits have not been demonstrated. Even if nutritional support has demonstrated clinical improvement, however, patients may choose not to maintain the necessary dietary supplementation to sustain their improvements.[16]

PATIENT CHARACTERISTICS. Age, anxiety and depression, and disturbances in cognition are patient characteristics that may affect the degree of compliance of COPD patients to therapeutic regimens. Most COPD patients are older (often over 60 years of age). This is a time of life when social roles may be altered (e.g., by retirement) and physical changes associated with aging become more pronounced (e.g., disorders in other body systems). Consequently, patients may have limited energy to invest in extensive training regimens, particularly if they must incorporate prescriptions for other illnesses into their lifestyle. In addition, COPD patients who are significantly disabled are frequently depressed or anxious.[47] Feelings of hopelessness and worthlessness can deter compliance with treatment programs,[36] as does fear of dyspnea.[48] There is evidence that some patients with COPD attempt to cope with their disease through the use of denial, repression, and isolation, limiting their ability to accept help or support from others.[15] Finally, neuropsychologic functioning may be altered in some COPD patients. Deficits may relate to hypoxemia, polycythemia, metabolic derangements, or drug effects. Memory, attention, and skill performance may be reduced; patients may simply be unable to comprehend or to remember their regimen.

EDUCATIONAL QUALITY. Better patient education may improve compliance and health outcomes in COPD. Presenting factual information to patients about their disease and its treatment may lead to changes in health beliefs and subsequently to changes in behavior. Some form of behavior modification is often needed, however, in addition to information about the disease if behavior change is to occur. Mazzuca[34] has reviewed 27 studies published between 1970 and 1981 that tested the impact of health education on compliance, physiologic status, and health outcomes in patients with chronic diseases. It was determined that educational programs with a behavioral emphasis lead to greater patient compliance than those with an emphasis on the presentation of factual information. Mazzuca concluded that patients need to know more about integrating therapies into their daily routines than about actual disease processes. Programs that include a self-management plan are more likely to improve the course of a chronic disease than those that only present medical facts and treatment rules. The effectiveness of behavior modification strategies in improving compliance has been supported in the general patient education literature.[19, 45]

BEHAVIOR MODIFICATION IN THE TREATMENT OF LUNG DISEASE

Kaplan and colleagues[28] have applied behavior modification techniques to the management of COPD. To increase compliance with an exercise program in COPD, they randomly assigned patients to one of five groups: behavior modification, cognitive modification, behavior-cognitive modification, attention only, or no treatment. Patients who received some form of behavior modification exercised more and achieved better results from exercise (well-being and exercise tolerance) than did patients who received attention only or no treatment. Greater gains in the treatment groups were observed in those who received the combined behavior modification and cognitive strategies (positive thinking and self-talk; see also Atkins and associates[4]). Efficacy expectations increased in both behavior modification groups. The study concluded that "increases in compliance with an exercise prescription (performance accomplishment) were associated with enhanced expectations for performing these behaviors in the future."[28]

Additional work in COPD has also been done in the development of the Quality of Well-Being Scale,[29] which is an outcome measure that has been specifically applied to assess the efficacy of COPD rehabilitation programs. This scale provides a means of quantifying physical functioning and general health status. The focus of the scale is on physical activity, social interactions, and general health. As noted previously, the scale does not consider patients' perceptions of the quality of their lives nor their general "satisfaction with life."

Although other applications of behavior modification in COPD have not been reported in the literature, we can nonetheless present some general guidelines for conducting needs assessments with individual patients and for employing specific behavior modification techniques in the treatment of COPD. These include the following:

1. Conducting a needs assessment to identify needs of individual patients in terms of motivation, response to treatment, and differences in perspective.
2. Applying selected behavior modification strategies, such as positive reinforcement, contingency contracting and goal setting, cognitive modification, self-assessment and feedback, relaxation training, and continued contact and follow-up.

Identification of Individual Differences Among Patients

Before instituting any treatment regimen, particularly one that requires active patient participation, clinicians need to be aware of the perspectives patients bring to the therapeutic interaction. This is especially important in COPD because of the variability of COPD patients in terms of their motivation to engage in self-care, their differences in responses to treatment, and their perspectives on self-care in the face of a progressively debilitating disease.

MOTIVATION. Outcome expectation and personal efficacy expectation influence behavior change. Patients must believe that performing the behavior will lead to some desired immediate or long-term outcome.[5, 6] For example, if patients do not find some symptomatic relief from bronchodilators, the likelihood of their adhering to a medication regimen may be reduced. Patients must also perceive that they can actually perform the behavior with enough skill and consistency to produce the desired outcome. Motivation is also enhanced by the presence of someone who can provide emotional and social support. This may be a significant other, a friend, or a home health worker who is involved in the rehabilitation process. If behavior modification is to be effective, a thorough needs assessment should be conducted to identify patient beliefs and situations that can either improve or inhibit effective behavioral performance. Tailoring the behavioral program while keeping these in mind enhances its effectiveness.

RESPONSE TO TREATMENT. Because there is enormous variability among COPD patients with respect to response to treatment, this variability should be considered when selecting a particular treatment regimen. Many patients may not be willing to expend the necessary effort to achieve small, relatively unrewarding benefits.[38] Thus, before behavior modification techniques are employed, the characteristics, responses, and desires of individual patients must be considered.

DIFFERENCES IN PERSPECTIVE. The perspective of the patient should also be examined, because patients may have different approaches to managing their disease. Three studies examining COPD patients' perspectives have been reported in the literature. Despite limited sample sizes, each has yielded valuable insight into the life of the COPD patient. Fagerhaugh[21] has interviewed 22 patients with emphysema about information regarding activities of daily living. It was concluded that patients carefully calculate potential energy expenditures in relation to any given activity and set rigid priorities about what activities to undertake. Included in these calculations are decisions about whether to follow or disregard prescribed medical regimens.

Barstow[8] summarized her discussions with a sample of patients with emphysema who attended breathing improvement classes. "Simplification of activities" and "pacing" were the two major coping techniques described by these patients. Modifications in personal hygiene practices were frequent, as were adjustments in eating, dressing, and socialization.

Carrieri and Janson-Bjerklie[13] asked COPD patients to describe the strategies they used to manage dyspnea. Planned decreases in overall activity, alterations in activities of daily living, and self-adjustments in medication were the most frequently used adaptive strategies. These three studies indicate that, despite medical advice, patients deliberately limit rather than increase their physical activities.

We are currently conducting a fourth study in an effort to identify the entire range of adaptive behaviors actually employed by COPD patients in daily living.[18] More than 250 incidents have been collected, encompassing a wide range of behavioral strategies in the areas of posture, activity modification, relaxation, breathing alterations, and planning for crises. Preliminary data suggest that patients repeatedly employ strategies that are not commonly mentioned in the pulmonary literature. For example, some patients have reported that they regularly practice self-induced gagging as a means of achieving mucous expectoration. Self-imposed social isolation and extremes in energy conservation (e.g., avoidance of physical activity) are also being reported.

Specific Behavior Modification Strategies

Once individual needs have been identified, various strategies can be used to promote behavior change either by enhancing self-efficacy or increasing outcome expectations. Although it is beyond the scope of this chapter to provide a detailed discussion of each, a brief description of some of the most common techniques is provided.

POSITIVE REINFORCEMENT. Reinforcement is the single most important part of the learning process.[33] It is also the broadest in its application, because reinforcements may be social, physical, or cognitive in nature. Basically, a person who is rewarded (reinforced) for a particular behavior in one instance will likely repeat that behavior when a similar situation is encountered in the future. However, the selection of effective reinforcers is as varied as are the individuals being reinforced. The key is to select the reinforcement that is meaningful to the particular individual. Considerable trial and error may be necessary in selecting the right reinforcer for a specific patient. Reinforcements are most effective when they follow the behavior immediately, although intermittent reinforcement is also an effective behavior modification technique.

CONTINGENCY CONTRACTING AND GOAL SETTING. An effective method employed in behavior modification is developing a contract that stipulates the specific behavior to be performed (e.g., walking two blocks per day) in return for some type of reward (reinforcement) that is contingent on the behavior being performed (e.g., watching a desired television program or having a cup of coffee). This technique was used successfully by Atkins and colleagues[4] in improving adherence to an exercise program by COPD patients. To be successful, the contract should include a behavior that is clearly specified and within the capability of the patient. The reward must be a desirable one, which is relatively immediate. Another form of the contract is goal setting, in which patients set goals for themselves according to clearly specified criteria. First, the goal should consist of a single behavior; second, the patient's likelihood of success should be relatively high; third, the patient's progress should be clearly documented; and fourth, a written record should be maintained. An example of a goal-setting contract is shown in Figure 57–2, in which a patient is asked to predict the degree of success (self-efficacy) and report actual success, along with any obstacles that may have interfered with goal achievement.

COGNITIVE MODIFICATION. Cognitive behavior modification, as described by Ellis[17] and Meichenbaum,[35] consists of helping

Lifestyle Weekly Contract

Name **Week of**

MY PLAN:

This week, I agree to do the following:

In accomplishing my goal, I think I will be:

not successful (0%)	a little successful (25%)	somewhat successful (50%)	rather successful (75%)	very successful (100%)

RESULTS:

In accomplishing my goal, I was:

not successful (0%)	a little successful (25%)	somewhat successful (50%)	rather successful (75%)	very successful (100%)

Obstacles that kept me from achieving my goal:

Figure 57–2. Example of a goal-setting contract for use in a lifestyle modification program.

patients identify their own negative thoughts and feelings and, through cognitive restructuring, replacing them with positive thoughts and feelings. This is done through positive "self-talk," in which patients make statements to themselves of a positive nature (e.g., "That was easy; walking one block was a piece of cake!"). It has often been found that cognitive modification is more effective when coupled with other behavior modification techniques that involve successful behavioral accomplishments.[7] Atkins and colleagues[4] found that combined cognitive and behavior modification was superior to cognitive modification alone.

SELF-ASSESSMENT AND FEEDBACK. An important means for enhancing behavior change is enabling patients to practice some form of self-monitoring, in which the results of their behavioral practices are evident to them. For example, Bass and coworkers[9] used at-home odometer readings on exercise bicycles to help patients monitor their daily progress. These self-assessments provide feedback to enhance self-efficacy. It should be noted that self-monitoring approaches are less effective than approaches that involve reinforcement.[19]

RELAXATION TRAINING. The use of relaxation training has been reported as a possible technique for reducing the anxiety associated with dyspnea.[15, 15a] Because it is generally used in conjunction with retraining of the breathing muscle, relaxation itself has not been extensively studied as an independent technique in COPD. Atkins and colleagues[4] incorporated relaxation training as part of their successful exercise training program. Progressive relaxation, as described by Jacobson,[27] involves relaxing one muscle group at a time (e.g., beginning with the toes and moving upward to the head and face). During the process, verbal suggestions may be given by the therapist to induce a sense of relaxation in future situations. The relaxation response, first described by Benson,[11] appears to be of special value in disorders involving some form of anxiety.[50]

CONTINUED CONTACT AND FOLLOW-UP. Although these are not specific therapies, continued contact and follow-up are important to ensure adherence with chronic, long-term regimens. A system of intermittent reinforcement should be incorporated into the follow-up plan to provide patients with the needed incentives to sustain their behavior change practices. Re-evaluation of progress and the setting of new goals are generally required as the disease process progresses. Without some method of sustained encouragement, many newly acquired behavioral practices may be abandoned by patients when behavioral treatment ceases.

RECOMMENDATIONS FOR BEHAVIORAL RESEARCH STUDIES

Behavioral research in COPD has been limited. Based on the research that has been done, we can conclude that patient education efforts that focus on presenting factual information on lung disease and its treatment can improve patient knowledge but do not necessarily change behavior. Furthermore, there is some evidence suggesting that the use of specific behavior modification techniques, such as contingency contracting and reinforcement, may lead to enhanced adherence with recommended treatments, such as exercise therapy.

It is not difficult to understand why more behavioral research has not been done in COPD. One reason may relate to treatment efficacy. Generally, the outcomes of COPD treatments are of limited clinical significance. Supplemental oxygen in hypoxemic patients is the only intervention shown by controlled trial to prolong life. Although smoking cessation may slow the rate of decline in pulmonary functions in patients with mild to moderate obstruction, little has been done to determine the most effective means of achieving cessation in COPD patients. The benefits of all other therapies are not related to improvements in pulmonary function but rather to the reduction of symptoms, improvement in functional abilities, and enhancement of the quality of life. Unfortunately, the latter improvements are variable, relatively small, and not readily predictable for any given patient. Until the efficacy of the various COPD treatment modalities has been clearly established, behavioral scientists may not be encouraged to apply behavior modification techniques in COPD, because the effectiveness of behavioral therapy depends on the efficacy of the behavior being promoted.

Because pulmonary function is rarely improved to any clinically significant degree on a permanent basis by any therapy, some investigators have turned to other outcome data, such as quality of well-being, as evidence of treatment success.[28] Usually these measures are determined by health care professionals rather than patients. Patients may have perspectives on "quality of life" that differ from those of health professionals. Further research is needed in this area.

We do not know what adaptations patients actually make to deal with their disease or whether these adaptations are congruent with those recommended by the health care team. Some coping skills have been identified, but more studies are needed that attempt to teach these skills to patients in an effort to bring about improvements in coping with COPD.

Finally, the potential benefits of prevention and early intervention require investigation. As noted by Parker and Lenfant,[45] it is surprising that there have been so few investigations directed at those populations at risk for acquiring lung disease. If it can be shown, for example, that the early use of bronchodilators reduces the decline in lung function in COPD, then intervention studies with a strong behavioral emphasis seem warranted.

REFERENCES

1. Andersen JB, Falk P. Clinical experience with respiratory resistive breathing training. Int Rehabil Med 1984; 6:183–185.
2. Anthonisen P, Riis P, Sogaard-Anderson T. The value of lung physiotherapy in the treatment of acute exacerbations in chronic bronchitis. Acta Med Scand 1964; 175:715–719.
3. Anthonisen NR, Wright EC, IPPB Trial Group. Bronchodilator response in chronic obstructive pulmonary disease. Am Rev Respir Dis 1986; 133:814–819.
4. Atkins CJ, Kaplan RM, Timms RM. Behavioral exercise programs in the management of chronic obstructive pulmonary disease. J Consult Clin Psychol 1984; 52:591–603.
5. Bandura A. Self-efficacy mechanism in human agency. Am Psychol 1982; 37:122–147.
6. Bandura A. Self-efficacy: Toward a unifying theory of behavioral change. Psychol Rev 1977; 84:191–215.
7. Bandura A. Social Learning Theory. Englewood Cliffs, NJ: Prentice-Hall, 1977.
8. Barstow RE. Coping with emphysema. Nurs Clin North Am 1974; 9:137–145.
9. Bass H, Whitcomb JF, Forman R. Exercise training: Therapy for patients with chronic obstructive pulmonary disease. Chest 1970; 57:116–121.
10. Belman MJ. Exercise in chronic obstructive pulmonary disease. Clin Chest Med 1986; 7:585–597.
11. Benson H. The Relaxation Response. New York: William Morrow, 1975.
12. Best JA, Bloch M. Compliance in the control of cigarette smoking. In: Haynes RB, Taylor DW, Sackett DL, eds. Compliance in Health Care. Baltimore: Johns Hopkins University Press, 1981, 202–222.
13. Carrieri VK, Janson-Bjerklie S. Strategies patients use to manage the sensation of dyspnea. West J Nurs Res 1986; 8:284–305.
14. Cherniack RM. Physical therapy. Am Rev Respir Dis 1980; 122:25–27.

15. Dudley DL, Glaser EM, Jorgenson BN, Logan DL. Psychosocial concomitants to rehabilitation in chronic obstructive pulmonary disease: Part I. Psychosocial and psychological considerations. Chest 1980; 77:413–420.
15a. Dudley DL, Glaser EM, Jorgenson BN, Logan DL. Psychosocial concomitants to rehabilitation in chronic obstructive pulmonary disease: Part II. Pyschosocial treatment. Chest 1980; 77:544–551.
16. Efthimiou J, Fleming J, Gomes C, Spiro SG. The effect of supplementary oral nutrition in poorly nourished patients with chronic obstructive pulmonary disease. Am Rev Respir Dis 1988; 137:1075–1082.
17. Ellis A. Reason and Emotion in Psychotherapy. New York: Lyle Stuart, 1962.
18. Elpern EH, Szidon JP, McNabb WL, et al. Critical incidents in self-management of chronic obstructive pulmonary disease. Am Rev Respir Dis 1987; 135:A–192.
19. Epstein LH, Cluss PA. A behavioral medicine perspective on adherence to long-term medical regimens. J Consult Clin Psychology 1982; 50:950–971.
20. Ewart C, Taylor CB, DeBusk RF. Increasing self-efficacy after heart attack: Effects of treadmill exercise. Presented at the Meeting of the American Psychological Association, Montreal, 1980.
21. Fagerhaugh SY. Getting around with emphysema. Am J Nurs 1973; 73:94–99.
22. Frownfelter DL. Chest Physical Therapy and Pulmonary Rehabilitation. Chicago: Year Book Medical Publishers, 1978.
23. Fulmer JD, Snider GL. ACCP-NHLBI National Conference on Oxygen Therapy. Chest 1984; 86:234–247.
24. Goldstein SA, Thomashow B, Askanazi J. Functional changes during nutritional repletion in patients with lung disease. Clin Chest Med 1986; 7:141–151.
25. Guyatt GH, Townsend M, Pugsley SO, et al. Bronchodilators in chronic air-flow limitation: Effect on airway function, exercise capacity, and quality of life. Am Rev Respir Dis 1987; 135:1069–1074.
26. Intermittent Positive Pressure Breathing Trial Group. Intermittent positive pressure breathing therapy of chronic obstructive pulmonary disease: A clinical trial. Ann Intern Med 1983; 99:612–620.
27. Jacobson E. Progressive Relaxation: A Physiological and Clinical Investigation of Muscular States and Their Significance in Psychology and Medical Practice. Chicago: University of Chicago Press, 1974.
28. Kaplan RM, Atkins CJ, Timms R. Validity of a quality of well-being scale as an outcome measure in chronic obstructive pulmonary disease. J Chron Dis 1984; 37:85–95.
29. Kaplan RM, Reis A, Atkins CJ. Behavioral issues in the management of chronic obstructive pulmonary disease. Ann Behav Med 1985; 7:5–10.
30. Krop HD, Block AJ, Cohen E. Neuropsychologic effects of continous oxygen therapy in chronic obstructive pulmonary disease. Chest 1973; 64:317–322.
31. Lertzman MM, Cherniack RM. Rehabilitation of patients with chronic obstructive pulmonary disease. Am Rev Respir Dis 1976; 114:1145–1165.
32. Make BJ, Paine R. Pulmonary rehabilitation for COPD patients. Hosp Pract 1987; 22:26–34.
33. Martin G, Pear J. Behavior Modification: What It Is and How To Do It. Englewood Cliffs, NJ: Prentice-Hall, 1978.
34. Mazzuca SA. Does patient education in chronic disease have therapeutic value? J Chron Dis 1982; 35:521–529.
35. Meichenbaum D. Cognitive Behavioral Modification: An Integrative Approach. New York: Plenum, 1977.
36. Mertens DJ, Shephard RJ, Kavanagh T. Long-term exercise therapy for chronic obstructive lung disease. Respiration 1978; 35:96–107.
37. Mohsenifar Z, Rosenberg N, Goldberg HS, Koerner SK. Mechanical vibration and conventional chest physiotherapy in outpatients with stable chronic obstructive lung disease. Chest 1985; 87:483–485.
38. Morgan AD, Peck DF, Buchanan DR, McHardy GJR. Effect of attitudes and beliefs on exercise tolerance in chronic bronchitis. Br Med J 1983; 286:171–173.
39. Moser KM, Bokinsky GE, Savage RT, et al. Results of a comprehensive rehabilitation program: Physiologic and functional effects on patients with chronic obstructive pulmonary disease. Arch Intern Med 1980; 140:1596–1601.
40. Mueller RE, Petty TL, Filley GF. Ventilation and arterial blood gas changes reduced by pursed lips breathing. J Appl Physiol 1970; 28:784–789.
41. Newton DA, Stephenson A. Effect of physiotherapy on pulmonary function. Lancet 1978; ii:228–230.
42. Nocturnal Oxygen Therapy Trial Group. Continuous or nocturnal oxygen therapy in hypoxemic chronic obstructive lung disease. Ann Intern Med 1980; 93:391–398.
43. Ormison L. Self-management strategies. In: Squyres WD, ed. Patient Education: An Inquiry Into the State of the Art. Dallas: Springer, 1980, 217–246.
44. Pardy RL, Rivington RN, Despas PJ, Macklem PT. The effects of inspiratory muscle training on exercise performance in chronic airflow limitation. Am Rev Respir Dis 1981; 123:426–433.
45. Parker SR, Lenfant C. Educational and behavioral approaches to the prevention and control of lung disease. In: Murray JF, Nadel JA, eds. Textbook of Respiratory Medicine. Philadelphia: WB Saunders, 1988, 2069–2098.
46. Paul G, Eldridge F, Mitchell J, Fiene T. Some effects of slowing respiration rate in classic emphysema and bronchitis. J Appl Physiol 1966; 21:877–882.
47. Sandhu HS. Psychological issues in chronic obstructive pulmonary disease. Clin Chest Med 1986; 7:629–642.
48. Shenkman B. Factors contributing to attrition rates in a pulmonary rehabilitation program. Heart Lung 1985; 14:53–58.
49. Sinclair DJM, Ingram CG. Controlled trial of supervised exercise training in chronic bronchitis. Br Med J 1980; 280:519–521.
50. Strider FD. Biofeedback and self-regulation therapies. In: Golden CJ, Alcaparras SS, Strider FD, eds. Applied Techniques in Behavioral Medicine. New York: Grune & Stratton, 1981, 87–100.
51. Thoresen CE, Kirmil-Gray K. Self-management psychology and the treatment of childhood asthma. J Allergy Clin Immunol 1983; 72:596–606.
52. Turner SA, Daniels JL, Hollandsworth JG. The effects of a multicomponent smoking cessation program with chronic obstructive pulmonary disease outpatients. Addict Behav 1985; 10:87–90.
53. Unger KM, Moser KM, Hansen P. Selection of an exercise program for patients with chronic obstructive pulmonary disease. Heart Lung 1980; 9:68–76.
54. Wilson DO, Rogers RM, Openbrier D. Nutritional aspects of chronic obstructive pulmonary disease. Clin Chest Med 1986; 7:643–656.
55. Yellowlees PM, Alpers JH, Bowden JJ, et al. Psychiatric morbidity in patients with chronic airflow obstruction. Med J Aust 1987; 146:305–307.
56. Zack MB, Palange AV. Oxygen-supplemented exercise of ventilatory and nonventilatory muscles in pulmonary rehabilitation. Chest 1985; 88:669–675.

Chapter 58

TREATMENT OF DYSPNEA WITH TRANQUILIZERS

Richard W. Light

The role of psychotropic drugs in the treatment of dyspnea remains to be defined.[20] It is known that there is a large variation in the exercise tolerance of patients with chronic obstructive pulmonary disease (COPD) who have a given level of pulmonary dysfunction. Several studies have shown that there is a relatively poor correlation between the exercise tolerance of patients with COPD and their level of pulmonary function. In general, the correlation coefficient between any measure of pulmonary function and the exercise tolerance is about 0.60,[4, 9, 17] which indicates that only about 36% of the variance in the exercise tolerance can be explained by the level of pulmonary dysfunction. For example, the maximal oxygen consumption of a patient with an FEV_1 of 1000 ml may vary from 800 to 2000 ml.[9] It is possible that the administration of psychotropic drugs could improve the exercise tolerance of patients with COPD and therefore improve the quality of their lives.

Psychotropic drugs could improve the exercise tolerance of patients with COPD by several mechanisms. First, a reduction in ventilatory drive might lead to increased exercise tolerance. If the $Paco_2$ increases because of a reduced drive, patients will require a lower minute ventilation to have the same $\dot{V}co_2$. Therefore, with the same level of minute ventilation, the patient can exercise at a higher workload. Second, these agents might reduce the oxygen consumption at any given level of exercise. Santiago and colleagues[23] reported that the administration of morphine to normal subjects reduced the resting $\dot{V}o_2$ and the oxygen consumption at any given workload. Third, the opiates might alter the central perception of breathlessness in the same way they alter the perception of pain. In this instance the patient would feel less discomfort for a given level of ventilation and would therefore be able to tolerate higher levels of ventilation for longer periods.

OPIATES

Opiates have been used since the late 19th century to relieve breathlessness associated with asthma,[19] pneumothorax,[18] and emphysema,[28] but their use was largely abandoned in the 1950s when their potential hazards to patients with COPD and respiratory failure was realized.[29] When opiates are given to normal individuals, both the hypercapnic and hypoxic responses are diminished.[23, 27] The ventilation at any given level of exercise is also reduced in normal subjects after they are given morphine[23] or codeine.[25] The degree of breathlessness is also reduced at any level of exercise, but the relationship between breathlessness and ventilation appears to be unaltered.[23, 25] Although one report[23] has demonstrated that the $\dot{V}o_2$ is decreased at a given level of exercise after the administration of morphine, a second report[25] has demonstrated no change in the $\dot{V}o_2$ after the administration of codeine.

Woodcock and colleagues[31] first studied the effects of opiates on the exercise tolerance of patients with COPD. After the acute administration of dihydrocodeine, 1 mg/kg, the breathlessness of 12 patients with COPD (mean FEV_1 = 0.73 L) was significantly reduced during exercise. Ventilation was also decreased during exercise, and the patients were able to walk 10% longer on a treadmill, the speed of which was increased logarithmically. At a given level of exercise their patients appeared to have a lower $\dot{V}o_2$ after codeine ingestion.[31]

We did a study that demonstrated that the acute administration of oral morphine markedly improved the exercise tolerance of patients with COPD.[10] Thirteen patients with a mean FEV_1 of 990 ml, whose exercise performance was limited by breathlessness, were studied on two separate days. On the main study day, the patients performed identical symptom-limited maximal exercise tests 60 minutes after receiving placebo and 60 minutes after the ingestion of morphine, 0.8 mg/kg. On the control day, the patients performed identical symptom-limited maximal exercise tests 60 minutes after receiving placebo twice. The order of the two test days was randomized and the patient did not know which medications were placebo, although the technicians did because an arterial line was inserted only on the day that the patients received morphine.

On the placebo day, the results from the two exercise tests were virtually identical. At rest after the patients received morphine, there was a significant decrease in the ventilation from 16.3 to 15.0 L/min ($P < 0.01$), whereas the $Paco_2$ increased nonsignificantly from 34.9 to 36.8 mm Hg.

Morphine had a dramatic effect on the exercise tolerance of our patients, as shown in Table 58–1. The mean maximal workload (Emax) increased 18.6%, from 78.5 to 93.1 watts ($P < 0.001$), and the duration of exercise increased 16% from 6.5 minutes to 7.5 minutes. Twelve of our thirteen patients achieved a higher workload after morphine ingestion (Fig. 58–1). The increase in exercise tolerance was not due primarily to a lower metabolic rate after morphine ingestion, because the $\dot{V}o_2$ increased by 19.3% and the $\dot{V}co_2$ increased by 13%. The increased exercise tolerance was not completely explained by an elevated $Paco_2$, since the ventilation at Emax was significantly higher ($P < 0.05$) following morphine ingestion. The increase in the ventilation was accomplished with a slightly higher respiratory rate and a slightly higher tidal volume.

Despite having higher ventilations and exercising for longer periods, our patients had nearly identical Borg scores at Emax after the two different exercise tests. This indicates that the ingestion of morphine reduced the discomfort associated with

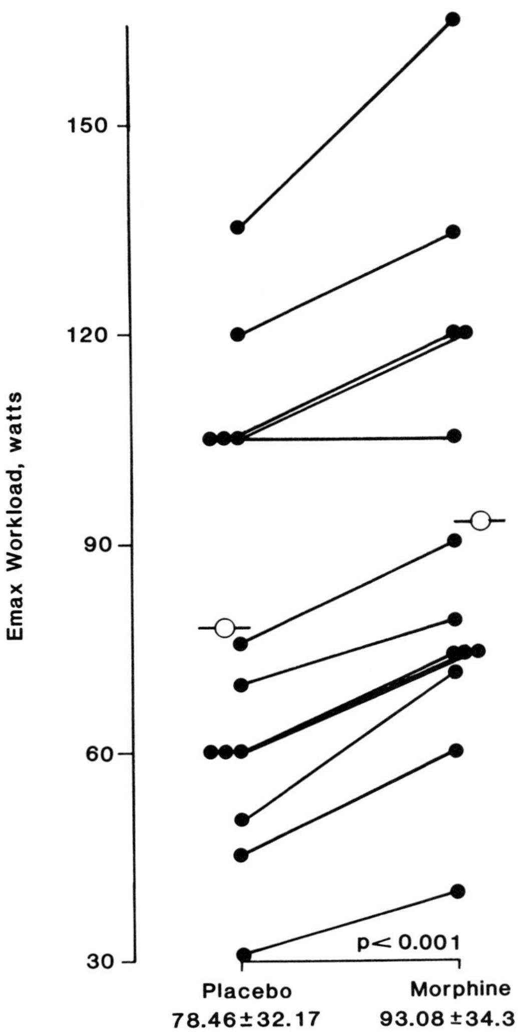

Figure 58–1. Maximal workload (Emax) achieved after the ingestion of oral morphine and placebo on the main study day.

a given level of ventilation. Indeed, when the relationship between the Borg scores and the ventilation was analyzed for the two different exercise tests, we found that the mean slope for this relationship for the exercise test after morphine (0.38 ± 0.25) was significantly lower than the mean slope before morphine (0.52 ± 0.34) ($P < 0.05$). In contrast, the mean slopes of the ventilatory response to exercise ($\Delta\dot{V}e/\Delta\dot{V}CO_2$) before (34.9 ± 7.1) and after (33.8 ± 6.9) were essentially identical. At Emax after morphine ingestion, there was a significant deterioration in the blood gases.

Data at the highest equivalent workload (Table 58–1) on the morphine day were compared to define better those factors responsible for the increased exercise tolerance after morphine ingestion. Since all patients exercised the same or more after morphine ingestion, the comparison was always the highest workload after placebo and the same workload after morphine.

There was no evidence that the ingestion of morphine decreased the metabolic requirements for a given level of exercise. There was no significant difference in the $\dot{V}CO_2$, and the $\dot{V}O_2$ was actually higher following morphine. At the same workload, the ventilation was significantly ($P < 0.05$) less after morphine, primarily because the respiratory rate was less ($P < 0.01$). As might have been expected, both the Borg score ($P < 0.001$) and the $P_{0.1}$ ($P < 0.01$) were significantly less after the patients received morphine. After morphine, the $PaCO_2$ was significantly ($P < 0.01$) higher and the PaO_2 was significantly ($P < 0.05$) lower, but the pH was unchanged because the increase in the $PaCO_2$ was counterbalanced by an increase in the base excess.

Although we performed no formal evaluation of mental function, it was obvious that morphine affected the mental function of the patients. Several patients were much more loquacious after morphine was ingested. Other patients were quieter, and some patients dozed intermittently between the administration of the morphine and the second exercise test. None of the patients were affected to the degree that they could not cooperate with the exercise tests.

To our knowledge, in only two controlled studies have opiates been administered to patients with COPD for a subacute period. Woodcock and colleagues[30] performed a double-blind placebo-controlled crossover study in which 16 patients with COPD received dihydrocodeine, 30 and 60 mg tid, and placebo each for 2 weeks. The patients had a mean FEV_1 of 0.75 and a mean $PaCO_2$ of 33.2. The results of this study were basically discouraging. Five of the patients who entered the study withdrew because of nausea and vomiting after taking dihydrocodeine. Of the 11 patients who completed the study, two were constipated and drowsy while taking dihydrocodeine, and two had symptoms of opiate withdrawal after the 60-mg dose was stopped. In the 11 patients who completed the study, the $PaCO_2$ was increased from 33.2 to 35.0 and 35.8 mm Hg with the 30-mg and 60-mg doses of dihydrocodeine, respectively. There was a marked improvement in subjective disability when the 30-mg dose was given but not when the higher dose was given. There was no significant difference in the distance walked in 6 minutes in any treatment period.[30]

A later study by the same group[3] compared 1-week trials of dihydrocodeine, 15 mg, or placebo 30 minutes before exercise as required, up to three times daily. They studied 18 patients with a mean FEV_1 of 0.83 L who took an average of 2.8 tablets per day. They reported that during the dihydrocodeine treatment week, the patients were more mobile (pedometer distance increased by 16%) and less breathless. At the end of each treatment period, the maximum distance walked on a treadmill was 16.5% higher and the breathlessness 11.8% less at equivalent distances while the patients were receiving dihydrocodeine. Though no adverse effects were reported, they did not measure blood gases and made no assessment of mental function.

There have been only a few other reports concerning the administration of opiates to patients dyspneic from lung disease. Robin and Burke[22] reported one patient in whom the administration of 3 mg of hydromorphone (Dilaudid) suppositories led to a dramatic reduction in dyspnea. Robin[21] has subsequently found that administration of the opiate in the form of a suppository is unacceptable to the patients. He presently uses a long-acting morphine preparation, 30 mg bid, and reports that he has treated six patients with this preparation for periods as long as 3 years. The administration of morphine resulted in a marked decrease in breathlessness, and the side effects have been tolerable. Two patients had small increases in the $PaCO_2$, and two patients have had difficulty with constipation.[21]

Several questions remain unanswered regarding the use of opiates for the treatment of breathlessness in patients with COPD. (1) What is the optimal opiate to use for this situation? (2) Can the improvement in exercise tolerance and breathlessness observed with acute studies be attained without significant alterations in mental function or other side effects such as constipation? (3) By what mechanism do opiates decrease dyspnea? Is the beneficial effect of opiates primarily due to a reduced sensation of breathlessness for a given level of ventilation or is it due to the elevation in the $PaCO_2$ such that less ventilation is required to eliminate a given amount of carbon dioxide? (4) Will many patients given the treatment for longer

TABLE 58–1. Data at Emax After Placebo Compared with Data at Emax After Morphine and at Highest Equivalent Workload After Morphine (Mean ± SD)

MEASUREMENT (unit)	PLACEBO (Emax)	MORPHINE (Emax)	MORPHINE (Highest Equiv)
Workload (watts)	78.5 ± 32.2	93.1 ± 34.3‡	78.5 ± 32.2
Exercise duration (minutes)	6.50 ± 2.05	7.54 ± 2.09‡	6.50 ± 2.05
$\dot{V}O_2$ (L/min)	0.88 ± 0.23	1.05 ± 0.29‡	0.94 ± 0.26*
$\dot{V}CO_2$ (L/min)	0.99 ± 0.35	1.12 ± 0.45†	0.95 ± 0.37
Ventilation (L/min)	41.7 ± 12.7	44.4 ± 12.8*	38.4 ± 11.5*
Respiratory rate	32.0 ± 4.5	32.5 ± 6.0	28.0 ± 4.83†
Tidal volume (L)	1.22 ± 0.42	1.26 ± 0.39	1.29 ± 0.45
Borg score	8.58 ± 2.31	8.67 ± 2.27	7.08 ± 2.35‡
$P_{0.1}$ (cm H_2O)	7.88 ± 3.45	8.23 ± 3.33	6.14 ± 2.08‡
$PaCO_2$ (mm Hg)	38.3 ± 8.51	43.5 ± 8.34‡	41.9 ± 7.83†
PaO_2 (mm Hg)	71.9 ± 15.5	65.8 ± 11.6*	66.7 ± 11.6*
pH	7.33 ± 0.05	7.30 ± 0.05‡	7.33 ± 0.05
HCO_3^- (mEq/L)	20.1 ± 3.38	21.4 ± 2.89*	21.6 ± 2.44*
SaO_2 (%)	91.4 ± 6.25	89.1 ± 6.30‡	89.9 ± 6.40†
Hbg (g/100 ml)	13.5 ± 1.76	14.8 ± 1.28†	14.7 ± 1.65†
CaO_2 (ml/100 ml)	17.1 ± 2.10	18.5 ± 1.85†	18.3 ± 2.32*
Heart rate	129.4 ± 21.2	134.1 ± 19.5	132.3 ± 19.7
Blood pressure	146.7 ± 23.9	145.2 ± 15.3	140.0 ± 15.3

*P <0.05.
†P <0.01.
‡P <0.001 (compared with placebo).

periods develop dangerous carbon dioxide retention? (5) Will tolerance to the beneficial effects of these drugs develop? (6) With the chronic administration of these drugs, will opiate addiction occur and will their sudden discontinuance lead to symptoms of opiate withdrawal? Until answers to these questions are forthcoming, the treatment of breathlessness with opiates in patients with COPD should be considered experimental.

BENZODIAZEPINES

With an uncontrolled study, Mitchell-Heggs and coworkers[13] rekindled interest in the use of psychotropic drugs for dyspnea when they reported in 1980 that daily administration of 25 mg of diazepam, a benzodiazepine, improved the breathlessness of four patients with severe breathlessness and COPD (FEV_1 of 0.7 to 1.3 L). The benzodiazepines tend to depress resting ventilation[1] and blunt ventilatory responses to hypercapnia and hypoxia.[1, 6]

However, subsequent controlled studies have failed to demonstrate any benefits of the chronic administration of benzodiazepines to patients with COPD. The administration of 25 mg daily for 2 weeks to 15 patients with COPD (mean FEV_1 = 0.73 L) had no effect on breathlessness and noticeably reduced exercise tolerance while producing considerable drowsiness.[32] The administration of clorazepate, 7.5 mg at bedtime, to five patients with severe COPD in a double-blind crossover study resulted in no improvement in exercise tolerance, arterial blood gases, self-rated breathlessness, or anxiety scores.[2] Likewise, the administration of alprazolam, 0.5 mg bid for 1 week, to 24 patients in a placebo-controlled crossover study resulted in no change in exercise tolerance or subjective sensations of dyspnea, although the PaO_2 tended to decrease and the $PaCO_2$ tended to increase.[12] In view of these studies, one must conclude that the benzodiazepines have no role in the treatment of breathlessness in patients with COPD.

PHENOTHIAZINES

Two different phenothiazines possibly could have a role in the treatment of patients with COPD. Prochlorperazine (Compazine) is a potent stimulant of the ventilatory response to hypoxia.[15] The administration of prochlorperazine in combination with morphine reverses the depression of the hypoxic response induced by morphine.[14] Although it has not been studied, it is possible that the combination of an opiate and prochlorperazine might be effective in treating dyspnea in COPD patients. This combination quite possibly would preserve the hypoxic response while decreasing the degree of discomfort associated with a given level of ventilation.

A second phenothiazine that might be considered for the treatment of dyspnea is promethazine (Phenergen). In normal individuals, the acute administration of promethazine, 25 mg by mouth, results in less breathlessness for a given level of ventilation.[24] In a placebo-controlled study of 18 patients with COPD, Woodcock and colleagues[32] demonstrated that the daily administration of 125 mg of promethazine for 2 weeks resulted in reduced breathlessness and improved exercise tolerance without altering lung function. However, the degree of improvement was small, and some patients experienced drowsiness.

More research is needed to define the place of phenothiazines in the treatment of breathlessness of patients with COPD. However, one must be careful in administering these agents on a long-term basis, since their administration can be associated with significant side effects, notably tardive dyskinesia.

OTHER PSYCHOTROPIC AGENTS

TRICYCLIC ANTIDEPRESSANTS. There is a high prevalence of depression in patients with COPD.[8] A reasonable hypothesis is that the alleviation of depression would benefit the patients. However, one double-blind placebo-controlled study of doxepin in 12 depressed patients with COPD demonstrated that it was ineffective in relieving the depression, and the patients actually felt better while they were receiving the placebo medication.[11]

MARIJUANA. Other agents that might be considered for the treatment of dyspnea in patients with COPD are the drugs belonging to the cannabis group. The active component of marijuana is delta-9-tetrahydrocannabinol (THC). Synthetic oral THC produces a dose-dependent bronchodilation.[26] If the primary mechanism by which opiates increase exercise tolerance is by altering the mental state of the individual, then these agents could prove useful. Marijuana appears to increase the hypoxic ventilatory response[16] and the hypercapnic ventilatory response[33] of normal subjects. However, marijuana appears to increase the metabolic rate and decrease the exercise tolerance of normal individuals and this effect may limit its usefulness. To my knowledge, no studies have evaluated the usefulness of cannabis in treating breathlessness in patients with COPD.

MEPERIDINE. The administration of meperidine (Demerol) to normal individuals affects ventilation in a manner very similar to that of the opiates. Resting ventilation is decreased[7] as are the ventilatory responses to hypercapnia and hypoxia.[5] No studies have been performed examining the effects of meperidine on the breathlessness or exercise tolerance of patients with COPD.

CONCLUSIONS

It remains to be determined whether any psychotropic drug has a role in the treatment of the dyspnea of patients with COPD. There appears to be no role for the benzodiazepines, as documented by controlled studies. Tricyclic antidepressants do not alleviate depression or improve exercise tolerance in depressed patients with COPD. The acute administration of opiates to patients with COPD results in a significant improvement in their exercise tolerance, probably by decreasing the respiratory drive and by decreasing the degree of discomfort for a given level of ventilation. However, there have been no studies of their effectiveness on a long-term basis, in which case one must worry about tolerance, addiction, and so on. Much more research is needed before firm conclusions can be made about the rightful place of tranquilizers in the treatment of dyspnea in patients with COPD.

REFERENCES

1. Catchlove RFH, Kafer EN. The effects of diazepam on respiration in patients with obstructive pulmonary disease. Anesthesiology 1971; 34:14–18.
2. Eimer M, Cable T, Gal P, et al. Effects of clorazepate on breathlessness and exercise tolerance in patients with chronic airflow obstruction. J Fam Pract 1985; 21:359–362.
3. Johnson MA, Woodcock AA, Geddes DM. Dihydrocodeine for breathlessness in "pink puffers." Br Med J 1983; 286:675–677.
4. Jones NL, Jones G, Edwards RHT. Exercise tolerance in chronic airway obstruction. Am Rev Respir Dis 1971; 103:477–491.
5. Kryger MH, Yacoub O, Dosman J, et al. Effect of meperidine on occlusion pressure responses to hypercapnia and hypoxia with and without external inspiratory resistance. Am Rev Respir Dis 1976; 114:333–340.
6. Lakshminarayan S, Sahn SA, Hudson LD, Weil JV. Effect of diazepam on ventilatory responses. Clin Pharmacol Ther 1976; 20:178–183.
7. Lambertsen CJ, Wendel H, Longenhagen JB. The separate and combined effects of chlorperazine and meperidine in normal men controlled at 46 mm Hg alveolar P_{CO_2}. J Pharmacol Exp Ther 1961; 131:381–393.
8. Light RW, Merrill EJ, Despars JA, et al. Prevalence of depression and anxiety in patients with COPD. Chest 1985; 87:35–38.
9. Light RW. Exercise, exercise testing and disability evaluation. In: George RB, Light RW, Matthay RA, eds. Chest Medicine. New York: Churchill Livingstone, 1983, 158–201.
10. Light RW, Muro JR, Sato R, et al. Effects of oral morphine on breathlessness and exercise tolerance in patients with chronic obstructive pulmonary disease. Am Rev Respir Disease 1989; 139:126–133.
11. Light RW, Merrill EJ, Despars J, et al. Doxepin treatment of depressed patients with chronic obstructive pulmonary disease. Arch Intern Med 1986; 146:1377–1380.
12. Man GCW, Hsu K, Sproule BJ. Effect of alprazolam on exercise and dyspnea in patients with chronic obstructive pulmonary disease. Chest 1986; 90:832–836.
13. Mitchell-Heggs P, Murphy K, Minty K, et al. Diazepam in the treatment of dyspnoea in the 'pink puffer' syndrome. Q J Med 1980; 49:9–20.
14. Olson LG, Hensley MJ, Saunders NA. The effects of combined morphine and prochlorperazine on ventilatory control in humans. Am Rev Respir Dis 1986; 133:558–561.
15. Olson LG, Hensley MJ, Saunders NA. Augmentation of the ventilatory response to asphyxia by prochlorperazine in man. J Appl Physiol 1982; 53:637–643.
16. Pavlin EG, Hornbein TF. Anesthesia and the control of ventilation. In: Handbook of Physiology. Section 3, The Respiratory System. Vol II, Control of Breathing. Bethesda, Md: American Physiological Society, 1986, 793–813.
17. Pineda H, Haas F, Axen K, Haas A. Accuracy of pulmonary function tests in predicting exercise tolerance in chronic obstructive pulmonary disease. Chest 1984; 86:564–567.
18. Powell DR, Hartley PH. Diseases of the Lungs and Pleurae. 5th ed. London: HK Lewis, 1911, 126–148.
19. Reigl F. Diseases of the respiratory organs. In Von Ziemsen H, ed. Cyclopedia of Medical Practice. Vol 4. London: Samson Law, 1876, 523–586.
20. Rice KL. Treatment of dyspnea with psychotropic agents (editorial). Chest 1986; 90:789–790.
21. Robin ED. Personal communication, 1989.
22. Robin ED, Burke CM. Single-patient randomized clinical trial. Opiate for intractable dyspnea. Chest 1986; 90:888–892.
23. Santiago TV, Johnson J, Riley DJ, Edelman NH. Effects of morphine on ventilatory response to exercise. J Appl Physiol 1979; 47:112–118.
24. Stark RD, Gambles SA, Lewis JA. Methods to assess breathlessness in healthy subjects: a critical evaluation and application to analyze the acute effects of diazepam and promethazine on breathlessness induced by exercise or by exposure to raised levels of carbon dioxide. Clin Sci 1981; 61:429–439.
25. Stark RD, Morton PB, Sharman P, et al. Effects of codeine on the respiratory responses to exercise in healthy subjects. Br J Clin Pharmacol 1983; 15:355–359.
26. Tashkin DP, Gong H Jr, Fligiel SEG. How the lungs are affected by marihuana smoking. J Respir Dis 1987; 8:87–107.
27. Weil JV, McCullough RF, Kline JS, Sodal IE. Diminished ventilatory response to hypoxia and hypercapnia after morphine in normal man. N Engl J Med 1975; 292:1103–1106.
28. West S. Diseases of the Organs of Respiration. Vol 1. 2nd ed. London: Charles Griffin, 1909, 200–217.
29. Wilson RH, Hoseth W, Dempsey ME. Respiratory acidosis. I. Effects of decreasing respiratory minute volume in patients with severe chronic pulmonary emphysema, with specific reference to oxygen, morphine and barbiturates. Am J Med 1954; 17:464–470.
30. Woodcock AA, Johnson MA, Geddes DM. Breathlessness, alcohol, and opiates. N Engl J Med 1982; 306:1363–1364.
31. Woodcock AA, Gross ER, Gellert A, et al. Effects of dihydrocodeine, alcohol, and caffeine on breathlessness and exercise tolerance in patients with chronic obstructive lung disease and normal blood gases. N Engl J Med 1981; 305:1611–1616.
32. Woodcock AA, Gross ER, Geddes DM. Drug treatment of breathlessness: contrasting effects of diazepam and promethazine in pink puffers. Br Med J 1981; 283:343–345.
33. Zwillich CW, Doekel R, Hammill S, Weil JV. The effects of smoked marijuana on metabolism and respiratory control. Am Rev Respir Dis 1978; 118:885–891.

Chapter 59

LUNG TRANSPLANTATION

Stanley B. Fiel **Joel D. Cooper**

In the decade following Medawar's demonstration of the immunologic basis of allograft rejection, interest in organ transplantation developed rapidly. Metras in France in 1950 and Hardin and Kittle in the United States in 1954 established the feasibility of canine lung transplantation.[12] Worldwide interest in human lung transplantation followed Hardy's attempt in 1963 to transplant a human lung.[6] Hardy's patient survived for 18 days, demonstrating not only that the operation was possible in humans, but also the ability of the transplanted lung to function.

During the 1960s and 1970s, successful lung transplantation lagged far behind that obtained in kidney, liver, and heart transplantation. During this period, 38 lung transplants were performed, but none of the recipients were restored to normal health for a significant length of time. A 23-year-old patient of Derom and coworkers,[4] who underwent right lung transplantation for advanced silicosis, was the only recipient discharged from the hospital. This patient left the hospital 8 months after transplantation but died shortly thereafter as a result of chronic rejection, sepsis, and bronchial stenosis. Primary respiratory failure, sepsis, or rejection caused the death of most patients within 2 weeks of transplantation. Of these first 38 transplants, only 9 patients survived more than 2 weeks, and 6 of these died in the first month as a result of bronchial anastomotic disruption.

In early experiments involving canine lung autotransplantation, animals were randomly assigned to a treatment group receiving standard immunosuppressants (azathioprine and prednisone) or to a control group receiving no immunosuppressants.[14] The treatment group showed significant bronchial complications, including ischemia, necrosis, and breakdown of the bronchial anastomosis. These adverse effects on bronchial healing were due entirely to prednisone; azathioprine did not adversely affect the healing of bronchial anastomoses. Subsequently it was shown that cyclosporin did not have a detrimental action on bronchial anastomotic healing.

Reitz and colleagues[16] were the first to achieve prolonged survival of heart-lung recipients (primates) using cyclosporin as the principal immunosuppressant. Transplantation of the heart and both lungs eliminated many of the factors contributing to failure of unilateral lung transplantation. Since all nonfunctional pulmonary tissue was replaced, the possibility of significant inequality of ventilation perfusion postoperatively was reduced. In addition, the risk of suppurative infection originating in a damaged area of parenchyma of the native lung was eliminated; consequently, there was no necessity to compromise the cyclosporin regimen.

In Reitz's work with primates, an effective immunosuppressant protocol was devised in which corticosteroids were not used. Tracheal anastomotic disruptures occurred even when corticosteroids were avoided; however, the introduction of an omental flap to reinforce the airway suture line has alleviated, if not eliminated, this problem.[5]

As of this writing, hundreds of heart-lung transplants and dozens of single- and double-lung transplants have been performed, with up to 70% survival two years after transplantation (Figs. 59–1 and 59–2). The shortage of suitable organ donors has limited all forms of transplantation, especially cardiopulmonary. Also during the last 10 years there has been a dramatic improvement in the outcome of cardiac transplantation, which has resulted in a large number of centers offering heart and heart-lung transplantation, so that competition for a scarce resource has further intensified.

Recent clinical advances have demonstrated that both single- and double-lung transplantation can succeed. The problems of infection and rejection, however, have not been eliminated and remain areas of major research activity. At present, unilateral lung transplantation is recommended for patients with restrictive disorders. Bilateral lung transplantation is generally performed for individuals with diseases in which air trapping, ventilation perfusion mismatch, or overflow of infection from the native lung to the transplanted lung represent substantial hazards. Cardiopulmonary transplantation is reserved for those patients with severe dysfunction of both the heart and the lungs (Table 59–1).

RECIPIENT EVALUATION AND SELECTION

Recipient selection significantly affects the outcome of lung transplantation. For this reason most centers now employ

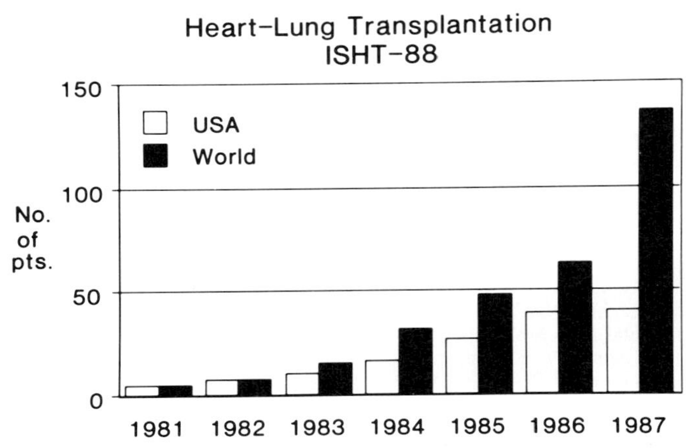

Figure 59–1. Number of heart-lung transplantations performed in the United States only versus around the world, from 1980 through 1987. (From Fragomeni LS, Kaye MP. The Registry of the International Society for Heart Transplantation: Fifth Official Report—1988. J Heart Transplant 1988, 7:249–253.)

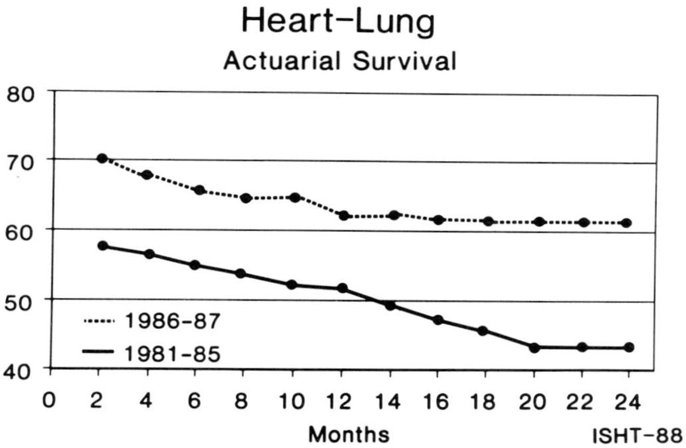

Figure 59–2. Actuarial survival curves for 1981 through 1985 and 1986 through 1987. (From Fragomeni LS, Kaye MP. The Registry of the International Society for Heart Transplantation: Fifth Official Report–1988. J Heart Transplant 1988, 7:249–253.)

strict selection criteria to improve the chances of a favorable outcome.[15] For pulmonary transplantation, patients are identified who are likely to die from lung disease within 2 years. These patients are usually oxygen dependent and have shown marked oxygen desaturation with exercise. They generally have had increasing oxygen requirements and hospitalizations during the preceding 12 months. Many of them have measurable deterioration in pulmonary function, and most have some degree of pulmonary hypertension. These prospective recipients are thoroughly evaluated, as shown in Table 59–2; patients with significant psychosocial problems are excluded, since patient compliance is essential to a satisfactory outcome.

Patients with bilateral pulmonary sepsis, either acute or chronic, are ill suited for single-lung transplantation, as the remaining infected lung would not only contaminate the transplanted lung but would serve as a focus for systemic infection following immunosuppression.[8] In patients with emphysema, it was initially feared that unilateral lung transplantation might result in hyperexpansion of the native lung with mediastinal shift and crowding of the transplanted lung. This has been demonstrated not to be the case. Ventilator-dependent patients are excluded from consideration for lung transplantation because they usually do not have sufficient stamina to permit rapid recovery postoperatively. Serologic screening will eliminate carriers of HIV or hepatitis B from further consideration.

Patients with end-stage fibrotic lung disease are the best candidates for single-lung transplantation.[8] The restrictive airway disease and increased vascular resistance in the native lung lead to preferential ventilation and perfusion in the transplanted lung, thereby avoiding ventilation-perfusion imbalance or any significant degree of wasted ventilation. Unfortunately, patients with end-stage pulmonary fibrosis are

TABLE 59–1. Available Cardiopulmonary Transplantation Procedures

PROCEDURE	INDICATION
Single-lung transplant	Pulmonary fibrosis Pulmonary hypertension
Bilateral lung transplant	Pulmonary fibrosis COPD Alpha$_1$-antitrypsin deficiency Cystic fibrosis Bronchiectasis
Heart-lung transplant	Eisenmenger's syndrome All of the above with significant cardiac dysfunction

TABLE 59–2. Recipient Criteria for Lung Transplantation

INDICATIONS

End-stage pulmonary insufficiency
Life expectancy 2 years or less
Increasing hospitalization
Cor pulmonale

CONTRAINDICATIONS

Absolute	Relative
Active malignant disease	Previous major thoracic surgery
Current corticosteroid use	Tracheostomy
Active nonpulmonary infection	Insulin-dependent diabetes mellitus
Renal or hepatic impairment	Allergy to trimethoprim-sulfamethoxazole
Multisystem failure	Fifty or more years old
Severe psychosocial disorders	
Hepatitis B or HIV	
Severe malnutrition	
Lack of compliance with therapies	

Notes: Central venous catheters, if necessary, should be placed on the left side (right side needed for areas for myocardial biopsies; jejunoscopy tubes are preferable to gastrostomy tubes). When these tubes are placed, the omentum should be spared (omentum is often used for wrapping the tracheal suture line). Large nasal polyps should be removed prior to surgery (nasal areas needed for bronchoscopy).

frequently treated with prednisone to retard the progress of the disease. Because of the adverse effect of corticosteroids on bronchial anastomotic healing, all transplant recipients must be weaned from prednisone at least 1 month before transplantation. Patients for double- and single-lung transplant should have no evidence of left ventricular dysfunction, coronary artery disease, or right ventricular failure as manifested by an RV fraction of $\leq 25\%$.

DONOR EVALUATION AND SELECTION

A lack of suitable donors is a major obstacle to pulmonary and cardiopulmonary transplantation. Only a small fraction of organ donors have lungs that remain suitable for transplantation. Generally the donor chest x-ray film must be clear, and the arterial oxygen tension must exceed 300 mmHg when 100% oxygen is administered, with 5-cm positive end-expiratory pressure. ABO compatibility is essential. It is also necessary to have a match of lung size between donor and recipient, though it is acceptable to place a slightly oversized lung in the patient.

To minimize ischemic injury to the lung, donors were at first limited to those families that would permit transfer of the donor to the hospital where the transplant was to be performed. Now the majority of donor lungs or heart-lungs are removed at the donor's hospital and transported to the recipient's hospital for transplantation.

The generally accepted criteria for donor selection are given in Table 59–3.

LUNG PRESERVATION

Although lung preservation techniques vary, the usual method is to immerse the lung or lung-heart graft in a Eurocollins solution at 4°C.[11] This simple technique usually has satisfactory results, with ischemic periods of up to 4 hours. Some centers use the technique of flushing with electrolyte solution, which is more routinely used in heart-lung transplantation. With refinement of the type of solution and use of different flush techniques, it is hoped that safe ischemic periods

TABLE 59–3. Donor Criteria in Lung Transplantation

Age less than 50 years
No acute pulmonary injury
No chronic pulmonary or heart disease
Normal chest radiograph
No fever or leukocytosis
Normal sputum Gram stain
Normal sputum culture
Blood group compatible with recipient
Negative antigen for HIV and hepatitis B
Thoracic size discrepancy $<10\%$
Acceptable pulmonary function at test ventilatory settings: $Po_2 >100$ torr at Fio_2 of 40%, IP <300 mmHg with normal tidal volume
Brain dead

may be extended up to 12 hours or longer and the donor pool thereby increased. An added margin of hemodynamic stability can be achieved by administration of L-thyroxine, 3 μg/kg, and methylprednisone, 15 mg/kg. The intravascular volume should be sufficient to promote an adequate diuresis without risking neurogenic pulmonary edema. Dopamine or an equivalent inotropic agent can be administered at rates up to 10 μg/kg/min to maintain the mean arterial pressure between 60 and 70 torr. Inspired oxygen is adjusted to maintain arterial oxygen saturation at no greater than 95% in order to minimize the risk of hyperoxic injury.

COORDINATION OF OPERATIONS

Coordination between the donor and recipient operations is necessary to minimize the organ's ischemic time. The most important need is to preserve the nerves within the chest—the phrenic and vagal nerves and the recurrent laryngeal nerve. The transplanted organs are denervated and, therefore, the longest length possible of recipient trachea is left, this being the only innervated airway to maintain a cough reflex. With a recipient whose heart will be used as a donor organ in another individual—the so-called domino procedure—special care must be taken.

OPERATIVE PROCEDURE

The technique for heart-lung transplantation is performed through a median sternotomy with the use of cardiopulmonary bypass.[7] The ventricles are excised at the atrial ventricular groove and discarded. The right atrium is preserved for subsequent anastomosis to the donor heart. The two lungs are removed separately, dividing the pulmonary arteries, veins, and bronchi on each side, lateral to the pericardium. The distal trachea and the remaining proximal stumps of the left and right main bronchi are dissected in the mediastinum, and the trachea is transsected just above the carina. A pleuropericardial window is fashioned on each side behind the phrenic nerve for subsequent passage of the lungs from the mediastinum into the pleural spaces. The donor heart-lung bloc is then placed in the recipient chest, and each lung is directed through the appropriate pleuropericardial window into the pleural space. The donor trachea is trimmed to two rings above the carina and anastomosed in end-to-end fashion to the recipient trachea. The donor aorta, transsected several centimeters above the aortic valve, is anastomosed in end-to-end fashion to the recipient aorta. The donor right atrium is incised from the inferior vena cava upward and medially to avoid injury to the SA node. The recipient right atrium is then anastomosed in "piggy-back" fashion to the recipient right atrium.

The technique for double-lung transplantation is derived from the heart-lung transplant procedure and similarly involves three anastomoses—the trachea, the common pulmonary artery (rather than the aorta), and the left atrium (rather than the right).[2] The procedure is performed through a median sternotomy with cardiopulmonary bypass. The left and right pulmonary veins are stapled and divided laterally to the staple lines. The right and left pulmonary arteries are similarly divided, followed by the right and left main bronchi, which are divided in the respective pleural spaces. Each lung is thus removed separately. The recipient trachea is subsequently divided just above the carina with excision of the carina and bronchial stumps. Pleuropericardial windows are made behind the phrenic nerve on either side by extending the opening through which the pulmonary veins enter the pericardium. The donor bloc consists of the two lungs attached by the distal trachea, the common pulmonary artery, and a cuff of left atrium containing the origins of the four pulmonary veins. The omentum is mobilized at the beginning of the procedure by extension of the sternotomy incision in the upper abdomen. The omentum is then brought through a fenestration made in the diaphragm and positioned behind the heart into the superior mediastinum. With the heart rotated forward, the double-lung bloc is placed behind the heart, and the lungs are directed through the pleuropericardial windows into the respective pleural spaces. The donor trachea is withdrawn into the superior mediastinum and anastomosed in end-to-end fashion to the recipient. The anastomosis is then completely wrapped with the omental pedicle. With the heart retracted forward, the back of the recipient atrium is incised and anastomosed to the cuff of donor left atrium. The operation is completed by anastomosing the common pulmonary artery of the recipient to that of the donor in end-to-end fashion. Very recently, bilateral lung replacement has been accomplished using a transverse thoracotomy and sequential replacement of each lung. This procedure has been associated with fewer complications than the double-lung procedure.

The technique for single-lung transplant utilizes a lateral thoracotomy and use of a left-sided double lumen endotracheal tube. The pulmonary artery and veins are divided between ligatures or a staple line close to the hilum of the lung. The bronchus is divided just proximal to the upper lobe bronchus. The omentum is mobilized through an upper abdominal midline incision. The bronchial anastomosis is performed first and is then wrapped with the omental pedicle. The pulmonary artery anastomosis is done next, followed by anastomosis of a cuff of donor left atrium to a cuff of recipient atrium, fashioned by connecting the two pulmonary venous stumps. The procedure is performed with standby cardiopulmonary bypass, which is usually not required.

PERI- AND POSTOPERATIVE MANAGEMENT

The general principles of peri- and postoperative care are similar to those used in other major thoracic procedures. Electrocardiographic, arterial, central venous, and pulmonary artery pressures should be continuously monitored. One-to-one nursing care and reverse isolation will limit exposure to nosocomial organisms and minimize the risk of opportunistic infection. Antacids should be given to prevent the formation of stress ulcers.

Mechanical ventilation should be provided at normal tidal and minute volumes. Inspired oxygen concentration is adjusted to maintain arterial oxygen saturation at no greater than 95% in order to minimize the generation of oxygen-free radicals and lessen the risk of hyperoxic lung injury. Peak airway pressure should be less than 30 to 40 cm of water to avoid disrupting the airway anastomosis. The recipient is weaned from mechanical ventilation as soon as spontaneous ventilation resumes.

Left atrial or pulmonary capillary wedge pressure should be maintained below 10 to minimize accumulation of extravascular lung liquid, since circulatory volume is a hazard to the transplanted lung. Low-dose inotropic agents are preferable to agents that increase vascular volume to maintain systemic perfusion pressure and cardiac output. Fluid intake, exclusive of blood products, should be limited to 1 liter per day per square meter of body surface area for the first 2 weeks after transplantation. Ultrafiltration should be used to alleviate fluid overload that is not responsive to diuretics.

Because denervation of the transplanted lung eliminates sensitivity to retained secretions, careful airway aspiration, avoiding trauma to the tracheobronchial anastomosis, is an essential aspect of perioperative care. Pulmonary physiotherapy to improve breathing, percussion, and drainage should be resumed in the intensive care unit and continued until no longer clinically indicated.

Daily monitoring in the intensive care unit should include a chest radiograph, standard assays of renal and hepatic function, and a complete blood count with differential. After discharge from intensive care, these tests are generally performed on a biweekly basis. Infection surveillance, begun in the ICU, is continued after discharge by means of weekly urinary and sputum cultures and measurements of serum titers to Epstein-Barr virus and cytomegalovirus. Daily Gram stains are also done, along with measures of respiratory function both in and out of the intensive care unit.

Patient education and physical rehabilitation are essential aspects of recovery and should begin as soon as possible.

IMMUNOSUPPRESSION

Cyclosporin is the principal agent for induction and maintenance of immunosuppression (Table 59–4). All patients generally receive a single dose of cyclosporin A and intravenous azathioprine (5 mg/kg and 1.5 mg/kg, respectively) immediately prior to transplantation. Early postoperative immunosuppression consists of oral cyclosporin, 10 mg/kg/day in divided doses. Doses are adjusted to give plasma cyclosporin trough levels of 150 to 200 mg/ml. Azathioprine is given at 1.5 mg/kg/day and is usually adjusted so as to keep the white blood cell count greater than 4000 and the platelet count normal. Antithymocyte globulin is usually given intravenously, at 10 to 15 mg/kg, for the first 3 to 5 days.

Some centers begin prednisone postoperatively, after the second week, at 0.5 mg/kg/day. The double-lung transplant recipients in Toronto have remained on higher doses of prednisone in an attempt to prevent the development of bronchiolitis obliterans. Corticosteroids generally are not used routinely in the first week or two, however, because they promote haphazard deposition of collagen in the healing bronchus, resulting in a 50% to 75% reduction in mechanical strength at the bronchial anastomosis and a delay in revascularization of the donor bronchus persisting up to 30 days following transplantation.

The dosages, actions, and interactions of immunosuppressant and other drugs must be learned by the recipient prior to discharge.

COMPLICATIONS

The complications usually associated with patients undergoing lung and heart-lung transplantation are summarized in Table 59–5. Complications can be divided into those that occur immediately and those that are delayed. The most important complications are described next.

REJECTION. The earliest histologic sign of acute pulmonary rejection is a perivascular, peribronchial mononuclear cell infiltrate. With increasing severity of rejection, the alveolar spaces become filled with proteinaceous material, type II pneumocytes, leukocytes, and erythrocytes, culminating in pulmonary capillary thrombosis and pulmonary infarction. The initial physiologic sequelae of pulmonary rejection are diminished pulmonary blood flow and impaired gas exchange across the graft.

The diagnosis of pulmonary rejection is frequently made on clinical grounds and is imprecise because the signs of rejection are similar to those of infection. The principal surveillance method is the chest radiograph; the initial radiologic manifestation is an alveolar infiltrate, which is often associated with arterial desaturation. The differential diagnosis includes pneumonia, fluid overload, inadequate graft preservation, and the reimplantation response (see later). The possibility of an infectious etiology also should be explored.

Following single-lung transplantation, quantitative perfusion scanning is useful in diagnosing rejection.[10] During the first month after transplantation, graft perfusion progressively increases; during rejection episodes, perfusion to the transplanted lung decreases significantly relative to baseline values.

When a clinical diagnosis of rejection is made, the patient receives three successive daily intravenous bolus doses of methylprednisone at 10 mg/kg; this treatment generally results in marked diminution of the rejection episode.

More accurate means of diagnosing rejection need to be devised, so that the patient can be treated specifically for rejection episodes rather than treated simultaneously for rejection, infection, and fluid overload. This problem has become more pressing as animal and human data have demonstrated that rejection of the lung may be observed without concomitant rejection of the heart.[5] A variety of cytoimmu-

TABLE 59–4. Immunosuppression Protocol for Heart-Lung Transplants

	CYCLOSPORIN A	AZATHIOPRINE	PREDNISONE	ATG
Initial	2–5 mg/kg/day	2 mg/kg/day	1 gram IV 125 mg IV q 8 hr × 3 doses	3–5 days (T cells 1%)
Maintenance	Increase according to creatinine + CyA level	2 mg/kg/day; adjust according to WBC + platelets	Discontinue	
Rejection				
Early (<1 month)	No change	No change	1 g IV daily × 3 days	3-5 days if severe
Late (>1 month)	No change	No change	Start or increase oral prednisone to 1 mg/kg/day tapered to 0.3 mg/kg/day or off over 2 weeks	

TABLE 59–5. Complications of Lung Transplantation

ACUTE	CHRONIC
ARDS/reimplantation	Infection
Tracheal anastomosis	Rejection
Hemorrhage	Coronary artery disease
Infection	Recurrence of the primary disease
Rejection	Bronchiolitis obliterans

nologic markers of pulmonary rejection have been proposed, but none are accurate enough to be routinely applied. The Papworth group and the Temple group have had encouraging results using systematic multiple transbronchial biopsy in heart-lung recipients for early detection of rejection.[14] Bronchoalveolar lavage also has been used to advantage.[15]

INFECTION. The majority of deaths occur during the augmented immunosuppression for acute rejection. These deaths have largely been caused by *Aspergillus,* cytomegalovirus, and gram-negative bacteria. Forty per cent of the patients receiving cyclosporin and 66% of the patients receiving azathioprine have died because of infection.[15] Most transplant patients are routinely treated prophylactically for *Pneumocystis* infection.

REIMPLANTATION RESPONSE. The reimplantation response is a transient, reversible defect in pulmonary gas exchange, compliance, and vascular resistance. It coincides with the radiologic appearance of interstitial edema, develops within a week of transplantation, and resolves within a month without any specific therapy. The cause is unknown; possible factors include ischemia, lymphatic interruption, surgical trauma, and denervation. It is important to distinguish among reimplantation response, pulmonary rejection, and infection.

OBLITERATIVE BRONCHIOLITIS. Bronchiolitis obliterans is a major cause of concern, especially because of its unpredictable response to treatment. The origin of this condition is unknown; abnormal mucociliary transport has been implicated, as have inability to clear foreign antigens, chronic infection secondary to viruses, pulmonary rejection, and cyclosporin toxicity.

AIRWAY ANASTOMOTIC HEALING. Airway anastomotic healing remains a major clinical problem.[2] It appears to be a more frequent and troublesome problem following double-lung transplantation, though there have been difficulties in single-lung as well as heart-lung transplantation. The apparent solution is either to augment the bronchial artery circulation directly or to decrease the length of the donor airway. The former could be achieved by reconnecting the bronchial circulation at the time of transplantation. Decreasing the length of the donor airway has been achieved in double-lung transplantation by performing two bronchial anastomoses. As noted earlier, sequential bilateral lung transplants through a single transverse incision have reduced or eliminated many of the postoperative complications associated with the double-lung transplant procedure.

PHYSIOLOGIC CONSEQUENCES

LUNG ISCHEMIA. In lung ischemia, the bronchial artery circulation is not reconstituted at the time of lung transplantation, leaving the donor bronchus devoid of native arterial circulation. The impact of ischemic injury to the lung has important consequences for the clinical outcome of lung transplantation. The effects of ischemic injury on lung function are, however, difficult to assess. During the early postoperative period, there may be faint infiltrates on the recipient's chest x-ray film, due, perhaps, to leakage of fluid and leukocytes to a capillary bed injured by ischemia.

DENERVATION. Denervation of the heart and lungs in allograft recipients is permanent. Recipients of lung transplants lose neural regulation of bronchomotor tone and develop anesthesia of the conducting airways. The latter has particular clinical importance. The absence of sensation slows the clearance of secretions and foreign bodies by cough and may predispose the patient to pulmonary infections that are often life threatening.[13]

BRONCHIAL CIRCULATION. Most of the bronchial arteries are severed when the heart and lungs are harvested, and they are not reconnected when the tracheal and major vascular anastomoses are constructed. Bronchial blood flow may not be entirely eliminated, however, since some of the bronchial arteries that arise from the coronary arteries may be preserved. Most of the bronchial venous system probably remains intact because it connects with the pulmonary circulation.

LYMPHATICS. Disruption of the pulmonary lymphatic system affects fluid balance in the lung, clearance of inhaled particles, and the traffic of immune cells to the lung. Since gas exchange in a well-preserved lung allograft becomes normal in only a few days, alternative patterns of lymphatic drainage must develop quickly. The mechanisms involved are at present poorly understood. Very little is known as well about the clearance of particles deposited on the gas-exchanging surface of the transplanted lung. Studies in animal models can be expected to provide information about the restoration of lymphatic flow in lung recipients.[1] Animal models have already demonstrated that the movement of immune cells between the immune system and lung seems to be restored within a few weeks of unilateral lung transplantation.[3]

CLINICAL RESULTS OF LUNG TRANSPLANTATION

The widest experience and longest follow-up thus far are for heart-lung transplantation. To date there have been over 785 heart-lung patients; their 2-year survival rate is over 60% and approaches 70% in some centers (see Fig. 59–2). There are fewer data on long-term survival at this point, but at 5 years the survival rate approaches 50%.

An informal world-wide registry maintained by one of the authors (J.D.C.) includes 209 single-lung transplants and 96 double-lung transplants performed between 1983 and 1990. Overall survival is 67% for single-lung and 61% for double-lung transplants. In the most recent 12 months, the program at Barnes Hospital has performed 23 single and 14 bilateral transplants. There was one hospital death and one late death.

As yet there are only limited data concerning the long-term changes in pulmonary function following unilateral transplantation. Improvements in vital capacity up to 44% have been recorded in patients with pulmonary fibrosis as early as 1 month after transplantation, with a plateau reached gradually during the ensuing months.[3] Diffusing capacity has improved similarly. Preferential perfusion of the graft has been confirmed by radionuclide studies. There also have been improvements in arterial saturation, generally reaching a plateau within 3 months of the transplant.

Bronchiolitis obliterans has been identified in up to 30% of Stanford University's initial group of cardiopulmonary recipients. Originally this complication was thought not to be encountered among recipients of isolated lung transplants, but in fact it has been reported in both single- and double-lung recipients. Transplant centers are now routinely following patients for airflow obstruction by means of outpatient spirometry. Routine transbronchial biopsies are also performed. These procedures, along with augmenting immunosuppression when pathologic criteria of rejection is met, appear to be decreasing the incidence of obliterative bronchiolitis.

In addition to pulmonary function improvement and better

arterial blood gases, there has been steady improvement in the exercise performance of transplant patients. While there is a need for long-term rehabilitation in these patients, functionally they are able to do all of the activities of daily living, and as time passes they frequently return to normal activity.

FUTURE CONSIDERATIONS

Issues and concerns that need to be addressed in the near future are (1) refinement of recipient selection criteria; (2) comparison of the surgical management of patients with different diseases, e.g., cystic fibrosis versus primary pulmonary hypertension versus pulmonary fibrosis; (3) the value of heart-lung transplantation with domino procedures versus single- and double-lung transplantation; (4) long-term postoperative management, including treatment of rejection and infection and prevention of recurrence of the original disease; (5) the quality of life following transplant; and (6) the pathophysiology of a denervated transplanted heart and/or lung.

It is not clear how extensive the cor pulmonale must be before a heart transplant becomes necessary.[9] In patients with cystic fibrosis, it is not known how much cyclosporin is absorbed nor how to manage enzyme replacement after transplantation. The financial issues related to transplantation are extremely important. The average cost for a heart-lung transplant is approximately $240,000, which does not include the maintenance cyclosporin cost of approximately $7,500 per year. This must be weighed against the cost of care for end-stage patients. For example, end-stage cystic fibrosis patients require hospitalization at a cost of about $20,000 per year. The cost is similar for other chronic diseases.

SUMMARY AND CONCLUSIONS

The results of pulmonary transplantation are encouraging thus far. Strict selection criteria for donors and recipients, attention to technical detail, and avoidance of perioperative corticosteroids have increased the likelihood of success following pulmonary transplantation. The use of an omental flap has resulted in a significant reduction of airway anastomosis problems.

The underlying pulmonary disease determines the appropriate transplant procedure. Unilateral lung transplantation is currently recommended mainly for patients with end-stage pulmonary fibrosis, double-lung transplantation for patients with obstructive lung disease and bilateral pulmonary sepsis, and heart-lung transplantation for patients with a combination of irreversible cardiac and pulmonary disease or bilateral pulmonary sepsis. Heart-lung transplantation has the most widespread acceptance at the present time, with the largest number of procedures performed. Transplantation is restricted in its use, however, because of the shortage of suitable donor organs and the lack of familiarity with the techniques for procuring and preserving donor hearts and lungs.

Development of a more reliable and accurate technique for the diagnosis of early allograft rejection would be an important step forward in this field.

Clinical and experimental evidence suggests that the adverse effects of pulmonary hypertension of the right ventricle may be reversed after normal pulmonary vascular resistance is restored. Lung transplantation is therefore a promising procedure for patients with primary pulmonary hypertension.

Considerably more clinical experience with single-lung, double-lung, and heart-lung transplantation is necessary before the relative long-term benefits of each can be established. It is clear, however, that transplantation of lung tissue for end-stage pulmonary disease can produce a degree of success similar to that achieved with other forms of transplantation. The majority of patients can be helped out of a crippling, restrictive lifestyle and can return to normal activities.

REFERENCES

1. Baldwin JC. Lung transplantation (editorial). JAMA 1988; 259:2286.
2. Cooper JD. Lung transplantation: a new era. Ann Thorac Surg 1987; 44:447.
3. Cooper JD, The Toronto Lung Transplant Group, et al. Unilateral lung transplantation for pulmonary fibrosis. N Engl J Med 1986; 314:1140.
4. Derom F, Barbier F, Ringoir S, et al. Ten-month survival after lung homotransplantation in man. J Thorac Cardiovasc Surg 1971; 61:835.
5. Griffith BP, Hardesty RL, Trento A, et al. Heart-lung transplantation: lessons learned and future hopes. Ann Thorac Surg 1987; 43:6.
6. Hardy JD, Webb WR, Dalton ML Jr, et al. Lung homotransplantation in man. JAMA 1963; 186:1065.
7. Jamieson SW, Stinson EB, Oyer PE, et al. Operative technique for heart-lung transplantation. J Thorac Cardiovasc Surg 1984; 87:930–935.
8. Kamholz SJ. Current perspectives on clinical and experimental single lung transplantation. Chest 1988; 94:390.
9. Lower RR. Heart-lung transplantation (editorial). Ann Thorac Surg 1984; 38:6.
10. Maurer JR. Unilateral lung transplant. Pulmon Perspect 1987; 4:4.
11. Montefusco CM. Lung transplantation. Surg Clin North Am 1986; 66:503.
12. Nelems JM, Rebuck AS, Cooper JD, et al. Human lung transplantation. Chest 1980; 78:569.
13. Patterson GA, Cooper JD, Goldman B, et al. Technique of successful clinical double lung transplantation. Ann Thorac Surg 1988; 45:626–633.
14. Penketh A, Higenbottam T, Hakim M, Wallwork J. Heart and lung transplantation in patients with end-stage lung disease. Br Med J 1987; 295:311.
15. Perelman MJ, Kapelanski DP. Pulmonary transplantation. Pulmon Crit Care Update 1988; 3:Lesson 28.
16. Reitz BA, Wallwork JL, Hunt SA, et al. Heart-lung transplantation: successful therapy for patients with pulmonary vascular disease. N Engl J Med 1982; 306:557.

Section IX

LONG-TERM CARE OF CHRONIC OBSTRUCTIVE PULMONARY DISEASE PATIENTS

Chapter 60

PREOPERATIVE EVALUATION AND PERIOPERATIVE CARE

Charles Mittman

Postoperative events that compromise lung function are the overwhelming cause of morbidity and mortality for all patients undergoing surgery. The patient with chronic obstructive lung disease is particularly at risk. This chapter reviews the pathophysiology of postsurgical complications, argues that the degree of risk can be estimated by preoperative evaluation, and summarizes approaches to reducing the risk once the physician has been alerted to the potential problem. Efforts to assess risk are clearly justified; in the high-risk patient, preventive therapy can reduce the risk, or a nonsurgical approach may be selected to deal with the patient's disease. If risk is judged to be low, the patient can be handled in a simpler, less costly fashion.

PATHOPHYSIOLOGY OF POSTOPERATIVE PULMONARY COMPLICATIONS

The sequence of postsurgical atelectasis, hypoxemia, and ventilatory failure is responsible for the bulk of morbidity and mortality in patients with chronic obstructive lung disease. For decades, it has been known that functional residual capacity (FRC) falls postoperatively.[14] This defect is proportional in magnitude to the proximity of the surgical incision to the thorax. The postoperative fall in FRC has many causes, including the direct effect of surgery on the lungs (if the chest has been opened or lung tissue removed), the effects of the surgical incision on chest wall expansion, muscle splinting to limit incisional pain, constricting dressings, respiratory muscle weakness because of anesthesia and analgesics, and, as recently shown, impaired diaphragm function.[7] The importance of respiratory muscle dysfunction in the pathogenesis of postoperative complications has been clearly documented.[13] The relationship between a fall in FRC and the risk of atelectasis is now understood with exposition of the concept of closing volume. Airways remain open if the lung tissue surrounding the airway is expanded sufficiently to apply a retraction force greater than the forces acting to collapse the airway. In young, healthy individuals, closing volume—the point at which airways begin to collapse—lies well below FRC. Closing volume increases with aging and development of emphysema. With loss of elastic recoil, at any given volume, lung tissue exerts weaker retractile forces on airways. Thus, in older patients and those with emphysema, closing volume may greatly exceed end-expiratory volume. The further fall in FRC after surgery exaggerates this tendency. Airways close, leading to atelectasis. Normally, microatelectasis is reversed by periodic deep, sighing respirations. Postoperatively, sighing occurs less frequently or not at all, further increasing the risk of development and progression of atelectasis. Analgesics, such as morphine, further interrupt the pattern of periodic sighing.[6]

Small airway closure and microatelectasis can set in motion a sequence of impaired airway clearance, secretion accumulation, further atelectasis, ventilation-perfusion mismatching, and hypoxemia. Progressive atelectasis is accompanied by fever and increasing oxygen consumption with progressive hypoxemia. This constellation of the "postoperative chest" can go on to ventilatory failure and even to death. The particular risk suffered by patients with chronic obstructive lung disease results directly from the central role in the etiology of these complications of an increased closing volume and impaired clearance of secretions. Although any patient undergoing surgery may experience this sequence, risks increase ten-fold with pre-existing lung disease.[32]

Beyond the immediate postoperative period, patients who have lung tissue removed surgically are at risk of suffering pulmonary hypertension, cor pulmonale, chronic ventilatory failure, and other effects of pulmonary insufficiency. The generous reserve capacity present in healthy lungs protects against this eventuality, even after pneumonectomy. Pre-existing lung disease may critically compromise this reserve capacity.

RISK ASSESSMENT

Efforts to predict (and prevent) postoperative complications date back over three decades. Gaensler and colleagues,[8] in 1955, and Miller and colleagues, in 1956,[18] showed that patients with reductions in expiratory flow rate indices were at risk of serious or fatal complications in the immediate postoperative period. This topic has been revisited frequently, in part in a futile search for the test or battery of tests that would accurately separate all patients who will develop a complication from those who could withstand surgery without any difficulty. Reflection will clarify why this goal is unrealistic. Not all complications stem from a pre-existing condition. Respiratory failure due to mucous stasis is directly related, but a postoperative myocardial infarction or the development of an antibiotic-resistant infection may be coincidental. A patient's ability to cope with the latter types of stresses will be influenced by the status of the cardiovascular/pulmonary system. Thus, prognosis will relate to measurable preoperative factors, such as flow rate indices. But the relationship could never be totally predictable. The same can be said for late-stage complications of chronic respiratory insufficiency. The less functional lung tissue present before surgery, the more likely will be the development of disabling impairment after surgery.[2] But it is unlikely that any test could be 100% predictive.

I am convinced by the wealth of clinical studies that even if not totally accurate, effective risk assessment can be done. This is not a uniformly held view. The issue of the use of spirometry for risk assessment before abdominal surgery has been recently reviewed.[12] Twenty-two reports in the literature were deemed by these investigators to offer objective evidence on the usefulness of spirometry. They concluded that every study failed to meet all their criteria for validity, which included a double-blind study design applied to patients with a spectrum of complications and a demonstration that spirometry actually benefited some patients. Fourteen of the twenty-two papers reviewed claimed predictive value for spirometry; eight reached an opposite conclusion. These latter papers and others have expressed such views as that risk could not be predicted[26] or that the process of sorting out high- from low-risk patients was not cost effective.[25] The authors of the review were not convinced by either the positive or negative studies and concluded that the predictive value of spirometry is unproven. Although a valid conclusion in a strict scientific sense, their analysis ignores the practitioner's need to use clinical studies to make operational decisions.

The basis for an operational recommendation to perform preoperative evaluation rests on two observations. First, if excess risk can be identified, steps can be taken to alleviate the hazard. Second, if risk is not increased, medical resources can be saved by not applying expensive diagnostic tests and therapy.[34] Key early studies included a demonstration by Dripps and Deming[4] that the "stir up" routine of physical therapy could reduce by over half the incidence of postoperative complications. Stein and Cassara[30] showed in 1970 that intensive treatment improved the risk after abdominal surgery. Patients shown to have significant obstructive defects did better if they had intensive presurgical preparation, including smoking cessation, bronchodilator therapy if needed, and training in deep breathing and coughing. Surgery was delayed until patients were thought to be optimally prepared. These patients, given intensive pre- and postoperative care, suffered a rate of complications one third of that seen in a similar group not prepared for surgery. Indeed, the treated patients with obstructive disease fared as well as a group with normal lung function.

Table 60–1 lists some of the kinds of tests shown to serve as predictors of complications in the postoperative period. This table is not meant to be a comprehensive summary of all studies of preoperative evaluation. Hundreds of papers have been published on this topic over the past 40 years. The reader is referred to recent reviews for a more comprehensive discussion of this literature.[9, 31, 32] The studies summarized here, as well as other published reports, show varying rates of complications in those testing abnormally. This is to be expected given the different tests studied, the various definitions of what constituted a complication (varying from the extremes of death to mild, transient, postoperative temperature elevation), the different types of surgery (abdominal, thoracotomy, lobectomy, pneumonectomy), and the different populations studied (percentage with COPD, age patterns, and so on).

Several points are worth noting. The value of a test can be expressed by four indices. Using the analogy of trying to fish colored balls out of a pond, the test sensitivity measures the effectiveness of netting the balls of interest. Did the test net all the abnormals? The test specificity is an equivalent measure for normals. Did the test leave behind all the normals? The predictive value measures how frequently a positive or negative test gives an accurate assessment. If the test is supposed to retrieve red balls, are there other colored balls in the net?

Since no single test can identify accurately all patients at risk of developing postoperative complications, it may be appropriate to use a two-stage approach to this problem. First, one applies a screening test, a broad net that will catch all or most of the individuals of interest. A screening test is acceptable even if it identifies some false-positive results. A negative result on such a screening test gives assurance that the risk of complications is very low. To be effective for screening, a test should have very high sensitivity and near 100% predictive value of a negative test. The predictive value of a positive result can be low. Early studies showed the value of measurements of expiratory flow rate in alerting physicians to the excess risk of complications in the postoperative period. These are valid screening tests if the level of performance selected to define the population at risk insures that those with a negative result are very unlikely to develop a problem.

Once screening has identified a group that includes all or most of those destined to have complications, further tests can be applied to sort out those truly at risk from the false-positive results. Several tests may be needed, since each individual test can fail to identify all those at risk (low sensitivity). Tests applied to the screened group should have a very high specificity and the predictive value of a positive test. A positive

TABLE 60–1. Assessment of Risk of Surgery

				USEFULNESS OF TEST			
						Predictive Value	
TEST CRITERIA	REF.	NO. PATIENTS/TYPE	SURGERY TYPE/ COMPLICATIONS	Sensitivity	Specificity	*Positive*	*Negative*
$FEV_1 < 2$ L	35	140/random	Thoracic/mortality	94	80	40	99
MVV < 50%	8	460/tuberculosis	Thoracic/mortality	92	96	40	99
	19	199/random	Thoracic/mortality	46	91	45	91
MEFR < 200 L/min	29	63/random	General and thoracic/ minor	95	78	70	97
$Paco_2 > 45$		30/MEFR < 200 L		24	100	100	36
$\dot{V}o_2$ max < 16 ml/kg/min	28	22/random (FEV_1 from 112 to 39% predicted)	Pulmonary/major	73	91	89	77
> 20 ml/kg/min			None	82	100	100	85

COMPLICATIONS
Minor: Cough, fever, atelectasis, severe dyspnea, elevated CO_2, pneumonia.
Major: Respiratory failure, myocardial infarction, arrhythmia requiring therapy, lobar atelectasis, pneumonia, pulmonary embolus, death.

test should indicate reliably that a complication is very likely. A fixed and elevated arterial P_{CO_2} carries a very high risk of postoperative mortality.[29] It was also shown years ago that the late complications of respiratory insufficiency could be predicted by tests of the adequacy of the pulmonary vascular bed.

A key refinement in this field came with the 1975 paper from Olsen and colleagues,[21] demonstrating that the post-thoracotomy FEV_1 could be predicted using a semiquantitative analysis of a lung scan. Their original suggestion that surgery is contraindicated if the projected postoperative FEV_1 is 800 ml or less has been subjected to repeated study. It remains a good guideline. Most recently, attention has focused on the use of exercise testing protocols to address the question of operability. Olsen[23] recently reviewed the literature on this topic. The current interest in formal exercise testing protocols is ironic. Prior to the application to this problem of objective tests of lung functions, some surgeons held that if their patient could accompany them on a walk up one flight of stairs, the patient could withstand thoracotomy. Van Nostrand and colleagues[35] showed that this was not a reliable test. Tests of oxygen consumption at maximal or near maximal exercise load predict mortality and morbidity after surgery.[22, 28] Patients who can sustain work loads above an oxygen consumption of 20 ml/kgm/min are good candidates for pulmonary resection.

Based on the available information in the literature, it is possible to recommend a scheme for risk assessment as shown in Figure 60–1. This is a general recommendation; details are influenced by the clinical condition of each patient and may be appropriately altered. The physician first should assess whether the patient's condition presents a potential for risk. Is a complication likely because of the presence of lung or neuromuscular disease, smoking, cough, advanced age, or obesity? Is upper abdominal or thoracic surgery planned? In any of these circumstances, spirometry is indicated. In the absence of such risk factors, one should be able to proceed to surgery with no further concern. An FEV_1 of more than two liters[35] or a maximal voluntary ventilation of more than 50% predicted[8, 19] is probably a good screening level to use to indicate that a complication is very unlikely. Patients falling below those cut-off points need further testing. For patients having abdominal surgery, the measurement of arterial CO_2 and, if lung function is questionable, an exercise protocol should sort out those truly at risk. If thoracotomy is contemplated, a perfusion lung scan should be performed to permit calculation of the projected postoperative FEV_1. The alternatives available for patients found to be at excessive risk include intensive pre- and postoperative care or use of a nonsurgical form of therapy.

TO OPERATE OR NOT

Guided by the fundamental principle that the first obligation of the physician is to do no harm, therapy decisions always

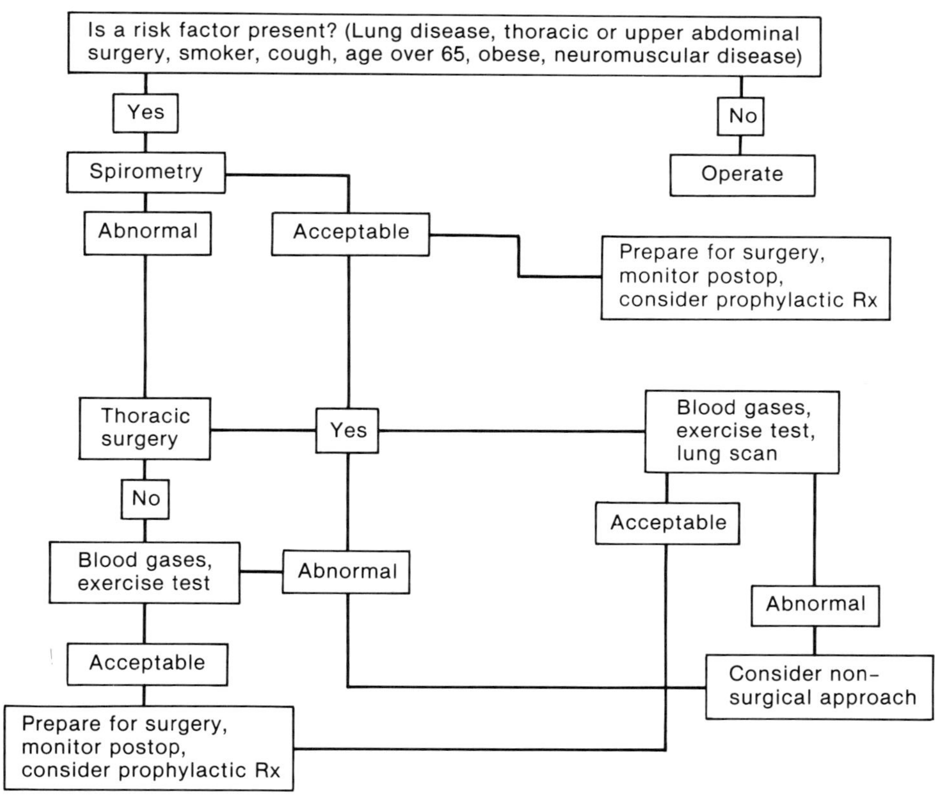

Criteria for Abnormal Risk Assessment

Spirometry: $FEV_1 < 2$ L, MVV < 50%
Blood gases: $P_ACO_2 > 45$ and fixed
Exercise test: V_{O_2} max > 15 ml/kg/min
Lung scan: Postop predicted $FEV_1 > 800$ ml

Figure 60–1. Preoperative Assessment of Operative Risk

involve a risk:benefit assessment. Most often this assessment is made instinctively; one's stream of thought need not pause to decide to administer penicillin for a pneumococcal pneumonia. So too, the decision to operate for a presumably resectable lung cancer in an otherwise healthy person is made in short order. Likewise, it is clear that in a patient with chronic respiratory failure, a central pulmonary lesion that would require a pneumonectomy cannot be treated surgically.

The risk:benefit assessment in the majority of patients falls between these extremes. Unfortunately, there is no exact equation or nomogram to apply in this region of the clinical spectrum. Affecting the decision are considerations of the likelihood of a fatal outcome in the immediate postoperative period or that resection will result in the patient being left as a respiratory cripple. Important in our assessment is the relative value of surgery versus other forms of therapy. Except in small cell cancers, chemotherapy offers no advantage. But it must be kept in mind that at least over an intermediate time interval (2 years), radiation therapy for nonsmall cell cancer may be as effective as resection, particularly for older patients.[11, 16, 27] The physician's view of acceptable risk may be quite different from the patient's. Boysen and colleagues,[3] in their studies of the usefulness of lung scans, accepted a 15% postoperative mortality after pneumonectomy to establish the cut-off point for the predicted postoperative FEV_1. McNeil and colleagues[16] took the obvious step of asking patients what was an acceptable risk. They explored risks of a fatal outcome ranging from 5% to 20% after lung resection. Most patients chose a less effective therapy rather than surgery, even when the risk was 5%. In patients not suited for extensive surgery, a limited resection can be an effective and acceptable alternative to radiation.[17]

MINIMIZING AN ELEVATED OPERATIVE RISK

When the decision has been reached to proceed with surgery in the presence of an increased risk, the fact that the physician is alerted to the potential for complications is the first defense. Forewarned, complications can be recognized earlier, including retention of secretions, fatigue of respiratory muscles, atelectasis, hypoxemia, and impending respiratory failure. Beyond early diagnosis, specific prophylactic and therapeutic measures play a role in insuring the best possible outcome after surgery.

SMOKING CESSATION

Smoking cessation triggers sequences of improvement in the tracheobronchial tree that span days to years. Patients with moderate smoking-induced injuries suffer abnormalities in tracheobronchial mucociliary clearance, accelerated rates of decline in lung function, and increased risk of developing lung cancer. On ceasing smoking, these abnormalities will return toward normal over a period of years.[33] Some tests of lung function may improve in several weeks to several months. Improvement in the signs of tracheobronchial irritation, as gauged by analysis of cells collected in sputum samples, occurs over a period of months.[19a] Exfoliated inflammatory cells begin to decrease in number promptly. Early reversal in the proliferative response to injury, as measured by the extent of metaplasia, is detectable after 3 months.

The time course and impact of these changes on the risk of postoperative complications has not been determined. The reduction in sputum volume that occurs over a matter of weeks suggests that patients would be better able to cope with surgery if they stopped smoking a month prior to the operation. Very few clinical situations offer this possibility. Abstinence for 1 or 2 days may have little real effect; it is routine to request this of our patients.

BRONCHODILATORS AND OTHER DRUGS

It should be obvious that maximal therapeutic benefit should be obtained from available cardiopulmonary drugs before subjecting a high-risk patient to surgery. The specifics of a maximally beneficial program will vary from patient to patient; details of achieving this goal are beyond the scope of this chapter. Corticosteroids may be needed if urgent surgery precludes the time-consuming selection of an optimal bronchodilator program. Many of these patients pose the additional problem of corticosteroid dependence and risk stress-induced steroid insufficiency. Ziment summarized these topics in 1984 in a well written and comprehensive review.[36]

PROMOTION OF DEEP BREATHING AND COUGH

If the postoperative syndrome of concern in these patients is initiated by atelectasis and retention of secretions, then prophylactic measures to reverse these problems should be effective. Using the "stir-up" routine to clear secretions, now so familiar, which Dripps and Waters[5] described in 1941, Dripps and Deming[4] demonstrated the value of this approach to the prevention of postoperative complications in 1946. As reviewed by Tisi in 1979,[31] numerous researchers have revisited this topic, always showing the beneficial effect of efforts to promote deep breathing and cough. If the efforts of a nurse or physical therapist to encourage patients with words and the laying on of hands is good, then the imperatives of modern medicine argue that a machine would be better. The literature is replete with evaluations of CO_2 inhalations, blow bottles, positive pressure breathing devices, insufflators, and incentive spirometers. After initial enthusiasm, most devices have been shown to be less effective than a trained, motivated nurse or therapist.[1] In the absence of that resource, the incentive spirometer appears to be an equivalent substitute. Devices that supply or add continuous positive airway pressure (CPAP) may be effective. For routine prophylaxis in the high-risk patient, the physician should opt for a machine only if an effective human alternative is unavailable.

Personal attention to the patient has obvious intangible advantages, and it insures that the patient will be observed frequently for signs and symptoms of an impending problem. The logistics of this aspect of care are best handled by the nurse who is in regular contact with the patient during the postoperative period. This assignment of responsibility is preferable to scheduled visits by a respiratory or physical therapist. In the absence of trained and enthusiastic nurses, the therapist may be the only effective choice.

Whether using physical therapy, an incentive spirometer, or CPAP, it is important to introduce the patient to the techniques to be used before surgery. The patient then can accept more readily the training and comprehend the importance of what will be a painful or unpleasant maneuver postoperatively. It is encouraging to find that practices reported by respiratory therapy departments in hospitals throughout the United States correspond generally to these recommendations.[20]

CONTROL OF PAIN

Control of pain is critical to the patient's ability to cooperate with measures to mobilize secretions. Analgesic doses should be timed to give maximal pain relief when physical therapy is administered. Where available, local or epidural anesthesia can be used, reducing the risk of respiratory depression. Physicians should examine their prescription practices with sensitivity to survey findings that suggest analgesics are given in inadequate doses in half of patients.

ANTIBIOTICS

The use of prophylactic antibiotics in these patients remains controversial. There is no objective evidence that they help in the postoperative period,[10] but they continue to be used. Use of a prophylactic antibiotic does not lessen the need for clinical surveillance; an infection may still develop. When this occurs in the patient given routine antibiotics, tests to determine drug susceptibility are critical.

OXYGEN

The patient care team must be sensitive to the subtle signs that can herald the development of hypoxemia. A change in mood or mental status may be the earliest sign. Supplemental oxygen, monitored by blood gas measurements, is called for; reversal of this problem may call for redoubled efforts to expand the lung and control and mobilize secretions. Bedside fiberoptic bronchoscopy may be needed if endotracheal suction fails.

VENTILATORY SUPPORT

Mechanical ventilation is life saving in the face of progressive ventilatory failure. Some have suggested continued ventilatory support during the postoperative period in the patient at high risk of development of this problem. Such prophylaxis is practiced in some centers for high-risk patients undergoing thoracotomy and upper abdominal surgery. It is routine practice for some after open heart surgery.[15] What little evidence exists suggests that it is not helpful.[24] Prolonged ventilatory support requires greater use of analgesics and sedatives but results in no discernible differences in the course of recovery. Thus, ventilatory support should be reserved for patients who develop respiratory failure unresponsive to other forms of therapy.

REFERENCES

1. Bartlett RH. Respiratory therapy to prevent pulmonary complications of surgery. Respir Care 1984; 29:667.
2. Boushy SF, Billing DM, North LB, Helgason AH. Clinical course related to preoperative and postoperative pulmonary function in patients with bronchogenic carcinoma. Chest 1971; 59:383.
3. Boysen PG, Block AJ, Olsen GN, et al. Prospective evaluation for pneumonectomy using the ^{99m}technetium quantitative perfusion lung scan. Chest 1977; 72:424.
4. Dripps RD, Deming MVH. Postoperative atelectasis and pneumonia. Ann Surg 1946; 124:94.
5. Dripps RD, Waters RM. Nursing care of surgical patients: the "stir-up." Am J Nurs 1941; 41:1.
6. Egbert LD, Bendixen HH. Effect of morphine on breathing pattern. JAMA 1964; 188:113.
7. Ford GT, Whitelaw WA, Rosenal TW, et al. Diaphragm function after upper abdominal surgery in humans. Am Rev Respir Dis 1983; 127:431.
8. Gaensler EA, et al. The role of pulmonary insufficiency in mortality and invalidism following surgery for pulmonary tuberculosis. J Thorac Surg 1955; 29:163.
9. Gass GD, Olsen GN. Preoperative pulmonary function testing to predict postoperative morbidity and mortality. Chest 1986; 89:127.
10. Harman E, Lillington G. Pulmonary risk factors in surgery. Med Clin North Amer 1979; 63:1289.
11. Hilton G. Present position relating to cancer of the lung: results with radiotherapy alone. Thorax 1960; 15:15.
12. Lawrence VA, Page CP, Harris GD. Preoperative spirometry before abdominal operations. Arch Intern Med 1989; 149:280.
13. Maeda H, Nakahara K, Ohno K, et al. Relationship to postoperative respiratory failure. Am Rev Respir Dis 1988; 137:678.
14. Marini JJ. Postoperative atelectasis: pathophysiology, clinical importance, and principles of management. Respir Care 1984; 29:516.
15. Matthay A, Wiener-Kronish JP. Respiratory management after cardiac surgery. Chest 1989; 95:424.
16. McNeil BJ, Weichselbaum R, Pauker SG. Fallacy of the five-year survival in lung cancer. N Engl J Med 1978; 299:1397.
17. Miller JI, Hatcher CR. Limited resection of bronchogenic carcinoma in the patient with marked impairment of pulmonary function. Am Thorac Surg 1987; 44:340.
18. Miller WF, Wu N, Johnson RL. Convenient method of evaluating pulmonary ventilatory function with a single breath. Anesthesiology 1956; 17:48.
19. Mittman C. Assessment of operative risk in thoracic surgery. Am Rev Respir Dis 1961; 84:197.
19a. Mittman C, Swan GE, Roby T. Early quantitative evidence of reversibility of tracheo-bronchial injury upon smoking cessation. Chest 1989; 96:2925.
20. O'Donohue WJ. National survey of the usage of lung expansion modalities for the prevention and treatment of postoperative atelectasis following abdominal and thoracic surgery. Chest 1985; 87:76.
21. Olsen GN, Block AJ, Swenson EW, et al. Pulmonary function evaluation of the lung resection candidate: a prospective study. Am Rev Respir Dis 1975; 111:379.
22. Olsen GN, Weiman DS, Bolton JW, et al. Submaximal invasive exercise testing and quantitative lung scanning in the evaluation for tolerance of lung resection. Chest 1989; 95:267.
23. Olsen GN. The evolving role of exercise testing prior to lung resection. Chest 1989; 95:218.
24. Pierson DJ, Lakshminarayan S. Postoperative ventilatory management. Respir Care 1984; 29:603.
25. Poe RH, Kallay MC, Dass T, Celebic A. Can postoperative pulmonary complications after elective cholecystectomy be predicted? Am J Sci 1988; 295:29.
26. Roukema JA, Carol EJ, Prins JG. The prevention of pulmonary complications after upper abdominal surgery in patients with noncompromised pulmonary status. Arch Surg 1988; 123:30.
27. Smart J. Can lung cancer be cured? JAMA 1966; 195:158.
28. Smith TP, Kinasewitz GT, Tucker WY, et al. Exercise capacity as a predictor of post-thoracotomy morbidity. Am Rev Respir Dis 1984; 129:730.
29. Stein M, Koota GM, Simon M, Frank HA. Pulmonary evaluation of surgical patients. JAMA 1962; 181:103.
30. Stein M, Cassara EL. Preoperative pulmonary evaluation and therapy for surgery patients. JAMA 1970; 211:787.
31. Tisi GM. Preoperative evaluation of pulmonary function. Am Rev Respir Dis 1979; 119:293.
32. Tisi GM. Preoperative identification and evaluation of the patient with lung disease. Med Clin North Am 1987; 71:399.
33. Tobin MJ, Suffredini AF, Grenvik A. Short-term effects of smoking cessation. Respir Care 1984; 29:641.
34. Torrington KG, Henderson CJ. Perioperative respiratory therapy. Chest 1988; 93:947.
35. Van Nostrand D, Kjelsberg MO, Humphrey EW. Preresectional evaluation of risk from pneumonectomy. Surg Obstet Gynecol 1968; 127:306.
36. Ziment I. Perioperative pharmacologic management. Respir Care 1984; 29:652.

Chapter 61

EVALUATION OF IMPAIRMENT AND DISABILITY IN PATIENTS WITH BRONCHITIS AND EMPHYSEMA

Kaye H. Kilburn

Impairment is a medically determined alteration in health status.[1] The term as customarily used means that there is a measurable loss of function. Thus, impairment ranges from changes in forced expiratory volume in 1 second (FEV_1) or vital capacity (VC), which are barely detectable by comparison with previous values in that individual or with predicted group values, all the way to life-threatening insufficiency of gas exchange. The American Thoracic Society (ATS) has defined impairment as "a functional abnormality which persists after appropriate therapy and with no reasonable prospect of improvement."[2]

Disability is defined legally as functional impairment sufficient to interfere with the patient's ability to do his or her usual job or perform other specific activities. Thus, in addition to the medical estimate or measurement of impairment, other information is required. This usually includes work characteristics, such as the duration of activities that produce dyspnea, recovery time usually available from such activities, average tolerated effort levels as well as dyspnea levels, the worker's motivation, and the likelihood of future medical problems. Also considered in disability are current and future economic dislocation, opportunities for retraining, and the condition of the job market, which in turn depends on local and even national economic factors. In brief, disability is impairment considered within the social milieu of employment.

Guidelines helpful in determining impairment for disability rating are published by the Social Security Administration,[3] U.S. Veterans Administration,[4] federal disability boards,[5] and worker's compensation boards in the various states beginning with Massachusetts and California in 1917.[6, 7] These guidelines should be consulted for details, rules, and procedures. The physician's input in the estimation of disability is important but is only part of the process. Obviously loss of lung capacity can be much better handled by a sedentary worker than by a lumberjack, stevedore, or construction laborer. Actually, disability should be defined for a specific job. It must be relevant to the particular program or regulation, that is, the policy that generated it. Thus, one will find specific disability criteria for railroad employees, social security disability, or a state's worker compensation.

For the physician doing examinations to help determine disability, perhaps the most broadly used definitions come from the American Medical Association (AMA) guidelines of 1965,[1] which define disability as an alteration of the capacity to meet personal, social, or occupational demands or to meet statutory or regulatory requirements.[7] Earlier guidelines refer to a reduction in or lack of ability to engage in gainful employment because of impairment. As the ATS committee on impairment and disability has pointed out, disability indicates the total effect of impairment on the patient's life.[2] This effect is determined by such factors as age, gender, education, economic and social environment, and the energy requirements of the patient's occupation. Thus, two persons with identical impairment may be differently affected in their life situation and thus in their disability. It is also obvious that disability may be complete or partial, permanent or temporary. It should be clear that disability may occur for reasons that have nothing to do with impairment as measured by standard tests of lung function, for example, because of disturbances in control of breathing, cardiovascular insufficiency, severe deconditioning, and bronchiectasis or infectious disease, particularly tuberculosis and acquired immunodeficiency syndrome (AIDS).

However, the first step in evaluation is to determine a worker's level of function compared with that of predicted healthy individuals and thus quantify his or her level of impairment. The second step is to measure functional decrements occurring across days, months, or years of exposure, whether the exposure is to cotton dust, foundry air, or cigarette smoke. Pulmonary function testing across brief intervals may provide important information regarding occupational asthma if airway responsiveness is demonstrated. It is also used in measurements of a group or population to determine how more subtle effects, caused by exposure to dusts or by ameliorated environmental conditions at work, are related to lung function.

METHODS

A wide range of methods are available to ascertain impairment but here the advice of the Greek philosophers is useful—the simplest is best. The breathing apparatus and heart are interdependent so that although we fragment function for descriptive and analytic purposes, the lung seldom shows a selective reduction of a single function. This is not to say that large differences in sensitivity do not exist or that the complaint of dyspnea may seem out of proportion to what can be measured. Rather, a large, expensive array of tests may contribute little information beyond that of a few relatively simple measurements.[8]

Methods of determining impairment should be accurate, sensitive, reproducible, and robust, that is, have a minimum of breakdowns. The methods used should be amenable to high speed data collection and handling for comparisons, quality checks, and reporting. Finally, it should be possible to create permanent records in a form that can be employed both for reporting to the individual and for assembling population data.[8]

Assessment of Dyspnea

A medical history should be carefully obtained to appraise the degree of dyspnea arising from activities that produce breathlessness and the presence of wheezing, cough, and sputum production. Dyspnea is essentially subjective and, like pain, remains a personal sensory phenomenon.[9] One subject will experience difficulty breathing with apparent calm acceptance, no dyspnea; another subject will show no outward signs of distress but will complain bitterly of shortness of breath.[10] How should one compare the responses of two such individuals who are poles apart? The approach that works best is to describe clearly the subject's complaints and separately describe what is observed, particulary evidence of distressed breathing.

Dyspnea is a universal human experience that must be interpreted in relation to the exertion that produces it. Dyspnea is abnormal only when it is exceptional, that is, beyond that usually experienced for the degree of exertion.[11] This makes description of stimuli that produce dyspnea important in the taking of a history. The dyspnea scales from the AMA Committee[1] (Table 61–1) in rating medical and physical impairment use class 1 to describe 0% impairment when dyspnea occurs consistent with the activity. Class 2 is for 10% to 20% impairment in which dyspnea does not occur at rest and seldom occurs during performance of the usual activities of daily living; for example, the patient can keep pace with persons of the same age and body build without breathlessness walking on the level but not on hills or stairs. Class 3 is for 25% to 35% impairment. Dyspnea does not occur at rest but does occur during activities of daily living. However, the patient can walk a mile at his own pace even though he cannot keep pace on the level with others of his same age and body build. In class 4, 50% to 70% impairment dyspnea occurs during such activities as climbing one flight of stairs or walking 100 yards on the level, with mild exertion, or even at rest.

Perhaps reflecting a different perspective or just the deliberations of another subcommittee, the dyspnea grades for classes of organic heart disease are worded somewhat differently. More impairment is attached to each class in that walking and climbing the stairs freely are mentioned, particularly in class 1 with its 0% to 15% impairment. The 20% to 45% of class 2 impairment resembles the percentages of class 2 for respiratory impairment. Class 3, 50% to 70%, defines walking more than two blocks on the level or climbing one flight of ordinary stairs, much more like class 4 in the respiratory impairment scale. In class 4, 80% to 95% impairment, activities of daily living beyond personal toilet produce discomfort. Finally, class 5 is added, which is dyspnea present on slight exertion, such as dressing or talking while at rest. Because walking and climbing stairs are almost universal experiences of daily life, it appears that four grades of dyspnea based on the effects of climbing two flights of stairs briskly without stopping as a 0 and one flight of stairs as 1 with 2, 3, and 4 as defined in the pulmonary dyspnea list above is practical. Despite much effort and some apparent relationships, little has been written about the correlation of grades of dyspnea with results of objective evaluations of respiratory function.

In general, however, dyspnea is perceived when the work of breathing is increased or respiratory muscle strength is decreased, resulting in less ventilation for the perceived effort. Both may be present in patients with airways obstruction.

MECHANICS OF BREATHING

Spirometry

Both experience and economy recommend spirometry as a first step in the measurement of lung functions for disability evaluations. The forced expiratory volume in 1 second (FEV_1), peak expiratory flow rate, the forced expiratory flow later in expiration at middle and lower volumes (FEF_{25-75} and FEF_{75-85}) are the measurements most frequently made. These standard measurements are more dependable than closing volume and

TABLE 61–1. Classes of Respiratory Impairment and Organic Heart Disease

RESPIRATORY IMPAIRMENT			
CLASS 1	**CLASS 2**	**CLASS 3**	**CLASS 4**
0% Impairment	**10%–20% Impairment**	**25%–35% Impairment**	**50%–70% Impairment**
When occurs, is consistent with the circumstances of activity.	Does not occur at rest and seldom occurs during performance of usual activities of daily living. The patient can keep pace with persons of same age and body build on the level without breathlessness, but not on hills or stairs.	Does not occur at rest but does occur during the usual activities of daily living. However, the patient can walk a mile at his own pace without dyspnea, although he cannot keep pace on the level with others of the same age and body build.	Occurs during such activities as climbing one flight of stairs or walking 100 yards on the level, on less exertion, or even at rest.
Spirometry (FEV_1)			
Not less than 85% of predicted.	70%–85% of predicted.	55%–70% of predicted.	Less than 55% of predicted.
CLASSES OF ORGANIC HEART DISEASE			
CLASS 1	**CLASS 2**	**CLASS 3**	**CLASS 4**
0%–15% Impairment	**20%–45% Impairment**	**50%–75% Impairment**	**80%–95% Impairment**
Walking, climbing stairs freely, and performance of usual activities of daily living do not produce symptoms.	Walking freely on the level, climbing at least one flight of stairs, and performance of usual activities of daily living do not produce symptoms.	Walking more than one or two blocks on the level, climbing one flight of ordinary stairs, or performance of usual activities of daily living produces symptoms.	Performance of any of the activities of daily living beyond the personal toilet or its equivalent produces increased discomfort.

closing capacity, which, because of excessive variability, are practically useless. Similarly, body plethysmography or measurements of airway resistance using pulsed flow provide precise information, but these methods are more complex and time consuming and are best used for sorting out difficult problems in subjects whose spirometry is normal.

The vital capacity and FEV_1 are basic and time-tested measurements. The calculation of midflow, FEF_{25-75}, and of flow at low volumes, FEF_{75-85}, provide additional sensitivity in detecting changes caused by air pollution and cigarette smoking. The correlation of FEV_1 with exercise capacity, as measured by maximal oxygen uptake, is very strong. It must be realized, however, that FEV_1 is a static test and does not measure fatigue or endurance. The maximal voluntary ventilation, if actually carried out for a minute, would be a reliable dynamic measurement. However, it is susceptible to errors when carried out for only 10 or 15 seconds or when calculated by multiplying the FEV_1 by 40. In addition, relationships of this sort can be utilized to better advantage in obstructive pulmonary disease than in other lung diseases.

Agreed upon methods for performing spirometry are described in the Occupational Health and Safety Administration's (OHSA) cotton dust standard[12] and in the report of the ATS's Snowbird Conference.[13] The test must be performed with the subject standing, wearing a nose clip, breathing into a volume measuring spirometer, which is accurately calibrated for volume and time and produces a permanent record. One may use water spirometers, piston or bellows types, such as the Ohio, and pneumotachygraphs, the latter integrating volume from the flow record. Heat sensor devices are unsatisfactory because they do not produce a record from which the shape of the curve and its component parts can be analyzed and they error in subjects with greatly reduced function. Thus, the equipment menu is restricted, and it must be selected to meet these criteria.

LUNG VOLUMES

The total thoracic gas volume (TGV) and the total lung capacity (TLC) are most useful measurements for emphysema. As the lung loses its internal tethering and increases in volume the TLC increases. As vital capacity and FEV_1 decrease, residual volume (RV) increases. The magnitude of the volume changes are detected best by measuring TLC. Residual volume, the difference between the TLC and the vital capacity, is slightly less sensitive, an unimportant difference because it can only be measured together with TLC. The RV/TLC ratio is almost always elevated above 140% when emphysema is present. The methods of measuring TLC include plethysmography, gas dilution, and planimetry of chest radiographs. Plethysmography has the advantage of an independent measurement that determines the amount of gas in the thorax by applying Boyle's Law. Thus, in a closed system at constant temperature, the product of pressure and volume within the system is constant. If the closed system is disturbed dynamically, then $P_1V_1 = P_2V_2$, and the equation can be solved. In the practical sense this is done by placing the subject in a chamber occluding the mouthpiece and having the subject make respiratory efforts against obstruction, thereby changing intrathoracic pressure and volume.

In the method requiring the dilution of gases the subject's lung is connected to a spirometer containing an accurately measured concentration and volume of test gas, usually helium. When the subject is turned to this system, usually at the end of a normal expiration, functional residual capacity (FRC) is measured after the system reaches equilibrium, that is, has diluted the test gas into the new volume and had its concentration remeasured. The new volume is then calculated. The disadvantage of this system is that it measures only thoracic gas spaces, which communicate with the airways. Thus, poorly ventilated zones, blebs, and bullae are measured incompletely or not at all.

Another method is to planimeter the standard 6-foot chest radiographs taken at full inspiration. Using the posteroanterior (PA) and lateral views, the areas of lung in both projections are summed and these areas are related to TLC via a regression equation.[15] The original coefficient of 0.86 correlating plethysmograph TGV and planimetry TGV can be improved if an effort is made to take the radiographs in full inflation, which means that the diaphragms must be below the ninth intercostal space, particularly on the PA radiograph. The measurement of TLC is increased in subjects with emphysema. It is also useful in subjects in whom volume loss or restriction has occurred due to interstitial fibrosis, diaphragmatic paralysis or eventration, chest wall weakness or deformity, pneumonectomy, or other disease. It is important to examine the chest radiographs and to estimate TLC before interpreting pulmonary function tests for the degree and type of impairment.

GAS EXCHANGE

Gas exchange is most easily measured by assessing the movement into the blood of carbon monoxide as a test gas. This diffusing capacity technique, devised by Maria Krogh in 1909,[15] has been perfected and automatized so that it can be done almost as quickly and simply as spirometry.[16, 17] It is highly correlated with alveolar volume and alveolar O_2 partial pressure. Diffusing capacity is adversely affected by inequality of ventilation, distribution of pulmonary blood flow, reduced volume of the pulmonary vascular bed, and reduction in blood hemoglobin concentration. It is most frequently decreased by ventilation-perfusion disproportion. Notwithstanding, it is a very sensitive test and useful in assessing impairment. It is most easily done using a single breath technique, which means a 10-second breath hold of a test gas containing carbon monoxide and helium. Carbon monoxide is measured with an infrared or a fuel cell analyzer. Helium, the other test gas, is measured for calculating the alveolar volume during the 10-second breath hold. In healthy subjects this rapid helium volume is 350 or 400 ml less than TLC. However, in the presence of airway obstruction and delayed equilibrium a smaller proportion is measured just as in the gas dilution methods for TLC using nitrogen or helium.

Originally, diffusing capacity had the disadvantage of inadequate population-derived prediction equations. However, not only has this problem been rectified but smoking-specific standards have been provided from a large, stratified, random population.[17] This information has increased the sensitivity of the diffusing capacity and its usefulness in classifying impairment. There is, however, still a larger individual variation of diffusing capacity in healthy subjects after adjusting for height and age so that the confidence intervals are wider than for vital capacity or FEV_1.

EXERCISE TESTING

The dynamic measurement of the capacity for exercise represents an unparalleled opportunity to correlate a subject's dyspnea with objective information. Perhaps the most useful measurement is the maximal oxygen uptake or the oxygen uptake during exercise at a pulse rate calculated as a percentage of maximal heart rate. Volumes have been written about exercise.[18–20] For obtaining steady state measurements a treadmill or bicycle is usually employed, although the Master's step test is also used.[21, 22] For most Americans walking on the treadmill is a more familiar procedure than bicycle riding. Computerized programs with rapid analysis of expired oxygen and carbon dioxide now make it possible to do exercise testing at multiple levels of work to approach a calculated submaximal pulse rate or oxygen uptake rapidly and precisely. The technique has been used extensively to assess coronary artery disease in which onset of pain or electrocardiographic disturbance is the stopping point. It is also useful in recognizing a deconditioned subject in whom the maximal heart rate is reached quickly.

In advanced obstructive lung disease the maximal oxygen uptake is reduced, the oxygen pulse is reduced greatly, the dead space to tidal volume ratio is increased, the alveolar-arterial oxygen difference widened, and the oxygen partial pressure of arterial blood reduced. Thus, the reasonably well-conditioned individual with obstructive lung disease experiences desaturation of arterial blood at an oxygen uptake well below the predicted maximal level. Perhaps the most useful observation from exercise testing in subjects with chronic obstructive lung disease is the level of exercise that produces dyspnea. The level is then related to the subject's job requirements. Even if this is done crudely as "light," e.g., desk and watchman; "medium," e.g., technician and mechanic; and "heavy," e.g., farmer, foundry and construction laborer, classification is useful.

The steady state diffusing capacity for carbon monoxide ($DL_{CO_{SS}}$), as described by Filley and coworkers,[23] combines oxygen uptake information with the transfer rate for carbon monoxide during exercise. The exercise $DL_{CO_{SS}}$ corresponds quite closely to the DL_{CO} single breath in all but deconditioned subjects. At a given workload it measures respiratory reserve capacity. The disadvantage of full exercise testing is that it requires several levels of graded exercise to approach maximal oxygen uptake at submaximal heart rate and thus requires more time and is more expensive than the preceding tests. It also requires provision for cardiopulmonary resuscitation should arrhythmia or collapse ensue during testing.

THE QUANTITATIVE EXPRESSIONS OF IMPAIRMENT

Comparisons to Determine Differences from Normal (Predicted) Values

The measurement of impairment implies comparison to a standard population considered to be normal. The first effort in this regard was that of Hutchinson,[24] who devised the spirometer, named the vital capacity, and published the first population-based vital capacity statistics in 1846. A hundred years later Baldwin and colleagues[25] provided pulmonary function values based on spirometry from a small group of hospitalized patients, and these remained the standard until a cooperative study by Kory and colleagues[26] provided new and higher values for normal. However, they did not segregate smokers from nonsmokers in selecting their healthy subjects. It remained for Morris and colleagues[27, 28] in 1971 and 1975 to provide comparison values for healthy nonsmoking individuals of both sexes based on a sizable population sample. In 1986, Miller and colleagues,[29] for the first time, provided smoking-specific comparisons providing an adjustment for smoking to apply when examining the effect of occupational or environmental factors that might influence function. Thus, they provided smoking-specific prediction equations for spirometry and for diffusing capacity[17] from the same probability sample of the Michigan population.

The height dependency of vital capacity and flows was established by Hutchinson in 1846.[24] He pointed out that vital capacity was directly related to height and inversely proportional to age in the range between 30 and 65 years. By 1920, West[30] had established simple prediction formulas for vital capacity but the modern era of pulmonary function testing dated from Baldwin and colleagues' 1948 work,[25] which introduced standard values. With height as the major predictor Hutchinson's observation of age dependence was confirmed. Thus, the standard predictive equations introduced by Baldwin and colleagues[25] were based on sex, height, and age. The confounding of the age factor by cigarette smoking or the increase in rate of decrement in smokers had been observed repeatedly during the modern period but was first measured by Miller and colleagues.[29] For nonsmokers, the Morris and Miller prediction equations yield practically identical results for vital capacity and flows. The addition of the years of smoking variable adjusts for its contribution and aids in analysis of occupational and environmental factors. That black people have somewhat smaller lungs than white people has been known since 1926[31] and confirmed in the U.S.[32] and Africa.[33] Although some have suggested that different predictive equations are needed, it is now clear that a satisfactory adjustment for blacks is to reduce the predictions based on white subjects by 12.5% for FVC, FEV_1, and flows and by 8% for diffusing capacity.[11]

If there were a generally useful formula for assessing impairment of working capacity applicable to obstructive pulmonary disease of both the small airways obstructive and emphysematous types it would be described here. It would be even better if the scheme were broadly applicable to chronic pulmonary diseases, including pulmonary fibrosis and asthma. Although measuring working capacity needed for a job is conceptually straightforward, it is not an easy concept to use in the workplace or to create an appropriate mockup in the laboratory. Beyond measuring the capacity for peak performance, endurance must be estimated. Unfortunately, schemes that begin with spirometry are numerically precise but fail to predict capacity for work except at the severe impairment end of the spectrum and even this has exceptions. Thus, what is proposed are recommendations that are workable in the majority of cases. It is pragmatic and guided by past experience, personal and collective,[1] but it must be tempered by skepticism and a willingness to listen, always to listen to the patient. For despite our sophisticated measurements, there is much in the complex adjustment of the human body to activity that can only be appraised by the subject's nervous system. Thus, the guiding principle is, when our measurements fit they may be accepted but when they do not *the illusion must be dismissed that measurements are infallible because they yield numbers.*

The population studies of spirometry have produced simple linear predictive equations that work across the age range 25 to 65 years for men and women. Thus, results on the subject being tested can and should be compared with the standard data and presented as percent predicted. Accepting 80% of predicted as approximately the 95% confidence interval of normal for FEV_1 and 40% of predicted as severe impairment,[2] an arbitrary apportionment of percent predicted is proposed. It is reasonable to assign slight impairment to the 79% to 65% range, moderate impairment to the 64% to 50% range, moderately severe impairment to the 49% to 40% range, and thus severe impairment to below 40%. Forced expiratory volume in 1 second is closely related to exercise capacity so that few subjects with FEV_1 below 1.5 L can exceed 20 ml/kg of oxygen uptake during exercise. For vital capacity severe impairment may be set at 50% of predicted and the lower end of normal again at approximately 80% with slight, 79% to 70%, moderate, 69% to 60%, and moderately severe, 59% to 50%.

The ratio FEV_1 to FVC is an excellent measure of obstruction, and a subject with a ratio of 40% is accepted as severely impaired, but even 60% represents slowing of expiration associated with dyspnea. The ratio is age dependent, decreasing from 80% to 70% from age 20 to 60 years as FEV_1 decreases more rapidly than FVC. Care must be taken to record all of the FVC or the ratio is artificially elevated. As the FEV_1/FVC ratio increases residual volume usually increases and with it the RV/TLC ratio increases.

A practical four-step approach (Fig. 61–1) is, step 1, to regard severe impairment as defined by an FVC of 50% predicted, and FEV_1 less than 40% of predicted, or an FEV_1/FVC less than 40% of predicted.[2]

Step 2 is to measure single breath diffusing capacity of the lungs ($DLco_{sb}$). If it is less than 40% of predicted severe impairment exists. Step 3 is to predict the "break point," defined as one of the following: (a) maximal oxygen uptake sustainable for the patient's usual job, (b) anaerobic threshold (the point at which as exercise increases minute ventilation rises out of proportion to the increase in oxygen uptake), (c) the point at which there is a drop in arterial oxygen tension with increase in exercise, or (d) when heart rate reaches 80% of the age predicted maximum rate. Thus, step 3 employs exercise consisting of 30 8-inch steps up and down in 60 seconds, monitoring arterial oxygenation with an ear oximeter. It can be used to estimate working capacity or impairment level. Thus, a subject who is able to walk briskly on level ground can usually complete the standard step test and achieve a maximal oxygen uptake of greater than 1.5 L/min. One who notes dyspnea walking at his peers' pace on level ground usually cannot complete the step test without becoming dyspneic and has a maximal oxygen uptake of less than 1.5 L/min.[11,21] A comprehensive exercise test, step 4, uses incremental measurements of oxygen uptake, minute ventilation, heart rate, and arterial blood oxygen tension at multiple levels to determine maximal O_2 uptake, anaerobic threshold, or O_2 consumption at 80% of maximal age-corrected heart rate, and arterial oxygen tension by sampling or by oximetry, requiring a fully equipped exercise laboratory.[20] The multiple steps of exercise and multiple analyses require a well-calibrated motor-driven treadmill or bicycle ergometer with repeated rapid measurements of ventilation and oxygen uptake, an electrocardiograph, and an ear oximeter. These are now usefully combined in computer-programmed devices, which set work increments at 100 KPM (kilopond-meter)/min power output for men or 50 KPM/min for small women or children.[20] Applying the concepts of this test to the workplace, about

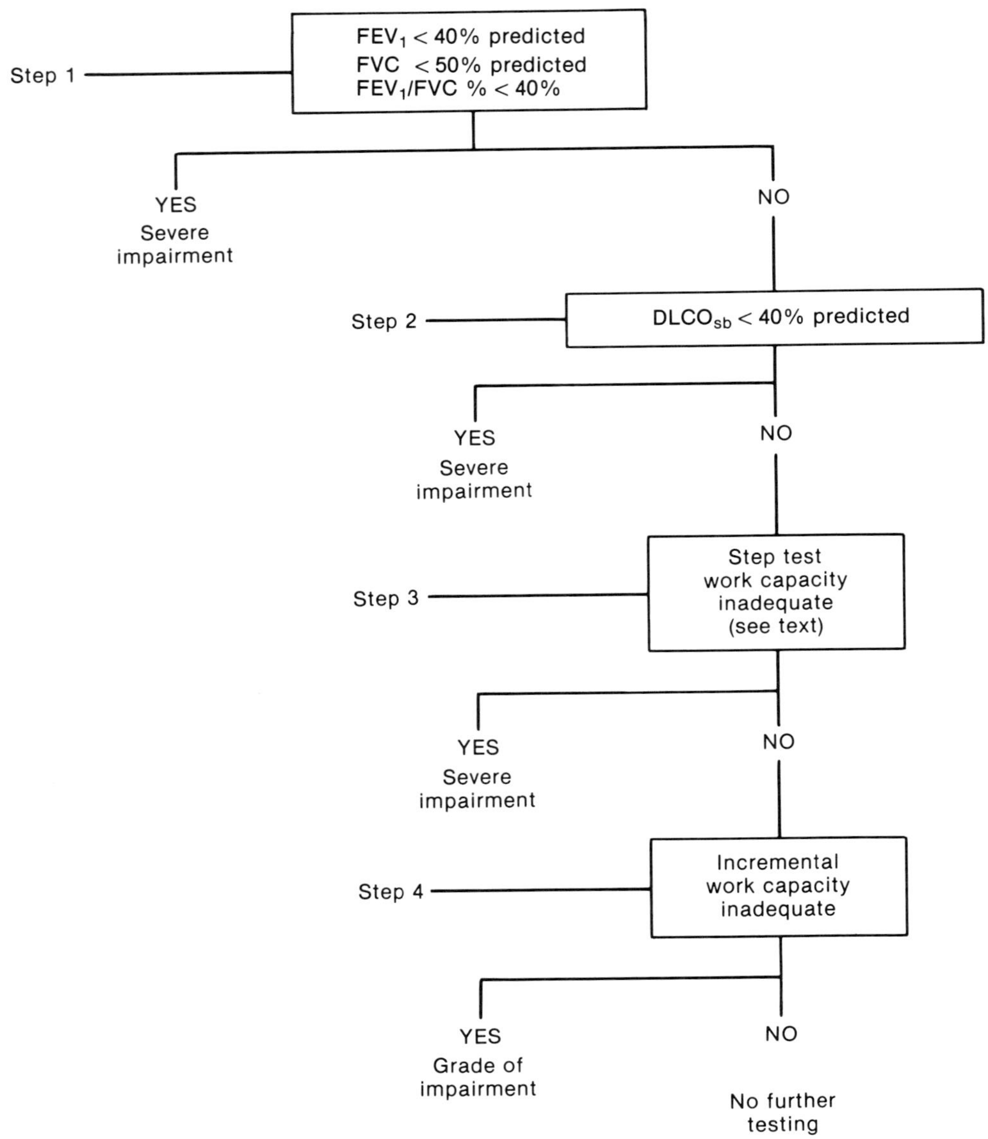

Figure 61–1. Four steps in impairment evaluation with decision criteria are (1) spirometry; (2) diffusing capacity for carbon monoxide, single breath; (3) step test; and (4) incremental working capacity, comprehensive exercise testing. Please see text for detailed explanation.

35% to 40% of maximal oxygen uptake can be sustained for 8 hours. If a maximal oxygen uptake of 2.5 L/min can be achieved in testing, then steady state work level, which requires an O_2 consumption of 1 L/min, can be carried for 8 hours.

Episodic worsening of ventilatory test performance from acute respiratory illness (flu and bronchitis), from asthma, or from work place exposures, such as to cotton dust, flour, toluene diisocyanate (TDI), trimellitic anhydride (TMA), and other chemicals must be sought by history and eliminated by repeat testing after removal of the adverse agents. Assessments of the response to bronchodilator as an alternative to challenge testing may be useful. Also bronchodilator reversal of the effect of short-acting chemicals, such as TDI, ozone, and nitrogen dioxide may assist in diagnosis. It is not clear whether such reversals of airway obstruction can be generalized to other situations.

CAUSATION

Genetic Factors

Alpha$_1$-antitrypsin or antiprotease deficiency is a risk factor increasing the likelihood of emphysema in homozygotes and decreasing the age at which it is recognized.[34–36] The risk for emphysema may increase in heterozygotes depending on their specific Pi phenotype.[34, 35] The synergistic effect of smoking in producing emphysema in antiprotease-deficient homozygotes is well known. Cigarette smoking may have a stimulating effect on neutrophil and macrophage proteases.[37, 38] Emphysema can result from lung digestion by cellular proteases in nondeficient antiprotease individuals.[40]

The evidence of genetic factors in chronic bronchitis is limited to exceptional disorders, such as tracheobronchomegaly and flabby airways, due to deficiency of tracheal and bronchial cartilage, as in the Williams-Campbell syndrome.[41] There are, however, studies of monozygotic twins with a chronic cough that have shown concordance exceeding that due to smoking habits. Kartagener syndrome, in which there is clear evidence for the absence of dynein side limbs on the microtubules of the cilia, leads to functional failure of the cilia and, as a consequence, to bronchiectasis or bronchiolectasis.[42, 43] Cystic fibrosis is a genetic disease manifested by disturbances of mucus, which over time alters a normal lung to one with dilated and cystic airways.[44, 45] Whether the viscoelastic properties of bronchial secretion are genetically controlled is still unclear. In addition, there may be defects of the immune system that interfere with defenses of the airway and heighten susceptibility to bacterial proteases. Asthma appears to be, in part, genetically determined[47] and is of major importance in association with other factors in producing chronic obstructive lung disease, at least in a segment of the affected population.

Air Pollution

Clearly, personal cigarette smoke is the air pollutant that contributes most to causing obstructive pulmonary disease. A smoker inhales 2 billion toxic particles per ml of smoke, thus, 70 billion particles per puff and about 1400 billion particles per cigarette smoked.[48] Consequences of this are so well known as to not require emphasis.

Occupational air pollution is important for its contribution to occupational asthma and to chronic bronchitis. New, exotic chemicals are being added yearly that can produce asthma at work: such natural products as cotton dust, wheat dust, flour, and red cedar dust and synthetic materials as TDI, TMA, and penicillin. Many chemicals and mixtures including silica in various forms and coal dust, diesel exhaust, and specific chemicals, such as ammonia, chlorine, phosgene, HCL and endotoxin[48] can cause occupational asthma or chronic bronchitis. Coal dust is important because it is the only occupational or environmental exposure with the proven capacity to cause emphysema, established by cohort studies.[49, 50] A review of occupational causes of lung disease is found in *Public Health and Preventive Medicine*.[51]

Environmental causes of chronic obstructive pulmonary disease are atmospheric or ambient air pollution of two major types: (1) the reducing type, from coal combustion, which is rich in sulfur oxides and fly ash particles and low in ozone and NO_2[52, 53] and (2) the oxidant type, most commonly seen in sun belt cities, particularly during the summer, where solar conversion of petroleum oxidation products yields ozone and nitrogen oxides in addition to SO_2. These toxic gases are inhaled adsorbed to particles with aerodynamic mean diameters below 10 μm from diesel and gasoline engine exhaust. There are chronic effects in children from both reducing and oxidant air pollution with the strongest correlations to respirable particles.[54]

DISABILITY: COMPLETING THE MEDICAL LEGAL EQUATION AND DECIDING HOW MUCH IMPAIRMENT CONSTITUTES DISABILITY

Job requirements, economic factors, personal motivation, the job market, and the possible effects of economic dislocation enter into the complex calculation of disability. Fortunately for the physician his contribution, the estimation of impairment as discussed earlier, is the more precise and not usually controversial. Described briefly are some of the factors that enter into disability evaluation. Although a number of schemes have been devised for estimating the oxygen cost of certain operations in industry or in a range of job categories, no substitute exists for a careful history and determination by the physician of the usual oxygen requirements for the job and the frequency and nature of episodic requirements above that level. For example, carrying tools and climbing ladders may be many times higher in oxygen requirement than is the job itself. If these episodic challenges are well spaced and there is time for recovery with little likelihood of emergencies requiring greater effort, they may be of only small consequence. In contrast, if considerable oxygen requirement or ventilatory capacity is needed immediately following ladder climbing or carrying in of tools the worker may be disabled, although he has plenty of capacity for the steady state part of his job. Use of treadmill exercise to determine work capacity or maximal oxygen uptake is useful in simulating the workplace but has its limitations. Direct observations of the patient at work may be required.

Motivation is varied in subjects being evaluated. A deeply ingrained work ethic will keep some individuals at work well after the average one has been disabled. Once again the patient's work history is of great importance. The number of jobs held, the duration of each job, and the satisfaction experienced on the job generally allow motivation to be appraised roughly after a few minutes of conversation. It is obviously important to consider the subject's wants and needs; for example, if a few months or 1 or 2 years of continuation of the patient's current job substantially improve the retirement stipend, then allowances should be made.

Regulatory and often legal issues complicate judgments concerning disability. The physician needs to have some knowledge of processes involved in state's worker compensa-

TABLE 61–2. A Comparison of Published Average Decrements in Forced Expiratory Ventilation in One Second (FEV_1) for Men

FEV_1 LITERS/YEARS	REFERENCE
1. 0.052 Smokers (miners)	Higgins ITT, Oldha PD. Ventilatory capacity in miners: A 5-year follow-up study. Br J Ind Med 1962; 19:65–76.
0.024 Nonsmokers	Higgins ITT. Tobacco smoking, respiratory symptoms and ventilatory capacity. Br Med J 1959; 1:325–329.
2. 0.025	Kory RC, Callahan R, Boren HG, Syner JC. The Veterans Administration-Army cooperative study of pulmonary function/clinical spirometry in normal men. Am J Med 1961; 30:243–258.
3. 0.024	Ferris BG, Anderson PO, Zinkmantel R. Prediction values for screening tests of pulmonary function. Am Rev Respir Dis 1965; 91:252–261.
4. 0.031	Rosenzweig JA, Atkins JA, Schrock LG. Ventilatory studies in a normal population after a seven year interval. Am Rev Respir Dis 1966; 94:74–77.
5. 0.026 (904) Smoking	Fletcher CM. Bronchial infections and reactivity in chronic bronchitis. J R Coll Phys Lond 1968; 2:183–190.
Age	
6. 0.032 25–34 0.041 55–64 (756)	Higgins ITT, Gilson, JC, Ferris BG, et al. IV Chronic respiratory disease in an industrial town: A nine-year follow-up study preliminary report. Am J Publ Health 1968; 58:16657–16676.
7. 0.042 Nonsmokers 0.070 Smokers 313 men age 50	Wilhelmsen L, Orha I, Tibblin G. Decrease in ventilatory capacity between ages 50 and 54 in representative sample of Swedish men. Br Med J 1969; 3:553–556.
8. 0.034	Howard P. A long-term follow-up of respiratory function symptoms and ventilatory function in a group of working men. Br J Ind Med 1967; 27:326–333.
9. 0.032 Age 25–64 pred	Morris JF, Koski A, Johnson LC. Spirometer standards for healthy nonsmoking adults. Am Rev Respir Dis 1971; 103:57–67.
0.031 15 year dec.	Morris JF, Koski A, Temple WP, et al. Fifteen years' interval spirometric evaluation of the Oregon predictive equations. Chest 1988; 93:123–127.
10. 0.023 for 25–75 years	Miller A, Thornton JC, Warshaw R, et al. Mean and instantaneous expiratory flows, FVC_1 and FEV_1: prediction equations from a probability sample of Michigan, a large industrial state. Bull Eur Physiopathol Respir 1986; 22:589–597.

tion laws, national railroad workers' programs, seamen's compensation, social security, and other programs. It is often useful to put the worker in contact with a counselor who can supplement the physician's information and review his legal rights. In a democratic society the decision to continue working belongs to the patient, not to the physician.

Factors such as economic dislocation and job market also enter into disability decisions. Workers in some trades, such as boilermakers or pipefitters, are accustomed to working anywhere within a large territory or region, whereas others are concerned if they live more than 5 miles from their work site. Job markets vary not only with economic and seasonal factors but also with technologic changes. It appears that in the past 40 years there have been particularly abrupt changes in apparent supply and demand for skilled labor. Certain long-time "stable" industries in the U.S., such as automobile and electronic manufacturing, have suffered from Asian competition.

Medical care requirements of patients, particularly those who need continuing care, are far easier for physicians to understand and plan for than are some of the aforementioned factors. It is clear that patients with airways obstruction benefit from medication and continuing care and need a dependable relationship with a physician or group of physicians. The care requirement for the young asthmatic man or woman may be quite different from that for a 55-year–old patient with emphysema who needs both periodic medical help with emergencies and continuous care. Clearly anticipation of the type, period, and necessity for care should be part of the physician's planning for disability action. Planning should include the possible complications that may occur, such as hospitalizations, the need for a breathing apparatus, or even oxygen at home.

The patient must be taught to live within the limitation of his disability. This means pacing work or energy use, foregoing activities that produce dyspnea, or doing them at a much slower pace. Supplemental oxygen may be required by some patients. The physician should develop the summary statement concerning impairment, progression, and prognosis, and a plan for meeting medical needs as the patient's disability worsens.

PROGNOSIS

It is clear from many studies that subjects who have left adverse occupational exposures or quit cigarette smoking have slower rates of functional loss. Cleaner work areas in "dirty" industries are often filled by ex-smokers who used seniority to reduce their occupational exposures. For populations, the yearly rate of fall or decrement of lung function has been precisely defined.[55] However, after substantial functional capacity is lost the rate of decline may decrease to nothing for years at a time. Clearly without knowing in detail where a given individual fits the physician must base prognosis on the mean for the group. Exacerbations of chronic bronchitis or bronchitic episodes may cause fluctuation in a patient's rate of decrement of function. Function is lost during the episode and may not be regained during convalescence. Common sense dictates removal of the patient from adverse exposures and avoidance of respiratory infections. Episodes of influenza and pneumonia are important stresses for the impaired individual. Similarly, prompt treatment, surveillance, and vigorous response by the physician are justifiable and prudent. Thus, in addition to stopping cigarette smoking and avoiding adverse occupational exposures, conservation of remaining function by minimizing respiratory infections is crucial.

The yearly measurement by spirometry of vital capacity and flows provides good indicators of prognosis (Table 61–2). After three or four yearly observations of FEV_1 the patient's rate of decrement of function can be estimated and the approximate time of crossing the critical level of impairment determined.[55] Many observers have noted that the FEV_1, the most stable of the predictive parameters, falls at a rate about 50% greater in the 55 to 64 age group than it does in subjects 30 years younger.[56] The correlation among the increasing degree of dyspnea and reduction in FEV_1 and midflow has been shown repeatedly since the early 1960s.[57]

Only a few longitudinal studies of patients with bronchitis have been completed. One by Gregory in Sheffield, England,[58] showed that the interval between onset of chronic bronchitis and disability from it, defined as loss of time from work for two consecutive winters, was 40 years for workers with an onset under 15 years of age, 10 years with an onset after age 40, and 2.3 years with the onset after age 60. Hypersecretion manifested by cough and phlegm may be present for years without accelerating the deterioration of function. However, in the age group older than 60 the appearance of cough and phlegm as chronic symptoms generally portends rapid reductions in functional capacity. The key is prospective studies of chronic bronchitis.

One such large study of 1136 British men 30 to 50 years old in the engineering works of London Transport and the Post Office Savings Bank from 1961 until 1969[55] provided longitudinal data on lung functions of employed subjects with the hypersecretory syndrome versus those with progressive airways obstruction caused by bronchitis. In some individuals the hypersecretory syndrome disappeared. Airways obstruction was irreversible but rarely caused disability before age 40.

Chronic bronchitis complicates the course of patients with asbestosis[61] and other interstitial lung diseases[62] when or after patients accelerate their rate of loss of lung volume. This accelerated group may need to be studied separately to estimate prognosis.

The prognosis of emphysema is more difficult to estimate because of a lack of firm clinical diagnostic criteria, its relative infrequency uncomplicated by chronic bronchitis, and the absence of suitable data comparing clinical information with lung pathology.[59] Part of this oversight could be corrected by correlating thoracic gas volume measured from the posteroanterior and lateral radiographs with the radiographic criteria. Studies comparing dyspnea radiographic changes with lung function may improve the ability of the physician to predict the course of emphysema with the Pi genotype.

REFERENCES

1. American Medical Association, Committee on Rating of Mental and Physical Impairment: Guides to the evaluation of permanent impairment. JAMA 1965; 194:177–190.
2. ATS Statement. Evaluation of impairment/disability secondary to respiratory disease. Am Rev Respir Dis 1982; 126:945–951.
3. Social Security Administration. Disability evaluation under social security: a handbook for physicians. HEW Pub No (SSA) 79–10089, 1979.
4. Code of Federal Regulations Pension Bonuses and Veterans' Relief, revised as of July 1977. Veterans Administration Schedule for rating disability, Section 6600 for bronchitis, 6603 for emphysema and 6802 for pneumoconiosis, September 1975.
5. Department of Labor. Standards for determining coal miners total disability or death due to pneumoconiosis. Fed Reg 1980; 45:13678–13712.
6. Ashford NA, Andrews RA. Workers' compensation. In: Rom WN, ed. Environmental and Occupational Medicine. Boston: Little, Brown, and Co., Inc., 1983.
7. Gaensler EA, Wright GW. Evaluation of respiratory impairment. Arch Environ Health 1966; 12:146–189.
8. Kilburn KH, Warshaw R. Pulmonary function testing for occupational epidemiology and disability. In: Wilson AF, ed. Pulmonary Function Testing Indications and Interpretations. New York: Grune & Stratton, Inc., 1985.
9. Comroe JH Jr. Dyspnea. Mod Conc Cardiovasc Dis 1956; 25:347–349.
10. Campbell EJM, Howell JBL. The sensation of breathlessness. Br Med Bull 1963; 36–40.
11. Kanarek DJ, Miller A. Respiratory impairment and disability. In: Miller A, ed. Pulmonary Function Tests in Clinical and Occupational Lung Disease. New York: Grune & Stratton, Inc., 1986.
12. United States Department of Labor, National Institute for Occupational Safety and Health. Cotton dust. Title 29. Code of Federal Regulations, Part 1910.1043 and 1910.1046a.
13. ATS Statement. Snowbird workshop on standardization of spirometry. Am Rev Respir Dis 1979; 119:831–838.
14. Harris TR, Pratt PC, Kilburn KH. Total lung capacity measured by roentgenograms. Am J Med 1971; 50:756–763.
15. Krogh M. Diffusion of gases through the lungs of man. J Physiol (Lond) 1914; 49:271–300.
16. Ogilvie CM, Forster RE, Blakemore WS, Morton JW. A standardized breath holding technique for the clinical measurement of the diffusing capacity of the lung for carbon monoxide. J Clin Invest 1957; 36:1–17.
17. Miller A, Thornton JC, Warshaw R, et al. Single breath diffusing capacity in a representative sample of the population of Michigan, a large industrial state. Am Rev Respir Dis 1983; 127:270–277.
18. American Heart Association. Exercise Testing and Training of Apparently Healthy Individuals: a Handbook for Physicians. New York: American Heart Association, 1972.
19. Wasserman K, Whipp BJ. Exercise physiology in health and disease. Am Rev Respir Dis 1975; 112:219–249.
20. Jones NL. Clinical Exercise Testing. Philadelphia: WB Saunders Company, 1988.
21. Master AM, Oppenheimer ET. A simple exercise tolerance test for circulatory efficiency with standard tables for normal individuals. Am J Med Sci 1929; 177:223–243.
22. Master AM, Rosenfeld I. Exercise electrocardiography as an estimate of cardiac function. Dis Chest 1967; 51:347–382.
23. Filley GF, MacIntosh DJ, Wright GW. Carbon monoxide uptake and pulmonary diffusing capacity in normal subjects at rest and during exercise. J Clin Invest 1954; 33:530–539.
24. Hutchinson J. On capacity of lungs and on respiratory functions with view of establishing a precise and easy method for detecting disease by spirometer. Tr Med-Chir Soc (Lond) 1846; 29:137.
25. Baldwin E deF, Cournand A, Richards DW Jr. Pulmonary insufficiency: physiological classification clinical methods of analysis standard values in normal subjects. Medicine 1948; 27:243–278.
26. Kory RC, Callahan R, Boren HG, Syner JC. The Veterans Administration-Army cooperative study of pulmonary function: I. Clinical spirometry in normal men. Am J Med 1961; 30:243–258.
27. Morris JF, Koski A, Johnson LC. Spirometric standards for healthy nonsmoking adults. Am Rev Respir Dis 1971; 103:57–67.
28. Morris JF, Koski A, Breese JD. Normal values and evaluation of forced end-expiratory flow. Am Rev Respir Dis 1975; 111:755–762.
29. Miller A, Thornton JC, Warshaw R, et al. Mean and instantaneous expiratory flows, FVC and FEV_1: Prediction equations from a probability sample of Michigan, a large industrial state. Bull Eur Physiopathol Respir 1986; 22:589–597.
30. West HF. Clinical studies on the respiration: VI. A comparison of various standards for the normal vital capacity of the lungs. Arch Intern Med 1920; 25:306–316.
31. Smillie WG, Augustine DL. Vital capacity of the negro race. J Am Med Assoc 1926; 87:2055–2058.
32. Schoenberg JB, Beck GJ, Bouhuys A. Growth and decay of pulmonary function in healthy blacks and whites. Respir Physiol 1978; 33:367–393.
33. Femi-Pearse D, Elebute EA. Ventilatory function in healthy adult Nigerians. Clin Sci 1971; 41:203–211.
34. Eriksson S. Pulmonary emphysema and $alpha_1$-antitrypsin deficiency. Acta Med Scand 1964; 175:197–205.
35. Ganrot PO, Laurell CB, Eriksson S. Obstructive lung disease and trypsin inhibitors in $alpha_1$-antitrypsin deficiency. Scand J Clin Lab Invest 1967; 19:205–208.
36. Hutchinson DCS, Barter CE, Cook PJL, et al. Severe pulmonary emphysema: a comparison of patients with and without $alpha_1$-antitrypsin deficiency. Q J Med 1972; 163:301–315.
37. Carrell RW, Jeppsson JO, Laurell CB, et al. Structure and variation of human $alpha_1$-antitrypsin. Nature 1982; 298:329–334.
38. Fera T, Abboud RT, Johal SS, Gibson N. Effect of smoking on functional activity of plasma $alpha_1$-protease inhibitor. Chest 1987; 91:346–350.
39. Damiano VV, Tsang A, Kucich U, et al. Immunolocalization of elastase in human emphysematous lungs. J Clin Invest 1986; 78:482–493.

40. Morrison HM, Kramps JA, Burnett D, Stockley RA. Lung lavage fluid from patients with $alpha_1$-proteinase inhibitor deficiency or chronic obstructive bronchitis: anti-elastase function and cell profile. Clin Sci 1987; 72:373–381.
41. Kilburn KH. Genetic aspects of chronic bronchitis. In: Freour P, Holland WW, eds. Chronic Obstructive Bronchopathies: The Link Between Theory and Practice. London: Kimpton Medical Publications, 1984.
42. Afzelius BA. A human syndrome caused by immotile cilia. Science 1976; 193:317–319.
43. Afzelius BA, Eliasson R. Flagellar mutants in man: on the heterogeneity of the immotile-cilia syndrome. J Ultrastruct Res 1979; 69:43–52.
44. Pedersen JT, Lykkegaard E, Faero O, Jacobsen L. Lung function in children and young adults with cystic fibrosis. Dan Med Bull 1974; 21:12–19.
45. Schwartz EE, Holsclaw DS. Pulmonary involvement in adults with cystic fibrosis. Am J Roentgenol Rad Ther & Nuc Med 1974; 122:708–718.
46. Meier HL, Heck LW, Schulman ES, MacGlashan DW Jr. Purified human mast cells and basophils release human elastase and cathepsin G by an IgE-mediated mechanism. Int Arch Allergy Appl Immunol 1985; 77:179–183.
47. Ishizaka K, Ishizaka T. The significance of immunoglobulin E in reaginic hypersensitivity. Ann Allergy 1970; 28:189–210.
48. Kilburn KH. Particles causing lung disease. Environ Health Perspect 1984; 55:97–109.
49. Ryder R, Lyons JP, Campbell H, Gough J. Emphysema in coal workers' pneumoconiosis. Br Med J 1970; 3:481–487.
50. Cockcroft A, Wagner JC, Ryder R, et al. Post-mortem study of emphysema in coalworkers and non-coalworkers. Lancet 1982: ii:600–603.
51. Last JM, ed. Occupational respiratory diseases. In: Maxcy-Rosenau Public Health and Preventive Medicine, 12 ed. Norwalk, CT: Appleton-Century-Crofts, 1986.
52. Bates DV. The health effects of air pollution: an update on current research. J Respir Dis 1980; 1:29–37.
53. Holland WW, Bennett AE, Cameron IR, et al. Health effects of particulate pollution: reappraising the evidence. Am J Epidemiol 1979; 110:527–659.
54. Kilburn KH, Warshaw R, Thornton JC, et al. Los Angeles smog reduces children's pulmonary function. JAMA, in press.
55. Fletcher C, Peto R, Tinker C, Speizer FE. The Natural History of Chronic Bronchitis and Emphysema. New York: Oxford University Press, 1976.
56. Higgins ITT, Gibson JC, Ferris BG Jr, et al. Chronic respiratory disease in an industrial town: a nine-year follow-up study preliminary report. Am J Public Health 1968; 58:1667–1676.
57. Higgins MW, Keller JB, Becker M, et al. An index of risk for obstructive airways disease. Am Rev Respir Dis 1982; 125:144–151.
58. Gregory J. A study of 340 cases of chronic bronchitis. Arch Environ Health 1971; 22:428–439.
59. Burrows B, Fletcher CM, Heard BE, et al. The emphysematous and bronchial types of chronic airways obstruction: a clinicopathological study of patients in London and Chicago. Lancet 1966; i:830–835.
60. Sutinen S, Christoforidis AJ, Klugh GA, Pratt PC. Roentgenologic criteria for the recognition of nonsymptomatic pulmonary emphysema: correlation between roentgenologic findings and pulmonary pathology. Am Rev Respir Dis 1965; 91:69–76.
61. Kilburn KH, Warshaw R, Thornton JC. Asbestos diseases and pulmonary symptoms and signs in shipyard workers and their families in Los Angeles. Arch Intern Med 1986; 146:2213–2220.
62. Roemmich W, Blumenfeld HL, Moritz H. Evaluating remaining capacity to work in miner applicants with simple pneumoconiosis under 65 years of age under title IV of public law 91-173. Ann NY Acad Sci 1972; 200:608–616.

Chapter 62

PSYCHOLOGIC, NEUROPSYCHOLOGIC, AND SOCIAL ASPECTS OF COPD

David E. Griffith Richard S. Kronenberg

The physiologic abnormalities associated with chronic obstructive pulmonary disease (COPD) are well recognized and are generally the primary focus of attention for physicians caring for these patients. Although improving physiologic parameters in COPD is unquestionably important, the more subtle but also very important psychologic and neuropsychologic problems and the social needs of these patients should not be ignored. The psychosocial aspects of COPD have been described in some detail[4, 10–13, 24, 41]; however, the incidence, prevalence, and particularly the management and prognosis of this aspect of COPD remain uncertain. Further, unless the clinician caring for these patients specifically makes an effort to seek out and alleviate their psychosocial dysfunction it will go unrecognized and probably adversely complicate any attempts at physiologic therapy. Chronic obstructive pulmonary disease patients, for example, may exhibit self-destructive behavior, such as continued cigarette smoking or medication noncompliance, or the avoidance of potentially satisfying strengthening physical activities. Anxiety and panic may also cause frequent physician visits or hospital admissions. Given that COPD is generally a progressive, irreversible process in which even physiologic treatment measures at present are only palliative, it seems quite surprising that more emphasis is not placed on psychosocial dysfunction in which the benefit to the patient may be more important than that of a small improvement in pulmonary function. The following discussion reviews what is known about the psychologic quality of life and neuropsychologic abnormalities in COPD patients with specific emphasis on available treatment modalities. We believe that the psychosocial disturbances in COPD patients are generally under recognized, under diagnosed, and largely untreated. More aggressive diagnosis and treatment of these disturbances may be a significant benefit to large numbers of COPD patients.

PSYCHOLOGIC DISTURBANCES

Chronic obstructive pulmonary disease is a progressive illness and it is not surprising that the disease shares many of the psychosocial disturbances common to other chronic illnesses. In fact the pattern of psychosocial disturbances in COPD is not specific or unique to that disease and does not allow differentiation psychologically of COPD patients from other groups of patients physically disabled by chronic disease.[9, 10] Casselith and colleagues[8] studied patients with a number of chronic debilitating illnesses that did not include COPD. The psychologic characteristics of these patients were fairly uniform with no pattern that was unique to any one disease. The severity of an individual patient's illness was more important than the specific type of illness in terms of correlating it best with the degree of psychologic disturbance.

Most clinicians have experience with patients with chronic illnesses in general and especially with COPD patients. Although there may be many similarities in the psychologic profiles of COPD patients and patients with other kinds of chronic illnesses, COPD is obviously a unique disease in terms of its pathogenesis. Chronic obstructive pulmonary disease develops and progresses slowly with many remissions and exacerbations and rarely becomes disabling before middle age. Yellowlees and coworkers[47] performed psychiatric evaluations of 50 patients with COPD and produced a profile of a typical patient. The "typical" COPD patient is a married man, middle aged or older, who has been ill for 5 to 10 years with impaired respiratory function. He has had multiple hospital admissions for exacerbations of COPD and has had at least one other significant illness requiring therapy. Altogether, he takes five different medications daily, producing both a major financial burden and problems with drug toxicity and noncompliance. He has a cigarette smoking history of 60 pack-years but has recently stopped smoking or at least markedly reduced his cigarette consumption. In terms of his psychologic profile, this patient tends to hyperventilate but has no obvious cognitive defect. He is anxious and depressed and both of these symptoms correlate with any concomitant use of alcohol. He avoids phobic situations, including taking showers, shaving, going to the toilet, riding elevators, or any situation where he might be alone or enclosed and not able to obtain medication or assistance. He generally will not go out without a companion and develops fear, hyperventilation, and panic if placed in situations associated with worsening airways obstruction.

A number of studies have examined the psychologic and personality characteristics of the COPD patient in more detail.[1, 2, 9, 17, 29, 31, 33, 47] The usual techniques used are standardized psychologic tests, Minnesota Multiphasic Personality Inventory (MMPI), clinical interviews, and self-reported symptom questionnaires. Agle and Baum[1, 2] studied 23 COPD patients who had symptoms of anxiety significant enough to interfere with their physiologic performance. These included unexplained tension, jumpiness, tremulousness, and feelings of impending doom. They found that most of their subjects had crippling degrees of depression with symptoms of sadness, tearfulness, lack of motivation, sense of worthlessness, suicidal ideation, and evidence of psychomotor retardation. These subjects also exhibited excessive body preoccupation out of proportion to an objective evaluation of their physical condition. There was also a high rate of alcohol use. This pattern of psychologic disturbance has been confirmed by other investigators.[31, 33, 47]

In addition to depression and anxiety, other common psychologic disturbances are hysteria, hypochondriasis, and a manipulative character disorder, along with dejection, anger, hostility, fatigue, and lack of vigor.[1, 2, 9, 17, 29, 31, 33, 47] Prominent personality traits in COPD patients include dependency, obstreperousness, obsessive behavior, and a tendency toward hysterical reaction.[2, 10, 33] Chronic obstructive pulmonary disease patients also perform poorly on measures of ego strength, reflecting an inability to cope with their changing life situation.[2] Coping mechanisms include denial, suppression, repression, and isolation.

Although these studies indicate a wide variety of psychologic problems in the COPD patient, there is no doubt that the most prevalent and consistent psychologic disturbance in these patients is depression. Aspects of COPD that might contribute to depression include limitation of daily activity, necessity of changing jobs, or even early retirement, inability to keep pace with companions, and the realization that the disease processes are progressive and irreversible. In general, the degree of depression does not correlate well with physiologic measurements, such as pulmonary function testing, blood gas values, and exercise capacity;[2, 7, 31] however alleviation of depression or anxiety may improve an individual patient's functional capacity.[2, 7] Anxiety, which tends to be related to dyspnea, is almost always accompanied by depression in these patients and may be an atypical presentation of depression.

We have said that the general pattern of psychologic disturbance in COPD is not particularly distinctive or characteristic but rather, with allowances for some differences in pathogenesis, is quite similar to that seen with other chronic illnesses. There is, however, one pervasive symptom of the disease that may produce an unusual or possibly unique psychologic disturbance and subsequent adaptation by the patient. That symptom is dyspnea. The physiologic basis of dyspnea is uncertain. An increase in dyspnea can be associated with any deviation from a relaxed or neutral state. That is, dyspnea may be associated with both activating (anxiety/anger) and nonactivating (depression/withdrawal) emotions that may trigger it or exacerbate it. The dyspnea, regardless of how it is produced, may itself further increase metabolic demands. This tends to exacerbate the patient's psychologic reaction, which in turn increases metabolic demand and produces a greater physiologic insufficiency. Thus, a vicious cycle is produced with a downward spiral of respiratory function that may incapacitate the patient and may be difficult to terminate (Fig. 62–1). In an investigation of 31 patients with COPD who were more breathless than would be predicted on the basis of their pulmonary function studies, Burns and Howell[7] noted a striking prevalence of psychologic disturbances, including depression, anxiety, and hysteria. The disproportionate dyspnea in these patients correlated with their psychologic disturbances. Significantly, the dyspnea improved with resolution of their psychologic difficulties.

Because of this link between psychologic disturbance and dyspnea, patients with COPD learn by experience to avoid strong feelings, to isolate themselves from psychosocial stimuli, and to use denial and repression to reduce the physiologic impact of external events. These patients attempt to avoid subjective distress or even extreme positive emotions, such as happiness, with the result that they live in what Dudley and colleagues have described as an "emotional straight jacket."[14] Patients also note that in attempting to adjust to life situations associated with their chronic and incapacitating disease they cannot overly express their feelings or deal with interpersonal conflicts without risking an exacerbation of their dyspnea. This

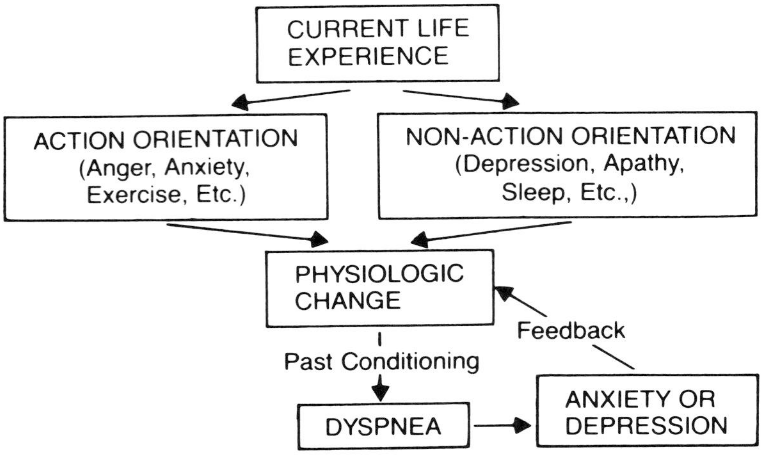

Figure 62–1. Postulated mechanism by which disability is produced and perpetuated in patients with COPD. Activating and nonactivating life changes lead to significant symptom production which, in turn, provides input for further changes in activation and further physiologic change. Symptoms are thereby perpetuated and exacerbated. (Reproduced with permission from Dudley DL. Psychophysiology of Perpetuation in Health and Disease. New York: Appleton Century-Crofts, 1969.)

rigid avoidance of affect only serves to perpetuate and worsen the problem, causing an increase in frustration, anger, and despair, which in turn cannot be dealt with by patient or physician. Because of their hesitancy to express anxiety or anger and because of a tendency to somatisize or even deny psychiatric symptoms, these patients may be especially difficult to interview and have trouble accepting psychiatric evaluation and therapy.

Another factor that may contribute to the difficulty in recognizing and treating psychologic problems, especially depression, in these patients is that many of the symptoms of depression overlap with those of COPD. Loss of appetite, sleep disturbance, lassitude, fatigue, and weight loss can be produced by the disease process of COPD or be caused by psychomotor retardation secondary to depression. Physicians may overlook a potentially dangerous depression in these patients by attributing it to symptoms caused by the patients' underlying disease. In this regard it should be pointed out that although the patterns of psychologic disturbance discussed earlier tend to be present in most COPD patients these patterns are by no means seen in all of them. A significant proportion of these patients show no significant psychologic disturbance.[31, 33] Moreover, there may be significant individual variability in specific characteristics, such as anger and hypochondriasis. Therefore, it is dangerous to generalize about psychologic problems in these patients, and psychologic testing may be worthwhile to evaluate or discover unexpected problems.

NEUROPSYCHOLOGIC FUNCTION

In addition to psychologic abnormalities, patients with COPD may demonstrate decreased mental functioning. A number of investigators have evaluated the cognitive ability of patients with COPD with varying degrees of hypoxia by performing a variety of neuropsychologic tests that assess cognitive, sensory, and motor ability[5, 18, 21–24, 26, 27, 30, 33, 37, 38, 44] (for a detailed discussion of the individual neuropsychologic tests, the reader is referred to the specific references cited). These studies have shown that COPD patients perform more poorly on neuropsychologic measures than do healthy control subjects and display a number of diverse cognitive abnormalities. The following discussion highlights pertinent aspects of these studies to evaluate possible etiologies of this impairment, specific cerebral function involved, and factors that may reverse or alter the progression of this impairment.

The unifying factor in patients with COPD and neuropsychologic dysfunction is hypoxemia. In fact, the loss of mental function found at high altitude in healthy individuals parallels that of hypoxemic COPD patients.[20] Impaired visual dark adaptation occurs at arterial oxygen tensions as high as 85 mm Hg. With further reduction in the arterial oxygen pressure ($Pa{O_2}$) to 60 to 45 mm Hg, impaired concentration and short-term memory and hyperventilation occur. With extreme hypoxemia, $Pa{O_2}$ of 35 to 45 mm Hg, lethargy, euphoria, irritability, hallucinations, impaired critical judgment, and muscular incoordination occur. With even further reduction of $Pa{O_2}$ to below 35 mm Hg, loss of consciousness occurs. Although most of these data were collected from young military recruits with acute exposure to hypoxia during training exercises, it is apparent that hypoxemia need not be extreme or severe to produce cerebral dysfunction. Admittedly, these observations represent the responses of neurons to abrupt changes in oxygen tension. Gradual or prolonged reduction of inspired oxygen may allow time for development of homeostatic mechanisms, which may tend to maintain normal brain function. These data also differ from the situation seen in COPD in that these subjects hyperventilated with the subsequent development of hypocapnic alkalosis and cerebral vasoconstriction. This is usually not the case in subjects with COPD.

Further evidence that hypoxia contributes to neuropsychologic dysfunction in COPD patients is provided by electroencephalogram (EEG) data.[5, 6] Slowing and disorganization in EEG patterns is characteristic of COPD patients. This pattern can be reversed with supplemental oxygen.[5, 6] Better neuropsychologic testing in some COPD patients has been associated with improvement in EEG pattern; however, the relationship between fast EEG waves and cognitive function remains uncertain.

In an important early cohort study, Krop and colleagues[30] evaluated the role of supplemental oxygen for neuropsychologic dysfunction. Patients underwent multiple neuropsychologic tests before and after either 1 month of standard management with continuous oxygen therapy or standard management with no supplemental oxygen. Neuropsychologic function was significantly depressed in the hypoxic patient group in proportion to the degree of hypoxemia. These neuropsychologic abnormalities consisted of simple motor dysfunction and perceptual motor performance dysfunction. After 1 month of therapy, the group treated with oxygen showed significant improvement in virtually all tests of neuropsychologic functioning. Statistically significant increases occurred in intelligence quotient (IQ), memory, and motor skills. The investigators concluded that hypoxia produced by obstructive lung disease is associated with impairment of neuropsychologic function and that this impairment is reversible following oxygen therapy.

Several subsequent studies have examined the neuropsycho-

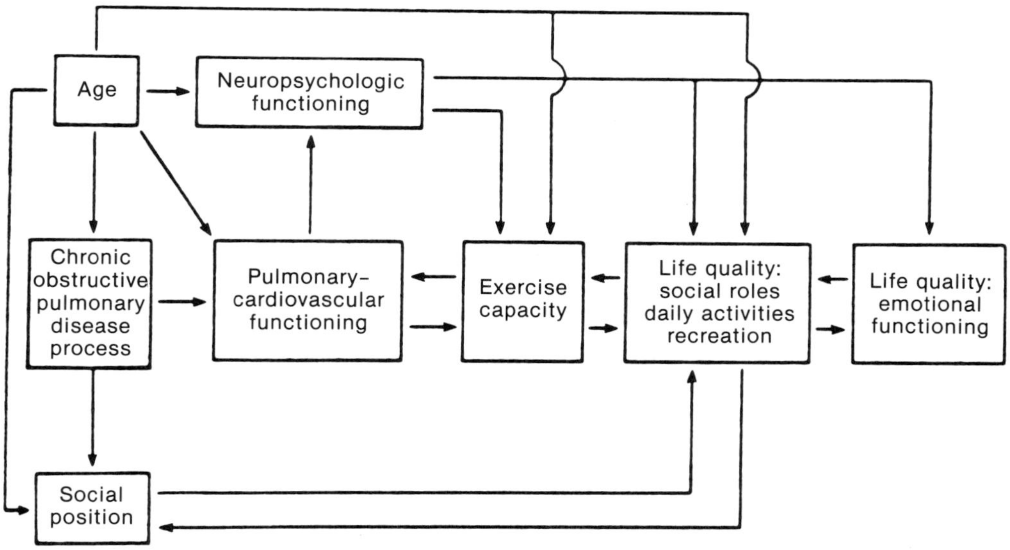

Figure 62–2. Interrelations of COPD and other variables affecting quality of life. (Reproduced with permission from McSweeny AJ, Grant I, Heaton RK, et al.: Arch Intern Med 1982; 142:473–478.)

logic status of large groups of COPD patients with a range of severity of hypoxia.[5, 8, 21–23, 26, 27, 37, 38, 44] These studies include two large multicenter trials involving several hundred patients.[21–23, 26, 37, 38] In general, patients score well on gross indicators of intellectual functioning. On more specific cognitive tasks, however, a wide range of subtle but definite neuropsychologic deficits are found. These abnormalities include altered or impaired alertness, attention, memory, problem-solving skills, language functioning, ability to acquire and retain new information, ability to form new concepts and think flexibly, performance of complex perceptual motor maneuvers, ability to engage in simple perceptual discriminations, and motor dexterity, strength, and quickness. These neuropsychologic deficits are common in chronic obstructive lung disease patients and are generally associated with hypoxemia, which may be mild.[22, 23, 26, 37, 38] This correlation, however, is subtle so that even though worsening neuropsychologic functioning is generally seen with worsening degrees of hypoxia, the overall decline in neuropsychologic testing accounted for by hypoxia is small. The observed cognitive dysfunctions do not correlate with either P_{CO_2} or pulmonary function testing.

In the two related large multicenter studies mentioned previously, administration of oxygen to hypoxemic COPD patients produced definite but "modest" improvement in neuropsychologic testing in contrast to the study cited earlier by Krop and colleagues,[30] in which a more significant benefit from supplemental oxygen was seen. The patients in the multicenter studies had baseline and follow-up testing done on room air, thus eliminating the possibility of short-term effects of oxygen. Significantly, patients who received continuous oxygen improved more on neuropsychologic testing than patients who received only nocturnal oxygen. The short-term beneficial effects of oxygen, presumably corresponding to improvement in the function of hypoxic neurons, are difficult to document. In a study evaluating the effects of acute oxygen exposure (20 minutes or 6 hours) on information processing in hypoxemic COPD patients, no significant impact on cognitive functioning occurred. This finding suggested that long-term effects of oxygen administration have a greater impact on neuropsychologic dysfunction.[44]

Although hypoxemia appears to be important in the development of neuropsychologic dysfunction in COPD patients, it is not the only factor involved (Fig. 62–2). Further, alleviation of hypoxemia improves but does not eliminate neuropsychologic dysfunction. Not all factors contributing to neuropsychologic deficits have been identified, but some inferences can be made. Age correlates in some studies with neuropsychologic function. Grant and colleagues[22] noted that 14% of healthy individuals had neuropsychologic morbidity and that their neuropsychologic profiles were remarkably similar to the COPD patients. They suggested that the neuropsychologic abnormalities seen in COPD may not be related to any specific brain pathologic finding but may, in fact, represent an exaggeration of the neuropsychologic decline of aging. The final neuropsychologic picture in COPD might then represent a contribution of specific deficits related to hypoxia on the one hand and acceleration of decline relating to aging on the other. In some circumstances polycythemia may also contribute to neuropsychologic dysfunction; however, in the setting of COPD it may in fact be protective, presumably related to maintenance of oxygen delivery to the brain.[22] At what level this protective effect might be overcome by deleterious effects of polycythemia, such as hyperviscosity, is unknown.

It is clear that neuropsychologic dysfunction is real in patients with COPD and that these cognitive deficits generally exist in the context of normal intellectual function. Probably many of these patients can appear neuropsychologically intact until confronted with some demand of adaptive functioning that exposes their impaired cognitive processes. However, beyond recognition of the problem, other conclusions are less reliable. The etiology or etiologies of the neuropsychologic dysfunction are unclear but appear to be at least partially due to hypoxemia. The mechanism of hypoxically induced neuropsychologic dysfunction may be several-fold. Although energy-producing pathways are not significantly affected by hypoxemia, oxygen administration may still improve the function of hypoxemic neurons with some short-term rapid onset neuropsychologic improvement.[20] However, more slowly appearing improvements in neuropsychologic function may reflect renewed synthesis of macromolecules critical to the maintenance of a neuron's physical/chemical integrity or formation of neurotransmitters.[20] Whether due to short-term or long-term effects or both, oxygen administration appears to alleviate at least some of the neuropsychologic impairment noted in hypoxemic COPD patients. Even "modest" improvement in neuropsychologic function with oxygen may be quite significant. Without oxygen therapy surviving patients would probably experience deteriorating mental function so that stable or slightly improved neuropsychologic functioning might actually reflect a significant treatment benefit.

QUALITY OF LIFE

The physiologic, psychologic, and neuropsychologic abnormalities of COPD combine to produce an overall deterioration in quality of life.[25, 33, 38] Not only do the limitations placed on physical activity and productive work require significant life adjustments, but decreased social, recreational, and sexual activities strain the patient's ability to maintain a sense of self-worth and a secure active role within a family. Several studies have demonstrated the adverse effect of COPD on the quality of life. A wide range of daily activities are negatively affected by COPD including emotional, social, and behavioral functioning (including self-care skills, mobility, and home management), as well as the ability to enjoy hobbies and recreational activities, sleep, and rest.[25, 33, 38] Sexual dysfunction may be present, particularly in male COPD patients, in the absence of other known causes of sexual problems.[19] Generally there is little or no direct correlation between variables that measure quality of life and either the Po_2 or pulmonary function.[33, 38] In terms of recent life events, COPD patients do not differ from control patients. Therefore, disturbances in the life quality of COPD patients do not appear related to major nonmedical changes in their personal lives.[38]

Quality of life abnormalities do correlate with neuropsychologic dysfunction and emotional or mood state.[33, 38] Socioeconomic position is also important in that the more affluent patients seem better able to cope with their disease, probably related to their ability to maintain more material resources. Patients in the lower socioeconomic strata may not seek medical help promptly, may be exposed to greater environmental hazards, and perhaps smoke more cigarettes.[33] In one study, current smokers, even though they were younger and had better pulmonary function testing than ex- or nonsmokers, had worse physical and psychosocial quality of life parameters and greater total mood disturbance than the ex- or nonsmokers.[38] The explanation for this finding is unclear.

Life quality, therefore, is not simply a function of the patient's cardiopulmonary and pathophysiologic status. Rather, in patients with COPD the ability to cope with disease is influenced by age, social position, and neuropsychologic status. Because of these findings patients with the poorest life quality are least likely to respond to traditional psychologic interventions.

Psychosocial assets are critical for COPD patients to maintain an adequate quality of life. They represent measures of the patient's overall ability to deal with his or her environment. Psychosocial assets can be broken down into the following categories:

1. Social support
   a. being in a setting in which one receives love
   b. being in a setting in which one is esteemed
   c. being in a mutually defensive system; if attacked, those around you will come to your aid.
2. Coping ability—the patient's ability to change environments to meet needs.
3. Adaptive ability—the patient's ability to adapt to existing environments.[13]

Chronic obstructive pulmonary disease patients with highly developed psychosocial assets exhibit effective interpersonal behavior; positive responses to group psychotherapy; protect themselves more efficiently from crippling symptoms, such as dyspnea; carry out treatment programs more carefully and responsibly; and may outlive their counterparts who are lacking such skills.[14, 15] Overall, patients with strong psychosocial assets are more responsive to rehabilitative efforts than are patients with few such assets.

Probably the single most important aspect of social support that contributes to strong psychosocial assets is a supportive husband or wife.[41] Family members are generally able to assist the COPD patient in coping with the adversities brought about by their illness; however, family members may also be severely and adversely affected by the patient's debilitating illness. Social, vocational, and recreational losses suffered by the patient may be paralleled by those suffered by family members. The spouse, particularly, may face changed roles and responsibilities at a time when intimacy and sexual relations are curtailed. Dealing with these changes in the family, maintaining communications, and supporting one another may severely strain the entire family's mechanisms for coping. Family members may endure almost as much reduction in quality of life and life satisfaction as the patient. Because of its important role in the support of the COPD patient, the family cannot be excluded in approaching proper psychosocial treatment for the patient.

DIAGNOSIS

Some investigators suggest thorough psychiatric and neuropsychologic evaluations for optimal management of COPD patients. We believe this approach is probably not necessary or cost effective in every patient with COPD. We also believe, however, that the psychologic and neuropsychologic aspects of COPD are frequently overlooked and in selected patients may be the most important contributors to the morbidity associated with their disease. Although not every patient may need extensive psychologic or neuropsychologic evaluation, it is clear that unless the primary physician explores these areas with specific lines of questioning, they will probably be missed, as patients will not usually volunteer this kind of information. A psychosocial history including inquiry into the patient's social, marital, sexual, vocational, and recreational status, is necessary. The patient's family may be helpful in this regard, although their perception of the patient's illness does not always coincide with that of the patient.

Aside from awareness and direct inquiry into psychologic and neuropsychologic areas, clues exist that may indicate which patients are having significant psychologic and neuropsychologic problems. Patients who should be targeted for more rigorous evaluation include:

1. Those with severely restricted lifestyle or regressive social behavior out of proportion to physiologic abnormalities.
2. Patients with frequent hospital admissions out of proportion to objective physiologic abnormalities.
3. Frequent and repetitive medication noncompliance.
4. Severe organic dysfunction.
5. Poor socioeconomic state.
6. Low psychosocial assets.
7. Substance (usually alcohol) abuse.

Awareness of these problems and the potential benefits of addressing them expands potential treatment modalities for COPD patients and possibly simplifies overall therapy in the group of patients who are the most difficult and frustrating for the physician to manage.

TREATMENT

The aim of treatment should be to maximize the patient's ability to cope with daily life and the changes brought about by the disease. The treatment plan should always focus on attainable goals and rewards, such as increased independence, increased exercise tolerance, and greater quality of life. Particular attention should be given to the following factors: the development of a useful working relationship with the patient; the recognition and treatment of major psychiatric disorders; the avoidance of pessimism; disengaging the dyspnea-anxiety cycle; the encouragement of optimal self care; and the provision for regular follow-up appointments.[2]

For hypoxemic patients with COPD, oxygen therapy has multiple benefits, including reduced polycythemia and pulmonary hypertension, lower mortality, reduced need for hospitalization, improved exercise tolerance, and increased activities of daily living.[3] Oxygen is a vital and integral part of both the physiologic and neuropsychologic management of severely hypoxemic patients ($Pa_{O_2} < 55$). As has been discussed previously, however, patients with "only" moderate or mild hypoxemia may also suffer neurophysiologic defects. The role of oxygen for this group of patients is less well defined. Hypoxemia appears to contribute to the neuropsychologic defects in these patients; however, it is by no means the only or even perhaps the most important factor contributing to their development. A confounding factor may be the tendency of some COPD patients to experience hypoxemia primarily at night. Although it appears that continuous oxygen therapy is more beneficial for neuropsychologic defects, there may be a role for nocturnal oxygen alone in selected patients who have hypoxemia only during sleep. Some evidence is available that patients with sleep apnea syndrome may have neuropsychologic deficits that improve with oxygen.[16] However, no studies are available that address the effect of nocturnal oxygen therapy on psychologic and neuropsychologic function in COPD patients who are only hypoxemic at night. Overall, the use of oxygen for severely hypoxemic patients is unquestionably beneficial, primarily for physiologic reasons. Although improved psychologic and neuropsychologic function may also ensue with a concomitant improvement in quality of life, the role of oxygen in improving neuropsychologic or psychologic function in moderately or mildly hypoxemic patients ($Pa_{O_2} >$ 55) is much less clear, and careful considerations of cost and effectiveness must be made before it is prescribed.

Medications, particularly bronchodilators, are an essential component in treating patients with COPD. It is intuitive that improvement of physiologic variables should also help psychologic and neuropsychologic function. As we have discussed, however, there is frequently not a good correlation between physiologic and nonphysiologic functioning in COPD patients. Further, bronchodilator medications can complicate or exacerbate underlying psychologic or neuropsychologic abnormalities (Table 62–1).[12, 43] Corticosteroids, for example, can be associated with frank psychosis, although this is rare in patients taking less than 40 mg of prednisone per day. The mental side effect symptoms of steroids can vary from mild euphoria accompanied by lessened fatigue and improved concentration to hypomanic symptomatology, e.g., flight of ideas, impaired judgment, insomnia, and increased appetite, to responses reflecting particular personality characteristics of the patient, e.g., increased anxiety, phobia, obsessive preoccupation, depression, or hypomania, and finally, frank psychosis. Premorbid personality or a previous history of mental illness may predispose patients to adverse reactions to steroids. Small doses of phenothiazines are usually effective in treating steroid psychosis. Some data also suggest an adverse affect of steroids on attention and memory, which appears related to dose.[42]

Other bronchodilator medications may also produce deleterious psychologic symptoms. $Beta_2$-agonists may produce anxiety, insomnia, paranoia, or hallucinations. Theophylline compounds may produce irritability, decreased ability to concentrate, anxiety, withdrawal, or hyperactivity. One postulated mechanism for the central nervous system side effects of theophylline is reduction in cerebral blood flow.[42, 48] Although the exact relationship of serum theophylline levels to cerebral blood flow is unknown, it is possible that theophylline contributes to hypoxia-related neuropsychologic defects. It seems clear that although physiologic parameters may improve with bronchodilator medication, these medications themselves may

TABLE 62–1. Some Psychiatric Symptoms Caused by Selected Pulmonary Drugs

DRUG	SYMPTOMS
Albuterol	paranoia, hallucinations
Antihistamines	anxiety, hallucinations, delirium
Atropine	confusion, memory loss, delirium, tactile, visual, and auditory hallucinations, paranoia
$Beta_2$ agonists	anxiety, insomnia
Cephalosporins	paranoia, confusion, disorientation
Chloramphenicol	memory impairment, confusion, depersonalization, hallucinations[41]
Corticosteroids	depression, mania, emotional lability, hallucinations, paranoia, catatonia
Cycloserine	depression, anxiety, confusion, hallucinations, paranoia, agoraphobia
Ephedrine	hallucinations, paranoia
Ethionamide	depression, psychosis
Gentamicin	confusion, hallucinations
Isoniazid	depression, anxiety, paranoia, hallucinations, confusion
Penicillin G procaine	hallucinations, disorientation, agitation, confusion, bizarre behavior
Phenylephrine	depression, hallucinations, paranoia
Pseudoephedrine	hallucinations, paranoia (more in children)
Theophylline	anxiety, withdrawal, hyperactivity

Reproduced with permission from Thompson WL, Thompson TL II. Adv Psychosom 1985; 14:136–148.

adversely affect psychologic and neuropsychologic functioning independent of their effects on improved physiologic functioning.

The role of psychotropic drugs, particularly anxiolytics and antidepressants, in treatment of the COPD patient remains unclear. The anxiolytics are particularly controversial, although they are frequently prescribed in COPD patients. Mitchell-Heggs and colleagues[34] gave "moderate" doses of diazepam in a single-blind, placebo-controlled trial to treat dyspnea in four "pink puffer" subjects. All experienced a reduction in dyspnea and improvement in effort tolerance, with no changes in resting blood-gas measurements. These investigators concluded that diazepam was safe in treating dyspnea in "pink puffers." Rosser and Guz[39] found a similar effect with benzodiazepines on breathlessness while also noting that the medication relieved anxiety. Conversely, Woodcock and coworkers,[45] in the placebo-controlled crossover trial of diazepam and promethazine for dyspnea in "pink puffers" found that 25 mg per day of diazepam produced significant drowsiness in 7 of 18 patients, with no effect on breathlessness and reduced exercise tolerance in the patient population as a whole, while promethazine reduced breathlessness and improved exercise tolerance.[45] These investigators concluded that diazepam was contraindicated for treatment of breathlessness in fixed airways obstruction.

If anxiolytics are prescribed, it seems appropriate to begin with smaller doses of short-acting benzodiazepines in order to minimize potential respiratory depression. It must be remembered that these drugs are intended for short-term amelioration of anxiety-related symptoms and not for unsupervised long-term use, which may be associated with drug dependency and eventual withdrawal symptoms. Prior to institution of anxiolytic therapy, anxiety symptoms associated with pulmonary disease should be clearly distinguished from anxiety-like symptoms associated with hypoxia. Lastly, anxiety about impending respiratory decompensation may in some cases be beneficial in that these patients may be more likely to take early appropriate therapeutic measures. Overall, these drugs are effective as anxiolytic agents but should be used judiciously with clearly established short-term goals for patients with COPD.

The role of antidepressants in the treatment of COPD is also unclear, although these agents may be of potential benefit. As noted previously, depressed patients tend to have low energy levels, loss of interest in usual activities, restlessness, agitation, and psychomotor retardation, all of which may be mistaken for symptoms of underlying lung disease and may interfere with compliance with bronchodilator medications. Most antidepressants have little or no effect on respiratory drive and, in fact, tricyclic antidepressants, especially protriptyline, may improve ventilation in some patients with sleep-related breathing disorders. Theoretically, anticholinergic antidepressants are of benefit because of the bronchodilating effect of anticholinergic agents, such as atropine. As with anxiolytics, it is prudent to begin therapy with antidepressant medications in small doses with gradual increases in the dose as tolerated by the patient.

The choice of relatively sedating (amitriptyline) or nonsedating (imipramine) tricyclic drugs can be made depending on the relative agitation or psychomotor retardation displayed by the patient. Yellowlees[48] described four COPD patients whose social and occupational functioning had deteriorated more than would be expected from their physiologic parameters. The psychosocial parameters in these patients improved remarkably to the point that they were "consistent with their degree of physical impairment" after institution of tricyclic antidepressant therapy. Of perhaps equal importance, a marked reduction in hospital admissions was seen in these patients following institution of the antidepressant therapy. Yellowlees points out that psychologic treatment with antidepressants is no panacea for COPD patients, and the overall role of antidepressants in a larger COPD population remains to be determined. A large placebo-controlled study to evaluate the role of tricyclic antidepressants in COPD patients is clearly warranted.

The precise role of psychiatric intervention is probably the least well defined of any treatment modality for COPD patients. Psychiatric intervention is unquestionably indicated in gross psychiatric disturbances, such as psychosis or attempted suicide; however, in the large numbers of less severely affected individuals it is of unclear benefit. Our feeling is that psychotherapy is probably underutilized but selection of patients for psychotherapy may be especially difficult. Because of somatization, neuropsychologic (cognitive) dysfunction, and general obstreperousness, the patients who need psychotherapy most may be the least likely to accept it. Similarly, these same qualities may impair a favorable response to psychotherapy. The primary caregiver can provide both counseling and support in the absence of direct psychiatric intervention. Routine and sometimes frequent office visits, even when the patient is doing well physiologically, can provide patients the opportunity to discuss emotional and psychosocial concerns with a trusted professional. The importance of this role for the physician cannot be overstressed and should not be abrogated because of the difficulty in dealing with these patients or the irreversibility of their physiologic abnormality.

PULMONARY REHABILITATION

A comprehensive pulmonary rehabilitation program may offer the most effective means of attaining improvement in overall psychosocial function for COPD patients. Several studies have demonstrated the benefit of this approach with regard to improved psychologic function and ability to perform activities of daily living in the absence of improved physiologic function.[1, 2, 17, 32] The major benefit of pulmonary rehabilitation may be in helping the patient overcome the fear of dyspnea that "locks" the patient in a phobic avoidance of activity. Patients can be reassured that some dyspnea is not necessarily dangerous or a harbinger of doom but is a natural response to effort that can be tolerated within limits. Patients in a rehabilitation program can be repeatedly exposed to small increments of the feared activity, i.e., exercise, while being protected and reassured by the presence of medical personnel who are closely monitoring their physical responses. This approach is similar to desensitization used in other phobias and allows the patient to develop confidence to continue physical activity without the presence of a physician.

Agle and Baum[2] identified seven factors in pulmonary rehabilitation associated with improved psychologic state and performance:[1]

1. Progressive exercise leading to a decrease in the fear of activity and dyspnea.
2. Education in self care leading to increased autonomy and control of symptoms.
3. Staff attitudes that care of the patient was worth the effort.
4. Setting of realistic goals leading to improved self esteem.
5. Clinical follow-up to consolidate gains.
6. Mutual support from group interactions.
7. Psychosocial factors within the patient that lead to strong motivation.

Although it is clear that exercise training is the core of pulmonary rehabilitation, it is not the only important aspect. Group or individual counseling, smoking cessation, instruction in breathing techniques, and consultation with a social worker may also add significantly to the overall benefit of the program.

Psychologic variables also predict outcome of rehabilitation effort. The patient's beliefs about the usefulness of therapy and exercise, fear of exertion, initial degree of depression, bodily preoccupation, and anxiety can predict response to rehabilitation better than an assessment of his or her initial pulmonary function.[36, 40] It is again noteworthy that those patients most likely to benefit from this form of therapy, i.e., those with the most severe psychosocial limitation, may be least likely to attain those benefits because of these psychosocial limitations.

REFERENCES

1. Agle DP, Baum GL, Chester EH, et al. Multidiscipline treatment of chronic pulmonary insufficiency. Psychological aspects of rehabilitation. Psychosom Med 1973; 35:41–49.
2. Agle DP, Baum GL. Psychological aspects of chronic obstructive pulmonary disease. Med Clin North Am 1977; 61:749–758.
3. Anthonisen NR. Long-term oxygen therapy. Ann Intern Med 1983; 99:519–527.
4. Block AJ. Neuropsychological aspects of oxygen therapy. Respiratory Care 1983; 28:885–888.
5. Block AJ, Castle JR, Keitt AS, et al. Chronic oxygen therapy. Treatment of chronic obstructive pulmonary disease at sea level. Chest 1974; 65:279–287.
6. Brezinova V, Calverley PMA, Flenley DC, Townsend HRA. The effect of long term oxygen therapy on the EEG in patients with chronic stable ventilatory failure. Bull Eur Physiopathol Respir 1979; 15:603–609.
7. Burns BH, Howell JBL. Disproportionately severe breathlessness in chronic bronchitis. QJ Med 1969; 38:277–294.
8. Cassileth BR, Lusk EJ, Strouse TB, et al. Psychosocial status in chronic illness. A comparative analysis of six diagnostic groups. N Engl J Med 1984; 311:506–511.
9. DeCencio DV, Leshner M, Leshner B, et al. Personality characteristics of patients with chronic obstructive pulmonary emphysema. Arch Phys Med Rehab 1968; 49:471–475.
10. Dudley DL, Glaser EM, Jorgensen BN, Logan DL. Psychosocial concomitants to rehabilitation in chronic obstructive pulmonary

disease. Part 1. Psychosocial and psychological considerations. Chest 1980; 77:413–420.
11. Dudley DL, Glaser EM, Jorgensen BN, Logan DL. Psychosocial concomitants to rehabilitation in chronic obstructive pulmonary disease. Part 2. Psychosocial treatment. Chest 1980; 77:544–551.
12. Dudley DL, Glaser EM, Jorgensen BN, Logan DL. Psychosocial concomitants to rehabilitation in chronic obstructive pulmonary disease. Part 3. Dealing with psychiatric disease (as distinguished from psychosocial or psychophysiologic problems). Chest 1980; 77:677–684.
13. Dudley DL, Sitzman J, Rugg M. Psychiatric aspects of patients with chronic obstructive pulmonary disease. Adv Psychosom Med 1985; 14:64–77.
14. Dudley DL, Verhey JW, Masuda M, et al. Long term adjustment, prognosis, and death in irreversible diffuse obstructive pulmonary syndromes. Psychosom Med 1969; 31:310–325.
15. Dudley DL, Pattison EM. Group psychotherapy in patients with severe diffuse obstructive pulmonary syndrome. Am Rev Respir Dis 1969; 100:575–576.
16. Findley L, Cubert K, Wilhoit S, et al. Nocturnal hypoxemia and cognitive functioning in sleep apnea patients [Abstract]. Am Rev Respir Dis 1985; 131(Suppl):A107.
17. Fishman DB, Petty TL. Physical, symptomatic and psychological improvement in patients receiving comprehensive care for chronic airway obstruction. J Chronic Dis 1971; 24:775–785.
18. Fix AJ, Golden CJ, Daughton D, et al. Neuropsychological deficits among patients with chronic obstructive pulmonary disease. Int J Neurosci 1982; 16:99–105.
19. Fletcher EC, Martin RJ. Sexual dysfunction and erectile impotence in chronic obstructive pulmonary disease. Chest 1982; 81:413–421.
20. Gibson GE, Pulsinell IW, Blass JP, Duffy TE. Brain dysfunction in mild to moderate hypoxia. Am J Med 1981; 70:1247–1254.
21. Grant I, Heaton RK, McSweeny AJ, et al. Brain dysfunction in COPD. Chest 1980; 77(suppl):308–311.
22. Grant I, Heaton RK, McSweeny AJ, et al. Neuropsychologic findings in hypoxemic chronic obstructive pulmonary disease. Arch Intern Med 1982; 142:1470–1476.
23. Grant I, Prigatano GP, Heaton RK, et al. Progressive neuropsychologic impairment and hypoxemia. Arch Gen Psychiatry 1987; 44:999–1006.
24. Greenberg GD, Ryan JJ, Bourlier PF. Psychological and neuropsychological aspects of COPD. Psychomatics 1985; 26:29–33.
25. Guyatt GH, Townsend M, Berman LB, Pugsley SO. Quality of life in patients with chronic airflow limitation. Br J Dis Chest 1987; 81:45–54.
26. Heaton RK, Grant I, McSweeny AJ, et al. Psychologic effects of continuous and nocturnal oxygen therapy in hypoxemic chronic obstructive pulmonary disease. Arch Intern Med 1983; 143:1941–1947.
27. Huppert FA. Memory impairment associated with chronic hypoxia. Thorax 1982; 37:858–860.
28. Jensen PS. Risk, protective factors, and supportive interventions in chronic airway obstruction. Arch Gen Psychiatry 1983; 40:1203–1207.
29. Kellner R, Samet JM, Pathak D. Hypochondriacal concerns and somatic symptoms in patients with chronic airflow obstruction. J Psychosomatic Res 1987; 31:575–582.
30. Krop HD, Block AJ, Cohen E. Neuropsychologic effects of continuous oxygen therapy in chronic obstructive pulmonary disease. Chest 1973; 64:317–322.
31. Light RW, Merrill EJ, Despars JA, et al. Prevalence of depression and anxiety in patients with COPD. Relationship to functional capacity. Chest 1985; 87:35–38.
32. Lustig FM, Haas A, Castillo R. Clinical and rehabilitation regime in patients with COPD. Arch Phys Med Rehab 1972; 53:315–322.
33. McSweeney AJ, Grant I, Heaton RK, et al. Life quality of patients with chronic obstructive pulmonary disease. Arch Intern Med 1982; 142:473–478.
34. Mitchell-Heggs P, Murphy K, Minty K, et al. Diazepam in the treatment of dyspnoea in the "pink puffer" syndrome. QJ Med 1980; 193:9–20.
35. Morgan AD, Peck DF, Buchanan D, et al. Psychological factors contributing to disproportionate disability in chronic bronchitis. J Psychosom Med 1983; 27:259–263.
36. Morgan AD, Peck DF, Buchanan DR, McHardy GJR. Effect of attitudes and beliefs on exercise tolerance in chronic bronchitis. Br Med J 1983; 286:171–173.
37. Prigatano GP, Parsons O, Wright E, et al. Neuropsychological test performance in mildly hypoxemic patients with chronic obstructive pulmonary disease. J Consult Clin Psychol 1983; 51:108–116.
38. Prigatano GP, Wright EC, Levin D. Quality of life and its predictors in patients with mild hypoxemia and chronic obstructive pulmonary disease. Arch Intern Med 1984; 144:1613–1619.
39. Rosser R, Guz A. Psychological approaches to breathlessness and its treatment. J Psychosom Med 1981; 25:439–447.
40. Rutter BM. The prognostic significance of psychological factors in the management of chronic bronchitis. Psychol Med 1979; 9:63–70.
41. Sandhu HS. Psychosocial issues in chronic obstructive pulmonary disease. Clin Chest Med 1986; 7:629–642.
42. Schraa JC, Dirks JD. The influence of corticosteroids in theophylline on cerebral function. Chest 1982; 82:181–185.
43. Thompson WL, Thompson TL II. Use of medications in patients with chronic pulmonary disease. Adv Psychosom Med 1985; 14:136–148.
44. Wilson DK, Kaplan RM, Timms RM, Dawson A. Acute effects of oxygen treatment upon information processing in hypoxemic COPD patients. Chest 1985; 88:239–243.
45. Woodcock AA, Gross ER, Geddes DM. Drug treatment of breathlessness: contrasting effects of diazepam and promethazine in pink puffers. Br Med J 1981; 283:343–346.
46. Yellowlees PM. The treatment of psychiatric disorders in patients with chronic airways obstruction. Med J Aust 1987; 147:349–352.
47. Yellowlees PM, Alpers JH, Bowden JJ, et al. Psychiatric morbidity in patients with chronic airflow obstruction. Med J Aust 1987; 146:305–307.
48. Young LD, Bowton D, Alford P, et al. Do medications reduce cerebral blood flow in COPD patients? Psychosomatics 1986; 27:240.

Chapter 63

RESPIRATORY CARE IN THE HOME

Michael L. Nochomovitz

The provision of a full range of health care services in the home is rapidly growing. The expenditures on homecare products and services in 1990 are projected by some analysts to exceed 9.0 billion dollars. These include nursing care services, durable medical equipment, infusion therapy, alimentation, and respiratory care. Nursing services account for the largest portion of these services (60% to 70%), while respiratory therapy equipment and services are expected to total almost 500 million dollars or more than 5% of this amount. The impetus for this unprecedented growth is technologic, economic, and social. Improvements in respiratory therapy equipment and availability of services have facilitated the provision of this category of care in the home. Changes in reimbursement of hospital services have further encouraged the development of alternate approaches. In addition to these factors the more educated patient increasingly elects to be cared for in the comfort and security of his or her own home rather than in a health care facility.

In the field of respiratory care, the use of home oxygen therapy in chronic obstructive pulmonary disease (COPD) and other cardiopulmonary disorders has increased in recent years. Following the landmark studies in the early 1980s a more knowledgeable medical community is familiar with the documented benefits of oxygen therapy and the indications for its use.[4, 5] The wider use of oximetry results in a greater awareness of hypoxemic conditions and the need for oxygen therapy. There is widespread acceptance by the lay public of patients using oxygen in public places. This has increased the vocational, occupational, and recreational activities of patients requiring treatment. Compliance among patients has also improved with increased familiarity with this treatment modality. Advances in our understanding of chronic respiratory failure have increased the use of assisted ventilation in the home in the form of negative and positive pressure devices.[13–15] Similarly, the availability of laboratories for the evaluation of breathing disorders during sleep has increased the number of patients receiving treatment for sleep apnea syndromes.[11, 12]

Cost-based reimbursement for Medicare hospitalizations has been replaced by a prospective payment system—Diagnostic Related Grouping (DRG), which discourages lengthy stays in hospital. Convalescence following acute illnesses is now unaffordable in the hospital setting. Prolonged stay in the hospital for ventilator-dependent patients is generally unacceptable to patients from an emotional and a psychologic standpoint when a viable homecare alternative exists.

DIAGNOSTIC RESPIRATORY CARE IN THE HOME

Much of what was considered to be firmly in the domain of in-patient care a few years ago in respiratory medicine is now becoming possible in the homecare setting. This change facilitates the management of patients who are quite ill in their home environment.

Considerable sentiment exists supporting the encouragement of physician home visits from patients and physician groups alike. At present specialized nursing care for clinical assessment of patients is more frequently used. Other diagnostic modalities specifically pertinent to respiratory care include home radiograms, arterial blood gases, and oximetry.

HOME X-RAYS. Portable films are routinely available in most larger communities in the U.S. Lateral films are usually not available, as patients may be too ill for this to be practical. In bedridden and/or homebound patients the portable x-ray machine may be extremely useful in ruling out pneumonia or heart failure. The suspicion of pneumonia does not per se necessitate transfer to a health care facility. In patients using positive pressure ventilation at home the suspicion of pneumothorax can also be evaluated on site.

ARTERIAL BLOOD GASES. Arterial blood gas samples are frequently drawn in the home and analyzed at a central laboratory. This practice facilitates the monitoring of patients with respiratory failure who may have previously been treated as in-patients. Given the availability of sophisticated nursing care, patients with exacerbations of chronic lung disease increasingly have the option of treatment at home in a familiar environment.

The availability of arterial blood gas procedures at home makes possible the monitoring of assisted ventilation in the form of negative and positive pressure devices. In patients on respirators gas exchange may be carefully monitored and interventions prescribed without necessitating hospitalization. This approach requires close cooperation between the physician and the home health care staff. It is to be expected that in those unfamiliar with this approach to high technology homecare extreme caution should be exercised in order to prevent misunderstandings and misinterpretations of physicians' orders. Careful documentation and frequent communication with the pulmonary physician or his or her designee is essential.

OXIMETRY. The federally mandated guidelines for long-term oxygen therapy have legitimized the use of oximetry at rest and during sleep to determine the need for home oxygen therapy. The technique is also a useful screening device for disorders of breathing during sleep. Conventional oximetry has been limited by the need for a stationary monitor or strip chart recorder, or both, and the lack of sufficient information to diagnose sleep apneas in a definitive manner.

Recent advances have resulted in the development of ambulatory monitors capable of checking oxygen saturation, electrocardiogram, and even other parameters, such as rib cage and abdominal motion. With suitable validation this modality could result in the evaluation of breathing disorders during sleep evolving into an ambulatory/home procedure. The equipment under investigation by a number of groups utilizes a portable recording device, an analog to digital replay unit, a report generation unit, and appropriate software for data processing.[36] Validation of the technique is required as well as consensus views on indications for use, relationship to conventional polysomnography, and reimbursement.

Therapeutic respiratory services in the home include inhalation therapy, oxygen therapy, and assisted ventilation, which consists of

1. Negative pressure devices.
2. Positive pressure ventilation.
3. Continuous positive pressure applied to the nose (Nasal CPAP).
4. Nasal ventilation.

INHALATION THERAPY

Inhalation of bronchodilators is prescribed via nebulizers for use in the home in cases of chronic obstructive airways disease, in which metered dose inhalers are viewed as being inadequate. Metered dose inhalers with the addition of spacer devices are suitable in most situations, with the required instruction in the physician's office or hospital preferably being supplemented by written/pictorial or video instruction.

Although a consensus exists regarding the efficacy of appropriately instructed metered dose inhalation, debilitated, incoordinated, or physically impaired patients would clearly benefit from the use of nebulizers. In patients with severe airways disease a case can be made for the use of nebulizers to achieve more predictable high-dose treatments in those with severe bronchospasm (Fig. 63–1). The availability of a nebulizer at home may save visits to the emergency room. Given the availability of a nebulizer, and the association with hospital care, communication with the patient's physician can result in an assessment of the severity of the condition and recommendations regarding the frequency of nebulized aerosol prior to a decision to present for care in an emergency department. In addition to the larger dose of medication administered a psychologic component probably exists for some patients in being reassured by the use of the nebulizer.

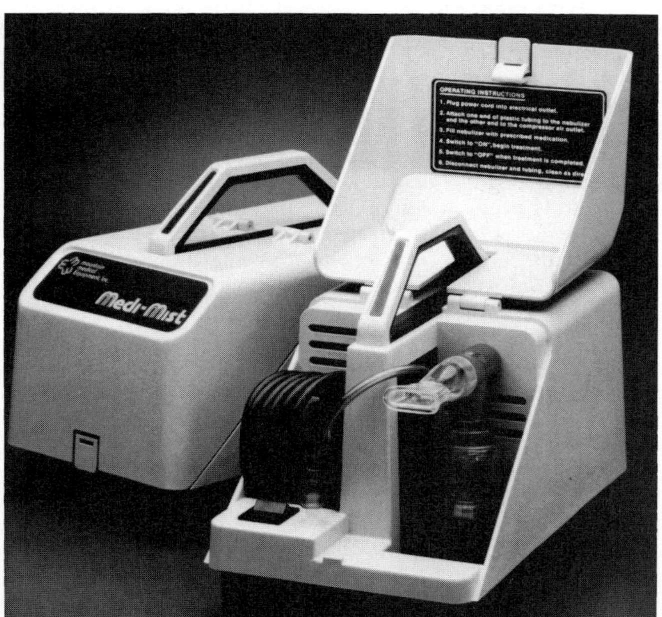

Figure 63–1. Hand-held nebulizer (Courtesy of Lincare Inc., Brookpark, Ohio).

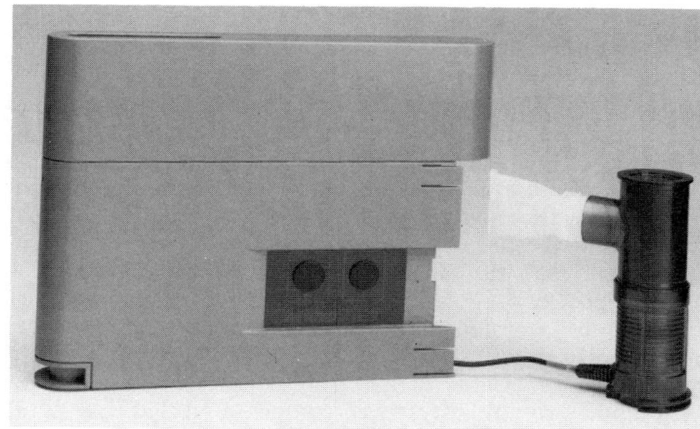

Figure 63–2. Portable nebulizer with rechargeable battery and AC use (Courtesy of Lincare Inc., Brookpark, Ohio).

The nebulizers are usually covered by third party payors for both rental and outright purchase. There is little in the way of servicing that is required of these devices, and they should be purchased rather than rented if their use is anticipated over a prolonged period. Careful instruction is required regarding their use and the measurement and mixing of medication for aerosol therapy. Unit dose medication in disposable containers is significantly more convenient but much more expensive. Elderly patients or those who have difficulty with fine motor movements would often benefit from this convenience if economically feasible. Newer nebulizers are now available that are rechargeable and extremely convenient for travel. Even patients comfortable with metered dose inhaler techniques who have a history of severe attacks of bronchospasm may achieve a sense of added security with the availability of a nebulizer at home or when traveling (Fig. 63–2).

HOME OXYGEN THERAPY

Background

Oxygen therapy is used in the home for a wide spectrum of patients with hypoxemia. Much of the data regarding the utility of oxygen has been collected from patients with COPD who make up the largest group requiring such therapy. For practical purposes the data regarding the benefit of oxygen therapy for hypoxic patients with COPD have been extrapolated to other chronically hypoxemic patients.

The prospect of preventing chronic hypoxia and its consequences led to studies of long-term oxygen therapy in COPD. The availability of portable liquid oxygen greatly facilitated the study of long-term home oxygen therapy and its long-term effect on the disease. In the first large study, patients received continuous (24-hour) oxygen for up to 2.5 years. The results suggested that a reduction occurred in the mortality of patients with cor pulmonale when compared with historical control subjects.[1] A subsequent cooperative study in the U.S.[2] demonstrated a lower mortality in patients receiving continuous oxygen therapy compared with nocturnal treatment only. The patients studied had arterial P_{O_2} values of not more than 55 mm Hg after intensive therapy or not more than 59 mm Hg plus either edema or hematocrit level of more than 55% or P. pulmonale on electrocardiogram (ECG). Neuropsychologic testing performed in patients receiving oxygen therapy in the Nocturnal Oxygen Therapy Trial (NOTT) study showed improvement in most tests and in the quality of life when all patients were considered regardless of the number of hours of O_2 therapy.

The only controlled home oxygen study to date, done by the Medical Research Council in the United Kingdom, studied COPD patients with hypoxic cor pulmonale randomized to 15 hr/d nasal oxygen therapy or no oxygen.[3] The oxygen group had a reduced mortality over 3 years in both men and women, although this effect only became evident in men after 500 days from starting the therapy. The grave prognosis for women has not been explained. Many patients receiving long-term O_2 therapy develop progressive hypercapnia, which is thought to be related to progressive airway obstruction or elimination of their hypoxic drive to breathe, or both. Patients with severe hypercapnia ($Paco_2 > 70$ mm Hg) have been followed for many months with relatively well-compensated acid base status and a functional ability appropriate for their degree of obstructive disease.[18, 21, 22, 34]

Oxygen Therapy During Sleep

Nocturnal oxygen therapy was hoped to offset the acute desaturation during sleep, which occurs even in healthy individuals. This phenomenon is thought to occur as a result of central hypoventilation and/or ventilation perfusion mismatch associated with sleep. It is particularly hazardous in hypoxemic COPD patients, who are closer to the steep portion of the oxyhemoglobin desaturation curve. Desaturation may result in a precipitous fall in oxygen tension, myocardial hypoxia, and arrhythmias.

A number of studies have been done showing a correlation between pulmonary hypertension and nocturnal desaturation in patients with COPD. Desaturation was associated with hypopnea, and supplemental oxygen prevented desaturation without alleviating breathing abnormalities. Reports have also been made of nocturnal oxygen therapy improving daytime somnolence, morning headache, and nocturnal arrhythmias in COPD patients who exhibit nocturnal desaturation without severe daytime hypoxemia. It has been suggested that years of nightly episodic pulmonary hypertension may determine which COPD patients develop cor pulmonale, although this issue remains to be resolved.

SLEEP APNEA. Studies of oxygen therapy in patients with sleep apnea have yielded inconsistent results. In one study obstructive apneas were prolonged, resulting in respiratory acidosis. Other studies have demonstrated a reduction in apneic time as well as reduced myocardial irritability.

Guidelines for Prescription of Home Oxygen Therapy

Although data regarding the efficacy of ambulatory oxygen exists only for COPD most investigators believe that the data should be applied for clinical purposes to other chronic hypoxemic respiratory and cardiac conditions.

Long-term oxygen therapy should be considered for only those patients whose general condition has been optimized to a stable baseline condition over a period of 2 to 3 weeks.[4, 23, 24] This practice does not preclude the use of short-term oxygen therapy while the patient's respiratory status improves with aggressive therapy. For purposes of reimbursement explicit guidelines exist for the prescription and use of long-term oxygen therapy. An arterial blood gas measurement on room air at rest showing a Po_2 of ≤ 55 mm Hg qualifies as hypoxemia by federal guidelines based on the NOTT study. This approach does not take into account variations in the Po_2 secondary to different degrees of ventilation, which would significantly alter the A-a gradient.

Arterial oxygen saturation documented by finger probe or ear oximetry is also accepted now by the Health Care Finance Administration (HCFA) as a determinant of tissue oxygenation. An oxygen saturation of $\leq 88\%$ has been established as the benchmark for hypoxia assuming a normal pH. Patients not qualifying for reimbursement by these criteria who have Po_2 values of > 55 mm Hg should be evaluated for evidence of tissue hypoxia, hypoxemia during exertion and sleep, and heart failure.[23]

Tissue hypoxia is defined as an Hct of $> 55\%$ or the presence of P. pulmonale on ECG as evidenced by a P wave of > 2 mm or peripheral edema. A drop in oxygen tension during sleep or exertion into the defined range would also qualify patients for therapy during that activity, e.g., sleep and exercise. The type of exercise or severity of exertion is not defined within the regulations. Similarly, as far as desaturation during sleep is concerned, the duration of desaturation is not specified. The level of desaturation is as defined for hypoxia, namely, a Po_2 of ≤ 55 mm Hg or desaturation to less than 88%.

Methods of Oxygen Administration

Oxygen Delivery Systems

COMPRESSED AIR CYLINDERS. Tanks of compressed air have been used in the home for many years. They are cumbersome and unattractive. They need to be well secured to prevent them from falling, which could conceivably result in explosion. These tanks are inexpensive and can deliver high flow rates depending on the flow regulator used. H or K cylinders have most typically been used and weigh 130 lbs with a capacity of more than 6.5 thousand L.

A smaller E cylinder is commonly employed for ambulation on a cart (Fig. 63–3). This weighs about 12 lbs and given a flow rate of 2 L/min a full E cylinder would last for approximately 5 hours. The E cylinder has been commonly used for ambulation by patients who use a concentrator as their stationary source of oxygen. Long tubing extending through the home attached to a large stationary reservoir should be discouraged. In addition to the inconvenience within the home having patients and family members at risk of tripping, the tubing may be easily kinked and the flow of oxygen compromised.

CONCENTRATORS. The oxygen concentrator utilizes a molecular sieve method to extract oxygen from atmospheric air. Concentrators have become more compact in the last few years and typically weigh 30 to 50 lbs (Fig. 63–4).

The device is usually electrically powered and is available from a wide range of manufacturers. The designs have been streamlined in some cases to blend in with furniture, and the noise level achieved in newer models is quite low. The services required with concentrators are reduced in the absence of having to refill a reservoir. Routine maintenance is required to ensure the reliability of the flow rate and the concentration of the oxygen. The cost of the concentrator to the patient, independent of third party reimbursement, is augmented by the electric bill associated with operating the machine.

The inspired flow of oxygen (FIo_2) depends on the flow rate and though rates of up to 5 L/min can be achieved, these would be at a reduced oxygen concentration. The clinical implications of these differences in concentration would not be consequential in the majority of situations in the home. The oxygen concentrator is clearly the method of choice for nonambulatory patients. A concentrator in the home is usually supplied with an E cylinder for ambulation. Ideally, liquid

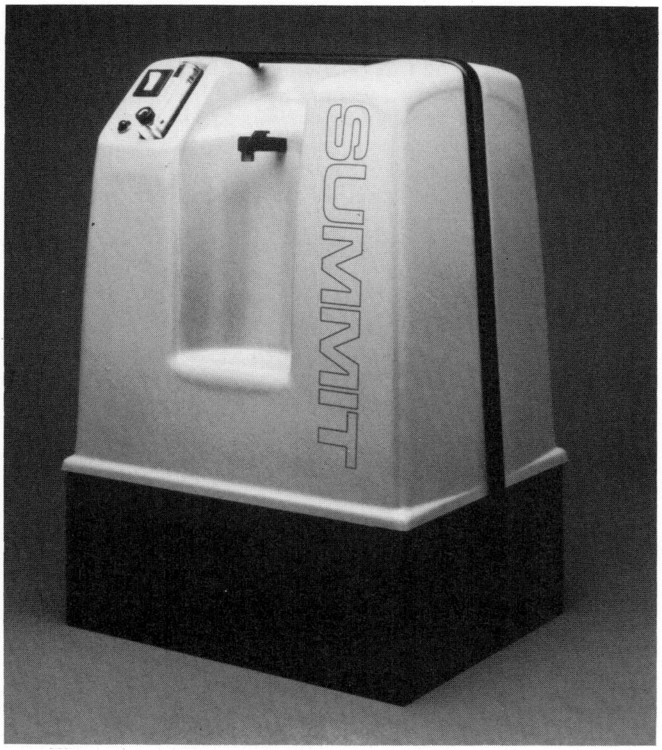

Figure 63–3. Oxygen concentrator for stationary use (Courtesy of Lincare Inc., Brookpark, Ohio).

oxygen would be available for portable use in addition to the concentrator to maximally facilitate ambulation. Durable medical equipment (DME) vendors may be reluctant to supply these two forms of oxygen therapy if they are not able to recover the cost of supplying the liquid oxygen as well. This will vary among vendors depending on their ability to supply liquid oxygen and the number of visits to the patient required to maintain an adequate supply of liquid oxygen.

Significant efforts are being expended to develop a portable concentrator that would be small and battery operated and greatly facilitate the delivery of long-term oxygen therapy. This can be expected to be the next major breakthrough in this field.

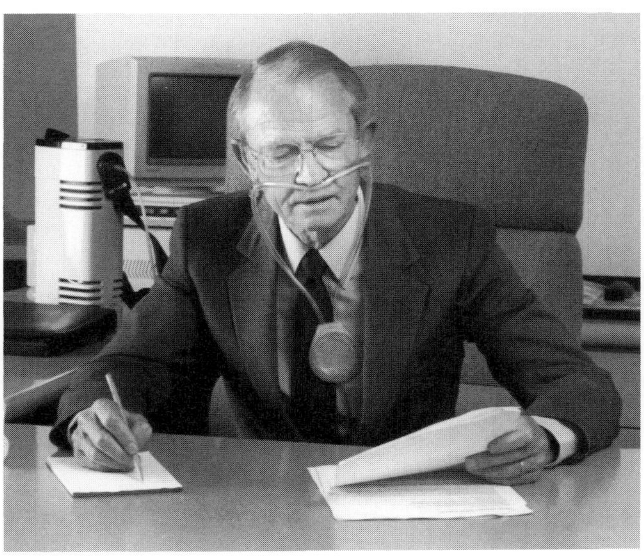

Figure 63–4. Oxygen-conserving device in the form of a pendant (Courtesy of Chad Therapeutics, Chatsworth, California).

LIQUID OXYGEN. Oxygen condensed into a liquid form allows for storage of a larger supply. Compared with compressed air cylinders much less filling would be required. Liquid oxygen is the most convenient for ambulatory use. Liquid oxygen does evaporate; therefore, occasional to intermittent use of a liquid reservoir may be wasteful. Patients utilizing liquid oxygen at home who are absent on vacation or during hospitalization may find their liquid oxygen supply depleted on their return home.

For the ambulatory patient liquid oxygen is extremely convenient and the modality of choice (Fig. 63–5). This form of oxygen is more expensive and under new HCFA regulations for reimbursement will tend to be used less frequently even though the patient's rehabilitative needs may best be served by this approach. The use of liquid oxygen should be encouraged when appropriate for ambulatory use. The expense of supplying liquid oxygen is less in the actual oxygen than in the need to maintain the supply of liquid oxygen in the home with periodic visits. These visits by the DME vendor are not reimbursed and must therefore be absorbed in the reimbursement for the oxygen itself.

Continuous (24-hour) oxygen therapy using liquid oxygen will become a rarity in the U.S. because of the number of visits required to supply the patient. The supply of liquid oxygen as an adjunct to nighttime concentrator use will be acceptable to vendors equipped to handle liquid oxygen (transportation, trained personnel). Patients may be directed away from utilizing liquid oxygen by some vendors wishing to use

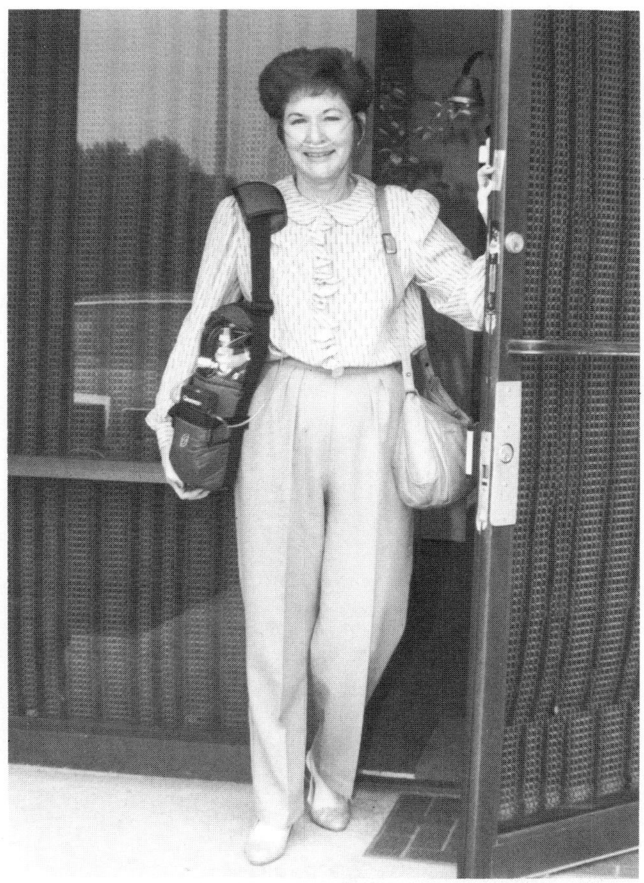

Figure 63–5. Patient using portable liquid oxygen with pulse delivery system for use during early inspiration (Courtesy of Chad Therapeutics, Chatsworth, California).

the modality incurring the least expense to them. The prescription of oxygen by the physician includes specifying the method of administration most advantageous to the patient's activity needs.

Oxygen Conservation Devices

RESERVOIR DEVICES. A number of cannula adaptations with oxygen reservoirs either at the nose or in the form of a pendant around the neck have been devised to conserve oxygen (Fig. 63–6). During exhalation oxygen is conserved in the reservoirs and inhaled with the next inspiration.[36]

These devices do conserve perhaps as much as 50% or 70% compared with standard nasal cannulae. The disadvantages include the frequent replacement of these devices and their unattractive appearance. This approach has not been widely used but may be utilized more with liquid oxygen. These devices would be attractive to suppliers wishing to limit the amount of oxygen employed or the number of home visits required to replenish a patient's supply. Patients wishing to use liquid oxygen and having to participate substantially in the payment for this therapy might also need to utilize these devices.

TRANSTRACHEAL OXYGEN. Considerable attention has been devoted to the development of the transtracheal method for long-term oxygen administration. The idea of administering oxygen through a cannula in the trachea is not new but the application in the present form has evolved over the last few years.[6, 31, 32]

A tracheocutaneous fistula is created with a series of catheters inserted between the tracheal rings. The tract matures over a period of 6 weeks at which time the patient is taught to replace the catheter, which is an 8F size with multiple ports for intratracheal oxygen flow.

The primary benefit of this technique is oxygen conservation with a significant reduction (up to 50%) in flow rates for patients requiring high-flow oxygen. Some patients view the transtracheal system as being cosmetically advantageous in their not having to display the conventional nasal cannula in public. A small oxygen cylinder will of course always be required. A minority of patients using nasal cannula have debilitating side effects, such as nasal crusting, chronic rhinitis, and impaired ability to smell. The last can usually be managed conservatively and it would be the unusual patient who would require an invasive procedure with the subsequent care involved to alleviate the symptoms listed previously.

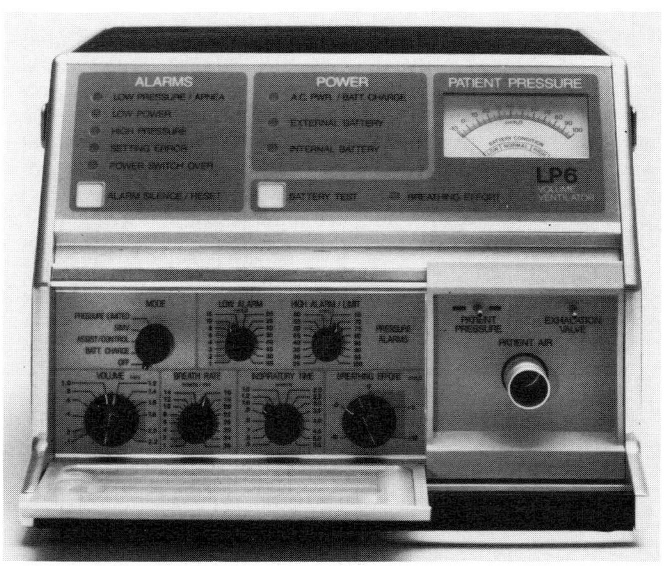

Figure 63–6. Portable positive pressure volume ventilator for use in the home (Courtesy of Lincare Inc., Brookpark, Ohio).

There are increasing reports of complications from the more widespread application of technique. Persistent cough, bronchospasm, infection, and subcutaneous emphysema are a few. Patients with copious sputum appear to have difficulty keeping the catheter patent. In addition, the expense of the procedure and the replacement catheters probably will make this modality less utilized in the future.

Transtracheal oxygen seems to be indicated mainly for patients requiring high flow oxygen to maintain adequate oxygenation (> 4 L/min).

PULSE DELIVERY SYSTEMS. Electronic demand delivery systems have become available that convey oxygen during the early part of the inspiratory phase.[6, 29, 33] Several of these devices have demonstrated oxygen savings of 2 to 1 and 3 to 1 over continuous flow systems. Data have suggested that the addition of pulsed oxygen therapy to a transtracheal catheter does not enhance oxygen conservation further. The cost effectiveness of these devices has yet to be demonstrated. The replacement of existing equipment would not seem to be reasonable at this time. With further demonstration of the economy and reliability of this equipment one can expect this approach to become widely used in the future.

Reimbursement for Oxygen Therapy

The majority of patients receiving long-term oxygen therapy at home are Medicare beneficiaries. Reimbursement for services provided for these patients is federally regulated. In many situations in the past other insurance carriers have used Medicare as a benchmark on which to model their reimbursement patterns for diagnostic or therapeutic modalities.

Oxygen and oxygen equipment is classified by HCFA as durable medical equipment (DME). Under a new plan implemented in 1989 home oxygen is reimbursed prospectively by a single monthly payment per patient for oxygen and the necessary equipment. This system is "modality neutral" with similar reimbursement for the different delivery systems.[5]

A small additional payment is made for portable equipment. Payment to the vendor is reduced for flow rates less than 1 L/min and increased for flow rates more than 3 L/min. The incentive for the vendor at this time is to provide the least expensive method of administration. The modalities of administration recommended by a particular vendor will vary depending on existing equipment. Vendors well equipped to supply liquid oxygen will use this modality to supplement the use of oxygen concentrators for ambulatory patients while continuous use of liquid oxygen will in all probability disappear.

The major negative impact of recent reimbursement modifications relates to the possible limitation of liquid oxygen. The extent of this impact will vary depending on location. Rural and other nonmetropolitan locations dependent on suppliers commuting long distances will be the areas least likely to have liquid oxygen available under a modality-neutral system. Many of the advances made over the last decades regarding the enhancement of lifestyle using liquid oxygen during ambulation, exercise, and recreational travel stand to be dissipated if the use of this modality is limited for an ambulatory patient.

ASSISTED VENTILATION

A range of technologies employing different physiologic principles can now be utilized in the home to assist or support ventilation in chronic respiratory diseases.[43] The home is the focus of these treatment modalities and there are as a result problems specific to the application and monitoring of these interventions, which bear consideration before committing to long-term home care. The issues are broadly categorized as

1. medical
2. social
3. psychologic
4. financial.

Before the introduction of any such technology in the home a medical decision must be made regarding the indications for assisted ventilation in each case. Given the medical appropriateness of the intervention the suitability of the social milieu is critical in determining the presence of the necessary family or external resource support to make introduction of the technology to the home feasible. Clearly the issues are of different magnitude for a noninvasive treatment, e.g., negative pressure ventilation, nasal ventilation, and nasal CPAP, than for an invasive, complex intervention, such as tracheostomy, with positive pressure ventilation and phrenic nerve pacing. In the last two examples an exquisitely receptive home and family environment should be in place before embarking on this route of care.

The psychologic issues need to be addressed early with the patient. Issues of assisted ventilation should be raised with all patients with severe neuromuscular disease or chronic respiratory failure at the time of the first office evaluation. The patients in whom long-term ventilatory support, particularly when tracheostomy and positive pressure ventilation are a distinct possibility, should be counseled and educated in this regard. The right to refuse this sometimes lifesaving intervention should be clearly stated together with a clear definition of the possible benefits of the treatment. Quality of life issues must be addressed so that patients can make decisions in an informed manner and evaluate their options appropriately. A multidisciplinary team knowledgeable in the various components of home ventilator care should be used to assess any patient who is a candidate for this care. The different devices employed for assisted ventilation are discussed in terms of the techniques of assisted ventilation and their physiologic principles of operation.

Negative Pressure Ventilation

IRON LUNG. A variety of negative pressure devices have been employed in the home to support or assist ventilation in patients with respiratory insufficiency. The iron lung, widely used in the poliomyelitis epidemics, was extremely cumbersome but effective. A few of these devices are still employed today by survivors of the polio epidemics who have become familiar with the device over the years. The device is rarely prescribed for homecare (in-patient) use for new patients.

CUIRASS/BODY WRAP/PONCHO. In later years negative pressure was applied to the anterior chest wall via a plastic shell (cuirass), which is custom-fit to the patient. Body wraps or ponchos that encircle the patient from the neck to the lower torso have been used. These negative pressure devices have been most widely used in neuromuscular diseases as well as in kyphoscoliosis.[10] They are usually inadequate for high quadriplegics.

The concept of negative pressure ventilation has been expanded to chronic respiratory failure patients, particularly those with COPD. The idea has been to rest the respiratory muscles and overcome respiratory muscle fatigue. A number of investigators have documented a lowering of P_{CO_2} and an increase in vital capacity following intermittent rest with a negative pressure device. Improved respiratory muscle strength and endurance have also been documented in this situation.[13–15]

The advantages of negative pressure devices relate to their ability to assist ventilation without the need for a tracheostomy. They are not complicated to operate and require minimal maintenance.

Some disadvantages exist. Upper airway obstruction may occur, particularly during sleep, because of asynchrony with the normal upper airway opening and closure mechanism. It is difficult to manage patients with copious secretions with a negative pressure device because coughing and postural drainage are not easily performed. The cuirass needs to fit extremely well, but fitting is extremely difficult in patients with chest wall deformities. The body wraps are warm and often uncomfortable. Depending on the degree of disability it may be cumbersome to get the patient into a body wrap or poncho. Negative pressure devices are compromised by severely reduced compliance of the chest wall. In patients with neuromuscular disease with loss of normal rib cage muscle activity the rib cage is known to become increasingly less compliant over time.

Application in the Home

Although patient education for use of negative ventilation may be done in the ambulatory setting or even in the home it is preferable to admit the patient to the hospital to familiarize him or her with the protocol for use of the particular device.

In addition to understanding the principle of the device the patient needs to have frequent measurements of exhaled tidal volume to determine the appropriate pressure settings for the machine. Arterial blood gas samples should be drawn to assess the precise effect on ventilation and oxygenation of the device. Once the patient's baseline has been established oximetry may be an appropriate method of monitoring at home.

Introduction to the device should be done slowly for a variety of reasons. The cuirass may hurt the chest wall if applied for too long at the outset. The patient may have difficulty breathing in synchrony with the device and be discouraged or frightened rapidly by the stridor associated with upper airway obstruction.

Positive Pressure Ventilation

Over the last 10 years a sophisticated service industry has developed around the utilization of positive pressure ventilation in the home.[7, 9, 44, 45] This has been facilitated by enhanced understanding of neuromuscular and chest wall diseases as well as the role of respiratory muscle fatigue in the pathogenesis of respiratory failure. The increased clinical recognition of the concept of long-term ventilation as a viable treatment option and the associated financial and social implications have encouraged patients and physicians to seek out the homecare option rather than indefinite nursing home stay.

Chronic positive pressure ventilation is utilized in the following patient groups:

- High quadriplegia
- Neuromuscular disease (Duchenne's muscular dystrophy, polio)
- Disorders of the chest wall (kyphoscoliosis)
- Central hypoventilation (congenital, idiopathic, acquired)
- COPD

Our own experience and that of others suggest that patients with COPD are among those least likely to experience satisfaction from long-term ventilation. This is in contrast to the patients with neuromuscular and chest wall diseases who frequently have advantageous outcomes in terms of correction of gas exchange abnormalities and an enhancement of daily living activities. The persistence of severe symptoms of dyspnea and the presence of chronic production of sputum are frequent features associated with patient dissatisfaction with this modality of treatment.

A variety of positive pressure ventilators are utilized with more than sufficient features to support ventilation in these patient groups. Whereas early models of portable positive pressure ventilators were pressure dependent, and later volume dependent but fixed rate, the current models provide a multiplicity of options. Assist control and intermittent mandatory ventilation (IMV) are now available on a number of machines that facilitate adjustment from hospital care to the home. Supplementary oxygen may be delivered and humidification may be achieved through a cascade device or an "artificial nose" placed directly in the circuit.

A backup ventilator is mandatory for high quadriplegics or totally ventilator-dependent patients. In patients who are capable of breathing for at least a short period of time off the respirator an Ambu bag may suffice. The newer ventilators can be powered by batteries capable of lasting for at least 1 hour in the event of power failure. In any event prior to discharge the local electric company as well as the police and fire departments should be informed of the patient's status in case of power outages or other emergency. The ventilator may be mounted on the back of a wheelchair on a platform to facilitate mobility.

The advantage of this method is that both the patient and family may be secure knowing that the positive pressure machine can be easily connected to support respiratory effort. This intervention frequently follows a prolonged period of severely impaired respiratory status that had resulted in a very unstable situation with poor sleep patterns and limitation on eating. The patient is usually not in immediate danger of succumbing from inability to breathe. Suctioning easily achieves clearance of secretions.

There are several disadvantages to the positive pressure ventilators. The patient obviously will need a tracheostomy, which requires changing and cleaning. The tracheostomy can itself cause increased secretions. A tracheostomy and a ventilator add another level of complexity to care at home. The patient requires a caregiver in the home at all times in case of emergencies.

TRACHEOSTOMY CARE. Patients with a chronic tracheostomy (and their caregivers and family) need to be skilled in cleaning and changing the tracheostomy tube. We recommend changing the tube once a month in the stable home-based patient. In most of our patients a cuffless tube is utilized, which facilitates speech on the ventilator. The tidal volume may be adjusted to compensate for the expected desired leak critical for speech.

NASAL CPAP. Numerous studies have documented that nasal CPAP is effective in the long-term treatment of obstructive sleep apnea and in the prevention of snoring.[39, 40] These conditions may coexist in patients with COPD or occur independently. The treatment is modulated by increasing the amount of positive pressure applied. The optimal pressures vary among patients. Nasal CPAP acts as a pneumatic splint preventing airway collapse. There are reports of the nightly need for CPAP becoming diminished after initial treatment. In today's clinical practice the pressure applied is titrated against oxygen saturation and degree of obstruction as monitored in a sleep laboratory. Daytime somnolence, polycythemia, and cor pulmonale appear alleviated in the patient in whom the treatment is tolerated.

Compliance with this treatment is a potential problem. The reasons include feelings of suffocation, nasal drying or rhinitis, ear pain, or conjunctivitis.

Advances in the design of the equipment required have resulted in a more silent device with better-fitting masks.

NASAL VENTILATION. Noninvasive intermittent positive pressure ventilation has been recognized as a method of improving the ventilation of patients with respiratory insufficiency. This technique has been applied via the mouth and through the nose with a tight-fitting mask.[8] The advantage of this approach is the ability to enhance ventilation and oxygenation via positive pressure administered into the airway without the need for a tracheostomy. A thermoplastic nasal mask is used, although this may have to be custom molded to ensure an adequate seal.

A conventional positive pressure ventilator is used with tidal volume and respiratory rate settings determined on the basis of measurements of oxygen saturation or arterial blood gas determinations. The limits of the ventilatory parameters are frequently determined by the patient's comfort and tolerance for the mask and the positive pressure being cyclically applied. The technique has been most frequently used in patients with kyphoscoliosis or neuromuscular disease.[8, 41, 42] However, we have utilized this approach in a limited number of patients with central alveolar hypoventilation and COPD.

Contraindications for this modality include an oropharyngeal muscle weakness inadequate for clearing oral secretions; an uncooperative or confused patient; an acute intrinsic lung disease requiring oxygen therapy; and a facial abnormality interfering with the interface. The greatest difficulties reported include discomfort from the mask pressure and leak into the eyes. Excessive leak around the mask renders the technique ineffective. The technique is a useful adjunct to the noninvasive alternatives to tracheostomy and positive pressure ventilation.

Other Devices

ROCKING BED. A rocking bed may be employed in the home for patients with respiratory insufficiency secondary to diaphragm paralysis with the availability of some other respiratory muscle activity. The bed is useful only when the patient is in bed. The device operates by tilting the patient to facilitate the descent of the diaphragm with gravity to effect inspiration. Expiration occurs with the head of the bed moving in the opposite direction toward the horizontal position and perhaps further. Rocking is said to promote bronchial hygiene. The bed operates on AC current only and it is cumbersome and not portable. The rocking bed does not appear to be a very useful method for patients with severe airway disease and has limited application in homecare today.

PNEUMOBELT. The pneumobelt consists of an inflatable bladder attached to a source of inflation, such as a portable positive pressure respirator. With each inflation the bladder is supposed to push the diaphragm upwards and effect expiratory movement. This usually requires more than 30 cm H_2O. The deflation of the belt results in inspiratory effort. The patient is required to sit close to upright (between 70 and 90 degrees) for effective use. This device has not proved to be very useful and is not widely utilized in the U.S. where more effective methods of assisting ventilation are now available.

PHRENIC NERVE PACING. Electrophrenic pacing has been used in a limited fashion to support or assist ventilation in patients with high quadriplegias and some central hypoventilation syndromes.[37]

The largest group of high quadriplegic patients still require the presence of a ventilator in the home, because the majority of cases reported do not achieve 24-hour support with the pacemaker. Patients who are high quadriplegics can be freed from the respirator for part of or the entire day. Speech is enhanced and vocational and recreational activities are facilitated. Phrenic nerve pacing is uncommon enough to be initiated only in a few centers where there is familiarity with the equipment, the implantation, and the postimplantation management of these unusual patients. Close follow-up by a specialty center is required and instruction regarding troubleshooting must be given to the patient's caregivers as well as to the local health care professionals who will be caring for the patient.

The prolonged hospitalization required by high quadriplegic patients for conditioning of the diaphragm following implantation of the pacemaker has in part resulted in very few of these patients being offered this procedure, which may greatly enhance their lives.

RESPIRATORY CARE DURING TRAVEL

An increasingly informed patient population with chronic respiratory disease has demanded better understanding of the illness and less restriction on recreational activities, such as travel. Patients with COPD and other chronic respiratory illnesses may have to undertake travel with a variety of respiratory devices. The most commonly used ones are aerosol nebulizers, oxygen, and devices for assisted ventilation.

The advent of portable rechargeable nebulizers (see earlier discussion) has made this a minor issue for patients and merely a question of acquisition. This type of "convenience" device will often have to be the patient's own financial responsibility depending on his or her insurance coverage.

Travel with oxygen within the U.S. is quite well defined although not necessarily easy. Public carriers, such as buses and trains, do not usually have restrictions on oxygen usage.

Air Travel

Travel on public carriers by air requires prior request by a physician for oxygen during flight. The format for this request varies according to the airline, each having its own specific documentation requirement. Oxygen used in flight is provided via a compressed air tank belonging to the airline. The oxygen is usually charged to the patient for each segment of the journey.

Patients who use continuous oxygen as a rule would expect to continue this therapy when traveling. Those with higher Po_2 levels who would not qualify for oxygen under normal circumstances may be advised by their physicians to use oxygen during flight because of the predictable drop on oxygen tension with ascent to cruising altitudes.[16] Although clear guidelines do not exist, some have advocated using available nomograms to prescribe oxygen for flight in those patients with sea level Po_2 of 68 or less when flying at 5000 feet. Hypoxic simulation tests advocated by some have not proven to be practical in this situation.[37]

Patients who are advised by their physicians to use oxygen during air travel need to use the oxygen supplied by the airline and cannot take their own equipment on board. Acceptance of the patient is also at the airline's discretion, since at this time airlines are under no legal obligation to provide this service. Patients need to be met on disembarkation with their own supply of oxygen if they are receiving continuous therapy. Similarly, on boarding a flight patients will usually not have any oxygen from the gate until they reach their seat on the aircraft, where a tank will be made available. During the flight the oxygen cannot be taken to the bathroom.

Cruise Ships

Some cruise ships do permit patients to use oxygen on board in the form of concentrator use in their cabin. For ambulatory utilization compressed air would technically be the most acceptable although storing sufficient amounts for a week-long cruise may be impractical. The status of liquid oxygen with the U.S. Coast Guard is unclear, although individuals should inquire from the cruise line regarding its use. This modality would clearly be the method of choice. Group travel in the form of cruises with medical supervision for patients with respiratory disease frequently minimizes these logistic problems for individual patients and should be encouraged. The cruise ship is particularly well suited for chronic respiratory patients with its well-defined environment and on-site recreational and entertainment activities. We have sponsored such cruises for the last few years. Our own experience has included patients with oxygen inhalation devices as well as positive pressure respirators. Respirators can be managed on board cruise lines only with the type of medical and technical support made available within such groups.

THE VENDOR—THE PHYSICIAN'S REPRESENTATIVE IN THE HOME

The DME supplier plays an increasingly important role in patient care. No longer does the vendor's role consist of simply delivering an apparatus. The reputable company is characterized by expertise in the management of high-technology equipment, the ability to assist in the patient education process at the time the therapy is introduced, and a system for communication with the physician regarding the nature of home visits and the information derived from them. The home visit report should now include a simple checklist of the patient's clinical status, e.g., pulse, blood pressure, and respiratory rate, as well as the patient's subjective assessment of his condition.

More complex information is required for the monitoring of patients using sophisticated respiratory assist devices. Billing practices also vary between companies, with some accepting assignment from Medicare and others (in the minority) requesting additional payment from patients, which in the case of liquid oxygen can amount to hundreds of dollars per month.

REFERENCES

1. Anthonisen NR. Hypoxemia and oxygen therapy. Am Rev Respir Dis 1982; 126:729–733.
2. Nocturnal Oxygen Therapy Trials. Continuous use of nocturnal oxygen therapy in hypoxemic chronic obstructive lung disease. Ann Intern Med 1980; 93:391–398.
3. Stuart Harris C, Bishop JM, Clark TJH, et al. Medical Research Council: long term domiciliary oxygen therapy in chronic hypoxic cor pulmonale. Lancet 1981; i:681–686.
4. Second Conference on Home Oxygen Therapy. Further recommendations for prescribing and supplying long term oxygen therapy. Am Rev Respir Dis 1988; 138:745–747.
5. O'Donohue WJ. New problems in home oxygen therapy. Am Rev Respir Dis 1989; 140:1813–1814.
6. Tiep BL, Christopher KL, Spofford BT, et al. Pulsed nasal and transtracheal oxygen delivery. Chest 1990; 97:364–368.
7. Mohr CH, Hill NS. Long term follow up of nocturnal ventilatory assistance in patients with respiratory failure due to Duchennes-type muscular dystrophy. Chest 1990; 97:91–96.
8. Bach JR, Alba AS. Management of chronic alveolar hypoventilation by nasal ventilation. Chest 1990; 97:52–57.
9. Alexander MA, Johnson EW, Petty J, Stauch D. Mechanical ventilation of patients with late stage Duchennes muscular dystrophy: management in the home. Arch Phys Med Rehab 1979; 60:289–292.
10. Splaingard ML, Frates RC, Jefferson LS, Rosen CL. Home negative pressure ventilation: report of 20 years of experience in neuromuscular disease. Arch Phys Med Rehab 1985; 66:239–242.

11. Motta J, Guilleminault C. Effects of oxygen administration in sleep-induced apneas. In: Guilleminault C, Dement WC, eds. Sleep Apnea Syndromes. New York: Alan R. Liss, 1978, 137–144.
12. Martin RJ, Sander MH, Pennock BE. Acute and long term ventilatory effects of oxygen administration in adult sleep apnea syndrome. Am Rev Respir Dis 1982; 125:175–180.
13. Cropp A, DiMarco AF. Effects of intermittent negative pressure ventilation on respiratory muscle function in patients with severe chronic obstructive pulmonary disease. Am Rev Respir Dis 1987; 135:1056–1061.
14. Gutierrez M, Beroiza T, Contreras G, et al. Weekly cuirass ventilation improves blood gases and inspiratory muscle strength in patients with chronic airflow limitation and hypercapnia. Am Rev Respir Dis 1988; 138:617–623.
15. Scano G, Gigliotti F, Duranti R, et al. Changes in ventilatory muscle function with negative pressure ventilation in patients with severe COPD. Chest 1990; 97:322–327.
16. Schwartz JS, Benowitz HZ, Moser KM. Air travel hypoxemia with chronic obstructive pulmonary disease. Ann Intern Med 1984; 100:473–477.
17. Henry JN, Krenis LJ, Cutting RT. Hypoxemia during aeromedical evacuation. Surg Gynecol Obstet 1973; 136:49–53.
18. Timms RM, Kvale PA, Anthonisen NR, et al. Selection of patients with chronic obstructive pulmonary disease for long-term oxygen therapy. JAMA 1981; 245:2514–2515.
19. Symposium on long-term oxygen therapy. Respir Care 1983; 28:857–930.
20. Fulmer JD, Snider GL. ACCP-NHLBI National Conference on Oxygen Therapy. Chest 1984; 86:234–274.
21. Pierson DJ. The toxicity of low-flow oxygen therapy. Respir Care 1983; 28:889–897.
22. West GA, Primeau P. Nonmedical hazards of long-term oxygen therapy. Respir Care 1983; 28:906–912.
23. Department of Health and Human Services Medicare Program. Coverage of oxygen for use in a patient's home. Final notice. Fed Reg 1985 (April 5); 50:13742–13750.
24. Petty TL. Problems in prescribing and supplying oxygen for Medicare patients. Am Rev Respir Dis 1986; 1343:340–341.
25. Levi-Valensi P, Weitzenblum E, Pedinielli J-L, et al. Three-month follow-up of arterial blood gas determinations in candidates for long-term oxygen therapy. Am Rev Respir Dis 1986; 133:547–551.
26. Kochansky M. Ear oximetry as a method of determining home oxygen prescriptions. Respir Care 1984; 29:1211–1220.
27. Nelson CM, Murphy EM, Bradley JK, Durie RH. Clinical use of pulse oximetry to determine oxygen prescriptions for patients with hypoxemia. Respir Care 1986; 31:673–680.
28. McDonald GJ. Long-term oxygen therapy delivery systems. Respir Care 1983; 28:898–905.
29. O'Donohue WJ Jr. Oxygen-conserving devices. Respir Care 1987; 32:37–42.
30. Tiep BL. New portable oxygen devices. Respir Care 1987; 32:106–112.
31. Heimlich HR. Respiratory rehabilitation with transtracheal oxygen system. Ann Otol Rhinol Laryngol 1982; 91:643–647.
32. Christopher KL, Spofford BT, Brannin PK, Petty TL. Transtracheal oxygen therapy for refractory hypoxemia. JAMA 1986; 256:494–497.
33. Block AJ. Intermittent flow devices: technically feasible, but rarely used. Chest 1984; 86:657–658.
34. Soffer M, Tashkin DP, Shapiro BJ, et al. Conservation of oxygen supply using a reservoir nasal cannula in hypoxemic patients at rest and during exercise. Chest 1985; 88:663–688.
35. Flenley DC. Long-term home oxygen therapy. Chest 1985; 87:99–103.
36. Decker MJ, Hoekje PL, Strohl KP. Ambulatory monitoring of oxygen saturation. Chest 1989; 95:717–722.
37. Nochomovitz ML, Peterson DK, Stellato TK. Electrical activation of the diaphragm. Clin Chest Med 1988; 9:349–358.
38. Gong H, Tashkin DP, Lee EY, Simmons MS. Hypoxia altitude simulation test. Am Rev Respir Dis 1984; 130:980–986.
39. Strohl KP, Redline S. Nasal CPAP therapy, airway muscle activation and obstructive sleep apnea. Am Rev Respir Dis 1986; 134:555–558.
40. Saunders MH. Nasal CPAP effect on patterns of sleep apnea. Chest 1984; 86:839–844.
41. Kerby GR, Mayer LS, Pingelton SK. Nocturnal positive pressure ventilation via nasal mask. Am Rev Respir Dis 1987; 135:738–740.
42. Leger P, Jennequin J, Gerard M, Robert D. Home positive pressure ventilation via nasal mask for patients with neuromuscular weakness of restrictive lung or chest wall disease. Respir Care 1989; 34:73–79.
43. Garay SM, Turino GM, Goldring RM. Sustained reversal of chronic hypercapnia in patients with alveolar hypoventilation syndromes. Am J Med 1981; 70:269–274.
44. Plummer AL, O'Donohue JR, Petty TL. Consensus report on problems in home mechanical ventilation. Am Rev Respir Dis 1989; 140:555–560.
45. O'Donohue JR, Giovanni RM, Goldberg AI. Long-term mechanical ventilation. Guidelines for management in the home and at alternate community sites. Chest 1986; 90(suppl):1–37.

Chapter 64

LONG-TERM CARE OF PATIENTS WITH CHRONIC BRONCHITIS AND EMPHYSEMA

W. Darlene Reid Richard L. Pardy

In the patient with established chronic obstructive pulmonary disease (COPD), long-term care has two essential components. The first is that once the severity of the illness is determined, the major objective is to treat the disease to the best of our ability and to teach the patient to function optimally within the confines of the disease. The second is that each patient must be managed individually, taking into account such factors as the severity of the illness, the facilities available, the patient's willingness to be involved in a comprehensive care program, the presence of other chronic illness, and the degree of family support.

It is therefore apparent that the subject of long-term care of the patient with chronic bronchitis or emphysema, or both, is an extremely broad field that has been the subject of a number of books and reviews.[12, 13, 40, 44, 48, 49, 53, 54, 65, 70, 79, 82, 86, 87, 97, 99] The major emphasis of this chapter is on three components of a long-term care program: patient education, exercise, and modification of activities of daily living. Before reviewing these areas, other components, dealt with in detail in previous or subsequent chapters, are very briefly reviewed.

COMPONENTS OF LONG-TERM CARE

Prevent Progression of Disease

Because the major cause of COPD is cigarette smoking, a primary goal is early detection of disease in cigarette smokers and cessation of smoking. Although only 5% to 25% of patients entering a smoking cessation program will stop permanently, major efforts to get patients with COPD to stop smoking are justified. Success with stopping smoking is more likely when the patient is given information on why he or she should stop, offered programs to help him or her stop, and given positive reinforcement by all members of the rehabilitation team.[39]

Avoidance of air pollutants in either work or local environments should be advised if these factors are contributing to progression of disease.

Prevent Complications

Respiratory tract infection may have a role in causing COPD and can produce acute exacerbations of emphysema and bronchitis. Although most respiratory tract infections cannot be prevented, patients with COPD are candidates for immunization with influenza and pneumococcal vaccines.[46, 62, 112]

Cor pulmonale may be prevented or ameliorated by the judicious use of oxygen to reduce pulmonary hypertension. Oxygen should be used as continuously as is practical, ideally 24 hours a day.[8] Controlled oxygen therapy in selected patients decreased mortality,[74] presumably by reducing pulmonary hypertension.[80]

The side effects of individual drugs used for the treatment of COPD and the interaction of such drugs with other medications should be avoided.[108] Therapy should be based on careful individual assessment and only drugs proven to be useful in the individual continued. Although inhaled sympathomimetic bronchodilators are uncommonly associated with side effects unless abused, methylxanthine preparations must be used judiciously to avoid side effects and interactions with other drugs and given in a dose that achieves therapeutic blood levels.

The severe and debilitating complications of long-term systemic corticosteroid therapy are well known to all practicing physicians.[105] The role of corticosteroids is controversial despite reports of improved spirometry in 13% to 29% of patients with stable COPD.[37, 45, 75, 98, 105, 107, 108] The best predictors of a significant response to oral corticosteroids in patients with COPD are sputum and blood eosinophilia and greater than 15% improvement in FEV_1 with inhaled beta-agonists.[108] Only patients responding to such therapy (improved spirometry) should be continued on it to minimize long-term complications—and then at the lowest dose associated with maintenance of any improvement obtained.[108]

Treat Reversible Components

Chest physical therapy consisting of postural drainage and percussion techniques is of proven benefit in clearing secretions and improving lung function, but only in patients with increased sputum production.

Expiratory airflow limitation caused by loss of elastic recoil, inflammation and fibrosis in airway walls, smooth muscle thickening and hyperactivity, and increased secretions in the airway lumen are important components of the pathophysiology of COPD. Appropriate choices of inhaled sympathomimetic, methylxanthine, and anticholinergic agent or corticosteroid, or both, should be made to increase airway diameter and decrease resistance to airflow. To determine appropriate medications for use in an individual patient, the response to such therapy, both symptomatic and objective (spirometric), should be documented. Only those drugs shown to result in improvement should be continued on a long-term basis. The importance of identifying the subpopulation of COPD patients with significant variability in spirometry over time or a significant improvement in response to bronchodilators, or both, is emphasized. This subpopulation has a better prognosis than patients with severe fixed airflow limitation[23] and this subgroup is more likely to benefit from corticosteroid therapy.[37, 45, 108]

Acute respiratory tract infection should be treated with antimicrobials. A Gram stain of the sputum is helpful in ensuring that there is infection, i.e., polymorphonuclear white blood cells, and may suggest an organism.

Think About the Pump

Dyspnea is the major symptom in all patients with COPD. It is prominent in patients with COPD because of increased airway resistance, mechanical impairment of the action of the respiratory muscles, and in some patients, respiratory muscle weakness.[3, 21, 59, 60, 64] Dyspnea is heightened when respiratory drives increase, as with exercise. Most of the measures so far discussed as part of a long-term care program are aimed at decreasing the load on the respiratory muscles in patients with COPD. Several new, promising therapies directed at improving the function of the respiratory muscles themselves are currently undergoing investigation and may in the future prove to be of benefit for the patient with COPD. Pilot studies in the areas of respiratory muscle training, respiratory muscle rest, and supplemental nutrition suggest that these therapies may have a future place in the long-term care of patients with COPD. They must all be considered experimental interventions at this point in time, and the precise indications for these therapies have yet to be clearly defined.

Patient Education, Exercise, and Modification of Activities of Daily Living

Patient Education

According to Lane and Evans,[63] "Patient education provides a vehicle for increasing self-management of chronic illness and promoting modifications of lifestyle which are considered important strategies for prevention." Many components of long-term pulmonary care demand a high degree of patient compliance, and some require major changes in lifestyle. Thus, patients need to understand the basic pathophysiologic changes that produce the symptoms and signs of the disease. They must also learn self-care and preventive measures to become more independent and able to cope with disease-related problems.

Patient education should entail a comprehensive ongoing program and a multidisciplinary approach with the patient participating actively. The health care team may involve a nurse, physiotherapist, occupational therapist, dietitian, social worker, psychologist, and respirologist. Input from each of these health professionals will vary according to the individual patient's needs.

The chronicity of COPD affects the patient's entire social and psychologic network, e.g., family, ability to work and provide financial support, household and leisure activities, interaction with friends, and ease in public. All these aspects should be dealt with in order to deliver successful comprehensive care.

Patient education sessions should provide information on the disease entity and self-management, a forum for COPD patients to share their coping strategies with each other, and an opportunity to identify each individual's specific needs and concerns regarding his or her condition. This information is best provided by both group and individual sessions with the different health professionals.

The content of the program should include information on the basic anatomy and physiology of the respiratory system, the pathophysiology of COPD, proper administration of medications, including oxygen, signs of infection, proper bronchial hygiene, nutrition, relaxation techniques,[42] exercise, and modification of activities of daily living.[20] Details of the content of patient education for COPD are described elsewhere.[5–7]

In the past, breathing retraining techniques had been prescribed as an essential component of patient education. Careful investigation has revealed that it is very difficult to alter the subconscious pattern of breathing in healthy individuals and the optimum pattern of breathing may be controlled within tighter constraints in the patient with COPD because of the pathologic and mechanical changes induced by disease.[68] Current findings do not support the use of "diaphragmatic," "abdominal,"[10, 96, 102] or "unilateral"[71] breathing techniques. Pursed-lip breathing and slowing of breathing frequency may be useful in stressful situations and during the implementation of relaxation techniques.[91]

There are several audiovisual productions that are available from local lung associations to assist in the presentation of learning material. Helpful publications for patient reading are issued by the lung associations as well.

Reports in the literature vary greatly regarding techniques for providing patient education; some simply issue a booklet containing pertinent information, others provide individual or group teaching sessions incorporating pre- and postteaching evaluations of the patient's knowledge,[20, 47] and some require the patient to be the primary member of the team in identifying his or her own needs and course of action.[31] The most successful programs are those that are interactive, providing ample opportunity for patient questions and re-evaluation of the patient's knowledge.

Although there are numerous reports in the literature touting the benefit of patient education programs, most reports are descriptive in nature, evaluating the impact of one program. Few studies contain an untreated control group or compare different teaching methods. Although the concept of patient education makes intuitive sense, much more needs to be done to identify patients most likely to benefit, what to reasonably expect from such programs, and the most effective methods to employ.

Exercise

Until the 1960s, the stress imposed by exercise was considered to be deleterious to patients with cardiopulmonary disorders. However, several reports in the sixties demonstrated the benefit of exercise training in the patient with COPD.[30, 83, 89] Since that time numerous investigators have examined the effect of whole body exercise training on different physiologic parameters in the COPD patient (Table 64–1). Although these reports present conflicting results regarding cardiovascular and skeletal muscle adaptation, the general consensus is that exercise training in COPD patients improves work tolerance[2, 14, 15, 27, 29, 32, 33, 43, 90, 109, 115] and the ability to perform functional activities.[79] Barach and colleagues[11] suggested that the progressive improvement in the ability to walk without dyspnea following training in COPD patients may be due to a physiologic response similar to that observed in athletes following a training program. Numerous studies have examined the mechanisms of improved exercise performance in COPD patients; however, these mechanisms are still not well understood. Possible mechanisms include increased aerobic capacity, increased respiratory muscle endurance, decreased sense of dyspnea, increased motivation, and improved efficiency.

Improved work tolerance[2, 14, 15, 27, 29, 32, 33, 43, 90, 109, 114, 115] and

TABLE 64–1. Effects of Exercise Training in Patients with COPD

CARDIOVASCULAR	
	Increased $VO_{2\,max}$ (*symptom-limited)[2, 15, 27, 29, 30, 33, 109]
	No change in HR at similar submaximal workloads[83, 109, 115]
	No change in cardiac output, stroke volume[2, 29, 33, 115]
RESPIRATORY	
	Increased tolerance of dyspnea[1, 79]
	No change in respiratory muscle endurance[16]
	Decrease in minute ventilation at similar workloads[29, 57, 89, 109]
	Increased mucociliary clearance[81, 116]
	Improvement in pulmonary function is debated[2, 14, 29, 43, 65, 104]
	Lowered pulmonary artery pressure is debated[2, 29, 33]
SKELETAL MUSCLE	
	Improvement in oxygen extraction[2, 33]
	No change in a-v O_2 content difference[29]
	No changes in skeletal muscle enzymes[15]
MAXIMAL WORKLOAD	
	Increased[2, 14, 15, 27, 29, 32, 33, 43, 90, 109, 114, 115]
	Improved efficiency—lower HR, $Vo_{2\,max}$ or increased anaerobic threshold[2, 14, 29, 57, 83, 89]
PSYCHOLOGICAL	
	Increased sense of well-being[1, 40, 76, 104, 115]
ACTIVITIES OF DAILY LIVING	
	Improvement[79]
	No change[24]

*Symptom-limited—$Vo_{2\,max}$ determined from maximal level of exercise terminated because of symptoms not because a plateau in oxygen consumption demonstrated. a-v O_2 = arterial-venous difference in oxygen content; $Vo_{2\,max}$ = maximal oxygen consumption; HR = heart rate.

decreased dyspnea[1, 79] have been documented in several reports examining the effects of exercise training in patients with COPD. However, the changes in skeletal muscle[15] and in the cardiovascular system[2, 29, 33, 83, 109, 115] found in healthy individuals have not been found consistently in patients with COPD. The inability of other investigators to find adaptive changes in the cardiovascular system or skeletal muscle may be attributed to a short training program. Alternatively, the intensity of training may have been too low to induce a physiologic response, the response too small to measure, or the tests used to measure the response inappropriate or insensitive.

Although an increase in respiratory muscle endurance in response to specific respiratory muscle training programs has been demonstrated in patients with COPD[85] and an increase in exercise performance found in association with the increased respiratory muscle endurance in some of these patients,[84, 85] the converse has not been found. That is, improved exercise performance after exercise training in patients with COPD was not associated with a change in respiratory muscle endurance.[16]

Increased motivation could account for an increase in the maximum exercise heart rate or minute ventilation achieved during an exercise test following a training program. A higher minute ventilation or heart rate in exercise would demonstrate that the patient was able to push himself or herself further into his or her age-predicted reserve capacity. Although greater motivation could account for improvements seen in some individuals,[33] neither a change in maximal heart rate nor minute ventilation has been consistently demonstrated to account for increases in exercise capacity.[14]

Increased efficiency seems to explain improved work tolerance following treadmill training in some patients with COPD.[14, 83, 89] However, it is not clear whether or not the benefits of treadmill walking are transferred to activities of daily living. This issue is discussed later (*see* Table 64–3).

Increased tolerance to dyspnea[1, 79] and improved sense of well-being[79] have been reported after exercise training programs. Dyspnea is very much dependent on the individual's perception of difficulty or distress with breathing.[59] The pathophysiology of this sensation is incompletely understood. Studies have permitted the quantification of dyspnea using psychophysiologic techniques.[3, 21, 59, 60, 69, 106] In both healthy subjects and patients with COPD exercise breathing oxygen was associated with a decrease in minute ventilation.[25, 26] In the healthy subjects dyspnea scores in exercise were also lower when breathing oxygen.[25] Similar scoring of dyspnea has not been used to assess the effects of exercise training in patients with COPD. A decrease in minute ventilation in exercise after training has been described in patients with COPD[29, 57, 89, 109] and might therefore explain decreased dyspnea in some cases. However, changes in breathing frequency, tidal volume, velocity of shortening or force output per breath of inspiratory muscles, or the proportion of time spent in inspiration per breath might equally account for reduced dyspnea after exercise training.[59, 60, 64]

An improved sense of well-being may be attributed to increased work tolerance, increased activities of daily living, and sense of accomplishment. A physiologic basis may exist, for instance, endorphin release, for a more positive outlook of patients with COPD following an exercise program.[78]

DESIGN OF A TRAINING PROGRAM. The extremely low exercise tolerance of the patient with COPD and the often relentless course of the disease precludes the use of training regimens designed for healthy individuals or cardiovascular patients. Nevertheless, similar principles of training should be applied. In design of an exercise training program, four principles of training should always be considered: overload, specificity of training, individual differences, and reversibility.[72] An *overload* needs to be applied to bring about a training response. The overload can be altered by varying frequency, duration, intensity, or a combination of these factors. Due to the *specificity of training*, maximal benefit will occur when the training techniques are similar to the functional outcome desired. It is obvious that training programs are optimized when they are planned to meet the *individual's needs and capacities*. The *reversibility principle* states that detraining will occur when a person is immobilized or decreases his or her activity level.

PRETRAINING EVALUATION. Before undertaking a training program, the patient should be adequately managed medically and be properly nourished. A pretraining evaluation is essential to screen for cardiovascular disease, to determine the specific needs of the patient, including the need for oxygen to prevent desaturation during exercise, and to determine the most appropriate training intensity. Although much has been written regarding the standardization of exercise testing for diagnostic purposes in patients with pulmonary disease, the use of exercise testing to design training programs for COPD patients is less well established.

Training should maximize functional performance during daily activities, and testing of those skills should mimic those activities as closely as possible. Evaluation should include testing of both the upper and lower extremities in addition to some kind of functional assessment. Functional assessment may be performed by administering an activity questionnaire[18, 19, 58] or by simulating functional activities.[111] A list of the advantages and disadvantages of different exercise testing modalities is shown in Table 64–2. Although progressive, incremental exercise tests are more time-efficient, a steady-state exercise test at a moderate submaximal level or a timed maximal walking distance test more closely simulates daily activities and thus may provide additional information.

Although evaluation of activities of daily living falls outside the realm of formal exercise testing, it is still an essential component for evaluation of COPD patients in determining the most appropriate training program. Standardized activity

TABLE 64–2. Comparison of Some Exercise Tests Used to Evaluate Patients with COPD

TESTING MODALITY	ADVANTAGES	DISADVANTAGES
Treadmill	—Well-defined workload —Easy to pace, and pace is determined by treadmill	—Not as functionally relevant as a 12-minute walk —More difficult to monitor than leg ergometer —Requires good balance
Leg Ergometer	—Well-defined workload —Easy to monitor	—Not as functionally relevant as walking —Pace determined by patient
Arm Ergometer	—Well-defined workload, although pace determined by patient —More functional because many daily activities require use of arms	—Difficult to monitor blood pressure during exercise —Very difficult to monitor
6 or 12-Minute Walk[73]	—Very functionally relevant —Requires minimal equipment	—Difficult to pace, i.e., test may be submaximal or patient may exceed optimal pace and stop short
Simulated Functional Activities	—More functionally relevant —Objective	—Difficult to standardize work rate and to quantitate workload
Functional Activities Questionnaire	—More functionally relevant	—Dependent on patient's perception of activity

questionnaires[18, 19, 58, 88] and analogue rating scales are used.[56] An alternative is to test functional activities by simulating them in the laboratory.[93, 111] Much work needs to be done to establish standard functional tests and to determine their reliability and validity.

Supervision and Monitoring

Most reports describe more success if the training program is supervised. This provides feedback to the patient and an opportunity to modify the program as the needs of the patient change. Supervision by the physiotherapist should be quite frequent initially and may then taper as the patient becomes more proficient in the exercise program. Successful programs have been conducted in hospitals, in outpatient departments, or at home.[24]

Heart rate and blood pressure should be monitored before, during, and after the supervised exercise training sessions. Monitoring the electrocardiogram is important in new patients to exclude arrhythmias. Monitoring of oxygen saturation may be extremely helpful in determining both the optimal intensity of exercise and the need for oxygen therapy. Similarly, the respiratory rate may also be a suitable guide to exercise intensity.[56]

Components of the Training Program

Training sessions should incorporate a warmup, a performance of an aerobic activity at a specific training intensity, and a cooldown period. Adequate warmup and cooldown not only ensure optimal performance but are safer and less stressful to the cardiovascular system. Thoracic mobility exercises[41] can be used for the warmup and cooldown. These include upper extremity and trunk exercises designed to promote flexibility of the trunk musculature. For the warmup, the thoracic mobility exercises can then be followed by very low-intensity exercise on the modality of choice for at least 2 to 3 minutes, followed by the training workload at a higher exercise intensity, and then the cooldown period, in which low-intensity exercise is performed for at least 3 to 5 minutes.

The exercise training *intensity* is usually extremely low in patients with COPD[4] compared with the workloads performed by healthy individuals and patients with cardiovascular disease. Age-predicted heart rate is not usually useful because the heart rate of patients with chronic respiratory disease is elevated with respect to oxygen consumption compared with the heart rate–oxygen consumption relationship in the healthy individual.[67] Monitoring heart rate is useful in detecting those patients who experience exercise-induced arrhythmias. Jones and colleagues[56] recommend that training be performed at 60% to 80% of the ventilatory capacity or equivalent heart rate. Carter and colleagues[27] attributed the success of their training program to the fact that patients were exercised to their ventilatory maximum rather than according to cardiovascular guidelines. However, probably the best indicator of exercise intensity during supervised and unsupervised training sessions may be the patient's sense of dyspnea and many recommend exercising at a level where breathing is not uncomfortable.

The patient's compliance to performance of exercise training is very much dependent on degree of comfort during exercise. One quantitative way of evaluating the patient's subjective response during training is the Borg rating scale of perceived exertion.[21] The patient may be advised to begin with exercise at a relatively low perceived intensity in order to familiarize himself or herself with exercise training but later train at moderate to high levels of perceived exertion.

The *duration of exercise* may initially have to be very short. A very short training duration[4, 72] or an interval program[56, 92] may be necessary for those patients with a very low exercise tolerance. An interval training program consists of high-intensity training workloads interspersed with low-intensity workloads or periods of rest. Ideally, one would like to aim for 25 to 30 minutes of exercise.

The specificity of training should be considered in selecting the most appropriate *modality or activity* for endurance training. Availability of equipment and climate are also important factors to consider (*see* Table 64–3). In most cases a combination of walking and possibly unsupported arm exercise are the most desirable training modalities.

Training should be performed three to five times per week. Less frequent training may produce no training effect, whereas more frequent training may not allow sufficient time for recovery. Progression of training intensity should be very slow in COPD patients.

Although exercise training has been suggested to be a very important component of a COPD long-term care program, more work needs to be done to further develop the most appropriate techniques. Definitive measures to evaluate the

TABLE 64–3. Advantages and Disadvantages of Different Modalities for Exercise Training in Patients with COPD

TRAINING MODALITY	ADVANTAGES	DISADVANTAGES
Treadmill	—Can be done indoors —Easy to monitor —Well-defined workload —Similar to walking —Pacing of treadmill can be used to demonstrate potential exercise tolerance if patient used self-pacing	—Can be boring —Patient requires good balance and coordination. Some may need to use handrails —Not identical to walking because pace determined by machine —Expensive for home purchase
Leg Ergometer	—Well-defined workload —Easy to monitor —Can be done in poor weather —Can provide strengthening of lower extremities —Relatively inexpensive	—Less functionally relevant than walking —Boring, and seat can be uncomfortable
Walking	—Interesting —Functional; requires the development of self-pacing	—Difficult in poor weather except can be done in local shopping centers —Difficult to monitor —Workload not as easy to quantitate
Arm Ergometer	—Well-defined workload —Easier to pace	—Requires careful progression in those with cardiac disease (↑ BP due to ↑ PVR) and COPD (may cause undue dyspnea and respiratory muscle fatigue)[28] —Less functional than unsupported arm exercise
Unsupported Arm Exercise	—Functionally relevant	—Workload is not standard or easy to quantitate —Need extra care for progression of exercise-reasons (see above)

BP = blood pressure; PVR = peripheral vascular resistance; ↑ = increased.

effectiveness of exercise training on activities of daily living need to be developed. Visual analogue scales,[56] detailed questionnaires,[18, 19, 88] and simulated work testing[111] are worth exploring to standardize methods of evaluating functional activities performed by COPD patients.

Modification of Activities of Daily Living

Developing strategies to modify the activities of daily living become more important with increasing disability.[101] Frustration, fear, and anxiety caused by increasing dyspnea may drain energy faster than the actual performance of tasks. Effort should be made to provide an atmosphere for training and evaluation that is pleasant and conducive to learning.[50] Assertiveness training is useful for enabling patients to develop positive techniques for asking their friends or spouse to assist them in these changes.[110] Renegotiating roles and responsibilities in household chores may pose great difficulties for both the patient, who may feel guilt, and the spouse, who may feel resentment.

Successful instruction in modifying daily activities will require several sessions and should include audiovisual aids and written handouts, and an opportunity to practice activities. Family members should be encouraged to attend, because they are often key in providing reinforcement. In addition to ways to modify the performance of stressful activities, adaptive equipment and hazards of products used during daily activities e.g., cleaning agents, should be discussed.

Decision-making is an integral part of modification of daily activities. The decisions made may indicate role reversal, the hiring of help, compromise or priority, and often, changing life-long habits. The patient must determine if a particular task is necessary and whether or not it can best be done by someone else. Often the entire approach to carrying out essential tasks must be reorganized.

The patient must learn to pace himself or herself to perform activities slowly and to stop before extreme fatigue occurs. Work should be simplified and large tasks should be divided into smaller components. On days when energy levels are higher the more taxing activities can be performed. Usually high-energy times are midmorning, midafternoon, and after meals have been well digested.

Clothes should be selected based on ease of putting on and comfort while wearing. Women should avoid wearing pantyhose and both men and women should avoid wearing anything tight around the abdomen or chest, such as belts, tight-fitting waistbands, or bras.

Bending over or reaching up using the upper extremities can markedly increase dyspnea and should be minimized. Chores should be carried out at a comfortable height or sitting. Rather than bending over, the patient could sit on a low stool during such activities as showering, gardening, or while reaching into low kitchen cupboards or refrigerator compartments. The use of pick-up tongs and slip-on shoes, and the carrying of objects with the use of a wheeled cart in the kitchen and around the house will help minimize stress on upper extremities.

The patient needs to learn how to organize activities in order to maximize comfort and safety. Patients with COPD are disabled and therefore are entitled to handicapped parking permits, which will enable them to park in more convenient locations. A CB radio in order to call for help if the car breaks down also may be useful.

Maintenance of some social activities is very important. Often, joining a club composed of other patients with respiratory disease can provide friends with things in common in addition to providing support.

More details regarding energy conservation techniques in activities of daily living are given in the booklet entitled "Around the Clock with COPD," an American Lung Association publication.[95]

SUMMARY

In this chapter we have summarized the effects of patient education, exercise training, and modification of activities of daily living in the long-term care of patients with COPD. Sufficient evidence exists for better quality of life and objective evidence exists for improvements in exercise capacity so that these therapies can be recommended as part of the comprehensive care of the patient with COPD. Deficiencies still exist, however. For example, we still do not know what components of an education program have the greatest chance of success, the best forum/teacher to employ, or how best to measure the response. Similarly, improved programs based on sound physiologic principles using tests and scoring outcome with variables appropriate to the patient with COPD and possibly preceded by nutritional assessment,[9, 34, 94] supplementation when necessary,[61, 66, 113] and incorporating respiratory muscle as well as limb muscle training[17, 84, 85] should lead to improvements in exercise training as part of long-term care of the patient with COPD.

It is not clear whether long-term care alters morbidity and mortality in COPD. This question can at least be partially answered if the definition and components of long-term care described earlier in this chapter are accepted and the results of clinical trials examined. Smoking cessation is successful in 5% to 25% of patients with COPD.[39] Smoking cessation slows the rate of decline in lung function with age.[22] Patients with more reversible airflow limitation by definition have a better response to bronchodilators. They also have a better response to oral corticosteroids[27, 45, 108] and have a better prognosis.[23] Such patients may not be included in some studies of patients with COPD since these patients have chronic asthmatic bronchitis.[23] Selected patients treated with oxygen have a reduced mortality.[8, 74, 80]

Other individual components of long-term care have not been examined for their effects on morbidity and mortality. However, such components as chest physical therapy,[38, 77] exercise (*see* Table 64–1), respiratory muscle training,[84, 85] nutrition,[17, 61, 113] modification of activities of daily living, and psychologic counseling[1, 35, 100] have achieved their immediate goals of improvements in clearance of secretions, exercise capacity, respiratory muscle performance, activities of daily living, quality of life, and lessening of anxiety and depression in selected patients. Several multicomponent programs have been associated with a decrease in the rate of hospital admissions after long-term care programs.[36, 52, 54, 65]

However, from studies to date, it would appear that only some patients benefit from long-term care programs. Those who do better are those with fewer feelings of anxiety and depression, those who are married, do not smoke, are strongly motivated, have less severe disease, and have strong family support.[1, 51, 103] Even so, most patients will respond to at least some parts of a long-term care program, such as those outlined in this chapter.

REFERENCES

1. Agle DP, Baum GL, Chester EH, et al. Multi-discipline treatment of chronic pulmonary insufficiency. 1. Psychologic aspects of rehabilitation. Psychosom Med 1973; 35:41–49.
2. Alpert JS, Bass H, Szucs MM, et al. Effects of physical training on hemodynamics and pulmonary function at rest and during exercise in patients with chronic obstructive pulmonary disease. Chest 1974; 66:647–651.
3. Altose M, Cherniack N, Fishman AP. Respiratory sensations and dyspnea. J Appl Physiol 1985; 58:1051–1054.
4. American College of Sports Medicine. Guidelines for Exercise Testing and Prescription. Philadelphia: Lea and Febiger, 1986, 72–75.
5. American Hospital Association, Staff Manual for Teaching Patients with COPD. Chicago, IL: American Hospital Association, 1982.
6. American Lung Association: Better Breathing Guide. New York: American Lung Association, 1982.
7. American Lung Association: Help Yourself to Better Breathing. New York: American Lung Association, 1982.
8. Anthonisen NR. Home oxygen therapy in COPD. Clin Chest Med 1986; 7:673–678.
9. Askanazi J, Weissman C, Rosenbaum SH, et al. Nutrition and the respiratory system. Crit Care Med 1982; 10:163–172.
10. Bake B. Effects of shape changes of the chest wall on distribution of inspired gas. Am Rev Respir Dis 1976; 114:1113–1120.
11. Barach AL, Bickerman HA, Beck AJ. Advances in treatment of non-tuberculous pulmonary disease. Bull NY Acad Med 1952; 28:353–384.
12. Bebout DE, Hodgkin JE, Zorn EG, et al. Clinical and physiological outcomes of a university hospital affiliated rehabilitation program. Respir Care 1983; 28:1468–1473.
13. Bell CW, Blodgett D, Goike CA, et al. Home care and rehabilitation in respiratory medicine. Philadelphia: JB Lippincott Co., 1984.
14. Belman MJ, Wasserman K. Exercise training and testing in patients with chronic obstructive pulmonary disease. Basics Respir Dis 1981; 10:1–16.
15. Belman MJ, Kendregan BA. Exercise training fails to increase skeletal muscle enzymes in patients with chronic obstructive pulmonary disease. Am Rev Respir Dis 1981; 123:256–261.
16. Belman MJ, Kendregan BA. Physical training fails to improve ventilatory muscle endurance in patients with chronic obstructive pulmonary disease. Chest 1982; 81:440–443.
17. Belman MJ. Exercise in chronic obstructive pulmonary disease. Clin Chest Med 1986; 7:585–597.
18. Bergner M, Bobbitt RA, Pollard WE, et al. The sickness impact profile: a development and final revision of a health status measure. Med Care 1981; 19:787–805.
19. Bergner M, Bobbitt RA, Pollard WE, et al. The sickness impact profile: a conceptual formation and methodology for development of a health status measure. Int J Health Serv 1975; 6:393–415.
20. Black LF, Mitchell MM. Evaluation of a patient education program for chronic obstructive pulmonary disease. Mayo Clin Proc 1977; 52:106–111.
21. Borg GAV. Psychophysical basis of perceived exertion. Med Sci Sports Exerc 1982; 14:377–381.
22. Bosse R, Sparrow D, Rose CL, et al. Longitudinal effect of age and smoking cessation on pulmonary function. Am Rev Respir Dis 1981; 123:378–381.
23. Burrows B. Course and prognosis in COPD. In: Hodgkins JE, Petty TL, eds. Chronic Obstructive Pulmonary Disease–Current Concepts. Philadelphia: WB Saunders Co., 1987; 268–278.
24. Busch AJ, McClements JD. Effects of a supervised home exercise program on patients with severe chronic obstructive pulmonary disease. Phys Ther 1988; 68:469–474.
25. Bye PTP, Esau SA, Walley KR, et al. Ventilatory muscles during exercise in air and oxygen in normal men. J Appl Physiol 1984; 56:464–471.
26. Bye PTP, Esau SA, Levy RD, et al. Ventilatory muscle function during exercise in patients with chronic airflow limitation. Am Rev Respir Dis 1985; 132:236–240.
27. Carter R, Nictra B, Clark L, et al. Exercise conditioning in rehabilitation of patients with chronic obstructive pulmonary disease. Arch Phys Med Rehabil 1988; 69:118–122.
28. Celli BR. Arm exercise and ventilation. Chest 1988; 93:673.
29. Chester EH, Belman MJ, Gahler RC, et al. Multidisciplinary treatment of chronic pulmonary insufficiency. III. The effect of physical training on cardiopulmonary performance in patients with COPD. Chest 1977; 72:695–702.
30. Christie D. Physical training in obstructive lung disease. Br Med J 1968; 2:150–151.
31. Clough P, Harnisch LA, Cebulski P, Ross D. Method for individualizing patient care for chronic obstructive pulmonary disease patients. Health Soc Work 1987; 12:127–133.
32. Cockcroft AE, Sanders MJ, Berry G. Randomized controlled trial of rehabilitation in chronic respiratory disability. Thorax 1981; 36:200–203.
33. Degre S, Sergysels R, Messin R, et al. Hemodynamic responses of physical training in patients with chronic lung disease. Am Rev Respir Dis 1974; 110:395–402.
34. Driver AG, McAlevy MT, Smith VL. Nutritional assessment of

patients with chronic obstructive pulmonary disease and acute respiratory failure. Chest 1982; 82:568–571.
35. Dudley DL, Glaser EM, Jorgenson B, et al. Psychosocial concomitants to rehabilitation in chronic obstructive pulmonary disease. Chest 1980; 77:413–420; 544–551; 667–684.
36. Dunham JL, Hodgkin JE, Nicol J, et al. Cost effectiveness of pulmonary rehabilitation programs. In: Hodgkin JE, Zorn EG, Connors GL, eds. Pulmonary Rehabilitation. Boston: Butterworth Publishers, 1984.
37. Eliasson O, Hoffman J, Trueb D, et al. Corticosteroids in COPD: a clinical trial and reassessment of the literature. Chest 1986; 89:484–490.
38. Faling LJ. Pulmonary rehabilitation—physical modalities. Clin Chest Med 1986; 7:599–618.
39. Fisher EB, Rost K. Smoking cessation: a practical guide for the physician. Clin Chest Med 1986; 7:551–565.
40. Fishman DG, Petty TL. Physical, symptomatic and psychological improvement in patients receiving comprehensive care for chronic airway obstruction. J Chronic Dis 1971; 24:775–785.
41. Frownfelter DLF. Chest Physical Therapy and Pulmonary Rehabilitation: An Interdisciplinary Approach. Chicago: Year Book Medical Publishers, 1987, 249–254.
42. Gaskell DV, Webber BA. Brompton Hospital Guide to Chest Physiotherapy. Oxford: Blackwell Scientific Publications, 1975, 22–26.
43. Guthrie AG, Petty TL. Improved exercise tolerance in patients with chronic airflow obstruction. Phys Ther 1970; 50:1333–1337.
44. Haas A, Pineda H, Haas F, et al. Pulmonary Therapy and Rehabilitation: Principles and Practice. Baltimore: Williams and Wilkins, 1979.
45. Harding SM, Freedman S. A comparison of oral and inhaled steroids in patients with chronic airways obstruction: features determining response. Thorax 1978; 22:214–218.
46. Health and Public Policy Committee, American College of Physicians. Pneumococcal vaccine. Ann Intern Med 1986; 104:118–120.
47. Hilton S. Controlled evaluation of the effects of patient education on asthma morbidity in general practice. Lancet, 1986; i:26–29.
48. Hodgkin JE, Farrell MJ, Gipson SR, et al. Pulmonary rehabilitation. Am Rev Respir Dis 1981; 124:663–668.
49. Hodgkin JE, Zorn EG, Connors GL, eds. Pulmonary Rehabilitation: Guidelines to Success. Boston: Butterworth Publishers, 1984.
50. Hopkins HL, Smith HD. Occupational Therapy, 7th ed. Philadelphia: JB Lippincott Company, 1988, 226–245.
51. Howard JE, Davies JL, Roghmann KJ. Respiratory teaching of patients: how effective is it? J Adv Nursing 1987; 12:207–214.
52. Hudson LD, Tyler ML, Petty TL. Hospitalization needs during an outpatient rehabilitation program for severe chronic airway obstruction. Chest 1976; 70:606–610.
53. Hudson LD, Pierson DJ. Comprehensive respiratory care for patients with chronic obstructive pulmonary disease. Med Clin North Am 1981; 65:629–644.
54. Johnson NR, Tanzi F, Balchum O, et al. Inpatient comprehensive pulmonary rehabilitation in severe chronic obstructive lung disease. Barlow Hospital study. Respir Ther 1980; 10:15–19.
55. Johnson NR, DeFlorio GP, Einstein H. Cost/benefit outcomes of pulmonary rehabilitation in severe COPD. Am Rev Respir Dis 1983; 127:111.
56. Jones NL, Berman LB, Bartkiewicz PD, Oldridge NB. Chronic obstructive respiratory disorders. In: Skinner JS, ed. Exercise Testing and Exercise Prescription for Special Cases. Theoretic Basis and Clinical Application. Philadelphia: Lea & Febiger, 1987, 175–187.
57. Kass I, Dyksterhuis JE, Rubin H, Patil KD. Correlation of psychophysiologic variables with vocational rehabilitation outcome in patients with chronic obstructive pulmonary disease. Chest 1975; 67:433–440.
58. Keller C. Predicting the performance of daily activities of patients with chronic lung disease. Percept Mot Skills 1986; 63:647–651.
59. Killian KJ, Campbell EJM. Dyspnea and exertion. Ann Rev Physiol 1983; 45:465–479.
60. Killian KJ, Jones NL. The use of exercise testing and other methods in the investigation of dyspnea. Clin Chest Med 1984; 5:99–108.
61. Knowles JB, Fairbarn MS, Wiggs BJ, et al. Dietary supplementation and respiratory muscle performance in patients with COPD. Chest 1988; 93:977–983.
62. LaForce FM, Eickhoff TC. Pneumococcal vaccine: the evidence mounts. Ann Intern Med 1986; 104:110–112.
63. Lane DS, Evans D. Measures and methods in evaluating patient education programs for chronic illness. Med Care 1979; 17:30–42.
64. Leblanc P, Bowie DM, Summers E, et al. Breathlessness and exercise in patients with cardiorespiratory disease. Am Rev Respir Dis 1986; 133:21–25.
65. Lertzman MM, Cherniack RM. Rehabilitation of patients with chronic obstructive pulmonary disease. Am Rev Respir Dis 1976; 114:1145–1165.
66. Lewis MI, Belman MJ, Dorr-Uyemura L. Nutritional supplementation in ambulatory patients with chronic obstructive pulmonary disease. Am Rev Respir Dis 1987; 135:1062–1068.
67. Loke J, Mahler DA, Man SFP, et al. Exercise impairment in chronic obstructive pulmonary disease. Clin Chest Med 1984; 5:121–144.
68. Loveridge BM. Breathing patterns in chronic obstructive pulmonary disease. In: Peat M, ed. Current Physical Therapy. St. Louis: CV Mosby Co., 1988, 57–60.
69. Mahler DA, Rosiello RA, Harver A, et al. Comparison of clinical dyspnea ratings and psychophysical measurements of respiratory sensation in obstructive airway disease. Am Rev Respir Dis 1987; 135:1229–1233.
70. Make BJ. ed. Pulmonary rehabilitation: Myth or reality? Clin Chest Med 1986; 7:519–540.
71. Martin CJ, Ripley H, Reynolds J, Best F. The distribution of ventilation. Chest 1976; 69:174–178.
72. McArdle WD, Katch FI, Katch VL. Exercise Physiology. Energy, Nutrition, and Human Performance. 2nd ed. Philadelphia: Lea and Febiger, 1986, 247–351.
73. McGavin CR, Artvinli M, Naoe H, McHardy GJR. Twelve minute walking tests for assessing disability in chronic bronchitis. Br Med J 1976; 1:822–823.
74. Medical Research Council Working Party. Long term domiciliary oxygen therapy in chronic hypoxic cor pulmonale complicating chronic bronchitis and emphysema. Lancet 1981; i:681–686.
75. Mendella LA, Manfreda J, Warren CPW, et al. Steroid response in stable chronic obstructive pulmonary disease. Ann Intern Med 1982; 96:17–21.
76. Mertens DJ, Shephard RJ, Kavanagh T. Long-term exercise therapy for chronic obstructive lung disease. Respiration 1978; 35:96–107.
77. Mohensifar Z, Rosenberg N, Goldberg HS, et al. Mechanical vibration and conventional chest physiotherapy in outpatients with stable chronic obstructive lung disease. Chest 1985; 87:483–488.
78. Morgan WP. Affective beneficence of vigorous physical activity. Med Sci Sports Exerc 1985; 17:94–100.
79. Moser KM, Bokinsky GE, Savage RT, et al. Results of a comprehensive rehabilitation program. Physiologic and functional effects in patients with chronic obstructive pulmonary disease. Arch Intern Med 1980; 140:1596–1601.
80. Nocturnal Oxygen Therapy Trial Group. Continuous or nocturnal oxygen therapy in hypoxemic chronic obstructive lung disease: a clinical trial. Ann Intern Med 1980; 92:391–398.
81. Oldenburg FA, Dolovich MB, Montgomery JM, Newhouse MT. Effects of postural drainage, exercise and cough on mucous clearance in chronic bronchitis. Am Rev Respir Dis 1979; 120:739–745.
82. O'Ryan JA, Burns DG, eds. Pulmonary Rehabilitation: From Hospital to Home. Chicago: Year Book Medical Publishers, 1984.
83. Paez PH, Phillipson EA, Masangkay M, et al. The physiologic basis of training patients with emphysema. Am Rev Respir Dis 1967; 95:944–954.
84. Pardy RL, Rivington RN, Despas PJ, et al. The effect of inspiratory muscle training on exercise performance in chronic airflow limitation. Am Rev Respir Dis 1981; 123:426–434.
85. Pardy RL, Reid WD, Belman MJ. Respiratory muscle training. Clin Chest Med 1988; 9:287–296.
86. Petty TL. Pulmonary rehabilitation. Basics Respir Dis 1975; 4:1–6.
87. Petty TL, ed. Intensive and Rehabilitative Respiratory Care. 3rd ed. Philadelphia: Lea and Febiger, 1982.
88. Phillips MA. A subjective ADL rating scale for the pulmonary rehabilitation patient. Occup Ther Health Care 1986; 3:79–88.

89. Pierce AK, Taylor HF, Archer RK, Miller WF. Response to exercise training in patients with emphysema. Arch Intern Med 1964; 113:28–36.
90. Pineda H, Haas F, Axen K. Treadmill exercise training in chronic obstructive pulmonary disease. Arch Phys Med Rehabil 1986; 67:155–158.
91. Reid WD, Loveridge BM. Review paper. Physiotherapy management of patients with chronic obstructive airways disease. Physiother Canada 1983; 35:183–195.
92. Reid WD, Warren CPW. Ventilatory muscle strength and endurance training in elderly subjects and patients with chronic airflow limitation: a pilot study. Physiother Canada 1984; 36:305–311.
93. Ries AL, Ellis B, Hawkins HW. Upper extremity exercise training in chronic obstructive pulmonary disease. Chest 1988; 93:688–692.
94. Rochester DF. Malnutrition and the respiratory muscles. Clin Chest Med 1986; 7:91–100.
95. Romaniuk KM. Around the Clock with COPD: Helpful Hints for Respiratory Patients. Connecticut: American Lung Association, 1984.
96. Sackner MA, Banks J, Silva G. Distribution of ventilation during diaphragmatic breathing in obstructive lung disease. Am Rev Respir Dis 1974; 109:331–337.
97. Sahn SA, Nett LN, Petty TL. Ten year follow-up of a comprehensive rehabilitation program for severe COPD. Chest 1980; 77:311–314.
98. Sahn SA. Corticosteroids in chronic bronchitis and pulmonary emphysema. Chest 1978; 73:389–396.
99. Sammer EA, Hodgkin JE, Zorn E, et al. Clinical and physiological response to comprehensive respiratory care. Respir Care 1979; 24:1207–1211.
100. Sandhu HS. Psychosocial issues in chronic obstructive pulmonary disease. Clin Chest Med 1986; 7:629–642.
101. Shanfield K, Hammond MA. Activities of daily living. In: Hodgkin JE, Zorn EG, Connors GL, eds. Pulmonary Rehabilitation: Guidelines to Success. Boston: Butterworth Publishers, 1984.
102. Shearer MO, Banks J, Silva G, Sackner MA. Lung ventilation during diaphragmatic breathing. Phys Ther 1972; 52:139–148.
103. Shenkman B. Factors contributing to attrition rates in a pulmonary rehabilitation program. Heart Lung 1985; 14:53–58.
104. Shephard RJ. Exercise and chronic obstructive lung disease. Exerc Sport Sci Rev 1976; 4:263–296.
105. Siegel SC. Corticosteroid agents: Overview of corticosteroid therapy. J Allergy Clin Immunol 1985; 76:312–320.
106. Silverman M, Barry J, Hellerstein H, et al. Variability of the perceived sense of effort in breathing during exercise in patients with chronic obstructive pulmonary disease. Am Rev Respir Dis 1988; 137:206–209.
107. Stokes TC, Shaylor JM, O'Reilly JF, et al. Assessment of steroid responsiveness in patients with chronic airflow obstruction. Lancet 1982; ii:345.
108. Theodore AC, Beer DJ. Pharmacotherapy for chronic obstructive pulmonary disease. Clin Chest Med 1986; 7:657–669.
109. Vyas MN, Banister EW, Morton JW, et al. Response to exercise in patients with chronic airways obstruction. 1. Effects of exercise training. Am Rev Respir Dis 1971; 103:390–400.
110. Walsh RL. Occupational therapy as part of a pulmonary rehabilitation program. Occup Ther Health Care 1986; 3:65–78.
111. Wilke NA, Sheldahl LM. Use of simulated work testing in cardiac rehabilitation: a case report. Am J Occup Ther 1985; 39:327–330.
112. Williams JH, Moser KM. Pneumococcal vaccine and patients with chronic lung disease. Ann Intern Med 1986; 104:106–109.
113. Wilson DO, Rogers RM, Openbrier D. Nutritional aspects of chronic obstructive pulmonary disease. Clin Chest Med 1986; 7:643–656.
114. Woolf CR. A rehabilitation program for improving exercise tolerance of patients with chronic lung disease. Can Med Assoc J 1972; 106:1290–1292.
115. Woolf CR, Suero JT. Alteration in lung mechanics and gas exchange following training in chronic obstructive lung disease. Dis Chest 1969; 55:37–44.
116. Zach MS, Purrer B, Oerwaldner B. Effect of swimming on forced expiration and sputum clearance in cystic fibrosis. Lancet 1981; ii:1201–1203.

INDEX

Note: Page numbers in *italics* refer to illustrations; page numbers followed by t refer to tables.